D1134691

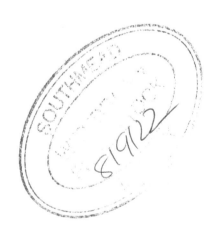

81922

Textbook of Medical Oncology

Fourth Edition

Edited by

Franco Cavalli, MD FRCP
Professor and Director
Oncology Institute of Southern Switzerland
Ospedale San Giovanni
Bellinzona, Switzerland

Stan B. Kaye, BSc MD FRCP FMedSci
CRUK Professor of Medical Oncology
Head of Section of Medicine
Institute of Cancer Research
Royal Marsden Hospital
Sutton, Surrey, United Kingdom

Heine H. Hansen, MD FRCP
Professor of Medical Oncology
The Finsen Center
Rigshospitalet
Copenhagen, Denmark

James O. Armitage, MD FRCP
The Joe Shapiro Professor of Internal Medicine
Section of Oncology Hematology
University of Nebraska Medical Center
Omaha, Nebraska, USA

Martine J. Piccart-Gebhart, MD PhD
Head of Medicine Department
Institut Jules Bordet
Université Libre de Bruxelles
Brussels, Belgium

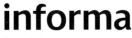

informa
healthcare

© 2009 Informa UK Ltd

First published in the United Kingdom in 2009 by Informa Healthcare, Telephone House, 69-77 Paul Street, London EC2A 4LQ. Informa Healthcare is a trading division of Informa UK Ltd. Registered Office: 37/41 Mortimer Street, London W1T 3JH. Registered in England and Wales number 1072954.

Tel: +44 (0)20 7017 5000
Fax: +44 (0)20 7017 6699
Website: www.informahealthcare.com

Although every effort has been made to ensure that all owners of copyright material have been acknowledged in this publication, we would be glad to acknowledge in subsequent reprints or editions any omissions brought to our attention.

Although every effort has been made to ensure that drug doses and other information are presented accurately in this publication, the ultimate responsibility rests with the prescribing physician. Neither the publishers nor the authors can be held responsible for errors or for any consequences arising from the use of information contained herein. For detailed prescribing information or instructions on the use of any product or procedure discussed herein, please consult the prescribing information or instructional material issued by the manufacturer.

A CIP record for this book is available from the British Library.
Library of Congress Cataloging-in-Publication Data

Data available on application

ISBN-10: 0 415 47748 4
ISBN-13: 978 0 415 47748 2

Distributed in North and South America by
Taylor & Francis
6000 Broken Sound Parkway, NW, (Suite 300)
Boca Raton, FL 33487, USA

Within Continental USA
Tel: 1 (800) 272 7737; Fax: 1 (800) 374 3401
Outside Continental USA
Tel: (561) 994 0555; Fax: (561) 361 6018
Email: orders@crcpress.com

Book orders in the rest of the world
Paul Abrahams
Tel: +44 (0)20 7017 4036
Email: bookorders@informa.com

Composition by Exeter Premedia Servies Private Ltd., Chennai, India
Printed and bound in Spain by Grafos SA.

Contents

Section III – Supportive Aspects

Contributors

Marc S. Ballas, MD MPH
NYU Cancer Center
NYU School of Medicine
New York, NY, USA

Susana Banerjee, MA MRCP
Specialist Registrar in Medical Oncology
Institute of Cancer Research and the Royal
Marsden Hospital
Department of Medicine
London, United Kingdom

Jean-Yves Blay, MD PhD
Professor of Medical Oncology
University Claude Bernard, Lyon I
INSERM Unit 590, Cytokine and Cancer
Centre Léon Bérard
Lyon, France

Clara D. Bloomfield, MD
Division of Hematology and Oncology
Department of Internal Medicine
The Ohio State University
Comprehensive Cancer Center
Columbus, OH, USA

Eduardo Bruera, MD
Palliative Care & Rehabilitation Medicine
The University of Texas
M.D. Anderson Cancer Center
Houston, TX, USA

Shirley H. Bush, MBBS
Palliative Care & Rehabilitation Medicine
The University of Texas
M.D. Anderson Cancer Center
Houston, TX, USA

John C. Byrd, MD
Division of Hematology and Oncology
Department of Internal Medicine
The Ohio State University
Comprehensive Cancer Center
Columbus, OH, USA

Ian Chau, MD MRCP
Department of Medicine
Royal Marsden Hospital
Sutton, Surrey, United Kingdom

Bertrand Coiffier, MD PhD
Hematology Department
Hospices Civils de Lyon
University Lyon 1
Lyon, France

Marco Colleoni, MD
Medical Senology Research Unit &
Division of Medical Oncology
Department of Medicine
European Institute of Oncology
Milan, Italy

Jesus Corral Jaime, MD
Medical Oncology Department
Lung Cancer Clinic
Virgen del Rocio University Hospital
Sevilla, Spain

David Cunningham, MD FRCP
Department of Medicine
Royal Marsden Hospital
Sutton, Surrey, United Kingdom

Gedske Daugaard, MD DMSc
Department of Oncology
Rigshospitalet
Copenhagen, Denmark

Ronald de Wit, MD PhD
Dept of Medical Oncology
Erasmus University Medical Center
Daniel den Hoed Cancer Center
Rotterdam, The Netherlands

Gianluca Del Conte, MD
Fondazione IRCCS
Istituto Nazionale dei Tumori
Milan, Italy

Silvia Dellapasqua, MD
Medical Senology Research Unit &
Division of Medical Oncology
Department of Medicine
European Institute of Oncology
Milan, Italy

Diana M. Eccles, MD
Department of Cancer Genetics
Academic Unit of Genetic Medicine
Wessex Clinical Genetics Service
Princess Anne Hospital
Southampton, United Kingdom

Alexander M.M. Eggermont, MD PhD
Department of Surgical Oncology
Erasmus University Medical Center
Daniel den Hoed Cancer Center
Rotterdam, The Netherlands

Elizabeth A. Eisenhauer, MD FRCPC
Investigational New Drug Program
NCIC Clinical Trials Group
Cancer Research Institute
Queen's University
Kingston, ON, Canada

Ferry A.L.M. Eskens, MD PhD
Medical Oncology Department
Erasmus University Medical Center
Rotterdam, The Netherlands

Martin F. Fey, MD
Department of Medical Oncology
Inselspital and Berne University
Berne, Switzerland

Rocío García-Carbonero, MD
Medical Oncology Department
GI Oncology Clinic
Virgen del Rocio University Hospital
Sevilla, Spain

Francesca Gay, MD
Divisione di Ematologia
Università di Torino
Azienda Ospedaliera S. Giovanni Battista
Torino, Italy

Richard D. Gelber, PhD
Department of Biostatistics and
Computational Biology
Dana-Farber Cancer Institute
Boston, MA, USA

Aron Goldhirsch, MD
Department of Medical Oncology
Department of Medicine
European Institute of Oncology
Milan, Italy

Martin Gore, PhD FRCP
Professor of Cancer Medicine
Institute of Cancer Research and the Royal
Marsden Hospital
Department of Medicine
London, United Kingdom

Heine H. Hansen, MD FRCP
Department of Medical Oncology
The Finsen Center
Rigshospitalet
Copenhagen, Denmark

Sandra J. Horning, MD
Division of Oncology
Department of Medicine
Stanford Comprehensive Cancer Center
Stanford, CA, USA

Andreas F. Hottinger, MD
Geneva University Hospital
Department of Oncology
Geneva, Switzerland

Jean François Larouche, MD
Department of Medicine
Division of Hematology and Oncology
Centre Hospitalier affilié universitaire de Québec
Québec, Canada

Marc Levivier, MD PhD
Centre Universitaire Romand de Neurochirurgie
University of Lausanne and University of Geneva
Switzerland

Lisa Licitra, MD
Head and Neck Medical Oncology Unit
Fondazione IRCCS
Istituto Nazionale dei Tumori
Milan, Italy

Guido Marcucci, MD
Division of Hematology and Oncology
Department of Internal Medicine
The Ohio State University
Comprehensive Cancer Center
Columbus, OH, USA

Anne Kirstine Moeller, PhD
Department of Oncology
Rigshospitalet
Copenhagen, Denmark

Krzysztof Mrózek, MD PhD
Division of Hematology and Oncology
Department of Internal Medicine
The Ohio State University
Comprehensive Cancer Center
Columbus, OH, USA

Franco M. Muggia, MD
NYU Cancer Center
NYU School of Medicine
New York, NY, USA

Antonio Palumbo, MD
Divisione di Ematologia
Università di Torino
Azienda Ospedaliera S. Giovanni Battista
Torino, Italy

Helle Pappot, MD
Department of Medical Oncology
The Finsen Center
Rigshospitalet
Copenhagen, Denmark

Wendy R. Parulekar, MD FRCPC
CIC Clinical Trials Group
Cancer Research Institute
Queen's University
Kingston, ON, Canada

Luis Paz-Ares, MD PhD
Chief of Medical Oncology
Virgen del Rocio University Hospital
Sevilla, Spain

Bodil Laub Petersen, PhD
Department of Pathology
Rigshospitalet
Copenhagen, Denmark

Isabelle Ray-Coquard, MD
Medical Oncology Department
Centre Léon Bérard
EA Unité Santé, Individu, Société 4129
Lyon, France

Darius Razavi, MD PhD
Institut Jules Bordet
Université Libre de Bruxelles
Brussels, Belgium

Alain Ronson, MD
Institut Jules Bordet
Université Libre de Bruxelles
Brussels, Belgium

Dirk Schrijvers, MD PhD
Ziekenhuisnetwerk Antwerpen (ZNA) - Middleheim
Lindendreef 1
Antwerp, Belgium

Cristiana Sessa, MD
Oncology Institute of Southern Switzerland
Ospedale San Giovanni
Bellinzona, Switzerland &
Fondazione IRCCS
Istituto Nazionale dei Tumori
Milan, Italy

Cora N. Sternberg, MD
Department of Medical Oncology
San Camillo Forlanini Hosp
Rome, Italy

Roger Stupp, MD
Centre Universitaire Romand de Neurochirurgie
University of Lausanne
Switzerland

Jaap Verweij, MD
Department of Medical Oncology
Erasmus University Medical Center
Daniel den Hoed Cancer Center
Rotterdam, The Netherlands

Damien C. Weber, MD
Geneva University Hospital and University of Geneva
Department of Radiation Therapy
Geneva, Switzerland

Meir Wetzler, MD
Leukemia Section
Department of Medicine
Roswell Park Cancer Institute
Buffalo, NY, USA

Rachel Wong, MBBS (HONS) FRACP
Department of Medicine
Royal Marsden Hospital
Sutton, Surrey, United Kingdom

Preface to the Fourth Edition

Since the publication of our third edition in 2004, we have seen an exciting acceleration in the pace of developments in medical oncology. Increasingly, we are building on the achievements of our mentors with conventional chemotherapy, to move into the new era of targeted systemic treatment. For this reason, we considered that the time could not be better for us to produce a fourth edition of our textbook.

We are delighted to welcome two new editors, Martine Piccart and James Armitage. They bring a wealth of expertise and experience across a range of clinical areas, including solid tumors and hematological malignancies. In addition, their key roles in European and US oncology help strengthen the global appeal and relevance of this edition.

We have undertaken an extensive revision of the third edition and therefore also welcome eight new authors. Drs. Muggia, Verweij, Blay, Bloomfield, Palumbo, Razavi, Stupp, Eggermont, and Eccles are all acknowledged experts in their respective fields, and we are most grateful for their input. As in the previous years, we are most pleased to enlist the help of young coworkers and extend our thanks to them for their enthusiasm. We see this generation as vital to the future of our specialty worldwide.

Our priority in this edition has been to reflect both the multidisciplinary nature of modern cancer treatment and the growing trend in systemic cancer therapy to bridge the gap between our improved understanding of the molecular basis of cancer and rational targeted treatment. Clearly, there is a long road to travel, but the trend toward cancer biomarker–driven "personalized" treatment is firmly on its way. At the same time, we have been determined not to neglect the chapters relating to overall patient care, recognizing the challenge that continues to face us, our patients, and their families.

We hope that this edition will be helpful to a range of individuals involved in medical oncology, particularly trainees as well as those involved in translational research.

We welcome comments; these are crucial for planning future editions.

Franco Cavalli
Stan B. Kaye
Heine H. Hansen
James O. Armitage
Martine J. Piccart-Gebhart

Color Plates

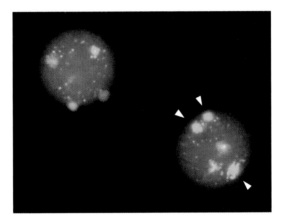

Figure 1.14 FISH. Interphase nuclei from leukemic cells analyzed with a DNA probe hybridizing to chromosome 7 (red dots) and a DNA probe recognizing sequences from chromosome 8 (green dots). One nucleus is normal with two copies of each chromosome, whereas one nucleus shows three green dots indicating trisomy 8, a common chromosomal abnormality in myeloid leukemias including MDS or CLL. *Source*: Courtesy of Dr. Martine Jotterand, CHUV, Lausanne. *See Page 20.*

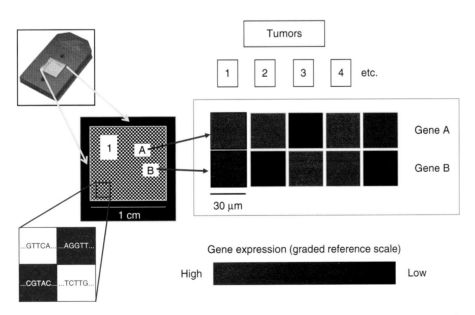

Figure 1.15 Gene expression profiling of tumors with cDNA microarrays or "chips." The chip is a small flat box (*upper left*), which in a rectangular chamber contains a siliconized surface loaded with single-strand nucleic acid sequences (*lower left*). These sequences represent either short, specific oligonucleotides or cDNA prepared from mRNA of various cells. Specific sequences are neatly arranged in rows and columns and are ready for hybridization with a sample composed of labeled single-stranded cRNA. A single chip may contain up to several 10,000 such sequences (representing genes, or so-called expressed sequence tags ESTs). After hybridization the chip surface can be read and the results expressed as quantitative estimates of gene expression, with respect to a scale of reference (*bottom center*). In this example mRNA from tumor 1 has been examined with the help of the chip. Gene A is overexpressed in this sample, and gene B is not expressed at all. Tumor 3 shows the reverse gene expression pattern, and the other samples all show distinct gene expression profiles. These raw data are then sorted with a number of strategies. Unsupervised clustering (explained in a terribly simplified fashion!) refers to a program that groups tumor samples according to similar or completely distinct expression profiles. In supervised clustering, additional information on the samples is fed in before sorting, for example, some clinical information. In the end, a limited number of genes can be pulled from such profiles which distinguish one tumor subgroup from another. *See Page 22.*

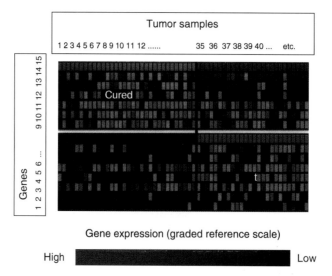

Figure 1.16 Microarray analysis of DLBCL. About one-half of patients with DLBCL are cured with CHOP-type chemotherapies and the other half relapse and often succumb to their disease. Although a number of clinicopathological parameters are available to create prognostic subgroups (International Prognostic Index), clinical and pathological information is inadequate for a neat distinction of these two subgroups. In this example, cases either cured or with an eventually fatal outcome were studied for their gene expression profiles. It turns out that DLBCL with a good prognosis displays a gene expression signature that is clearly different from the profile that lights up in lymphoma cells from eventually fatal cases. Although the microarrays used in this experiments offered thousands of genes for analysis, a neat prognostic distinction of the two clinical DLBCL subgroups can be made with a restricted and selected group of genes (horizontal rows), in fact no more than 15 genes. *Source*: Modified after Ref. 68. *See Page 23.*

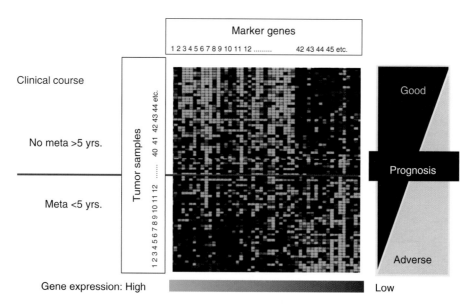

Figure 1.17 cDNA microchip analysis (so-called supervised classification on prognosis gene expression signatures) of samples from women with early node-negative breast cancer. In this example, tumor tissue samples from women with T1-2 N0 stage early breast cancer were analyzed with microarrays. For data analysis, cases were split: those who remained disease-free for at least 5 years and those who relapsed within 5 years after diagnosis and primary treatment (so-called supervised clustering analysis of chip data). The established clinical and biological prognostic parameters in breast cancer (T stage, N stage, receptor status, etc.) did not permit prediction with any accuracy as to which women would remain disease-free or relapse. In the molecular analysis, genes have been ordered according to their correlation with the two clinical prognostic patient groups. The microchip analysis lights up gene expression profiles that clearly differ between tumors treated successfully and those cases that had relapsed within 5 years after diagnosis. In women with no evidence of metastases after 5 years of follow-up, genes with low expression cluster to the upper left of the panel (lighting up in green), and overexpressed genes (depicted in red) are grouped in the upper right sector of the panel. The reverse pattern or expression profile is seen in the group of women who had relapsed. *Source*: Modified after Ref. 69. *See Page 24.*

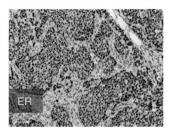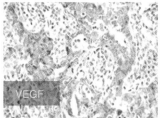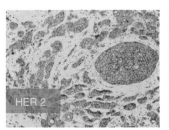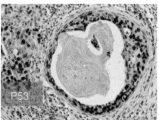

Figure 1.18 Immunohistochemical analysis of gene expression in breast cancer. Invasive-ductal breast cancer sections staining with diagnostic antibodies recognizing (*from left to right*) estrogen receptors (nuclear; ER), vascular endothelial growth factor (VEGF), HER2 (membrane bound), and p53 (nuclear). The section stained with p53 also shows noninvasive ductal carcinoma in situ (DCIS; *right*). The stromal cells in between the tumor cells are mostly negative. *Source*: Courtesy of Prof. H.J. Altermann, Pathologie Länggasse, Berne. *See Page 24*.

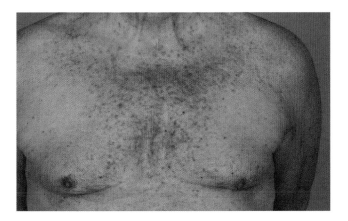

Figure 3.7 Typical example of EGFR inhibitor induced skin rash. *See Page 46*.

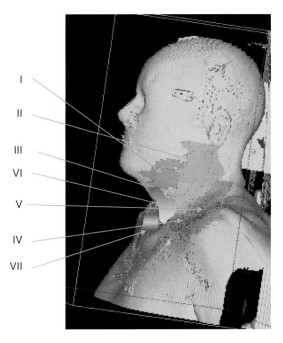

Figure 7.3 Lymph node regions in the head and neck. *See Page 127*.

(A)

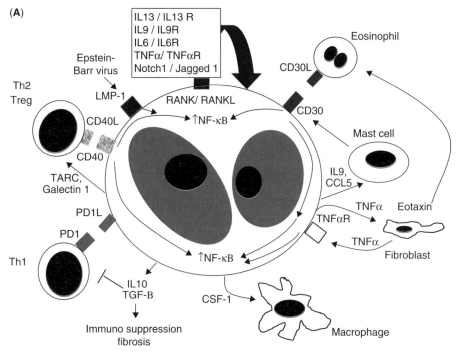

IL13 / IL13 R
IL9 / IL9R
IL6 / IL6R
TNFα/ TNFαR
Notch1 / Jagged 1

Epstein-
Barr virus

Th2
Treg

LMP-1

CD40L

CD40

TARC,
Galectin 1

PD1L

PD1

Th1

IL10
TGF-B

Immuno suppression
fibrosis

RANK/ RANKL

↑NF-κB

↑NF-κB

CSF-1

Eosinophil

CD30L

CD30

Mast cell

IL9,
CCL5

TNFα

TNFαR

TNFα

Eotaxin

Fibroblast

Macrophage

(B)

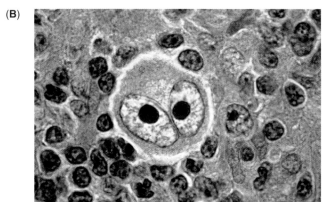

Figure 14.1   Hodgkin Reed-Sternberg cell and its microenvironment: **(A)** interactions that result in immunosuppression and favor survival; **(B)** photomicrography. *Abbreviations*: IL13, Interleukin-13; IL13R, Interleukin-13 receptor; IL9, Interleukin-9; IL9R, Interleukin-9 receptor; IL6, Interleukin-6; IL6R, Interleukin-6 receptor; NF-κB, Nuclear Factor kappa B; RANK, receptor activator for NFκB; LMP, latent membrane protein; TARC, thymus and activation regulated chemokine; PD1, programmed death-1; TGF-B, transforming growth factor beta; CSF, colony stimulating factor; TNF, tumor necrosis factor; CCL5 also known as RANTES (regulated on activation, normal T-cell expressed and secreted). *See Page 264.*

(A)

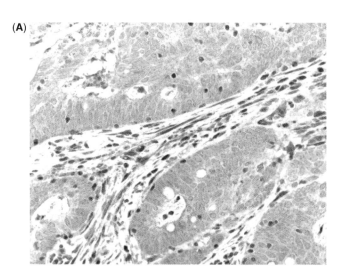

Figure 22.6   **(A)** Immunohistochemistry, colon tumor block stained with antibodies to hMSH2 showing loss of nuclear staining in tumor tissue and normal (brown) staining in stromal cells. *See Page 387.*

Molecular Biology of Cancer

Martin F. Fey

INTRODUCTION

Research into the molecular and cellular biology of cancer has given us remarkable insights into the molecular basis of neoplasia, such as disordered cell proliferation, disturbed differentiation, and altered cell survival as well as disruption of normal tissue, invasion, and metastasis. Human cancer results mostly from gene mutations in its cells of origin which confer a biological advantage to these cells. Today, knowledge about molecular mechanisms of carcinogenesis has become far more than just a playground for experimental biology. Molecular markers are now available for improving cancer diagnosis and classification. At the therapeutic level, the identification of aberrant molecular pathways in cancer cells provides the basis for molecularly targeted therapy. It is, therefore, essential for clinicians caring for cancer patients to understand the molecular and cellular basis of neoplasia.

CLONAL CELLULAR ORIGIN AND THE SOMATIC MUTATION THEORY OF CANCER CELLS
Somatic Mutation Theory of Cancer and Tumor Clonality

A clone is defined as a population of cells derived through mitotic division from a single somatic cell of origin. This definition neither implies that a clonal population of cells must necessarily be genetically or phenotypically homogeneous nor does it infer that a cell clone must be cancerous (1). Initially, cancer arises from a single somatic cell present in normal tissue, which during mitosis acquires gene mutations (somatic mutations) suitable for turning it into an early founder cell of a clonal tumor (Fig. 1.1). Such mutations need to provide a biological advantage to that cell and its progeny as otherwise clonal expansion would not occur. A mutation knocking out a gene that is absolutely essential for the function of the cell is likely to kill it rather than turn it into a founder cell of a cancer clone. A totally innocuous mutation in a gene of no interest to a particular cell would fail to alter its biological behavior, and thus, it provides no basis for neoplastic transformation. It turns out that most gene mutations that succeed in driving a cell into a neoplastic transformation severely alter cell proliferation, cell differentiation, cell survival, and other vital functions.

A single gene mutation is not enough to found a tumor. Rather, molecular carcinogenesis requires a sequential series of different yet linked mutational hits in at least two or more critical genes in the same cell (Fig. 1.2) (2,3).

As that cell and its progeny continue to proliferate in a clonal fashion, daughter cells will subsequently acquire additional mutations, and will grab yet new selection advantages such as proliferative drive, escape from cell death programs (apoptosis), etc. Such cells would establish subclones which may in turn become parent clones themselves. Therefore clonality assessment provides a snapshot of the clonal composition of a tumor at the time of analysis, but the clonal composition of neoplasms may change over time as tumors progress.

Cancer Stem Cells

The recent concept of cancer stem cells adds significant information to the established principles of the origin of a clonal tumor. One assumes that mutations leading to cancer would occur in rare cells that are long-term residents in the respective tissue, for example, in colon mucosa or in the bone marrow. To become a "mother cell" of a tumor, a mutated cell would not only have to proliferate and expand clonally, but it also needs to self-renew and acquire additional mutations. Cancer would thus originate from long-lived uncommon tissue stem cells with the ability for self-renewal, that is, a typical feature of a stem cell. When mutated, such a cell becomes a cancer stem cell. The quiescence of these cells and their inherent resistance to drugs may account for a considerable amount of treatment failures in clinical oncology. Stem cells including cancer stem cells tend to be more resistant to cytostatic drugs, radiation, and perhaps to some of the "newer" targeted agents than more mature (cancer) cells from the same clone or tissue. Ideally, cancer treatment would have to target cancer stem cells while sparing normal stem cells within the body's tissues (4–6).

Normal colonic mucosa and colon cancer provide a good example of our yet incomplete notion of how cancer stem cells may play a role in tumorigenesis. Colonic epithelium is replaced every 5 days. Stem cells are thought to reside at the bottom of colon crypts where they are responsible for tissue renewal. During asymmetric division, colon stem cells undergo self-renewal and generate cells that migrate up the crypt and differentiate to form specific cell types in colon mucosa. Colon stem cells therefore must harbor the genetic programs that determine the structure and function of the specific regions or sections in the gut. There is evidence to support the notion that these cells, when they develop critical gene mutations, may turn into colon cancer stem cells yielding cancers with multiple differentiated cell types. Mutations in the adenomatous polyposis coli (APC) gene placed on chromosome 5 may be an early event in

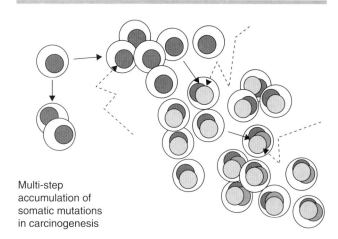

Multi-step
accumulation of
somatic mutations
in carcinogenesis

Figure 1.1 The somatic mutation theory of cancer. At mitosis a cell may acquire a somatic mutation (solidline) conferring a selection advantage over other cells. This provides the basis for clonal expansion of that cell and its progeny. Some of its daughter cells may acquire yet other somatic mutations (dottedlines) providing additional selection advantages. In the end, cancer presents as a clonal tumor composed of related yet distinct subclones. This concept neatly incorporates the more recent data on the role of cancer stem cells as the earliest precursor cells of many if not all tumors.

this chain of events (Fig. 1.2). Mutant APC may lead to an increased rate of crypt fission, crypt branching, and budding and thus pave the way to the development of adenomas, morphologically recognizable forerunners of invasive colon cancer (5).

Stem cell biology is best characterized in the hematopoietic system. Cancer stem cells are evident in leukemia, for example, in chronic myelogenous leukemia (CML). The ABL kinase inhibitor imatinib mesylate in CML has provided a radically new approach of a targeted "molecular" therapy against a human cancer. Nevertheless, residual disease may persist after CML treatment even in complete responders. In vitro studies indicate that although inhibition of the BCR-ABL kinase may kill most cells within a CML clone, it does not appear to affect CML stem cells. The unique molecular features of cancer stem cells must therefore be

defined to provide targets for therapeutic intervention that would hit "at the heart of the matter." A number of molecular pathways are particularly active in cancer stem cells. For example, the nuclear factor κ B (NFκB) pathway is constitutively active in acute myeloid leukemia (AML) stem cells but silent in normal hematopoietic stem cells, rendering the former selectively susceptible to drugs that would interfere with this pathway (6,7).

The Clinical Relevance of Assessing Tumor Clonality

Assessment of tumor clonality at the molecular level is usually not necessary as a routine diagnostic procedure. The histological diagnosis of breast or colorectal cancer, for example, is usually very accurate, and formal proof that a given tumor is clonal (as invariably it will be) is not necessary. However, in selected instances, assessment of the clonal composition of cellular proliferations in biopsy material may be of direct practical importance.

The diagnosis of lymphoid neoplasms and lymphoproliferative syndromes is routinely based on morphology, immunohistochemistry, and immunophenotyping. These techniques will succeed in establishing the precise diagnosis of a clonal lymphoid neoplasm of either B- or T-cell origin in perhaps 90–95% of all cases. However, molecular analysis of clonality may be helpful in the remaining rare cases where morphology and related techniques fail to distinguish a neoplastic clonal population of lymphoid cells from a reactive polyclonal assembly of lymphoid elements, as seen in an inflammatory infiltrate. This is particularly troublesome for T-cell proliferations (5–7% of all lymphoid malignancies), or natural killer cell tumors (<2%) where no reliable immunohistochemical markers of clonality are available. *Clonal antigen receptor gene rearrangements* are well-established clonal markers in the vast majority of B- or T-cell neoplasms, and their absence in a lymphoproliferation would strongly support the presence of a polyclonal and hence reactive process (8–10). The detection of a clonal cell population derived from either B- or T-cell lineage is almost always abnormal and often associated with a malignant neoplastic proliferation (Fig. 1.3).

The germline immunoglobulin (Ig) and T-cell receptor (TCR) gene loci contain many different variable (V), diversity (D), and joining (J) gene segments, which are

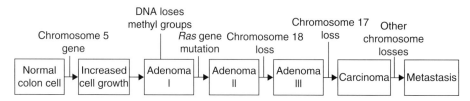

Figure 1.2 Colon cancer—a model disorder for stepwise accumulation of somatic mutations. The morphological cascade leading from normal colonic mucosa to advanced colon cancer is governed by stepwise accumulation of somatic mutations in many different genes. The gene on chromosome 5 known as the adenomatous polyposis coli/familial adenomatous polyposis (APC/FAP) tumor suppressor gene is an early gatekeeper in colorectal carcinogenesis, possibly at the colon crypt (cancer) stem cell level. The gene lost on chromosome 18q is the SMAD4 gene, encoding a protein involved in the transforming growth factor β (TGFβ) signaling pathway, which normally provides a growth-inhibiting differentiation signal to the cell. The gene deleted on chromosome 17 is the p53 tumor suppressor gene. The order in which these somatic mutations hit the cells and their composition may vary between individual cases.

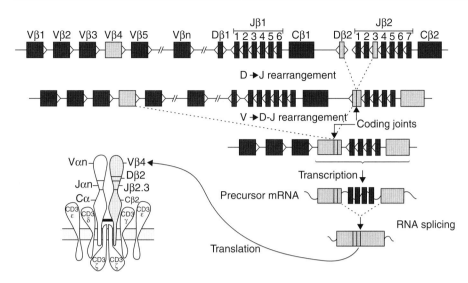

Figure 1.3 Antigen receptor gene rearrangement. Schematic diagram of sequential rearrangement steps, transcription, and translation of the *TCR*β gene as an example. In this example, first a Dβ2 to Jβ2.3 rearrangement occurs, followed by a Vβ4 to Dβ2–Jβ2.3 rearrangement, resulting in the formation of a Vβ4–Dβ2–Jβ2.3 coding joint (VDJ joining). The rearranged *TCR*βgene is transcribed into precursor mRNA, spliced into mature *TCR*β mRNA, and finally translated into a TCRβ protein chain. The two extrachromosomal TRECs that are formed during this recombination process are indicated as well; they contain the D–J signal joint and V–D signal joint, respectively. *Source*: Adapted from Ref. 8.

rearranged during early lymphoid differentiation. V–D–J rearrangements are mediated via a recombinase enzyme complex where proteins called RAG1 and RAG2 play a key role by recognizing and cutting the DNA at recombination signal sequences located downstream of the V gene segments, at both sides of the D gene segments, and upstream of the J gene segments. Functionally rearranged Ig and TCR genes result in surface membrane expression of Ig, TCRαβ or TCRγδ molecules.

The detection of single Ig light-chain protein expression in a lymphoproliferation (Igκ or Igλ, but not both) has long been used to discriminate between reactive (polyclonal) B lymphocytes (normal Igκ or Igλ ratio: 0.7–2.8) versus aberrant (clonal) B lymphocytes with Igκ or Igλ ratios of >4.0 or <0.5. In the vast majority of mature B-cell malignancies, single Ig light-chain expression can support the clonal origin of the malignancy. The same principle, however, is not readily applicable to T-cell lymphoproliferations, particularly if suspect lymphoproliferative disorders are intermixed with normal (reactive) lymphocytes.

In contrast to the antibody-based techniques, molecular techniques are broadly applicable for the detection of clonally rearranged Ig/TCR genes. Their detection by polymerase chain reaction (PCR) requires precise knowledge of the rearranged antigen receptor gene segments in order to design appropriate primers at opposite sides of the junctional regions. In routine PCR-based clonality studies, the distance between the primers should be <1 kb, preferably <500 bp, and in formalin-fixed tissues where DNA is much degraded, preferably <300 bp. This is particularly important to discriminate between PCR products from monoclonal versus polyclonal Ig/TCR gene rearrangements. The main advantages of PCR techniques are their speed, the low amounts of DNA required, the possibility to use DNA of lower quality, and the relatively good sensitivity of 1–5%. Consequently, PCR techniques allow the use of small biopsies (e.g., fine-needle aspiration biopsies) or of formaldehyde-fixed paraffin-embedded archival material with low-quality DNA, that is partly degraded into small fragments.

Although molecular clonality studies can be highly informative, several limitations and pitfalls might hamper the interpretation of the results:

- Ig and TCR gene rearrangements are not necessarily restricted to B- and T-cell lineages, respectively. Cross-lineage TCR gene rearrangements occur relatively frequently in immature B-cell malignancies, not only in precursor B-ALL (>90% of cases), but also in AMLs, and mature B-cell malignancies might contain TCR gene rearrangements.
- Reactive lymph nodes can show reduced diversity of the Ig/TCR gene repertoire caused by predominance of several antigen-selected subclones (oligoclonality). In particular, lymph nodes or blood samples of patients with an active EBV or CMV infection can show a restricted TCR repertoire or TCR gene oligoclonality. Also, immunosuppression is frequently associated with restricted TCR repertoires, for example, in transplant patients. Recovery from transplantation and hematological remission are followed by restoration of the polyclonal TCR repertoire.
- False-positive PCR results are a problem, if no adequate analysis of the obtained PCR products is performed to discriminate between monoclonal, oligoclonal, or polyclonal PCR products. False-negative results occur because of improper annealing of the applied PCR primers to the rearranged gene segments. First, precise detection of all different V, D, and J gene segments would require many different primers, which is practical. Consequently, family primers, which specifically recognize most or all members of a particular V, D, or J family, or consensus primers are designed, which recognize virtually all V and J gene segments of the locus under study. Family primers and consensus primers are optimal for a part of the relevant Ig/TCR gene segments, but show a lower homology to others. This may eventually lead to false-negative results, particularly in Ig/TCR genes with many different gene segments. The second problem is somatic

hypermutations in rearranged Ig genes of germinal center and postgerminal center B-cell malignancies.

- Clonality does not as such imply malignancy. This applies to B- or T-cell proliferations in immunodeficiency syndromes, such as in patients with human immunodeficiency virus (HIV) infections or patients with congenital immunodeficiency. In organ transplant recipients, clonal B-cell lymphoproliferations might develop and often regress upon withdrawal of immunosuppression. B-cell clones have also been reported in autoimmune diseases, such as in Sjögren's syndrome. Finally, benign monoclonal gammopathies are sometimes associated with clonal B-cell proliferations. Benign clonal T-cell proliferations may be seen in a variety of benign cutaneous diseases.

In a number of tumors, clonality analysis helps to clarify the molecular pathology of a disorder, although it is not necessary in clinical practice.

- Analysis of Ig gene rearrangement patterns in Reed–Sternberg cells isolated from nodular lymphocyte-predominant Hodgkin's lymphoma suggested that this particular lymphoma is a monoclonal extension of B cells, particularly germinal-center B cells at the centroblastic stage of differentiation (11).
- Sequential analysis of Ig or TCR gene rearrangement patterns permits to trace the clonal evolution of a lymphoma over time. Examples are the clonal relationship between chronic B-cell lymphocytic leukemia and secondary high grade B-cell lymphoma in Richter's syndrome, or follicular lymphoma with transformation into a secondary high-grade lymphoma (12).
- In patients with head and neck cancer, solitary lung nodules composed of squamous cell carcinoma may either represent a new primary tumor or metastases. Obviously in such tumors no antigen receptor gene rearrangements can be expected. Analysis of tumor-specific genetic alterations was, therefore, performed with the help of *polymorphic microsatellite markers* that may discern such clonal relationships (Fig. 1.4). It appears that solitary nodules of squamous cell carcinoma in the lung in patients with known head and neck cancers are more likely to represent a metastasis than an independent lung cancer (13,14). Likewise, microsatellite analysis could be applied to any patient with multiple tumors where clonal tumor relationships are not clear on clinical, radiological, or histological grounds.

In summary, the vast majority of tumors seen in our patients are of clonal origin, which is of course in perfect accordance with the somatic mutation theory of cancer. Assessment of clonality may occasionally be useful in cancer diagnostics, particularly molecular immunogenotyping of lymphoproliferative lesions where the distinction between polyclonal/reactive and clonal/neoplastic processes might otherwise be difficult or impossible.

Types of Gene Mutations Seen in Cancer

Genetic information is contained in double-stranded DNA (Fig. 1.5). Genes are transcribed into mRNA and eventually the encoded protein is produced. In the molecular alphabet

words are called codons composed of three letters or nucleotides each. Each codon encodes either an amino acid and/or specifies a function such as a start signal or a stop signal for transcription. Any alteration in the order of these

(A) Point polymorphisms (creating 2 alleles at a given locus)

● Restriction enzyme cutting site: present or absent

(B) Variable number of tandem repeat (VNTR) minisatellites ▲

(C) Microsatellites

CACACACACACACACACACA
CACACACACACA
CACACACACACACACACACACACACACA

(D) Single nucleotide polymorphisms (SNPs)

GAGTCTGCGCGCTATCAGGCCTGTGTCCATAGTT
AAGTCTGCGCGCTATTAGGCCTGTGTCCATAGTC

Figure 1.4   DNA polymorphisms. DNA polymorphisms are variations in the nucleotide sequence of DNA. Most of them are functionally silent. Polymorphic alleles are present in the constitutional DNA of each individual and passed on in the germline to the progeny. DNA polymorphisms are widely used genetic markers tagging particular allelic chromosomal regions similar to signposts along roads or motorways. Several different types of DNA polymorphisms are illustrated in this figure where DNA fragments are schematically illustrated as bars. (a) Point polymorphisms are created through variations in the DNA sequence that form new restriction enzyme sites (drak gray circle) or destroy a preexisting cutting site (restriction fragment length polymorphisms, RFLP). The length of a DNA fragment is, therefore, defined through the spacing between two specific enzyme-cutting sites. This type of polymorphism is called a bimorphism as only two alleles are possible (a longer and a shorter one). Although popular for genetic analyses in the early days of genetics, this type of polymorphism has lost much of its importance for molecular genetic diagnostics. (b) The length of a DNA fragment may be determined by insertion of variable numbers (VN) of tandem repeats (TR) or minisatellites. Minisatellites are composed of short nucleotide sequence blocks (perhaps 20mer to 30mer of length) that are aligned one after another as repeat motifs (drak gray triangles). This polymorphism may, thus, create many different alleles in a population depending on the number of TR inserted. A given individual may of course only harbor two alleles in a diploid set of chromosomes, one inherited by the father and one inherited by the mother. (c) Microsatellites have become a most widely used type of polymorphism. Similar to VNTR, microsatellites are composed of variable numbers of short nucleotide repeat units, for example, dinucleotides (CACACA in this example), or trinucleotides. Their numbers determine the length of PCR fragments amplified through specific primers placed at sequences flanking the repeat units. Many different alleles may occur in a given population. (d) Single nucleotide polymorphisms (SNPs, pronounced "snips") are variations in single base pairs of the DNA that change from one chromosome to the other. There are about 3 million SNPs randomly distributed throughout the genome, which represent 90% of all variations in the human genome. SNPs are nowadays among the most widely used markers, particularly because SNP patterns can now be investigated very efficiently with microchips ("snip chips") that cover most of the genome with a marker density of 300–1000 bp. A SNP profile can distinguish patients who would otherwise be indistinguishable, for example, by linking the polymorphism to the fact of whether a patient tolerates a drug or not for genetic reasons.

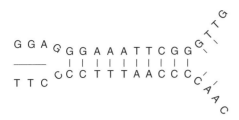

Figure 1.5 Nucleic acid hybridization. Two single strands of nucleic acids may form a stable double-strand through base-pairing provided their nucleotide sequences are complementary. In the genetic code the purine base adenine (A) can only form bonds with the pyrimidine base thymine (T) in DNA or uracil in RNA, and the purine base guanine (G) can only team up with the pyrimidine base cytosine (C). Bonds between G and T or A and C (*left part*) are not possible. Much of molecular biology really boils down to the simple finding that two single strands of nucleic acids may bind to each other very specifically provided their nucleotide sequences (the molecular alphabet) are complementary. This is a fundamental principle of molecular biology which you ought to remember when you struggle with the PCR and other molecular diagnostic tests, or when you are lost in the jungle of gene mutations, DNA mismatch repair, etc.

nucleotides may scramble the genetic code. This is relevant since cancer is essentially a molecular disorder of cells and their genes. The somatic mutation theory of cancer predicts that gene mutations are crucial in carcinogenesis, because genetic mutations may activate genes inappropriately or inactivate genes which are needed in the normal life of a cell. Somatic mutations are acquired at mitosis whereas germline gene mutations are passed on to an individual from a parent or occur *de novo* at meiosis.

A survey of the *diverse types of gene mutations* encountered in cancer, and examples of how they disturb gene function is assembled in Table 1.1. It displays a message written according to the principles of the genetic code where each "letter," that is, an amino acid in a protein chain or a genetic function, is represented by a nucleotide triplet in the DNA sequence. Various types of DNA mutations altering the message are indicated in the corresponding column and classified as to whether they represent "activating" mutations (i.e., mutations that lead to inappropriate activity of the gene) or "inactivating" mutations (i.e., silencing the gene). Additional molecular mechanisms that are not presented in Table 1.1 are the following:

Telomeres, the physical ends of linear chromosomes cannot be fully replicated by "conventional" DNA polymerases. In the absence of a specialized replication mode for the chromosomal tips, a chromosome would lose telomere repeats with each cell division. An enzyme complex, *telomerase* is able to compensate such telomere loss by adding appropriate nucleotides to chromosomal 3′ ends. In most human somatic cells, telomerase activity is repressed, whereas in the vast majority of human tumors, telomerase is reactivated. Therefore, an attractive approach to cancer therapy could be the inhibition of telomerase in tumor cells to shorten their survival, perhaps with little deleterious effect on most normal cells. The precise impact on differences between telomerase activity in human normal and cancer cells is still controversial, but the connection between telomerase activity and human carcinogenesis is intriguing (15).

A new molecular principle has recently been discovered in chronic lymphocytic leukemia (CLL). CLL often shows deletions in chromosome 13q, but no classical tumor suppressor genes were found at this locus. Instead, a cluster of two microRNA genes, *MIRN15A* and *MIRN16-1*, is located exactly inside the minimal region of genetic loss at 13q14, and both genes are deleted or downregulated in the majority of 13q- CLL samples (16). MicroRNAs are small noncoding RNA molecules distinct from but related to small interfering RNAs (siRNAs). These small 19–24-nucleotide (nt) RNAs are transcribed as parts of longer molecules named pri-miRNA, several kilobases (kb) in length, that are processed in the nucleus into hairpin RNAs of named pre-miRNA by double-stranded RNA-specific ribonuclease. The hairpin RNAs are transported to the cytoplasm, where they are digested by a second double-stranded RNA-specific ribonuclease. In animals, single-stranded microRNA binds specific messenger RNA (mRNA) through sequences that are significantly, though not completely, complementary to the target mRNA, mainly to the 3′ untranslated region. Bound mRNA remains untranslated, resulting in reduced levels of the corresponding protein. Alternatively, in some case, bound mRNA can be degraded, resulting in reduced levels of both the corresponding transcript and the protein. Today the number of microRNAs, including those electronically cloned, is growing fast. Current collective evidence strongly indicates a role for microRNAs in hematological cancers and solid tumors.

Patients with a myelodysplastic syndrome (MDS) with deletion of chromosome 5q (the 5q- syndrome) have severe macrocytic anemia, normal or elevated platelet counts, normal or reduced neutrophil counts, erythroid hypoplasia in the bone marrow, and hypolobated micromegakaryocytes. They may progress to AML, although more slowly than other forms of MDS. The 5q- MDS shows a remarkable response to treatment with the thalidomide analogue lenalidomide. Patients with 5q- MDS do not have biallelic gene deletions within a common deleted region (CDR) on 5q and no point mutations. Rather the 5q- syndrome is caused by *protein haplo-insufficiency*, which is a loss of only one allele at a given locus, implicating reduced protein expression from the remaining single allele, that is, a reduction in gene dosage (17). Partial loss of function, or haplo-insufficiency of a gene called *RPS14* recapitulates the phenotype of the 5q- syndrome, that is, an erythroid maturation block with preservation of megakaryocyte differentiation. Decreased expression of *RPS14*, a component of the 40S ribosomal subunit, results in an accumulation of the 30S pre-rRNA species with a concomitant decrease in 18S/18SE rRNA levels, which is consistent with reports that *RPS14* is specifically required for the processing of 18S pre-rRNA.

CHROMOSOMAL TRANSLOCATIONS IN HEMATOLOGICAL MALIGNANCIES AND SARCOMAS

A chromosomal translocation creating the Philadelphia (Phi) chromosome was the first clonal karyotype abnormality or marker chromosome firmly linked to a human cancer, CML (Fig. 1.6a). Ever since this observation was made in 1960 by Nowell and Hungerford in Philadelphia (hence its

Table 1.1   Types of Gene Mutations Seen in Malignant Tumors
You have discovered mice in your kitchen which you would like to eliminate. In analogy to the genetic code, you write up a call for help (the message) using three-letter words (to mimic codons or nucleotide triplets in the genetic code). The start of the message is indicated by the triplet *AUG*, the universal initiation codon of transcription. One of the three triplets *UAA* or *UAG* or *UGA* (stop codons in the genetic code) indicates where the message stops, similar to a period in writing

DNA wild (i.e., normal) type sequence	Description	Comments
5′ *AUG* HUE AND CRY AND GET THE CAT *UAA* 3′ DNA sequence alterations seen in cancer	Wild type DNA sequence or message	*AUG* is the universal initiation codon of transcription *UAA/UAG/UGA* are stop codons
5′ *AUG* HUE AND CRY AND GET THE **B**AT *UAA* 3′	Point mutation	Altered, but still functional message *Example* *ras* gene point mutation in AML
AUG HUE AND CRY AND GET THE **RAT** *UAA*	Point mutation	Missense mutation. Gene inactivation
AUG HUE AND CRY AND **FRY** THE CAT *UAA*	Substitution of one codon for another	Missense mutation. Gene inactivation
AUG HUE AND CRY A^ND^GE TTH ECA TUA A	Deletion of more or fewer than three nucleotides	Frameshift mutation throwing the 3′ part of the message out of context. Insertion of extra nucleotides (more or fewer than three) into a codon yields a similar problem. Gene inactivation *Example* NPM mutation in AML
AUG HU^E AND CRY AND GET THE C^AT *UAA*	Deletion	Range of deletion may be between loss of a few nucleotides and loss of an entire chromosome. Loss of function *Example* Normal allele in tumor suppressor genes, for example p53
AUG HUE AND CRY *UAA* ^AND GET THE CAT UAA^	Premature insertion of stop codon	Truncated or abolished message. Gene inactivation. *Example* FAP gene mutation in familial ade- nomatous polyposis colon cancer
1) *AUG* HUE AND CRY AND GET THE **MAT** *UAA* 2) *AUG* HU^E AND CRY AND GET THE C^AT *UAA*	Point mutation on allele 1; Deletion of wild type message in allele 2 (LOH)	Typical mutational pattern of a classical tumour suppressor gene. LOH = loss of heterozygosity due to loss of allele 2 *Example* p53 tumor suppressor gene
A) *AUG* HUE AND CRY AND GET THE CAT UAA B) *AUG* AND PUT THE DOG OUT *UAA* A-B) *AUG* HUE AND CRY AND PUT THE DOG OUT *UAA*	Messages A and B from different genes A-B fusion gene/message	Chromosomal translocation producing a fusion gene composed of parts from gene A and B. Altered message with new meaning. *Example* BCR-ABL fusion gene in CML

GET THE CAT
       GET THE CAT
       GET THE CAT
 AUG HUE AND CRY AND GET THE CAT *UAA*
       GET THE CAT
       GET THE CAT
       GET THE CAT
	Gene amplification	Increase in allelic copy number of a gene or a part thereof, mostly leading to inappropriate overexpression of the protein. Gain of function
		 Example
		 HER2/neu in breast cancer

AUG HUE AND CRY AND GET THE CAT **AND GET THE CAT** *UAA*	Internal tandem duplication of an exon or genetic material in a gene	Partial duplication of message or parts thereof within a gene. Gene activation *Example* Internal tandem duplication of the FLT3 gene in AML
AUG HUE AND CRY AND GET THE CAT *UAA Message copies in cells with deficient DNA mismatch repair mechanisms:* *AUG* HUE AND CRY AND **P**ET THE CAT *UAA* *AUG* **S**UE **(AND CRY AND GET)** THE CAT *UAA* *AUG* HUE AND CRY AND GET **HUM PTY DUM PTY** *UAA*	Deficient DNA mismatch repair genes	Mutations in DNA mismatch repair genes may contribute to genetic instability and lead to errors at DNA copying throughout the genome *Example* Replication-error-positive (RER⁺) tumors, for example hereditary non-polypo¬sis colon cancer (HNPCC) syndrome
C^meth^pG C^meth^pG C^meth^pG *AUG* HUE AND CRY AND GET THE CAT *UAA* C^meth^pG C^meth^pG C^meth^pG **AUG HUE AND CRY AND GET THE CAT UAA**	Hypermethylation of C residues in CpG rich sequences	Hypermethylation of cytosine C residues (often in CG-rich sequences, so-called CpG islands) in or near a gene (e.g., in the promoter) can shut off or activate a gene

name), the characterization of chromosomal translocations has given us remarkable insights into both the molecular pathology of many different hematological neoplasms as well as unprecedented knowledge about the contribution of many genes to normal cellular physiology (18–20). Chromosomal translocations creating fusion genes occur regularly in many (but not all) leukemias as well as in a variety of sarcomas including small round cell tumors

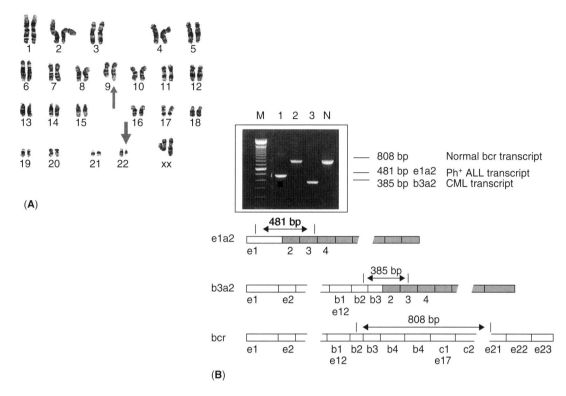

(A)

(B)

Figure 1.6 Chromosomal translocations—the Philadelphia chromosome in CML at the chromosome and molecular level. (a) A karyotype is prepared from cultured leukemic cells of a female CML patient (XX). In the mitotic figures, the individual chromosomes can be identified. Chromosomes are numbered according to their size (No. 1 is the longest chromosome in the human karyotype, No. 22 the shortest one). Each chromosome shows a typical banding pattern seen on light microscopy. The small abnormal chromosome to the right of the normal chromosome 22 (red arrow) represents the Philadelphia chromosome composed from parts of chromosome 9 and chromosome 22. As this translocation is reciprocal, a second abnormal chromosome (where parts from chromosomes 22 are added to chromosome 9) is seen next to the normal chromosome 9 (pale red arrow), but this is not relevant for the pathology of CML. *Source*: Courtesy of Dr. Martine Jotterand, Lausanne. (b) The most frequent types of transcripts from the BCR-ABL fusion genes seen in Phi+ leukemias are shown. Open boxes indicate exons from the BCR gene and shaded boxes exons from the ABL gene. PCR primers are depicted as black vertical lines. Exons are numbered. Phi+ ALL often shows the e1a2 transcript composed of exon 1 from the BCR gene joined to exon 2 of the ABL gene. This transcript may be detected by RT-PCR using a primer on BCR exon 1 and a primer on ABL exon 3 yielding a 481 bp fragment. One of the most frequent transcripts seen in CML is the b3a2 transcript. Here the BCR primer is placed onto exon b2 (=e13) present in the M-BCR (Fig. 1.10) and the ABL primer recognizes sequences from exon 3. The result is a 385 bp PCR fragment. The normal nontranslocated BCR gene produces a 808 bp fragment using BCR primers b2/e13 and e21. Use of this primer pair would yield no signal from any Phi+ chromosome because annealing sites for the e21 primer would all be replaced by ABL sequences. RT-PCR amplicons are electrophoresed on an agarose gel and visualized as discrete bands (*top inset*). Their molecular size may be identified with the help of a molecular weight marker with multiple fragments differing in size by 100 bp (M). N is a normal leukocyte sample, and cases 1–3 are Phi+ ALL with transcript e1a2 (1), a myeloid leukemia with a normal 808 bp BCR transcript and no evidence of a BCR-ABL fusion transcript (2), and a CML with transcript b3a2, respectively. The specificity of the primers used and the identification of the PCR fragment size in the gel suffice for the molecular diagnosis. Nowadays, however, the PCR fragments are often sequenced to determine their exact nucleotide sequence and the result compared with published sequence maps from the BCR and the ABL genes. *Source*: Courtesy of Dr. E. Oppliger Leibundgut, Berne.

(peripheral/primitive neuroectodermal tumors), but are rare in carcinomas. Recurrent balanced chromosomal rearrangements are strongly associated with distinct tumor entities, and there is compelling evidence that they represent early events in malignant transformation (18).

Molecular Biology of Chromosomal Translocations

Chromosomal translocations may basically lead to two types of gene alterations (Fig. 1.7):

1. A gene residing on one chromosome (chromosome A) may be juxtaposed to regulatory sequences of another completely unrelated gene on a different chromosome (chromosome B). The gene from chromosome A may

still retain an intact internal organization, but it ends up in a different genetic environment that drastically alters its expression. This type of translocation is most frequently seen in the lymphomas (Fig. 1.7). A classical example is Burkitt's lymphoma where the c-*myc* oncogene on chromosome 8 is translocated near the Ig heavy-chain gene locus on chromosome 14q32. As in B cells, Ig gene loci are actively transcribed as a part of normal B-cell function, Ig heavy chain gene promoter and enhancer sequences will constitutively activate their new neighbor, the c-*myc* oncogene. As a result transcription and translation of this oncogene are greatly enhanced. Overproduction of the c-*myc* protein, which is a transcription factor, will in turn activate other genes downstream and profoundly alter the

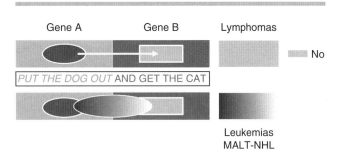

Figure 1.7   The principle of chromosomal translocations. Chromosomal translocations may place an intact gene into a new genetic neighborhood. The result is usually untimely or otherwise inappropriate expression of its normal protein product (*top panel*). Fusion genes composed of parts from two different chromosomes may yield abnormal fusion proteins (also termed chimeric proteins) that do not occur in normal cells (*bottom panel*).

proliferation and survival characteristics of these lymphoma cells.

2. A different set of chromosomal translocations create unique fusion genes. In this type of translocation, unrelated parts of different genes, which originally reside on completely different chromosomal loci, are brought together to form a new unique fusion gene. This type of translocation most commonly occurs in leukemias, male germ cell cancers, and in some sarcomas. The classic citation in this respect is the Phi chromosome in CML (Figs. 1.6 and 1.7). Typically, parts of a gene (but not the entire gene) on one chromosome are joined to parts of another gene (again not the entire gene) from a partner chromosome. The resulting fusion gene takes regulatory sequences and some of the exons from one partner chromosome and the rest of its exons and intronic sequences from the other chromosome. Transcription of this fusion gene results in an abnormal fusion or hybrid messenger RNA composed of sequences from both genes and the same will be true for the fusion protein. Such fusion genes contribute to leukemia if their product is able to change the life of the cell to its advantage. Clever experiments have shown that the BCR-ABL fusion gene (the molecular equivalent of the Phi chromosome in CML) can be introduced into normal hematopoietic stem cells of mice. In a bone marrow transplant model, these manipulated stem cells may repopulate the marrow of the experimental animals after marrow-ablative treatment. However, the resulting hematopoiesis is not normal but resembles a murine myeloproliferative syndrome reminiscent of human CML. Such experiments provide direct proof that fusion genes and their abnormal protein products contribute to leukemogenesis, even if perhaps a single molecular hit is not always sufficient to create a full-blown leukemia.

Classical examples of various malignancies and their typical translocations are listed in Table 1.2. Most partner genes involved in such translocations operate in molecular pathways essential for cell proliferation, differentiation, and cell death. The BCR and ABL genes are protein kinases that typically operate in signal transduction. Many genes involved in chromosomal translocations are transcription factors. Some partner genes in chromosomal translocations are receptors that, similar to protein kinases, may be involved in signal transduction and cell differentiation. Acute promyelocytic leukemia (APL) is the prime example for this type of translocation as it involves the retinoic acid receptor α. Genes regulating programmed cell death, apoptosis, may also be involved, for example, *bcl*-2.

A largely unsolved riddle is the molecular mechanism by which such translocations are created (18,21). As for most gene fusions no specific initiating factors have been found, chromosomal instability, a common feature of many cancer cells, may perhaps create translocations simply by chance, and one may assume that DNA double-strand breaks are required for most chromosome aberrations that produce fusion genes. A concept with a relatively firm basis is gene translocation through illegitimate genetic recombination and recombinase errors in B lymphoid cells. There is good reason to assume that this applies to lymphoid neoplasms where one of the partner genes involved is an antigen receptor gene. Reshuffling, juggling, and recombination of gene segments from antigen receptor genes are normal physiological events that are crucial to create functional Ig or TCR genes (Fig. 1.3). Recombinases required for antigen receptor gene rearrangements operate through the "diagnosis" of specific recognition sequences conveniently placed near the gene segments of interest. It so happens that some of these sequences can also be found near oncogenes, for example, near the *bcl*-2 oncogene. Although in a B cell the Ig genes are being rearranged, a recombinase could pick by error a *bcl*-2 oncogene sequence instead of an Ig gene sequence and join it to an Ig gene locus. Inappropriate activation of *bcl*-2, an antiapoptotic gene under the influence of an Ig gene promoter, would provide the cell with a distinctive survival advantage over normal lymphocytes.

The fact that chromosomal translocations are consistently associated with specific tumor types supports the assumption of cell lineage-specific mechanisms of tumorigenesis (22). At least one of the two partners of fusion genes is often active in a cell lineage-specific biological playground. The BCR-ABL chimeric gene product does not transform nonhematopoietic cell types (e.g., NIH 3T3 fibroblasts), but does confer growth factor independence and inhibition of apoptosis in hematopoietic cell culture systems. Its lineage specificity may also depend on the type of its promoter. BCR-ABL expression under the BCR gene promoter has devastating effects on many cell types whereas expression of the same fusion gene under a metallothionein promoter specifically leads to leukemia in mice. The APL-specific PML-RARα fusion protein exerts growth suppression and cell death in nonhematopoietic and many hematopoietic cell lines, but the myeloid environment is tolerant to these toxic effects, and myeloid cells gain an advantage from this chimeric protein. Lineage-specific expression of an oncogene may also be achieved if it is placed under the control of a gene that is normally active in this cell type. An example is c-*myc* overexpression

Table 1.2 Selected Examples of Chromosomal Translocations in Hematological Malignancies and Sarcomas

Neoplasm	Karyotype	Gene A	Gene B	Comments
B-cell lymphomas Follicular NHL	t(14;18)(q32;q21)	18q21 *bcl-2* gene (B-cell lymphoma gene 2) *Anti-apoptosis* gene	14q32 Ig heavy-chain gene	Overexpression of *bcl-2* prevents apoptotic death in transformed B cells. The t(14;18) is also seen in some normal B cells indicating that by itself it is not sufficient for full neoplastic transformation
Mantle cell NHL (and some other B-cell lymphomas)	t(11;14)(q13;q32)	11q13 *bcl-1* locus harboring the PRAD1 oncogene/ cyclin D1/CCND1 gene *Cell cycle regulator*	14q32 Ig heavy-chain gene	Overexpression of cyclin D1
Burkitt's NHL	t(8;14)(q24;q32)	8q24 c-*myc* oncogene *Transcription factor*	14q32 Ig heavy-chain gene	In a transgenic mouse model, overexpression of c-*myc* was shown to yield lymphoma. In endemic BL sequences far upstream of c-*myc* join into the Ig gene region whereas in sporadic BL sequences within the first intron and exon of c-*myc* are involved
B-cell leukemias Childhood B-cell precursor ALL (favorable prognosis)	t(12;21)(p13;q22)	12p13 Tel gene/ETV-6 gene Translocation Ets leukemia Ets (E26 avian erythroblastosis virus transformation-specific protein) translocation variant gene 6 *Transcription factor*	21q22 AML1 gene or PEBP2αB gene (human homologue of the DNA-binding α-subunit of the heterodimeric polyomavirus enhancer core binding protein PEBP2$\alpha\beta$) or CBFA2 gene (core binding factor A2) *Transcription factor*	Fusion gene. This translocation is usually not seen in routine karyotypes, but only on molecular analysis (FISH or PCR). The TEL gene is frequently rearranged in a wide variety of hematological neoplasms. The TEL/AML1 fusion gene is the most common gene rearrangement in childhood ALL, but rare in adult ALL
T-cell neoplasms Ki1+/CD30+ anaplastic T-cell NHL	t(2;5)(p23;q35)	2p23 ALK gene (anaplastic lymphoma kinase) *Tyrosine protein kinase*	5q35 NPM gene (nucleophosmin gene) *Nuclear phosphoprotein* involved in ribosome assembly	Fusion gene
Acute and chronic myeloid leukemias CML (and Phi+ ALL)	t(9;22)(q34;q11) Philadelphia chromosome	9q34 c-*abl* oncogene *Tyrosine protein kinase* involved in signal transduction	22q11 BCR gene *Serine/threonine protein kinase* involved in signal transduction	Fusion gene The BCR-ABL fusion protein p210 shows increased tyrosine protein kinase activity, confers growth factor independence, and inhibits apoptosis. Imatinib mesylate (or Glivec[R]) inhibits this fusion protein. In Phi+ ALL breaks often occur in the first intron of the BCR gene (m-BCR), and the fusion protein is somewhat smaller (p185 or p190) than in CML
AML FAB M2 with maturation	t(8;21)(q22;q22)	8q22 ETO gene (for eight twenty-one) or MTG8 gene *Transcription factor*	21q22 AML1 gene or PEBP2αB gene (human homologue of the DNA-binding α-subunit of the heterodimeric polyomavirus enhancer core binding protein PEBP2$\alpha\beta$) or CBFA2 gene (core binding factor A2) *Subunit of a transcription factor*	Fusion gene
APL	t(15;17)(q22;q21)	15q22 PML gene (promyelocytic leukemia) *Transcription factor*	17q21 RARα gene (retinoic acid receptor α gene) *Receptor involved in cell differentiation*	Fusion gene

(Continued)

Table 1.2 Selected Examples of Chromosomal Translocations in Hematological Malignancies and Sarcomas (*Continued*)

Neoplasm	Karyotype	Gene A	Gene B	Comments
Treatment-related AML	Abnormal 11q23 and various partner chromosomes	Various partner genes	11q23 MLL gene (mixed lineage leukemia) ALL-1 gene HRX/HTRX gene (human homologue of the Drosophila trithorax gene) *Transcription factor*	Mostly fusion genes. MLL is among the most promiscuous oncogenes in human leukemia, but the fusion partners do not appear to contain a common motif. 11q23 abnormalities occur particularly in treatment-related AML after exposure to epipodophyllotoxins targeting topoisomerase II and in infant ALL
Sarcomas				
Ewing sarcoma and related small round cell tumors including peripheral/ primitive neuroectodermal tumors	t(11;22)(q24;q12)	11q24 FLI-1 gene (friend leukemia integration site 1, associated with virus-induced murine erythroleukemia) *Transcription factor*	22q12 EWS gene (Ewing sarcoma gene) *Transcription factor*	Fusion gene

in Burkitt's lymphoma under the influence of an Ig gene promoter in B cells.

Clinical Relevance of Detecting Chromosomal Translocations in Hematological Neoplasms

The molecular dissection of chromosomal translocations has provided new diagnostic tools in hematological oncology and in the difficult diagnosis of certain types of sarcomas. Molecular analysis might be used at diagnosis for staging, during patient follow-up, and for the detection of contaminating malignant cells in hemopoietic stem cell harvests used in autologous stem cell transplantation. It must be stressed, however, that the molecular detection of karyotype abnormalities does not replace cytogenetics. Careful cytogenetic analysis of lymphomas and leukemias is still indispensable to provide a valuable survey of their karyotypes. None of the molecular methods used in clinical pathology provides this type of unbiased screening over genetic alterations in cancer. Rather, molecular techniques may specifically complement karyotyping as further outlined below.

Most of the chromosomal translocations are now amenable to specific amplification by the PCR. The beauty of this concept is that in a chromosomal translocation, the molecular area where partner genes meet is a unique hybrid sequence specific for a leukemia or a lymphoma cell and absent in normal cells. In a few translocations such as the t(14;18) in follicular lymphoma, DNA may be used as the starting material for the PCR (12, 23, 24). However, PCR amplification of translocation genes is only successful if both gene partners break and reassemble within precisely defined molecular breakpoints or in breakpoint cluster areas for which specific primers may be designed. This is indeed the case for follicular lymphoma, but in many other lymphomas and leukemias, breakpoints may vary on at least one of the partner genes. Reverse transcription PCR (RT-PCR) starting from fusion mRNA overcomes this problem in a very elegant way. As the splicing of primary RNA transcripts eliminates all intronic sequences, the fusion gene mRNAs are small and handy and offer sequences

suitable for the design of PCR primers (Fig. 1.8). In practice, RNA is extracted from leukemic cells, subjected to reverse transcription, which produces a cDNA copy from the fusion gene mRNA of interest which is enriched through PCR amplification. The PCR detection of chromosomal translocations is highly specific and much quicker than karyotyping. An alternative detection technique is the fluorescent in situ hybridization (FISH) that is described later in this chapter.

In practice, many leukemias can now be typed at the molecular level, which is valuable because specific cytogenetic abnormalities are of considerable prognostic significance and information on the karyotype is increasingly being used to design custom-tailored treatment programs. The prime example is APL. This leukemia has a good prognosis and the detection of the specific t(15;17) accurately predicts whether a case suspected to represent APL on morphology really will respond to differentiation therapy with all-transretinoic acid (ATRA). Myeloid leukemias that resemble APL on morphology but lack this specific molecular abnormality are very unlikely to respond to ATRA (25–27).

Molecular techniques can also be used for lymphoma staging. In patients with follicular lymphoma, occult involvement of the bone marrow, which is not detectable by light microscopy of smears or biopsies, can be traced by PCR amplification of the t(14;18). It is not quite clear at present whether in clinical stage I or II follicular lymphoma the detection of occult marrow involvement (molecular stage IV) would really have an impact on clinical management (12,23,28).

Another chief interest of molecular karyotyping in leukemia and lymphoma is the possibility for highly sensitive molecular follow-up and the detection of minimal residual disease (MRD) (8,28). Remission in cancer patients is defined as the absence of any detectable tumor using available diagnostic methods. In the leukemias, hematological remission requires the demonstration of a normal bone marrow on morphology as well as the return to normal peripheral blood cell counts. Unfortunately, hematological remission is no guarantee for cure as

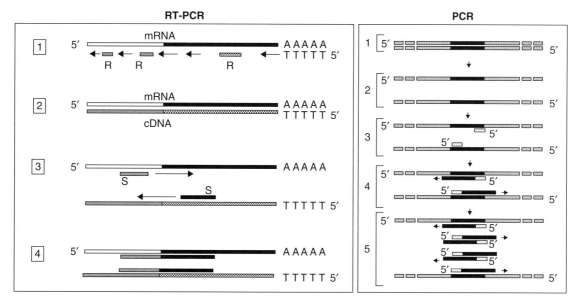

Figure 1.8 The principle of the PCR and RT-PCR. Right panel: (1) A double-stranded DNA sample contains a region of interest (black) for PCR amplification. (2) In an initial step, DNA is heated to separate the two complementary strands. (3) In order to amplify the black excerpt, some DNA sequence information on its flanking regions is necessary. This information is used to prepare primers (short oligonucleotide sequences of about 20–25 nt) that are complementary to specific and unique sequences on the respective single strands of DNA (small dotted boxes). Under suitable conditions (temperature, time, and salt concentrations in the tube being the most critical), the primers anneal specifically to their complementary sequences on the DNA strands. (4) Annealed primers provide the starting signal for a DNA polymerase (Taq polymerase) to synthesize a new DNA strand along the template strands with nucleotides provided in the reaction mix (arrows). It is essential that the new strand extends into the region of the other primer. This will in turn guarantee that in a next round of PCR, each primer will find a suitable sequence to anneal not only to the original "mother" template but also on the newly formed short PCR fragments. (5) Each PCR round or cycle runs sequentially through steps 2–4 and the technique thus permits exponential amplification of the fragment of interest (black). Typically PCR steps take anything between 10 sec to several minutes each. Usually 25–45 PCR cycles are performed and provide $2n$ amplification, where n is the number of cycles. After 30 cycles, this means a lot of identical fragments! The PCR product may be visualized by gel electrophoresis and identified through its molecular size, or it may be sequenced. Left panel: (1) Instead of DNA the starting material is single-stranded RNA extracted from a leukemia cell with a chromosomal translocation. The fusion mRNA is therefore composed of sequences from one chromosome (empty box) joined to sequences from another chromosome (black box). mRNA typically has a poly(A) tail at its 3′ end. The first step of the RT-PCR reaction is to copy the mRNA strand into a complementary DNA strand (cDNA strand). Two types of primers may be used to direct this synthesis: either a poly(dT) primer that anneals with the poly(A) tail of the mRNA molecule or random primers composed of nonspecific redundant sequences with a high likelihood of finding a sequence on the mRNA strand where they may anneal (gray and dotted boxes marked R). Thus, they provide the starting signals for the unidirectional synthesis of a cDNA strand (arrows) directed by the enzyme reverse transcriptase (RT). (2) The result is a nucleic acid double strand with one strand representing the original fusion mRNA and the other one the newly synthesized cDNA strand. Subsequently, the technique follows the principle of the PCR as shown in the right panel. (3) Heating separates the two strands. A specific set of primers is now used to target nucleic acid sequences of interest. Both primers (gray and black small boxes marked S) are specific for sequences flanking the fusion area where exons transcribed from either partner chromosome were spliced together. These primers are used to synthesize complementary DNA copies from the mRNA and the cDNA templates, respectively. Synthesis of these strands is directed by a polymerase, usually heat-stable Taq polymerase. (4) The result of this round is the production of two copies of fusion cDNA sequences, which along with the original templates, are amenable to further rounds of specific PCR amplification.

malignant cells in the bone marrow may go undetected if present below the 1–5% threshold. Specific amplification of chromosomal fusion genes provides a sensitive method for the detection of minimal residual leukemia or lymphoma. The sensitivity of detecting occult malignant cells in normal tissue varies between 1×10^4 and 1×10^6. There is a price to pay, however, for such high detection sensitivity. The PCR has a risk of false-positive results through amplification of contaminant nucleic acid fragments. RT-PCR may be false-negative if at the time of sampling malignant cells do not express the critical fusion gene.

A number of interesting correlations between PCR typing data and clinical parameters have been worked out in the literature:

* Patients with AML characterized by t(8;21) have an excellent long-term prognosis after chemotherapy although PCR monitoring may demonstrate that varying levels of detectable t(8;21) transcripts persist in long-term remission (29).
* In contrast, APL patients in stable long-term remission invariably show negative PCR results. The reappearance of the PCR-detected t(15;17) almost always heralds

clinical relapse (26,27). The question of whether molecular APL relapse during ongoing hematological remission ought to be retreated at an early stage (before relapse becomes apparent on bone marrow morphology or clinically) is currently unresolved.

- Patients with t(14;18)-positive follicular lymphoma who achieve molecular remission during the first year of their treatment enjoy a significantly longer failure-free survival than those who do not. In some series, serial PCR analysis to determine molecular response in this lymphoma apparently correlates well with outcome (12,24).

- In ALL antigen receptor gene rearrangements provide unique leukemia- and case-specific molecular tags amenable to PCR (Fig. 1.3). In each leukemic clone, an Ig or TCR gene is a unique marker because specific variable (V), diversity (D), and joining (J) sequences are selected from a large pool to form a specific rearranged gene through VDJ joining. Deletions of germline nucleotides and insertion of small numbers of extra nucleotides into the recombination site add to molecular diversity. Such clone-specific sequences can be amplified by PCR and distinguished from the background originating from normal lymphoid cells. Clonal evolution may, however, jeopardize this elegant strategy of snooping for minimal residual leukemia, as specific rearrangement patterns may change over time. Interesting but conflicting results have been obtained from prospective PCR analyses of minimal residual ALL in children. Molecular signs of residual leukemia in remission may persist over several years after stopping chemotherapy, which perhaps suggests that complete eradication of the leukemic clone may not be a strict prerequisite for cure. On one hand, a single positive PCR result early in remission does not necessarily indicate impending relapse. On the other hand, negative PCR results in remission do not guarantee durable remissions (8,30).

- High-dose chemotherapy and transfusion of autologous hematopoietic stem cells are often used in the treatment of lymphoma and leukemia. Although patients are intensively pretreated before stem cell harvest, such harvests may still be contaminated with malignant cells having escaped treatment. The reinfusion of such tumor cells may contribute to relapse. A variety of methods are valuable to reduce or eliminate such contaminating tumor cells, including purging of stem cell harvests or positive enrichment for CD34+ stem cells. A control over the efficacy of such maneuvers may nevertheless be valuable. It turns out that the demonstration by PCR of the absence or presence of follicular lymphoma cells with a translocation t(14;18) in stem cell harvests is probably clinically relevant. In patients where no contaminating lymphoma cells are detected by PCR, disease-free survival seems to be much increased over those patients in whom residual lymphoma is detected in the marrow (27,31).

CHROMOSOMAL LOSS AND THE CONCEPT OF TUMOR SUPPRESSOR GENES

In 1969, a seminal article appeared in the journal *Nature*. (32) It described suppression of the malignant behavior of cultured tumor cells when they were fused with certain nonmalignant cells. Interestingly, loss of chromosomes in hybrid cells was associated with reversion to malignancy. It was argued that the normal cells fused to the malignant cells would contribute "something" that would suppress their malignant character, and that this "something" was again lost when certain chromosomes were eliminated from the hybrids.

Two years later, an equally interesting observation was reported. Knudson noted that a rare tumor, retinoblastoma, occurred in two different epidemiological settings: in patients without a family history (sporadic cases), tumors were mostly unilateral whereas in patients with a positive family history (indicating hereditary predisposition), retinoblastomas were often bilateral and associated with other rare tumors such as soft tissue sarcomas. Knudson argued that a concept of two genetic "hits" affecting both copies of a gene would provide a simple explanation covering both clinical patterns (Fig. 1.9) (33,34). In patients with sporadic tumors, a first genetic "hit" knocks out one retinoblastoma gene allele in a somatic cell from the retina. The remaining allele suffices for normal gene function and therefore no immediate biological effect would be noted. Destruction in the same cell of the second allele (a second hit at a later stage) completely knocks out the gene and a malignant tumor develops. Both hits represent somatic genetic events striking sequentially at the same cell. In patients with hereditary cancer predisposition, the first hit is inherited from a parent or occurs de novo in the germline. A germline gene alteration is thus present in all cells (not just the retina) throughout the life of the individual, but it remains silent at the phenotypic level. However, through a second hit in a somatic cell, in the retina or elsewhere, the remaining normal allele may also be inactivated. The combination of a predisposing germline hit and a second somatic hit in the same cell provides the basis for tumor development. In contrast to sporadic cases, only one somatic hit is required in familial cases which explains their higher risk for bilateral retinoblastomas and tumors outside the eye.

Observations from cell biology, epidemiology, and clinical genetics were eventually brought together through the molecular cloning of the retinoblastoma (Rb) gene to provide a comprehensive picture of how Rb inactivation contributes to cancer (35,36). For a start it was noted that in some retinoblastomas, a part of chromosome 13 at band q14 was missing. This provided a first clue to the chromosomal localization of the putative gene. In the next step, polymorphic DNA markers mapped to 13q14 were used to visualize fragments from maternal and paternal chromosome 13q copies separately (Fig. 1.4). Although constitutive DNA from normal cells showed two alleles, tumor DNA showed loss of heterozygosity (LOH), that is, loss of one band. This did not by itself identify the affected gene but genetic mapping helped to narrow down its position on chromosome 13q14 at the molecular level. Eventually the Rb gene was cloned based on the knowledge of its location with no prior information on its sequence (this is termed "positional cloning"), and its structure, mRNA, and protein product were fully characterized. The Rb gene contains over 27 exons spanning about 200 kb of DNA on chromosome 13. It encodes a nuclear phosphoprotein of approximately 105 kDa termed p105-Rb. Rb protein is a cell growth

Sporadic
tumors

Tumor syndromes
with hereditary
predisposition

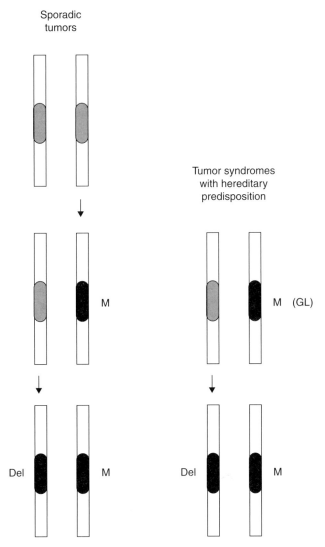

Figure 1.9 Mutations in tumor suppressor genes in hereditary and sporadic cancers. Two allelic chromosomes are depicted (white bars) containing a tumor suppressor gene (shaded boxes). In patients with sporadic tumors, a somatic cell is hit at mitosis by a first mutation (e.g., a point mutation) in one copy of the tumor suppressor gene (left panel: black box indicated by M). Such a recessive mutation does not exert an appreciable impact on the behavior of the cell as long as the normal chromosome copy is still intact. However, if the gene allele on that other chromosomal copy (arrow) is also inactivated in a second step in the same cell (indicated by a second black box labeled M), both alleles of the tumor suppressor gene are knocked out through sequential two-step inactivation. Patients from families with hereditary cancer predisposition are one step ahead in this schedule. The first mutation is inherited in the germline (GL) and thus present in all cells of the body (right panel: black M). A somatic cell, therefore, requires just a single hit to eliminate the remaining normal gene copy (arrow) for full inactivation of the tumor suppressor gene.

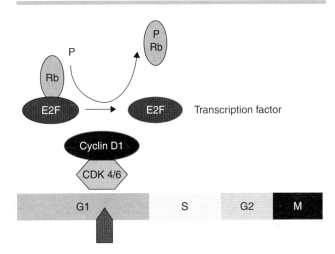

Figure 1.10 The role of the retinoblastoma (Rb) protein in the cell cycle. The cyclin D1/cyclin-dependent kinase (CDK) 4/6 complex phosphorylates the Rb protein. In its hypophosphorylated form (*left*), it is able to bind the transcription factor E2F. Once phosphorylated, Rb must release E2F that will further activate the cell cycle via its enforcement of transcription of downstream genes (not shown). The cell thus overcomes the restriction point in G1 (arrow).

is mostly a small mutation somewhere in the gene, for example, a point mutation or a small deletion that nevertheless precludes the production of a functional Rb protein from that allele. The second hit is the complete or almost complete loss of the remaining normal chromosome. In fact, this second hit was first noted in the karyotypes of Rb patients and identified with polymorphic DNA markers as LOH, whereas the detection of small first hit mutations only became possible once the gene had been cloned and sequenced.

The Rb gene as well as other tumor suppressor genes contribute to cancer through loss of function in contrast to many oncogenes where genetic hits induce gene activation (gain-of-function mutations). Elegant proof for this concept has come from gene knockout experiments. Mice that lack both copies of tumor suppressor genes, for example, p53$^{-/-}$ mice, are particularly prone to developing cancers compared with their normal or heterozygous litter mates (e.g., p53$^{+/+}$ mice or p53$^{+/-}$ mice, respectively). The simplest definition of tumor suppressor genes, therefore, describes genes that contribute to cancer through inactivation and loss-of-function mutations, regardless of their diverse functional or biological roles (Table 1.3). This definition implies that unequivocal demonstration of inactivating mutations is crucial. The function of tumor suppressor gene products is extremely diverse, but a common theme is that these genes represent potential bottlenecks in a wide range of different cellular pathways or key points in many complex cellular pathways regulating cell proliferation, differentiation, apoptosis, as well as cell survival and response to genetic damage. The wide range of different functional properties, thus, precludes the use of functional criteria in defining these genes.

Tumor suppressor genes are frequently inactivated in cancer, including common cancers such as colorectal carcinoma, breast, and prostate cancer as well as lung cancer.

suppressor retaining the cell in a resting state. It sequesters the E2F family of transcription factors that, if let loose, would activate several genes encoding S-phase functions in the cell cycle (Fig. 1.10).

Cloning of the Rb gene obviously provided the tool to look at molecular retinoblastoma genetics. The first hit

Table 1.3 Examples of Human Tumor Suppressor Genes and Hereditary Cancer Syndromes

Gene	Locus	Function	Sporadic tumor types with inactivation of the gene	Associated hereditary tumor syndromes
APC or FAP gene	5q21	Involved in regulation of apoptosis, possibly cellular adhesion and in signal transduction via binding to and sequestration of β-catenin. Blocks activation of *myc*-transcription in response to growth factors (the *myc* oncogene would induce cell division)	Sporadic colorectal cancer (early mutations in premalignant lesions, gatekeeper role)	APC or FAP Large gene with mostly frameshift or non-sense mutations. Protein truncation assays are therefore suitable for mutation search
BRCA1 (Breast cancer 1)	17q21	Nuclear proteins implicated in transcriptional regulation Components of DNA damage response pathways	Rare in sporadic breast cancer	Familial breast cancer syndromes with breast, ovarian, and prostate cancer (BRCA1) Excess of male breast cancer Large gene with mostly frameshift or non-sense mutations. Protein truncation assays therefore suitable for mutation search
hMSH2, hMLH1 and others	2p15 3p21	DNA mismatch repair (MMR)	Rare sporadic colorectal cancers with somatic MMR mutations. Absence of microsatellite instability in colorectal carcinoma is probably a good indicator for the absence of HNPCC	HNPCC and other tumors HNPCC may be indirectly detectable through search for instable microsatellite repeats in cancers (RER+ tumors; mutator phenotype) hMSH2 and hMLH1 mutations account for 90% of familial cases
NF1 gene	17q11	Neurofibromin with *ras* GAP activity involved in signal transduction via the *ras* pathways	Neurofibromas	von Recklinghausen's neurofibromatosis Many mutations detectable in protein truncation test
p16$^{INK4A/MTS1}$	9p21	Cyclin-CDK inhibitor in the cell cycle	T-cell neoplasms, gliomas, melanoma, urinary bladder cancer, mesothelioma, and others	Familial melanoma and familial pancreatic cancer (mutations in exon 1α and exon 2)
p53 gene	17p13	Transcription factor, checkpoint control at the G1/S-phase of the cell cycle with induction of G1 cell cycle arrest and/or induction of apoptosis after DNA damage "Guardian of the genome"	Many different types of tumors	Li–Fraumeni syndrome with sarcomas, breast cancer, brain tumors, and others Mutations clustered in the DNA binding domain (exons 5–8)
Retinoblastoma gene (Rb)	13q14	Transcription factor binding protein Represses transcription of S phase genes	Retinoblastoma, soft tissue sarcomas, osteosarcomas, small cell lung cancer	Familial retinoblastoma Mutations scattered over gene

Hematological neoplasms seem to be less frequently affected, but inactivation of tumor suppressor genes may contribute to clonal evolution of leukemias or lymphomas, for example, in blast crisis of CML or in transformation of follicular lymphoma to secondary high-grade lymphoma.

The p53 gene as a transcription factor and cellular gatekeeper for growth and division is a typical tumor suppressor gene (37–41). It is frequently inactivated in human cancer by the characteristic two-step mechanism. Mice nullizygous for the gene (p53$^{-/-}$) are more susceptible to γirradiation or to carcinogens used for the induction of tumors. Thus, there is clear evidence that inactivation of p53 is associated with cancer. Small p53 mutations in cancers are mainly seen in the DNA-binding domain of the protein and result in its defective contact with DNA which p53 needs to assume its proper role as a transcription factor. The mutational spectra at the p53 gene locus provide a strong case for the carcinogenic role of diverse environmental agents, and it has been claimed that the frequency and type of p53 mutations can act as molecular dosimeters for carcinogen exposure. In lung cancer, the prevalent type of mutations are G:C to T:A transversions (substitutions of a purine for a pyrimidine or vice versa) related to adducts of benzo(a)pyrenes from cigarette smoke. In contrast, colon cancers show G:C to A:T transitions (substitutions of one purine for another purine or one pyrimidine for another pyrimidine), particularly at CpG sequences. This is consistent with mutagenesis by endogenous deamination mechanisms rather than exogenous carcinogens.

What is the normal role of p53? If a cell has suffered some damage to its genetic material, for example, through irradiation or carcinogens, DNA damage must absolutely be recognized *before* the two strands divide and get copied. p53 comes in at this stage as the guardian of the genome (Fig. 1.11). It spots DNA damage and prevents the cell from propagating potentially serious typing errors in its DNA sequence. As a consequence, normal or wild-type p53 is upregulated in the cell. One of its mediators is the p21 cell cycle brake that will interfere with cyclin/cyclin-dependent kinase complexes in G1 and stop the cell from getting past the restriction point (see cell cycle). Either the cell must repair the damaged double strands or it will be eliminated

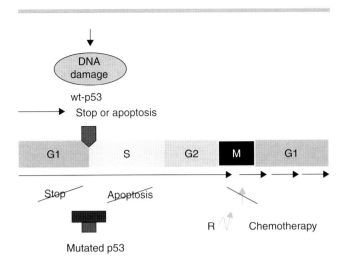

Figure 1.11 p53—guardian of the genome. DNA damage activates the wild-type p53 protein (wt-p53). This will stop the cell in G1, and it may only proceed in the cycle if it manages to repair any DNA damage. Alternatively, it may be eliminated via apoptosis. In many cancers p53 is inactivated through mutations (*bottom part*). Damaged cells may, therefore, copy their DNA and propagate errors in its genetic message. Also, cells with inactivated p53 become less sensitive to chemotherapy or radiotherapy.

via apoptotic pathways. The interference of p53 with apoptosis may be mediated via its effect on the apoptosis-related gene BAX, which counteracts *bcl*-2. It should come as no surprise that p53 has its regulators too. The mdm2 protein inhibits p53 and leads to its degradation, thus limiting the duration of cell cycle arrest induced by p53 (40).

Inactivating p53 gene mutations are among the most frequent in human cancer and associated with adverse prognosis as well as reduced sensitivity to chemotherapy and radiotherapy as shown for breast or colorectal cancer. Replacement of the wild-type gene in tumor cell lines reverts their malignant behavior in the culture dish. In preliminary but remarkable clinical experiments, injection of normal p53 gene contained in a retroviral expression vector into lung cancer lesions refractory to conventional chemo-radiotherapy led to tumor cell apoptosis and tumor regression in a few patients (42). These clinical experiments, therefore, serve as proof of principle that the restoration of wild-type p53 may result in control of tumor growth in patients with p53-deficient cancers.

MOLECULAR GENETICS OF HEREDITARY CANCER PREDISPOSITION SYNDROMES

Several epidemiological and clinical arguments support the view that cancer may occur in a hereditary setting. Cancer patients may have a strong positive family history with relatives affected either by the same type of tumor or by other tumors. Multiple cancers (e.g., bilateral breast cancer or a combination of breast and ovarian cancer) in the same individual are particularly strong indicators of genetic predisposition. Hereditary cancers show a clear trend to present at an unusually early age when compared with sporadic

Table 1.4 Clues to Hereditary Cancer Predisposition from Clinical History

Bilateral tumors in paired organs (e.g., bilateral breast cancer)
Multiple different tumors in the same patient
Unusually early age at presentation (e.g., breast cancer in a 25–30-year-old women)
Relatives in the family affected with cancer
• with the same type of tumor
• with different types of tumor
• with unusual patterns of presentation (e.g., male breast cancer)
• with tumors at an usually early age of onset

Note: The family history must be obtained with care and precision. A quick superficial enquiry as to whether "there was someone with cancer in the family or not" may often fail to uncover the whole story. It is essential to draw a precise pedigree, and the patient may sometimes need help from other family members to reconstruct the genealogy of their kindred. Cancer diagnoses should be obtained as precisely as possible, including the age of onset of cancer in each patient.

cancers. The chance that a major gene mutation is segregating in a family where cancer is diagnosed is influenced by the proportion of relatives affected by relevant cancers and by the ages of onset (Table 1.4). However, the modern small (nuclear) family provides limited scope for the expression of a genetic cancer trait, particularly in sex-restricted types of tumors.

Many cancer predisposition genes follow the genetic pattern of the tumor suppressor genes described earlier. In a cancer family, a recessive germline mutation is inherited or it occurs de novo at meiosis in one gene copy only. It usually has no immediately apparent phenotypic effect. If in a cell a second somatic mutation knocks out the other normal allele, the complete lack of gene activity and the absence of the gene product can profoundly alter the biology of that cell and contribute to cancer development (43,44).

An increasing number of cancer predisposition genes have now been cloned (Table 1.3). Initially, two ways have been taken to find new hereditary cancer genes. Large families in which individuals with and without a cancer diagnosis were well characterized at the phenotypic level were used for genetic linkage analysis. This genetic hunt for a gene responsible for a hereditary disorder initially almost always resembled blindman's buff where luck rather than ingenious logic decided on success or failure. Constitutional DNA samples were taken from all individuals of these families, including healthy subjects and cancer patients, typed with highly polymorphic genetic markers, mostly variable-number-of-tandem-repeat markers or microsatellites that mapped to defined chromosomal localizations (Fig. 1.4). Highly polymorphic markers show a great number of different alleles passed down through a pedigree in a Mendelian fashion. If a particular allele of a polymorphic marker was shown to be handed on through the pedigree along with the phenotype of the disease, that is, the cancer, it was said to be "linked" to the putative gene locus. This first round indicated the chromosomal region where the suspected gene was localized, for example, chromosome 5 in familial adenomatous polyposis (FAP) families. This approach was more problematic in cancer than in other hereditary disorders, mainly because the phenotypic expression of the altered gene (i.e., the development of a cancer) is not always clearly apparent in early life. In a family with severe cystic fibrosis or hemophilia, it is usually easy to decide in early childhood whether an individual is clinically affected or not. In contrast, a cancer phenotype in a hereditary setting may nevertheless appear during later life. Any member of a "cancer" family may develop a sporadic cancer, for example, sporadic breast cancer or colon cancer, that is unlinked to the genetic trait, but cannot be distinguished histologically from a tumor where hereditary predisposition plays a strong role. Linkage analyses were fruitful in the detective work to trace hereditary cancer genes. For example, the hunt for the hereditary breast cancer gene BRCA1 started in this way (44). In 1990, linkage of early-onset familial breast cancer to chromosome 17q21 was reported. It took another 4 years of hard work in this competitive field to clone the BRCA1 gene and to characterize it in detail. Nowadays, the gene is well characterized and tests are available to screen candidate families for germline mutations in constitutional DNA.

Another strategy to find hereditary cancer genes was to examine tumor DNA for LOH at particular genetic loci. Data from cytogenetic analysis of tumors helped to select appropriate molecular markers. Acquired chromosomal deletions in cancers are excellent clues to the presence of tumor suppressor genes, and precise mapping of such deletions narrows down the chromosomal region of interest. An interstitial deletion on chromosome 5q seen in a patient with Gardner's syndrome (a hereditary disorder related to FAP) thus paved the way to localize the FAP/APC gene to the long arm of this chromosome (43). The cloning of the retinoblastoma gene was another example of this strategy, as deletions of chromosome 13 were apparent in tumor cells.

Once a tumor suppressor gene is cloned, its mutational patterns can be examined both in sporadic tumors as well as in individuals from cancer families. Patients with classic hereditary cancer syndromes almost invariably show germline mutations of relevant cancer predisposition genes in their constitutional DNA. In addition, their tumors often show LOH with loss of the corresponding normal chromosome (the second hit according to Knudson). The pattern of germline mutations may vary greatly between families. Many of the genes are large (e.g., the BRCA genes or the FAP/APC gene), and for these reasons molecular analysis to look for family-specific mutations may be cumbersome. Automated DNA sequencing of PCR products, the DNA chip technology, and other assays such as protein truncation tests now offer the possibility to screen families with hereditary cancers for germline mutations in presymptomatic individuals. Direct DNA sequencing is currently the most thorough and specific way of searching for mutations, and its use has been great facilitated through the advent of high-throughput genetic sequencer machinery and computer programs. DNA microchips containing sequences of entire genes of interest permit automated sensitive detection of mutations. Some mutations although quite diverse may still produce a common defect at the protein level. If the gene product is a truncated protein created through a nonsense mutation that inserts a premature stop codon or a frameshift mutation, this may be assessed by a protein truncation test without the need for gene sequencing. Most mutations in the FAP/APC gene can be detected this way, and the same is true for many BRCA1 gene mutations, or for some germline mutations in DNA mismatch repair (MMR) genes affected in hereditary nonpolyposis colorectal cancers (HNPCC) (43,44).

Germline mutations in constitutional DNA of clinically unaffected family members signal a risk for one or several types of cancer to develop. Unfortunately, in most cancer predisposition syndromes, the clinical management of those family members found to be at risk is still unclear. Presymptomatic molecular diagnosis of hereditary cancer is therefore associated with difficult ethical decisions. In addition, family members who opt for presymptomatic molecular diagnosis may have had harrowing personal experience of the disease in close relatives. Among the measures to be discussed are serial screening for early diagnosis of cancers (e.g., mammography in women at risk for breast cancer), prophylactic surgery of the organ at risk (prophylactic bilateral mastectomy), removal of premalignant lesions (e.g., total colectomy in FAP/APC), or chemoprevention.

SIGNAL TRANSDUCTION AND ITS DISTURBANCES IN CANCER

Imagine you are sitting in a cinema watching a film on the screen. The optical signals captured by the retina are transferred into signals suitable for transport along the optic nerves to the appropriate areas of the brain. Here, the visual messages are further modulated for you to become aware of what is happening on the screen. Simultaneously, the sound track of the picture produces a different type of signals taken up via the auditory channels, but eventually optical and acoustic signals are amalgamated in your central nervous system. This in turn will elicit your reactions to what you are seeing and hearing (perhaps you like the movie or perhaps you don't). These complicated multistep processes may be likened to signal transduction in a cell that receives signals from its extracellular environment and transfers them into the nucleus to elicit a biological response. Due to the complicated structure of mammalian cells including compartmentalization of the nucleus and other elements within the cell, there are multiple barriers between the cell's genetic material and its extracellular environment. Thus, signal transduction pathways are essential to establish and maintain contact between the nucleus and the outside world of a cell.

Signals to which a cell would like to react may come in different forms. Hormones, cytokines, or growth factors are among the most important. Specific cell surface receptors span the plasma membrane and bind individual signal molecules also known as their ligands, for example, a hormone or a growth factor. Receptors are often arranged as a transmembrane device. The external moiety binds the ligand arriving from the extracellular area, and the part at the inner surface of the cell membrane is activated. The intracellular part of a receptor may have protein kinase or another enzymatic activity that is suitable to pass on the signal downstream, although the actual primary messenger (the hormone or the growth factor) never actually enters the cell. Protein kinases or other proteins with enzymatic activity in turn activate further chains of messenger cascades until the original message is passed on to the nucleus in a way suitable to elicit a response. In the nucleus, a transcription factor may be activated and may regulate a specific gene. The ultimate goal of signal transduction pathways is not simply to transport a message to the nucleus, but rather to elicit a specific well-timed biological response and to modify gene transcription to alter cellular behavior on demand.

Signal transduction problems in cancer are not only important, but also highly complex. It seems sufficient, therefore, to give some examples and not even try to review this subject in a comprehensive manner. Figure 1.12 shows excerpts of the epidermal growth factor signal transduction pathway (leaving out many details) where alteration of critical steps may contribute to cancer (40,45,46). It also illustrates the points where drugs may interfere with these pathways.

The HER2 or *neu* oncogenic protein (also known as c-*erb*B2 oncogene) is another example of a transmembrane growth factor receptor (47,48). Upon its activation, its internal moiety displays tyrosine kinase activity. HER2 is amplified and overexpressed in a variety of cancers, notably breast cancer, and associated with aggressive clinical behavior of such neoplasms. An antibody (trastuzumab) directed against this oncogene is now in clinical use and has been found to exhibit specific therapeutic activity in breast cancers with marked overexpression of the HER2/neu oncogene. Assessment of HER2/neu expression status on breast cancer biopsies through immunohistochemistry has, therefore, widely been incorporated into diagnostic routine in many pathology departments to provide a predictive marker for appropriate use of trastuzumab.

Another player in a signal transduction line, the *ras* oncogene, is frequently altered in cancer (49). The discovery of activating *ras* oncogene mutations in a bladder carcinoma was the first identification of an activated oncogene in human cancer. Other types of cancers followed, notably acute myeloblastic leukemia, lung cancer, and gastrointestinal carcinomas. In all these cancers, constitutive activation of *ras* through point mutations mimics chronic stimulation by the corresponding lineage-specific growth factors. The *ras* oncogene is activated in cancer through point mutations in specific codons that confer resistance of the active *ras*-GTP complex to GAP. GAP is an enzyme that accelerates the conversion of active *ras*-GTP into the inactive *ras*-GDP form. *ras* oncogene point mutations, therefore, do their trick by maintaining *ras* in its active *ras*-GTP form. Insight into the normal structure and function of *ras* has yielded an interesting (albeit still experimental) strategy for cancer treatment. In order to work properly, *ras* needs to be attached to the inner cellular membrane. This is achieved through farnesylation of the protein brought about by the enzyme farnesyltransferase. Inhibitors of *ras* farnesylation may therefore be therapeutically useful in cancer because they specifically interfere with the increased activity of this important second messenger and help to shut down *ras* signaling in the absence of growth factors (Fig. 1.12).

Several cancers show inappropriate expression of protein kinases, for example, tyrosine protein kinases that are involved in signal transduction at some stage, but do not belong to the receptor-type kinases. The BCR-ABL fusion protein in CML is an example (50). The blockade of the abnormal tyrosine kinase activity exerted by the BCR/ABL fusion protein in CML is now possible with the help of a small molecule, imatinib mesylate (or Glivec®). Imatinib

mesylate has revolutionized the therapy for this disease, as the drug achieves a very high rate of lasting remissions at the cost of very little toxicity. Gefitinib (Iressa®) is an inhibitor of the epidermal growth factor receptor (EGFR)-type kinase (Fig. 1.12) and was hailed as a new treatment for lung cancer (51). In spite of promising early clinical data, phase III trials combining gefitinib with chemotherapy in nonsmall cell lung cancer failed to come up with a distinct therapeutic advantage. One of the reasons for this failure was probably the fact that patients were not selected by molecular profiles (possibly predicting response to or resistance to gefitinib) but by conventional clinical and routine histological criteria. Indeed, subsequent large-scale studies in lung cancer using a single agent approach with both erlotinib (Tarceva®) and gefitinib have demonstrated the benefit of treatment in defined subsets of lung cancer patients (see later chapter on lung cancer).

The history of gefitinib shows that at the clinical level, molecular therapy must stand its test in clinical trials just as much as "old-fashioned" cytotoxic treatment, and extrapolation of exciting in vitro results to cancer patients is not justified without careful clinical studies. Nevertheless, such "small molecules" that specifically interfere with important molecular pathways in cancer cells show much promise, and their clinical use requires clinical oncologists to get at least a basic grasp of the molecular pathology of human cancer.

CELL CYCLE IN CANCER

Cellular proliferation, cell differentiation, and cell death are normal biological processes under strict control of a variety of modulating systems. In order to maintain law and order in this essential part in the life of a cell, there must be rules to replicate by, but these control mechanisms may be overthrown in cancer. Research into cell cycle biology is, therefore, inextricably linked with experimental cancer research, and clinical application of news from the experimental bench is starting to see the light of day (52,53).

A cell might rest "outside" the cycle in a phase termed G0 (many cancer cells, particularly cancer stem cells do!). An appropriate signal (e.g., a growth factor or another mitogenic signal) might change this state and drive the cell toward division. In G1 (for Gap1) the preparatory steps for subsequent DNA synthesis are undertaken. The cell must overcome a checkpoint in G1, the restriction point, before it is allowed to start DNA synthesis (Fig. 1.13). Small proteins called cyclins operate as activators in this phase and help to shorten G1. Cyclins cannot work alone but need partners, the cyclin-dependent kinases (CDK) to exert their effect. Cyclin-CDK complexes activate yet other partners downstream through phosphorylation (an all important mechanism of activating proteins in biology!). A famous partner is the retinoblastoma (Rb) protein. In a resting cell, it is almost devoid of phosphate groups (hypophosphorylated), and in this state it binds transcription factors, notably E2F (Fig. 1.10). It can thus block the cell from getting out of G1. The cyclin D1-CDK4/6 partnership now adds phosphate groups to the Rb protein that in turn must release the E2F transcription factor from captivity. Transcription factors exert profound effects on other genes that they either activate or deactivate to help the cell overcome

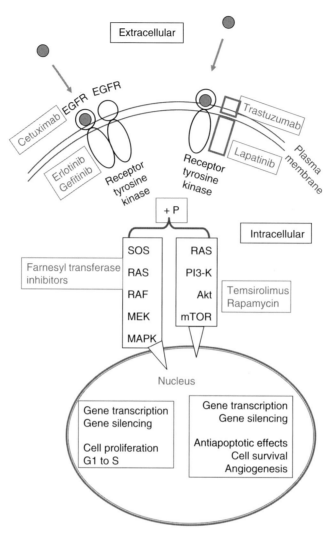

Figure 1.12 Signal transduction and the epidermal growth factor receptor (EGFR) pathway. This cartoon shows excerpts from an important signal transduction pathway that transmits an external signal into the nucleus of the cell. A growth factor, a hormone, or a cytokine—a ligand (epidermal growth factor in this example)—binds to the extracellular domain of its receptor. Receptor proteins are usually placed in a transmembrane position with the receptor portion protruding to the extracellular area. The intracellular domain of the protein assumes a different function. Upon reaction of the ligand with the receptor, a signal is transferred across the plasma membrane to the internal cytoplasmic domain of the receptor protein. This domain is often an enzyme, for example, a tyrosine protein kinase as in this example. It is activated through autophosphorylation which in turn may switch on several next steps. A variety of activated cytoplasmic effector proteins travel to the nucleus and act on gene transcription. Alterations of different steps and players may be tightly linked to cancer (see main text). EGFR is a transmembrane tyrosine kinase receptor protein from a family of four related proteins (HER1-4), also known as the ErbB tyrosine-kinase receptor family. Different ligands ("signals from the outside world") can bind to the extracellular part of these receptors, except for HER2 which does not have the capacity to interact with an external ligand. Receptor-ligand binding induces formation of receptor protein dimers, either homodimers (EGFR-EGFR) or heterodimers (HER2-EGFR). In contrast to HER1, 3, and 4, HER2 may dimerize with EGFR in the absence of a specific HER2 ligand. Receptor mutations or overexpression in tumors can also induce dimerization, hence activation, in the absence of ligands. Activation of the receptor leads in turn to activation of intracellular kinases. Their autophosphorylation triggers a series of intracellular pathways, where other proteins are placed in an assembly line where turn by turn they are activated through phosphorylation (+P) (e.g., SOS-RAS-RAF-MEK-MAPK). Depending on the pathway activated, the end result may differ. The SOS-RAS-RAF-MEK-MAPK pathway eventually induces cell cycle progression and cell proliferation, whereas the PI3-K-AKT pathway sends out antiapoptotic and prosurvival signals. A tight multistep control of such processes is essential for the life and death of a cell, and in contrast to equally redundant bureaucratic procedures in government administration, signal transduction, complicated as it may seem, actually works. Antibodies (e.g., cetuximab) block the extracellular part of their target protein, and small molecules (e.g., erlotinib) block the tyrosine kinase activity of the intracellular part. Note that the graphic presentation deliberately boils down this complicated field to a few key features. *Abbreviations*: Akt, enzyme Ak transforming factor, a serine-threonine kinase (also known as protein kinase B); EGFR, epidermal growth factor receptor; MAPK, mitogen-activated protein kinase; MEK, mitogen extracellular signal kinase; P, phosphorylation (i.e., the main effect produced by kinases with the help of ATP); PI3-K, phosphoinositide 3-kinase, a lipid kinase; RAF, receptor activation factor; RAS, rat sarcoma enzyme, a G-protein (guanine nucleotide exchange factor) inhibited by farnesyl transferase inhibitors; SOS, son-of-sevenless, a kinase (name derived from Drosophila gene nomenclature), which helps to release GDP (guanosine diphosphate) from the *ras* protein.

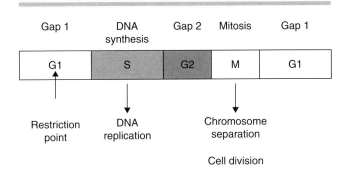

Figure 1.13 The cell cycle. The cell cycle is divided into several phases. In G1 (gap 1) the cell is resting, and further progression is blocked unless it overcomes the restriction point. Under the influence of growth-stimulating signals, the restriction point may be overcome and the cell's machinery prepares for DNA synthesis. DNA is replicated in S phase. After a second short gap (G2), the cells enters mitosis where chromosomes separate. Two daughter cells are produced, which enter their own G1 phases each. Cells may also rest outside the cell cycle in a state called G0 (not shown) from whence they may reenter the cell cycle via G1.

the G1 checkpoint and enter S phase. After that there is nothing to stop it from moving on. Most importantly the cell will become independent from growth factors and from cyclin-CDK complexes as it proceeds on its way toward mitosis. DNA synthesis will now ensue in S phase, and after a second short interval termed G2, the cell will divide in mitosis. The daughter cells will either stay in an active cycling state or rest in G0.

Several players in this scenario may contribute to cancer if inappropriately activated or inactivated. In mantle cell lymphoma, the cyclin D1 gene on chromosome 11 may be translocated to the Ig heavy-chain gene locus on chromosome 14 (54). Overexpression or untimely expression of cyclin D1 under the influence of the Ig locus may contribute in an oncogenic fashion to the malignant behavior of the neoplastic B cells present in this disorder. Certain types of nonsmall cell lung cancer show amplification of the cyclin D1 gene. Also, a DNA sequence variant in the cyclin D1 gene that modulates splicing of cyclin D1 mRNA and is responsible for the formation of a variant cyclin D1 transcript and the production of a cyclin D1 protein with increased stability has been observed (cyclins normally are very short lived and their action in the cell cycle is therefore restricted in time). Presence of this variant transcript in patients with nonsmall cell lung cancer appears to be associated with shorter survival and increased risk of relapse. The Rb pathway is a coherent unit almost universally targeted in cancer. The retinoblastoma gene is a classical tumor suppressor gene where loss of function clearly contributes to neoplastic behavior of a cell. Inactivated Rb cannot hold E2F in check, and "free" E2F, therefore, manages to activate downstream genes in an uncontrolled fashion. The Rb gene is inactivated in a variety of hereditary and sporadic tumors, in retinoblastoma (of course!), sarcomas, small cell lung cancer, and others.

The cell cycle needs brakes to keep its activating players under control, notably the cyclin–CDK complexes. A variety of cyclin-dependent kinase inhibitors (CKIs) have

been described by now. CKI proteins are usually designated with numbers indicating their molecular size. p21, for example, is a 21 kDa CKI protein. Some CKI are specialized to deal with particular cyclin–CDK complexes (mostly with those operating in G1) and others are more universal in their action. CKIs are often mutated or their expression altered in cancer. The p16 gene located on chromosome 9p21 is homozygously deleted in a variety of solid tumors and T-cell neoplasms. Inactivating germline p16 mutations have been found in families with melanoma and pancreatic cancer. If the gene is intact, its expression in cancer may still be blocked via another mechanism, that is, gene methylation of CpG residues at its 5′ end (methylation is a common mechanism in biology to switch off genes or blocks of genes). Inactivation of this G1 cell cycle brake in a tumor would therefore set the stage for continuous tumor cell cycling, which may well contribute to the malignant behavior of such cells. The universal CKI p27 may also be inactivated in cancer, but in a different fashion. The gene is almost always normal in cancer cells and so is p27 mRNA production. Some cancers, however, produce p27 mRNA but no p27 protein. It appears that these cells possess a mechanism of putting the p27 cell cycle brake out of order by destroying the protein. Such tumors, for example, colon or breast cancers, behave more aggressively at the clinical level than tumors with a normal p27 pathway (55,56).

A survey of the sections on tumor suppressor genes, the cell cycle, and signal transduction in cancer shows that these fundamental principles of biology are in fact inextricably intertwined. Cancer results from genetic plays in this highly complicated and gigantic biological internet. Thus, errors may be inserted in one program or another, wrecking the p16 or the *ras* files, or slipping in typing mistakes in the spelling check.

MOLECULAR DIAGNOSTICS IN CANCER

Molecular diagnosis of cancer requires that suitable diagnostic material must be obtained. This is not trivial. Rather, it is essential that clinicians harvesting biopsies, blood samples, or body fluids are aware of the methodological principle of a molecular test they would like to order.

The PCR in Cancer Diagnosis

Among the many methods now available in molecular genetics, the PCR has become the front-runner for diagnostic purposes (Fig. 1.8). It offers the unique possibility to amplify small specific gene segments or RNA fragments for rapid analysis; results are often available within the same day of material harvest. In many instances, PCR makes do with damaged material or even archival specimens where nucleic acids are ill preserved. The PCR product is a DNA fragment of specific sequence and length (usually in the range of a few dozen to several hundred base pairs) amplified either from DNA or in the case of RT-PCR from cellular RNA. As the PCR fragment specificity is defined through the sequence specificity of the primers, it may suffice for proper identification to visualize the PCR fragment on gel electrophoresis where its molecular size can be estimated (Fig. 1.6). If this is not sufficient, the fragment may be sequenced (automated nowadays). This will yield

Table 1.5 Diagnostic Use of PCR in Pathology and Oncology/Hematology

(a) Molecular alterations in tumors detectable by PCR or RT-PCR
- Point mutations, base pair insertions, and other small mutations
- Chromosomal translocations
- Small base pair deletions
- Loss of heterozygosity (LOH; microsatellite markers)
- Gene expression analysis by RT-PCR or by competitive semiquantitative RT-PCR or by real-time PCR (TaqMan PCR)

(b) Application of PCR technology to diagnostic problems in cancer

PCR detection of diagnostic molecular markers	Detection of germline mutations in cancer families
	Detection of occult cancers through amplification of molecular markers in body fluids (e.g., *ras* gene mutations from stool in colorectal carcinoma or microsatellite markers from urine in bladder cancer)
	Diagnosis of specific cancers t(15;17) in APL; t(8;21) in AML with maturation. Clonal analysis of lymphoproliferations by immunogenotyping and others
Detection of prognostic or predictive markers in a cancer	Various chromosomal translocations in hematological neoplasms
	Mutated oncogenes or tumor suppressor genes in solid tumors p53 gene mutations in breast cancer. LOH at various loci in colon cancer (including allelotyping)
Tumor staging	Occult marrow involvement in lymphoma (e.g., t[14;18] in follicular lymphoma)
	Involvement of cerebrospinal fluid with lymphoid leukemia or lymphoma (clonal antigen receptor gene rearrangements)
	Examination of resection margins in surgical specimens for occult carcinoma (e.g., neck dissection tissue in head-and-neck carcinoma tagged by p53 mutations)
	Occult lymph node metastases of various cancers undetectable by histology (e.g., detection of carcinoembryogenic antigen mRNA by RT-PCR to assess nodal status in colorectal cancer considering that lymphoid cells do not express CEA)
Patient follow-up after treatment (MRD)	Sensitive PCR detection of specific chromosomal translocations in leukemia or lymphoma
	Detection of contaminating tumor cells in bone marrow or hematopoietic stem cell harvests used for autologous stem cell transplantation

precise information on DNA sequence variants or gene mutations contained, such as activating oncogene point mutations, or inactivating small deletions in a tumor suppressor gene. Automated sequencing of PCR products has now become the most widely used approach in molecular diagnostics.

Applications of PCR-based techniques are listed in Table 1.5. Although generally presented in many articles as simple and elegant, PCR detection of many molecular markers needs very careful quality control and a lot of experience in technical troubleshooting. Interpretation of its results in a clinical context requires a critical mind that should not be overruled by the notion that it is better simply because it is "molecular biology." The clinical relevance of many molecular markers must still be demonstrated, and this is best achieved in prospective clinical trials where molecular diagnostics are applied to well-defined patient populations and incorporated into controlled treatment programs.

Fluorescent In Situ Hybridization (FISH)

PCR methods, as described above, usually start from nucleic acids extracted from a biopsy specimen. In clinical pathology it may be useful to match morphology with molecular data. This may be achieved by the FISH technique (57–60). FISH is a method to identify chromosomal abnormalities in mitotic figures or interphase nuclei at the single cell level with the help of molecular probes tagged by various fluorescent dyes (Fig. 1.14). Multicolor FISH may detect several different abnormalities in parallel. FISH may be used to detect *known* chromosomal abnormalities using specific DNA probes, and the technique does not present the type

of nonbiased survey on the chromosome status that karyotyping provides (recent technical developments aim at overcoming this final limitation). Considering that chromosomal abnormalities are of unique prognostic importance in many hematological cancers, the incorporation of FISH diagnostics into routine is attractive. The technique is particularly appealing to the study of solid tumors where

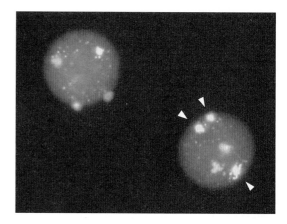

Figure 1.14 FISH. Interphase nuclei from leukemic cells analyzed with a DNA probe hybridizing to chromosome 7 (red dots) and a DNA probe recognizing sequences from chromosome 8 (green dots). One nucleus is normal with two copies of each chromosome, whereas one nucleus shows three green dots indicating trisomy 8, a common chromosomal abnormality in myeloid leukemias including MDS or CLL. *Source:* Courtesy of Dr. Martine Jotterand, CHUV, Lausanne. *See Color Plate on Page ix.*

conventional cytogenetic techniques often fail for a variety of reasons (failure of setting up tumor cell cultures, unsatisfactory mitotic figures, etc.). In CLL, FISH may detect chromosomal aberrations in about 80% of cases; these data are clinically relevant: for example, patients with deletions on chromosome 13q stand a much better chance of long-term survival than those with, say, a deletion on chromosome 17p (60). FISH is also accepted as one of the gold standard assays to detect amplification of the HER2/*neu* gene in breast cancer, as an alternative to immunohistochemistry.

Comparative genomic hybridization (CGH) detects chromosome copy number changes genomewide (58). Genomic DNA isolated from tumor and normal control cells (mostly lymphoid cells) labeled with different fluorochromes are hybridized to normal metaphase chromosomes prepared as in conventional karyotyping. Differences in fluorescence ratio along metaphase chromosomes of tumor versus normal cells quantitatively indicate changes in the DNA sequence copy number in the tumor genome. More recently, array-based CGH (aCGH) has been established, where microarrays of genomic sequences replace the metaphase chromosomes as hybridization targets. The main advantage of aCGH is the ability to perform chromosome copy number analyses with much higher resolution than was ever possible using chromosomal CGH. CGH is mainly a research tool, with so far little established routine use in cancer diagnostics.

Genetic Tumor Analysis with Polymorphic DNA Markers

Human DNA contains a great number of highly polymorphic markers in its introns, with often ill-defined biological roles, but undeniably useful for molecular diagnostics (Fig. 1.4). Informative markers, particularly microsatellites composed of di-, tri-, or tetranucleotide base pair repeats, and single nucleotide polymorphisms (SNPs), are now precisely mapped with suitably narrow spacing to cover the entire genome. Most individuals are constitutionally heterozygous for such markers, which simply means that the paternal and the maternal allele can be detected (i.e., visualized) separately on molecular analysis. If one allele carries a critical gene mutation, the SNP marker would thus label that allele and thus indirectly point to the presence of the mutation (which as such can or must not be detected). If an SNP-labeled allele is linked to a phenotype, for example, a pharmacogenetic profile of an individual, it might suffice for diagnostic purposes to trace the polymorphism rather than the actual gene and its mutation. Polymorphic markers can also be used to compare constitutional (normal) DNA and tumor DNA from the same patient (61,62). SNPs and microsatellites are easily amenable to semi-automated PCR typing and to DNA microarrays analysis, allowing for comprehensive genome surveys on the extent and localization in tumors of chromosomal or allele deletions (LOH, or uniparental disomy, UPD) and new microsatellite alleles created at mitosis (a mirror of genetic instability). Such analyses known as molecular allelotyping have been conducted in a variety of human cancers, including lung, prostate, and breast carcinomas as well as lymphocytic leukemias. From a diagnostic point of view, this technology provides an alternative to the cytogenetic detection of chromosomal deletions. For example, karyotyping of CLL is not always easy and the beauty of allelotyping

with batteries of informative microsatellites or SNPs is that DNA from resting cells, or even degraded DNA from archival samples, can be used.

Clinical Interest in the DNA Microchip Technology

The human genome sequence is now available, virtually complete. Why should oncologists bother about this data bank? Until now most research in molecular carcinogenesis has been directed at discovering and characterizing single "cancer" genes. Virtually all established diagnostic techniques in molecular cancer pathology suffer from the limitation that they only tell us what we are specifically looking for. It may well be that a chosen molecular marker may be less relevant than another one which was not ordered by the clinician or was not considered by the pathologist. Colon cancer is an example that illustrates this issue. For example, patients with stage III colon cancer seem to derive more benefit from adjuvant therapy if their tumors retain a wild-type K-*ras* sequence (55,56). Interestingly, colon cancer with a wild-type K-*ras* status will also derive particular benefit from EGFR-targeted treatment (see later chapter on colon cancer). Colon cancers with microsatellite instability may be less aggressive than tumors with stable microsatellites. Retention of 18q alleles in microsatellite-stable tumors and mutations of the gene for type II TGF-β1 receptor in node-positive microsatellite-instable colon cancers both point to a more favorable prognosis after adjuvant chemotherapy. A glance at this literature shows that in most articles, the molecular marker of interest was carefully studied, and one or the other additional gene included in the analysis, but no such study provided an overall appraisal of all molecular markers of potential clinical value in this cancer. The established molecular diagnostic techniques are mostly too laborious to permit the comprehensive screening of a tumor biopsy sample for all possible types of genetic markers.

A new approach would be to screen cancer specimens for all possible "gene" problems; that is, to obtain individual comprehensive cancer gene expression profiles at the RNA expression level (also known as "signatures"). This is now possible with microarray gene profiling (63,64). In contrast to the study of single genes and their proteins, molecular tumor profiling is a large-scale analysis of gene expression in a tumor using the DNA microarrays (Fig. 1.15). DNA microarrays typically consist of rows and rows of oligonucleotide sequence strands or cDNA sequences lined up in dots on a silicon chip or glass slide (63–66). Oligonucleotide sequences or cDNAs on the chip permit specific hybridization to labeled mRNAs of interest extracted from a biopsy. Arrays can accommodate up to 30,000 specific sequences on a single chip, chosen either randomly or deliberately "biased" to represent theme parks of genes typically expressed in a cell type of interest, for example, "lymphoid genes" in B cells ("lymphochip") (66).

The lymphochip is a cDNA microarray containing selected genes preferentially expressed in lymphoid cells (67,68). Analysis of gene expression in various lymphoid malignancies yields an orderly picture of gene expression patterns in particular types of lymphoma, reflecting both lineage characteristics, stage of maturation of lymphoid cells, and proliferation signatures. Diffuse large B-cell lymphoma (a clinically heterogeneous group of lymphomas

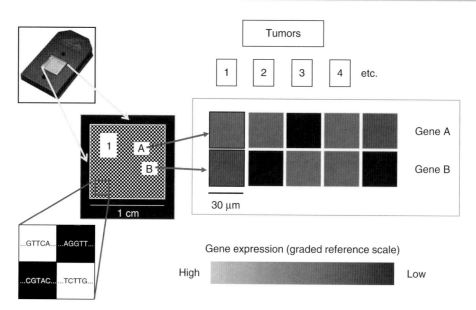

Figure 1.15   Gene expression profiling of tumors with cDNA microarrays or "chips." The chip is a small flat box (*upper left*), which in a rectangular chamber contains a siliconized surface loaded with single-strand nucleic acid sequences (*lower left*). These sequences represent either short, specific oligonucleotides or cDNA prepared from mRNA of various cells. Specific sequences are neatly arranged in rows and columns and are ready for hybridization with a sample composed of labeled single-stranded cRNA. A single chip may contain up to several 10,000 such sequences (representing genes, or so-called expressed sequence tags ESTs). After hybridization the chip surface can be read and the results expressed as quantitative estimates of gene expression, with respect to a scale of reference (*bottom center*). In this example mRNA from tumor 1 has been examined with the help of the chip. Gene A is overexpressed in this sample, and gene B is not expressed at all. Tumor 3 shows the reverse gene expression pattern, and the other samples all show distinct gene expression profiles. These raw data are then sorted with a number of strategies. Unsupervised clustering (explained in a terribly simplified fashion!) refers to a program that groups tumor samples according to similar or completely distinct expression profiles. In supervised clustering, additional information on the samples is fed in before sorting, for example, some clinical information. In the end, a limited number of genes can be pulled from such profiles which distinguish one tumor subgroup from another. *See Color Plate on Page ix.*

despite their morphological similarity) can be split into subtypes with gene expression profiles typical of either germinal center B cells or activated B cells. Diffuse large B-cell non-Hodgkin's lymphoma (DLBCL) expression signatures differ markedly between patients who had been cured and those who eventually relapsed (68). The promise is that such expression profiles or signatures offer more precise prognostic information than established prognostic factors, such as the International Prognostic Index in NHL (Fig. 1.16), and eventually translate into concepts of refined differentially targeted therapy.

Likewise, one invasive-ductal breast cancer specimen may look deceptively similar to another on histology, but the fate of the two women may be totally different. This is because of inherent biological differences of the two tumors hidden in their genome, which may be elusive to morphological examination. Variation in gene transcription programs governed by specific somatic gene alterations account for much of the biological diversity in human tumors. The study of gene expression patterns in human breast cancer specimens displays distinct molecular portraits or gene expression profiles providing molecular "fingerprints." (69) Tumors may be clustered by sharing gene expression patterns, and it is likely that such subgroups comprise clinically distinct subtypes or entities of breast cancers. It also turns out that the overall gene expression pattern of a breast cancer case is by and large retained in

its metastases. Figure 1.17 shows an analysis where T1-2 N0 tumors, which had or had not relapsed within 5 years after diagnosis and primary treatment, show clearly distinct gene expression profiles, respectively. Breast cancers of the basal-like cell type, which often express neither hormone receptors nor HER2 ("triple-negative breast cancer") cannot be readily identified by histology, but exhibit specific gene expression profiles detectable on microarray analysis (70).

A few words of caution on the chip technology are warranted. Currently, molecular diagnostics with DNA microarrays do not displace time-honored diagnostic tools such as morphology and related techniques, as the demands on bioinformatics to handle the impressive data flow are considerable and costs are still excessive (63,65). The clinical relevance of this technology and the new data it creates will undoubtedly need to be refined and tested in appropriate clinical trials. Although global gene expression profiling of cancers with the DNA chip technology is now a reality, the detailed characterization of single genes and their proteins with a possible role in the molecular pathology of cancers is far from being an old hat. New strategies to detect and characterize human proteins in biological material (including clinical specimens) are now mandatory and indeed on the horizon. As a concept, proteomics are on their road to provide a new wave of fascinating data with a great potential for cancer medicine, since, similar to

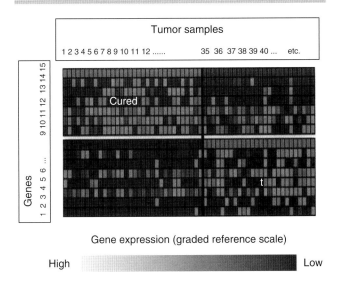

Gene expression (graded reference scale)

High   Low

Figure 1.16 Microarray analysis of DLBCL. About one-half of patients with DLBCL are cured with CHOP-type chemotherapies and the other half relapse and often succumb to their disease. Although a number of clinicopathological parameters are available to create prognostic subgroups (International Prognostic Index), clinical and pathological information is inadequate for a neat distinction of these two subgroups. In this example, cases either cured or with an eventually fatal outcome were studied for their gene expression profiles. It turns out that DLBCL with a good prognosis displays a gene expression signature that is clearly different from the profile that lights up in lymphoma cells from eventually fatal cases. Although the microarrays used in this experiments offered thousands of genes for analysis, a neat prognostic distinction of the two clinical DLBCL subgroups can be made with a restricted and selected group of genes (horizontal rows), in fact no more than 15 genes. *Source:* Modified after Ref. 68. *See Color Plate on Page x.*

cDNA microchips, proteomic analysis provides a survey of protein production in a tumor specimen, hence specific protein production signatures.

Immunocytochemical and Immunohistochemical Analysis of Diagnostic Cancer Biopsies

In diagnostic practice, pathologists often choose to look at the protein product of a gene through immunohistochemistry or immunocytochemistry rather than bothering about the detection of DNA or RNA alterations in a tumor. The immunohistochemical detection of proteins produced by oncogenes or tumor suppressor genes on tissue sections through appropriate (monoclonal) antibodies has become a logical extension of the molecular analyses that initially led to the characterization of these genes and their products.

- Many mutations inactivating the p53 tumor suppressor gene lead to the formation of more stable (albeit non-functional) p53 protein. As the half-life of the wild-type protein is very short, it usually does not provide a strong signal on immunohistochemistry. The consequence of many p53 gene mutations is the accumulation in a cell of inactive p53 protein with increased half-life. Intensive staining of tumor cells with an appropriate p53

antibody may therefore be taken to indicate the presence of p53 gene mutations although the correlation is not strict. In clinical practice, immunohistochemical detection of p53 is performed much more frequently than gene sequencing. Many clinical studies linking p53 gene mutants with clinical outcome in tumor patients are based on immunohistochemistry rather than gene analysis (Fig. 1.18).

- Amplification of the HER2/*neu* oncogene and its overexpression in breast cancer is thought to represent an adverse prognostic factor. More importantly, HER2/neu overexpression quantified in a standardized immunohistochemistry assay is a predictive factor to decide whether a woman with breast cancer stands a chance of benefiting from treatment with a monoclonal antibody, trastuzumab, directed against the HER2/neu protein. For all practical purposes, HER2 is often always detected by immunohistochemistry rather than by FISH analysis of HER2 gene amplification (Fig. 1.18).

Clinical Validation of Predictive Markers in Cancer

"Traditional" cancer treatments were geared toward interfering with abnormal proliferation of cancer cells, and hence many cytostatic drugs interfere with DNA synthesis, the mitotic apparatus, or block gene transcription in a nonspecific fashion. Likewise, radiotherapy interferes with basic cellular mechanisms, which are not specific for cancer cells. The unwelcome problem of such biologically "broad" shots against cancer cells is toxicity to normal tissues, particularly those with a high fraction of cycling cells, such as the bone marrow or mucosal epithelia. Advances in our understanding of the molecular pathology of cancer have, therefore, been hailed particularly with the notion that biomarkers will define target molecules which in turn will permit the development of "targeted cancer therapies." (71–73) Such drugs are indeed available, mostly antibodies ("mabs") or small molecules ("nibs"), that may block pathways or molecules important for cancer cells, in a more or less specific way. The concept of targeted therapy implies that cancer cell heterogeneity must be taken into account and that we need predictive markers to anticipate whether a tumor would stand a reasonable chance of responding favorably to a particular drug (46).

A predictive marker tells us the potential outcome of a patient with a given tumor upon specific treatment, whereas a prognostic marker simply provides information on the natural history of the disease, mostly independent of treatment. A prognostic marker may also be a predictive marker. For example, the expression of estrogen receptors in breast cancer implies a better prognosis, at the same time indicating endocrine responsiveness. Some markers have prognostic value but do not guide treatment choices, though others are predictive but not prognostic. For example, CD20 expression in malignant lymphoma has as such no prognostic value, but its presence indicates that the tumor may respond to treatment with an anti-CD20-antibody, rituximab.

In an ideal world, a predictive marker molecule detected in a tumor biopsy would identify a molecular feature of that tumor that neatly predicts its response to a specific drug. Tumors that do not express the marker would stand little or no chance of responding to the treatment

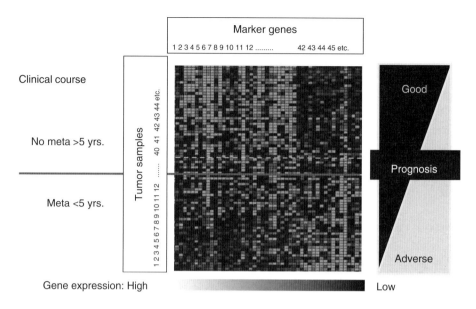

Figure 1.17 cDNA microchip analysis (so-called supervised classification on prognosis gene expression signatures) of samples from women with early node-negative breast cancer. In this example, tumor tissue samples from women with T1-2 N0 stage early breast cancer were analyzed with microarrays. For data analysis, cases were split: those who remained disease-free for at least 5 years and those who relapsed within 5 years after diagnosis and primary treatment (so-called supervised clustering analysis of chip data). The established clinical and biological prognostic parameters in breast cancer (T stage, N stage, receptor status, etc.) did not permit prediction with any accuracy as to which women would remain disease-free or relapse. In the molecular analysis, genes have been ordered according to their correlation with the two clinical prognostic patient groups. The microchip analysis lights up gene expression profiles that clearly differ between tumors treated successfully and those cases that had relapsed within 5 years after diagnosis. In women with no evidence of metastases after 5 years of follow-up, genes with low expression cluster to the upper left of the panel (lighting up in green), and overexpressed genes (depicted in red) are grouped in the upper right sector of the panel. The reverse pattern or expression profile is seen in the group of women who had relapsed. *Source*: Modified after Ref. 69. *See Color Plate on Page x.*

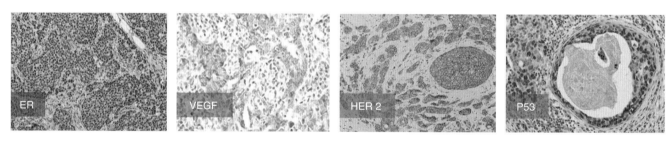

Figure 1.18 Immunohistochemical analysis of gene expression in breast cancer. Invasive-ductal breast cancer sections staining with diagnostic antibodies recognizing (*from left to right*) estrogen receptors (nuclear; ER), vascular endothelial growth factor (VEGF), HER2 (membrane bound), and p53 (nuclear). The section stained with p53 also shows noninvasive ductal carcinoma in situ (DCIS; *right*). The stromal cells in between the tumor cells are mostly negative. *Source*: Courtesy of Prof. H.J. Altermann, Pathologie Länggasse, Berne. *See Color Plate on Page xi.*

that could be avoided in such marker-negative cases. There are a few examples, where this system truly works, notably the BCR-ABL-positive leukemias. Any leukemia expressing the BCR-ABL fusion kinase stands an excellent a priori chance of responding to imatinib mesylate (50). However, the detection of the BCR-ABL fusion gene by PCR does not guarantee that a beneficial response may be upheld over time, as molecular mechanisms inducing drug resistance eventually turn up, where specific mutations in the BCR-ABL gene eventually abolish the effectiveness of

imatinib mesylate. Unless specifically sought after, these mutations, for example, the tyrosine kinase T315I-mutation, will not be detected. Marker detection needs a reliable predictive test with clinically validated and reproducible results. The detection of HER2 in breast cancer samples only predicts response to trastuzumab, if a high expression level of the protein is detected immunohistochemically or if gene amplification is demonstrated with a suitable FISH assay (47). It is not sufficient if a pathologist uses any kind of anti-HER2 antibody, identifies a number of positive cancer cells, and then labels the case as "HER2" positive, suggesting that anti-HER2 treatment should be installed. Instead tests should be used that had been validated in prospective clinical trials run to demonstrate the effectiveness of the drug, and any deviation from such practice implies treading on slippery ground.

In summary, diagnostic molecular pathology is a land of plenty with many choices. PCR methods, FISH and CHIPS, or tissue immunostaining with monoclonal antibodies were all developed through advances in molecular basic cancer research. They clearly overcome the technical boundaries of traditional diagnostic methods. However, in times of severe financial restraints in most health services new expensive molecular methods need to be validated carefully with respect to their clinical impact. If properly demonstrated, however, the advantages may be very considerable. As pointed out in the introduction, knowledge about molecular mechanisms of carcinogenesis has become far more than just a playground for experimental biology.

REFERENCES

1. Wainscoat JS, Fey MF. Assessment of clonality in human tumor: a review. Cancer Res 1990; 50: 1355–60.
2. Wood LD, Parsons DW, Jones S et al. The genomic landscapes of human breast and colorectal cancers. Science 2007; 318: 1108–13.
3. Dionigi G, Bianchi V, Rovera F et al. Genetic alteration in hereditary colorectal cancer. Surg Oncol. 2007; 16(Suppl 1): S11–15.
4. Boman BM. Cancer stem cells: a step toward the cure. J Clin Oncol 2008; 26: 2795–99.
5. Boman BM, Huang E. Human colon cancer stem cells: a new paradigm in gastrointestinal oncology. J Clin Oncol 2008; 26: 2828–38.
6. Jordan CT, Guzman ML, Noble M. Mechanisms of disease. Cancer stem cells. New Engl J Med 2006; 355: 1253–61.
7. Savona M, Talpaz M. Getting to the stem cell of chronic myeloid leukaemia. Nat Rev Cancer 2008; 8: 341–50.
8. van Dongen JJ, Langerak AW, Brüggemann M et al. Design and standardization of PCR primers and protocols for detection of clonal immunoglobulin and T-cell receptor gene recombinations in suspect lymphoproliferations: report of the BIOMED-2 Concerted Action BMH4-CT98-3936. Leukemia 2003; 17: 2257–317.
9. van der Velden VH, Hochhaus A, Cazzaniga G et al. Detection of minimal residual disease in hematologic malignancies by real-time quantitative PCR: principles, approaches, and laboratory aspects. Leukemia 2003; 17: 1013–34.
10. Walsh SH, Rosenquist R. Immunoglobulin gene analysis of mature B-cell malignancies: reconsideration of cellular origin and potential antigen involvement in pathogenesis. Med Oncol 2005; 22: 327–41.
11. Küppers R, Yahalom J, Josting A. Advances in biology, diagnostics, and treatment of Hodgkin's disease. Biol Blood Marrow Transpl 2006; 12: 66–76.
12. Bahloul M, Asnafi V, Macintyre E. Clinical impact of molecular diagnostics in low-grade lymphoma. Best Pract Res Clin Haematol 2005; 18: 97–111.
13. Leong PP, Rezai B, Koch WM et al. Distinguishing second primary tumors from lung metastases in patients with head and neck squamous cell carcinoma. J Natl Cancer Inst 1998; 90: 972–7.
14. Nagel S, Borisch B, Thein SL et al. Somatic mutations detected by mini- and microsatellite DNA markers reveal clonal intratumor heterogeneity in gastrointestinal cancer. Cancer Res 1995; 55: 2566–870.
15. Cosme-Blanco W, Chang S. Dual roles of telomere dysfunction in initiation and suppression of tumorigenesis. Exp Cell Res 2008; 314: 1973–9.
16. Calin GA, Croce CM. MicroRNA signatures in human cancers. Nat Rev Cancer 2006; 6: 857–66.
17. Ebert BL, Pretz J, Bosco J et al. Identification of RPS14 as a 5q-syndrome gene by RNA interference screen. Nature 2008; 451: 252–3.
18. Mitelman F, Johansson B, Mertens F. The impact of translocations and gene fusions on cancer causation. Nat Rev Cancer 2007; 7: 233–45.
19. Gilliland DG. Molecular genetics of human leukaemias: new insights into therapy. Semin Hematol 2002; 39: 6–11.
20. Gilliland DG, Jordan CT, Felix CA. The molecular basis of leukemia. Hematology Am Soc Hematol Educ Program 2004: 80–97.
21. Greaves MF, Wiemels J. Origins of chromosomal translocations in childhood leukaemia. Nat Rev Cancer 2003; 3: 639–49.
22. Barr FG. Translocations, cancer and the puzzle of specificity. Nat Genet 1998; 19: 121–24.
23. Mendinges CM, Meijerink JP, Mensink EJ et al. Lack of correlation between numbers of circulating t(14; 18)-positive cells and response to first-line treatment in follicular lymphoma. Blood 2001; 98; 940–44.
24. Hirt C, Schüler F, Dölken G. Minimal residual disease (MRD) in follicular lymphoma in the era of immunotherapy with rituximab. Semin Cancer Biol 2003; 13: 223–31.
25. Grimwade D, Howe K, Langabeer S et al. Establishing the presence of the t(15;17) in suspected acute promyelocytic leukaemia: cytogenetic, molecular and PML immunofluorescence assessment of patients entered into the M.R.C. ATRA trial. Brit J Haemat 1996; 94: 557–73.
26. Mistry AR, Pedersen EW, Solomon E et al. The molecular pathogenesis of acute promyelocytic leukaemia: implications for the clinical management of the disease. Blood Rev 2003; 17; 71–97.
27. Reiter A, Lengfelder E, Grimwade D. Pathogenesis, diagnosis and monitoring of residual disease in acute promyelocytic leukaemia. Acta Haematol 2004; 112: 55–67.
28. Summers KE, Davies AJ, Matthews J et al. The relative role of peripheral blood and bone marrow for monitoring molecular evidence of disease in follicular lymphoma by quantitative real-time polymerase chain reaction. Br J Haematol 2002; 118: 563–6.
29. Guerrasio A, Rosso C, Martinelli G et al. Polyclonal haemopoiesis associated with long-term persistence of the AML1-ETO transcript in patients with FAB M2 acute myeloid leukaemia in continuous clinical remission. Br J Haematol 1995; 90: 364–8.
30. Cazzaniga G, Biondi A. Molecular monitoring of childhood acute lymphoblastic leukemia using antigen receptor gene rearrangements and quantitative polymerase chain reaction technology. Haematologica 2005; 90: 382–90.
31. Gribben JG, Freedman AS, Neuberg D et al. Immunologic purging of marrow assessed by PCR before autologous bone marrow transplantation for B-cell lymphoma. New Eng J Med 1991; 325: 1525–33.
32. Harris H, Miller OJ, Klein G et al. Suppression of malignancy by cell fusion. Nature 1969; 223: 363–8.
33. Knudson AG jr. Mutation and cancer: statistical study of retinoblastoma. Proc Nat Acad Sci USA 1971; 68: 820–3.
34. Knudson AG. Hereditary cancer: theme and variations. J Clin Oncol 1997; 15: 3280–7.
35. Cavenee WK, Dryja TP, Phillips RA et al. Expression of recessive alleles by chromosomal mechanisms in retinoblastoma. Nature 1983; 305: 779–84.
36. Leiderman YI, Kiss S, Mukai S. Molecular genetics of RB1-the retinoblastoma gene. Semin Ophthalmol. 2007; 22: 247–54.

37. Levine AJ. p53, the cellular gatekeeper for growth and division. Cell 1997; 88: 323–31.

38. Wahl G, Vala O. Genetic instability, oncogenes and the p53 pathway. Cold Spring Harbour Symp Quant Biol 2000; 65: 511–20.

39. Feng Z, Hu W, Rajagopal G et al. The tumor suppressor p53: cancer and aging. Cell Cycle 2008; 7: 842–7.

40. Toledo F, Wahl GM. Regulating the p53 pathway: in vitro hypotheses, in vivo veritas. Nat Rev Cancer 2006; 6: 909–23.

41. Kuribayashi K, El-Deiry WS. Regulation of programmed cell death by the p53 pathway. Adv Exp Med Biol. 2008; 615: 201–21.

42. Roth JA, Nguyen D, Lawrence DD et al. Retrovirus-mediated wild-type p53 gene transfer to tumors of patients with lung cancer. Nat Med 1996; 2: 985–91.

43. Lynch HT, Lynch JF, Lynch PM et al. Hereditary colorectal cancer syndromes: molecular genetics, genetic counseling, diagnosis and management. Fam Cancer 2008; 7: 27–39.

44. Blackwood A, Weber BL. BRCA1 and BRCA2: from molecular genetics to clinical medicine. J Clin Oncol 1998; 16: 1969–77.

45. Bussink J, van der Kogel AJ, Kaanders JHAM. Activation of the PI3-K/Akt pathway and implications for radioresistance mechanisms in head and neck cancer. Lancet Oncol 2008; 9: 288–96.

46. Ciardiello F, Tortora G. EGFR antagonists in cancer treatment. New Engl J Med 2008; 358: 1160–74.

47. Hudis C. Trastuzumab – mechanism of action and use in clinical practice. New Engl J Med 2007; 357: 39–51.

48. Hicks DG, Kulkarni S. HER2+ breast cancer: review of biologic relevance and optimal use of diagnostic tools. Am J Clin Pathol. 2008; 129: 263–73.

49. Downward J. Targeting RAS signaling pathways in cancer therapy. Nat Rev Cancer 2003; 3: 11-22.

50. Druker BJ, Talpaz M, Resta DJ et al. Efficacy and safety of a specific inhibitor of the BCR-ABL tyrosine kinase in chronic myeloid leukemia. New Engl J Med 2001; 344: 1031–37.

51. Sridhar SS, Seymour L, Shepherd FA. Inhibitors of epidermal growth factor receptors: a review of clinical research with a focus on non-small lung cancer. Lancet Oncol 2003; 4: 397–406.

52. Sherr CJ. G1 phase progression: cycling on cue. Cell 1994; 79: 551–5.

53. Gali-Muhtasib H, Bakkar N. Modulating cell cycle: current applications and prospects for future drug development. Curr Cancer Drug Targets 2002; 2: 309–36.

54. Fernàndez V, Hartmann E, Ott G et al. Pathogenesis of mantle-cell lymphoma: all oncogenic roads lead to dysregulation of cell cycle and DNA damage response pathways. J Clin Oncol 2005; 23: 6364–9.

55. Steeg PS, Abrams JS. Cancer prognostics: past, present and p27. Nat Med 1997; 3: 152–4.

56. Ahnen DJ, Feigl P, Quan G et al. Ki ras mutation and p53 mutation overexpression predict the clinical behaviour of colorectal cancer: a Southwest Oncology Group Study. Cancer Res 1998; 58: 1149–58.

57. Tibiletti MG. Interphase FISH as a new tool in tumor pathology. Cytogenet Genome Res 2007; 118: 229–36.

58. Bayani J, Squire JA. Comparative genomic hybridization. Curr Protoc Cell Biol 2005; Chapter 22: Unit 22.6 137–44.

59. Sreekantaiah C. FISH panels for hematologic malignancies. Cytogenet Genome Res 2007; 118: 284–96.

60. Döhner H, Stilgenbauer S, Benner A et al. Genomic aberrations and survival in chronic lymphocytic leukemia. New Engl J Med 2000; 343: 1910–16.

61. Novak U, Oppliger Leibundgut E, Hager J et al. A high resolution allelotype of B-cell chronic lymphocytic leukemia (B-CLL). Blood; 2002; 100: 1787–94.

62. Kawamata N et al. Molecular allelotyping of pediatric acute lymphoblastic leukaemias by high-resolution single nucleotide polymorphism oligonucleotide genomic microarray. Blood 2008; 111: 776–84.

63. Fey MF. Impact of the Human Genome Project on the clinical management of sporadic cancers. Lancet Oncol 2002; 3: 349–56.

64. Quackenbush J. Microarray analysis and tumor classification. New Engl J Med. 2006; 354: 2463–72.

65. Sotiriou C, Piccart M. Taking gene-expression profiling to the clinic: when will molecular profile signatures become relevant for patient care? Nat Rev Cancer 2007; 7: 545–53.

66. Staudt L. Molecular diagnosis of the hematologic cancers. New Engl J Med. 2003; 348: 1777–85.

67. Alizadeh AA, Eisen MB, Davis RE. Distinct types of diffuse large B-cell lymphoma identified by gene expression profiling. Nature 2000; 403: 503–11.

68. Shipp MA, Ross KN, Tamayo P et al. Diffuse large B-cell lymphoma outcome predicted by gene-expression profiling and supervised machine learning, Nat Med 2002; 8: 68–74.

69. van 't Veer LJ, Dai H, van de Vijver MJ et al. Gene expression profiling predicts clinical outcome of breast cancer. Nature 2002; 415: 530–6.

70. Rakha EA, Reis-Filho JS, Ellis IO. Basal-like breast cancer: a critical review. J Clin Oncol 2008; 26: 2568–81.

71. Papadopoulos N, Kinzler KW, Bert Vogelstein B. The role of companion diagnostics in the development and use of mutation-targeted cancer therapies. Nat Biotechnol 2006; 24, 985–95.

72. Croce CM. Oncogenes and cancer. New Engl J Med 2008; 358: 502–11.

73. Letai AG. Diagnosing and exploiting cancer's addiction to blocks in apoptosis. Nat Rev Cancer 2008; 8: 121–32.

2

Principles of Systemic Therapy

Franco M. Muggia and Marc Ballas

HISTORICAL OVERVIEW

The history of cancer chemotherapy is usually traced to the sensational December 2, 1943, incident (1) that occurred at the harbor of Bari, Italy. An air raid destroyed 17 allied ships including one containing mustard "bombs" (being stored as possible retaliation to the threat of chemical warfare): exposed personnel experienced the marrow hypoplasia and involution of lymphoid tissue previously reported with sulfur mustard gas during World War I (2). In fact, the medicinal studies of the related nitrogen mustard by U.S. governmental agencies in concert with biomedical researchers at academic institutions such as Yale had already started in 1942 (3–5) and was further catalyzed by the search for effective drugs against chronic infections including tuberculosis (6). This constellation of events led to the creation of the U.S. National Institutes of Health and the National Cancer Institute (NCI) that were to play a pivotal role in launching the era of anticancer chemotherapy. These government entities had the ability to sponsor scientific exchanges with other national and international institutions functioning largely unencumbered by profit motives. They succeeded as a clearing house of ideas to combat cancer in spite—in retrospect—of the rather primitive understanding of neoplastic growth and its molecular biology.

With the support of Congress, constituted as part of the U.S. government's Public Health Service, the NCI organized programs for the identification of drugs useful in cancer treatment. Activity against carcinogen-induced L1210 and P388 leukemias in mice became a criterion for selectivity of a drug against these rapidly dividing tumor cells without irreparably harming the host (7). A number of drugs related to nitrogen mustard and biochemically designed antimetabolites were shown to have clinical activity, and in spite of the shortcomings of random screening, successes could be claimed against some human malignancies (8). Collaboration with other governmental agencies (e.g., the Department of Agriculture) and the pharmaceutical industry also led to the selection of useful natural products, such as the vincas, camptothecins, and taxanes, the first one mostly developed by the industry and the last two through the perseverance of NCI-sponsored investigations. Another landmark achievement was the identification of antitumor properties of 5-fluorouracil (5-FU) and its eventual potential in the treatment of breast and gastrointestinal cancers by Heidelberger and colleagues (9).

SYSTEMIC TREATMENT MODALITIES: 21ST CENTURY TERMINOLOGY

Paul Ehrlich's introduced the word chemotherapy at the beginning of the 20th century (10). NCI programs designed to identify "magic bullets" against cancers therefore adopted the term "chemotherapy." Anticancer drugs introduced since nitrogen mustard became synonymous with chemotherapy and largely predated the more sophisticated therapies based on molecular targets. Recently, the term chemotherapy has taken the connotation of a nonspecific cytotoxic treatment that does not or barely distinguish between normal and malignant cells in achieving their eradication. This distorted view of their scientific, albeit largely empiric development, has resulted in an unfortunate pejorative meaning of chemotherapy. Chemotherapy drugs are often linked to toxic events and their intolerance is reinforced by their use in hopeless circumstances when all other treatments are exhausted. It is unwarranted to introduce new terminology, but it is worth revisiting the original concepts to reiterate the term as applying to a chemical molecule that is exerting a direct antitumor effect.

Endocrine therapy deserves special identification as a systemic approach for hormone-dependent tumors, which developed nearly in parallel with chemotherapy. Although its basis was initially empirical, the identification of hormone receptors in tumors rendered such agents the prime example of "molecular targeting" and underscored the importance of identifying and measuring the molecular targets, especially in selected patients who might benefit from such intervention.

So what about the newer terms molecularly "targeted" therapies and "biologicals"? The problem with this terminology is that chemotherapy drugs, even if introduced by an empirical process of selection—often based on vague notions of their targets—were later found to be truly molecularly targeted. For example, the camptothecins were known to be tumor selective (11) before their only target, topoisomerase I, was identified (12). In other instances, particularly pertaining to antimetabolites, the targets were quite precisely identified, and differential effects between tumor and normal cells spurred their development. As early as 1957, Heidelberger patented 5-FU and directed it against gastrointestinal cancers (9). However, drugs developed against a particular molecular target, such as against ras, turn out to have a vast array of actions that make these compounds hardly molecularly selective (13). To avoid this dilemma and to encompass molecules such as monoclonal antibodies that may have immunological and well as direct antitumor effects, the word biological is often used. All three terms are worth utilizing in describing systemic therapy with greater precision (Table 2.1a), until newer more acceptable terminology is developed. We include gene therapy for completeness, although to date this has been a local modality. Table 2.1b–e lists the major drug classes and their most common indications.

Problems with these terminologies are readily apparent from the examples given: (1) the camptothecin derivatives, topotecan and irinotecan, are chemotherapeutic drugs that are precisely molecularly targeted as their actions are only mediated through topoisomerase I (14); (2) trastuzumab is the most successful example of a molecularly targeted agent because patients are selected for treatment by testing for overexpression or amplification of the Her2 growth factor receptor (15)—very much the same way endocrine therapy of breast cancer is linked to the presence of estrogen

Table 2.1a   Terminologies Describing Systemic Therapy of Cancer

Terminology	Description (Table 2.1b–e)	Example(s)
Chemotherapy	Molecule exerting a direct antitumor effect	Cisplatin, topotecan (Table 2.1b)
Endocrine therapy	Interference of hormone-dependent growth	Tamoxifen in ER+tumors (Table 2.1c)
Molecularly targeted	Treatment selected because of known target	Trastuzumab in Her2 therapy overexpressed tumors (Table 2.1d)
Biological therapy	Therapy indirectly affecting tumors	Bevacizumab via antiangiogenesis
Gene therapy	Therapy delivering genetic information (e.g., to normalize or sensitize cancer cells)	None (systemic)
Immunotherapy	Utilization of host-effector mechanisms	Rituximab (Table 2.1e)

Abbreviation: ER, estrogen receptor positive.

Table 2.1b–e   Drugs Currently Useful in the Systemic Therapy of Cancer (see also Appendix)

Category	Indications	Features of class, drug
(b) Chemotherapy		
Alkylating drugs		Cumulative bone marrow depression
Chlorambucil	CLL, NHL, hairy cell	Use in solid tumors largely replaced
Cyclophosphamide	NHL, breast	Activated by liver microsomes
Ifosfamide	NHL, sarcoma	Activated by liver microsomes
Melphalan (PAM)	Multiple myeloma	Use in solid tumors largely replaced
Nitrogen mustard	Hodgkin's lymphoma (HL)	Replaced by oral derivatives in all other indications
NU: carmustine, semustine	Brain tumors, NHL, HL, multiple myeloma	Delayed cumulative thrombocytopenia and nonhematologic toxicities limit their use
Platinums: *cis-* and carboplatin	Germ cell, ovary, lung, H&N, sarcoma	Analogs attenuate cisplatin severe emesis and toxicities other than BM-related ones
Oxaliplatin	Colon and other GI	Neurotoxicity acute and cumulative
Other		
Dacarbazine (DTIC)	Melanoma	Useful mainly in cutaneous disease
Temozolomide	Same and brain tumors	Oral drug, same activation as dacarbazine
Mitomycin C	Anal cancer	Bioreductive radiosensitization
Antifolates		Interfere with folates as cofactors
Methotrexate	Choriocarcinoma	Dihydrofolate reductase inhibition
Pemetrexed	Mesothelioma, NSC lung	Thymidylate synthase (TS) inhibition; therapeutic index (TI) improved
Antimetabolites		Utilize metabolite activation pathways
Cytarabine	AML	Arabinose instead of ribose in nucleoside
Gemcitabine (dFdC)	Pancreas, breast, ovary, NSC, bile duct	Triphosphate incorporated into DNA; inhibition of ribonucleotide reductase
	Colon, breast, gastric	TS inhibition, RNA incorporation
5-FU	Colon, breast, gastric	Oral prodrug of 5FU
Capecitabine	CLL	Deaminase inhibitor: immunosuppression
Fludarabine	CML	Not used except for ↓WBC acutely
Hydroxyurea	AML, MDS	Histone deactelase (HDAC) inhibition
AzaC, decitabine 6MP, 6TG	ALL	Incorporation into DNA

(Continued)

Table 2.1b–e Drugs Currently Useful in the Systemic Therapy of Cancer (see also Appendix) (*Continued*)

Category	Indications	Features of class, drug
Mitotic inhibitors		Affect mitotic spindles; tubulin binding
Vincristine	ALL, children tumors	Dose-limiting neurotoxicity
Vinblastine	HL	Replaced in other tumors by vinorelbine
Vinorelbine	Breast, NSC lung	Dose-limiting BM toxicity
Docetaxel	Breast, NSC lung, H&N	Dose-limiting BM toxicity; alopecia
Paclitaxel	Breast, NSC lung, ovary	Dose-limiting neurotoxicity; alopecia
Topoisomerase binders		Damage via binding of enzyme impeding
Topo I: irinotecan	Colon, SC lung	DNA religation at break site
Topotecan	Ovary, SC lung	Prodrug of SN-38; biliary excretion
Topo II: dauno-, ida-	AML	Minimal GI toxicity; mostly BM toxicity
	Breast, sarcomas	Cumulative heart damage, alopecia
Doxo-, epirubicin	Breast, AML	Cumulative heart damage, alopecia
Mitoxantrone	Germ cell; NHL, HL	Cumulative heart damage, alopecia
Etoposide		Dose-limiting BM toxicity; alopecia
Miscellaneous		Variably defined mechanisms of action
Bleomycin	Germ cell, HL	Pulmonary and cutaneous toxicities
Dactinomycin	Children tumors	Radiation "recall" first described
(c) Endocrine therapy		
LHRH agonists	Breast (premenopausal), prostate	Transient increase in gonadal hormones when first administered
Tamoxifen	Breast	Selective estrogen receptor modulation
Aromatase inhibitors	Breast	Inhibit androgen to estrogen conversion
Antiandrogens	Prostate	Androgen receptor modulation
Miscellaneous		
Several cytotoxics	Breast	Ovarian function suppression
Glucocorticoids	Breast, prostate	Gonadal and adrenal function suppression
Ketoconazole	Prostate	
Progestins	Breast, endometrium	Inhibition of steroidgenesis
Androgen, estrogen	Breast, prostate	Progesterone receptor; indirect effects? Special circumstances—under study
(d) "Targeted" therapy		
Erlotinib	Lung, pancreas	EGFR TKI
Gefitinib	Lung in responders	EGFR TKI
Sunitinib	Renal cell, GIST	VEGFR TKI, PDGFR TKI
Sorafenib	Renal cell, HCC	VEGFR TKI, PDGFR TKI, raf
(e) Immunotherapy*		
Interferon alpha	Melanoma, KS, RCC	May act via nonimmune mechanisms
Rituximab	NHL, CLL	Anti-CD20, antibody also used as radioimmunoconjugate with 90Yttrium, 125I
Tici-, ipilumimab	Melanoma	Anti-CTLA4 antibody
Interleukin 2	RCC	Combined with LAK cells

*Vaccine immunostimulants not included.

Abbreviations: ALL, acute lymphocytic leukemia; AML, acute myelocytic leukemia; NSC, non small cell; BM, bone marrow; H&N, head and neck carcinoma; SC, small cell; CLL, chronic lymphocytic leukemia; HL, hodgkin's lymphoma; MDS, myelodysplastic syndrome; KS, Kaposi's sarcoma; NHL, non hodgkin's lymphoma; TKI, tyrosine kinase inhibitor; EGFR, epidermal growth factor receptor; PDGFR, platelet-derived growth factor receptor; VEGFR, vascular endothelium growth factor receptor.

and/or progesterone receptors in cancer cells—but may be working in part by immunological means (16); (3) bevacizumab inhibits neovascularization via binding to vascular endothelial growth factor A (VEGFA) (17), but some of its therapeutic efficacy may derive from normalization of a tumor's interstitial pressure[18] or directly when tumors express the VEGF receptors (19); and (4) similarly, rituximab's remarkable effect against lymphomas (20) may be by directly targeting the tumor cells expressing CD20 or by activating effector mechanisms (21).

A simpler view consistent with the history of drug development holds that "targeted therapies" were developed with a molecular target in mind, whereas "cytotoxic chemotherapies" were identified through empiric screens looking at cytotoxicity and outcome in preclinical models. Nevertheless, even these empiric approaches were mostly directed to rapid proliferation (later recognized to be mostly a flawed concept) and to DNA damage.

RATIONALE FOR SYSTEMIC THERAPY

Systemic therapy for cancer under the rubric of chemotherapy was first introduced for the treatment of leukemia and lymphoma, whereas the treatment of "solid tumors" focused on surgery, radiation, and, whenever applicable, endocrine interventions that were known to influence the course of breast, endometrial, and prostate cancers. Gradually, experimental systemic therapy provided some palliative benefits and at varying pace it became incorporated into the treatment strategy for particular cancers. Skipper and Schabel from Southern Research Institute and under contract from the NCI developed the rationale for "curative" approaches in murine leukemias and then in solid tumor mouse models (22). These models introduced the concept of "log-cell kill" that translated into the clinic for the need of earlier interventions to achieve complete responses (CRs) and additional treatments beyond the level of detectable disease (e.g., micrometastases). These studies were widely held as the basis for the implementation of adjuvant therapies in solid tumors where combination chemotherapies were beginning to achieve CRs. In fact, adjuvant therapy of cancer began to be successfully applied against breast cancer in the 1970s and became the focal point for similar studies in other common malignancies of the gastrointestinal and pulmonary tracts (10). Table 2.2 illustrates how the introduction of systemic therapies influenced the outcome of specific cancers with varying degrees of success and at markedly different speed. These examples underline the importance of biology and drug discovery in subsequent achievements, with clinical trials (directed to adjuvant or metastatic situations, see below) and strategies being subservient to basic knowledge of a disease. However, clinical oncologists have long understood the importance of testing novel treatment strategies on the heels of any discovery: carefully conducted clinical experiments take time and are the essential sequel to any basic discovery. Recent drug development finally breaking through the resistance of kidney and hepatocellular cancers to systemic therapy and the restraining effect of tyrosine kinase inhibitors such as imatinib mesylate and sunitinib on the growth of the notoriously chemorefractory metastatic gastrointestinal stromal tumor (GIST) underscore the importance of biology in catalyzing the eventual key role of systemic therapies in the treatment of these cancers when they are beyond curative surgery.

The evolution of systemic therapy in these cancers not only reflect the impact of knowledge of tumor biology, but also underscore that empirically derived therapy could be shown through clinical trials to play a role in the treatment of a cancer, even with rudimentary knowledge of tumor biology. It should be noted, however, that the more accessible a tumor is for study, such as is the case of hematologic malignancies, the more tailored the systemic treatments may become. In solid tumors, a similar evolution is rapidly taking place during the beginning of this century: for example, a molecular classification of breast cancers is increasingly determining the kind of systemic therapy to be applied and the subsets to be studied in clinical trials in both adjuvant (when there is no evident disease present after surgery) and metastatic settings. In colon cancer, the molecular changes underlying the evolution from a normal colonic epithelium to preneoplastic changes, to adenomas, and subsequently to invasive and later metastatic adenocarcinoma were first articulated by Kinzler and Vogelstein (75); these served not only to emphasize a role for screening, but also to consider their influence on treatment interventions. In fact, increasingly we note that molecular features such as microsatellite insta-

bility (76,77) and k-ras mutations (78) may determine the systemic therapy to be used in both adjuvant (after surgical resection) and metastatic settings. Epithelial ovarian cancer and lung cancers are almost universal targets of systemic treatments after surgery because they are mostly diagnosed at advanced stages. Varying degrees of success with treatments among histologic subtypes, reflecting differing etiologies and biology served to emphasize the importance of molecular biology in determining outcome, mostly in relation to "platinum-based" therapies. A recent development, based on our understanding of the importance of DNA repair mechanisms to overcome lethality from platinum-DNA adducts, renders future selection of systemic therapies in these diseases dependent in part on the function of BRCA genes and the expression of ERCC1 (79–81).

The rationale for the concept of "adjuvant" systemic therapy in lieu of the more difficult treatment of metastatic disease is challenged when systemic treatment is sufficiently effective that the policy of surveillance—deferring treatment after surgery for most patients so as to treat only those that eventually manifest metastases—yields an equivalent outcome to adjuvant treatment of all patients (64). In testicular cancer of the seminomatous type, a particularly radiosensitive malignancy that most commonly presents in clinical stage I, the question is one of "prophylactic" retroperitoneal radiation—a procedure known to improve outcome over surgery alone since the 1940s (82)—or substituting it by two cycles of systemic carboplatin, and long-term results of a clinical trial comparing these policies have recently been presented and debated (83,84).

The outcome of cancers arising in the uterine cervix or of head and neck origin is more dependent on our ability to control locoregional disease than to the containment of distant metastases. However, as both local and systemic treatments are refined, a close interplay between surgery, radiation, and systemic therapy is likely to represent the principal direction of modern therapeutics. Concomitant chemotherapy and radiation have generally yielded more positive results than the sequential use of these modalities (85). In locally advanced laryngeal cancer, the most important role played by the use of radiation and chemotherapy was the preservation of the larynx without compromising the results of surgery (86). Preservation of function and lessening of morbidity are also major rationales for the use of systemic therapy in locally advanced breast cancer, childhood solid tumors, and bone and soft tissue sarcomas.

Immunotherapy also deserves special mention as a systemic intervention. For years, discouraging aspects of systemic therapies for cancer have been the development of drug resistance, the nearly uniform failure to eradicate neoplastic cells even if one achieves a CR from a systemic treatment, and the frequent lack of correlation between objective responses and overall outcome. Attempts at nonspecifically "boosting" antitumor immunity have been forthcoming for several decades, with only occasional suggestions of success. Immunologic effects of drugs and radiation have been shown to enhance the recognition of the immune system (via dendritic cells) of tumor antigens leading to long lasting immunity (87,88). This knowledge and the availability of powerful immune reagents (as well as better immune monitoring) may enhance the reliability of these approaches and our ability to overcome the shortcomings of current systemic approaches.

Table 2.2 Tracing the Impact of Systemic Therapy: Highlights in Selected Cancers

Disease: Intervention (Dates) (Refs.)	Comments
Breast cancer	
a. Endocrine +/– chemotherapy activity (1950–1970) (23–25)	Cooperative groups lead studies in advanced disease and then focus on adjuvant treatments
b. Node positive adjuvant studies (1960, 1970–1980); node negative adjuvant studies (1980): clear benefit (26–28)	
c. Primary chemotherapy (neoadjuvant) studies (1985) (29)	
d. Her2 as a prognostic factor and target (1990–1999)	
e. Trastuzumab adjuvant trial (2004): dramatic gain (30,31)	
Colon cancer	
a. 5-FU activity against metastases (1957–1970) (32) but no clear advantage over observation as adjuvant (33)	VA adjuvant studies: interpreted as negative and flawed
b. All screened drugs (1970–1998): no activity (34,35)	
c. Studies of 5-FU with levamisole, leucovorin, or portal vein infusion (1990–2004): modest survival benefit (36–39). rekindles interest	Mayo Clinic and NSABP efforts
d. Irinotecan and oxaliplatin add to 5-FU's activity, and FolFOx becomes standard (2004) (40,41)	Activity of platinums and camptothecins
e. Bevacizumab and antibodies to EGFR added to chemotherapy: improved outcomes (2004–present) (42–45)	Impact of "Biologicals" gains from surgery on metastases
Lung cancer (nonsmall cell)	
a. Minimal impact of chemotherapy in advanced disease (1960–2000); stages I, II: negative studies (46)	Cooperative groups: initial focus on small cell; on nonsmall cell focus on precise staging + systemic treatment
b. Combined modality studies with surgery and radiation: stages IIIA and IIIB benefit (1990–2000) (49)	
c. Positive adjuvant cisplatin trial (2004) (47,48,50)	Gains with platinum-based chemotherapy and targeted drugs dispel pessimism
d. EGFR, antiangiogenesis as targets (2003–2008) (51–54)	
Ovarian cancer	
a. Alkylating agent era (1950–1972)	Brief remissions and minimal improvement with combinations
b. Nonplatinum combinations (1972–1980) (55)	
c. Cisplatin (1979): advantage over combinations (56)	Cisplatin and the less toxic carboplatin: steady strides including ip delivery
d. Carboplatin (1986) and paclitaxel (1996): to date standard treatment in early and advanced stages (57,58)	Modest improvement with taxanes, liposomal doxorubicin, gemcitabine, and topotecan
e. Impact of intraperitoneal (ip) cisplatin meta-analysis (2006) (59–61)	
f. Wide testing of targeted therapies, especially bevacizumab	Activity of bevacizumab
Testis cancer	
a. Actinomycin D, alkylating, and vinca : CRs (1950s–1970s) (62)	Response emulates choriocarcinoma
b. Vinblastine + bleomycin regimen (1970–1972) (63)	Curative in nearly ¼
c. Introduction of cisplatin and integration to b (64)	With cisplatin cures from 60–90% (67)
d. Cisplatin-based chemotherapy and focus on cisplatin failures: high-dose, ifosfamide, taxanes (65)	Focus now is in (1) how to avoid resistance; (2) new agents (66)
Prostate cancer	
a. Castration applied since 1930s; acid phosphatase (68)	Androgen dependence
b. Estrogens and later antiandrogens in palliation (1960–1990s) (69,70); PSA to monitor disease (1980s) (71,72)	Failures: hormonal independence
c. Chemotherapy trials showing improved outcomes (quality of life; later survival) (2000–2006)	Impact of mitoxantrone + prednisone; docetaxel
d. "Targeted" therapies through understanding of hormonal independence mechanisms (73,74)	Ongoing exploration of molecular targets

With our expanding body of knowledge and therapeutic armamentarium focused on human neoplasia, we also have witnessed the dissemination of pseudoscientific treatments based on poorly conceived or poorly documented, often sweeping, concepts that claim to boost the immune system, provide "antioxidant" protection, specifically starve tumor cells from detrimental nutrients. These pseudoscientific fads ranged from harmless, nonspecific ways to enhance quality of life and overcome noxious effects of our therapies, to downright dangerous natural products spiked with anticoagulants and high-dose estrogens (89), and even to harmful immune "boosters" contaminated by viruses such as HIV and hepatitis (90). "Hypothesis generating" concepts should remain hypothesis generating until backed by clinically tested well-documented trials (and not a series of anecdotes). More sophisticated technically driven innovations also deserve mention as they increasingly compete with the application of systemic therapies. Ablation of liver metastases employing radiofrequency ablation or cryoablation (among several other techniques) has achieved a role in the management of colon cancer metastatic to the liver complementary or in lieu of resection (91). These and other technical feats that result from stereotactic delivery of radiation to a metastatic site appeal to patients and their therapists. However, we should expect that the compilation of results in a particular disease setting be held to the same scrutiny and level of evidence demanded of systemic therapies.

TREATMENT REGIMENS: PRINCIPLES OF COMBINATIONS, PHARMACOLOGY, DOSE SCHEDULE, AND SUPPORTIVE CARE

The development of treatment regimen is a complex enterprise that most often follows sequentially on the heels of a prior regimen that had been adopted in a prior clinical trial. During the latter part of the 20th century, clinical investigators followed basic principles for the development of drug combinations, always hopeful that such regimens would result in improved outcome and avoid the emergence of drug resistance by analogy to antibiotics in the anti-infectious field. These "clinical" principles included (1) single agent activity against the cancer in question (this concept drove most phase II studies with single agents as a necessary step for their eventual integration into the "standard regimen," (2) minimally overlapping toxicities (ever mindful to the need of avoiding dangerous levels of bone marrow suppression before the era of hematopoietic growth factor support), and (3) differing mechanisms of action—this was an impetus for new drug discovery—rather than analogue development that was commonplace at the beginning of the chemotherapy era (92). These concepts still provide useful guidelines to current regimen development algorithms; however, increasingly the principles have been expanded, in one dimension, current regimens should include pharmacologic backup, exploration of dose schedules, and reliance on supportive care measures to minimize toxicities, and in another dimension, we now seek the integration of drug effects not only on the tumor cells, but also on the host and the tumor microenvironment (see next paragraph).

Mathematical modeling of what may represent synergistic, additive, and subadditive effects between two drugs have received much attention (93) and are obviously exponentially more complex as one examines the effect of three drugs in combination. In evolving "rational" treatment regimens, drug combination strategies were designated as sequential or concurrent biochemical blockades primarily applicable to antimetabolites or other forms of complementary blockade that included other forms of DNA damage (94). The hallmarks of neoplasia by Hanahan and Weinberg (95) have been used to illustrate the range of targets to which we direct our current treatments. Within this new view, it may be useful to consider analogous concepts for certain drug combinations: for example, vertical blockade may refer to combined treatments of a molecule directed against a ligand with a molecule that inhibits receptor action (e.g., bevacizumab with sorafenib) (96) and horizontal blockade to the combination of a drug directed against the tumor cells and the endothelium (e.g., a taxane) coupled with a drug directed to the pericytes (e.g., imatinib mesylate) (97).

Whether used as a single agent or as part of a combined regimen, *pharmacological principles* need to be broadly considered, particularly because clinical situations have become inordinately complex: most patients are usually on a number of nonantineoplastic medications and profound ethnic variations in drug metabolism and tolerance have emerged. Pharmacokinetics and pharmacodynamics of anticancer drugs appear within several chapters; here we wish to mention the importance of knowing whether a drug is metabolized by the cytochrome p450 enzymatic machinery or is a substrate of a particular isoform, how much a role does renal excretion play, and pharmacodynamic effect of age—among others—in drug dosing. Studies addressing pharmacology in the presence of hepatic or renal dysfunction have been instituted in the development of recent anticancer drugs. In addition, the validity of dosing all anticancer drugs by per-square-meter base rather than on a strictly weight basis or on flat dosing has been increasingly questioned. Examples of flat dosing perhaps being advantageous may be found in studies looking at the oral 5-FU prodrug, capecitabine; the proteasome inhibitor, bortezomib (98); and the new generation vinca alkaloid, vinorelbine (99). In particular, with capecitabine, adherence to the dose schedule that was approved by the FDA and dose its modification in the presence of toxicities has been problematic, clinicians have been guided by practical considerations and titration to patient tolerance that are likely counterproductive (100). Moreover, the package insert prescribed dose reductions because of toxicity as opposed to shortening the days of drug administration run the risk of resulting in totally inadequate dose levels of the active drug.

The dose schedule of a given regimen is generally derived from the phase I, II, and III studies carried out to demonstrate drug efficacy and obtain an indication. In adjuvant settings with curative implications, one should not deviate from these prescribed "package-insert" regimens without good reasons. In the treatment of metastatic disease, the situation is more complex: regimens gain approval for having demonstrated efficacy often based on surrogate end points (e.g., prolongation of progression-free survival) and less commonly on improved overall survival. Moreover, the results may be achieved at a cost of considerably greater toxicity or are only applicable to the subset of patients entered into the trial. Finally, many more studies and regimens are available for the metastatic setting than for adjuvant studies; this results in greater latitude in what becomes "standard" treatment and what dose schedule of a regimen to use. There is no substitute for experiencing a particular regimen in rendering such a treatment useful and safe for a patient in need of palliative treatment. Increasingly, the approaches to metastases of common cancers have established a hierarchy of treatments beyond first line, extending all the way to second and third and occasionally beyond. This situation occurs not only because of the availability of a number of competing treatments with differing mechanisms of action and reasonable therapeutic indices, but also in view of our better ability to assess the disease and its progression under the preceding treatment, more easily allowing subsequent interventions. Although innumerable palliative treatments directed to a particular patient have raised issues of their appropriateness, one must recognize that these are most often because of early detection of progression and not the result of truculence or poor judgment on the part of the therapist. Risk-benefit issues, often including economic considerations, are addressed in a later section.

Dose intensity retrospective calculations were initially introduced by Hryniuk and coworkers (55) to emphasize the importance of dose in achieving optimal results. Eventually, the assumptions that each drug in a combination contributed equally to such outcome were deemed too simplistic, but the concept of dose density modeled by Norton and Simon (101) was prospectively tested in clinical trials of metastatic breast cancer (102) and attained validation. Of course, growth factors to accelerate myelopoiesis had become available and permitted the safe administration of myelosuppressive regimens on every 2 weeks rather than every 3 weeks. Filgrastim and peg-filgrastim have been widely used in developing regimens that maximize dose density and dose rate, although proof of their superiority over conventional regimens lacking these growth factors must be obtained in every specific instance (103). Nevertheless, dose dense regimens, regardless of proof of superiority, do lead to early completion of the treatment course that may be preferred logistically (such as in preoperative situations). Currently these agents are advocated routinely to avoid febrile neutropenia, if the likelihood of such development for a given regimen exceeds 20% (104).

Other *supportive care measures* during drug treatment may have subtle effects on outcome associated with a given treatment regimen that are not so easily expected or quantified. The recent adverse outcomes in association with concomitant administration of erythropoietic agents to ameliorate fatigue from chemotherapy (105) and with calcium/magnesium repletion to prevent neuropathy during oxaliplatin (106) are general and specific examples, respectively. However, it is possible that beneficial effects may extend beyond their anticipated "supportive care" effects. Although speculative, one may hypothesize that the improved outcome in ovarian cancer trials following the introduction of HT3 blockers to avoid platinum emesis is a result to complete the treatment as well as to tolerate better subsequent treatments (107). A more current example is the use of metformin to treat hyperglycemia with IGF1-R directed antibodies—metformin as a drug has its own antitumor effects and may be additive to the regimen under study (108).

A KEY QUESTION: SEQUENTIAL VS. COMBINATION?

In the third section we pointed out the advantage of concomitant versus sequential treatment when chemotherapy is given in combination with radiation in certain cancers such as those arising in the head and neck area. The advantage of a such combined approach was further derived from several trials in locally advanced cancers of the uterine cervix. Historically, such combined radiation + drug approaches were limited to agents thought to be radiosensitizers; such combinations had radiotherapy as the main stay of treatment along with doses of the relevant drug(s)—such as 5-FU—at the beginning and at the end of treatment (109). Both efficacy and side effects increased in the combination compared to radiotherapy alone. As more effective agents such as cisplatin became available, the combinatorial effect proved beneficial to enhance local tumor control and to augment overall tumor eradication. In other tumor types, such as breast, esophageal, lung cancers, pancreatic, and anorectal, combinations of chemotherapy and radiation have been examined in multiple trials with regard to timing of the two modalities (85). The idea of sequencing emerged to avoid side effects, as both morbidity and occasionally excess mortality were associated with concomitant administration. Although trial design has been quite variable, in many of these different tumor types the concomitant effect has generally proved more effective. The drugs that have "synergized" with radiation include the platinums and 5-FU already cited, as well as taxanes, vinca alkaloids, gemcitabine, and mitomycin C.

Concomitant systemic therapy with radiation is attractive conceptually and this extends beyond the use of cytotoxic agents. In rectal cancer, Willet et al. published on a small experience suggesting that bevacizumab enhanced the results of radiation and chemotherapy (18). Experience in breast cancer, both preclinically and clinically, supports the use of trastuzumab in Her2 overexpressing tumors concomitantly with radiation (110). EGFR inhibition, similarly, enhances the antitumor effects of radiation in head and neck cancers (111). Trastuzumab also overcomes mechanisms of radiation resistance. All these considerations support the concomitant approach over sequential use of chemoradiation.

With chemotherapy and with combinations of "targeted" therapies, however, the case for combined versus sequential must be reconsidered in nearly all instances where combinations have been developed and established. Traditionally, multiagent chemotherapy was mostly developed for the treatment of leukemia, lymphomas, and breast cancer in the 1960s and widely established its value in clinical trials in the 1970s. The current situation is much more complex. Multiple agent combinations have often been reduced to doublets, and even such two-drug combinations are often not persuasively more effective than sequential single agents. The trend of shedding drugs from multidrug combinations of borderline efficacy in the treatment of cancers of the bladder, breast, lung, and ovary, as examples, began in the early 1980s and has resulted in the use of doublets in many instances. This has permitted optimal dosing of drug combinations and has furthermore fostered the integration of the newer "targeted" drugs into such regimens. In colon cancer, this situation did not apply because up to the 1990s 5-FU given alone or with "biochemical modulators" such as leucovorin was the only drug with efficacy against this disease and multiple attempts at combination regimens including drugs such as nitrosoureas, mitomycin C, other alkylating agents, and cisplatin resulted in enhanced toxicity with no increased efficacy (34).

Adequately powered clinical trials showing an advantage of a combination over single agents have been published recently to gain approval of an additional agent for metastatic breast cancer. As background in this setting, the study by Sledge et al (112). failed to show that paclitaxel + doxorubicin was superior in progression-free survival to either single agent. Subsequently, however, capecitabine received full approval for treatment of breast cancer when it showed an advantage in combination with docetaxel over docetaxel alone (113); an approval for gemcitabine was also obtained when gemcitabine combined with paclitaxel proved superior in progression-free survival to paclitaxel alone (114). In both these instances, a substantial number of these patients did not cross over to receive the other drug and begged the question of whether the more toxic combination would be superior to the optimal use of the sequential single agents.

A similar scenario has been seen in the treatment of ovarian cancer both in first-line trials (Table 2.3) and when it recurs after an interval of 6 months or greater from the last platinum-based induction treatment (Table 2.4). This last situation is considered operationally as defining a "platinum-sensitive" recurrence—that is, a situation where a platinum such as cisplatin or carboplatin would yield the best outcome. Table 2.4 shows the results of randomized trials that show the contribution to the outcome of adding a specific nonplatinum drug to carboplatin in comparison to the platinum alone (or in the instance of ICON4, also to other platinum-based combinations). Only in the largest randomized trial was there a difference in survival, but overall the contribution of the second drug, although seemingly statistically significant was still quite modest. In first-line setting, no differences were noted in the two trials (attributed in part to preemptive crossover) examining platinum + paclitaxel combination when it was compared to another doublet before widespread availability of the taxane upon failure of first-line treatment.

TYPES OF INTERVENTION (COMBINED MODALITY, INDUCTION, CONSOLIDATION, MAINTENANCE)

Surgery and radiation have traditionally come to play complementary roles in targeting local control of the disease when it is beyond cure by either modality alone. Examples of such complementary role include radiation of the pelvis following hysterectomy for "high or intermediate risk" stage I endometrial cancer, preoperative or postoperative radiation for rectal cancer beyond stage I, postoperative radiation in high Gleason score prostate cancer, radiation of the surgical scar in advanced mesothelioma. These complementary indications have been absorbed into "combined modality" as systemic therapies increasingly play a role either preoperatively or as an adjuvant to surgery, or as chemoradiation instead of radiation alone in other circumstances. Combined modality treatment is currently being tested or has become preferred in locally advanced cancers of various head and neck sites, rectum,

stomach, cervix, and prostate. In stage IIIB nonsmall cell lung cancer, definitive chemoradiotherapy alone with no further surgery has demonstrated equal efficacy to postoperative chemoradiotherapy combination. In endometrial cancer, it is the pelvic radiation that is being eliminated, as chemotherapy has taken more of an adjuvant role in situations associated with high probability of recurrences. Combined modality treatment of either resectable or locally advanced inoperable pancreatic cancer has been the subject of several trials but it is controversial whether chemoradiation has an advantage in either situation over no further treatment or chemotherapy alone, respectively.

In childhood malignancies, such as rhabdomyosarcomas, Ewing's sarcoma, other bone and soft tissue sarcomas, Wilms' tumors, neuroblastomas, and non-Hodgkin's lymphomas, combined modality has long been established but trials are ongoing to reduce the need for radiation and to study its long-term effects on normal growth as systemic therapy improves. This toxicity-reduction objective is behind many ongoing clinical trials in situations where high cure rates have been achieved.

The terminology to describe the application of various nonsurgical therapies reflects the underlying concepts of how they are used: initial treatment with drugs or radiation is referred to as *induction*, and this is followed by *consolidation* when another form of treatment is applied as part of the initial plan and delivered without intervening relapse. Consolidation with radiation was a commonplace postoperative treatment in many conditions where local relapse was frequent. However, postoperative radiation of kidney cancer, endometrial cancer, and uterine leiomyosarcomas, among others, was associated with fewer local recurrences but no difference in overall survival because it had no effect on distant metastases. Consolidation can also be achieved with delivery of intracavitary radiation—as has been done in ovarian cancer albeit without success and also by giving additional drugs—a maneuver also without success in ovarian cancer. *Maintenance* is the use of a drug or drug regimen given as induction and then continued beyond the achievement of a maximal response or evidence of persistent disease. Maintenance is the rule in situations where only partial responses or disease stabilization is achieved. However, it can also be used after CR if the risk for recurrence is notoriously high—for example, after a clinical CR following induction chemotherapy for stage IIIC ovarian cancer. This situation has a median relapse-free survival of 18–24 months. One study by the GOG showed that every 4-weekly paclitaxel extended the median relapse-free survival by 7 months in patients receiving 12 additional treatments compared to those who received only 3 additional treatments (124).

CLINICAL TRIALS, MEASURES OF OUTCOME, QUALITY OF LIFE, AND TOXICITY

Phase I and phase II trials provide the initial building blocks of systemic therapy and are increasingly designed to establish pharmacokinetic parameters, and in the case of "targeted therapies" validation of pharmacodynamic end points to ensure that the target has been reached. Phase III trials were of various kinds such as exploratory, explanatory, or confirmatory, that is, to set a new standard

Table 2.3 Paclitaxel/Platinum Combinations in Randomized First-Line Advanced Ovarian Cancer Trials

Trial	Treatment regimens	No. of patients	Percentage of early crossover	Progression-free survival (mo)	Overall survival (mo)
GOG-132 (115)	Paclitaxel (135 mg/m², 24 hr) and cisplatin (75 mg/m²)	201	22	14.2	26.6
	Cisplatin (100 mg/m²)	200	40	16.4	30.2
	Paclitaxel (200 mg/m², 24 hr)	213	23	11.2*	26
MRC-ICON3 (116)	Paclitaxel (175 mg/m², 3 hr) and carboplatin AUC 6	478	23	17.3	36.1
	Carboplatin AUC 6	943	25	16.1	35.4
	Paclitaxel (175 mg/m², 3 hr) and carboplatin AUC 6	232	23	17	40
	Cyclophosphamide (750 mg/m²) and doxorubicin (75 mg/m²) and cisplatin (75 mg/m²)	421	20	17	40
GOG-111 (117)	Paclitaxel (135 mg/m², 24 hr) and cisplatin (75 mg/m²)	184	None	18	38
	Cyclophosphamide (750 mg/m²) and cisplatin (75 mg/m²)	202	None	13*	24*
OV-10 (118)	Paclitaxel (175 mg/m², 3 hr) and cisplatin (75 mg/m²)	162	None	15.5	35.6
	Cyclophosphamide (750 mg/m²) and cisplatin (75 mg/m²)	161	4	11.5*	25.8*

*Statistically significant (p ≤ 0.05) differences versus other arms.
Source: Adapted from Physician Data Query (www.cancer.gov).

Table 2.4 Example of Combinations vs. Single Agents in "Platinum-Sensitive" Ovarian Cancer Recurrence

Eligibility	Platinum regimen	Patient no.	Comparator	Comments on outcome (Ref.)
Platinum sensitive	Cisplatin + doxorubicin + cyclophosphamide		Paclitaxel	Randomized phase II; CAP superior PFS, OS (119)
Platinum sensitive	Carboplatin + epirubicin	190	Carboplatin	Powered for response differences; OS 17 vs. 15 m (120)
Platinum sensitive	Carboplatin + gemcitabine	356	Carboplatin	PFS 8.6 m vs. 5.8 m OS 18 m vs. 17 m (121)
Platinum sensitive	Cisplatin or carboplatin + paclitaxel	802	Single or nontaxane + platinums	PFS 11 m vs. 9 m OS 24 m vs. 19 m (122)
Platinum sensitive	Carboplatin + pegylated liposomal doxorubicin	104	None	PFS 9 m, median OS 32 m (123)

treatment (125). Clinical trials—particularly randomized phase III trials—are the main source of information for systemic treatments given under various circumstances. Not only do they provide information about relative efficacy, but they are also repositories of vast amounts of toxicity data collected in a uniform way. Both acute and long-range effects are within the scope of clinical trials. For example, serial studies by the GOG have clearly documented renal toxicities associated with cisplatin to remarkably increase as one goes from 75 mg/m² per cycle to a dose of 100 mg/m² per cycle. Studies done by the national surgical adjuvant breast and bowel project (NSABP) and other cooperative groups have also documented that escalating doxorubicin dose beyond 60 mg/m²/cycle is not associated with improved outcome in breast cancer adjuvant settings; similarly, escalating cyclophosphamide beyond

600 mg/m²/cycle is counterproductive. A systemic therapy applied under specific circumstances to be approved by regulatory agencies must provide evidence of survival advantage or an appropriate surrogate such as progression-free survival over a similar outcome following standard therapy, or having similar efficacy while improving quality of life. As therapeutic regimens become more complex and are approved for various lines of treatment, the use of surrogate end points becomes inevitable for newer upfront regimens to be established as survival may be influenced by a number of variables after the study regimen is applied. Rarely, information on the impact of systemic therapies can be gleaned by studying large population-based data collections such as SEER and Medicare. Chapter 4 (by Parulekar, Eisenhauer, and Gelber) expands on the design, execution, and analysis of clinical trials.

RISK/BENEFIT RATIO

In the application of any systemic therapy, the risk/benefit ratio is an underlying theme that underscores the validity of its use for specific circumstance at hand. Such issues are often discussed in the context of patients who have comorbidities or who have failed multiple other therapies and therefore do not fulfill the criteria that is inherent in the use of a certain regimen. Under these special circumstances, clinical trials offer little further insight. Ultimately, one proceeds with the treatment based on the therapist's individual experience and after thorough information of both risks and potential benefits.

In some instances, the trial itself "pushes the envelope" in testing treatments that have inherent greater risks but a greater potential for achieving long-term benefit. Trials during the 1990s greatly expanded the exploration of high-dose chemotherapy in breast cancer that had very adverse prognostic features such as more than 10 positive lymph nodes at the outset. A major criticism of this approach, however, was that comparative studies were not done because of the inherent assumption that only the ratio was being tested, and therefore if the risk could be diminished, the benefit was indisputable. Comparative trials, however, failed to show improved benefits from this approach.

Economic factors are also often brought to this equation in the application of systemic therapies. However, economic factors may be arbitrarily set and are, therefore, often spurious or of secondary importance in decision making. This statement does not necessarily imply the endorsement of measures regardless of cost or excluding prioritization of treatments based on costs; however, such decisions should probably be made at levels beyond those of an oncology service.

A GLIMPSE INTO THE FUTURE

Therapeutic advances are occurring at an accelerated pace, but quantum leaps in tumor eradication and survival are often coupled with insight into tumor biology that had been acquired prior to the introduction of a new agent. The saga of imatinib mesylate and its effect on chronic myelogenous leukemia comes to mind: it followed decades of delineation of chromosomal changes and then identification of the bcr-abl oncogene (126). As an important sideline in its development, documenting that imatinib is a receptor tyrosine kinase (RTK) that inhibited c-kit in nanomolar concentrations led to discovering its beneficial effects in patients with metastatic GIST (127). Such findings stimulated development of other RTKs that have found their way into oncologic treatment. The remarkable effects of the antibody to the VEGF on improving outcome in colon, lung, breast, and likely ovarian cancers capped three decades of antiangiogenic research by the pioneering efforts of Judah Folkman (128), subsequently joined by many others. The anti-VEGF antibody, bevacizumab, the anti-CD20 antibody, rituximab (129), and the anti-Her1 antibody, trastuzumab (130), are examples of monoclonal antibody technology that became established in therapeutics nearly three decades after the Nobel Prize in medicine was awarded for such development (131). Finally, one of the most

remarkable therapeutic achievements, the development of platinum drugs, followed empiric observations (92). It should not be lost on us that deciphering the remarkable selectivity of these agents for certain tumors may open the way for additional breakthroughs. Moreover, once the systemic therapy is remarkably curative, it revolutionizes the overall approach to the disease.

Looking back at our successes indicates that though we must continue to seek the "lock and key" approach to overcome a neoplastic transformation, answers for most of our common forms of neoplasia will continue to come from multiple approaches. Expecting that all treatment will be "targeted" and that all our current cytotoxic treatments will play no role in the ensuing decades is likely to prove an erroneous prediction. "Personalized medicine" has become a favorite expression, but it is likely to be less about personalization and more about evolving logical strategies that can increasingly provide better outcomes through insight of tumor biology, diagnosis, and therapeutic trials.

REFERENCES

1. Hirsh J. An anniversary for cancer chemotherapy. JAMA 2006; 296: 1518–20.
2. Krumbaar EB. Role of the blood and the bone marrow in certain forms of gas poisoning. 1. Peripheral blood changes and their significance. JAMA 1919; 72: 39–41.
3. Goodman LS, Gilman A. The pharmacological basis of therapeutics (Section XV). In: Drugs Used in the Chemotherapy of Neoplastic Disease, 2nd edn. New York: The Macmillan Company, 1958: 1414–50.
4. Goodman LS, Wintrobe MM, Dameshek W et al. Nitrogen mustard therapy. JAMA 1946; 132: 126–32.
5. Rhoads CP. Nitrogen mustard in the treatment of neoplastic disease. JAMA 1946; 131: 656–8.
6. Zubrod CG. Chemical control of cancer. Proc Natl Acad Sci (USA) 1972; 69: 1042–7.
7. Skipper HE. Cancer chemotherapy is many things: G.H.A. Clowes Memorial Lecture. Cancer Res 1971; 31: 1173–9.
8. Zubrod CG. Agents of choice in neoplastic disease. In: Sartorelli AC, Johns DG, eds. Antineoplastic and Immunosuppressive Agents I. New York: Springer Verlag, 1974: 1–11.
9. Heidelberger C, Chaudhari NK, Danenberg P et al. Fluorinated pyrimidines: a new class of tumor inhibitory compounds. Nature 1957; 179: 663–6.
10. DeVita VT Jr, Oliverio VT, Muggia FM et al. The drug development and clinical trials program of the Division of Cancer Treatment, National Cancer Institute. Cancer Clin Trials 1979; 2: 195–216.
11. Muggia FM, Creaven PJ, Hansen HH et al. Phase I clinical trial of weekly and daily schedules of camptothecin (NSC 100880): Correlation with preclinical studies. Cancer Chemother Rep 1972; 56: 515–21.
12. Liu LF, Depew RE, Wang JC. Knotted single-stranded DNA rings: a novel topological isomer of single-stranded circular DNA formed by E. coli omega protein treatment. J Mol Biol 1976; 106: 439–52.
13. Reuter CWM, Morgan MA, Bergmann L. Targeting the ras signaling pathway: a rational, mechanism-based treatment for hematologic malignancies? Blood 2000; 96: 1656–69.
14. Hsiang YH, Liu LF. Identification of mammalian DNA topoisomerase I as an intracellular target of the anticancer drug camptothecin. Cancer Res 1988; 48: 1722–6.
15. Slamon D, Leyland-Jones B, Shak S et al. Use of chemotherapy plus a monoclonal antibody agains HER2 for metastatic

breast cancer that overexpresses HER2. N Engl J Med 2001; 344: 783–92.

16. Disis ML, Gooley TA, Rinn K et al. Generation of T-cell immunity to the Her-2/neu protein after active immunization with anti Her-2/neu peptide vaccines. J Clin Oncol 2002; 20: 2624–32.

17. Gasparini G, Longo R, Toi M et al. Angiogenic inhibitors: a new therapeutic strategy in oncology. Nat Clin Pract Oncol 2005; 2: 562–77.

18. Willett CG, Duda DG, di Tomaso E et al. Complete pathological response to bevacizumab and chemoradiation in advanced rectal cancer. Nat Clin Pract Oncol 2004; 10: 145–7.

19. Schmidt M, Voelker HU, Kapp M et al. Expression of VEG-FR-1 (Flt-1) in breast cancer is associated with VEGF expression and with node-negative tumour stage. Anticancer Res 2008; 28: 1719–24.

20. McLaughlin P, Grillo-Lopez A, Link B et al. Rituximab chimeric anti-CD20 monoclonal antibody therapy for relapsed indolent lymphoma: half of patients respond to a four-dose treatment program. J Clin Oncol 1998; 16: 5825–33.

21. Cartron G, Dacheux L, Salles G et al. Therapeutic activity of humanized anti-CD20 monoclonal antibody and polymorphism in IgG Fc receptor FcgammaRIIIa gene. Blood 2002; 99: 754–8.

22. A memorial issue for Dr. Frank M. Schabel Jr containing articles prepared for the symposium on dose-response relationship in clinical oncology. 13th International Congress of Chemotherapy. Vienna, Austria, August 1983. Cancer 1984; 4(Suppl 6): 1132–1238.

23. Muggia FM, Cassileth PA, Ochoa M Jr et al. Treatment of breast cancer with medroxyprogesterone acetate. Ann Int Med 1968; 68: 328–77.

24. Segaloff A. Hormonal therapy of breast cancer. Cancer Treat Rev 1975; 2: 129–35.

25. Greenspan EM, Fieber M, Lesnick G et al. Response of advanced breast carcinoma to the combination of the antimetabolite, methotrexate and the alkylating agent, thio-TEPA. J Mt Sinai Hosp 1963; 30: 246–67.

26. Bonadonna G, Brussamolini E, Valagussa P et al. Combination chemotherapy as an adjuvant treatment in operable breast cancer. N Eng J Med 1976; 294: 405–10.

27. Zambetti M, Valagussa P. Sequential or alternating doxorubicin and CMF regimens in breast cancer with more than three positive nodes. JAMA 1995; 273: 542–7.

28. Fisher B, Redmond C, Wickerham DL et al. Doxorubicin-containing regimens for the treatment of stage II breast cancer. The National Surgical Adjuvant Breast and Bowel Project experience. J Clin Oncol 1990; 8: 1483–96.

29. Bonadonna G, Veronesi U, Brambilla C et al. Primary chemotherapy to avoid mastectomy in tumors with diameters of three centimeters or more. J Natl Cancer Inst 1990; 82: 1539–45.

30. Romond EH, Perez EA, Bryant J et al. Trastuzumab plus adjuvant chemotherapy for operable HER2-positive breast cancer. N Engl J Med 2005; 353: 1673–84.

31. Smith I, Procter M, Gelber RD et al. 2-year follow-up of trastuzumab after adjuvant chemotherapy in HER2-positive breast cancer: a randomised controlled trial. Lancet 2007; 369: 29–36.

32. Ansfield FJ, Schroeder JM, Curreri AR. Five years clinical experience with 5-fluorouracil. JAMA 1962; 181: 295–9.

33. Higgins G, Humphrey E, Juler G et al. Adjuvant chemotherapy in the surgical treatment of large bowel cancer. Cancer 1976; 38: 1461–7.

34. Muggia FM. Closing the loop: providing feedback on drug development (Editorial). Cancer Treat Rep 1987; 71: 1–2.

35. Moertel CG. Chemotherapy for colorectal cancer. N Eng J Med 1994; 330: 1136–42.

36. Petrelli N, Herrera L, Rustum Y et al. A prospective randomized trial of 5-fluorouracil versus 5-fluorouracil and high-dose leucovorin versus 5-fluorouracil and methotrexate in previously untreated patients with advanced colorectal carcinoma. J Clin Oncol 1987; 5: 1559–65.

37. Petrelli N, Douglass HO Jr, Herrera L et al. The modulation of fluorouracil with leucovorin in metastatic colorectal carcinoma: a prospective randomized phase III trial. Gastrointestinal Tumor Study Group. J Clin Oncol 1987; 7: 1419–26.

38. Moertel C, Fleming TR, Macdonald JS et al. Fluoruracil plus levamisole as effective adjuvant therapy after resection of stage III colon carcinoma: a final report. Ann Intern Med 1995; 122: 321–6.

39. Wolmark N, Rockette H, Fisher B et al. The benefit of leucovorin-modulated fluorouracil as post-operative adjuvant therapy for primary colon cancer: results from National Surgical Adjuvant Breast and Bowel Project protocol C-03. J Clin Oncol 1993; 11: 1879–87.

40. de Gramont A, Figer A, Seymour M et al. Leucovorin and fluorouracil with or without oxaliplatin as first-line treatment in advanced colorectal cancer. J Clin Oncol 2000; 18: 2938–47.

41. Douillard JY, Cunningham D, Roth AD et al. Irinotecan combined with fluorouracil compared with fluorouracil alone as first-line treatment for metastatic colorectal cancer: a multicentre randomised trial. Lancet 2000; 355: 1041–7.

42. Hurwitz H, Fehrenbacher L, Novotny W et al. Bevacizumab plus irinotecan, fluorouracil, and leucovorin for metastatic colorectal cancer. N Engl J Med 2004; 350: 2335–42.

43. Sargent DJ, Patiyil S, Yothers G et al. End points for colon cancer adjuvant trials: observations and recommendations based on individual patient data from 20,898 patients enrolled onto 18 randomized trials from the ACCENT Group. J Clin Oncol 2007; 25: 4569–74. Epub 2007 Sep 17.

44. Goldberg RM, Sargent DJ, Morton RF et al. Randomized controlled trial of reduced-dose bolus fluorouracil plus leucovorin and irinotecan or infused fluorouracil plus leucovorin and oxaliplatin in patients with previously untreated metastatic colorectal cancer: a North American Intergroup Trial. J Clin Oncol 2006; 24: 3347–53.

45. De Roock W, Piessevaux H, De Schutter J et al. KRAS wild-type state predicts survival and is associated to early radiological response in metastatic colorectal cancer treated with cetuximab. Ann Oncol 2008; 19: 508–15. Epub 2007 Nov 12.

46. Hansen HH, Muggia FM, Andrews RJ et al. Intensive combined chemotherapy and radiotherapy in patients with non-resectable bronchogenic carcinoma. Cancer 1972; 30: 315–24.

47. Legha SS, Muggia FM, Carter SK. Adjuvant chemotherapy in lung cancer: review and prospects. Cancer 1977; 39: 1415–24.

48. Holmes EC, Hill LD, Gail M. A randomized comparison of the effects of adjuvant therapy on resected stages II and III non-small cell carcinoma of the lung. The Lung Cancer Study Group. Ann Surg 1985; 202: 335–41.

49. Le Chevalier T, Arriagada R, Quoix E et al. Radiotherapy alone versus combined chemotherapy and radiotherapy in unresectable non-small-cell lung carcinoma. Lung Cancer 1994; 10(Suppl 1): S239–44.

50. Non-small cell lung cancer collaborative group. Chemotherapy in non-small cell lung cancer: a meta-analysis using updated data on individual patients from 52 randomised clinical trials. BMJ 1995; 311: 899–909.

51. Pérez-Soler R, Chachoua A, Hammond LA et al. Determinants of tumor response and survival with erlotinib in patients with non-small-cell lung cancer. J Clin Oncol 2004; 22: 3238–47.

52. Shepherd FA, Pereira J, Ciuleanu TE et al. Erlotinib in previously treated NSCLC. N Engl J Med 2005; 353: 123–32.

53. Kris MG, Natale RB, Herbst RS et al. Efficacy of gefitinib, an inhibitor of the epidermal growth factor receptor tyrosine kinase, in symptomatic patients with non-small cell lung cancer: a randomized trial. JAMA 2003; 290: 2149–58.

54. Sandler A, Gray R, Perry MC et al. Paclitaxel-carboplatin alone or with bevacizumab for non-small-cell lung cancer. N Engl J Med 2006; 355: 2542–50. Erratum in: N Engl J Med 2007; 356: 318.

55. Levin L, Simon R, Hryniuk W. Importance of multiagent chemotherapy regimens in ovarian carcinoma: dose intensity analysis. J Natl Cancer Inst 1993; 5: 1732–42.

56. Piccart MJ, Speyer JL, Wernz JC et al. Advanced ovarian cancer: three-year results of a 6-8 month, 2-drug cisplatin-containing regimen. Eur J Cancer Clin Oncol 1987; 23: 631–41.

57. du Bois A, Lück HJ, Meier W et al. A randomized clinical trial of cisplatin/paclitaxel versus carboplatin/paclitaxel as first-line treatment of ovarian cancer. J Natl Cancer Inst 2003; 95: 1320–9.

58. Ozols RF, Bundy BN, Greer BE et al. Phase III trial of carboplatin and paclitaxel compared with cisplatin and paclitaxel in patients with optimally resected stage III ovarian cancer: a Gynecologic Oncology Group study. J Clin Oncol 2003; 21: 3194–200.

59. Alberts DS, Liu PY, Hannigan EV et al. Intraperitoneal cisplatin plus intravenous cyclophosphamide versus intravenous cisplatin plus intravenous cyclophosphamide for stage III ovarian cancer. N Engl J Med 1996; 335: 1950–5.

60. Markman M, Bundy BN, Alberts DS et al. Phase III trial of standard-dose intravenous cisplatin plus paclitaxel versus moderately high-dose carboplatin followed by intravenous paclitaxel and intraperitoneal cisplatin in small-volume stage III ovarian carcinoma: an intergroup study of the Gynecologic Oncology Group, Southwestern Oncology Group, and Eastern Cooperative Oncology Group. J Clin Oncol 2001; 19: 1001–7.

61. Armstrong DK, Bundy B, Wenzel L et al. Intraperitoneal cisplatin and paclitaxel in ovarian cancer. N Engl J Med 2006; 354: 34–43.

62. Jacobs EM, Muggia FM. Testicular cancer: risk factors and the role of adjuvant chemotherapy. Cancer 1980; 45: 1782–90.

63. Bosl GJ, Gluckman R, Geller NL et al. VAB-6: an effective chemotherapy regimen for patients with germ-cell tumors. J Clin Oncol 1986; 4: 1493–9.

64. Williams SD, Stablein DM, Einhorn LH et al. Immediate adjuvant chemotherapy versus observation with treatment at relapse in pathological stage II testicular cancer. N Engl J Med 1987; 317: 1433–8.

65. Loehrer PJ Sr, Lauer R, Roth BJ et al. Salvage therapy in recurrent germ cell cancer: ifosfamide and cisplatin plus either vinblastine or etoposide. Ann Intern Med 1988; 109: 540–6.

66. Bokemeyer C, Oechsle K, Honecker F et al. Combination chemotherapy with gemcitabine, oxaliplatin, and paclitaxel in patients with cisplatin-refractory or multiply relapsed germ-cell tumors: a study of the German Testicular Cancer Study Group. Ann Oncol 2008; 19: 448–53. Epub 2007 Nov 15.

67. Stoter G, Koopman A, Vendrik CP et al. Ten-year survival and late sequelae in testicular cancer patients treated with cisplatin, vinblastine, and bleomycin. J Clin Oncol 1989; 7: 1099–104.

68. Chua DT, Veenema RJ, Muggia FM et al. Acid phosphatase levels in bone marrow: Value in detecting early bone marrow metastasis from carcinoma of the prostate. J Urol 1970; 103: 462–6.

69. Crawford ED, Blumenstein BA, Goodman PJ et al. Leuprolide with and without flutamide in advanced prostate cancer. Cancer 1990; 66(Suppl 5): 1039–44.

70. Eisenberger MA, Blumenstein BA, Crawford ED et al. Bilateral orchiectomy with or without flutamide for metastatic prostate cancer. N Engl J Med 1998; 339: 1036–42.

71. Tannnock IF, Osoba D, Stockler MR et al. Chemotherapy with mitoxantrone plus prednisone or prednisone alone for symptomatic hormone-resistant prostate cancer: a Canadian randomized trial with palliative endpoints. J Clin Oncol 1996; 14: 1756–64.

72. Pinsky PF, Andriole G, Crawford ED et al. Prostate-specific antigen velocity and prostate cancer gleason grade and stage. Cancer 2007; 109: 1689–95.

73. Soloway MS, Schellhammer PF, Smith JA et al. Bicalutamide in the treatment of advanced prostatic carcinoma: a phase II multicenter trial. Urology 1996; 47(Suppl 1A): 33–7; discussion 48–53.

74. Petrylak DP, Tangen CM, Hussain MH et al. Docetaxel and estramustine compared with mitoxantrone and prednisone for advanced refractory prostate cancer. N Engl J Med 2004; 351: 1513–20.

75. Kinzler KW, Vogelstein B. Lessons from hereditary colorectal cancer. Cell 1996; 87: 159–70.

76. Jover R, Zapater P, Castells A et al. The efficacy of adjuvant chemotherapy with 5-fluorouracil in colorectal cancer depends on the mismatch repair status. Eur J Cancer 2008; Aug 21.

77. Vilar E, Scaltriti M, Balmaña J et al. Microsatellite instability due to hMLH1 deficiency is associated with increased cytotoxicity to irinotecan in human colorectal cancer cell lines. Br J Cancer 2008; Oct 21.

78. De Roock W, Piessevaux H, De Schutter J et al. KRAS wild-type state predicts survival and is associated to early radiological response in metastatic colorectal cancer treated with cetuximab. Ann Oncol 2008; 19: 508–15. Epub 2007 Nov 12.

79. Rottenberg S, Nygren AO, Pajic M et al. Selective induction of chemotherapy resistance of mammary tumors in a conditional mouse model for hereditary breast cancer. Proc Natl Acad Sci USA 2007; 104: 12117–22.

80. Liu X, Rottenberg S, Pajic M et al. Somatic loss of BRCA1 and p53 in mice induces mammary tumors with features of human BRCA1-mutated basal-like breast cancer. Proc Natl Acad Sci USA 2007; 104: 12111–6.

81. Borst P, Rottenberg S, Jonkers J. How do real tumors become resistant to cisplatin. Cell Cycle 2008; 7: 1353–9.

82. Boden GL, Gibb R. Radiotherapy and testicular neoplasms. Lancet 1951; 2: 1195–7.

83. Powles T, Robinson D, Shamash J et al. The long-term risks of adjuvant carboplatin treatment for stage I seminoma of the testis. Ann Oncol 2008; 19: 443–7. Epub 2007 Nov 28.

84. Aparicio J, Germà JR, García del Muro X et al. Risk-adapted management for patients with clinical stage I seminoma: the Second Spanish Germ Cell Cancer Cooperative Group study. J Clin Oncol 2005; 23(34): 8717–23.

85. Baer L, Muggia FM, Formenti SC. Platinum compounds and radiation. In: Bonetti A, Howell SB, Leone R, Muggia FM, eds. Platinum and Other Heavy Metal Compounds in Cancer Chemotherapy. Humana Press, 2009: Chapter 25, 211–24.

86. Hong WK, Lippman SM, Wolf GT. Recent advances in head and neck cancer—larynx preservation and cancer chemoprevention: the Seventeenth Annual Richard and Hinda Rosenthal Foundation Award Lecture. Cancer Res 1993; 53: 5113–20.

87. Formenti SC, Demaria S. Effects of chemoradiation on tumor-host interactions: the immunologic side. J Clin Oncol 2008; 26: 1562–3.

88. Apetoh L, Ghiringhelli F, Zvitvogel L. Calreticulin dictates the immunogenicity of anti-cancer chemotherapy and radiotherapy. Med Sci 2007; 23: 257–8.

89. Oh WK, Kantoff PW, Weinberg V et al. Prospective, multicenter, randomized phase II trial of the herbal supplement,

PC-SPES, and diethylstilbestrol in patients with androgen-independent prostate cancer. J Clin Oncol 2004; 22: 3705–12. Epub 2004 Aug.

90. Curt GA, Katterhagen G, Mahaney FX Jr. Immunoaugmentative therapy. A primer on the perils of unproved treatments. JAMA 1986; 255: 505–7.

91. Ravikumar TS, Kaleya R, Kishinevsky A. Surgical ablative therapy of liver tumors. Cancer: Principles and Practice of Oncology Updates 2000; 14: 1–12.

92. Muggia FM. Introduction. Platinum compounds: the culmination of the era of cancer chemotherapy. In: Bonetti A, Howell SB, Leone R, Muggia FM, eds. Platinum and Other Heavy Metal Compounds in Cancer Chemotherapy. Humana Press, 2009: Chapter 1, 1–10.

93. Wampler GL, Carter WH Jr, Campbell ED et al. Relationships between various uses of antineoplastic drug-interaction terms. Cancer Chemotherapy & Pharmacology 1992; 31: 111–17.

94. Capizzi RL, Keiser LW, Sartorelli AC. Combination chemotherapy—theory and practice. Semin Oncol 1977; 4: 227–53.

95. Hanahan D. Weinberg RA. The hallmarks of cancer. Cell 2000; 100: 57–70.

96. Azad NS, Posadas EM, Kwitkowski VE et al. Combination targeted therapy with sorafenib and bevacizumab results in enhanced toxicity and antitumor activity. J Clin Oncol 2008; 26: 3709–14.

97. Bergers G, Song S, Meyer-Morse N et al. Benefits of targeting both pericytes and endothelial cells in the tumor vasculature with kinase inhibitors. J Clin Invest 2003; 111: 1287–95.

98. Hamilton A, Eder JP Pavlick AC et al. Proteasome inhibition with bortezomib (PSC341): a phase I study with pharmacodynamic end points using a day 1 and day 4 schedule in a 14-day cycle. J Clin Oncol 2005; 23: 6107–16.

99. Wong M, Balleine RL, Blair EY et al. Predictors of vinorelbine pharmacokinetics and pharmacodynamics in patients with cancer. J Clin Oncol 2006; 24: 2448–55.

100. Ratain MJ. Dear Doctor: We really are not sure what dose of capecitabine you should prescribe for your patient (Editorial). J Clin Oncol 2002; 20: 1434–5.

101. Norton L, Simon R. Tumor size, sensitivity to therapy, and design of treatment schedules. Cancer Treat Rep 1997; 61: 1307–17.

102. Citron ML, Berry DA, Cirrincione C et al. Randomized trial of dose-dense versus conventionally scheduled and sequential versus concurrent combination chemotherapy as postoperative adjuvant treatment of node-positive primary breast cancer: first report of Intergroup Trial C9741/Cancer and Leukemia Group B Trial 9741. J Clin Oncol 2003; 21: 1431–9.

103. Green MD, Koelbl H, Baselga J et al. A randomized double-blind multicenter phase III study of fixed-dose single-administration pegfilgrastim versus daily filgrastim in patients receiving myelosuppressive chemotherapy. Ann Oncol 2003; 14: 29–35.

104. Crawford J. Once-per-cycle pegfilgrastim (Neulasta) for the management of chemotherapy-induced neutropenia. Semin Oncol 2003; 30(4 Suppl 13): 24–30.

105. Bohlius J, Langensiepen S, Schwarzer G et al. Recombinant human erythropoietin and overall survival in cancer patients: results of a comprehensive meta-analysis. J Natl Cancer Inst 2005; 97: 489–98, 2005.

106. Gamelin L, Boisdron-Celle M, Morel A et al. Oxalipaltin-related neuropathy: interest of calcium-magnesium infusion and no impact on its efficacy. J Clin Oncol 2008; 26: 1188–9.

107. Muggia FM. Sequential single agents as first-line chemotherapy for ovarian cancer: a strategy derived from the results of GOG-132. Int J Gynecol Cancer 2003; 13(Suppl 2): 156–62.

108. Yauger BJ, Gorden P, Park J et al. Effect of depot medroxyprogesterone acetate on glucose tolerance in generalized lipodystrophy. Obstet Gynecol 2008; 112: 445–7.

109. Windschitl HE, O'Connell MJ, Wieand HS et al. A clinical trial of biochemical modulation of 5-fluorouracil with N-phosphonoacetyl-L-aspartate and thymidine in advanced gastric and anaplastic colorectal cancer. Cancer 1990; 66: 853–6.

110. Pegram MD, Konecny GE, O'Callaghan C et al. Rational combinations of trastuzumab with chemotherapeutic drugs used in the treatment of breast cancer. J Natl Cancer Inst 2004; 96: 739–49.

111. Haddad Ri, Shin DM. Recent advances in head and neck cancer. N Engl J Med 2008; 359: 1143–54.

112. Sledge GW, Neuberg D, Bernardo P et al. Phase III trial of doxorubicin, paclitaxel, and the combination of doxorubicin and paclitaxel as front-line chemotherapy for metastatic breast cancer: an intergroup trial (E1193). J Clin Oncol 2003; 21: 588–92.

113. Miles D, Vukelja S, Moiseyenko V et al. Survival benefit with capecitabine/docetaxel versus docetaxel alone: analysis of therapy in a randomized phase III trial. Clin Breast Cancer 2004; 5: 273–8.

114. Albain KS, Nag SM, Calderillo-Ruiz G et al. Gemcitabine plus paclitaxel versus paclitaxel monotherapy in patients with metastatic breast cancer and prior anthracycline treatment. J Clin Oncol 2008; 26: 3950–7.

115. Muggia FM, Braly PS, Brady MF et al. Phase III randomized study of cisplatin versus paclitaxel versus cisplatin and paclitaxel in patients with suboptimal stage III or IV ovarian cancer: a Gynecologic Oncology Group study. J Clin Oncol 2000; 18: 106–15.

116. The ICON Collaborators. Paclitaxel plus carboplatin versus standard chemotherapy with either single-agent carboplatin or cyclophosphamide, doxorubicin, and cisplatin in women with ovaraian cancer: the ICON3 randomized trials. Lancet 2002; 360: 505–15.

117. McGuire WP, Hoskins WJ, Brady MF et al. Cyclophosphamide and cisplatin compared with palcitaxel and cisplatin in patients with stage III and stage IV ovarian cancer. N Eng J Med 1996; 334: 1–6.

118. Piccart MJ, Bertelsen K, James K et al. Randomized intergroup trial of cisplatin-paclitaxel versus cisplatin-cyclophosphamide in women with advanced epithelial ovarian cancer: three-year results. J Natl Cancer Inst 2000; 92: 699–708.

119. Cantù MG, Buda A, Parma G et al. Randomized controlled trial of single-agent paclitaxel versus cyclophosphamide, doxorubicin, and cisplatin in patients with recurrent ovarian cancer who responded to first-line platinum-based regimens. J Clin Oncol 2002; 20: 1232–7.

120. Bolis G, Scarfone G, Giardina G et al. Carboplatin alone vs carboplatin plus epidoxorubicin as second-line therapy for cisplatin- or carboplatin-sensitive ovarian cancer. Gynecol Oncol 2001; 81: 3–9.

121. Pfisterer J, Plante M, Vergote I et al. Gemcitabine plus carboplatin compared with carboplatin in patients with platinum-sensitive recurrent ovarian cancer: an intergroup trial of the AGO-OVAR, the NCIC CTG, and the EORTC GCG. J Clin Oncol 2006; 24: 4699–707.

122. Parmar MK, Ledermann JA, Colombo N et al. Paclitaxel plus platinum-based chemotherapy versus conventional platinum-based chemotherapy in women with relapsed ovarian cancer: the ICON4/AGO-OVAR-2.2 trial. Lancet 2003; 361: 2099–106.

123. Ferrero JM, Weber B, Geay JF et al. Second-line chemotherapy with pegylated liposomal doxorubicin and carboplatin is highly effective in patients with advanced ovarian cancer in late relapse: a GINECO phase II trial. Ann Oncol 2007; 18: 263–8.

124. Markman M, Liu PY, Wilczynski S et al. Phase III randomized trial of 12 versus 3 months of maintenance paclitaxel in patients with advanced ovarian cancer after complete response to platinum and paclitaxel-based chemotherapy: a

Southwest Oncology Group and Gynecologic Oncology Group trial. J Clin Oncol 2003; 21: 2460–5.

125. Carter SK. The strategy of cancer treatment. In: Muggia FM, Rozencweig M, eds. Clinical Evaluation of Anticancer Therapy. Boston: Martinus Nijhoff Publishers, 1987: 211–16.

126. O'Brien SG, Guilhot F, Larson RA et al. Imatinib compared with interferon and low-dose cytarabine for newly diagnosed chronic-phase chronic myeloid leukemia. N Engl J Med 2003; 348: 994–1004.

127. Desai J, Shankar S, Heinrich MC et al. Clonal evolution of resistance to imatinib in patients with metastatic gastrointestinal stromal tumors. Clin Cancer Res 2007; 13: 5398–405.

128. Hanahan D. Weinberg RA. Retrospective: Judah Folkman (1933–2008). Science 2008; 319: 1055.

129. Grillo-Lopez AJ. Rituximab (Rituxan/MabThera): the first decade (1993–2003). Expert Rev Anticancer Ther 2003; 3: 767–79.

130. Slamon DJ, Leyland-Jones B, Shak S et al. Use of chemotherapy plus a monoclonal antibody against HER2 for metastatic breast cancer that overexpresses HER2. N Engl J Med 2001; 344: 783–92.

131. Wu AH. A selected history and future of immunoassay development and applications in clinical chemistry. Clin Chim Acta 2006; 369: 119–24.

3

Principles and Examples of Cancer (Cell) Specific Therapies

Ferry A. L. M. Eskens and Jaap Verweij

INTRODUCTION

Over the past decades, systemic cancer treatment has greatly relied on the use of cytotoxic chemotherapy. For principles of such treatment see chapter 2.

Cytotoxic chemotherapy exerts its activity by targeting the various steps of the nuclear DNA replication process and cancer cell proliferation, but because of a lack of cell selectivity it not only kills cancer cells but also affects normal cells and tissues, resulting in a wide spectrum of sometimes life threatening side effects. In other words, although cytotoxic chemotherapy can be considered as targeted therapy in a sense, a striking lack of selectivity for cancer cells remains a major drawback.

In recent decades, biological and molecular research has unraveled a large number of processes that play important and specific roles in carcinogenesis and cancer growth. In contrast to the nuclear DNA replication processes inhibited by cytotoxic chemotherapy, the majority of these processes are located either in the cellular cytoplasm, at the cell membrane, or even in the extracellular environment. It has been shown that in normal cells and under physiological conditions the relevance of these processes is less obvious and sometimes even absent, and therefore these processes are considered more cancer (cell) specific. If it were possible to specifically target and inhibit any of these processes, this would hopefully leave normal cells and tissues largely unaffected, thereby circumventing most of the cumbersome side effects usually related to nonspecific cytotoxic chemotherapy. Therefore, designing such specific inhibitory agents has been one of the challenges in the development of a new generation of drug treatments that we, in view of the above, prefer to refer to as cancer (cell) specific anticancer therapy, rather than using the more misleading term "targeted therapy" (Fig. 3.1).

Unfortunately, it is also a reality that the majority of human epithelial cancers are not driven by a single aberrant cancer (cell) specific process, and therefore cancer (cell) specific therapy that inhibits one specific process is still very unlikely to become a curative treatment option for the majority of cancer patients. Trying to target multiple different processes will also, to a small extent, affect normal cells, but the total resultant of this will still be the occurrence of undesired side effects. Current knowledge and clinical experience have indeed shown convincingly that the very complex biology of human cancer poses a formidable challenge for the design of cancer (cell) specific anticancer agents (Fig. 3.2).

BASIC PRINCIPLES

Cancer (Cell) Specific vs. Nontargeted Therapy

In contrast to cytotoxic chemotherapy, most cancer (cell) specific anticancer agents have been rationally designed, following the recognition and structural and functional characterization of a specific target. Irrespective of their exact localization, these targets are usually proteins encoded by mutated genes, or dysregulated receptors and signaling proteins; their presence and usually uncontrolled activity directly or indirectly leads to autonomous cell proliferation.

The molecular mechanism of action of most cancer (cell) specific agents is based upon often reversible, functional inhibitory interaction between a target and the specific agent, and as such is expected to selectively affect cancer cells and leave normal cells largely unaffected. Based upon their mechanism of action, the majority of these agents do not induce acute cell death, and cancer cells are rather inhibited in their autonomous growth or transformed into a state of quiescence.

Dosing Aspects

As cancer (cell) specific therapy often relies on reversible target inhibition, the optimal dosing strategy will likely have to be different from that of cytotoxic therapy. Whereas the latter exerts anticancer activity in a steep dose-dependent manner and therefore is administered at the highest tolerable dose, in cancer (cell) specific therapy a "saturation" of the target is pursued, and this can frequently be obtained (at least in preclinical models) at doses that are far below the highest tolerable dose. It has indeed been shown that in many of these models, target inhibitory and anticancer effects are not dose dependent (Fig. 3.3). To obtain optimal target inhibition, however, a certain minimum concentration of the drug is required; if at such a "threshold" concentration complete receptor binding is obtained, further escalation of the dose will not lead to additional target inhibition, but most likely will only add unnecessary toxicity. The optimal biological effect dose (OBD) of molecular targeted therapy therefore is the equivalent of the maximum tolerated dose (MTD) of cytotoxic therapy and is the dose that should be aimed at. To define the dose that exerts optimal target inhibition, it is thus crucial to assess as reliably as possible this pharmacodynamic effect. A problem that is discussed later in this chapter is that at present it is often difficult to define optimal target inhibition and thus the OBD.

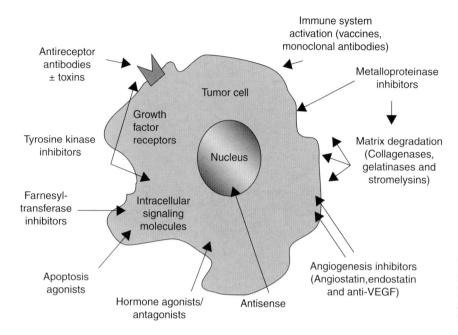

Figure 3.1 Overview of different cancer cell specific therapies that either target the cell membrane, the cytoplasm, or intranuclear processes. *Abbreviation*: VEGF, vascular endothelial growth factor.

Mechanism of Target Inhibition

Once a cancer (cell) specific target has been identified, in theory various approaches can be explored to inhibit its activity. There are in essence three approaches that have received a lot of attention:

- Antisense oligonucleotides or ribozymes that can serve to inhibit RNA transcription and receptor synthesis;
- Specific monoclonal antibodies targeting either the receptor or the ligand;
- Competitive inhibition at the phosphorylation binding domains of the intracellular site of the receptor once ligand–receptor interaction has occurred.

The last two approaches have been explored most extensively and therefore will be discussed in more detail when reviewing the various cancer (cell) specific agents.

Drug Scheduling

As mentioned, the goal of cancer (cell) specific therapy is to induce optimal target inhibition with subsequent optimal tumor growth inhibition. For reasons of clarity and presentation it is presumed here that tumor growth is dependent on the activity of only one target, but as already mentioned before, this probably is an oversimplification of the real-life tumor biology. As target inhibition of a growth factor does not likely induce cell-kill but rather leads to growth inhibition, clinically this activity is likely to induce tumor growth delay or tumor stasis rather than regression of tumor size. As the receptor–drug interaction is reversible, interruption of drug exposure may lead to restored ligand–receptor interaction with subsequent reactivation of the target, enabling

cells to restore their normal function and proliferative activity, and resulting in tumor regrowth. Cancer (cell) specific therapy therefore is often also referred to as cytostatic therapy.

For many of the targets it is currently not convincingly known if optimal inhibition truly has to be continuous or whether similar activity can be achieved by intermittent treatment. From current clinical experience with some of the orally available cancer (cell) specific cytostatic agents it remains unclear if intermittent treatment has a negative impact on clinical activity. Whatever the outcome of these discussions, an important element of the resulting treatment, be it continuous or semi-continuous, is that optimal target inhibition and thus optimal treatment compliance is of crucial importance. To achieve this, drugs that can be given safely for prolonged periods of time without the onset of major side effects interfering with chronic drug dosing must be developed. This can be achieved by parenteral formulations with a long half-life, but for optimal patient convenience, oral formulations may be preferred.

Anticancer Activity

Preclinical studies have shown that cancer (cell) specific agents induce tumor growth inhibition rather than tumor regression. Importantly, optimal growth inhibition was often obtained in case of minimal (residual) disease activity. Even though clinical studies have shown that patients with advanced metastatic disease may benefit from cancer (cell) specific treatment, it is conceivable that an even greater benefit can be achieved among those with minimal residual disease after surgery, raditotherapy and/or, cytoreductive chemotherapy. Another important consideration is to

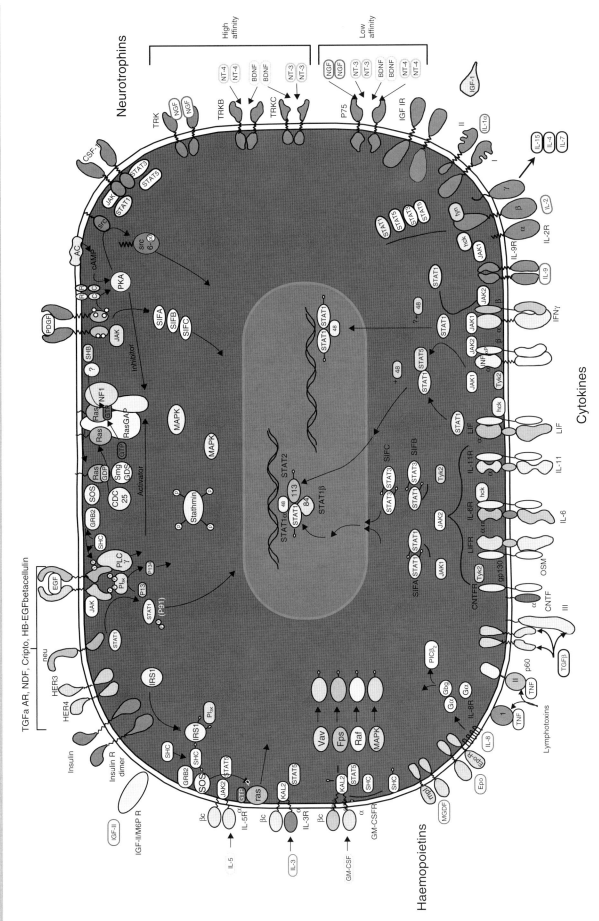

Figure 3.2 Cancer cell surface receptors; which one is crucial in cancer growth?

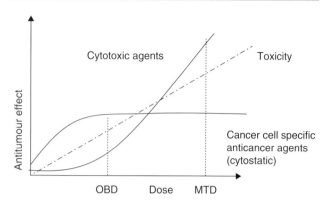

Figure 3.3 Dose-response curves of cancer cell specific and cytotoxic agents. *Abbreviations*: MTD, maximal tolerable dose; OBD, optimal biological dose.

combine cancer (cell) specific treatment with conventional cytoreductive treatment or radiotherapy. This conceptual approach is supported by the notion that in many model studies such combinations showed either additive or even synergistic activity.

CLASSES OF CANCER (CELL) SPECIFIC THERAPIES

There are various cancer (cell) specific processes that could be interesting targets for the development of specific inhibitory agents. Once again, and as mentioned before, these targets belong to a variety of different locations, namely at the cellular membrane, in the intracellular cytoplasm, in the nucleus, or in the cancer cell environment.

- Targets at the membrane of the cancer cell involve
  ○ transmembrane growth factor receptors
  ○ stromal invasion factors
- Targets in the cellular cytoplasm involve
  ○ intracellular signal transduction processes
- Targets in the cellular nucleus involve
  ○ specific DNA and RNA transcriptional processes
  ○ cell cycle-dependent kinases
  ○ histone deacetylases
  ○ spliceosome
- Targets outside the cancer cell involve
  ○ tumor-related blood vessels
  ○ cell-to-cell signaling

In the following chapter, we summarize the available information without the aim to be complete, as the field is continuously evolving.

Transmembrane Targets on the Cell Surface
Signal Transduction Inhibitors
Protein tyrosine phosphorylation was discovered in the early 1980s, and subsequently, it was recognized to play a key role in the regulation of essential processes such as cell cycle, cell metabolism, cell growth, and cell proliferation.

Protein tyrosine phosphorylation is a process that is located at the inner cell surface of various transmembrane growth factor receptors of which the ErbB family of epidermal growth factor receptors (EGFRs) was the first to be identified. The ErbB family consists of the four members ErbB1/EGFR, ErbB2/HER-2, ErbB3, and ErbB4 (Fig. 3.4). These receptors share a common structure that consists of an extracellular ligand-binding domain, a single transmembrane helix, and a cytoplasmic domain. The last consists of a protein kinase domain and a tightly attached regulatory segment or domain that can be phosphorylated.

Following ligand–receptor interaction, the binding of ATP to the cytoplasmic regulatory segment of the protein kinase domain induces receptor homo- or heterodimerization. The subsequent tyrosine kinase activation will activate multiple downstream effector pathways that ultimately lead to various cellular responses.

A central role in the activation of some important mitogenic downstream effector pathways is the phosphorylation of cellular Ras. In addition, and taken as an example to illustrate the enormous diversity of effects and interactions, the activation of other, less-defined pathways through increased EGFR tyrosine kinase activity is responsible for an increased production and secretion of factors that can also induce tumor-related angiogenesis.

The regulation and inhibition of tyrosine kinase activity is exerted through different mechanisms. Inhibitory protein tyrosine phosphatases can dephosphorylate the regulatory segment related to the tyrosine kinase domain, whereas ligand–receptor interaction as such induces a rapid endocytosis and subsequent degradation of both the receptor and ligand.

In many human epithelial cancers increased expression of EGFR has been found, correlated with tumor aggressiveness and poor clinical outcome. This relationship is even stronger when constitutively activated EGFR due to some typical mutations is present. The current prognostic role of EGFR in various epithelial malignancies and the prediction of efficacy of specific inhibitory agents is strongly related to this mutational status (1,2). Whatever the exact underlying pathophysiological mechanisms for the relation between EGFR expression and clinical outcome, inhibiting uncontrolled EGFR tyrosine kinase activity has been a target for the development of specific anticancer agents for a relatively long period, using either monoclonal antibodies or small-molecule tyrosine kinase inhibitors (Table 3.1).

Meanwhile, as positive data have been obtained, these results are described in slightly more detail.

Monoclonal antibodies specifically target the extracellular domain of EGFR and competitively inhibit normal ligand–receptor interaction (Fig. 3.5).

Cetuximab is a human:murine chimeric antibody that is in the most advanced stages of clinical development. Randomized clinical studies with intravenous cetuximab given in combination with chemotherapy or radiotherapy have shown promising anticancer activity in colorectal and squamous head and neck cancer (3–6). In addition, single-agent studies in colorectal cancer patients that had become refractory to cytotoxic chemotherapy also showed positive results (7). In this category of patients, Ras mutational status

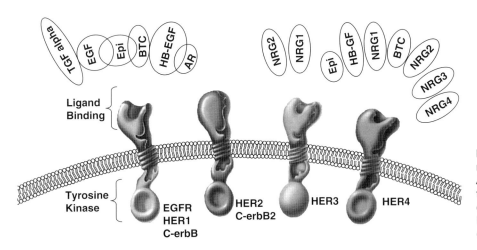

Figure 3.4 ErbB family of transmembrane receptors and their natural ligands. *Abbrevations*: TFG, transforming growth factor; EGF, epidermal growth factor; Epi, epiregulin; NRG, Neuregulin; HB-EGF, heparin binding-EGF; AR, Amphiregulin; BTC, beta cellulin.

Table 3.1 Signal Transduction Inhibitors Targeting EGFR in Clinical Trials

Drug	Target	Clinical development
Monoclonal antibodies		
Cetuximab	ErbB1/EGFR	Approved
Panitumumab	ErbB1/EGFR	Approved
Trastuzumab	ErbB2/HER-2	Approved
Nimotuzumab	ErbB1/EGFR	Phase II
MDX-447	ErbB1/EGFR	Phase II
Pertuzumab	ErbB2/HER-2	Phase II
Matuzumab	ErbB1/EGFR	Phase I
Tyrosine kinase inhibitors		
Gefitinib	ErbB1/EGFR	Approved
Erlotinib	ErbB1/EGFR	Approved
Imatinib	KIT, PDGFR, BCR-ABL	Approved
Lapatinib	ErbB1/EGFR	Approved
Vandetanib	ErbB1/VEGFR	Phase III
BIBW 2992	ErbB1/ErbB2	Phase II
CP-724,714	ErbB2	Phase II
CI-1033	ErbB1/ErbB2	Phase II
PKI-166	ErbB1/EGFR	Phase I
AV-412	ErbB1/ErbB2	Phase I
EKB-569	ErbB1/ErbB2	Phase II
HKI-272	ErbB1/ErbB2	Phase II
GW2016	ErbB1/ErbB2	Phase I
JNJ 26483327	ErbB1/VEGFR-3	Phase I

predicted clinical benefit, again underscoring the complex interactions between transmembrane receptor activation and downstream signaling pathway activation. Diarrhea and skin rash have been described as the most prominent side effects, of which skin rash is considered to be predictive for an increased response rate in patients with colorectal cancer (8).

Panitumumab is a fully human antibody that has also demonstrated favorable outcomes in refractory colorectal cancer, and more monoclonal antibodies are currently being evaluated in clinical trials. The pattern of side effects of these antibodies is showing large overlap, though skin rash in particular is considered to be a strong signal of biological activity. Topical treatment as well as the use of corticosteroids and antibiotics have been successful in the management of drug-induced skin rash.

The monoclonal antibody trastuzumab that specifically targets ErbB-2 or Her-2 is discussed in detail in chapter 5.

Small-molecule tyrosine kinase inhibitors of EGFR and other members of the ErbB family are also in advanced stages of clinical testing (Fig. 3.6). Gefitinib and erlotinib were the first compounds to be developed and demonstrated clinical activity in phase I and II trials in patients with NSCLC. Therefore, large randomized Phase III trials with gefitinib and erlotinib in combination with two different regimens of cytotoxic chemotherapy in patients with advanced NSCLC were performed. Unfortunately, all these studies failed to show any clinical benefit (9–12). As patients in these studies were not selected for EGFR expression or more specifically, mutational status of EGFR, and drug–drug interactions were not adequately assessed prior to exploring these combinations in large clinical trials, the results of the trials were disappointing. In chemotherapy refractory patients with EGFR expressing NSCLC, single-agent therapy with erlotinib, however, was able to significantly improve survival and quality of life (13). In addition to gefitinib and erlotinib, a large number of new EGFR tyrosine kinase inhibitors are currently undergoing clinical testing.

In contrast to monoclonal antibodies that specifically target either EGFR or Her-2, many of the more recently

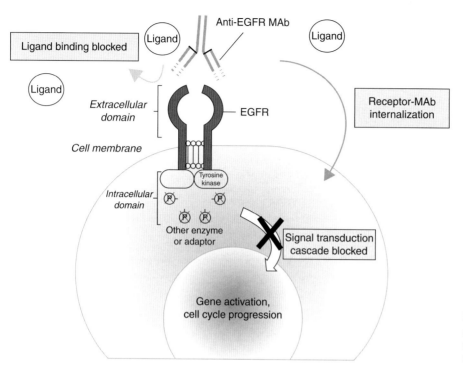

Figure 3.5 EGFR inhibition via monoclonal antibodies blocking ligand binding. *Abbreviations*: EGFR, epidermal growth factor receptor; MAb, monoclonal antibody.

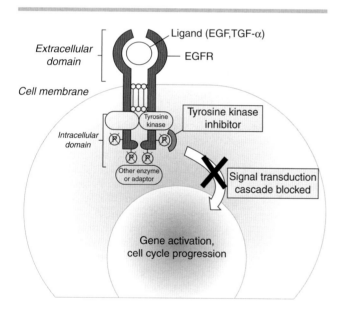

Figure 3.6 EGFR inhibition via tyrosine kinase inhibitors. *Abbreviations*: EGFR, epidermal growth factor receptor; TGF-α, transforming growth factor α.

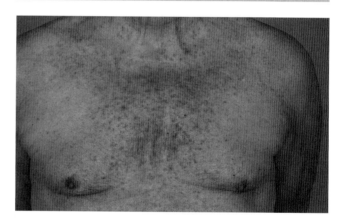

Figure 3.7 Typical example of EGFR inhibitor induced skin rash. *See Color Plate on Page xi.*

developed tyrosine kinase inhibitors block activity of both receptors (as well as that of other tyrosine kinases), thereby possibly increasing clinical relevance. In almost all studies with EGFR tyrosine kinase inhibitors diarrhea and skin rash have been reported as the most prominent side effects and have been dose limiting in early clinical studies (Fig. 3.7). Whether this skin rash correlates with EGFR inhibition and/or might predict antitumor activity is much less clear than for the monoclonal antibodies and currently remains a matter of debate.

The small-molecule tyrosine kinase inhibitors that are mainly directed at inhibiting activity of ErbB2/HER-2 will also be discussed in more detail in chapter 5.

Apart from the ErbB family of receptors, many other transmembrane receptors depend on tyrosine kinase activity and are considered to be of interest for the development of specific inhibiting agents.

The insulin-like growth factor receptor (IGFR) plays an important role in cell proliferation and inhibition of apoptosis, and an increased expression of this receptor as well of its natural ligand, insulin-like growth factor (IGF), has been found to be correlated with worse outcome in some epithelial cancers. Insulin is another ligand of IGFR, and the cross talk that exists between the insulin receptor and IGFR induces the activation of a complex pathway of intracellular signal transductions where the phosphatidylinositol-3-kinase (PI 3-kinase) pathway and the mitogen-activated protein (MAP) kinase pathway play central roles in a way comparable to their role following the activation of EGFR. Activation of these pathways is a crucial phenomenon in cell proliferation and tumor growth. Inhibiting the IGFR therefore is considered to be another rational and cancer (cell) specific approach that merits attention, and specific inhibitory monoclonal antibodies such as IMC-A12, AMG479, R1507, and CP 751,871 have been developed. Early clinical studies with these antibodies, either as single agent or in combination with cytotoxic chemotherapy are currently ongoing (14).

Chronic myeloid leukemia (CML) and gastrointestinal stromal tumors (GISTs) are two unique disease entities, as their tumor growth is driven by only a single genetic defect. This hallmark distinguishes them from almost all other human epithelial cancers that, as mentioned before, depend on a complex of genetic abnormalities. In CML the Philadelphia chromosome resulting from a t(9,22) reciprocal translocation and in GIST the *KIT* proto-oncogene, respectively, are the unique driving forces for tumor growth. These genetic defects encode for the BCR-ABL fusion protein and KIT transmembrane receptor, respectively, that both harbor a constitutively activated tyrosine kinase. Imatinib mesylate (Gleevec, Glivec) is a specific inhibitor of the tyrosine kinase activity of ABL kinase, the BCR-ABL fusion protein, KIT, and the PDGF receptor (PDGFR) and therefore has been considered a rational treatment option for CML and GIST. In a Phase I study in GIST, imatinib yielded surprisingly high response rates that were subsequently confirmed in large randomized Phase III studies, showing an impressive positive impact on overall survival (15). Imatinib therefore is now considered standard of care for first-line treatment of unresectable GIST. In CML imatinib was superior to the combination of interferon-α and low-dose cytarabine with regard to several cytogenetic and clinical end points, and therefore is also considered now to be the standard of care (16,17).

Downstream Signaling

In mammalian cells, three *ras* genes coexist, namely H-*ras*, K-*ras*, and N-*ras*, encoding for H-Ras, K-Ras, and N-Ras protein, respectively. Ras proteins localize to the inner surface of the cellular membrane and once converted from an inactive Ras.guanosine 5′-diphospate (Ras.GDP) into the active Ras.guanosine 5′-triphosphate (Ras.GTP) conformation plays a crucial role in the intracellular transduction of various growth-promoting signals that originate from activated cell surface receptors. Signals transduced by Ras are

those coming from the EGFR and the PDGFR, from cytokines such as interleukin-2 and -3, from granulocyte-macrophage colony stimulating factor and from hormones such as insulin and IGF. Through various downstream effector pathways, most signals transduced by Ras lead to cellular proliferative responses through increased nuclear gene transcription activity. In addition to this, the activation of the RhoB effector pathway is thought to play an important role in actin cytoskeleton organization whereas the activation of the phosphatidylinositol 3-kinase pathway regulates cell survival through inhibition of apoptosis (Fig. 3.8).

Cellular activity of Ras is balanced by intracellular activation and inactivation through the activity of GTPase activating protein (GAP), which degrades activated Ras. GTP back into the inactive Ras.GDP conformation. In the absence of continuous growth factor stimulation Ras.GTP is rapidly reverted into Ras.GDP. Ras proteins are synthesized as soluble inactive proteins on free ribosomes. Prior to being localized to the inner surface of the cellular membrane, Ras has to undergo a series of posttranslational modifications of which farnesylation is the first and rate-limiting step. This addition of a farnesyl moiety from farnesyl diphosphate to the sulfur atom of the cysteine locus of the carboxy-terminal tetrapeptide CaaX of Ras is exerted through the enzyme farnesyl transferase (FT).

Although FT has a high specificity for farnesylation of Ras, other mammalian proteins also depend on farnesylation through FT for their cellular functions. Although this principle has been used to demonstrate target inhibition of specific farnesyl transferase inhibitors (FTIs), its diversity could also be part of the explanation for the difficulties encountered in the development of FTI (18,19).

Among the various and mutually interactive intracellular signaling pathways downstream from Ras, the Raf kinase pathway plays a pivotal role in tumorigenesis through subsequent activation of a series of downstream pathways, of which the PI 3-kinase pathway and the MAP kinase pathway are most important. The PI 3-kinase pathway is another pathway that is directly activated following the activation of various transmembrane receptors and/or Ras, and subsequently activates a number of distinct pathways, such as the mammalian polypeptide kinase target of rapamycin (mTOR) that is important for cell proliferation and survival. All these separate pathways have been recognized as specific targets for inhibition (Fig. 3.9). Specific PI 3-kinase inhibitors such as BGT 226 and BEZ235 have been developed and are undergoing early clinical trials, whereas specific mTOR inhibitors such as temsirolimus, everolimus, sirolimus, rapamycin, and derivatives such as RAD 001 are in a more advanced stage of clinical testing. Temsirolimus is the lead compound of this class and has gained regulatory approval for the treatment of some types of renal-cell cancer (20). As activated expression of mitogen-activated protein kinase/EAK-kinase (MEK) has been found in various human tumor types, inhibition of the MAPK/ MEKK pathway by specific protein kinase inhibitors has been the target for the development of a new class of antitumor agents that are now being tested in clinical studies.

Cyclin-dependent kinases play important roles in the subsequent steps of a normal cell cycle. The overexpression of some of these serine/threonine kinases or cyclin-dependent kinases leads to aberrations in cell cycle regulation that result in uncontrolled cell proliferation. The development

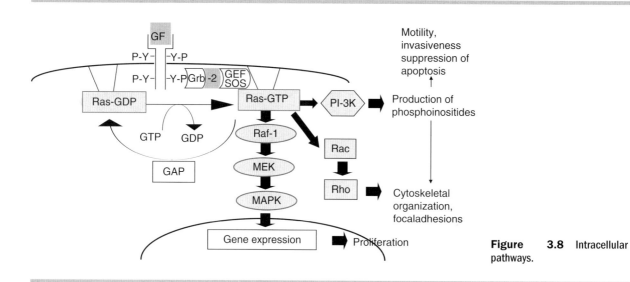

Figure **3.8** Intracellular signaling pathways.

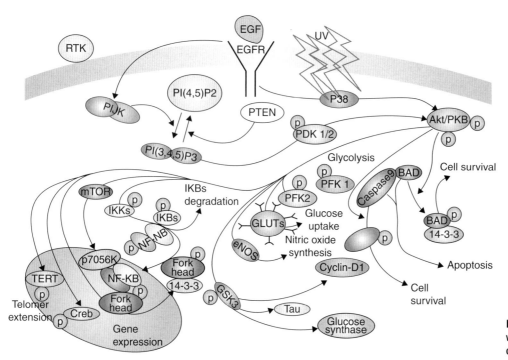

Figure 3.9 The complex pathways and potential interactions of downstream signaling pathways.

of pharmacologic inhibitors or modulators of deregulated cyclin-dependent kinases therefore could be a promising new treatment strategy. At least three specific cyclin-dependent kinase inhibitors (seliciclib, RGB 286638, and AZD 5438) have entered clinical trials.

Inhibitors of Stromal Invasion

In addition to newly formed blood vessels sprouting toward the growing tumor, the tumor itself secretes various factors that increase the invasive phenotype. Tumor hypoxia is essential for these processes, and hypoxia-induced factor 1

(HIF-1) plays a pivotal role in increased tumoral expression of Met, which is another tyrosine kinase dependent transmembrane receptor. When Met is activated through binding of its natural ligand hepatocyte growth factor (HGF), and even more so when mutations in this receptor induce increased or autonomous signaling activity, the stromal invasiveness of the tumor increases dramatically and favors metastases development. Many details of this phenomenon still need to be elucidated (21). Currently, two approaches are being explored in early clinical studies with compounds that inhibit this signaling pathway; small-molecule tyrosine kinase inhibitors of Met such as XL880, Xl-184, Pf 2341066,

JNJ 38877605, SU11274, and monoclonal antibodies target-ing the Met ligand HGF such as AMG 102. To date, only early clinical studies have been performed, and apart from toxicity data no results are available yet.

Targets in the Cellular Nucleus

Although the cellular nucleus and the processes involved in DNA replication have always been considered to be the target of nonspecific cytotoxic chemotherapy, it is increas-ingly recognized that these processes can be a target for (cancer cell) specific targeting agents. Examples of these intranuclear targets are transcriptional processes of onco-genes, the nuclear spliceosome that plays a role in the tran-sition from pre-messenger RNA (pre- mRNA) to messenger RNA, and the process of histone deacetylation; specific inhibitors of this latter process (HDACi) induce hyperacety-lation of histones that modulate chromatin structure and gene expression resulting in growth arrest, cell differentia-tion, and apoptosis of tumor cells. Whereas CI-994, LBH 589, Depsipeptide or FK228, CHR 3996, belinostat, and MS-275 are HDACi currently undergoing early clinical studies, the HDACi vorinostat is approved for the treatment of cutaneous T-cell lymphoma.

Targets Outside the Cancer Cell

Angiogenesis Inhibitors

Under physiological circumstances angiogenesis is a strictly regulated process with only temporary and localized bursts of activity in situations such as embryogenesis, hair growth, wound healing, and in the female reproductive cycle. The phenotypical antiangiogenic status is the result of sup-pressed vascular endothelial growth factor (VEGF) expres-sion and a functional predominance of a number of naturally occurring antiangiogenic factors such as trombospondin-1, endostatin, angiostatin, and interferon-α and -β.

In cancer however, a proangiogenic phenotype exists. As a result of a growing imbalance between antiangiogenic and proangiogenic factors, an increased and uncontrolled proliferation of endothelial cells occurs with the subsequent formation of new blood vessels. In cancer, these new blood vessels often have an inferior quality and are more leaky than normal blood vessels. Newly formed vessels sprout into the extracellular matrix (ECM) following the degrada-tion of the basement membrane surrounding the endothe-lial cells. Various vascular cell adhesion molecules such as the integrins αvβ3 play a role in this process by directing the endothelial cells of newly formed vessels in the direction of the tumor. Growing blood vessels can supply the tumor with oxygen and essential nutrients and are a port of entry for tumor cells to spread throughout the body and form metastases. In tumors reaching the size of approximately $1\,mm^3$ local hypoxia induces the expression of HIF-1 and HGF that induce a so-called angiogenic switch resulting in increased angiogenesis and tumor invasiveness.

Tumor-related angiogenesis is a multistep process that is stimulated through various proangiogenic factors that can be detected in the direct vicinity of tumor cells.

Being the predominant proangiogenic factor, VEGF has the most specific endothelial proliferative effects (22). The VEGF family consists of various isoforms and is secreted by tumor cells and stromal factors such as endothelial cells,

epithelial cells, mesothelial cells, and leukocytes. VEGF binds with high affinity to the extracellular domain of two homologous endothelial cell receptors, VEGFR-1 or flt-1 and VEGFR-2 or FLK-1/KDR. In addition to this, the bind-ing of VEGF to VEGFR-3, which is primarily located on lymph vessels, induces lymphangiogenesis, another impor-tant process in metastasis development (Fig. 3.10).

VEGFR-2 plays a dominant role in tumor-related angiogenesis. Following ligand–receptor interaction, VEGF receptor tyrosine kinase activity is stimulated, inducing a cascade of downstream intracellular signals that induce endothelial cell proliferation and the formation of new blood vessels. VEGF has little or no effect on quiescent endothe-lial cells of mature blood vessels. Other proangiogenic fac-tors that have been identified are among others basic fibroblast growth factor (bFGF), platelet-derived growth factor (PDGF), and IGF, each with their own endothelial receptor.

As the correlation between VEGF expression and increased angiogenic activity, tumor aggressiveness, meta-static potential, and poor clinical outcome has been recog-nized in many human tumors, inhibiting angiogenesis has been an important focus of drug development over many years. Inhibiting endothelial cell proliferation is likely to be restricted to tumor areas, and thus it is conceivable to develop agents that will cause less systemic side effects. Besides, endothelial cells are genetically stable and not likely to develop resistance.

As angiogenesis is a multistep process, involving secretion and activity of growth factors or ligands, ligand–receptor interactions, receptor tyrosine kinase activity, endothelial cell proliferation, and endothelial cell–ECM interaction, each of these steps can be considered as a target for agents with specific inhibiting effects. In addition, so-called vascular disrupting agents (VDA) have been developed and are able to damage the endothelium of established tumor-related vasculature, thereby selectively destroying the existing blood vessels of solid tumor.

Anti-VEGF(R) Antibodies. Bevacizumab is a recombi-nant humanized monoclonal antibody that targets VEGF with high affinity. By binding VEGF prior to its attachment to any of the natural receptors, ligand–receptor interaction and subsequent angiogenic activity are inhibited. Based upon the experience of a vast number of clinical studies, detailed information on both side efffects and efficacy has been obtained, although many questions remain unan-swered. The spectrum of drug related side effects has been found to be completely different from that seen with cyto-toxic anticancer therapy and includes hypertension, protei-nuria, thromboembolic complications, bleeding, and, to a lesser extent, gastrointestinal perforations. Hypertension is the most frequent side effect, but this phenomenon can be managed in the majority of cases by using conven-tional antihypertensive medication. Proteinuria, although frequently observed, has almost never been dose limiting and has always been found to be completely reversible after dose reduction or drug discontinuation. When bevaci-zumab is not given in a period of about six weeks preced-ing or following surgery, the risk of bleeding complications or wound repair problems appears to be negligible. Although bevacizumab use has induced a number of bowel perforations, the number of fatalities has been very small.

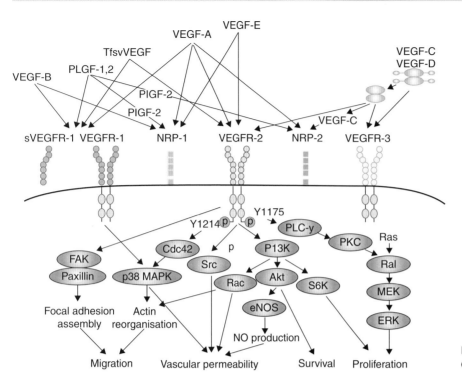

Figure 3.10   VEGF and VEGFR induced intracellular signaling pathways and their crosstalk.

Risk factors for this side effect are recent abdominal operations, radiotherapy, or underlying bowel disease. With regard to clinical activity, large randomized Phase III studies have clearly shown benefit in first and second line treatment of metastatic colorectal cancer and first-line treatment of metastatic breast cancer, nonsmall cell lung cancer (NSCLC), and renal cell cancer (23–29). In all situations except for renal cell cancer, bevacizumab was combined with cytotoxic chemotherapy. Apart from smaller studies in metastatic renal-cell carcinoma, bevacizumab given as single-agent therapy has never resulted in relevant clinical benefit in solid tumors. In renal cell cancer, combining interferon with bevacizumab seems to have clinical activity exceeding that of single-agent interferon (30). Because bevacizumab has to administered frequently and intravenously, the subsequent development step may be the development of a VEGF targeting antibody that can be administered subcutaneously (Aflibercept that is currently being explored) or maybe even orally (Table 3.2).

Apart from antibodies that block VEGF, antibodies that specifically block VEGFR-2 can also proof useful. These antibodies are currently undergoing clinical trials (31).

VEGF Receptor Tyrosine Kinase Inhibitors. Another way to inhibit VEGF induced angiogenesis is by blocking receptor tyrosine kinase activity of the activated endothelial VEGF receptor. This activity initiates the intracellular downstream signal cascade that leads to endothelial cell proliferation.

A large number of orally available small-molecule inhibitors of VEGF receptor tyrosine kinase activity (some also inhibiting other receptor tyrosine kinases) have been developed, all of which could be safely administered to patients, even for prolonged periods of time (Table 3.3).

Table 3.2   VEGF(R) Targeting Antibodies in Clinical Trials

Drug	Target	Clinical development	Side effects
Bevacizumab	VEGF	Approved	Hypertension Proteinuria Thromboembolism Bleeding Fatigue GI perforation
VEGF-Trap (Aflibercept)	VEGF	Phase III	Hypertension Proteinuria Chest pain fatigue
IMC-1121B	VEGFR	Phase I	Ongoing study
CDP 791	VEGFR	Phase I	Ongoing study

Although the antibody bevacizumab has a very specific target, some VEGF receptor tyrosine kinase have a more broad spectrum inhibitory activity and downregulate the tyrosine kinase activities of PDGF, c-Kit, RET, and the intracellular Raf/Ras signal transduction pathway. Apart from this, VEGF tyrosine kinase inhibitors that simultaneously inhibit EGFR have been developed, and these agents are increasingly being referred to as broad spectrum tyrosine kinase inhibitors. Based on the positive results of large randomized clinical studies, the broad spectrum tyrosine kinase inhibitors sunitinib and sorafenib have now been registered for routine use, sunitinib in first-line metastasic renal cell cancer and second line gastrointestinal stroma tumors treatment, and sorafenib in first-line metastatic hepatocellular and second line metastatic renal-cell cancer treatment, respectively (32–35). In contrast to the bevacizumab

Table 3.3 VEGFR Tyrosine Kinase Inhibitors in Clinical Trials

Drug	Target kinase	Clinical development
SU11248 (Sunitinib)	VEGFR-2, VEGFR-3, PDGFR, c-Kit	Approved
Bay 43-9006 (Sorafenib)	VEGFR-2, VEGFR-3, PDGFR, c-Kit, RAF/RAS	Approved
PTK787/ZK22854 (Vatalanib)	VEGFR-1, VEGFR-2, c-Kit, PDGFR	Phase III
ZD6474 (Vandetanib)	VEGFR-2, EGFR	Phase III
AG-013736 (Axitinib)	VEGFR-1, VEGFR-2, VEGFR-3, c-Kit, PDGFR	Phase III
AZD2171 (Cediranib)	VEGFR-1, VEGFR-2, VEGFR-3, c-Kit, PDGFR	Phase III
GW 786034 (Pazopanib)	VEGFR-1, VEGFR-2, c-Kit, PDGFR	Phase III
AMG-706 (Motesanib)	VEGFR-2, VEGFR-3, PDGFR, c-Kit, RET	Phase III
CP-547, 632	VEGFR-2, FGF	Phase II
AV-951	VEGFR-1, VEGFR-2, VEGFR-3, c-Kit, PDGFR	Phase II
XL-184	VEGFR-2, MET, RET	Phase II
ABT-869	VEGFR-2, VEGFR-3, PDGFR, c-Kit	Phase II
SU14813	VEGFR-2, VEGFR-3, PDGFR, c-Kit	Phase II
BMS-582664 (Brivanib)	VEGFR-2, VEGFR-3, FGFR	Phase I
Bay 57-9352 (Telatinib)	VEGFR-2, VEGFR-3, PDGFR, c-Kit	Phase I
AEE788	VEGFR-2, EGFR	Phase I

trials, all these studies explored single-agent treatment with tyrosine kinase inhibitors. To date, combinations with cytotoxic agents have yielded toxicity problems and randomized Phase III trials have been scarce (36). This is strikingly different from the data available on bevacizumab, and yet poorly understood. With regard to side effects, the patterns observed with bevacizumab and most of the small-molecule tyrosine kinase inhibitors seem to be largely overlapping, with hypertension and proteinuria being predominant. However, the spectrum of side effects of the broad spectrum tyrosine kinase inhibitors seems to be more diverse, with gastrointestinal toxicity, skin toxicity, thyroid dysfuntion, and cardiac functional impairment as emerging entities (37,38). Currently, a large number of both broad spectrum as well as more selective VEGF tyrosine kinase inhibitors such as Vandetanib (ZD6474), Vatalanib (PTK787), Axitinib (AG-013736), Cediranib (AZD2171), Motesanib (AMG-706), Telatinib (Bay 57-9352), AV-951, Pazopanib (GW786034), SU14813, CP-547,632, and others are in different stages of clinical development. Interesting biological activity and hints of clinical activity have been observed.

Inhibitors of Endothelial Cell Proliferation. Endostatin, angiostatin, and thrombospondin-1 are naturally occurring inhibitors of endothelial cell proliferation and migration (Table 3.4).

Though endostatin is a structural homologue of a fragment from collagen XVIII, angiostatin is a fragment of plasminogen. The gene for both compounds has been cloned, and recombinant humanized derivatives have undergone extensive clinical testing. Unfortunately, the promising results that were observed in preclinical studies have not been substantiated in clinical trials, and the development of these compounds has at best been sustained

Thrombospondin-1 is a large glycoprotein with proangiogenic and antiangiogenic properties, the latter being exerted when thrombospondin is bound to the endothelial CD-36 receptor, inducing apoptosis of actively proliferating endothelial cells. Naturally occurring thrombospondin is a very large molecule that is not suitable for pharmaceutical development, but as its antiangiogenic properties are restricted to the N-terminal region, various structural modifications have been made, leading to compounds with highly conserved antiangiogenic properties that can be administered subcutaneously. Some of these compounds are currently in Phase I and II studies.

Thalidomide and its derivative lenalidomide are inhibitors of endothelial cell proliferation through largely unknown mechanisms of action, although the reduction of tumor necrosis factor-alpha (TNF-α) has been proposed as mechanism. Promising anticancer activity has been seen in multiple myeloma, myelodysplastic syndrome, AIDS related Kaposi sarcoma, and, to a lesser degree, renal cell carcinoma, but the role in many other more frequently occurring tumor types thus far has not been established (39,40).

Agents Inhibiting the Formation of New Blood Vessels. Actively proliferating endothelial cells that are about to form new blood vessels express the integrin $\alpha v\beta 3$ that interacts with various glycoproteins of the ECM surrounding tumor cells. The endothelial cell–matrix interaction plays a role in directing the endothelial cells through the ECM. As actively proliferating endothelial cells express integrins, whereas quiescent cells do not, inhibiting these integrins by means of antibodies or small-molecule antagonists could inhibit the formation of new blood vessels without affecting established blood vessels (Table 3.5).

Vitaxin or Medi-522, a monoclonal antibody, and cilengitide, a small-molecule inhibitor of $\alpha v\beta 3$ are in clinical development and have shown excellent clinical tolerability and interesting antitumor results in gliomas (41).

Vascular Disrupting Agents. Vascular disrupting agents (VDA) are able to occlude or destroy the established vasculature of tumors (42). Most VDA do so by disrupting the microtubule structure of the endothelial cells. As the endothelium from tumor vasculature differs from that of

Table 3.4 Direct Inhibitors of Endothelial Cell Proliferation in Clinical Trials

Drug	Target	Clinical development
ABT-510	Endothelial CD-36	Phase II
Angiostatin	Various	Phase II
Endostatin	Various	Phase III
Thalidomide/lenolidamide	Reduction of TNF-α production	Approved

Table 3.5   Agents Targeting the Formation of New Blood Vessels in Clinical Trials

Drug	Target	Clinical development
Medi-522	Integrin αVβ3	Phase II
Cilengitide	Integrin αVβ3	Phase II

Table 3.6   Vascular Disrupting Agents in Clinical Trials

Drug	Target	Clinical development
Combretastatin A4	Endothelial tubulin	Phase III
ASA404	Endothelial tubulin	Phase III
ZD6126	Endothelial tubulin	Phase II
DMXAA	Induction of TNF-α	Phase II
AVE8062A	Endothelial tubulin	Phase I
NPI-2358	Endothelial tubulin	Phase I
EPC2407	Endothelial tubulin	Phase I

Table 3.7   Proposed End Points of Early Clinical Studies with Systemic Anticancer Agents

	Cytotoxic chemotherapy	Cancer cell specific therapy
Phase I studies	1. *Acute toxicity*	1. *Acute toxicity*
		2. *Delayed toxicity*
	2. *Maximum Tolerated Dose*	3. *Optimal biologic effect dose*
	Defined by:	Defined by:
	Toxicity	Target AUC
		Inhibition of cellular target
		Inhibition of surrogate marker
Phase II studies	1. *Antitumor activity*	1. *Antitumor activity*
	Defined by:	Defined by:
	Tumor regression rate	Time to progression
		Surrogate marker inhibition
	2. *Delayed toxicity*	2. *Delayed toxicity*

normal blood vessels, small-molecule VDAs that specifically recognize tumor vasculature can have tumor-specific antivascular effects (Table 3.6). PET scan analysis in studies with some of these small-molecule VDAs have shown reversible changes in tumor perfusion, changes in the perfusion of the spleen and kidney, though specific DEMRI kinetic parameters (K^{trans}) varied significantly in the tumor but not in the normal tissues (43,44).

Most of the small-molecule VDAs are tubulin inhibitors, including CA4P, ZD6126, AVE8062, OXi-4503, NPI-2358, MN-029, and EPC2407, and clinical studies with these compounds are currently ongoing.

Within the complex process of angiogenesis, several sequential steps can be determined that all play a well-determined role in this process. Although specific inhibition of each of these isolated steps has shown to be feasible, some doubt remains as to whether full inhibition of angiogenesis can be reached with the inhibition of one single step. To optimally inhibit angiogenesis, it is probably necessary to inhibit two or more (sequential?) steps of the process, and therefore combining two or more antiangiogenic agents, combining antiangiogenic agents with stromal invasion inhibitors, or combining antiangiogenic agents with VDAs may be required.

PRACTICAL IMPLICATIONS ON STUDY DESIGN
Study Methodology: Phase I Studies
The design of Phase I studies in the clinical development of cytotoxic anticancer agents is aimed at safety, defined in terms of acute dose-limiting toxicity (DLT) and the MTD, which usually is the highest but one dose level. As most cytotoxic agents show a steep dose-response relation, the MTD is the highest safe dose that is recommended for further activity testing in single-agent Phase II studies (Fig. 3.3).

For cytostatic agents such end points may only be applicable if preclinical studies have shown a recognizable pattern of acute side effects, which is not always the case. In contrast, as prolonged or even continuous treatment is

often necessary to obtain optimal target inhibition, describing long-term or late-onset toxicity is important. To enable this, patients should ideally be treated for prolonged periods of time, which is often difficult to achieve in the typical end-stage of disease Phase I population. Therefore, performing Phase I trials with these agents in patients with relatively indolent diseases will imply a change in the selection of patients for clinical studies.

As indicated, defining the optimal biological effect dose (OBD) rather than the MTD may be the primary end point for Phase I studies with cytostatic agents (Table 3.7). Assessing this biologic effect requires information on the level of target inhibition by the drug dose administered. Optimally, this would be done in repeated tumor biopsy specimens, but as these are cumbersome procedures for patients, this is often difficult to perform. Alternatively, one tries to determine these biological effects in more easily accessible tissues such as leukocytes, skin biopsies, scalp or eyebrow hairs, or oral mucosa scrapings, assuming that the effects in these tissues could serve as surrogate for the effect in the tumor. This biomarker analysis has been performed in a very large number of trials, and has been able to indicate biological effects for many different classes of agents; VEGFR tyrosine kinase inhibitors have been associated with (often dose-dependent) changes in plasma levels of VEGF (increasing) or plasma levels of soluble VEGFR-2 (decreasing), decreased phosphorylation of the EGFR has been repeatedly observed in skin samples following exposure to various EGFR tyrosine kinase inhibitors, and a decrease in farnesylation of surrogate proteins in buccal scrapings was demonstrated following exposure to specific farnesyl transferase inhibitors. Although there are examples of success, often we lack possibilities in pursuing this in a meaningful and truly predictive way. Dynamic enhanced magnetic resonance imaging (DEMRI) and positron emission tomography (PET) are among the various noninvasive biomarker analytical techniques that are being explored to assess changes in tumor blood flow and tumor viability, respectively following the administration of angiogenesis inhibitors (45–47). Similarly there have been efforts to project knowledge on plasma drug concentrations in animal models yielding adequate effects on a tumor to the human situation. Clearly this approach also suffers from a lot of uncertainties. Whatever the procedure, one can safely conclude that for optimal assessment of pharmacodynamic and pharmacokinetic effects more sophisticated methods will have to become available, with a very close cooperation between preclinical and clinical research groups being here of crucial importance.

Enriching early clinical studies with the preferred enrollment of patients that are most likely to benefit from a new cancer agent is something that might seem to be attractive from various perspectives; the number of patients for whom the experimental treatment is not useful will be minimized, thereby preventing disapointments from their perspective, and the registrational pathway of a new agent will be considerably shortened if based upon a smaller number of patients the tumor types most likely to be of further interest can be selected. The big question is how to select these tumor types, and practically this means that predictive factors or surrogate markers for response are actively being looked for. Recent examples of these markers were increased expression of the EGFR in many epithelial tumor types such as NSCLC and colorectal cancer.

Study Methodology: Phase II Studies

Phase II studies with classical cytotoxic anticancer agents are designed to screen for antitumor activity, and the number and dimension of tumor regressions are usually taken as end point. Well-defined response criteria exist (48).

For the development of cytostatic agents, inducing growth inhibition rather than tumor regression, assessing the latter will almost certainly lead to an underestimation of antitumor activity, and therefore other end points will have to be used in these studies. Time to progression could serve this purpose, but as a consequence Phase II studies using this end point should be randomized, possibly with a placebo control group. If preclinical studies have shown synergistic activity of a cytostatic agent with cytotoxic chemotherapy, it is also conceivable to use a similar design comparing TTP on cytotoxic therapy with TTP on cytotoxic therapy combined with a cytostatic agent. Another alternative is to assess antitumor activity through the so-called randomized discontinuation design (49). In this design all patients are treated for a predefined period of time, after which the patients that did not progress are randomized to continue treatment or to stop (or to receive a placebo treatment). This design enables one to determine whether slow tumor growth is attributable to the study drug or to a naturally slow-growing tumor. The effect on biomarkers such as serum tumor marker levels or target inhibition in skin biopsies or leukocytes can also serve as surrogates of clinical activity in the absence of tumor regression. This could also serve to correlate pharmacokinetic with pharmacodynamic results in larger groups of patients. However, one should realize that the induction of biological activity does not necessarily translate into clinical activity.

Additional issues dealing with the design of phase I, II, and III studies with both cytotoxic and cytostatic anticancer agents are dealt with in greater detail in chapter 4.

OTHER POSSIBLE APPLICATIONS OF MOLECULAR TARGETED THERAPY

Up to now, cancer (cell) specific therapy has been administered to patients with advanced malignant disease. However, because of cytostatic mechanism of action, it is unlikely that optimal clinical efficacy will be achieved under these circumstances. Although it has been demonstrated in a large number of clinical studies that combining molecular targeted agents with either cytotoxic chemotherapy or radiotherapy can have additive or even synergistic anticancer activity, it still remains questionable whether the application of these agents would not be more efficacious in a situation of minimal residual disease, such as in the one obtained following optimal surgical debulking and/or optimal cytotoxic chemotherapy. Also an optimal effect of cancer (cell) specific therapy will often require administration for prolonged periods of time, and therefore oral treatment devoid of dose-limiting side effects is strongly preferred. As it is likely that more than one molecular target will be relevant in a specific tumor, it is conceivable that in the future combinations of target inhibiting agents will have to be considered if optimal growth inhibition is to be achieved. Currently, however, combining various classes of targeted agents has mostly been explored in early clinical studies of patients with advanced malignant disease. In early breast cancer, a large adjuvant trial exploring the sequence or the combination of two antiHER-2 therapies, namely trastuzumab and lapatinib, has started recruitment in 2007.

The question whether large groups of healthy persons should be treated with molecular targeted agents in the setting of chemoprevention cannot be answered adequately at this moment. Especially in these cases, defining the target or targets of a tumor that is not (yet) clinically present and that should be inhibited will be of crucial significance. Once again, an agent that combines various specific target inhibiting capacities within one tablet or capsule would be preferable from a theoretical point of view.

CONCLUSION

The development and introduction of cancer (cell) specific therapy has fundamentally changed our way of thinking of cancer. It is very well possible that within the next few years human tumors will be characterized with regard to their key genetic or molecular targets, after which a highly "individualized" therapy will be selected. After decades of nonselective trial-and-error treatment this development means nothing less than a fundamental breakthrough in anticancer therapy.

REFERENCES

1. Paez J, Janne P, Lee J et al. EGFR mutations in lung cancer: correlation with clinical response to gefitinib therapy. Science 2004; 304: 1497–500.
2. Lynch T, Bell D, Sordella R et al. Activating mutations in the epidermal growth factor receptor underlying responsiveness of non-small-cell lung cancer to gefitinib. N Engl J Med 2004; 350: 2129–39.
3. Cunninham D, Humblet Y, Sinet S et al. Cetuximab monotherapy and cetuximab plus irinotecan in irinotecan-refractory metastatic colorectal cancer. N Engl J Med 2004; 351: 337–45.

4. Van Cutsem E, Nowacki M, Lang I et al. Randomized phase III study of irinotecan and 5-FU/FA with or without cetuximab in the first-line treatment of patients with metastatic colorectal cancer (mCRC): the CRYSTAL trial. J Clin Oncol 2007; 25(18S Suppl): abstract 4000.

5. Vermorken J, Mesia R, Vega V et al. Cetuximab extends survival of patients with recurrent or metastatic SCCHN when added to first line platinum based therapy—results of a randomized phase III (extreme) study. J Clin Oncol 2007; 25(18S Suppl): abstract 6091.

6. Bonner J, Harrari P, Giralt J et al. Radiotherapy plus cetuximab for squamous-cell carcinoma of the head and neck. N Engl J Med 2006; 354: 567–78.

7. Jonker D, O'Callaghan C, Karapetis C et al. Cetuximab for the treatment of colorectal cancer. N Engl J Med 2007; 357: 2040–8.

8. Perez-Soler R, Saltz L. Cutaneous adverse effects with HER1/EGFR-targeted agents: is there a silver lining? J Clin Oncol 2005; 23: 5235–46.

9. Giaccone G, Herbst R, Manegold C et al. Gefitinib in combination with gemcitabine and cisplatin in advanced non–small-cell lung cancer: a phase III trial—INTACT 1. J Clin Oncol 2004; 22: 777–84.

10. Herbst R, Giaccone G, Schiller J et al. Gefitinib in combination with paclitaxel and carboplatin in advanced non–small-cell lung cancer: a phase III trial—INTACT 2. J Clin Oncol 2004; 22: 785–94.

11. Herbst R, Prager D, Hermann R et al. TRIBUTE: a phase III trial of erlotinib hydrochloride (OSI-774) combined with carboplatin and paclitaxel chemotherapy in advanced non-small-cell lung cancer. J Clin Oncol 2005; 23: 5892–9.

12. Gatzemeier U, Pluzanska A, Szczesna A et al. Phase III study of erlotinib in combination with cisplatin and gemcitabine in advanced non-small-cell lung cancer: the tarceva lung cancer investigation trial. J Clin Oncol 2007; 25: 1545–52.

13. Shepherd J, Rodrigues Pereira J, Ciuleanu J et al. Erlotinib in previously treated non-small-cell lung cancer. N Engl J Med 2005; 353: 123–32.

14. Haluska P, Shaw H, Batzel G et al. Phase I dose escalation study of the anti insulin-like growth factor-I receptor monoclonal antibody CP-751,871 in patients with refractory solid tumors. Clin Cancer Res 2007; 13: 5834–40.

15. Demetri G, von Mehren M, Blanke C et al. Efficacy and safety of imatinib mesylate in advanced gastrointestinal stromal tumors. N Engl J Med 2002; 347: 472–80.

16. O'Brien S, Guilhot F, Larson R et al. Imatinib compared to interferon and low-dose cytarabine for newly diagnosed chronic-phase chronic myeloid leukemia. N Engl J Med 2003; 348: 994–1004.

17. Peggs K, Mackinnon S. Imatinib mesylate-the new gold standard for treatment of chronic myeloid leukemia. N Engl J Med 2003; 348: 1048–50.

18. Harousseau J, Lancet J, Reiffers J et al. A phase 2 study of the oral farnesyltransferase inhibitor tipifarnib in patients with refractory or relapsed acute myeloid leukemia. Blood 2007; 109: 5151–6.

19. Fenaux P, Raza A, Mufti G et al. A multicenter phase 2 study of the farnesyltransferase inhibitor tipifarnib in intermediate- to high-risk myelodysplastic syndrome. Blood 2007; 109: 4158–63.

20. Hudes G, Carducci M, Tomczak P et al. Temsirolimus, interferon alfa, or both for advanced renal-cell carcinoma. N Engl J Med 2007; 356: 2271–81.

21. Sattler M, Salgia R. c-Met and hepatocyte growth factor: potential as novel targets in cancer therapy. Curr Oncol Rep 2007; 9: 102–8.

22. Ferrara N, Alitalo K. Clinical applications of angiogenic growth factors and their inhibitors. Nat Med 1999; 5: 1359–64.

23. Hurwitz H, Fehrenbacher L, Novotny W et al. Bevacizumab plus irinotecan, fluorouracil, and leucovorin for metastatic colorectal cancer. N Engl J Med 2004; 350: 2335–42.

24. Kabbinavar FF, Schultz J, McCleod H et al. Addition of bevacizumab to bolus fluorouracil and leucovorin in first-line metastatic colorectal cancer: results of a randomized phase II trial. J Clin Oncol 2005; 23: 3697–705.

25. Giantano BJ, Catalano PJ, Meroplo MJ et al. Bevacizumab in combination with oxaliplatin, fluorouracil, and leucovorin (FOLFOX4) for previously treated metastatic colorectal cancer: results from the eastern cooperative oncology group study E3200. J Clin Oncol 2007; 25: 1539–44.

26. Miller KD, Wang M, Gralow J et al. Paclitaxel plus bevacizumab versus paclitaxel alone for metastatic breast cancer. N Engl J Med 2007; 357: 2666–76.

27. Sandler A, Gray R, Parry MC et al. Paclitaxel-carboplatin alone or with bevacizumab for non-small-cell lung cancer. N Engl J Med 2006; 355: 2542–50.

28. Manegold C, von Pawel J, Zatloukal P et al. Randomised, double-blind multicentre phase III study of bevacizumab in combination with cisplatin and gemcitabine in chemotherapy-naïve patients with advanced or recurrent non-squamous non-small cell lung cancer (NSCLC): BO17704. J Clin Oncol 2007; 25(18S Suppl): abstract LBA7514.

29. Yang J, Haworth L, Sherry R et al. A randomized trial of bevacizumab, an antivascular endothelial growth factor antibody, for metastatic renal cancer. N Engl J Med 2003; 349: 427–34.

30. Escudier B, Pluzanska A, Koralewski P et al. Bevacizumab plus interferon alfa-2a for treatment of metastatic renal cell carcinoma: a randomised, double-blind phase III trial. Lancet 2007; 370: 2103–11.

31. Youssoufian H, Hicklin DJ, Rowinsky EK. Monoclonal antibodies to the vascular endothelial growth factor receptor-2. Clin Cancer Res 2007; 13: 5544s–8s.

32. Escudier BA, Eisen T, Stadler WM et al. Sorafenib in advanced clear-cell renal-cell carcinoma. N Engl J Med 2007; 356: 125–34.

33. Llovet J, Ricci J, Mazzaferro V et al. Sorafenib in advanced hepatocellular carcinoma. N Engl J Med 2008; 359: 378–90.

34. Motzer RJ, Hudson TE, Tomczak P et al. Sunitinib versus interferon alfa in metastatic renal-cell carcinoma. N Engl J Med 2007; 356: 115–24.

35. Demetri GD, van Oosterom AT, Garrett CR et al. Efficacy and safety of sunitinib in patients with advanced gastrointestinal stromal tumour after failure of imatinib: a randomised controlled trial. Lancet 2006; 368: 1329–38.

36. Hecht JR, Trarbach T, Jaeger E et al. A randomized, double-blind, placebo-controlled, Phase III study in patients (Pts) with metastatic adenocarcinoma of the colon or rectum receiving first-line chemotherapy with oxaliplatin/5-fluorouracil/leucovorin and PTK787/ZK 222584 or placebo (CONFIRM-1). J Clin Oncol 2005; 23(16S Suppl): LBA3.

37. Rini B, Tamaskar I, Shaheen P et al. Hypothyroidism in patients with metastatic renal cell carcinoma treated with sunitinib. J Natl Cancer Inst 2007; 99: 81–3.

38. Chu T, Rupnick M, Kerkela R et al. Cardiotoxicity associated with tyrosine kinase inhibitor sunitinib. Lancet 2007; 370: 2011–19.

39. Dimopoulos M, Spencer A, Attal M et al. Lenalidomide plus dexamethasone for relapsed or refractory multiple myeloma. N Engl J Med 2007; 357: 2123–32.

40. Melchert M, Kale V, List A. The role of lenalidomide in the treatment of patients with chromosome 5q deletion and other myelodysplastic syndromes. Curr Opin Hematol 2007; 14: 123–9.

41. Nabors L, Mikkelsen T, Rosenfeld S et al. Phase I and correlative biology study of cilengitide in patients with recurrent malignant glioma. J Clin Oncol 2007; 25: 1651–7.

42. Siemann D, Bibby M, Dark G et al. Differentiation and definition of vascular-targeted therapies. Clin Cancer Res 2005; 11: 416–20.

43. Galbraith S, Maxwell R, Lodge M et al. Combretastatin A4 phosphate has tumor antivascular activity in rat and man as demonstrated by dynamic magnetic resonance imaging. J Clin Oncol 2003; 21: 2831–42.

44. Anderson H, Yap J, Miller M et al. Assessment of pharmacodynamic vascular response in a phase I trial of Combretastatin A4 phosphate. J Clin Oncol 2003; 21: 2823–30.

45. Liu G, Rugo H, Wilding G et al. Dynamic contrast-enhanced magnetic resonance imaging as a pharmacodynamic measure of response after acute dosing of AG-013736, an oral angiogenesis inhibitor, in patients with advanced solid tumors: results from a phase I study. J Clin Oncol 2005; 23: 5464–73.

46. Morgan B, Thomas A, Drevs J et al. Dynamic contrast-enhanced magnetic resonance imaging as a biomarker for the pharmacological response of PTK787/ZK 222584, an inhibitor of the vascular endothelial growth factor receptor tyrosine kinases, in patients with advanced colorectal cancer and liver metastases: results from two phase I studies. J Clin Oncol 2003; 21: 3955–64.

47. De Geus-Oei, van der Heijden H, Visser E et al. Chemotherapy response evaluation with 18F-FDG PET in patients with non-small cell lung cancer. J Nucl Med 2007; 48: 1592–8.

48. Therasse P, Arbuck SG, Eisenhauer E et al. New guidelines to evaluate the response to treatment in solid tumors. J Natl Cancer Inst 2000; 92: 205–16.

49. Rosner G, Stadler W, Ratain M. Randomized discontinuation design: application to cytostatic antineoplastic agents. J Clin Oncol 2002; 20: 4478–84.

4

Principles of Clinical Trials

Wendy R. Parulekar, Elizabeth A. Eisenhauer, and Richard D. Gelber

INTRODUCTION

Clinical trials are experiments conducted on human subjects for the purpose of evaluating one or more therapeutic interventions. Observational studies on cancer patients can generate knowledge about cancer behavior, biologic determinants of outcome, and hypotheses about therapeutic benefit. However, observational studies cannot control for factors that might influence outcome. Only through clinical trials can therapeutic interventions be reliably assessed. All aspects of the study rationale, objectives, design, treatments, data requirements, statistical justification, and analysis plan are detailed in the protocol document. As a clinical trial is an experiment, it must begin with a hypothesis or question: What are the toxic and/or biologic effects of a treatment or intervention? What effect does an intervention have on rates of tumor response, or on time to relapse, progression or death? To be successful, a study must clearly define the primary question and outcome measure(s) of interest, utilize an appropriate design and sample size to address the question, and collect and analyze data according to prespecified criteria. Increasingly clinical studies are enriched by the addition of secondary end points including quality of life and biomarker studies. Furthermore, studies conducted on human subjects must comply with international standards of ethical review and conduct. Finally, at the conclusion of each trial the interpretation of its results should be undertaken in the context of preexisting knowledge in the particular clinical setting studied. This chapter addresses all such aspects of clinical trials in cancer patients.

INTERNATIONAL STANDARDS AND HARMONIZATION

Today clinical cancer research takes place in an international arena. For this process to be effective, those engaged in clinical cancer research require a common "language" to describe trial outcomes. In the 1970s, the World Health Organization (WHO) initiated a series of international meetings to standardize the reporting of cancer study results and their recommendations, "Reporting Results of Cancer Treatment," were published in 1981 (1). Included in it were sections regarding reporting of baseline patient data, treatment delivery, toxic effects (WHO toxicity criteria), objective response, time-to-event results, and general guidelines on reporting trial results.

The WHO recommendations were widely adopted but with time were found wanting in certain areas. The toxicity criteria were limited and did not allow for descriptions of many toxic effects of treatment. An initiative by the U.S. National Cancer Institute (USNCI) in 1982 led to the creation of "Common Toxicity Criteria (CTC)," which has undergone several revisions, most recently to CTCAE v 3.0 (http://ctep.cancer.gov/forms/CTCAEv3.pdf), to respond to the need for expanded toxicity categories. WHO Response Criteria were modified by many research groups to accommodate individual needs, which led to noncomparable definitions for response in some situations. To address this issue, the International Working Party developed a revised set of tumor measurement guidelines, the "RECIST" criteria (2) that have been widely adopted. Further, another International Working Group developed standard response criteria for lymphomas(3) (see section "End points").

The *Guideline for Good Clinical Practice* (http://www. ich.org/LOB/media/MEDIA482.pdf) is the product of an international collaboration of regulatory agencies to achieve harmonized standards and requirements for the registration of medicinal products internationally (International Conference on Harmonization or ICH). This effort, which applies broadly to pharmaceutical development in all areas of medicine, has been underway since 1989. Topics for guideline development include quality, safety, efficacy, and statistical considerations in clinical trials. As each topic is identified, several formal steps of discussion and development take place, which culminate in a final guideline recommended for adoption by government regulatory agencies.

ETHICAL CONSIDERATIONS

International standards have also evolved with respect to the ethical conduct of trials and the protection of human subjects in medical research. The Nuremberg Code (1947) and the Declaration of Helsinki (1964) defined principles to govern biomedical research and protect the rights, safety, and well-being of trial subjects. Specifically delineated were issues of informed consent and its voluntary nature, the need for scientific rigor in the rationale and design of the proposed investigation, balance in the potential risks and benefits of the investigation, and the obligation to truthfully report results. Other jurisdictions have elaborated on these principles, in some cases defining regulations governing the conduct of clinical research. The *Guideline for Good Clinical Practice* reaffirms the principles of the Declaration of Helsinki. It also details the process of ethical committee review of research, the content of consent forms, the obligations of the investigator and the sponsor in clinical trials, the required elements of clinical research protocols, and the documents which must be in place prior to beginning a clinical trial.

The ethical issues associated with Phase I cancer trials have received special attention because the study population is believed to be a vulnerable one: being comprised of individuals with a stage of disease for which standard or curative therapy has been exhausted. In this setting it is the task of the investigator to assure that the process of consent does not overemphasize the potential benefits of an untested treatment but instead conveys in lay language the true goal of the Phase I trial: to determine dosing recommendations for further study, often using toxicity information as a guide (vide infra). Although often unstated, the goals of the patient may be at variance with this. Thus there are challenges to ethical committees, educators, and investigators to be cognizant of this special area of concern and to train physicians in the skills required to discuss the benefits and risks of enrolling patients on Phase I studies (4).

Ethical issues are also relevant for randomized clinical trials in which the choice of treatment is determined by a chance mechanism (5,6). A distinction is made between the roles of physician investigator whose primary responsibility is the welfare of the patient, and that of the clinical scientist who also has an interest in conducting clinical research. Some have argued that these roles are in conflict when the care of individual patients is at stake, thus making randomized trials inherently unethical. Others argue that applying therapies without substantial evidence concerning their safety and effectiveness is unethical and that the most valid way to obtain unbiased evidence is from randomized studies. A balance is required between the benefit/risk for individual patients versus the value of the trial to future patients. The oversight of research by an independent ethical review committee helps to assure this balance. When in doubt, the concerns for the individual patient should take precedence over the concerns for the study. Respect for the patients as individuals is also a central aspect of ethical conduct in clinical research.

THE PROTOCOL DOCUMENT

A carefully conceived and executed protocol document is essential for conducting a high-quality clinical trial. The elements of the protocol document are listed in Table 4.1. Unless the essential elements are defined clearly before the commencement of the trial, the potential for obtaining biased and uninterpretable results exists. For example, bias can occur if dose reductions and procedures to be followed in case of toxic reactions are not specified. Regulatory authorities consider the protocol to be the definitive prospective plan for the clinical trial.

DATA MANAGEMENT AND QUALITY CONTROL

Good data management practices for conducting a high-quality clinical trial must be the responsibility of trained data managers rather than busy clinicians (7). Assurance that informed consent was obtained, that proper verification of eligibility criteria prior to patient enrollment was carried out, and recording of treatment information are the first steps. Data monitoring of studies and quality control audits are fundamental aspects of the *Guideline for Good Clinical Practice*. Data fraud in biomedical research is rare, but when it occurs the loss of confidence in clinical trials can be devastating. Protocols must therefore be designed in such a way that they are feasible to conduct with good quality control standards.

THE CLINICAL TRIAL PARADIGM

To understand the statistical principles for the design and analysis of clinical trials, it is important to distinguish between the observed outcomes obtained from the study and the effects that the treatment might produce in the larger target population. This distinction is illustrated in Figure 4.1. The protocol document defines the patient *population* of interest. The clinical trial recruits a *sample* of opportunity. The study end points obtained from the selected sample are recorded and the results are summarized using statistical methods to *describe* the observed results obtained in the sample and to *infer* what the true treatment effect might be in the patient population based on the observed results. The lower portion of Figure 4.1 illustrates

Table 4.1 Elements of the Protocol Document

Protocol section	Description
Study schema	Pictorial summary of the essential elements of the study design. This should be simple and logical and reflect the study objectives
Background and rationale	Description of current state of knowledge that justifies the planning and conduct of the trial
Objectives	Few in number and achievable with the proposed study design
Patient population	Clearly defined and ideally homogeneous cohort. Eligibility and ineligibility criteria should be easily verifiable at the time of patient enrollment, and the rationale for the criteria should be consistent with the study objectives
Treatment allocation	Randomization used to avoid bias in comparative trials, stratification to achieve prognostic factor balance or to prospectively define intended subgroup analyses. Discussion of placebo control group, crossover plan, etc.
Treatment	Description of treatment administration, schedule, duration, potential toxicities, dose modification criteria
Follow-up procedures	Patient visit schedules, clinical and laboratory data to be obtained
End points	Standardization and quantification of criteria for the evaluation of treatment effects. Definition of primary and secondary end points for analysis
Statistical considerations	Review and justification of study design, presentation of sample size determinations, description of monitoring policies and plans for interim analyses, and outline of data analysis plan
Forms submission	Simple, efficient, and comparable schedules for all treatment arms. Discussion of special quality control procedures
Informed consent	Description of study rationale and objectives, risks, benefits, alternative treatments (including no additional therapy), and statement of the right to withdraw in terms that can be understood by the patients

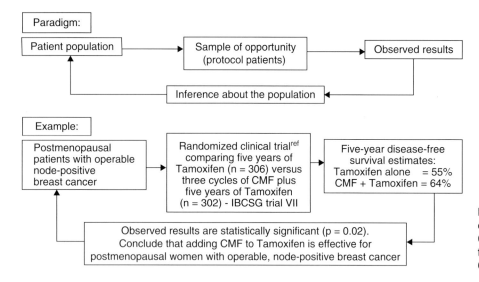

Figure 4.1 Clinical trial paradigm and example for a Phase III trial. *Abbreviations*: CMF, cyclophosphamide, methotrexate, and fluorouracil; IBCSG, International Breast Cancer Study Group. *Source*: From Ref. 8.

an example for a Phase III study (8). In this case the 5-year disease-free survival percents provide the descriptive estimates summarizing the study results and the *p* value provides the statistical inference indicating that the observed results could be expected only 2 times out of 100 if the two treatments were actually equally effective for the patient population.

The observed result from a clinical trial is a combination of the average true effect of treatment for the patient population, systematic error (or bias), and random error (or variability). The objectives of clinical trial methodology are (1) to minimize biases that might produce observed treatment effects that are distortions of the real impact of treatment, and (2) to control the variability of the trial estimates by evaluating an adequate sample size to detect treatment effects that might be reasonably expected. All of the principles of clinical trials discussed below are designed to achieve one or both of these objectives.

END POINTS

Explicit descriptions of the end points of clinical trials are important if results are to be properly interpreted. The study end point quantifies the effect of the treatments being studied. It can consist of (1) a quantitative (discrete or continuous) measurement on each patient at a particular point in time, or "longitudinally," that is, several times throughout the follow-up time; (2) the observation of whether or not a particular event has taken place; or (3) the time elapsed between a prefixed time point (such as randomization or initiation of treatment) and the moment when a certain event occurs.

An example of a continuous outcome belonging to category (1) is the measurement of bone mineral density at the end of treatment. The emotional well-being of a patient assessed at predetermined times on a scale with multiple levels is an example of a longitudinal quantitative measure with "categorical" outcomes. Examples of outcomes

of type (2), frequently referred to as "events," are disease progression within 1 year, objective response to treatment, or the occurrence of some toxic reaction. The outcomes in category (3) are usually called "survival times," but the final event which defines the time interval does not have to be death (in fact, progression-free and disease-free survival are common end points). Not all patients will have had the event of interest by the time of the data analysis. The "survival time" of these patients is only known up to a lower bound (the latest time that they were observed as not having had the event), and these "survival times" are called "censored." The presence of censored observations complicates the analysis of the trial data. In particular, the reported results may be subject to bias if the chance of censoring is related to treatment, for instance if some patients never returned for later visits ("lost to follow-up") because of toxic effects or worsening of their health.

The choice of the end point of interest must be specified during the design phase of the trial as it affects the selection of the statistical techniques for the analysis of the results, and the sample size required to properly evaluate treatments. The following section discusses several other types of outcomes frequently evaluated in cancer clinical trials: toxic effects, tumor response, biomarkers, quality of life, and economic measures.

Toxic (Adverse) Effects

Toxicity is an important measurement in cancer clinical trials as most therapeutic interventions in cancer cause significant morbidity. Toxicity criteria describe adverse effects in categories and grades with Grade 0 meaning "normal" or "none" and Grade 4 meaning life-threatening toxicity. The most commonly used criteria in cancer trials are the Common Toxicity Criteria developed by the USNCI. The original version contained 49 toxicity terms grouped into 18 categories. Modifications have added new terms to categorize new effects of treatment and to allow for more comprehensive reporting. In 2003, version 3.0 of the criteria (now called Common Terminology Criteria for Adverse Events or CTCAE) was launched. CTCAE v 3.0 contains more than 200 adverse event terms grouped into 28 categories (http://ctep.cancer.gov/forms/CTCAEv3.pdf).

Adverse event terms include toxic effects of treatment, symptoms of disease, or other medical events. Most trials require a baseline assessment to document symptoms or residual toxic effects from previous treatment and then periodic assessments over the course of the therapy. In general, toxicity is reported in tabular form as the worst grade for each effect for each patient. Duration of toxic effects and relationship to study treatment may also be described. In randomized trials, comparison of toxic effects between treatment arms is an important component of the analysis.

Objective Tumor Response

Tumor response refers to the description of objective change in measured disease during the course of therapy. As noted above, many variations from the original WHO criteria developed in the decades since their publication, which led to confusion in interpretation of trial results (9). In fact, the application of varying response criteria can lead to strikingly different conclusions about the efficacy of the same regimen (10). In response to these problems, an International Working Party was formed in the mid-1990s to standardize and simplify response criteria. New criteria, known as the Response Evaluation Criteria in Solid Tumors (RECIST criteria), were published in 2000 (2). Like earlier criteria, RECIST response assessment requires baseline measurement of malignant lesions and then periodic reevaluations to determine the maximal degree of shrinkage (if any) or growth of the overall tumor burden. Unlike earlier criteria in which tumor assessments were based on the sum of the products of bidimensional measurable lesions, the RECIST criteria define measurable disease on the basis of only a single diameter and determine the tumor burden by summing the longest diameters of measurable lesions.

Using the RECIST definitions, a complete response (CR) requires the disappearance of all evidence of disease. Partial response (PR) is a 30% or more decrease in the sum of longest diameters of measurable lesions. Progressive disease (PD) is at least a 20% increase in sum of longest diameters of measurable lesions or the appearance of new disease. Stable disease (SD) is a state that does not meet either PR or PD criteria. In addition, CR and PR must be confirmed by repeat measurements no less than four weeks after the first set of measurements were performed. Non-measurable lesions must disappear for CR status. In trials where objective response is an end point, patients are assigned a "best response" to therapy on the basis of the above definitions and a response rate is reported.

Objective response is generally utilized only in Phase II studies, as a primary end point, where it can provide an objective measure from which decisions can be taken regarding further study of the drug or regimen. Thus, it is used as a surrogate measure of efficacy—a sufficiently high response rate can indicate that the regimen under study has the potential to improve survival. However, the fact that a regimen can produce responses is not proof that it will also improve survival: that requires testing in an appropriately designed study.

Biomarkers

The term "biomarker" has been defined as a "characteristic that is objectively measured and evaluated as an indicator of normal biologic processes, pathogenic processes or pharmacologic responses to a therapeutic intervention (11)." "Biomarker" thus means many things and the actual meaning depends on the clinical setting in which the term is applied. For example, biomarkers include laboratory or imaging measures of molecular changes in tumors in response to drug treatment (so-called pharmacodynamic effects); change in tumor size (objective response); blood, urine, or radiologic findings associated with early cancer detection, prognostic indicators or predictors of treatment effect. A prognostic (bio)marker is one that provides information about the outcome of an individual who is marker positive, in the absence of therapy or when treated with empiric therapy. A predictive (bio)marker is one that predicts the *differential* efficacy of a particular therapy based on marker status (12). Finally, a biomarker may be defined in a regulatory environment as a surrogate end point for clinical benefit in the drug approval process (13).

Biomarkers guide drug discovery and development by contributing to target selection and assessment of its modulation in preclinical and early clinical studies. The increased understanding of the molecular basis of cancer has led to the use of the term "biomarker" as a synonym for the molecular properties of cells such as gene and gene products (mRNA and proteins). It has also led to the integration of biomarkers in the clinical trial design as an aid to the selection of drug dose and schedule (Phase I), demonstration of drug activity (Phase II), evaluation of drug efficacy in a randomized setting (Phase III), including the use as a means of selecting patient populations most likely to benefit.

A major challenge to the use of biomarkers in preclinical and clinical studies relates to the issue of assay methodology. Although drug and assay development may occur in parallel, there exists an urgent need to standardize the methodologies and reporting of biomarker assay results in all phases of clinical trial research. Examples of these requirements include descriptions of specimen handling and reagent preparation as well as data regarding assay sensitivity, specificity, and reproducibility.

Quality of Life (QOL), Health Related Quality of Life (HRQOL), and Patient-Reported Outcomes (PROs)

The U.S. Food and Drug Administration (FDA) stated that efficacy with respect to overall survival and/or improvements in QOL might provide the basis for drug approval (14). QOL represents a broad construct encompassing all aspects of a person's well-being. HRQOL is more specific representing an individual's perceptions of how an illness and its treatment affect, at a minimum, the physical, mental, and social aspects of his or her life. Recently, the assessment of HRQOL has been further refined to consider patient-reported outcomes (PROs), a measurement of any aspect of a patient's health status that comes directly from the patient, without the interpretation of the patient's responses by a physician or anyone else (15). In clinical trials, a PRO instrument can be used to measure the impact of an intervention on one or more aspects of patients' health status, ranging from the purely symptomatic (response of a headache) to more complex concepts (e.g., ability to carry out activities of daily living), to extremely complex concepts such as HRQOL (16). Including PRO measurements in clinical trials is relevant only if there is a clear hypothesis to be tested and a methodology and analysis plan prospectively defined. For example, for patients with advanced disease, PROs may be measured to document the palliative benefits of therapies given to patients who are symptomatic.

Health Related Quality of Life and PRO measurements can be analyzed using univariate, multivariate, or longitudinal methods. Univariate analyses are used to compare group means based on individual scales. Multivariate analyses can adjust these mean values for multiple factors such as treatment, patient characteristics, and disease status. Longitudinal analyses evaluate change over time based on assessments taken at multiple time points. Statistical issues concerning how to handle dropouts and missing QOL assessments must be considered (17).

Quality-adjusted survival is an end point that considers both quality and quantity of life. Generally, this end point represents a patient's survival time weighted by utility values ranging from zero (as bad as death) to one (perfect health) and reflecting patient preferences for time spent in a particular health state. One approach to evaluating quality-adjusted survival time within clinical trials is the Quality-adjusted Time Without Symptoms of disease or Toxicity of treatment method (Q-TWiST) (18,19). To apply the Q-TWiST method, clinical health states that can occur during the course of the patients' treatment and follow-up are defined to reflect changes in clinical status that may be associated with changes in QOL. For example, one clinical health state may be associated with toxicity caused by treatment (Tox), another associated with disease progression (Prog), a third associated with the development of late sequelae such as cardiac dysfunction (LS), and a fourth representing a relatively good state of health associated with none of the above (TWiST). The second step is to use a nested sequence of Kaplan-Meier curves to partition the overall survival time of each treatment group separately. The areas between these curves provide estimates of the average amount of time patients spend in each of the defined clinical health states. The third step is to compare the overall quality-adjusted survival between the two treatment groups using a variety of weights for the health states. Sensitivity analyses based on threshold utility plots indicate the utility weights for which one treatment would be preferred to another. Patient-derived utility weights can also be incorporated in a Q-TWiST analysis (20). In cancer medicine, Q-TWiST has been used to evaluate adjuvant therapies for breast cancer (21,22), interferon treatment for melanoma (23), bone marrow transplant for childhood acute myeloid leukemia (24), and therapies for advanced disease (25).

Cost-Effectiveness Analysis (CEA)

There is an increasing emphasis on cost savings and cost containment in providing medical services and therapies. Methodological and statistical issues relating to this initiative must be considered (26). Economic evaluation involves analysis of alternative strategies considering both health improvements and financial resource implications. CEA is the accepted method of economic evaluation of health care alternatives, according to the report by the U.S. Panel on Cost-Effectiveness in Health and Medicine (27). It compares two different approaches by considering the ratio of incremental costs divided by incremental effectiveness (measured in units of quality-adjusted life years [QALYs]). Collecting individual patient cost data and measuring QALYs longitudinally represent challenges for the conduct of economic evaluations alongside clinical trials (28).

ANALYSIS OF CLINICAL TRIAL RESULTS

The choice of the analysis method for the clinical trial data depends on the end point to be analyzed. The two most common measures of treatment effect encountered are based on the proportion of events and the survival distribution.

Proportion of Events

The proportion of events is defined as the ratio between the number of patients in a group for whom an event has been observed and the total number of patients in that group. When computed for the sample of trial patients, this ratio is an estimate of the true proportion of events that one would observe if the treatment were to be assigned to the whole patient population represented by the sample. As an estimate based on a limited number of patients, the ratio will vary around the true population proportion if the trial were repeated many times.

The analysis of a trial whose end point is a proportion of events usually produces a *point estimate*, a *confidence interval*, and a statistical *test of hypothesis* about the population proportion. A point estimate is the observed proportion of successes, computed within each patient subgroup in the trial (e.g., within each treatment arm). A confidence interval for the population proportion of successes is a pair of values (p_1, p_2) such that the population proportion can be expected to fall within the interval with a given *level of confidence*. The precise interpretation of a confidence interval is that if one were to repeat the trial a large number of times (on different samples of patients) and compute a 95% confidence interval for the population proportion from each of the trials, then approximately 95% of the resulting intervals would actually contain the *true* population proportion. Confidence intervals can be generated, which have any level of confidence between 0% and 100%. The width of the interval will become larger as the required level of confidence increases, including the entire range between 0 and 1 in order to achieve a 100% level of confidence. This is obviously not very informative. A confidence level of 95% is standard practice.

A test of hypothesis consists of a statistical procedure designed to give an answer to the following kind of questions: "Can we reject the hypothesis (*null* hypothesis) that the two proportions of events p_A and p_B for treatments A and B applied to the whole patient population are identical?" Other questions that may be answered are "Can we reject the hypothesis that the proportion of events in a specific treatment arm is at least 20%?" The statistical theory of hypothesis testing in clinical trials involves specifying an *alternative hypothesis* and an admissible *type I error* (or α *[alpha] level*). The type I error is the probability of rejecting the null hypothesis when it was actually true. A type I error of 5% is commonly accepted. The definition of the alternative hypothesis involves choosing the direction of the treatment difference to be considered "extreme" in the testing procedure. Suppose response to treatment is taken as the "event" of interest, and that p_E and p_C are the response rates corresponding to experimental therapy and control therapy, respectively. If the possibility that $p_E < p_C$ is not at all clinically interesting, then $p_E > p_C$ would be the alternative hypothesis of interest. Such an alternative hypothesis is called "one-sided" to distinguish it from the "two-sided" alternative hypothesis "$p_E \neq p_C$," which will reject the null hypothesis whenever the evidence from the trial is either in the direction $p_E < p_C$ or in the direction $p_E > p_C$. In the context of Phase III clinical trials the use of two-sided alternative hypotheses is highly recommended, as it is possible that a promising experimental therapy could actually prove to be *less* effective than the standard therapy. A statistical test is said to *reject the null hypothesis at the level of significance 100α percent* if the value of a quantity computed from the data (the "test statistic") falls within a given interval (the "rejection region"). Such intervals contain all the values of the test statistic that are considered to be "too extreme," where being "extreme" is defined by the specified alternative hypothesis and the level of significance.

An alternative and equivalent way of conducting a test of hypothesis is the computation of a *p* value. A *p* value is the probability that a value for the test statistic equal to or more extreme than the one observed can be obtained *if the null hypothesis is assumed to be true*. Rejection of the null hypothesis is then declared whenever the *p* value is smaller than the preassigned value of the type I error α, usually set at 5%.

Survival Data

When the end point is a survival time, the population characteristic of interest is the *survival distribution* rather than just the number of events. A survival distribution is the probability distribution of the variable "survival time,"

and it quantifies the probability that a randomly selected patient survives (or, more generally, "does not have an event") until a given time point. There is one such probability for each time point, and one can plot the survival curve (or probability of surviving) versus the time axis.

Just as with the proportion of events, survival distributions obtained from an individual trial can only provide an *estimate* of the true population distribution. The estimated curve (the equivalent of the point estimate) will also vary around the real population distribution. The Kaplan-Meier method(29) is the statistical approach most frequently used to estimate the survival distribution. An example of a Kaplan-Meier estimate of a survival function is shown in Figure 4.2. Some key features to look for and related questions to ask when examining a survival plot are listed below:

- the units on the vertical axis (does the probability of survival shown range from 0 to 1, or is the scale truncated?);
- the scale of the vertical axis (are the survival curves drawn according to log scale or a linear scale?);
- the units on the horizontal scale (over what length of time does the survival curve extend?);
- the amount of follow-up time available for the sample used to plot the curves (how many patients remain at risk to be included in the analysis at the tails of the curves?).

The plot in Figure 4.2 shows a linear vertical scale ranging from 0% to 100%, a horizontal scale extending to 24 months from date of randomization, and a reasonable number of patients at risk at 2 years (the median follow-up was 1 year at the time of the data cutoff, because the treatment difference at the first interim efficacy analysis was so significant that the IDMC recommended release of study results earlier than anticipated) (30).

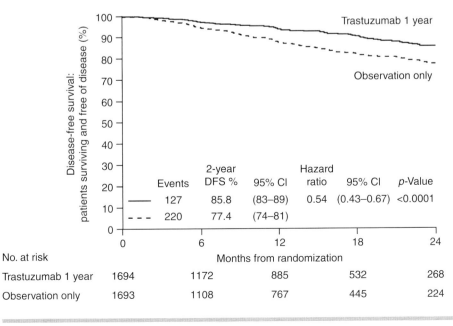

Figure 4.2 Kaplan-Meier estimates of the two disease-free survival distributions for the 1-year trastuzumab (Herceptin®) group and for the observation only group from the Herceptin Adjuvant (HERA) Trial. (30) The median follow-up of patients for this analysis is 1 year; the Independent Data Monitoring Committee (IDMC) released results earlier than anticipated because the treatment difference at the first interim analysis was so significant. Also shown are the estimated percentages of patients surviving disease-free at 2 years from randomization, the 95% confidence intervals for these estimates, the logrank *p* value for the treatment comparison, and the number of patients who remain at risk over time. The hazards ratio estimate—comparing the risk of an event in the trastuzumab group to the risk of an event in the observation only group—is 0.54 (95% confidence interval, 0.43–0.67) indicating a 46% reduction in the risk of an event with the trastuzumab treatment. *Abbreviations*: DFS, disease free survival; CI, confidence interval.

	Events	2-year DFS %	95% CI	Hazard ratio	95% CI	p-Value
——	127	85.8	(83–89)	0.54	(0.43–0.67)	<0.0001
- - -	220	77.4	(74–81)			

No. at risk

Trastuzumab 1 year	1694	1172	885	532	268
Observation only	1693	1108	767	445	224

Tests of hypothesis can be conducted on survival distributions. Equality of the survival distributions corresponding to two treatments is the hypothesis ordinarily tested in clinical trials having a survival end point. Such a test is conducted by computing a test statistic called the *logrank* statistic. This test is most powerful under the assumption that the ratio of the logarithm of the two true survival distributions is constant over time, which is not true if, for instance, the two survival curves cross or there is a plateau in one or both of the curves. Cure rate models might be more appropriate for the latter situation. Multiple regression analysis techniques are available to account for the effect of prognostic factors in the analysis of both proportions of events [logistic models (31)] and survival distributions [proportional hazards models (32)]. All of the above statistical methods are discussed in standard textbooks and are also readily available in statistical packages.

DEVELOPMENT AND EVALUATION OF NEW THERAPEUTIC APPROACHES

As noted at the beginning of this chapter, clinical trials are experiments conducted on human subjects, which address therapeutic questions. An important role of some studies is to amass the safety and efficacy information necessary to license a new therapeutic, though there are also numerous clinical trials conducted without that specific goal in mind. In Europe, the Committee for Medicinal Products for Human Use (CMPH) of the European Medicines Agency (EMEA) has provided important notes for guidance on conducting studies in cancer patients for the purpose of evaluating new anticancer medicines.[a]

In general, before any new drug can be licensed for approval randomized data demonstrating efficacy (progression-free or relapse-free survival, overall survival, palliation) must be demonstrated. In the United States, the Code of Federal Regulations describes similar criteria, though as of 1992 there is an additional provision to allow accelerated approval based on surrogate end points reasonably likely to predict clinical benefit.

The approval in these circumstances may be based on nonrandomized data, but the approval is contingent on there being a commitment to perform a randomized study to confirm clinical benefit (for a review see Ref. 33).

Traditionally, clinical trials are divided into three stages or phases: I, II, and III. In addition, recently in the United States, the Food and Drug Administration created the designation of "Phase 0" trials which are exploratory first-in-human trials that are designed to speed up the development of promising drugs by establishing very early on whether the drug or agent behaves in human subjects as was anticipated from preclinical studies (34). Phase I and II trials are most easily differentiated from each other within the context of the development of a new agent or therapeutic maneuver, where clear goals are articulated for each trial phase and decisions about the continued

evaluation of the new agent are made at the conclusion of phase I and II studies.

However, the concepts described here also apply to the evaluation of "old" drugs in new combinations, although within this context trials may combine the goals of phase I and II studies within a single protocol. The principles in the design and analysis of Phase III trials described below have identical application in the comparative study of new versus standard therapy and in the comparative evaluation of two or more standard therapeutic approaches.

Preclinical Data

The preclinical evaluation of any new drug should provide data on drug mechanism of action, pharmacology, toxicology, and efficacy. Essential pharmacokinetic (PK) data includes information regarding absorption, distribution, metabolism, and excretion for single and repeated drug administration schedules.

In compliance with international regulations, toxicology data, both acute and chronic, must be available from two animal species with data from the most sensitive species used to guide selection of the starting dose in subsequent Phase I studies (see ICH Guidelines M3, S4, S4A, S6, S7A, S7B on this topic at www.ich.org).

Biomarker studies should also be completed to give information about the molecular pharmacodynamic effects ("proof of principle") of the drug in tumor and normal tissues (35). Early identification of novel biomarkers in the drug discovery process is recommended to allow for the development and validation of bioanalytical methods prior to the commencement of clinical studies (36). When the molecular target of interest is also expressed in noncancerous tissue, then drug effect in those tissues can be studied and correlated with the changes seen in tumor tissue. These data may be used to guide dose selection in clinical studies when tumor sampling may not be feasible.

Regardless of the mechanism of action of any drug, antitumor efficacy in appropriate preclinical models must be demonstrated as a prerequisite for evaluation in clinical studies. Accepted efficacy end points for molecularly targeted agents include tumor shrinkage or inhibition of tumor growth (growth delay). The relationship between optimal antitumor effects in models and pharmacological exposure to drug with biomarker/target changes in tissues is an important piece of information to guide clinical development.

Finally, preclinical evidence of predictive tumor markers is important to garner: Is the drug effect limited to tumors of certain histologies? With specific molecular changes? These data, too, will guide clinical development.

Phase 0 Trials

As noted above, Phase 0 trials are a relatively new entity in cancer drug development. The goals of these studies are to establish drug specific biomarker assay methodology and feasibility in limited numbers of patients as a means of guiding subsequent drug development and ultimately, compressing timelines for new agent approval and enabling early identification of therapeutic failures (37). Other Phase 0 trials may be directed to selecting the better of two analogues for Phase I development on the basis of PK profile,

[a]See CMPH/EMEA Note for Guidance: Evaluation of Anticancer Medicinal Products in Man at http://www.emea.europa.eu/pdfs/human/ewp/020595en.pdf and http://www.emea.europa.eu/pdfs/human/ewp/2799408en.pdf

absorption characteristics, or other attributes. Limiting the number of dose levels and patients under evaluation lessens the need for extensive preclinical pharmacological and toxicology data. An example of a possible Phase 0 clinical trial involves the preoperative setting for patients with early breast cancer. A molecularly targeted agent at a predefined dose would be given in the short time period between the diagnostic biopsy and definitive surgery. Drug target modulation can be evaluated using pre- and post-treatment tumor biopsies, for example, altered levels of the active (phosphorylated) form of a protein. Inclusion of functional imaging studies can be considered as another measure of drug effect, for example, changes in tumor metabolism or vascularity and blood flow using serial PET scans or dynamic contrast enhanced (DCE) MRI examinations respectively. In addition to pharmacodynamic data, rigorous PK data collection is an essential part of Phase 0 clinical trial conduct. In June 2008, a special series of reports on Phase 0 trials in oncology was published by the American Association of Cancer Research (38), which highlights some of the special issues associated with these trials.

Phase I Trials

Goal and Primary End Point of Phase I Trials

Except when Phase 0 trials are undertaken, Phase I trials are the first clinical studies of a new agent or new therapeutic approach. Because of the toxic nature of many cancer therapies, Phase I trials are conducted in cancer patients who have failed standard therapy, rather than in normal volunteers. The *major goal* of Phase I trials is to determine the recommended dose of the agent(s) under study in the schedule administered (39). Secondary goals include description of toxic effects, PKs, determination of target inhibition (if appropriate), and documentation of any antitumor effects (i.e., response).

Using the data from the preclinical studies, a starting dose and dose escalation scheme are selected and applied to limited cohorts of patients until a predefined end point is met. The traditional end point used in Phase I studies of cytotoxic chemotherapy has been the maximum tolerated dose (MTD) which is based on toxicity assessment using standard criteria such as CTCAE v 3.0. Choice of this end point is based on the existence of a relationship between dose, efficacy, and toxicity seen in animal models, and to from historical analysis of clinical studies, thus allowing the use of toxicity as a surrogate of activity. Furthermore, for many agents, particularly cytotoxic drugs, but not exclusively, the mechanism of normal tissue toxicity is the same as that for the antitumor effects. The MTD is achieved when a predefined proportion of patients at a specific dose level develop serious toxicities (otherwise known as dose-limiting toxicities or DLTs) beyond which further dose escalation is not possible. The dose selected for further testing, the recommended Phase II dose (RPTD) is generally one dose level below the MTD.

Patient Selection

As Phase I trials evaluate therapies of unknown efficacy and potentially serious toxicity in patients with a life-threatening disease, there has been much written on the ethical considerations and patient selection criteria for these studies (39).

In general, only those patients who have exhausted treatments that offer an improvement in survival or cure rates should be enrolled. Furthermore, when the route of elimination and toxic effects in humans is unknown, patients entering Phase I trials should have adequate hepatic, renal, and hematologic function. The consent process should clearly outline the goals of the trial and that both benefit and toxicity are unknown. As dose levels approach the recommended Phase II dose, it is common practice to enroll "better risk" patients with characteristics more typical of those who might receive the drug in Phase II trials. In this way, the recommended dose will be assessed in a population similar to that in which it will be applied.

Phase I Trial Design

In broad terms, the design of a Phase I trial involves treating small cohorts of patients at ever-increasing doses of the drug(s) until toxic effects, or another end point, stops further escalation. Phase I trial design is guided by the principles of efficiency and minimization of exposure of participants to doses that are subtherapeutic or too toxic. There is debate about whether doses should be increased within individual patients: to do so may confuse acute versus cumulative toxic effects, but some believe this caution is not warranted (40). Three elements determine the duration of the trial and the total number of patients enrolled (1): the starting dose (2), the escalation method employed, and (3) the number of patients enrolled at each dose level.

The starting dose is derived from preclinical toxicology of the most sensitive species (e.g., 1/10 the mouse equivalent LD10 or 1/3 of the lowest nontoxic dose in the most sensitive species if nonmurine).

Multiple dose escalation schemes have been proposed and can be classified as those that are "rule based" and those that are "statistically based." The most widely used rule-based design from a historical perspective is the modified Fibonacci escalation. Using this, after an initial doubling of dose, each higher escalation steps has ever-decreasing relative dose increments until a fixed dose ratio is reached (e.g., dose increases of 100%, 65%, 50%, 40%, and 30–35% thereafter). Dose escalation continues until the MTD is reached, usually defined as the dose producing DLT in 2 of 3 or 2–3 of 6 patients. The next lower dose level is the recommended Phase II dose (RPTD).

Problems with the Fibonacci including its inefficiency and treatment of too many patients at subtherapeutic levels (41) have given rise to a number of different escalation approaches and suggestions for changing the number of patients enrolled at low doses (42,43).

Novel rule-based designs, focus on doubling the dose in successive patient cohorts until an "event" occurs which switches the escalation to a more conservative (e.g., fixed proportion) approach. The "event" may be the observation of a toxic effect (accelerated titration designs) or the achievement of a PK end point (e.g., 40% of the predicted AUC at the MTD, based on animal pharmacological studies) (44). Simulation techniques have shown that accelerated titration escalation is safe with the accrual of one patient per dose level switching to conservative escalation once DLT in one patient or Grade 2 toxicity in two patients had been seen (40). Similarly, pharmacologically guided dose escalation has been successfully applied to some trials but not others (45). Limitations of this latter method relate to wide inter-patient variability in PK seen with some compounds, problems with measuring or detecting blood levels, and the fact that some compounds in man have active metabolites not seen in animals.

The second approach to more efficient dose escalation has been statistically based. Examples include the Continual Reassessment Method (CRM) and modified CRM (46,47), and Escalation with Overdose Control (EWOC)(48) among others. These methodologies estimate MTD at the outset of the trial and utilize toxicity data accumulated throughout the study to refine the hypothetical dose-toxicity curve and update the MTD estimate. Dose levels, which are often preassigned, may be adjusted on the basis of the revised MTD estimates. The goals of these methodologies are to provide rapid, safe escalation to doses close to, but not surpassing, the MTD and to give a more precise estimate of the MTD at the end of the trial. Most practical experience has accumulated with the modified CRM method, which in addition to the dose-escalation process described above, usually involves enrollment of only one patient per dose level in the early stages of the trial. This method appears safe, treats more patients at or near the MTD, and enrolls fewer patients overall (49). However, it does not always shorten the duration of Phase I trials, likely due to the waiting period between dose levels to observe for drug related toxicity.

The enrollment of only one patient per dose level, particularly at the lowest doses of a Phase I trial, has become a frequent and apparently safe approach and is often included in the novel escalation schemes mentioned above. This approach could be problematic if wide inter-patient variability in toxicity is expected (such as for antifolates) when factors other than dose can contribute to the severity of toxicity (50), or when end points other than toxicity are used (e.g., pharmacodynamic measures), where more than one patient per dose level is required to assess the end point of interest appropriately.

Nontoxicity End Points: Pharmcodynamic and Pharmacokinetic End Points

Because many novel agents target intracellular or extracellular molecules that may be inhibited at doses below those maximally tolerated, the use of toxicity as the primary end point in Phase I trials of these drugs has been questioned (51,52). Furthermore, some evidence of proof of concept that these drugs are affecting their putative target is an important aspect of their early clinical development. Although toxicity may, in some cases, be mechanism based [e.g., rash from epidermal growth factor receptor (EGFR) inhibitors (53)], more direct evidence of target perturbation is often desired.

Although a direct assessment of target modulation is an attractive primary end point from a theoretical point of view, using this as the only guide for dose escalation decisions poses challenges. These include the availability of a validated assay to assess target effect in tumor (or normal) tissue as well as prior knowledge of the degree of modulation or inhibition of the target needed for dose selection (when laboratory assay methods are used to assess target effect). In addition, more patients will be required per dose

level using this approach as the tissue sampling required pre- and posttreatment may not be satisfactory in all enrolled patients. If functional imaging methods are the basis of assessment of target effect of drug, there are also challenges in determining standard methods, interpretation, and access to imaging technology. Finally, even if measurement of target effect is possible, observations on the toxic effects of the drug must still be made and, should these be severe, their observation immediately overrides any rules for escalation based on target modulation.

Pharmacokinetic (PK) measures may also be used as a primary end point for dose selection. The use of PK for this purpose requires that there are robust preclinical data linking PK measures with drug effect on target and efficacy, preferably in vivo. An example where this was used was in the Phase I study of cetuximab, a chimeric antibody directed against the epidermal growth factor receptor. In the Phase I study, no MTD was defined, so a dose range was recommended on the basis of PK data consistent with serum antibody concentrations above 200 nmol/L. This concentration of drug was associated with optimal antitumor activity in preclinical models (54). Subsequent studies demonstrated an inhibition of epidermal growth factor receptor (EGFR) activity in a surrogate tissue (skin) in patients treated with the optimal dose of cetuximab based on PKs (55).

Despite interest in assessing target modulation, in a recent review of Phase I trial design for molecularly targeted agents, toxicity and to a lesser extent PK data were the most frequently used end points to guide Phase II dose recommendation (56). In part, this is because often toxicity is mechanism based (and thus serves as a marker of drug effect). Furthermore, selection of the highest tolerable dose will minimize the chance of the dose being too *low* for target modulation or inhibition.

However, regardless of the "primary" end point for dose determination, the final dose recommendation very often is the result of multiple inputs: toxicity, PK, and when at all possible, proof of concept molecular studies. Indeed this approach to Phase I design of molecular targeted agents was recently concluded to be a sensible one to draw together all available data (57).

Phase II Trials
Goal and Primary End Point of Phase II Trials

Once the recommended dose and schedule for a new therapy is available, Phase II trials may begin. The primary goal of these trials is to screen the new agent or regimen for efficacy and to estimate the level of activity. Through this, Phase II single agent trials may provide guidance regarding the future development strategy of the drug or combination. The traditional measure of drug efficacy has been objective tumor regression defined by standard criteria such as RECIST (2). Objective response is the only end point for single agent Phase II trials that has reliably been shown to identify agents that, in later studies, are shown to improve survival. Although not all agents causing responses increase survival, some do. Other end points that used Phase II trials can include measures of tumor progression, tumor marker response [e.g., ovarian and prostate cancers (58–60)] feasibility, PKs, toxicity, and the early exploration of the possible molecular predictors of effect through appropriate biomarker studies.

When objective response is the primary end point, the single agent Phase II trial of a new drug determines if the experimental agent has a response rate above a targeted value deemed critical for pursuing the agent further. The target response rate is often set at 20% but this may vary depending on the tumor type and the patient population under evaluation. For example, a response rate of 15% might be of interest in a tumor such as melanoma, but a higher rate of 30% might be a more realistic target value in untreated breast cancer, which is responsive to numerous agents. Of major importance in this type of trial is the need to minimize the chance that a *truly* active agent is erroneously rejected. That is, the trial design should attempt to limit the probability of a false negative result (type II error). False positive conclusions about the activity of a new drug will be uncovered by its further evaluation following the initial Phase II trial. However, if a false negative conclusion leads to the rejection of the new agent, there may not be another trial conducted to provide the true information.

Combination Phase II trials are similar in the sense that they are designed to determine the activity of a combination regimen against a target level of activity. For example, a new multi-drug regimen in breast cancer might only proceed into Phase III trials if in Phase II it produces response rates superior to a prespecified target value determined based on standard combination therapy results. However, other factors, primarily toxic effects, will be important to the decision about the regimen's future. Thus, in this setting, not only efficacy, but also toxicity, is estimated and both parameters are important in the decision to pursue the regimen further.

Patient Selection

Entry criteria for Phase II studies vary according to the agent and tumor type under investigation. In general, patients with measurable, advanced disease are eligible. Extensive prior therapy, poor performance status, and high tumor burden may impact negatively on response rates and such patients may be excluded from these studies. The requirement for minimal or no prior therapy is somewhat controversial especially in tumor types where the disease is treatable even in the advanced state. In such situations (so-called window trials), patients may be entered onto study as long as they are followed closely and offered standard therapy upon patient request, at physician discretion, or once progression has been demonstrated. For Phase II studies of molecularly targeted therapy, correlative studies using tumor or other surrogate tissue may be included as part of study design. In these situations the eligibility criteria must clearly state whether availability of tissue, whether from previous diagnostic surgery or collected in fresh biopsies, is a requirement for study entry.

Phase II Trial Design

As noted above, an important aspect of the design of Phase II studies is the need to limit the risk of false negative conclusions and to provide an adequate estimate of activity in positive studies. The other major consideration that affects design is the desire to limit exposure of excessive numbers of patients to truly ineffective treatment. These competing requirements—to have enough patients to be

sure that the agent is truly inactive before it is rejected, but not so many that excessive numbers of patients receive inactive therapy—have led to trial designs having two or more sequential stages of accrual. Should insufficient activity be seen after the first stage, the study will be terminated, only continuing to the end of the second (or third) stage if sufficient numbers of responding patients are noted.

A number of such multistage designs have been described, which utilize objective tumor response as the primary end point (61–63). The sample size for a Phase II trial depends on the specification of a number of parameters that differ according to the tumor type, patient population, and the drug under evaluation. These parameters include target levels of activity and the two desired error limits. The α error is a measure of the probability of accepting an inactive drug (false positive result) and the β error a measure of the probability of rejecting a truly active drug (false negative result). The multistage designs "reject" an agent and stop the trial early if too few responses are seen at the end of the first stage. The numbers of consecutive nonresponding patients that must be enrolled to reject a drug depends on the target response rate hypothesized to be of interest. The lower the response rate of interest, the greater the number of consecutive failures needed to conclude that the agent does not meet the hypothetical level of activity. Alternatively, to decrease the risk of false negative conclusions (i.e., decrease the type II error or β) the sample size in the first stage must be increased.

An example of a multistage design, the Gehan design (61), focuses primarily on the elimination of drugs having a level of activity less than a prespecified amount, often 20%, which in practice translates into accrual of 14 patients and terminating the study if no responses are seen. This number is based on the fact that the probability of observing 0/14 responses when the true response rate is 20% is <0.05 [(1 − 0.20)(14) < 0.05]. If the agent passes the first stage, more patients are entered according to the level of presumed therapeutic effectiveness and the desired level of error (β). In the example given of 14 patients in the initial stage, the observation of one response will lead to an expansion of 11 additional patients to obtain a power of 90%, and an expansion of 45 additional patients to obtain a 95% power. Table 4.2 shows examples of sample sizes for Phase II trials using the Gehan design with varying target response rates of interest and β errors.

Table 4.2 Sample Sizes for the Initial Cohort in Phase II Trials Using the Gehan Design (61)

Target minimum Response rate (%)	Number of patients in first stage if	
	$\beta = 0.05$	$\beta = 0.10$
5	59	45
10	29	22
15	19	15
20	14	11
25	11	9
30	9	7
35	7	6
40	6	5
45	6	4
50	5	4

Both the Fleming (62) and the Simon (63) designs require that two "target" levels of activity be hypothesized: a lower response rate (p_0) below which there would be no interest in pursuing the agent further, and a higher response rate (p_1) representing a level of activity of definite interest. In the Fleming design, the trial is terminated at the end of the first stage if extreme results are observed in either direction: that is, if the evidence supports either the hypothesis that the agent's activity is less than p_0 or that the regimen has definite activity above p_1. It will only continue to the second stage if neither of these conditions is met. At the end of the second stage, recommendations to accept or reject the drug for further investigation are again made on the basis of the final observed number of responses. Table 4.3 illustrates the Fleming design using as hypotheses p_1 of 20–40% and p_0 of 5–20% in various combinations.

A problem with the Fleming design is that, when the criteria for high activity are met, the trial will stop early, but there is often a desire in clinicians to continue accrual to broaden experience with the agent and obtain a better estimates of activity. In an attempt to address this, Simon (63) has published the "optimal two-stage early rejection design." This design continues enrolment when activity is seen at the end of the first stage.

Other Phase II design options deserve comment. The first is one in which examination of another end point besides response is incorporated in a multivariate approach. Zee and colleagues have examined the utility of considering both response and early progression in decisions about early study termination (64,65). This approach presumes that an agent with excessive rates of early progression will not have a great deal to contribute, even if it produces occasional responses. Both the number of early progressors and responders are evaluated at the early stopping point and the decision to continue accrual depends on the frequency of both end points.

Furthermore, "randomized Phase II trials" are being seen more commonly (66). Usually the term randomized is used in the context of large sample size, Phase III trials adequately powered to make comparisons between treatment arms (see section "Phase III trials"). However, in the Phase II setting, there are some circumstances when it may be advantageous to randomize patients. The first instance is when two or more investigational regimens are available for study. Randomizing between regimens is a convenient way to accrue similar patient populations to simultaneous trials but there is no intent to compare outcomes as each arm has their own stopping rules. The second type of randomized Phase II trial has been dubbed a "pick the winner" design. Patients are randomized to two or more potentially active regimens and the design is focused on

selecting the one most likely to be superior by a prespecified amount. Scenarios where this may be logical are when two doses or schedules of the same drug are pitted against each other to derive data allowing the selection of the "winning" regimen to go into further study against standard therapy. Such trials are not adequately powered to determine the superior regimen, rather the statistical calculation allows for reasonable certainty that if one of the regimens is truly more active by a prespecified degree (e.g., 15% higher response rate), the probability is high that it will be declared the winner and selected for further study. This strategic approach has been used in trials comparing various methods of administration of the cytotoxic agent topotecan (67). Finally, randomized Phase II trials may assign patients to either a standard versus an investigational therapy and then evaluate an efficacy measure (response, proportion progression-free at a fixed time point, progression free survival). This design may be used in a *noncomparative* manner where the activity level in the standard arm will allow greater confidence in interpretation of the results in the experimental arm, as it provides information about the patient population entered on the study. Alternatively, such a design may be used with *comparative* intent, having higher alpha levels than is usual in Phase III trials. This is most frequently applied when nonresponse end points are used (see below) (68,69).

Challenges in Phase II Trials of Novel Noncytotoxics

Use of Response End Point. For molecularly targeted agents that may inhibit growth as their primary mechanism of action (i.e., cytostatic rather than cytotoxic), from a theoretical perspective, objective response may not provide a useful signal of drug activity. These agents will need to prove their worth by prolonging survival, but short of large randomized trials, are there other end points besides response which may be used to screen these drugs for promising evidence of efficacy in small patient samples? A variety of alternative end points have been considered for use in nonrandomized Phase II trials including change in rate of rise of tumor marker levels, functional imaging, measures of target inhibition and rates of stable disease or its opposite, clinical progression rates, or a continuous measure of tumor size (51,52,69,70). However, all of these options remain infrequently used so it is difficult to assess their utility in identifying truly active drugs (71). Furthermore, designs that rely on measures of progression (PFS or proportion progression free) carry with them the bias of patient selection, which hampers the interpretation of results from single arm studies. Thus the use of randomized

---

Table 4.3 Examples of Fleming Design (62) and Stopping Rules for Phase II Trials

p_0 (%)	p_1 (%)	α	Power (1 - β)	Number of patients			First stage		End of study	
				First stage	Second stage	Total	Reject drug ≤resp	Accept drug ≥resp	Reject drug ≤resp	Accept drug ≥resp
5	20	0.058	0.865	15	15	30	0	4	3	4
10	30	0.031	0.839	15	15	30	1	5	6	7
20	40	0.037	0.801	20	15	35	4	9	11	12

designs as noted earlier, or a randomized discontinuation design have been suggested when progression end points are believed to be most appropriate. The randomized discontinuation design randomizes patients archiving a minimum period of stable disease on a new agent to continue or discontinue the drug and comparers the progression-free survival following randomization (72). A challenge to the use of this design relate to the potential large number of patients treated in the inception cohort to acquire sufficient numbers to randomize (68).

Some investigators have chosen to avoid the problem of identifying the activity of noncytotoxics in Phase II by moving them directly from Phase I to Phase III trials. This approach may be justified when the preclinical data are compelling and if early stopping rules are part of the randomized study design. The most appropriate stopping rule for this circumstance is one which would require early evidence that the experimental arm is more active than control (e.g., fewer patients progressing at a fixed time point), rather than the more common stopping rule based on extreme results (see section "Interim analysis stopping boundaries and data safety monitoring boards"). This design may also be referred to as a "seamless" Phase II–III trial. Studies with designs of this nature are underway and their efficiency and utility will be known in the next 5–10 years.

Incorporation of Biomarkers. The Phase II setting provides an opportunity to explore molecular targets and strategies of patient enrichment (73). If prior knowledge of a biomarker that may predict drug activity exists, then the Phase II study may be enriched with patients with the (presumed) predictive characteristic. As this is usually not known prior to commencement of the Phase II study, a more practical approach would be to use a standard Phase II design and prioritize correlative studies as part of study conduct. This would mandate the availability of an adequate tumor specimen (diagnostic or freshly sampled) as an eligibility criterion for all patients who are entered on the study. Prospective declaration of a predictive biomarker to be tested in the study would allow one to focus on a particular hypothesis and assay methodology. Another strategy would be to characterize the molecular profiles of tumor specimens from responders and nonresponders to a particular therapy. Comparisons of the molecular profiles of these groups might lead to a hypothesis of a predictive biomarker that could be further evaluated in another Phase II study or be incorporated as a stratification factor in a Phase III trial.

Interpretation of Results of Phase II Trials

At the conclusion of a "positive" Phase II trial, the overall response rate should be reported along with the appropriate 95% confidence intervals. RECIST guidelines advocate that the denominator should include all eligible patients regardless of their evaluability. Indeed, particularly in randomized Phase II designs, some would argue that an intent to treat analysis is required which would include all patients, not just those eligible. Modifications to the size of the denominator can have a substantial effect on the estimates of activity. Phase II reports should include details about the population studied, especially with respect to those

characteristics known to affect response. Finally, as some have shown, independent review of imaging to verify responses will decrease response rates substantially (74). Each of these elements will have an impact on the final response rate and thus the enthusiasm with which results are greeted.

Phase III Trials
Goal and End Point of Phase III Trials

Phase III clinical trials *compare* one or more experimental therapies with the best standard therapy or competitive therapies. When there is no effective standard therapy a placebo treatment may be the comparator. End points for a Phase III trial are selected to reflect comparative efficacy among treatments and include time-to-event information, tumor response, toxicity, quality of life, or other measures of treatment effectiveness.

Patient Selection

As Phase III trials are often the basis for widespread use of a new treatment approach, patients enrolled in the trial should be representative of the patients for whom the treatment will be used in practice. The patient risk profile should be such that the benefits are likely to outweigh the risks for study participants. Enrollment of patients with an exceptionally good prognosis may dilute the ability of the trial to detect treatment differences as the event rate will be lower than anticipated. Patients who might be at increased risk to suffer toxic effects of treatment—for example, those with compromised hematology, liver, renal, or cardiac function—may be excluded from the trial. The eligibility and ineligibility criteria should be clearly described to identify the population to which the observed results might apply.

Generally speaking, eligibility criteria for Phase III trials that are inclusive and broad based are preferred, enabling results to be extrapolated to a larger population, and providing the opportunity to study treatment effects across a variety of subpopulations. Recently, there has been an emphasis on recruiting special populations—minority races, female sex, and elderly—to clinical trials, so that treatment effects can also be evaluated within these groups. Although pediatric malignancies are very rare, a large percentage of pediatric oncology patients are enrolled in clinical trials. The opportunity for cure must be balanced against the risk of long-term treatment sequelae for the pediatric population.

Randomization, Stratification, Minimization, and Blinding

One of the main objectives of a Phase III trial design is to eliminate systematic biases that could influence the comparison of the treatments. Bias can arise in many different ways, ranging from the selection process of the patients to be assigned to the different treatments, to the lack of proper follow-up, to the imbalance of the distribution of prognostic factors or of treatment delivery among the arms. One way to reduce bias is to make sure that a proper *randomization* procedure is used to generate comparable patient groups (75). Randomization consists of the use of a chance mechanism to assign patients to the treatments, and it ensures that each patient in a study has the same opportunity of being assigned to the therapies in the trial. It makes the treatment groups "alike on the average" with respect to all factors (known or unknown) that may affect the end points of the trial. Neither the doctor nor the patient should know in advance which of the treatments will be assigned. Thus, randomization eliminates the possibility that the preferences of patients or clinicians will influence the constitution of the treatment groups. Simple randomization by chance can result in an unbalanced number of treatments being assigned. *Random permuted block randomization* assigns patients to treatments within blocks so that after a specific number of assignments have been made (e.g., after every fourth or eighth treatment assignment) the number of patients assigned to each treatment is the same. A balanced assignment of patients to treatments is the most statistically efficient use of a fixed number of randomized patients. However, there might be advantages for an *unbalanced* randomization in which the allocation of patients to treatments is unequal—such as making a trial more acceptable by having a twofold chance of getting the experimental arm.

A strategy often used to further reduce potential bias is a *stratified randomization* plan. Patient subgroups (called *strata*) are defined with respect to a set of prognostic factors that may influence the outcome, and randomization is carried out separately within each stratum to guarantee balance among treatment groups. Stratification is helpful especially in small trials, or in the early stages of larger trials. A random permuted block design within strata can assure prognostic factor balance across treatments within strata. It is important, however, to avoid including too many strata in the design, as this will reduce the trial's efficiency. A process known as *minimization* has also been used to balance treatment groups with respect to prognostic factors (76). To use minimization, the prognostic factors of the patients in each treatment group are accounted for during the accrual period of the study. As each new patient is identified for enrollment, the sum of prognostic factors corresponding to those of the new patient is calculated for each treatment group. The patient is assigned to the treatment which would minimize the difference between prognostic factors in each treatment.

An additional safeguard against bias is the design of a *blinded* trial, that is, one in which patients are not aware of the treatment to which they have been assigned. Such trials (when feasible) are termed *single blinded*. A *double blinded* trial is one in which neither the patient nor the physician know the treatment assignment. Blinded trials require that the physical aspect of the treatments be the same, and this is not always possible. Also, toxic effects clearly associated with one or more of the treatments may make blinding impossible. Blinding, however, is particularly valuable in trials for which the end point is subjective, such as pain relief. Blinding is also useful to improve compliance with treatment administration and to enhance the chances that the frequency and intensity of follow-up examinations are the same for both treatment groups. In addition, accurate assessment of the true extent of additional toxicity associated with treatment can only be assessed if the trial is blinded. *Placebo controlled* trials use an inert substance packaged to resemble the experimental drug in place of the active treatment in order to blind the study.

The lack of proper follow up, as well as more general issues of compliance, can seriously bias the conclusions from a trial. These issues may include the unwillingness/ inability of a patient to fill out a form, the failure to follow a patient for study end points, or the discontinuation of the randomized treatment. All of these issues generate missing data, either in the usual sense (e.g., a missing form) or in the general meaning of not being able to observe the outcome that one is really interested in for each patient. We will comment below on what is known as the "intent-to-treat" approach to the analysis and the interpretation of data arising from clinical trials.

Two by Two Factorial, Crossover, and Equivalence (Noninferiority) Studies

Several specialized types of designs are available to improve the efficiency of Phase III clinical trials. *Two by two factorial designs* (77,78) use all randomized patients to investigate two treatment interventions simultaneously within the same trial. For example, to evaluate the effects of treatments A and B, patients would be randomized to one of four groups: treatment A, treatment B, both, or neither. The effect of treatment A would be estimated by comparing all patients who received treatment A with those who did not receive treatment A, stratifying the analysis according to whether or not treatment B was also received. Estimating the effect of treatment B would be done in the same way. Two by two factorial designs are most appropriate when there is no preexisting knowledge suggesting a strong interaction between the effects of the two test treatments. In contrast to the three arm study (treatment A, treatment B, and neither), the 2×2 design provides an estimate of the treatment interaction. Factorial designs are underutilized in Phase III cancer clinical trials.

In *crossover designs* (79), each patient receives each study treatment sequentially during different time periods. Patients are randomized to receive either treatment A during the first period followed by treatment B during the second period, or the reverse order of treatment administration. The comparison of treatment effects is conducted within each patient and the results accumulated across all patients. This type of design is useful if a distinct end point can be measured within each time period to reflect the treatment effect obtained in that period, or if it is possible to administer two treatments and elicit a preference from the patient. Crossover designs are very efficient because each patient provides his or her own control and the interpatient variability of the response is reduced. However, a period effect (difference in treatment response associated with the period of evaluation) or a period-treatment interaction (different treatment response associated with the period during which each treatment is received) will reduce the efficiency of the design and complicate the interpretation of results. The pharmaceutical industry has favored these designs on the basis of their efficiency, although the FDA has discouraged them due to the potential for confounding. The designs discussed above should not be confused with studies that allow patients who experience progressive disease though receiving one treatment to receive the alternative therapy at the time of progression. These studies might be more acceptable to doctors and patients because patients who fail their first treatment have an opportunity to receive the second, but the crossover portion of the protocol is not intended to provide a direct comparison of treatments.

Another frequently used design is the *equivalence* (or *noninferiority*) trial (80,81). In contrast to the usual *superiority* trial design which seeks to provide evidence against the null hypothesis (to demonstrate superiority of one treatment over another), the equivalence trial seeks to "prove" the null hypothesis by collecting evidence against the possibility that the experimental treatment is really worse than the standard. Because a clinical trial can never fully guarantee that the two treatments are exactly equal, the goal is to demonstrate that the new treatment is not likely to be inferior to the old by an amount that is considered to be medically unacceptable. These designs are useful if the new treatment is less toxic, less costly, more convenient than the old, and would be recommended on these grounds as long as efficacy was not compromised too much. The sample sizes for equivalence trials are ordinarily larger than for superiority trials, because the magnitude of treatment inferiority that would be tolerable is usually very small. In addition, the inferiority threshold stated in the study design influences the hypothesis testing result; if someone disagrees with the choice of this threshold, the conclusions of the study might be disputed. Thus, noninferiority trial designs should be used sparingly, only when the therapeutic question cannot be addressed by a superiority design.

Sample Size Determination for Phase III Trials

All quantities evaluated on trial patients constitute *estimates* of the corresponding characteristics of the patient population, and as such they are subject to variability. Patients enrolled in a trial are only a (usually very small) portion of the potential population of patients that one has in mind when designing the study. If the same trial were to be conducted twice (on two different samples of patients), it would be very unlikely for the numerical values of any measure used to quantify treatment effect (such as the proportion of patients still alive after 5 years) to be identical for the two trials. The *precision* of an estimate defines how close it is likely to be to the true (unknown) population value, and depends on the sample size of the trial.

The sample size determination depends on several factors: the end point of interest, the goal of the data analysis, assumptions about the true variability of observations, specification of the magnitude of treatment differences of interest, the size of acceptable statistical errors (Type I and Type II), the availability of subjects in the eligible population, and the cost of running the trial. For a time-to-event end point, the sample size is based on the number of events observed at the time of analysis; additional assumptions about the event rate, the accrual period and the subsequent follow-up interval are thus required to determine the number of patients to enroll. Occasionally sample sizes are based on the number of patients needed to obtain a 95% confidence interval for the difference between two treatments, which is no wider than a specified amount. Most often the sample size is determined such that the final test of hypothesis will have a prespecified *power* $(1 - \beta)$. The power of a test is the probability that the test will reject the null hypothesis if the true treatment effect difference is bigger than a prespecified clinically worthwhile amount (i.e., when a specific alternative hypothesis is true). The power of 80% or better is commonly used. Specifying the alternative hypothesis for the analysis of proportions involves making an assumption about the event rate for the traditional treatment (usually based on previous knowledge), and specifying the smallest clinically relevant difference in event rate between such therapy and the new treatment under investigation. Together with the selected type I error of the test (traditionally 5%), these quantities determine the minimum number of patients that must be recruited in each arm. Table 4.4 shows the required sample sizes per treatment group for a variety of situations (82).

For survival analyses the determination of the sample size is computed similarly. A survival distribution can be summarized by its median survival time, which is the time point at which 50% of the patients are still alive. Alternatively, the probability of survival at a given time point (e.g., at 5 years) can be used. An assumption (again, based on previous knowledge) must be made about the median survival corresponding to the traditional therapy, as well as the smallest clinically relevant difference in median survival between the two treatments. The desired power of the test and its type I error must also be provided. On the basis of these quantities, the required number of patients who might have an event of interest can be determined. A sufficient number of patients must be enrolled

Table 4.4 Number of Patients Per Treatment for a Comparative Trial Based on Proportions (Assuming a Two-sided False-positive Rate of 5% and Equal Allocation of Patients to Each Treatment)

Magnitude of clinically important differences between proportions			Sensitivity or power			
r_1		r_2	0.5	0.7	0.8	0.9
10%	vs.	15%	375	579	725	957
10%	vs.	20%	117	176	219	286
10%	vs.	30%	40	58	71	92
10%	vs.	40%	22	31	38	48
40%	vs.	45%	791	1245	1573	2093
40%	vs.	50%	210	324	407	538
40%	vs.	60%	58	86	107	139
40%	vs.	70%	27	40	48	62

For more extensive tables see Ref. (82) (Table A.3).

Table 4.5 Sample Size for a Survival End Point Illustrating the Role of Accrual Period and Additional Follow-up Time. Number of Patients Per Treatment to Detect an Improvement in Median Survival from 12 to 18 Months (Level of Significance = 0.05; Power = 0.80)

Years of accrual	Years of additional follow-up		
	1	2	3
1	150	117	104
2	132	110	103
3	122	107	102

and followed for a long enough period of time to enable the required number of events to be observed. Studies in populations of patients at low risk of an event, therefore, require enrollment of many more patients than studies in high-risk populations. The anticipated event rate, the accrual rate, the accrual period, and the follow-up period are specified to determine the total number of patients required. Tables such as the one shown in Table 4.5 are then available to illustrate the required sample size (83,84).

Interim Analysis Stopping Boundaries and Data Safety Monitoring Boards

One of the recent advances in the statistical design of randomized clinical trials has been the development of procedures that facilitate interim analysis of study data without increasing the risk of obtaining a false-positive result based on multiple looks at the data. Flexible group sequential methods are now available to allow early stopping of trials if interim results indicate either a striking advantage for one treatment over the other, or no difference at all (85–87). Software is also available to design sequential stopping boundaries (88). The characteristics of the sequential design must be established prior to initiation of the trial and any data analysis. If boundaries are altered to fit the observed data, the protection against an inflated false-positive error rate is violated.

Almost all Phase III clinical trials are currently conducted under the guidance of a Data Safety Monitoring Board [also called Independent Data Monitoring Committee (IDMC) in the ICH GCP guidelines]. Principles defining the composition, independence, and responsibilities of this board have been described by the U.S. National Cancer Institute (89) and Food and Drug Administration (90). Essentially, interim results and safety monitoring data are periodically presented to the Board (consisting of independent scientists and patient representatives), and the board advises the study investigators on the continued viability and ethical conduct of the trial. In this way, investigators who are participating in the trial are not exposed to interim study results that might bias their participation. The committee is charged with protecting the interests of patients in the study (both current and future patients) and assuring that the study continues to meet the highest ethical standards for clinical trial conduct. This includes taking into consideration new information that might have become available from other studies.

Biomarker Studies in Phase III Trials

Biomarker studies are increasingly incorporated into the design and conduct of Phase III trials as a means of exploring the molecular basis of cancer behavior and response to therapy. If sufficient criteria are met, biomarkers can be classified as being prognostic or predictive (12).

The first step in determining the utility of a biomarker may involve a retrospective analysis of the clinical database compiled in a Phase III study. Using available tumor/tissue specimens collected on study, the presence or absence of the molecular target of interest is determined and measured in a quantitative or qualitative fashion. Using an appropriate assay and cut points for assay results, specimens are classified as marker positive/negative or high/low. Comparison of the outcome of all patients classified as marker positive to the outcome of those designated marker negative will yield an estimate of the prognostic value of the marker. Comparison of the outcomes of patients with known marker status when treated with/without a particular therapy will provide information regarding the predictive value of the marker for that therapy. Due to the possibility that a biomarker is both prognostic and predictive, all subgroups as defined by patient and treatment status are compared. The appropriate statistical methodology is required for these types of subgroup analyses (see section "Subgroup analysis").

This strategy was utilized in a study examining the relationship between molecular changes in a DNA repair gene (biomarker) and response to therapy and outcome in patients with a type of brain tumor (glioblastoma) who were previously enrolled in a Phase III study comparing radiotherapy with or without the addition of an oral chemotherapy agent known as temozolomide. The Phase III study demonstrated a statistically and clinically significant survival advantage with the use of combined therapy compared to radiotherapy alone (91). Retrospective analysis of patients with tumor biopsy specimens assessable for this genetic alteration showed that the presence of the biomarker was independently associated with prognosis and appeared to predict a greater benefit from combined radiotherapy and temozolomide compared to radiotherapy alone. The latter result was not statistically significant in a multivariate analysis, most likely due to the lack of power to test for interactions in the subgroup analyses (92). This example demonstrates the exploratory nature of retrospective analyses and the challenges associated with such analyses. In addition to power issues, patient selection bias may also influence results as patient and disease characteristics in the group for whom tumor samples are available may be different than those for whom samples could not be retrieved.

A more rigorous approach to retrospective validation of a biomarker in the context of a Phase III randomized study involves collection of tumor samples in sufficient numbers of patients in each treatment arm and knowledge of the assay techniques and algorithms which will be used for the analyses. The biological hypotheses of interest and the sample sizes needed to test these hypotheses must be declared prospectively. This approach was used to test a multigene assay as a prognostic biomarker in tamoxifen-treated, node negative breast cancer (93) and in general, may be considered when there are ethical and logistical constraints to launching a prospective randomized Phase

III study to test the clinical utility of a biomarker. Special mention is needed regarding the concepts of training and test sets. A training set comprises data from which the prognostic or predictive biomarker is derived. The test set refers to another set of data required to validate the biomarker role previously identified. Independence of both data sets minimizes the chance of reaching the wrong conclusion regarding the importance of the biomarker and is an important aspect of these types of analyses.

Incorporation of biomarkers into Phase III clinical trial design can also be done in a prospective fashion. A biomarker may be used as an eligibility criterion, thus enriching the patient population for study of a new agent of combination of agents. This type of design was used to investigate the efficacy of trastuzumab in early and advanced breast cancer (30,94,95). Trastuzumab is an antibody directed against the extracellular domain of the HER2 receptor. This receptor is overexpressed in approximately 20% of patients with breast cancer and is associated with a poor prognosis (96–98). Only patients with HER2 positive disease were eligible for inclusion in the pivotal Phase III studies. The strategy of limiting recruitment to those patients with a biomarker of interest may result in a smaller sample size needed to detect important treatment effects of a specific therapy and may also prevent premature declaration of failure for those agents with modest but clinically important efficacy in selected populations (but no detectable efficacy in unselected populations). Disadvantages to this strategy include the need for in-depth understanding of the drug mechanism of action and the availability of an accurate and reproducible assay prior to study commencement. Finally, the exclusion of patients without the biomarker of interest may lead to an incomplete understanding of drug effects and the potential patient population who might benefit from a particular therapy.

Prospective clinical trial designs for predictive marker validation have been described by Sargent et al. and can be classified as indirect or direct assessments (12). All require biomarker status determination prior to randomization. In the indirect assessment strategy, the patient population is split into marker positive and negative groups followed by randomization to the standard and experimental therapies in both groups. The statistical methods for analysis vary for this type of study and include a test for interaction between marker status and treatment or a formal comparison between the treatment effects in each marker group.

In the *direct assessment* design, the randomization is between use of the marker to determine therapy versus determination of therapy independent of marker status. The primary outcome comparison is between the group of patients in the marker-based arm versus the group of patients in the nonmarker-based arm.

An example of the *indirect assessment* clinical trial design is found in a North American Intergroup lung cancer protocol (N0723). This planned study will evaluate the prognostic and predictive role of EGFR status as defined by fluorescent in situ hybridization (FISH) analysis. In this study, EGFR status will be determined in all patients. Those with EGFR positive tumors will be randomized to receive EGFR targeted therapy with a small molecule tyrosine kinase inhibitor versus treatment with pemetrexed chemotherapy. Those with marker negative disease will be randomly allocated to receive the same agents. Thus this design will utilize an indirect marker assessment strategy to determine the clinical utility of EGFR status.

A variation on the prospective marker validation designs described above is utilized in the MINDACT trial (EORTC 10041/BIG 03/04). This trial seeks to determine the clinical utility of a genomic-based score for risk stratification and treatment allocation in 6000 patients with node negative breast cancer (99). Previous data had demonstrated that the genomic biomarker profile outperformed several clinical methods of risk assessment commonly used in clinical practice such as the Nottingham Prognostic Index, the St. Gallen criteria, and the Adjuvant! Software (100). In the MINDACT study, patients will have their risk of disease recurrence estimated by the genomic signature as well as by histopathological features using the Adjuvant! online program. Those patients with high-risk disease according to both methods will be treated with chemotherapy; low-risk disease will be treated with endocrine therapy. Those patients with discordant results will undergo randomization to use of either the genomic score or clinicopathologic features to guide therapeutic decisions. Using this design, The MINDACT trial is the first to evaluate prospectively the value of a microarray-based prognostic marker and to test the feasibility of its clinical application.

Challenges for the Future

The links between clinical trials research and bench sciences should continue to be strengthened. Randomized clinical trials should be conducted with the prospective creation of a pathology tissue bank and imbedding of translational biological questions whenever possible to be used to evaluate current and future markers that might predict treatment outcomes. Not only is it important to determine whether or not a treatment is effective, it is also important to determine those patients for whom the magnitude of the effect might be largest. Biological correlates of treatment effectiveness are likely to be extremely important for tailoring treatments for specific patient populations in the future.

Phase IV Trials

The term "Phase IV clinical trial" usually refers to a clinical trial designed to monitor a new drug after it has been approved to be marketed. The goals of the monitoring usually relate to adverse effects as well as additional large-scale, long-term studies of morbidity and mortality. Another goal of these trials is the identification of subsets of patients for whom the drug performs particularly well. This can be very important for marketing purposes, as well as for further developments of the drug. For example, the results of these trials may form the basis for a label change.

INTERPRETING THE RESULTS OF TRIALS

Guidelines for reporting clinical trials are designed to assure the reader of the quality of the study and to improve the accurate interpretation of the results (101). A consensus has been published on the consolidation of standards for reporting trials (CONSORT statement) (102,103). These guidelines are used by many medical journals.

Intention-to-Treat Analysis

Randomization in Phase III trials is intended to reduce systematic bias that could confound treatment comparisons. Excluding patients from data analysis can, however, defeat the purpose of randomization and introduce bias. For example, in a trial comparing chemotherapy versus no chemotherapy, excluding patients who do not complete chemotherapy could leave only the "healthiest" patients in the chemotherapy group, although all patients would be included in the no-chemotherapy group. Even if the trial were randomized, it is clear that those patients who remain after the exclusion are not comparable between the two groups. The *intention-to-treat principle* calls for including all patients in the primary data analysis according to their randomized treatment. The intention to use chemotherapy is compared against the intention not to use chemotherapy. Although the treatment effect estimated from the trial could be diluted by including noncompliant patients, the potential for bias introduced by patient exclusion is a greater concern. Intention-to-treat analysis has, therefore, become standard for the primary evaluation in comparative clinical trials.

Interpreting the *p* Value and the Role of Confidence Intervals

The interpretation of *p* values is often a source of confusion. The *p* value resulting from a statistical test of hypothesis is *not* the probability that the two treatments are equivalent (or different), but rather a measure of the strength of the evidence against the null hypothesis. The distinction between statistical and clinical significance should also be clear: *p* values have nothing to do with the quantification of *treatment effect*, which is measured by the difference in response rates, or in median survival between the treatment arms. To illustrate this point consider two clinical trials, each designed to compare the effect of two treatments, and suppose that the results of the two trials are summarized in the table below.

	Observed response (%)		*p* Value
	Rate for arm A	Rate for arm B	
Trial 1	20	30	0.3
Trial 2	20	30	0.03

The conclusion that the two treatments compared in the first trial do not differ in effect, although the two treatments compared in the second trial do differ, is wrong. In fact, the large *p* value in the first trial is because of the fact that the trial was not powerful enough to detect the difference in response rate, that is, its sample size was probably too small. The point estimates and 95% confidence intervals for the difference in response rates provide a more informative summary of the estimated magnitude of the treatment effect difference. These estimates for arm B versus arm A are +10% (−10% to +30%) for trial 1 and +10% (+3% to +17%) for trial 2. In both studies, the observed response for treatment B is 10% higher than for treatment A, but the 95% confidence interval for the difference includes 0% in trial 1 (hence the *p* value is greater than 0.05) but does not include 0% in trial 2 (hence the *p* value is less than 0.05). The confidence interval provides a range of plausible values for the difference in response rate based on the observed data.

In Phase III cancer clinical trials the treatment effects realistically sought after can be quite small. However, even moderate benefits can be of real clinical importance because of the large number of patients that a change in therapy might potentially affect. The detection of a small clinically relevant difference in response can require quite large sample sizes.

Subgroup Analysis

Given the resources and effort required to conduct a clinical trial, it is current practice in most reported clinical trial analyses to not only estimate overall treatment effects, but also to estimate treatment effects and test hypotheses within different subsets of patients. The use of such subset analyses, however, is quite controversial, and it is one of the more troublesome aspects of clinical trial analysis and interpretation (104).

The statistical concerns include the issue of inflating the "alpha levels" as a result of repeated testing, that is, the possibility that significant results will emerge by chance alone when one examines multiple subgroups of patients. Evaluating treatment effects separately for multiple patient subgroups increases the risk of obtaining spurious positive results. Furthermore, if the overall result is statistically significant, there is a high probability that randomly selected subgroups of patients will produce strikingly different outcomes just by chance alone. For example, if the overall observed size of the treatment effect is two standard deviations, there is a one in three chance that one randomly selected subset of half of the patients will produce an observed effect of three standard deviations (highly statistically significant) whereas the other half will produce an observed effect of only one standard deviation (not at all statistically significant) (105).

Another major concern is the lack of statistical power to detect treatment effects within smaller subgroups of patients, producing false negative results. Most clinical trials are designed to have enough power to evaluate the treatment effect only for the whole study population. Results from subset analyses, therefore, should always be presented and interpreted with caution.

Subgroup analyses should be prespecified in the original study protocol, so that they can be considered "a priori" analyses as opposed to "post hoc" (or data-derived) analyses. This, however, may not always be possible, as new scientific knowledge derived from other trials may become available during the conduct of the study. The statistical plan can be amended, but only before the data analysis is performed. Prespecifying the subgroup analyses to be performed can reduce the temptation to over-analyze the data in search for statistical significance. Subgroups should only be defined according to pretreatment characteristics and not, for example, on compliance or outcome variables.

In subgroup analyses treatment effects are usually computed within groups of patients defined with respect to the value of a covariate of interest to explore the possible interaction of the magnitude of treatment effect and that covariate. A recently developed method is the Subpopulation

Treatment Effect Pattern Plot (STEPP), which is a display of treatment effects computed within overlapping subpopulations of trial patients defined with respect to a variable of interest (106–108). By displaying the pattern of treatment effect differences along a continuum of values for a covariate (e.g., age, or quantitative assessment of estrogen receptor), STEPP illustrates whether the magnitude of treatment benefit differs according to values of the covariate. This avoids the problems of either selecting one or more cut points to categorize the covariate, or relying on parametric models that imply a specific relationship.

Subgroup analyses are frequently performed and reported in the clinical literature because they assist physicians in using study results in their clinical practice, by allowing the assessment of treatment effects within "relevant" patient subpopulations. Identifying the best possible treatment for the individual patient involves estimating the therapeutic effect for that patient, so that treatment benefit is maximized and the potential unnecessary side effects are minimized from unnecessary treatment reduced to a minimum. Subgroup analyses also can more generally help raise questions for further research. Despite the challenges associated with performing and reporting subgroup analyses (104), "when subgroup analyses are properly conducted, presentation of their results can be informative, avoiding any presentation of subgroup analyses because of their history of being over interpreted is a steep price to pay for a problem that can be remedied by more responsible analysis and reporting."(109)

Meta-analysis

Meta-analysis is an analysis of the combined results of several separate studies to increase the statistical power for detecting treatment effects (110). Unfortunately, the magnitude of treatment effects (especially improvement in overall survival) obtained from many currently available cancer therapies is relatively small, and only large trials are likely to achieve statistical significance. For example, it requires over 3000 patients to be followed for an average of 5 years to obtain an 80% power to achieve statistical significance if the true treatment effect is an increase in 5-year overall survival from 50% to 55%. The lack of statistical significance in undersized studies builds the impression that the treatment is ineffective. Controversy arises when a few trials achieve statistical significance while several other trials do not. A properly conducted meta-analysis can identify whether modest, but real, treatment effects exist.

A meta-analysis proceeds in four steps. First, the research question is defined. For example, what is the evidence that adjuvant tamoxifen improves survival for patients with operable breast cancer? Second, a literature review is conducted and investigators in the field are contacted to identify all relevant studies. Because there is a higher likelihood for positive studies to be published, relying only on published reports can result in publication bias (111). Third, the appropriate studies are identified and the data obtained. Such data can be summary measures from published reports or individual patient data (IPD) from the study investigators. The IPD approach is preferred because unpublished studies can be included, data quality control checks can be performed, and greater flexibility in the analysis can be achieved. Fourth, the statistical analysis to combine the separate studies is carried out, and the results are interpreted.

The term "overview" has been suggested to describe a specific type of meta-analysis conducted using strict guidelines to reduce systematic bias. Overviews are based exclusively on properly randomized clinical trials. All available randomized trials (both published and unpublished) that investigate the therapeutic question of interest are included. All patients are evaluated according to their randomized treatment assignment (intention-to-treat analysis). Estimates of treatment effects based on comparing like patients within each individual study are obtained, and then statistical methods are used to combine these separate treatment effect estimates into an overview result (112).

Meta-analyses, despite the substantial increase in statistical power, cannot answer all questions concerning the worth of a given treatment. In particular, the overall estimates of the magnitude of treatment effect obtained from the entire cohort of patients may be misleading. The magnitudes of treatment effects estimated in the overview are based on an "arithmetic construction" that ignores quantitative interactions between the treatment effect and patient characteristics or concomitant therapies (113,114). In addition, "indirect comparisons" of treatment effects obtained from different trials are influenced by the characteristics of these trials. For example, comparing the magnitude of the tamoxifen effect obtained from trials that used 5 years of treatment versus that obtained from trials that used 1 year of treatment is not as valid as a direct randomized comparison of 5 versus 1 year of tamoxifen.

Meta-analysis of cancer clinical trials is a very powerful procedure that stimulates international collaboration, helps to resolve controversies that arise from apparently contradictory results of undersized trials, and focuses attention on major unanswered questions. Nevertheless, well-conducted, large-scale randomized clinical trials continue to be the basis for evaluating the worth of new therapies and regimens for cancer patients.

Can Clinical Trials Be the Treatment of Choice for Patients with Cancer?

The fact that a relatively small percentage of oncology patients participate in randomized clinical trials has substantially slowed progress in improving the use of current therapies and developing new treatment approaches. Several studies have explored reasons for this low participation (115–117). Although moderate improvements in outcome for common diseases can save many lives, individual trials often do not enroll enough patients to provide reliable evidence to detect these effects. Efforts must be made to make participation in clinical trials more widely acceptable. Patient advocacy groups are recognizing the important role played by a vibrant cancer clinical research effort. More progress can be made only if clinical trials become the treatment of choice for many more patients with cancer (118).

ACKNOWLEDGMENTS

We thank Marco Bonetti for his work on the first edition of this chapter and Shari Gelber for her contributions to editing the current edition.

REFERENCES

1. Miller AB, Hoogstraten B, Staquet M et al. Reporting results of cancer treatment. Cancer 1981; 47: 207–14.

2. Therasse P, Arbuck SG, Eisenhauer EA et al. New guidelines to evaluate the response to treatment in solid tumors (RECIST Guidelines). J Natl Cancer Inst 2000; 92: 205–16.

3. Cheson BD, Pfistner B, Juweid ME et al. Revised response criteria for malignant lymphoma. J Clin Oncol 2007; 25: 579–86.

4. Agrawal M, Emaneul EJ. Ethics of phase I oncology studies: reexamining the arguments and data. JAMA 2003; 290: 1075–82.

5. Hellman S, Hellman D. Of mice but not men, problems of the randomized clinical trial. N Engl J Med 1991; 324: 1585–9.

6. Passamani E. Clinical trials, are they ethical? N Engl J Med 1991; 324: 1589–92.

7. McFadden E. Management of Data in Clinical Trials, 2nd edn. New York: John Wiley & Sons, 2007.

8. International Breast Cancer Study Group. Effectiveness of adjuvant chemotherapy in combination with tamoxifen for node-positive postmenopausal breast cancer patients. J Clin Oncol 1997; 15: 1385–93.

9. Tonkin K, Tritchler D, Tannock I. Criteria of tumor response used in clinical trials of chemotherapy. J Clin Oncol 1985; 3: 870–5.

10. Baar J, Tannock I. Analyzing the same data in two ways: a demonstration model to illustrate the reporting and misreporting of clinical trials. J Clin Oncol 1989; 7: 969–78.

11. Biomarkers Definitions Working Group. Biomarkers and surrogate endpoints: Preferred definitions and conceptual framework. Clin Pharmacol Ther 2001; 69: 89–95.

12. Sargent DJ, Conley BA, Allegra C et al. Clinical trial designs for predictive marker validation in cancer treatment trials. J Clin Oncol 2005; 23: 2020–7.

13. Cummings J, Ward TH, Greystoke A et al. Biomarker method validation in anticancer drug development. Br J Pharmacol 2008; 153: 646–56.

14. Shaughnessy JA, Wittes RE, Burke G et al. Commentary concerning demonstration of safety and efficacy of investigational anticancer agents in clinical trials. J Clin Oncol 1991; 9: 2225–32.

15. Bren L. The importance of patient-reported outcomes: it's all about the patient. FDA Consumer Magazine, November–December, 2006.

16. FDA Draft Guidance: Patient-Reported Outcome Measures: Use in Medical Product Development to Support Labeling Claims. U.S. Department of Health and Human Services, Food and Drug Administration, February 2006. www.fda.gov/CDER/GUIDANCE/5460dft.pdf [Accessed 19 August 2008].

17. Bernhard J, Gelber RD (guest editors). Workshop on missing data in quality of life research in cancer clinical trials: practical and methodological issues. Stat Med 1998; 17: 511–793.

18. Goldhirsch A, Gelber RD, Simes RJ et al. For the Ludwig Breast Cancer Study Group, Costs and benefits of adjuvant therapy in breast cancer: a quality-adjusted survival analysis. J Clin Oncol 1989; 7: 36–44.

19. Gelber RD, Cole BF, Gelber S et al. The Q-TWiST method. In: Spilker B, ed. Quality of Life and Pharmacoeconomics in Clinical Trials, 2nd edn. Philadelphia: Lippincott-Raven, 1996: 437–44.

20. Kilbridge KL, Cole BF, Kirkwood JM et al. Quality of life adjusted survival analysis of high-dose adjuvant interferon alpha-2b for high-risk melanoma patients using intergroup clinical trial data. J Clin Oncol 2002; 20: 1311–18.

21. Fairclough DL, Fetting JH, Cella D et al. Quality of life and quality adjusted survival for breast cancer patients receiving adjuvant therapy. Qual Life Res 1999; 8: 723–31.

22. Cole BF, Gelber RD, Gelber S et al. Polychemotherapy for early breast cancer: an overview of the randomized trials with quality-adjusted survival. Lancet 2001; 358: 277–86.

23. Cole BF, Gelber RD, Kirkwood JM et al. Quality-of-life-adjusted survival analysis of interferon alfa-2b adjuvant treatment of high-risk resected cutaneous melanoma: an Eastern Cooperative Oncology Group study. J Clin Oncol 1996; 14: 2666–73.

24. Parsons SK, Gelber S, Cole BF et al. Quality-adjusted survival after treatment for acute myeloid leukemia in childhood: a Q-TWiST analysis of the Pediatric Oncology Group Study 8821. J Clin Oncol 1999; 17: 2144–52.

25. Cole BF, Gelber RD, Gelber S et al. A quality-adjusted survival (Q-TWiST) model for evaluating treatments for advanced stage cancer. J Biopharm Stat 2004; 14: 111–24.

26. Neymark N, Kiebert W, Torfs K et al. Methodological and statistical issues of quality of life (QOL) and economic evaluation in cancer clinical trials: report of a workshop. Eur J Cancer 1998; 34: 1317–33.

27. Gold M, Russel L, Siegel J et al. Cost-effectiveness in Health and Medicine. New York: Oxford University Press, 1996.

28. Shis Y-C, Halpern MT. Economic evaluations of medical care interventions for cancer patients: how, why, and what does it mean? CA Cancer J Clin 2008; 58: 231–44.

29. Kaplan EL, Meier P. Nonparametric estimation from incomplete observations. J Am Stat Assoc 1958; 53: 457–81.

30. Piccart-Gebhart MJ, Procter M, Leyland-Jones B et al. Trastuzumab after adjuvant chemotherapy in HER2-positive breast cancer. N Engl J Med 2005; 353: 1659–72.

31. Cox DR. The Analysis of Binary Data. London: Methuen Press, 1972.

32. Cox DR. Regression models and life-tables (with discussion). J R Stat Soc Series B Stat Methodol 1972; 34: 187–220.

33. Johnson JR, Williams G, Pazdur R. End points and United States Food and Drug Administration approval of oncology drugs. J Clin Oncol 2003; 21: 1404–11.

34. Guidance for Industry, Investigators and Reviewers, Exploratory IND Studies. http://www.fda.gov/CDER/guidance/7086fnl.htm [Accessed July 2008].

35. Gelmon K, Eisenhauer EA, Harris AL et al. Anticancer agents targeting signaling molecules and cancer cell environment: Challenges for drug development? J Natl Cancer Inst 1999; 91: 1281–7.

36. Lee JW, Weiner RS, Sailstad JM et al. Method validation and measurement of biomarkers in nonclinical and clinical samples in drug development: a conference report. Pharm Res 2005; 22: 499–511.

37. Kummar S, Kinders R, Rubinstein L et al. Compressing drug development timelines in oncology using phase "0" trials. Nature Rev Cancer 2007; 7: 131–9.

38. See articles in CCR Focus (series). Clin Cancer Res 2008; 14: 3657–97.

39. ASCO Special Article, Critical role of phase I clinical trials in cancer treatment. J Clin Oncol 1997; 15: 853–9.

40. Simon R, Freidlin B, Rubinstein L et al. Accelerated titration designs for phase I clinical trials in oncology. J Natl Cancer Inst 1997; 89: 1138–47.

41. Von Hoff DD, Turner J. Response rates, duration of response and dose response effects in phase I studies of antineoplastics. Invest New Drugs 1991; 9: 115–22.

42. Arbuck SG. Workshop on phase I design. Ninth NCI-EORTC New Drug Development Symposium, Amsterdam, March 12, 1996. Ann Oncol 1996; 7: 567–73.

43. Eisenhauer EA, O'Dwyer PJ, Christian M et al. Phase I clinical trial design in cancer drug development. J Clin Oncol 2000; 18: 684–92.

44. Collins JM, Grieshaber BA. Pharmacologically guided phase I trials based upon preclinical development. J Natl Cancer Inst 1990; 82: 1321–6.

45. Graham MA, Kaye SB. New approaches in preclinical and clinical pharmacokinetics. In: Workman P, Graham MA, eds. Cancer Surveys, Volume 17: Pharmacokinetics and Cancer Chemotherapy. New York: Cold Spring Harbor, 1993: 27–49.

46. O'Quigley J, Pepe M, Fisher L. Continual reassessment method: a practical design for phase I clinical trials in cancer. Biometrics 1990; 46: 33–48.

47. Goodman SN, Zahurak ML, Piantadosi S. Some practical improvements in the continual reassessment method for phase I studies. Stat Med 1995; 14: 1149–61.

48. Babb J, Rogatko A, Zacks S. Cancer phase I trials: efficient dose escalation with overdose control. Stat Med 1998; 17: 1103–20.

49. Siu LL, Rowinsky EK, Clark GM et al. Dose escalation using the modified continuous reassessment method (MCRM) in phase I clinical trials: a review of the San Antonio experience (abstract). Ann Oncol 1998; 9(Suppl 2): 127.

50. Seymour L, Eisenhauer E. A review of dose-limiting events in phase I trials: antimetabolites show unpredictable relationships between dose and toxicity. Cancer Chemother Pharmacol 2001; 47: 2–10.

51. Eisenhauer EA. Phase I and II trials of novel anticancer agents: endpoints, efficacy and existentialism. The Michel Clavel lecture. Ann Oncol 1998; 9: 1047–52.

52. Eckhardt SG, Eisenhauer E, Parulekar WR et al. Developmental therapeutics: Successes and failures of clinical trial designs of targeted compounds. In: Perry MC, ed. American Society of Clinical Oncology Educational Book. American Society of Clinical Oncology, 2003: 209–19.

53. Baselga J, Rischin D, Ranson M et al. Phase I safety, pharmacokinetic, and pharmacodynamic trial of ZD1839, a selective oral epidermal growth factor receptor tyrosine kinase inhibitor, in patients with five selected solid tumor types. J Clin Oncol 2002; 20(21): 4292–302.

54. Baselga J, Pfister D, Cooper MR et al. Phase I studies of anti-epidermal growth factor receptor chimeric antibody C225 alone and in combination with cisplatin. J Clin Oncol 2000; 18: 904–14.

55. Albanell J, Codony-Servat J, Rojo F et al. Activated extracellular signal-regulated kinases: association with epidermal growth factor receptor/transforming growth factor expression in head and neck squamous carcinoma and inhibition by anti-epidermal growth factor receptor treatments. Cancer Res 2001; 61: 6500–10.

56. Parulekar WR, Eisenhauer EA. Phase I trial design for solid tumor studies of targeted, non-cytotoxic agents: Theory and practice. J Natl Cancer Inst 2004; 96: 990–7.

57. Booth CM, Calvert AH, Giaccone G et al. Endpoints and other considerations in phase I studies of targeted anticancer therapy: recommendations from the task force on Methodology for the Development of Innovative Cancer Therapies (MDICT). Eur J Cancer 2008; 44: 19–24.

58. Bubley GJ, Carducci M, Dahut W et al. Eligibility and response guidelines for phase II clinical trials in androgen-independent prostate cancer: recommendations from the prostate-specific antigen working group. J Clin Oncol 1999; 17: 3461–7.

59. Scher HI, Halabi S, Tannock I et al. Design and end points of clinical trials for patients with progressive prostate cancer and castrate levels of testosterone: recommendations of the prostate cancer clinical trials working group. J Clin Oncol 2008; 26: 1148–59.

60. Rustin GJ, Quinn M, Thigpen T et al. Re: New guidelines to evaluate the response to treatment in solid tumors (ovarian cancer). J Natl Cancer Inst 2004; 96: 487–8.

61. Gehan EA. The determination of the number of patients required in a preliminary and a follow-up trial of a new chemotherapeutic agent. J Chronic Dis 1961; 13: 346–53.

62. Fleming TR. One-sample multiple testing procedure for phase II clinical trials. Biometrics 1982; 38: 143–51.

63. Simon R. Optimal two-stage designs for phase II clinical trials. Control Clin Trials 1989; 10: 1–10.

64. Zee B, Melnychuk D, Dancey J et al. Multinomial phase II cancer trials incorporating response and early progression. J Biopharm Stat 1999; 9: 351–63.

65. Dent S, Zee B, Dancey J et al. Application of a new multinomial phase II stopping rule using response and early progression. J Clin Oncol 2001; 19: 785–91.

66. Simon R, Wittes RE, Ellenberg SS. Randomized phase II clinical trials. Cancer Treat Rep 1985; 69: 1375–85.

67. Hoskins P, Eisenhauer E, Beare S et al. A randomized phase II study of two schedules of topotecan in previously treated patients with ovarian cancer. J Clin Oncol 1998; 16: 2233–7.

68. Gray R, Manola J, Saxman S et al. Phase II clinical trial design: methods in translational research from the Genitourinary Committee at the Eastern Cooperative Oncology Group. Clin Cancer Res 2006; 12: 1966–9.

69. Korn EL, Arbuck SG, Pluda JM et al. Clinical trial designs for cytostatic agents: are new approaches needed? J Clin Oncol 2001; 19: 265–72.

70. Karrison TG , Maitland ML, Stadler WM et al. Design of phase II cancer trials using a continuous endpoint of change in tumor size: application to a study of sorafenib and erlotinib in non–small-cell lung cancer. J Natl Cancer Inst 2007; 99: 1455–61.

71. El-Maraghi R, Eisenhauer EA. Review of phase II trial designs used in studies of molecular targeted agents: outcomes and predictors of success in phase III. J Clin Oncol 2008; 26: 1346–54.

72. Kopec JA, Abrahamowicz M, Esdaile JM. Randomized discontinuation trials: utility and efficiency. J Clin Epidemiol 1993; 46: 959–71.

73. Simon R. Re-examination of the design of early clinical development trials for molecularly targeted drugs. In: Perry MC, ed. American Society of Clinical Oncology Educational Book. American Society of Clinical Oncology, 2006: 126–9.

74. Gwyther SJ, Gore ME, ten Bokkel Huinink W et al. Results of independent radiological review of over 400 patients with advanced ovarian cancer treated with topotecan (Hycamtin) (Abstract). Proc Am Soc Clin Oncol 1997; 16: 351a.

75. Zelen M. The randomization and stratification of patients to clinical trials. J Chronic Dis 1974; 27: 365–75.

76. Pocock SJ, Simon R. Sequential treatment assignment with balancing for prognostic factors in the controlled clinical trial. Biometrics 1975; 31: 103–15.

77. Pocock S. Clinical Trials: A Practical Approach. New York: John Wiley & Sons, 1983.

78. Peterson B, George SL. Sample size requirements and length of study for testing interaction in a 2 x k factorial design when time-to-failure is the outcome. Control Clin Trials 1993; 14: 511–22.

79. Brown BW. The crossover experiment for clinical trials. Biometrics 1980; 36: 69–79.

80. Blackwelder WC. "Proving the null hypothesis" in clinical trials. Control Clin Trials 1982; 3: 345–53.

81. Piaggio G, Elbourne DR, Altman DG et al. for the CONSORT Group. Reporting of noninferiority and equivalence randomized trials: an extension of the CONSORT statement. JAMA 2006; 295: 1152–60.

82. Fleiss JL. Statistical Methods for Rates and Proportions, 2nd edn. New York: John Wiley & Sons, 1981.

83. George SL, Desu MM. Planning the size and duration of a clinical trial studying time to some critical event. J Chronic Dis 1974; 27: 15–24.

84. Freedman LS. Tables of the number of patients required in clinical trials using the logrank test. Stat Med 1982; 1: 121–9.

85. O'Brien PC, Fleming TR. A multiple testing procedure for clinical trials. Biometrics 1979; 35: 549–56.

86. Lan KKG, DeMets DL. Discrete sequential boundaries for clinical trials. Biometrika 1983; 70: 659–63.

87. Pampallona S, Tsiatis AA. Group sequential designs for one-sided and two-sided hypothesis testing with provision for early stopping in favor of the null hypothesis. J Stat Plan Inference 1994; 42: 19–35.

88. EaSt Version 5.0: Software for the design, simulation and interim monitoring of flexible clinical trials. Cambridge, MA: Cytel Software Corporation, 2007.

89. Smith MA, Ungerleider RS, Korn EL et al. Role of independent data-monitoring committees in randomized clinical trials sponsored by the National Cancer Institute. J Clin Oncol 1997; 15: 2736–43.

90. FDA Draft Guidance for Clinical Trial Sponsors on the Establishment and Operation of Clinical Trial Data Monitoring Committees. U.S. Department of Health and Human Services, Food and Drug Administration, November, 2001. www.fda.gov/cber/gdlns/clindatmon.pdf [Accessed 19 August 2008].

91. Stupp R, Mason WP, van den Bent MJ et al. Radiotherapy plus concomitant and aduvant temozolomide for glioblastoma. N Engl J Med 2005; 352: 987–96.

92. Hegi ME, Diserens A-C, Gorlia T et al. MGMT gene silencing and benefit from temozolomide in glioblastoma. N Engl J Med 2005; 352: 997–1003.

93. Paik S, Shak S, Tang G et al. A multigene sssay to predict recurrence of tamoxifen-treated, node-negative breast cancer. N Engl J Med 2004; 351: 2817–26.

94. Slamon DJ, Leyland-Jones B, Shak S et al. Use of chemotherapy plus a monocloncal antibody against HER2 for metastatic breast cancer that overexpresses HER2. N Engl J Med 2001; 344: 783–92.

95. Romond EH, Perez EA, Bryant J et al. Trastuzumab plus adjuvant chemotherapy for operable HER2-positive breast cancer. N Engl J Med 2005; 353: 1673–84.

96. Slamon DJ, Clark GM, Wong SG et al. Human breast cancer: correlation of relapse and survival with amplification of the HER-2/neu oncogene. Science 1987; 235: 177–82.

97. Seshadri R, Firgaira FA, Horsfall DJ et al. Clinical significance of HER-2/neu oncogene amplification in primary breast cancer. J Clin Oncol 1993; 11: 1936–42.

98. Pritchard KI, Shepherd LE, O'Malley RP et al. HER2 and responsiveness of breast cancer to adjuvant chemotherapy. N Engl J Med 2006; 354: 2103–11.

99. Cardoso F, Van't Veer L, Rutgers E et al. Clinical application of the 70-gene profile: the MINDACT trial. J Clin Oncol 2008; 26: 729–35.

100. Buyse M, Loi S, van't Veer L et al. Validation and clinical utility of a 70-gene prognostic signature for women with node-negative breast cancer. J Natl Cancer Inst 2006; 98: 1183–92.

101. Zelen M. Guidelines for publishing papers on cancer clinical trials: responsibilities of editors and authors. J Clin Oncol 1983; 1: 164–9.

102. Begg C, Cho M, Eastwood S et al. Improving the quality of reporting of randomized controlled trials: the CONSORT (consolidation of standards for reporting trials) statement. JAMA 1996; 276: 637–9.

103. Moher D, Schultz KF, Altman DG, for the CONSORT Group. The CONSORT statement: revised recommendations for improving the quality of reports of parallel-group randomized trials. Lancet 2001; 357: 1191–94.

104. Wang MS, Lagakos SW, Ware JH et al. Statistics in medicine—reporting of subgroup analyses in clinical trials. N Engl J Med 2007; 357: 2189–94.

105. Peto R. Statistical aspects of cancer trials. In: Halnan KE, ed. Treatment of Cancer. London: Chapman and Hall, 1982: 867–71.

106. Bonetti M, Gelber RD. A graphical method to assess treatment – covariate interactions using the Cox model on subsets of the data. Stat Med 2000; 19: 2595–609.

107. Bonetti M, Gelber RD. Patterns of treatment effects in subsets of patients in clinical trials. Biostatistics 2004; 5: 465–81.

108. Regan MM, Gelber RD. Using clinical trial data to tailor adjuvant treatments for individual patients. Breast 2007; 16: S98–104.

109. Lagakos SW. The challenge of subgroup analyses–reporting without distorting. N Engl J Med 2006; 354: 1667–9.

110. Glass GV. Primary, secondary and meta-analysis of research. Educational Researcher 1976; 5: 3–8.

111. Begg CB, Berlin JA. Publication bias: a problem in interpreting medical data. J R Stat Soc [Ser A] 1988; 151: 419–63.

112. Early Breast Cancer Trialists' Collaborative Group. Treatment of Early Breast Cancer, Volume 1: Worldwide Evidence 1985–1990. Oxford: Oxford University Press, 1990.

113. Gelber RD, Goldhirsch A, Coates AS. For the International Breast Cancer Study Group, Adjuvant therapy for breast cancer: understanding the overview. J Clin Oncol 1993; 11: 580–5.

114. Coates AS, Goldhirsch A, Gelber RD. Overhauling the breast cancer overview: are subsets subversive? Lancet Oncol 2002; 3: 525–6.

115. Taylor KM, Margolese RG, Soskolne CL. Physicians' reasons for not entering patients in a randomized clinical trial of surgery for breast cancer. N Engl J Med 1984; 310: 1363–7.

116. Ford JG, Howerton MW, Lai GY et al. Barriers to recruiting underrepresented populations to cancer clinical trials: a systemic review. Cancer 2008; 112: 228–42.

117. Albrecht TL, Eggly SS, Gleason ME et al. Influence of clinical communication on patients' decision making on participation in clinical trials. J Clin Oncol 2008; 26: 2666–73.

118. Gelber RD, Goldhirsch A. Can a clinical trial be the treatment of choice for patients with cancer? (editorial). J Natl Cancer Inst 1988; 80: 886–7.

5

Breast Cancer

Marco Colleoni, Silvia Dellapasqua, and Aron Goldhirsch

EPIDEMIOLOGY/ETIOLOGY

Breast cancer is one of the most common types of cancer, accounting for about 26% of new cancer cases among women. Incidence rates decreased from 2001 to 2004 after increasing since 1980. The disease is very rare before the age of 20, seldom occurs below 30 years of age, and its incidence rate rises up to the age of 50 years. In postmenopausal women, the rate of increase slows down, although the incidence continues to rise. Breast cancer is the leading cause of cancer death between ages 20 and 59 years. However, breast cancer mortality rates have declined in recent years, reflecting improvements in early detection and treatment (1,2).

Geographical variation of incidence and mortality are described. Interestingly, migrating populations adjust incidence rates to that of host countries within a couple of generations, underlining the importance of risk factors related to environment and lifestyle beyond genetically inherited factors (3).

Recognized breast cancer risk factors include age, ethnicity, estrogen exposure, abnormal proliferation of breast tissue (atypical hyperplasia or in situ carcinoma), radiation exposure, family history/genetic predisposition, and lifestyle factors, such as obesity, alcohol consumption, and lack of exercise (4). Table 5.1 lists some of the main risk factors associated with an increased breast cancer risk. Additional endocrine and lifestyle-related risk factors include early menarche, late menopause, nulliparous/delayed first pregnancy, no/short duration breastfeeding, use of oral contraceptives, and hormone replacement therapy. Interventions on lifestyle are difficult to study and are likely to influence outcome, if at all, only after a long period of time.

The rapid growth of DNA-based tests has raised complex questions about medicolegal and ethical issues related to genetic screening, its accuracy, impact, and consequences upon individuals and their families. In addition, the possible intervention strategies for breast cancer prevention in women who have tested positive are either without any proof of efficacy, controversial, or still under investigation. Several general approaches have been proposed: lifestyle modifications, prophylactic mastectomy and/or oophorectomy, intensified screening, and chemoprevention (Table 5.2).

Specific Risk Factors

Overall, inherited *genetic susceptibility* accounts for only about 5–10% of breast cancers.

Susceptibility genes include *BRCA1* (20–40% of hereditary breast cancers), *BRCA2* (10–30%), *TP53* (<1%), *PTEN* (<1%), *ATM, CHK2, STK11* (<1%), and Fanconi's Anemia genes (1%) (5). *BRCA1* and *BRCA2* are associated with hereditary breast cancer in younger age groups, increased incidence of familial ovarian cancer (*BRCA1* and *BRCA2*), and male breast cancer (*BRCA2*). The lifetime breast cancer risk among women with *BRCA1/2* varies from 56% to 80–85% (6). Several mutations in *BRCA1/2* occur with a higher frequency among individuals of Ashkenazi (East European) Jewish descent, with three predominant mutations in *BRCA1* (185delAG and 5382insC) and *BRCA2* (6174delT) accounting for the majority of germline mutations (7). A two-hit model has been proposed to explain the mechanism by which breast cancer can arise in BRCA1/2 carriers. The first hit represents loss of the wild type BRCA1 or BRCA2 allele, resulting in an increased rate for subsequent genomic events. A second event increasing proliferation of the partially malignant clone may lead to selection of cells with additional mutations in genes that facilitate tumor progression (8). BRCA1-related breast cancer features include earlier age at onset, medullary features, higher proliferation, poor differentiation, estrogen receptor (ER) and progesterone receptor (PR) negative, HER-2-negative, EGFR-positive, often with basal-like phenotype, and more lymphocytic infiltration than sporadic cancers. BRCA2-related breast cancer features include lower mitotic counts and expression of ER/PR. Despite the association with adverse prognostic characteristics, BRCA1/2-associated breast cancers have prognoses similar to or better than sporadic tumors of similar stage (9).

A history of breast cancer is a contraindication for the use of many *oral contraceptives* (10). At least four studies (11–14) found no increased contralateral breast cancer risk among women who used oral contraceptives. The Women's Contraceptive and Reproductive Experiences study reported no association with breast cancer risk (15) whereas the Collaborative Group on Hormonal Factors in Breast Cancer found a modest increased risk with recent oral contraceptive use (16).

Hormone replacement therapy (HRT) with estrogens in combination with progesterone, used to relieve menopausal symptoms, is associated with increased breast cancer risk (17–20). For women with a history of breast cancer, HRT is contraindicated. Two randomized clinical trials investigated the use of HRT in breast cancer survivors, and although the HABITS study showed a significant increased risk of recurrence and was terminated early (21), a trial in Sweden found no association (22). Several observational

Table 5.1   Risk Factors (Except Age) Associated with Risk of Invasive Breast Cancer

Major risk factors increasing risk >2 times (in descending order)
- Evidence of mutated BRCA 1 or BRCA 2
- CHEK2 (also known as CHK2): (*CHEK2(*)1100delC, a truncating variant that abrogates the kinase activity*) approximately twofold increase of breast cancer risk in women and a tenfold increase of risk in men
- Premenopausal breast cancer in mother and sister
- In situ cancer—ductal or lobular or atypical hyperplasia in breast biopsy
- Premenopausal breast cancer in mother or sister; bilateral breast cancer in first relative
- Hyperplasia without atypia in breast biopsy

Minor risk indicators or factors increasing risk ≤2 times
- Postmenopausal breast cancer in first degree relative
- Obesity in women above 50 years
- Excess radiation to the chest wall or breast in history
- Alcohol consumption
- Nulliparous or delayed first pregnancy
- No breast feeding or short duration breast feeding of children
- Prolonged use of estrogens (contraceptive and/or hormone replacement)

studies showed no increased risk of recurrence or increased mortality associated with HRT use among breast cancer survivors (23–25).

Environmental factors are thought to explain a large proportion of breast cancer incidence. Exposure to ionizing radiation, especially at a young age, is associated with an increased breast cancer risk. Hodgkin's disease survivors who received supra-diaphragmatic radiation have an increased breast cancer risk. Cigarette smoking is a controversial risk factor for breast cancer (26) whereas soy food intake (27), dietary vitamin D (28), and sunlight (29) may have a protective effect. Although most environmental factors have not been convincingly found to influence breast cancer risk, environmental exposure in combination with genetic predisposition, age at exposure, and hormonal milieu might have a cumulative effect on breast cancer risk (30).

DIAGNOSIS/SCREENING

More than 85% of newly diagnosed breast cancers are detected as a lump in the breast. In about 80% of these, a thickening of part of the breast is felt by the patient. Hemorrhagic/stained nipple discharge, nipple retraction, and erosion are less frequent. In about 10% of cases breast cancer is diagnosed as an overt metastatic disease.

Early detection of breast cancer through breast self-examination, clinical examination, and radiological imaging techniques, mainly screening mammography, increases chances of long-term survival. Breast self-examination and clinical examination can diagnose breast cancer by findings such as a suspicious lump in the breast or in the axilla. Mammography screening may reduce breast cancer mortality in certain populations with a beneficial effect that persists even after long-term follow-up (31). Screening mammography can detect noncancerous lesions as well as in situ and invasive breast cancers that are smaller than those detected by other means (Fig. 5.1). It is therefore associated

Table 5.2   Interventions for Prevention of Breast Cancer for Women at High Risk (as Identified by DNA Examination, Linkage Studies, or Other Features in Table 4.1)

Lifestyle modifications
- Increased physical activity.
- Reduced dietary fat. Difficult to study. Might be most important in preadolescent and adolescent girls. Investigation in these age groups are warranted.
- Reduced alcohol consumption. About 4% of the breast cancers in developed countries are attributable to alcohol.

Prophylactic mastectomy
- Offered to women with hereditary cancers (especially for the BRCA 1 and BRCA 2 carriers) after proper genetic counseling.
- Data on the efficacy of this approach are insufficient.
- Several case reports exist of the development of breast cancer following total mastectomy. Breast tissue is left behind even after radical mastectomy.

Intensive screening
- Some advocate regular mammography for BRCA 1 and BRCA 2 carriers starting at 25 (experimental).
  Might not be appropriate with current means because mammography is not very efficient in young age and frequently repeated, close mammographies for a long period of time might be detrimental.
- Development of non-ionizing imaging technology: MRI and PET require additional investigations to allow recognition of early malignant features. Ultrasound imaging is currently not considered sufficiently accurate.

Chemoprevention
- *Tamoxifen.* The first drug proven to reduce breast cancer incidence in four randomized placebo-controlled trials. Its use was based upon the experience in adjuvant trials (39% reduction of incidence in contralateral breast cancer). The first report on benefit from its use as chemoprevention was based upon data from the BCPT of the NSABP on 13,388 study participants. Only tumors with endocrine responsive disease responded to treatment. Side effects of tamoxifen, especially increased risk of endometrial cancer, thromboembolic complications (including deaths from such complication), and teratogenicity are important in evaluating its potential role as a preventive drug.
- *Raloxifene.* Another selective estrogen receptor modulator (SERM) with estrogen-like effects on bone (increase in bone mineral density) and on lipid (decrease in total and LDL cholesterol levels) metabolism, but not on endometrium. In placebo-controlled studies, primarily conducted to control osteoporosis, there was a significant reduction of breast cancer.
- *Retinoids* have a potential role in preventing breast cancer through their effect on several transcription factors, among which TGF-B (which is antiproliferative on breast cancer cells). Fenretinide (4 hydroxyphenyl-retinamide or 4-HPR) is a retinoid which has been investigated in a placebo-controlled trial (in node-negative breast cancer).
- *Vitamin D* analogs are good candidates for a prevention trial. Side effects of such agents on calcium metabolism are, however, a major impediment.

with more diagnostic testing, surgeries, radiotherapy, and anxiety. Some of the screen detected cancers might never become clinically relevant so that their diagnosis and treatment constitutes overdiagnosis and overtreatment. Main limits of screening mammography are false negatives (related to the sensitivity of the test), false positives (related to the specificity), overdiagnosis (true positives that will

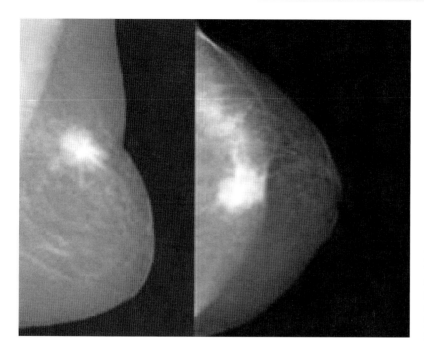

Figure 5.1 Mammography of a 65-year-old women who noticed a lump in her breast. Clinical examination revealed a 2.5 cm lump with skin fixation and no ulceration. On pathological examination there was an invasive ductal carcinoma pT1c (2 cm) pN1 (1 out of 34), steroid hormone receptors were both positive (80% and 60%, for estrogen and progesterone receptors, respectively).

not become clinically significant), and radiation risk. Screening mammography is more likely to miss cancers in women with radiographically dense breasts, as well as cancers that are rapidly growing. Screening mammography can detect subclinical breast cancer and has been proven particularly effective in reducing breast cancer mortality in women above the age of 50, despite a significant number of false positive cases, whereas its use below the age of 50 is controversial because of lower incidence of the disease and lower efficacy of mammographic evaluation of the premenopausal breast.

HISTOPATHOLOGY

A complete pathological evaluation of all breast lesions is the most important step for establishing a correct diagnosis. In case of breast cancer lesions, additional assessment of tumor biological features is fundamental for defining the treatment approach.

Main Histotypes of Breast Carcinoma
Noninvasive Breast Carcinoma
Ductal carcinoma in situ (DCIS) is a heterogeneous pathologic condition in which malignant breast epithelial cells arise and proliferate in the ducts but do not invade the surrounding stroma. The incidence of DCIS is increasing, and a greater proportion of diagnoses are made in asymptomatic patients, often by calcifications on mammography (Fig. 5.2). DCIS is multifocal in about 30% of cases, mainly in the same breast. Treatment goal in DCIS is to control local disease and prevent subsequent development of invasive cancer. No data from randomized trials compare mastectomy and breast-conserving therapy for DCIS treatment. A large randomized trial comparing lumpectomy with

lumpectomy plus radiotherapy showed lumpectomy plus radiotherapy to be a more effective treatment. Comedo necrosis and surgical margin involvement are predictors of risk of recurrence. The five-year risk of local recurrence after lumpectomy and radiotherapy is approximately 8%. In local relapses after breast-conserving therapy, the chance of an invasive component is approximately 50%. The mortality rate due to breast cancer in patients who had breast-conserving therapy is between 0.3% and 0.5%. The incidence of axillary node metastasis is very low (2–6%) and probably due to an invasive component not recognized at the time of the pathological examination of the specimen. Axillary dissection is not routinely recommended (32).

Lobular carcinoma in situ (LCIS) is a proliferative lesion limited to one or more mammary lobules without invasion of the basement membrane. Many pathologists refused to use the term carcinoma for a noninvasive lesion and coined various definitions, such as *epitheliosis, small cell neoplasia,* and *lobular neoplasia.* Recently the term *lobular intraepithelial neoplasia (LIN)* has gained consideration in defining this risk factor associated with development of invasive breast cancer (ductal or lobular). The reason for the high frequency (10–15% at 10 years; overall risk might reach 50%) of subsequent development of invasive ductal cancers remains unclear. This neoplasia occurs mainly in premenopausal women, and is multicentric in 50–70% of the cases. The diagnosis is often made on occasional removal of breast tissue.

Noninvasive "lobular" proliferations are divided into atypical lobular hyperplasia (ALH) and LCIS. In ALH a terminal duct lobular unit is colonized by small discohesive cells, the colonized units are not expanded, and their lumina are not obliterated by this proliferation. Conversely, LCIS is comprised of a population of cells with similar cytomorphological characteristics, but the colonized structures are expanded and the lumina lost. These lesions

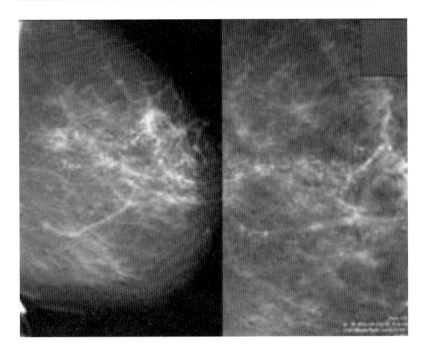

Figure 5.2 Particular mammographic images of a 60-year-old woman with ductal carcinoma in situ (DCIS). Imaging disclosed irregular, diffuse, and clustered microcalcifications. A quadrantectomy without axillary clearance was performed. On pathological examination DCIS of intermediate grade, of micropapillary type with necrosis and microcalcifications (Imaging with the courtesy of Dr. Enrico Cassano, European Institute of Oncology).

likely represent a temporal continuum, with LCIS evolving from ALH, and the terms lobular neoplasia or, more recently, in situ lobular neoplasia are used to encompass both lesions. The cytological similarities between lobular neoplasia in situ and infiltrating lobular carcinoma suggest a temporal continuum extending to invasive disease. Both ALH and LCIS frequently resemble infiltrating lobular carcinoma with respect to expression of biological markers, being ER and PR positive, and HER-2 and p53 negative (33).

Invasive Breast Carcinoma
Infiltrating ductal carcinoma is the most common type of breast cancer (67.9%, five-year relative survival 79%), followed by lobular carcinoma (6.3%, five-year survival 84%) and medullary carcinoma (2.8%, five-year survival 82%). Other types include mucinous (colloid) adenocarcinoma (2.2%, five-year survival 95%), comedocarcinoma (1.4%, five-year survival 87%), Paget's disease (nipple and other breast) (1.1%, five-year survival 79%), papillary carcinoma (0.9%, five-year survival 95%), tubular adenocarcinoma (0.7%, five-year survival 96%), and inflammatory carcinoma (0.5%, five-year survival 18%). Other rare types of invasive cancers include adenoid-cystic carcinoma, apocrine carcinoma, and carcinoma with squamous metaplasia. These types of cancer might require some specific adjustment of the treatment program (34).

Other Nonmalignant and Malignant Breast Diseases
Several pathological nonmalignant conditions present with single or multiple breast lumps or with symptoms and signs that simulate breast cancer.

Fibrocystic mastopathy occurs more often between 30 and 55 years of age and is frequently identified by women as multiple lumps in one or both breasts. Mammographic patterns of multiple areas of fibrosis and cysts are typical, representing a difficult background for evaluation of an underlying malignant neoplasia. Another associated pathological entity is sclerosing adenosis, which may appear in younger ages. There is uncertainty whether this condition may lead to an increased breast cancer risk: the overall increased risk of 1.86 of developing breast cancer was more likely to have resulted from the selection of patients than from the real malignant potential of the disease. Proliferation with cell atypia upon pathological assessment is, however, associated with an increased breast cancer risk, especially in the presence of a positive family history.

Fibroadenoma presents as one or more mobile, indolent lumps, commonly in women between 20 and 25 years of age. Fibrocystic mastopathy is occasionally associated.

Intraductal papilloma usually presents in larger ducts as a mobile lump, often associated with hematic/stained nipple discharge, and requires surgical removal. Galactography might be necessary for localization of the node. Cell atypia are found in about a quarter of papillomas. Multiple intraductal papillomas carry a higher breast cancer risk, although the risk is much lower for solitary central papillomas.

Other malignant diseases of the breast might simulate breast cancer:

Phyllodes tumor (previously recognized as cystosarcoma phyllodes) is a rare fibroepithelial neoplasm of the breast with a very variable, but usually benign, course. It presents often in adolescence as a breast mass. Pathological examination shows epithelial and mesenchymal components and defines the grade of malignancy. Treatment requires a wide surgical removal, which often results in a total mastectomy. High-grade or recurrent disease might require radiation therapy and systemic treatments.

Sarcoma usually presents as a large fast growing, painless mass. Histopathological features and clinical behavior are similar to sarcomas of other organs.

Malignant lymphoma is a very rare presentation, usually of B-cell type. Its evaluation and treatment follow guidelines for this type of disorder.

Prognostic and Predictive Factors

Prognostic factors are patient or tumor characteristics that can be used to assess the baseline prognosis, helping in the estimation of costs/benefits for a treatment. Predictive factors are patient or tumor characteristics that can be used to predict a response to a given treatment, allowing a better use of available approaches. Both aspects must be taken into consideration when evaluating patients with newly diagnosed breast cancer in order to formulate the best treatment decision making.

The histological type of disease has a very limited prognostic value: most common breast cancer histotypes are treated using similar decision algorithms. Some specific histological types might, however, require specific therapeutic considerations: medullary, pure mucinous, and adenoid-cystic carcinomas are associated with favorable prognosis. Emphasis must be given to several other biological features of the disease, which provide the most significant information on prognosis and on prediction of response to a given antineoplastic treatment (35–55).

An increasing number of prognostic and predictive factors are currently being investigated. A list of established or putative prognostic and predictive variables is provided in Table 5.3. Table 5.4 lists the most important features with prognostic relevance which influence treatment choice.

A novel approach to determine prognosis was attempted using gene-expression profiling to predict disease outcome beyond clinical and histologic criteria. Multigene signatures using cDNA microarrays were found to correlate with clinical outcome (56,57), and to retain independent prognostic value in multivariate prognostic models, yet this approach requires further prospective validation. Two of these multigene signatures, namely Oncotype DX [based on 21 genes by RT-PCR (58)] and MammaPrint (based on a 70 gene-expression profiling) are currently being prospectively tested in well-powered randomized clinical trials (59,60).

CLINICAL PRESENTATION/STAGING
Definition of Stage and General Therapeutic Consequences

Most patients with breast cancer are diagnosed with operable disease, with a disease confined to the breast and the ipsilateral axillary lymph nodes. The extension of the disease from the breast to the overlying skin (with or without ulceration) or the underlying chest wall (T4) or to locoregional nodes (other than ipsilateral axillary nodes) are classified as locally advanced disease. Overt metastases to other organs are referred to as metastatic disease.

The current multidisciplinary approach to operable disease involves the sequential use of surgery, adjuvant systemic therapy and, in case of breast conservation or very high risk for local recurrence, radiation therapy to the remaining ipsilateral breast or to locoregional area after mastectomy.

In case of locally advanced disease, systemic treatment represents the primary approach, followed, after achievement of response, by surgery and radiation therapy, in order to achieve freedom of disease.

Metastatic breast cancer is a chronic disease requiring specific strategies to control the disease progression and related symptoms (61). The choice of treatment in this context should follow the principle of "the least toxic therapy available for a maximal avoidance of disease symptoms."

Major attention should, therefore, be given to the design of a comprehensive treatment strategy for every stage of the disease. Staging procedures should thus follow algorithms, which focus on assessment of prognosis and adequacy of local disease control (for operable disease), and specific therapeutic consequences (also for advanced disease).

Beyond the efforts for accurate staging, the design of a comprehensive treatment strategy requires the definition of breast cancer biological characteristics, in particular ER and PR expression, HER-2/neu overexpression or amplification, proliferation index, tumor grade, vascular/lymphatic invasion, as well as patients features such as age, menopausal status, comorbid conditions/concomitant therapies, and potential degree of patient's frailty.

Staging

An attempt to provide some prognostic estimation and the possibility to compare results from different clinical trials was performed by grouping of patients according to the anatomical extent of the disease. The most widely used staging system is the one adopted by both the Union International Contre le Cancer (UICC) and the American Joint Committee on Cancer (AJCC), based on the tumor, nodes, metastases (TNM) system (62). This system, recently reviewed as shown in Table 5.5, is suboptimal since it lacks consideration of several biological features available today; however, it is still important for uniformity of reports from series and trials.

The AJCC staging system (http://cancernet.nci.nih. gov) provides a strategy for grouping patients with respect to prognosis. Therapeutic decisions are formulated in part according to staging categories but primarily according to tumor size, lymph node status, ER and PR levels in the tumor tissue, HER-2/neu status, menopausal status, and the general health of the patient.

The AJCC has designated staging by TNM classification (63). This system was modified in 2002 and classifies some nodal categories as stage III that were previously considered stage II (64). As a result, survival by stage for case series classified by the new system will appear superior to those using the old system (65).

TNM Definitions

Definitions for classifying the primary tumor (T) are the same for clinical and for pathologic classification. If the measurement is made by physical examination, the examiner will use the major headings (T1, T2, or T3). If other measurements, such as mammographic or pathologic measurements, are used, the subsets of T1 can be used. Tumors should be

Table 5.3   Prognostic Factors in Patients with Breast Cancer

Factor	Remarks
Histopathological factors	
Tumor size	Best information if pathologically determined.
	Direct relationship between increased tumor size and worse prognosis.
Axillary lymph node status	Most important prognostic variable. Several lymph nodes (about 10) must be examined to correctly estimate prognosis.
	Negative axillary sentinel lymph node biopsy (SNB) is now accepted as allowing avoidance of axillary dissection.
	Micro-metastatic disease in sentinel lymph nodes is prognostically relevant but it is still currently a subject for research.
Internal mammary lymph node status	Site of the primary tumor might influence outcome. Internal mammary nodes involvement is an important prognostic factor, but their dissection did not improve prognosis. SNB can also be applied to the internal mammary chain, although the therapeutic implications of sentinel-node involvement in this area are less certain and are largely experimental.
Vascular invasion	Extensive peritumoral vascular invasion was considered to elevate risk category.
Histological grade	Histological grade (composed of several features indicating more less resemblance to non malignant breast tissue) is prognostically relevant. Nuclear grade is considered to be the most important component. Mitotic count might be the best predictor of prognosis.
Estrogen and progesterone receptor status	Estrogen (ER) and progesterone (PR) receptor content in the primary tumor are powerful markers to predict endocrine responsiveness in their presence and cytotoxic responsiveness in their absence.
	Most clinical data use a different grouping which combines receptor-absent disease with that expressing low receptor levels (so called receptor-negative). The central importance of the steroid hormone receptors emphasizes the absolute necessity to measure ER and PgR report results in a standardized quantitative manner (e.g., percent of cells stained), and use quality-assured procedures in experienced laboratories instead of reporting merely positive or negative receptor status (often adopting arbitrary cutoffs).
	Gene-expression profiling studies support a clear separation of steroid hormone receptor-absent disease as an entity distinct from disease showing low or higher levels of receptor, while some clinical studies already provide empirical data that receptor-absent disease is different from that with even low levels of receptor expression.
Cell proliferation indexes	
Thymidine labeling	Measured on unfixed tumor material.
	Higher values indicated worse prognosis.
Flow cytometry (S-phase)	Measured on fixed material. Determination of proportion of cells in S phase.
	Higher values indicate worse prognosis and chemotherapy response.
Ki-67	Measured on fixed material. Higher percentage of stained cells indicate worse prognosis and chemotherapy response.
Receptors (growth factors or growth regulators, including oncogenes)	
Epidermal growth factor receptor (EGFR, c-erbB-1)	Measured mainly on unfixed material.
	Higher percentage might predict worse prognosis.
HER2/*neu* (c-erbB-2)	Measured on fixed material.
	Higher expression might predict worse prognosis.
	Predictor of response to trastuzumab. Predictor of response to anthracycline combination chemotherapy, and for resistance to tamoxifen or CMF combination chemotherapy.
IGF-IR (Insulin-like growth factor receptor)	Measured in the serum.
	Lowering of its serum levels was seen during treatment with tamoxifen.
Somatostatin receptor	Presence in the tumor indicated better prognosis.
Tumor suppressor genes	
p53	Although p53 protein accumulation and gene mutation were implicated in resistance to chemotherapy, the clinical value of these findings remains controversial.
bcl-2	Bcl-2 protein may be involved in apoptosis regulation and therefore to response to cytotoxics or endocrine therapy.
nm23	Reduced expression of *nm*23 in the tumor was associated with high metastatic potential, thus with worse prognosis.
Miscellaneous	
Heat shock protein (hsp 27)	Expressed in a variety of environmental and pathophysiological stressful condition and thought to be involved in protein–protein interactions (among which also oncogen products).
	High concentrations of hsp 27 in tumor cells was associated with worse prognosis.
pS2	Estrogen-regulated cysteine-rich protein (subset of ER?).
	Predicted response to endocrine therapy.
Tumor growth factor	Expression of TGF-α in tumor tissue was associated with worse prognosis.
Cathepsin D	Increased concentrations in tumor tissue correlated with worse prognosis.
Urokinase-plasminogen activator (uPA) and Plasminogen activator-inhibitor (PAI-1)	Proteases determined on frozen tissue.
	Increased levels (as measured on tissue extracts using ELISAs) indicate dire prognosis in node-negative and node-positive disease. In contrast, patients with low uPA/PAI-1 and ER showed a particularly good prognosis.
Cyclic AMP-binding proteins	Regulatory subunits of c-AMP protein-dependent kinase.
	Increased concentration in tumor tissue correlated with worse prognosis.
Angiogenesis	Neoplastic microvessel density is directly associated with prognosis. Vascular endothelial growth factor (VEGF) and its receptor seem also to be associated with prognosis and susceptibility to drugs which affect angiogenesis.
Laminin receptor	Receptors to adhesive structural glycoprotein.
	Increased concentration in tumor cells was associated with worse prognosis.
Cyclin E	Deregulated expression might correlate with survival but results are preliminary.
Tumor cells in bone marrow and circulating blood	Isolated tumor cells or micrometastases in bone marrow were shown to be prognostically important, even years after diagnosis.

Table 5.4 List of Important Features with Prognostic Relevance and Which Influence Treatment Choice and Patients' Preferences

Patient and clinical-related features	Tumor-related
• Age	• Nodal status
• Menopausal status	• Pathological tumor size
• Estimated duration of tumor growth	• Multicentricity
• Clinical presentation	• Clear margins of the tumor after resection
• Imaging presentation (multicentricity)	• Histopathological features (histological type, grade, vessel invasion, intraductal component)
• Results of liver, renal, and marrow function tests	• Estrogen (and progesterone) receptor content in the primary tumor
• Additional imaging for chest and skeleton (useful at baseline for accurate comparison during follow-up—in case of symptomatic events)	• HER2/neu expression in the primary tumor
• A baseline marker (e.g., CA 15-3 CEA) (useful at baseline for accurate comparison during follow-up in case of symptomatic events)	• A marker of proliferation
	• Additional pathological and biological factors (Table 5.3)

measured to the nearest 0.1 cm increment. Patients with pN3a and pN3b disease are considered operable. Patients with pN3c disease are considered inoperable.

Primary Tumor (T)

- TX: Primary tumor cannot be assessed
- T0: No evidence of primary tumor
- Tis: Intraductal carcinoma, lobular carcinoma in situ, or Paget's disease of the nipple with no associated invasion of normal breast tissue
  Tis (DCIS): Ductal carcinoma in situ
  Tis (LCIS): Lobular carcinoma in situ
  Tis (Paget): Paget's disease of the nipple with no tumor (Paget's disease associated with a tumor is classified according to the size of the tumor.)
- T1: Tumor not larger than 2.0 cm in greatest dimension
  T1mic: Microinvasion not larger than 0.1 cm in greatest dimension
  T1a: Tumor larger than 0.1 cm but not larger than 0.5 cm in greatest dimension
  T1b: Tumor larger than 0.5 cm but not larger than 1.0 cm in greatest dimension
  T1c: Tumor larger than 1.0 cm but not larger than 2.0 cm in greatest dimension
- T2: Tumor larger than 2.0 cm but not larger than 5.0 cm in greatest dimension
- T3: Tumor larger than 5.0 cm in greatest dimension
- T4: Tumor of any size with direct extension to (a) chest wall or (b) skin, only as described below
  T4a: Extension to chest wall (including ribs, intercostal muscles, and serratus anterior muscle but not pectoral muscle)

T4b: Edema (including peau d'orange) or ulceration of the skin of the breast, or satellite skin nodules confined to the same breast
T4c: Both T4a and T4b
T4d: Inflammatory carcinoma (diffuse brawny induration of the skin of the breast with an erysipeloid edge, due to tumor embolization of dermal lymphatics with engorgement of superficial capillaries, usually without an underlying palpable mass; radiologically there may be a detectable mass and characteristic thickening of the skin over the breast)

Regional Lymph Nodes (N)

- NX: Regional lymph nodes cannot be assessed (e.g., previously removed)
- N0: No regional lymph node metastasis
- N1: Metastasis to movable ipsilateral axillary lymph node(s)
- N2: Metastasis to ipsilateral axillary lymph node(s) fixed or matted, or in clinically apparent ipsilateral internal mammary nodes in the *absence* of clinically evident lymph node metastasis
  N2a: Metastasis in ipsilateral axillary lymph nodes fixed to one another (matted) or to other structures
  N2b: Metastasis only in clinically apparent ipsilateral internal mammary nodes and in the *absence* of clinically evident axillary lymph node metastasis
- N3: Metastasis in ipsilateral infraclavicular lymph node(s) with or without axillary lymph node involvement, or in clinically apparent ipsilateral internal mammary lymph node(s) and in the *presence* of clinically evident axillary lymph node metastasis; or, metastasis in ipsilateral supraclavicular lymph node(s) with or without axillary or internal mammary lymph node involvement
  N3a: Metastasis in ipsilateral infraclavicular lymph node(s)
  N3b: Metastasis in ipsilateral internal mammary lymph node(s) and axillary lymph node(s)
  N3c: Metastasis in ipsilateral supraclavicular lymph node(s)

Pathologic Classification (pN)

Classification is based on axillary lymph node dissection with or without sentinel lymph node (SLN) dissection. Classification based solely on SLN dissection without subsequent axillary lymph node dissection is designated (sn) for sentinel node, for example, pN0(I+) (sn).

- pNX: Regional lymph nodes cannot be assessed (e.g., not removed for pathologic study or previously removed)
- pN0: No regional lymph node metastasis histologically, and no additional examination for isolated tumor cells (ITCs: single tumor cells or small cell clusters <0.2 mm, usually detected only by immunohistochemical (IHC) or molecular methods but that may be verified on hematoloxylin & eosin (H&E) stains, which do not usually show evidence of malignant activity, such as proliferation or stromal reaction)
- pN0(I-): No regional lymph node metastasis histologically, negative IHC

Table 5.5   TNM Classification of Breast Cancer (TNM UICC, 6th Edition) (Changes with Respect to the Previous Classification)

TNM$_{UICC}$, 5th edition	TNM$_{UICC}$, 6th edition
Regional lymph nodes: (iii) Level III (apical axilla): lymph nodes medial to the medial margin of the pectoralis minor muscle including those designated as subclavicular, infraclavicular, or apical	*Regional lymph nodes:* (iii) Level III (apical axilla): apical lymph nodes and those medial to the medial margin of the pectoralis minor muscle excluding those designated as subclavicular or infraclavicular
Some *M1* referred to "regional" lymph node metastases (supraclavicular), while reference to infraclavicular lymph node metastases was ambiguous (...any other...)	*New:* Infraclavicular (subclavicular) (ipsilateral) and supraclavicular (ipsilateral) are considered as Regional Lymph Nodes
Clinical classification *Primary tumor (T):*	*Primary tumor (T):*
Tis: Carcinoma in situ: intraductal carcinoma, or lobular carcinoma in situ, or Paget's disease of the nipple with no tumor	Tis: Carcinoma in situ: Tis *(DCIS)* Ductal carcinoma in situ Tis *(LCIS)* Lobular carcinoma in situ Tis *(Paget)* Paget's disease of the nipple with no tumor
Regional lymph nodes (N): N2: Metastasis to ipsilateral axillary node(s) fixed to one another or to other structures	*Regional lymph nodes (N):* N2: Metastasis in *fixed* ipsilateral axillary node(s) or in clinically apparent ipsilateral internal mammary lymph node(s) in the absence of clinically evident axillary lymph nodes metastasis *New:* N2a: Metastasis in axillary lymph node(s) fixed to one another or to other structures N2b: Metastasis only in clinically apparent internal mammary lymph node(s) in the absence of clinically evident axillary lymph nodes metastasis
N3: Metastasis to ipsilateral internal mammary lymph node(s)	N3: Metastasis in ipsilateral infraclavicular lymph node(s) with or without axillary lymph node involvement or in clinically apparent ipsilateral internal mammary lymph node(s) in the presence of clinically evident axillary lymph node metastasis; or metastasis in ipsilateral supraclavicular lymph node(s) with or without axillary or internal mammary lymph node involvement *New:* N3a: Metastasis in infraclavicular lymph node(s) N3b: Metastasis in internal mammary and axillary lymph nodes N3c: Metastasis in supraclavicular lymph node(s)
Pathological classification *Regional lymph nodes (N):* Low axillary lymph nodes resection will ordinarily include six or more lymph nodes	*Regional lymph nodes (N):* Low axillary lymph nodes resection will ordinarily include six or more lymph nodes. *If the lymph nodes are negative, but the number ordinarily examined is not met, classify as pN0* *New:* Examination of one or more sentinel lymph nodes may be used for pathological classification. If classification is based solely on sentinel-node biopsy without subsequent axillary lymph node dissection it should be designated (sn) for sentinel node, e.g.,pN1(sn)
pN0: No regional lymph nodes metastasis	pN0: No regional lymph nodes metastasis[a]
pN1a: Only Micrometastasis (none larger than 0.2 cm)	pN1mi: Micrometastasis (larger than 0.2 mm, but none larger than 2 mm in greatest dimension)
pN1: Metastasis to movable ipsilateral axillary node(s)	pN1: Metastasis in 1–3 ipsilateral axillary node(s) and/or in ipsilateral internal mammary nodes with microscopic metastasis detected by sentinel lymph node dissection but not clinically apparent
pN1bi: Metastasis to one to three lymph nodes, any more than 0.2 cm and all less than 2.0 cm in greatest dimension	pN1a: Metastasis in one to three axillary lymph node(s), including at least one larger than 2 mm in greatest dimension pN1b: *Internal* mammary lymph nodes, with microscopic metastasis detected by sentinel lymph node dissection but not clinically apparent pN1c: Metastasis in one to three axillary lymph nodes and *internal* mammary lymph nodes, with microscopic metastasis detected by sentinel lymph node dissection but not clinically apparent
pN1bii: Metastasis to four or more lymph nodes, any more than 0.2 cm and all less than 2.0 cm in greatest dimension	pN2: Metastasis in four to nine ipsilateral axillary lymph nodes, or in clinically apparent ipsilateral *internal* mammary lymph node(s), in the *absence* of axillary lymph node metastasis pN2a: Metastasis in four to nine axillary lymph nodes including at least one that is larger than 2 mm pN2b: Metastasis in clinically apparent *internal* mammary lymph node(s), in the *absence* of axillary lymph node metastasis

(Continued)

Table 5.5 TNM Classification of Breast Cancer (TNM UICC, 6th Edition) (Changes with Respect to the Previous Classification) (*Continued*)

TNM$_{UICC}$, 5th edition	TNM$_{UICC}$, 6th edition
	New:
	pN3: Metastasis in 10 or more ipsilateral axillary lymph nodes; or in ipsilateral *infraclavicular* lymph nodes or in clinically apparent ipsilateral *internal* mammary lymph nodes, in the *presence* of one or more positive axillary lymph nodes; or in more than three axillary lymph nodes with clinically negative microscopic metastasis in *internal* mammary lymph nodes; or in ipsilateral *supraclavicular* lymph nodes
	pN3a: Metastasis in 10 or more axillary lymph nodes (at least one larger than 2 mm) or metastasis in *infraclavicular* lymph nodes
	pN3b: Metastasis in clinically apparent *internal* mammary lymph node(s), in the *presence* of positive axillary lymph node(s); or metastasis in more than three axillary lymph nodes and in *internal* mammary lymph nodes with microscopic metastasis detected by sentinel lymph node dissection but not clinically apparent.
	pN3c: Metastasis in *supraclavicular* lymph node(s)
pN2: Metastasis ipsilateral of axillary lymph nodes that are fixed to one another or to other structures	*Not considered*
Grading: Histopathological grading referred to the degree of differentiation	*Grading*: Histopathological grading. Reference indicated as Elston CW & Ellis IO, Histopathology 1991.

[a]Cases with only isolated tumor cells (ITC) in regional lymph nodes are classified as pN0. ITC are single tumor cells or small clusters of cells not more than 0.2 mm in greatest dimension. That are usually detected by immunohistochemistry or molecular methods but which may be verified on H&E stains. ITCs do not typically show evidence of metastatic activity e.g., proliferation of stromal reaction.

- pN0(I+): No regional lymph node metastasis histologically, positive IHC, and no IHC cluster larger than 0.2 mm
- pN0(mol-): No regional lymph node metastasis histologically, and negative molecular findings (RT-PCR, reverse transcriptase-polymerase chain reaction)
- pN0(mol+): No regional lymph node metastasis histologically, and positive molecular findings (RT-PCR)
- pN1: Metastasis in one to three axillary lymph nodes, and/or in internal mammary nodes with microscopic disease detected by SLN dissection but not clinically apparent
  pN1mi: Micrometastasis (larger than 0.2 mm but not larger than 2.0 mm)
  pN1a: Metastasis in one to three axillary lymph nodes
  pN1b: Metastasis in internal mammary nodes with microscopic disease detected by SLN dissection but not clinically apparent
  pN1c: Metastasis in one to three axillary lymph nodes and in internal mammary lymph nodes with microscopic disease detected by SLN dissection but not clinically apparent (If associated with more than three positive axillary lymph nodes, the internal mammary nodes are classified as pN3b to reflect increased tumor burden.)
- pN2: Metastasis in four to nine axillary lymph nodes, or in clinically apparent internal mammary lymph nodes in the *absence* of axillary lymph node metastasis to ipsilateral axillary lymph node(s) fixed to each other or to other structures
- pN2a: Metastasis in four to nine axillary lymph nodes (at least one tumor deposit larger than 2.0 mm)
- pN2b: Metastasis in clinically apparent internal mammary lymph nodes in the *absence* of axillary lymph node metastasis
- pN3: Metastasis in ten or more axillary lymph nodes, or in infraclavicular lymph nodes, or in clinically apparent ipsilateral internal mammary lymph node(s) in the *presence* of one or more positive axillary lymph node(s); or, in more than three axillary lymph nodes with

clinically negative microscopic metastasis in internal mammary lymph nodes; or, in ipsilateral supraclavicular lymph nodes

pN3a: Metastasis in ten or more axillary lymph nodes (at least one tumor deposit larger than 2.0 mm); or, metastasis to the infraclavicular lymph nodes

pN3b: Metastasis in clinically apparent ipsilateral internal mammary lymph nodes in the *presence* of one or more positive axillary lymph node(s); or, in more than three axillary lymph nodes and in internal mammary lymph nodes with microscopic disease detected by sentinel lymph node dissection but not clinically apparent

pN3c: Metastasis in ipsilateral supraclavicular lymph nodes

Distant Metastasis (M)
- MX: Presence of distant metastasis cannot be assessed
- M0: No distant metastasis
- M1: Distant metastasis

AJCC Stage Groupings

Stage 0	Tis, N0, M0
Stage I	T1 (including T1mic), N0, M0
Stage IIA	T0, N1, M0 or
	T1 (including T1mic), N1, M0 or
	T2, N0, M0
Stage IIB	T2, N1, M0 or
	T3, N0, M0
Stage IIIA	T0, N2, M0 or
	T1 (including T1mic), N2, M0 or
	T2, N2, M0 or
	T3, N1, M0 or
	T3, N2, M0
Stage IIIB	T4, N0, M0 or
	T4, N1, M0 or
	T4, N2, M0
Stage IIIC	Any T, N3, M0
Stage IV	Any T, Any N, M1

ROLE OF SURGERY/RADIOTHERAPY

Treatment of Breast Cancer

The global strategy in approaching a patient with limited disease confined to the breast and ipsilateral axillary nodes has drastically changed in the past 30 years. Currently, the following treatments should be discussed:

- Breast surgery should be offered to patients presenting with tumors confined to the breast, not involving skin or muscle, and at most accompanied by palpable lymph nodes in the ipsilateral axilla. For large, isolated lesions (in relationship to the size of the breast), primary systemic therapy should be considered to allow breast conservation.
- Postoperative radiation therapy is generally indicated for all patients undergoing breast-conserving surgery. Postoperative radiation to the chest wall after total mastectomy or more extensive surgery is strongly recommended only for patients who have a very high risk for locoregional recurrence (>20%).
- Adjuvant systemic therapy should be considered for all patients with invasive breast cancer.

Surgical Procedures

Surgery has a prominent role to eliminate overt disease, when confined to the mammary gland and to ipsilateral axillary nodes. Table 5.6 illustrates the various surgical procedures. Breast conservation and total mastectomy with axillary clearance have been demonstrated to produce equivalent survival results in multicenter, randomized clinical trials (66). Decisions regarding the type of local therapy should be made after discussion with the patient taking into account her preferences. Breast conservation, defined as complete tumor excision followed by whole breast irradiation, should be offered as preferred therapy to most women with operable breast cancer.

Proper surgical technique contributes to cosmetic results, which are enhanced if incisions are placed appropriately (including a separate incision for axillary dissection), no sutures are placed in the substance of the breast, and complete hemostasis is obtained. For accurate pathological evaluation, orientation of the intact, excised specimen and avoidance of diathermy allow evaluation of excision margins. Re-excision should be performed if pathological excision margins are smaller than a few millimeters. This

Table 5.6 Common Surgical Procedures for Breast Cancer Treatment

Surgical procedure	Definitions and remarks
Radical mastectomy	• *En bloc* removal of the breast and overlying skin as well as the pectoralis major and minor muscles. Includes a total axillary clearance. • Might still be a reasonable treatment for patients with large, bulky tumors involving pectoralis muscles, for whom the use of primary systemic therapies are contraindicated.
Extended radical mastectomy	• *En bloc* removal of the internal mammary lymph nodes chain and vessels through thoracotomy. Involves also the resection of a portion of the sternum and adjacent ribs (second to fourth), breast and overlying skin, as well as the pectoralis major and minor muscles. Includes also a total axillary clearance. • This procedure has no indications.
Modified radical mastectomy	• Also named total mastectomy with axillary lymph node dissection and preservation of the pectoralis major muscle. Not as precisely defined as radical mastectomy. Variations were introduced according to the procedure used to dissect or not the pectoralis minor muscle (with or without its preservation, including the neurovascular bundle). Axillary dissection is variably performed to include clearance of I, II, and III axillary lymph node level. • Used by many who prefer some degree of dissection of the pectoralis minor to optimize axillary lymph node clearance.
Total mastectomy (+axillary clearance)	• Removal of the entire breast, the overlying skin, and the pectoralis muscle fascia, without the removal of pectoralis muscles. The additional axillary clearance is not included in the procedure, thus if performed, it should be specifically mentioned. • Currently the total mastectomy and axillary clearance are often performed as an alternative to breast conservation procedures when the latter is contraindicated or not applied due to patient's preference.
Subcutaneous mastectomy	• Removal of the breast tissue preserving the skin envelope and the nipple-areolar complex. • This procedure has a controversial role in the treatment of invasive cancer since about 10–15 percent of breast tissue is left behind.
Breast preservation procedures	• These procedures are usually completed with axillary lymph node clearance and radiation therapy.
• Tumorectomy, lumpectomy	Removal of the tumor with grossly clear margins. Also referred to as wide excision to distinguish from diagnostic lumpectomy.
• Quadrantectomy	*En bloc* removal of the tumor within a quadrant of breast along with pectoralis major muscle fascia and overlying skin.
Breast reconstruction after mastectomy (immediate or delayed)	• Using either local tissue and submuscular implant, or a myocutaneous flap (latissimus dorsi or transverse rectus abdominis flap) with or without implant of prosthesis. • Usually requires two or more surgical interventions. The timing of these procedures is controversial. • Connective tissue reactions towards silicon implants were described, and influence patients' acceptance
Sentinel-node biopsy	Axillary staging through the pathologic evaluation of the first lymph node that drains the tumor area (sentinel-node biopsy) was tested to avoid extensive surgery on a negative axilla. The proper technique to use should include lympho-scintigraphy and as an alternative blue-dye injection. An extensive pathology work-up and training is required for an accurate and reproducible result.

might also help in identifying multiple cancer foci (either intraductal or invasive).

The conserved breast should receive whole breast irradiation. Routine irradiation of the dissected axilla or other draining lymph node regions usually does not improve local control and increases morbidity (67).

Total mastectomy may be preferred to breast conservation in several cases (Table 5.7). Aspects such as short life expectancy and a small endocrine responsive tumor might lead to considering less than mastectomy without irradiation to the conserved breast, however no group was identified to allow avoidance of radiation to the conserved breast (68). New technologies, such as partial, intraoperative breast irradiation, are currently investigated, and represent promising treatments for the future.

Axillary lymph node dissection is preferred to removal of level I and II axillary lymph nodes and remains the standard of care for invasive breast cancer, especially for women with palpable nodes in the axilla, multicentric disease, or large tumors (>3 cm). It provides significant prognostic information, and controls nodal metastases and disease progression in the axilla. An axillary staging through the pathological evaluation of the first node draining the tumor area (sentinel-node biopsy, SNB) was tested to avoid extensive surgery on a negative axilla, and was found to be proper for routine use, when the size of the tumor does not exceed 2–3 cm (69). The technique to use, extent of the pathological work-up, and training required for an accurate and reproducible surgery are heterogeneous and must adhere as much as possible to described methods (70).

Axillary lymph node dissection is not required for the management of DCIS; however, during the last decade, sentinel lymph node biopsy has been increasingly used to exclude the presence of axillary metastases (when invasive disease is present within the DCIS). This approach should be considered when there is an increased probability for the presence of invasive breast cancer within the DCIS (71).

Radiation Therapy After Surgery

Radiation therapy remains an important component of the management of breast cancer. In the past, chest wall irradiation after mastectomy was routinely carried out in most women, especially in node-positive disease. Randomized trials demonstrated that, despite the significant reduction in local recurrence, only a modest influence on systemic relapse and overall survival (OS) in patients with high-risk disease could be obtained (72,73). Central review of data from 20,000 women from 40 randomized trials of radiotherapy for early breast cancer was performed: breast cancer mortality was reduced ($p = 0.0001$) but other, particularly vascular, mortality was increased ($p = 0.0003$), and overall 20-year survival was 37.1% with radiotherapy versus 35.9% in the control arm ($p = 0.06$) (74).

The largest effect on systemic disease and subsequent improved survival was observed in two trials of patients at high-risk of recurrence, when radiation therapy to the chest wall was delivered together with systemic therapy. Controversies exist, however, concerning the adequacy of surgery and systemic treatment (low-dose regimen chemotherapy and short tamoxifen duration) delivered in these trials. Recent analysis of the Danish and the EORTC trials has cast doubt on the traditional perception that radiotherapy is of most benefit to patients with higher risk of relapse (e.g., ≥4 positive nodes). In these trials, indeed, the highest survival benefit was seen among patients with one to three positive nodes, while the reduction in locoregional recurrences was largest in patients with more advanced cancer (75).

Radiation therapy to the conserved breast after proper tumor surgery reduces the incidence of relapse in the ipsilateral breast. Breast radiation is usually performed using supervoltage equipment to 4500–5000 cGy in doses of 80–200 cGy/day, through fields tangential to the chest wall. Increasing the dose to the primary site to 6000 cGy or 60 Gy (boost) is often performed, using either electron beam or interstitial implantation. The role of routine boosting is imprecise although the role of a boost was recently described particularly in younger patients (76). Disease control in the conserved breast with radiation therapy is dependent upon several features, including multicentricity, total tumor excision, presence of extensive intraductal component, and vessel invasion.

Radiation therapy confined to fields less than the whole breast (partial breast irradiation, PBI) has been investigated using a number of different techniques. Long-term safety, efficacy, and issues about treatment of relapse in the breast following PBI require further evaluation. At present, PBI should be confined to prospective clinical trials (77).

Table 5.7 Conditions under Which Breast Conservation Procedure Should Not Be Advised for Local Control of Disease

Condition	Remarks
• Large tumor relative to the size of the breast	• Precludes an acceptable cosmetic result.
• Gross multifocal disease	• Breast relapse rate is high despite radiation therapy. Extensive intraductal component (EIC = when at least 25% of the tumor area) was associated with high breast relapses after radiation therapy (especially after tumorectomy). • Central tumors or Paget's disease of the nipple are not a contraindication for breast conservation.
• Extensive malignant type diffuse microcalcifications are present on mammography	• Does not allow a proper, patient-reassuring follow-up.
• Prior high-dose radiation therapy has been given to the region	• Prior radiation therapy (e.g., previous malignant lymphomas), or concomitant pathological condition which does not allow curative radiation of the breast without risk of severe toxic effects (e.g., collagen-vascular disease, or significant cardiac or pulmonary insufficiency).

Several issues associated with local disease control still need to be clarified. For instance, screening-detected cancers or very small tumors are still treated in the same way as symptomatic cancers of the breast, despite the fact that data on the adequacy of their treatment with surgery alone are either not available or controversial (78).

The clinical relevance of clear surgical margins for breast conservation is controversial. The failure rate in cases of unclear margins, with either in situ or invasive cancer, is increased despite radiation therapy, but the magnitude of this increase is not well defined.

The adequacy of radiation therapy to the breasts of young women is an issue for debate. The local failure rate following radiation therapy is higher for younger women, but several features other than age have also been associated with this increased risk.

Elderly patients derive similar benefits from proper radiation therapy as younger women. Logistics are often, however, more complex for patients of more advanced age resulting in a higher burden of treatment. Cost–benefit considerations for elderly women are likely to yield different results.

Some long-term side effects of radiation therapy remain unknown as a result of the lack of proper longitudinal studies designed to identify late sequelae (79). Efforts are made to improve late toxicity from the known interaction between radiation and drugs, like anthracyclines or taxanes commonly employed in the adjuvant setting (80).

Integration of radiation therapy and systemic adjuvant chemotherapy is a matter of controversy. Attempts to complete the local treatment by delivering radiation therapy immediately after surgery have conflicted with the logical approach of starting systemic treatment without delay. Delivering the two modalities simultaneously can result in an unsatisfactory outcome. In contrast, the International Breast Cancer Study Group (IBCSG) has shown for the first time in randomized trials (trials VI and VII) that the incidence of breast recurrence in the conserved ipsilateral breast within five years of follow-up was similar whether there was no radiotherapy delay, or there was a delay of three or six months to allow for completion of cytotoxic adjuvant therapy (81). Concurrent radiation therapy and *classical* CMF (cyclophosphamide, methotrexate, and 5-fluorouracil) was attempted omitting radiation on the days in which i.v. MF is administered. This approach seems feasible and represents a reasonable approach to shorten the overall adjuvant treatment period. Controversy exists on the timing of radiation therapy with respect to tamoxifen due to some reports on increased risk of lung fibrosis when the two modalities are combined (82).

Follow-up After Local Treatment

Follow-up after local treatment for breast cancer has the primary role to identify recurrences of breast cancer and/or second primary cancers. Relapses after early breast cancer have highest rates within the first five years following primary treatment, but patients remain at risk for the rest of their lives. Second, it may recognize local complications after breast surgery and radiation therapy and long-lasting side effects of treatment (83). Finally, it may exert a psychosocial function, since early breast cancer patients frequently face a burden of anxiety and depression due to their worries about recurrence (84).

Limits of follow-up include costs (in terms of patient/physician time and monetary costs), anxiety (no testing procedures have optimal sensitivity nor specificity), and the fact that recurrent breast cancer is not a curable disease. Of note, early institution of "salvage" therapy is not more efficacious than using the "salvage" therapy at a future time point in the disease course, with the exception of locoregional recurrences.

Controversies exist about routine use of laboratory tests and imaging procedures, which rarely identify metastatic disease in asymptomatic patients. More than 75% of all breast cancer recurrences are heralded by symptoms, often detected by patients, or by findings on physical examination, in particular for locoregional recurrences.

Two randomized trials were conducted in Italy to investigate the role of intensive follow-up. In the first of such trials, comparing intensive follow-up (physical examination, annual mammography, biannual chest x-ray, and bone scan) versus clinical follow-up (physical examination and mammography), an earlier detection of recurrences was shown in the intensive follow-up group, with no difference in the five-year overall mortality (85). In the second trial, comparing intensive surveillance (physician visits, bone scan, liver ultrasound, chest x-ray, and laboratory tests) versus control (only clinically indicated tests + yearly mammogram), there were no differences in terms of OS, time to detection of recurrence, and quality of life in the two groups (86).

The 2006 ASCO-recommended investigations in breast cancer surveillance include

- history, physical examination, and patient education regarding symptoms of recurrence (every 3–6 months for the first three years, then every 6–12 months for the next two years, then annually)
- genetic counseling (in women at high risk for familial breast cancer syndromes)
- breast self-examination (monthly)
- mammography (yearly).

Insufficient data exist so far to recommend routine use of the following tests in asymptomatic patients: blood tests, chest x-ray, bone scan, liver ultrasound/computed tomography, PET scan, and breast MRI (87). The latter exam, however, is thought to be useful as an adjunct to mammography in the follow-up of BRCA 1–2 mutation carriers or for patients who have been treated for breast cancer and have not been elected to undergo bilateral mastectomy (88–90). Alkaline phosphatase is the most sensitive test in cases of overt metastatic disease (91). The role of circulating tumor markers such as CEA and CA15-3 for early detection of metastatic disease was defined as potentially useful, although the clinical utility of routine serial determination is still being investigated due to lack of sensitivity and specificity (92).

SYSTEMIC TREATMENT
Adjuvant Systemic Therapy

Many breast cancer patients who remain disease free after local and regional treatment eventually relapse and die as a result of, or with, overt metastases. The current hypothesis ascribes the failure to obtain freedom from disease to occult micro-metastatic disease already present at the time of diagnosis and first surgery. After observations of tumor regression after oophorectomy, adjuvant systemic therapy had initially been applied as ovarian ablation. Systemic adjuvant chemotherapy was later introduced as a result of response rates of measurable metastases to cytotoxic agents, the hypothesis being related to an attempt to kill cells that detach during surgery, which were considered to be responsible for the development of overt metastases. This hypothesis of perioperative migration of cells with metastatic potential has been abandoned in favor of the one attributing overt metastases to micro-metastatic disease at the time of primary diagnosis. Newer hypotheses include the organization of micro-metastatic disease within its environment, forming structures with proper stroma and vascularization, which become important features to consider for the development of novel treatment strategies.

Almost all knowledge about the benefits of adjuvant systemic treatment has derived from randomized trials which were designed to define treatment benefit in terms of disease free survival (DFS) or OS. Two main types of treatments have been investigated in the past few decades: endocrine therapies and cytotoxic drugs (administered as single- or multiple-agent regimens), or their combination. These treatments were found to be effective in prolonging DFS and OS as compared to locoregional treatment only. More recently, trials have investigated new therapeutics directed toward specific targets, such as trastuzumab, in the attempt to improve further treatment outcome. Adjuvant therapy averts relapse in one-third of the patients who would have relapsed without its use, resulting in a death rate reduction by about one-fifth. Cumulative estimates after 5–15 years of follow-up indicate that the benefit in terms of reduction of the risk of death is about 7–12% (OS percentage increases at 10 years from 40% to 50%) in node-positive and 2–5% in node-negative breast cancer (OS percentage increases at 10 years from 79% to 84%). Newer trials that compare a newer adjuvant systemic therapy with the best available treatment, are likely to yield smaller differences, which might however be medically and humanly relevant, thus requiring a larger sample size.

As a result of these sample size considerations, summing up of the results in an overview or meta-analysis from individual trials, which compared one therapy with another, has become the most powerful tool for identifying treatment outcome differences. The latest update of this international collaborative effort was performed in 2005. The overview was specifically carried out to identify a real treatment effect from a given adjuvant treatment, providing less information about the magnitude of treatment effects, due to heterogeneity of selection criteria and treatments in the various trials (93).

- Tamoxifen was found to be effective in the adjuvant treatment of patients with operable breast cancer at any stage and at any age, the magnitude of treatment effect being related with ER expression. Five-year treatment duration is reasonable although the debate on longer durations is awaiting publication from recently completed trials.
- Chemotherapy was effective in improving DFS and OS in all groups, the largest magnitude of treatment effect

being observed in ER-poor/negative disease independently of age.
- Ovarian ablation was found to be effective in patients less than 50 years of age, presenting at any stage of operable disease.

The choice of adjuvant treatment is based on results from clinical trials and evaluation of risk factors derived from disease and patient-related features (Table 5.8). Expert consensus meetings, such as those held in St. Gallen (Switzerland) since 1978, attempt to define general principles based upon available evidence and expert opinion to guide the treatment choice for women with early breast cancer. Since 2005, a fundamental change was made in the algorithm for selection of adjuvant systemic therapy for early breast cancer, in that endocrine responsiveness of the cancer was given a primary importance in the selection of systemic therapy. Three categories were acknowledged: highly endocrine responsive (high expression of both ER and PR in a majority of tumor cells), incompletely endocrine responsive (lower expression of ER and/or PR), and endocrine nonresponsive (complete absence of both ER and PR). The degree of endocrine responsiveness contributes, together with an assessment of the level of risk of relapse, to a decision about whether endocrine therapy alone may be sufficient: highly endocrine responsive tumors in patients at low risk of relapse may be suitable for endocrine therapy alone, while chemotherapy may be required for patients with highly endocrine responsive tumors in case of intermediate- or high-risk, and for patients with incompletely endocrine responsive tumors. Much as steroid hormone receptors are targets for endocrine therapies, the presence of HER-2 on the cell surface is an effective target for trastuzumab. Moreover, it was acknowledged that axillary lymph node involvement did not automatically define high risk, so that intermediate risk included both node-negative disease (if some features of the primary tumor indicated elevated risk) and patients with one to three involved lymph nodes without additional high-risk features. Table 5.9 summarizes the St. Gallen risk categories for patients with operated breast cancer. Treatment choice recommendations for each subpopulation defined by these factors were made. Table 5.10 describes available types of systemic adjuvant therapies based upon baseline prognosis and features influencing treatment outcome.

Chemotherapy Regimens and Their Toxicities

Historical developments and trials as well as clinical practice led to the availability of several types of chemotherapeutic regimens proven or presumed to be effective adjuvant therapies. It is recognized that there are two general levels of cytotoxic therapy regimens. Treatment with four courses of AC (doxorubicin and cyclophosphamide) was shown to be equivalent to six courses of classical CMF (94). Several regimens and schedules such as Canadian CEF (cyclophosphamide, epirubicin, fluorouracil), CAF regimen (95), dose-dense doxorubicin, paclitaxel, and cyclophosphamide (96), and to some extent also tailored FEC (fluorouracil, epirubicin, and cyclophosphamide) (97) and docetaxel, doxorubicin, and cyclophosphamide (TAC) (98) have been shown in comparative trials to yield superior results, though at the cost

Table 5.8 Adjuvant Systemic Therapies and Some Relevant Treatment Concepts Investigated in Randomized Clinical Trials

Treatments	Results and remarks
Ovarian ablation	• Overview results showed an estimated relative reduction in the odds of relapse or death of 26% and a reduction in the odds of death of 25%.
	• The reduction in relapses associated with the use of ovarian ablation appeared late during follow-up.
	• Chemotherapy-induced amenorrhea was also found to be associated with improved DFS in trials of adjuvant cytotoxic therapies. It is unlikely that the main therapeutic effect of adjuvant chemotherapy in premenopausal patients is exclusively due to ovarian suppression. Improved DFS was seen in patients who had ER-positive tumors, and was observed also in patients who resumed menses after an amenorrhea lasting several months.
	• Current trials investigate ovarian suppression with GnRH analogs and its combination with chemotherapy.
Perioperative cytotoxic therapy of short duration	• Overview data showed a slight reduction of relapses.
Preoperative chemotherapy	• Preoperative chemotherapy with four courses of adriamycin and cyclophosphamide (AC) yielded similar results to the postoperative use of the same regimen (NSABP trial B-18).
	• Several regimens were tested as preoperative chemotherapy in early breast cancer including some new agents and approaches. The advantage of evaluating primary tumor responses to preoperative chemotherapy was used for the definition of new administration modalities (e.g., continuous infusion of 5-fluorouracil given with intermittent 4-epirubicin and cisplatin with an estimated response rate of 98%).
Adjuvant prolonged chemotherapy	• For recurrence, polychemotherapy produced substantial and highly significant proportional reductions both among women aged under 50 at randomization (35%) and among those aged 50–69 (20%). Adjuvant polychemotherapy produces an absolute improvement of about 7–11% in 10-year survival for women aged under 50 at presentation with early breast cancer, and of about 2–3% for those aged 50–69. Most investigated regimens in surgery-controlled trials were CMF-type; compared with CMF alone, anthracycline-containing regimens produced somewhat greater effects on recurrence and mortality. The benefits of adjuvant chemotherapy within 10 years outweigh the burdens especially for younger women (<50 years old) and among older women (50–69 years) to a lesser degree when the size of the benefit in terms of quality-adjusted survival was evaluated.
	• Multidrug regimens were found to be superior to single drugs (alkylating agents).
	• The use of anthracyclines instead of methotrexate in trials in which the two regimens were compared (i.e., CEF vs. *classical* CMF or CAF vs. *classical* CMF) showed a significant improvement of DFS at cost of increased toxicity.
	• An alternating regimen with doxorubicin followed by CMF compared with the same drugs given in a sequence starting with CMF resulted in an advantage for the doxorubicin-first regimen.
	• Two major trials examined four courses of paclitaxel after four cycles of AC, but the interpretation of these results has been made difficult by the confounding of duration, receptors and the concurrent administration of tamoxifen compared with AC alone. The effect was exclusively observed in the subpopulation with ER-negative disease.
	• A trial which investigated a dose reduction showed a significant decreased treatment effect for patients treated with the lower dose.
Adjuvant Tamoxifen	• Overview data showed that Tamoxifen reduced the annual odds of recurrence or death by 26% and the odds of death by 14% (summary effect of trials with 1, 2, or 5 years Tamoxifen). Tamoxifen was effective in patients with tumors classified as estrogen receptor positive. Contralateral breast cancer risk was reduced by approximately 35%.
	• Different doses of tamoxifen have not been compared. The recommended dose is 20 mg/day.
	• Treatment duration trials with tamoxifen show that the duration of 5 years should be recommended until further information will be available from ongoing studies. Reduction of odds of recurrence or death in trials of 5 years duration were 42% and 22%, respectively.
	• Different endocrine therapies using progestins (e.g., medroxyprogesterone acetate), and *older* aromatase inhibitors (aminoglutethimide) were insufficiently investigated.
Adjuvant aromatase inhibitors	• Initial adjuvant endocrine therapy with the aromatase inhibitors anastrozole or letrozole was tested in large trials against tamoxifen and found to significantly reduce relapse among postmenopausal women with endocrine responsive disease.
	• Sequential adjuvant endocrine therapy using exemestane or anastrozole after 2–3 years of tamoxifen to complete 5 years of endocrine therapy significantly improved treatment outcome.
	• Letrozole was tested against placebo after completion of about 5 years of adjuvant tamoxifen. A significant advantage in disease-free survival was observed. OS was also significantly better in the subgroup of patients with node-positive disease at diagnosis, but not for the cohort with node-negative disease. Several issues of safety (bone fractures, cardiac, and vascular disease as well as changes in blood lipids) require further study.
	• The most recent revision of the ASCO Technology Assessment concluded that optimal hormonal therapy for a postmenopausal woman with ER-positive breast cancer should include an aromatase inhibitor.
	• For patients at low risk of relapse or with comorbidity raising concern on the safety of aromatase inhibitors, adjuvant tamoxifen alone remains a reasonable alternative, and may be the only economically viable option in many situations.

(Continued)

Table 5.8 Adjuvant Systemic Therapies and Some Relevant Treatment Concepts Investigated in Randomized Clinical Trials (*Continued*)

Treatments	Results and remarks
Adjuvant chemo-endocrine therapies	• The Overview showed that for patients above 50, chemo-endocrine therapy (with tamoxifen) compared with chemotherapy alone reduced the annual odds of recurrence by 28% and the odds of death by 20%. Similarly, when compared to tamoxifen alone, the reductions in odds were 26% and 10%, respectively. • Combined chemo-endocrine therapies with tamoxifen and an anthracycline-based regimen yielded better DFS than endocrine therapy alone in patients with ER-positive tumors. The combination of tamoxifen with CMF-type regimens was superior to tamoxifen alone in trials using the *classical* CMF regimen. • Laboratory studies have demonstrated that chemotherapy cell kill was inhibited in the presence of tamoxifen. Clinical data also suggested a negative interaction between cytotoxics (alkylating agents and 5-fluorouracil) and tamoxifen, and this issue is still under study. The Intergroup trial 0100, showed the superiority of sequential over concurrent administration of AC and tamoxifen for postmenopausal women with node-positive (42% with ≥4 N+), receptor-positive (ER or PgR) disease.
High-dose chemotherapy	• A dose-intense regimen using several drugs on a weekly schedule for 16 weeks was found to significantly improve DFS and OS when compared to six courses of CAF. • High-dose chemotherapy with peripheral blood progenitor cell or bone marrow support remains investigational, since definitive results from ongoing clinical trials are not yet available and results from early trials failed to detect a significant advantage for high-dose chemotherapy.
Dose-dense chemotherapy	• Another concept recently examined in a large randomized trial is that of dose density. Patients receiving treatment on a two-weekly rather than a three-weekly schedule to the same total dose showed superior DFS and OS. These data must be taken into account with the additional cost of the growth factors required when deciding whether a particular patient should receive chemotherapy in a dose-dense fashion.
Adjuvant trastuzumab	• Trastuzumab has recently been demonstrated to lead to dramatic improvements in DFS when used in the adjuvant therapy setting in combination with or following chemotherapy.

Table 5.9 Definition of Risk Categories for Patients with Operated Breast Cancer (Modified from St. Gallen 2007)

Risk category	
Low risk	Node-negative, and all of the following features: pT[a] ≤2 cm, and Grade 1[b], and Absence of extensive peritumoral vascular invasion[c], and ER and/or PR expressed,and Her-2/neu gene neither overexpressed nor amplified, and Age[d] ≥35 years
Intermediate risk	Node-negative, and at least one of the following features: pT[a] >2 cm, or Grade 2–3[b], or Presence of extensive peritumoral vascular invasion, or ER and PR absent, or Her-2/neu gene overexpressed or amplified, or Age[d] <35 years Node-positive (one to three involved nodes), and: ER and/or PR expressed, and Her-2/neu gene neither overexpressed nor amplified
High risk	Node-positive (one to three involved nodes), and: ER and PR absent, or Her-2/neu gene overexpressed or amplified Node-positive (four or more involved nodes)

[a]pT, pathological tumor size (i.e., size of the invasive component).
[b]Histologic and/or nuclear grade.
[c]Peritumoral vascular invasion defined intermediate risk for node-negative disease, but did not influence risk category for node-positive disease.
[d]Patients with breast cancer at young age have been shown to be at high risk of relapse.

of greater complexity, cost, or toxicity. These more intensive regimens may be preferred in patients at higher risk.

Specific Chemotherapy Regimens

Cyclophosphamide, Methotrexate, and 5-Fluorouracil (CMF), Adriamycin and Cyclophosphamide (AC) and Flurouracil, Adriamycin (Epirubicin), and Cyclophosphamide (FAC or FEC). CMF, with M and F given on days 1 and 8 every four weeks, and C given orally on days 1–14, was initially the most widely investigated regimen on which efficacy data were obtained. It is still considered a proper treatment for patients with node-negative disease for whom chemotherapy is an appropriate choice (99), especially in conditions in which doubt has been raised on inferior therapeutic

Table 5.10   Choice of Treatment Modalities (Modified from St. Gallen 2007)

	Highly endocrine responsive	Incompletely endocrine responsive	Endocrine nonresponsive
HER-2 negative	ET (consider adding CT according to risk)	ET (consider adding CT according to risk)	CT
HER-2 positive	ET + Herceptin + CT	ET + Herceptin + CT	Herceptin + CT

Abbreviations: ET, endocrine therapy; CT, chemotherapy.

yield. The CMF regimen and an anthracycline-based combination such as doxorubicin (Adriamycin) and cyclophosphamide (AC) are considered to have similar treatment effects for patients with node-positive disease. Overview data and individual trials which compared classical CMF to an anthracycline-based regimen substituting methotrexate with either epirubicin (CEF) or adriamycin (CAF) showed an advantage in terms of treatment outcome for the anthracycline-treated patients at the cost of increased toxicity. During the 2007 St. Gallen meeting, four courses of AC or six courses of classical CMF were considered acceptable in patients with highly (but at high risk of relapse) or incompletely endocrine responsive HER-2-negative disease.

Subgroup analyses and data from several trials in which duration chemotherapy was one of the variables, indicate that in older premenopausal patients (above the age of 40) three courses of *classical* CMF might yield similar results to six courses (100). Acute toxicity of the CMF regimen includes gastrointestinal side effects, nausea/vomiting, mucositis, conjunctivitis, diarrhea and, in about 40% of the patients, alopecia. Toxic effects of anthracyclines include hematological and mucosal toxicity, nausea/vomiting, alopecia (almost universal), skin pigmentation, and cumulative cardiac toxicity. FAC and FEC (day 1 every 21) are usually used for six courses. No direct comparison of these regimens with classical CMF is available. The use of higher epirubicin dose was associated with a significant improvement of treatment outcome (DFS and OS) among patients with node-positive breast cancer (101). Subjective toxicity and objective tolerance are dependent upon treatment duration. One of the most recent trials designed to test the shorter versus longer treatment duration of a single chemotherapy regimen is the French study of FEC for six versus three courses. Longer treatment appeared more effective; it was entirely uncertain to which extent this result was due to the endocrine effects of the longer duration treatment in this premenopausal population.

CEF (Canadian), CAF (Intergroup), and Tailored FEC. More intensive anthracycline-based regimens are either used with drugs delivered on a *CMF-like* schedule (oral C and day 1 and 8 administration of i.v. drugs), or in a toxicity-tailored fashion. The first type includes the Canadian CEF (102) and the CAF regimen (95), and both were proven to be superior to classical CMF. The toxicity-tailored FEC yielded superior results even when compared to high-dose, marrow-supported chemotherapy. The use of all these combinations is associated with a high degree of myelosuppression leading to the use of either prophylactic antibiotics or marrow stimulating growth factors (G-CSF). This aspect of using cytotoxic combinations with anthracyclines (plus cyclophosphamide and fluorouracil) with G-CSF led

to a small but significant increase in the incidence of acute myelogenous leukemia (AML) or myelodysplastic syndrome (MDS), their incidence being sharply elevated in more intense regimens (103,104). These acute leukemia risk estimates need to be taken into account, especially for patients with node-negative disease.

Taxanes. Two major trials have examined four courses of paclitaxel after four cycles of AC, and both showed a significant improvement in treatment outcome. The U.S. Intergroup trial accrued 3121 patients and showed that four courses of paclitaxel after four courses of AC improved treatment outcome compared with four courses of AC alone. The five-year DFS and OS were 70% versus 65% and 80% versus 77%, respectively, differences which were both statistically significant (105). The NSABP B-28 trial had a similar design and accrued 3059 patients. The five-year DFS and OS percentages were 76% versus 72%, and 85% versus 81%, respectively, statistically significant only for DFS (106). Subgroup analysis, based upon whether the patients received tamoxifen after chemotherapy or not, yielded conflicting results and might indicate that the effect of adding paclitaxel is less evident in patients with tumors expressing hormone receptors who received tamoxifen after chemotherapy. The interpretation of these data is also difficult due to the confounding treatment effects of different durations. One of the most interesting approaches to increase the yield of the sequential combination was through administration of the drugs every two weeks instead of every three weeks (dose-dense) with the aid of G-CSF. One U.S. Intergroup trial tested this approach in a trial, which accrued 2005 patients. The results showed, after a median follow-up time of 36 months, that dose-dense treatment improved DFS (RR 0.74; $p = 0.010$), and OS (RR 0.69; $p = 0.013$). Four-year DFS was 82% for the dose-dense regimens and 75% for the standard dose (107). The results of this trial need confirmation, especially in a comparison with those regimens proven, in clinical trials, to be more effective than classical CMF (i.e., CEF or CAF). The combination of docetaxel, adriamycin, and fluorouracil (TAC) was proven to be superior to FAC (both regimens given on day 1 every 21 days) in the recent Breast Cancer International Research Group (BCIRG) trial (98).

Three additional trials failed to show a clear-cut benefit for taxane-based chemotherapy. The MA.21 trial, conducted by the National Cancer Institute of Canada, compared CEF, AC followed by paclitaxel, and dose-dense EC followed by paclitaxel in node-positive and high-risk node-negative women with breast cancer. Results of an interim analysis showed that recurrence rates were highest among patients treated with the conventionally timed taxane-containing regimen (108). The BIG 2-98 trial, conducted in

2887 node-positive patients: at five years median follow-up, a hazard ratio for docetaxel-containing versus nondocetaxel-containing regimens of borderline significance (109). Finally, in the TACT (Taxotere as Adjuvant Chemotherapy) trial, it was established that docetaxel-based sequential chemotherapy overall was not superior to anthracycline-based therapy of equivalent duration both for disease-free and overall survival (110).

Several tens of thousands additional women with operable breast cancer have been included in randomized clinical trials investigating the role of taxanes that have yet to report results. The St. Gallen expert consensus meeting in 2007 concluded that taxane combinations are effective in the adjuvant setting but especially in cohorts of patients with endocrine nonresponsive or incompletely responsive tumors. Exploratory analyses to identify those for whom the addition of a taxane-containing regimen might be superfluous has not been attempted. The question on how best to schedule taxanes seemed to favor weekly administration of paclitaxel, or the three-weekly docetaxel, but must be best studied within the context of optimal ER, PgR, and HER-2 determination.

Trastuzumab (Herceptin™)

Her-2/neu overexpression/amplification occurs in approximately 25% of breast cancers and is considered both a prognostic factor and a therapeutic target for trastuzumab, a humanized monoclonal antibody directed against the HER-2/neu protein extracellular domain. Trastuzumab therapy prolongs survival of patients with metastatic HER-2/neu-overexpressing breast cancer both alone and combined with chemotherapy. Four large, randomized, clinical trials and one smaller randomized trial of adjuvant trastuzumab have been conducted, all reporting an increased DFS and OS, leading to the FDA approval of trastuzumab in the adjuvant setting. The *NSABP B-31* trial compared four cycles of AC followed by four cycles of paclitaxel (P) (AC→P, arm 1) with AC→P plus 52 weeks of trastuzumab (H) beginning with the first cycle of P (AC→PH, arm 2). The *Intergroup N9831* trial compared four cycles of AC followed by 12 weekly doses of paclitaxel (AC→P, arm A) with AC→P followed by 52 weeks of H beginning after P (arm B) and with AC→P plus 52 weeks of H beginning with the first P cycle (arm C) (111). The joint statistical analysis showed 261 events in the control arms (arms 1 and A) and 133 in the investigational arms (arms 2 and C) (HR 0.48; 95% CI 0.39–0.59; $p = 2 \times 10^{-12}$), with an absolute difference in DFS rate of 12% at three years and 18% at four years. There was a 33% lower mortality hazard ($p = 0.015$) with the addition of trastuzumab. An unplanned comparison of arms B and C suggested that delayed administration of trastuzumab may be less effective than concurrent administration (112).

The Breast International Group (BIG) Herceptin® Adjuvant (HERA) trial (113) was a multicenter, randomized, controlled trial comparing one year or two years of trastuzumab given every three weeks with observation in patients with HER-2/neu-positive early breast cancer who had completed locoregional therapy and at least four cycles of neo-/adjuvant chemotherapy. At the first planned interim analysis comparing one year of trastuzumab versus observation, after a median follow-up of one year, 127 events

were observed in the trastuzumab group and 220 in the observation group (HR 0.54; 95% CI 0.43–0.67; $p < 0.0001$), with an absolute difference in the DFS rate at two years of 8.4% (85.8% vs. 77.4%). There were 89 distant recurrences in the trastuzumab group and 171 in the observation group (HR 0.49; 95% CI 0.38–0.63; $p < 0.0001$). Overall survival in the two groups was not significantly different. After a median follow-up of two years, one year of treatment with trastuzumab after adjuvant chemotherapy showed a significant OS benefit: 59 deaths were reported for trastuzumab and 90 in the control group (HR for risk of death with trastuzumab vs. observation alone, 0.66; 95% CI 0.47–0.91; $p = 0.0115$) (114).

The Breast Cancer International Research Group *BCIRG-006 trial* compared three arms of adjuvant systemic therapy in node-positive and node-negative patients whose tumors had Her-2/neu gene amplification by FISH: (a) AC followed by trastuzumab plus docetaxel chemotherapy (A→TH), (b) docetaxel and carboplatin plus trastuzumab (TCH), and (c) AC followed by docetaxel alone (A→T) as the control arm. At the interim analysis the risk for disease recurrence was 51% (95% CI 35–63%) lower in the A→TH arm ($p = 4.8 \times 10^{-7}$) and 39% (95% CI 21–53%) lower in the TCH arm ($p = 0.00015$) (115).

Finally, the Finnish *FinHer trial* showed a significant advantage of a short-term administration of adjuvant trastuzumab. Patients were randomized to docetaxel every three weeks for three doses versus nine weeks of vinorelbine, both combined with weekly trastuzumab for nine weeks alone in patients with HER-2/neu-positive breast. All patients subsequently received three cycles of low-dose FEC. At a median follow-up of three years, the short course of adjuvant trastuzumab was effective in preventing breast cancer recurrences (HR, 0.46; $p = 0.0078$) (116).

In contrast, the French *PACS-04 trial* failed to show a benefit for trastuzumab. In this small trial, women aged <65 years with node-positive early breast cancer were randomized to six cycles of adjuvant FEC100 (fluorouracil, epirubicin, and cyclophosphamide) or ED (epirubicin and docetaxel), and subsequently to observation only or one year of trastuzumab in case of HER-2-positive tumors. There was a trend toward efficacy of trastuzumab during the first 18 months, however at the four-year evaluation no significant differences in DFS and OS were observed between the trastuzumab and the observation arms (117).

Ovarian Ablation and Ovarian Endocrine Function Suppression

For premenopausal women with endocrine responsive disease, ovarian function suppression (with goserelin) with or without tamoxifen appeared to be at least as effective as CMF chemotherapy alone. The addition of tamoxifen to goserelin is more effective than goserelin alone at least in the presence of chemotherapy (118). The sequential use of goserelin following CMF appeared better than either modality alone in patients with node-negative disease, at least in subset analyses for women with ER-positive breast cancer and those younger than 40 years (119). Bilateral oophorectomy followed by tamoxifen was effective among patients with tumors overexpressing HER-2 compared with no adjuvant therapy (120).

Aromatase Inhibitors in Postmenopausal Patients

Inhibition of aromatase is an important approach for reducing growth stimulatory effects of oestrogens in postmenopausal women with hormone-dependent breast cancer. The new generation of aromatase inhibitors has shown an acceptable toxicity profile and three molecules have been studied in the adjuvant setting (121). The *Arimidex, Tamoxifen, Alone or in Combination (ATAC) trial* compared five years of tamoxifen, five years of anastrozole, or five years of both agents given in combination. A significantly improved DFS, time to recurrence (TTR), and time to distant recurrence (TDR) was shown for anastrozole over tamoxifen with a similar OS, the absolute difference in four-year DFS being 2.4% (86.9% with anastrozole vs. 84.5% with tamoxifen) (122,123). At a median follow-up of 100 months, the significant advantage for anastrozole over tamoxifen for DFS (HR 0.85; 95% CI 0.76, 0.94; $p = 0.003$), TTR (HR 0.77; 95% CI 0.67, 0.88; $p = 0.0001$), TDR (HR 0.84; 95% CI 0.72–0.98; $p = 0.027$), and CLBC (OR 0.6; 95% CI 0.42, 0.85; $p = 0.004$) was maintained. Absolute differences for anastrozole and tamoxifen increased over time (TTR 2.7% at five years and 4% at nine years). Breast cancer deaths were nonsignificantly fewer with anastrozole than tamoxifen but there was no difference in OS (124).

The *BIG 1–98 trial* compared five years of letrozole, five years of tamoxifen, two years of tamoxifen followed by three years of letrozole, or two years of letrozole followed by three years of tamoxifen. The first analysis was conducted comparing five years of either tamoxifen or letrozole: after a median follow-up of 51 months, DFS favored letrozole over tamoxifen, with significant benefits to letrozole for TTR and TDR, but with no significant benefit to OS. The absolute difference in four-year DFS was 2.9% (87.5% in the letrozole group, 84.6% in the tamoxifen group) (125,126). The *IES study* randomized women who had completed 2–3 years of tamoxifen to receive exemestane or further tamoxifen for a total of five years of treatment. At 55.7 months median follow-up, the trial showed an improvement in DFS but no significant difference in OS with exemestane. Time to contralateral breast cancer (HR 0.57, 95% CI 0.33–0.98) TTR (HR 0.70, 95% CI 0.58–0.83), and TDR (HR 0.83, 95% CI 0.71–0.99) were also significantly improved with exemestane (127,128).

The National Cancer Institute of Canada *MA.17 trial* randomized 5187 postmenopausal women who had completed approximately five years of tamoxifen to receive five years of letrozole or five years of placebo. At 30 months median follow-up, women who received letrozole after five years of tamoxifen experienced significantly longer DFS but not OS. Subgroup analyses revealed an OS benefit with letrozole in the node-positive group (HR 0.61; 95% CI 0.38–0.98; $p = 0.04$) and in those who received more than five years of tamoxifen (HR 0.56; 95% CI 0.33–0.97, $p = 0.04$) (129).

Given the positive results of aromatase inhibitors given either upfront, sequentially, or as an extended treatment, the latest ASCO Technology Assessment report suggests that the "optimal adjuvant hormonal therapy for a postmenopausal woman with receptor-positive breast cancer should include an aromatase inhibitor either as initial therapy or after treatment with tamoxifen. Of course, women with breast cancer and their physicians must weigh the risks and benefits of all therapeutic options."

Treatment of Elderly Patients

About 50% of all newly diagnosed breast cancers occur in women over 65 years. Comorbid conditions and compromised functional status contribute to the tendency to exclude elderly women from randomized clinical trials. Adjuvant therapies for elderly patients are therefore extrapolated from results of trials conducted in a younger population, and tamoxifen or cytotoxics, if suitable, should therefore be considered depending upon the woman's physiological age and psychological needs. The chance of obtaining long-term benefit from adjuvant therapies is limited as a result of the shorter life expectancy. Elderly women, however, do as well as younger patients for locally and regionally confined disease stages, but have a worse prognosis in metastatic disease. Adjuvant treatments might thus yield a long enough time period without symptoms of relapse and toxicity of treatments.

Results from the CALGB/CTSU 49907 trial, which compared capecitabine versus either AC or CMF in elderly breast cancer patients, have been recently presented. After a median follow-up of two years, patients randomized to capecitabine were 2.4 (95% CI 1.5–3.8) times more likely to experience an relapse free survival (RFS) event ($p = 0.0003$) and 2.1 (95% CI 1.2–3.7) times more likely to die ($p = 0.02$) (130).

Treatment of Male Breast Cancer

The incidence of male breast cancer is <1% of that for women and its presentation usually requires a modified radical mastectomy for local control because of involvement of the pectoralis muscle fascia. Lymph node involvement and ER status (positive in about 85% of the cases) have prognostic relevance similar to that of female breast cancer (131). Hormonal ablative therapy is associated with a 50–60% response rate in advanced disease, but no reports are available on adjuvant use. Tamoxifen is considered the first choice both in advanced disease and adjuvant setting, but as for antiandrogens, gonadotropin-releasing hormone (GnRH) analogues, and oestrogens, which are also effective in advanced disease, no information is available on its efficacy to reduce relapse and prolong survival. The use of aromatase inhibitors in patients with gonadal suppression is probably effective too, but information, mainly related to aminoglutethimide, is scarce. Adjuvant therapies (chemotherapy followed by tamoxifen, or tamoxifen alone) are usually prescribed extrapolating results from breast cancer trials in women. Radiation therapy to the chest wall and regional node sites is often delivered due to higher risk of local recurrence.

Quality-of-Life Considerations and Adjuvant Therapies

The burden of side effects of adjuvant systemic treatments has been considered by patients and physicians to be overwhelming. However, very few clinical trials focused on quality-of-life aspects of adjuvant treatments. Typically benefits in clinical trials are described in terms of DFS and OS. Quality-of-life aspects were, however, considered using two different approaches:

- Measuring patient perceptions of a specific quality-of-life-related item (e.g., perception of well-being, sensation of nausea, or tiredness) at a given time. It has been shown that the effect of cytotoxic treatments is transient and minor compared to patients' adaptation following diagnosis and surgery for breast cancer.

- Comparing two treatments (used in the trial by random allocation) which differ from each other substantially in terms of objective or subjective toxicity, and in terms of freedom from relapse. Comparisons are based upon the estimation of the time spent without symptoms of recurrent disease and toxic effects of therapy (TWiST) (132). Periods of time with symptoms of disease or toxic effects of treatment can be downweighted according to patient's perceptions allowing an estimation of quality-adjusted TWiST (Q-TWiST). This avoids methodological difficulties related to measurement of health states or perceptions of quality of life, focusing upon comparison of time periods which allow a personal interpretation for each individual patient.

- Patient preferences for adjuvant treatment assessed through her own perception on how much benefit from the treatment experienced in the past, makes the treatment worthwhile (trade-off: benefit in terms of improved prognosis paid for with a burden of side effects). Despite methodological difficulties (patients tend to justify their past treatment), patients indicated a large acceptance for a small potential benefit.

Patterns of Relapse After Adjuvant Systemic Therapy and Response to "Salvage Treatment"

Patients who relapse during or soon after adjuvant systemic therapy (within 6–12 months of its cessation) tend not to respond to a similar systemic therapy used in the adjuvant setting, and have a dire prognosis. In contrast, patients who develop metastases long after cessation of adjuvant treatment tend to have an excellent response, especially if the sites of recurrent disease are local, regional, or in soft tissues. Prognosis after adjuvant systemic therapy is dependent upon several factors, including site of relapse, time interval between diagnosis and appearance of metastatic disease, and several other tumor and host-related features such as ER. Current new technology, based on gene-expression profiles, might be very useful in defining prognosis, patterns of response to available treatments. Some information exists on the fact that genes involved in cell cycle, DNA replication, and chromosomal stability are consistently elevated in the various poor prognostic groups of patients. The consistent biological and clinical associations with gene-expression profiles might be helpful for tailoring new therapies.

Preoperative Therapy

The term "locally advanced breast cancer" refers to disease stages presenting as infiltration of the underlying muscles in the presence of a large primary tumor (T3b), extensive edema of the skin over the breast, skin ulceration, inflammatory cancer of the breast, satellite nodes on the skin, fixed axillary nodes, parasternal nodes, and edema of the arm. Some of the patients who present with locally advanced disease might have a slow growing neoplasia, but most patients have a very aggressive disease, with five-year

survival rates varying from 0% to 36%. Prognosis is worse for patients with inflammatory breast cancer (five-year probability of being alive about 30%) than with locally advanced breast cancer (five-year probability of being alive more than 70%; log-rank test, $p < 0.0001$). The treatment strategy includes primary chemotherapy, surgery (if feasible), and radiation therapy, leading to some improvement in outcome. High-dose chemotherapy (with or without colony-stimulating factors and bone marrow or peripheral committed precursors of blood cell support), or a dose-intense treatment with continuous or weekly drug administrations yielded a significant tumor regression in a large proportion of patients. Intensive systemic treatments are usually considered for patients with inflammatory breast cancer. In a large randomized trial a comparison between a dose-dense regimen with EC (plus G-CSF) and a CEF combination chemotherapy (with antibiotics), yielded similar results (133). Patients with a slow-growing, locally advanced breast cancer might obtain significant benefit, in terms of control of disease, from systemic endocrine therapy, radiation therapy, and low-dose chemotherapy. Weekly anthracyclines as well as continuous infusion fluorouracil regimens were used. The choice of treatment should thus take into account several factors indicative of tumor aggressiveness (i.e., history of growth, proliferation markers) and potential endocrine responsiveness. Assessment of responsiveness to preoperative therapy may in the future be useful in selection of postoperative adjuvant therapy.

Treatment of Metastatic Disease

Overt metastases indicate a chronic, incurable disease. Treatments are defined by their efficacy to provide palliation. An important feature influencing treatment choice relates to the heterogeneous course of the disease, with survival varying from a few weeks to more than 10 years. Overall, median duration of survival exceeds two years. Thus, the choice of treatment should account for extent of the disease, related symptoms, and estimation of survival, aiming to increase the total duration of the time with no/few disease-related symptoms, with lowest costs in terms of side effects. Systemic therapies, radiation, or surgery should be discussed for this purpose in a multidisciplinary setting.

The choice of treatment should also take into consideration certain indicators of aggressiveness of the disease and predictors of response. Shorter DFS, low/no ER expression in tumor cells, multiple organ involvement, and a short time interval from completion of previous adjuvant therapy are indicators of aggressive disease and short survival. Host-related factors (performance status) also influence the prognosis being associated with lower response rates and shorter duration of response.

The subjective attitude of the patient and the physician toward systemic treatment is one of the major factors that influence choice and acceptance of a therapeutic program, but only a few studies took such factors into consideration. Personal preference and considerations about quality of life, rather than data from clinical trials, should guide the treatment choice. Time to expected response to treatment is also a feature that may influence the choice of therapy: endocrine manipulations require an average of 6–12 weeks, whereas chemotherapy might influence

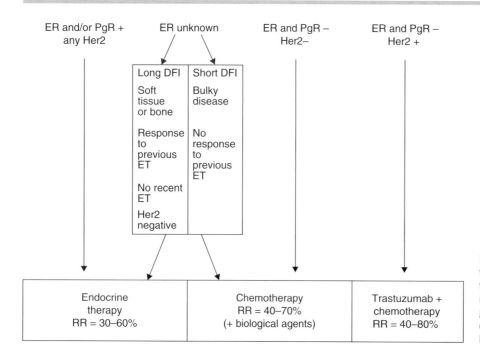

Figure 5.3 Algorithm of features (predictive factors) used for selection of type of initial systemic therapy for patients with metastatic disease. *Abbreviations*: ER, estrogen receptor; PgR, progesterone receptor; ET, endocrine therapy; DFI, disease free interval; RR, response rate.

disease symptoms within a shorter time. An algorithm which accounts for several features may aid the selection of the type of initial systemic therapy for patients with metastatic disease (Fig. 5.3).

The question of whether asymptomatic patients with metastatic disease should receive immediate systemic therapy upon detection of metastatic spread is a matter of controversy: treatment is usually offered immediately after diagnosis of metastases, attempting to defer the appearance of symptoms.

Before starting systemic therapy it is important to evaluate, with the least bothersome diagnostic method available (e.g., radiological assessment to sites of bone pain, assessment of single hepatic lesions by ultrasonography, etc.), most measurable sites of disease, providing the basis for an accurate evaluation of response. The use of tumor markers such as CEA or CA15-3 is valuable only within the context of the clinical situation. The usefulness of assessing objective responses in advanced breast cancer is controversial. Although objective response obtained by chemotherapy is associated with subjective palliation, many patients with stable disease, and even 33% of patients with progressive disease, experience significant pain relief. Measurable objective response is an important tool for assessing the effectiveness of antineoplastic drugs. It is, however, the evaluation of the impact of therapy upon the patients' quality of life, through the definition of symptom relief, drugs side effects, anxiety and depression, personal relations, physical performance, sense of well-being, and efforts to cope with the disease, which determines its usefulness.

Endocrine Therapy for Metastatic Disease

Endocrine treatments are usually well tolerated, enhancing their acceptability as a therapeutic option. In general,

endocrine therapies are offered to a patient with metastatic disease knowing that:

- About one-third of an unselected patient population is likely to respond to endocrine (or hormone) therapy; median duration of response is 8–14 months. Chances of response are higher when the tumor is rich in ER (50–60% response rate). Responses are more likely to occur in patients with prolonged DFS, with metastatic presentation of soft tissue or bone alone.
- Response to one endocrine therapy predicts a higher chance of effectiveness with subsequent hormonal manipulations.
- Discontinuation of an endocrine therapy such as estrogens, progestins, and tamoxifen at the time of disease progression (usually after a response) might induce a subsequent response. The mechanism for this *withdrawal response* phenomenon is not clearly understood.
- Starting of some hormonal manipulations may be accompanied by an exacerbation of cancer-related symptoms (*flare*). This might appear within hours or days, and last for several days or weeks. Flare might be associated with an increase of serum tumor markers, alkaline phosphatase, and hypercalcaemia. The incidence of this phenomenon is between 3% and 9%, and is likely to be followed by an objective response to therapy. Flare has been observed after the start of therapy with estrogens, tamoxifen, androgens, and progestins, but has been only anecdotally suspected after aromatase inhibitors.

Endocrine therapies have developed to encompass several types of endocrine-related mechanisms of controlling tumor growth and proliferation. Many of the mechanisms are related to suppression of estrogens or estrogen-mediated growth stimulation. Other pathways for cytostatic and cytocidal activity include direct cytotoxicity on tumor cells and growth factor-mediated effect (e.g., inducing expression of transforming growth factor TGF-beta, reducing expression of insulin-like growth factor I or IGF-I). Response to endocrine treatments is mostly predicted by the concentration of steroid hormone receptors, which determination depends upon several tumor and patient-related factors: sampling method, tumor cellularity, organ site of the neoplastic tissue, sex, menopausal status, day of cycle (for premenopausal women), pregnancy and lactation, and drug administration (e.g., steroid hormones). The method of determination is crucial for identifying overexpression of estrogen and progesterone receptors (ER and PgR): ligand-binding assay (LBA), which was historically first developed for commercial use, does not identify all endocrine responsive tumors, and currently immunohistochemical (IHC) method is recommended. ER and PgR overexpression in more than 1% of the tumor cells confers some endocrine responsiveness to the tumor (134).

Table 5.11 displays the summary data on endocrine treatments. Ovarian ablation for premenopausal women with breast cancer remains a relevant treatment option, especially if added to tamoxifen (135). Other forms of surgical endocrine ablation, adrenalectomy and hypophysectomy, were abandoned in the mid-1980s. Although estrogens and androgens are still used by some as a tertiary endocrine treatment, their relatively frequent toxic effects led to their substitution with less toxic compounds.

The most widely used endocrine therapy is tamoxifen. The drug binds by competition to the estradiol receptor, altering the effects of the receptor-hormone complex and resulting in reduced proliferation and growth. An additional mechanism of growth inhibition was ascribed to tamoxifen-induced TGF-beta production. In recent years use of aromatase inhibitors in postmenopausal patients has significantly increased. For premenopausal patients standard endocrine treatments includes ovarian function suppression plus tamoxifen. The question of whether for postmenopausal patients aromatase inhibitors should be considered the primary endocrine therapy or should it be tamoxifen with the alternative drug being given subsequently, if indicated, has been a matter of debate, but starting with an aromatase inhibitor might represent the most relevant choice. The optimal sequence of endocrine therapy for postmenopausal women will have to await further research. HER-2/neu overexpression may predict response to endocrine therapy with nonsteroidal aromatase inhibitors.

Tamoxifen is usually administered in the daily dose of 20 mg. Its half-life after a continuous administration exceeds 200 hr, and blood levels remain detectable for 6–12 weeks after treatment ends. Tamoxifen is a relatively nontoxic treatment, and its chronic use, mainly in the adjuvant setting, has been associated with certain rare side effects. Thrombophlebitis has been observed in 13% of the patients. Some protective effect upon postmenopausal-associated bone loss as a result of its oestrogenic effect on some target tissues was also described. Long-term use of tamoxifen has been reported to be associated with an increased incidence of endometrial cancer (two- to four-fold). Other antiestrogens with different toxicity profile, different pharmacokinetics or biological effects are currently being tested (Table 5.11).

Aromatase inhibitors have been extensively developed in recent years. These compounds block steroid hydroxylation and cleavage enzymes, causing a deficient production of estrogens in peripheral tissues (those less selective inhibit

Table 5.11 Endocrine Treatments Tested in Trials of Advanced Breast Cancer

Therapy	Menopausal status	Response rate (%)	Range (%)	Remarks on treatment results
Oophorectomy	Pre	35	12–55	In ER+ selected patients response rate might exceed 50%; more effective in women over 35 years of age
Adrenalectomy	Post	32	23–46	In series of patients with ER+ tumors response rate was over 60%
Hypophysectomy		36	22–58	Until the 1980s also used for pain relief which was obtained in 70% of the patients—unrelated to endocrine mediated tumor response
Estrogens	Post	26	15–38	Mainly diethylstilbestrol (DES). During the last decade used in trials evaluating recruitment of cancer cells preceding cytotoxics
Androgens	Post	21	10–38	Fluoxymestrone tested until recently with cytotoxics or as single endocrine agent
Tamoxifen	Post	32	16–52	Most widely used endocrine agent
Tamoxifen	Pre	30	20–45	Some trials in premenopausal patients used a dose of 40–120 mg/day
Tam withdrawal		8		22% stable disease
Toremifene		29		Toremifene: similar to tamoxifen. Only 5% response rate in tamoxifen-refractory tumors
Faslodex		20	17–20	Estrogen Receptor Downregulators (Fulvestrant)
Progestins	Post	30	9–67	Medroxyprogesteron acetate Megestrol acetate
Aromatase inhibitors		32	16–43	Exemestane (FCE 24304) (type I) Fadrozole (CGS 16949A) (type II) Letrozole (CGS 20267) (type II) Anastrozole (ZD1033) (type II)
GnRH analogs	Pre	36	32–45	Buserelin Goserelin Leuprolide D-Trp-6 GnRH analog
Antiprogestins		12	–	RU486; other antiprogestins for potential testing: Org31806 and ZK112993
Antiprogestins		10	–	Mifepristone
Antiandrogens		3–5	–	Cyproterone; Flutamide, OH-Flutamide

steroidogenesis in the adrenal glands too). In trials for patients with advanced and endocrine responsive disease, use of either anastrozole or letrozole has been shown to yield some advantage in terms of treatment outcome as compared to tamoxifen (136,137). Anastrozole and letrozole were compared, in postmenopausal patients with advanced disease, to progestins, demonstrating similar or superior efficacy and a favorable toxicity profile. Between steroidal aromatase inhibitors, exemestane may be considered a treatment option. Use of ovarian suppression with aromatase inhibitors has been only marginally investigated.

Progestins are an effective therapy in metastatic breast cancer. Their effectiveness is related to a receptor-mediated mechanism, as well as via interference in the pituitary–ovarian and the pituitary–adrenal axes (138). The largest therapeutic effect is obtained with high doses. Side effects include mainly weight gain, water retention, and other toxicities related to some glucocorticoid effects of these compounds. High-dose progestins may follow as a third line treatment, or find indication if some of the side effects of these drugs on appetite and mood are desirable.

Fulvestrant is an ER antagonist, which has no known agonist (estrogenic) effect and downregulates the ER protein. In two Phase III clinical trials fulvestrant was as effective and as equally well tolerated as anastrozole for the treatment of postmenopausal women with advanced and metastatic breast cancer (139,140). In retrospective analyses, mean duration of response was significantly greater for fulvestrant compared with anastrozole. Fulvestrant may offer certain benefits compared with daily oral dosing regimens, as the injection is given monthly.

Corticosteroids induce responses in breast cancer. In a study by Minton et al. (141), objective responses to prednisolone were seen in 14% of patients, and 21% achieved stable disease for at least six months. Corticosteroids provide palliation, especially for bone pain and dyspnea, and are therefore particularly useful for terminal care. Side effects related to chronic administration are difficult to control and include cushingoid appearance, diabetes mellitus, water retention, atrophic changes of the skin and vessels, gastric and duodenal bleeding with or without ulcers, and osteoporosis.

Analogues of luteinizing hormone-releasing hormone (LHRH) show a significant antineoplastic activity, especially in premenopausal women. Their use has significantly reduced surgical ovarian ablation. These analogues of the decapeptide that is intermittently secreted in regular pulses by the hypothalamus cause release of LH and FSH (luteinizing and follicle-stimulating hormones) until exhaustion inducing the suppression of endocrine ovarian function and a lowering in estradiol. Use of these compounds is associated with minimal toxic effects, partially related to their parenteral route of administration. Amenorrhea occurs on average within 40 days and menses resume usually within 80 days of cessation of therapy.

Estrogens are rarely used today because of their side effects (nausea/vomiting, water retention, and cardiovascular damage). They are still rarely used as a fourthline hormonal therapy in older patients with no cardiovascular contraindications. Available compounds are diethylstilboestrol (5 mg, three times daily), ethinyl estradiol (1 mg, three times daily), or Premarin (2.5 mg, three times daily). Withdrawal response is estimated to occur in one-third of the patients who progress after therapy with oestrogens.

Androgen therapy may lead to significant palliation despite some undesired side effects, which are only partially reversible: masculinization, hoarseness, hirsutism, a masculinelike boldness, acne, and seborrhea. The most used compound is fluoxymesterone acetate (30 mg/day). The use of the compound, which does not cause water retention, may have an indication in elderly women with congestive heart failure.

Combinations of endocrine therapies were tested in several clinical trials, the results of which are not conclusive. Combinations of endocrine therapies (as opposed to their sequential use) are still being investigated.

Chemotherapy for Metastatic Disease

Cytotoxic agents are usually used for all patients whose aggressive disease requires a fast objective tumor regression. Overall response rates to chemotherapy are reported to range from 40% to 90%, with complete responses in 5–10%. The median time to maximal response varies between 7 and 14 weeks (maximum 16 months). The median duration of response to chemotherapy ranges from 6 to 12 months. Some patients are described as having been in response for more than a decade. Whether the use of chemotherapy also prolongs survival is a matter of controversy. It is postulated that some improvement in OS is limited to patients with aggressive tumors, as opposed to those with less rapidly progressive disease. The most significant factor related to improvement of survival, as well as of quality of life, is response to treatment.

Factors that predict a high response rate are the following: good performance status; single or two sites of metastatic disease, especially in soft tissue; prior hormonal therapy; high proliferation index (limited evidence).

Factors that predict a longer duration of response and survival are good performance status; single or two sites of disease, especially in soft tissue and nodular lung metastases; prior endocrine therapy, or response to endocrine manipulations.

Factors predictive for a decreased chance of response and for shorter duration of response and survival are prior chemotherapy and/or radiation therapy, bone and visceral metastases, low blood lymphocyte counts. Age, menopausal status, and steroid hormone receptor status do not influence response rate or duration of response to chemotherapy.

The most frequently used drugs include cyclophosphamide, doxorubicin, methotrexate, 5-fluorouracil, epirubicin (all used in first-line regimens), paclitaxel, docetaxel, vinorelbine, mitomycin C, and mitoxantrone. Table 5.12 displays the summary results of several Phase II trials, which defined the objective response rates to various agents usually employed for metastatic disease (the first group in Table 5.12). Several agents were found to be active in the treatment of the disease but did not enter the current armamentarium of compounds used in current therapies (the second group in Table 5.12).

Combination of cytotoxics demonstrated a higher response rate in the majority of the trials as compared with a single agent. The overall yield of a combination, compared with the same drugs given sequentially, is, however, still controversial, especially when the most effective compounds are used (142). The population with liver and lung metastases (i.e., disease sites with a dire prognosis

Table 5.12 List of Cytotoxic Agents and Data on Effectiveness in Metastatic Breast Cancer

Agent	Remission rate overall %	Remission rate pretreated %	Remission rate not pretreated, not heavily pretreated %
Chlorambucil	17	–	–
Capecitabine	25	20	36
CBDCA	15	4	35
Cyclophosphamide	33	22	36
Doxorubicin (adriamycin)	32	29	43
4-Epiadriamycin	39	33	71
Etoposide (oral)	27	22	35
Gemcitabine	26	18	37
Liposomal Doxorubicin	30	26	43
Mitoxantrone	21	7	27
5-Fluorouracil	27	15	28
Melphalan	20	4	25
Methotrexate	28	17	26
MitomycinC	22	22	–
Platinum	21	8	52
Taxol (paclitaxel)	56	48	62
Taxotere (docetaxel)	67	–	67
Thiotepa	29	–	25
Vinblastine	21	0	–
Vincristin	19	10	8
Vinorelbine	35	20	50

resulting from rapid progression) might benefit when treated with the combination. On the other hand, the sequential use of single agents had some advantages for less aggressive disease presentations such as soft tissue and bone metastases. A cooperative study randomized patients to receive paclitaxel and doxorubicin both given as a combination and sequentially. Although response rate and time-to-progression were both better for the combination, survival was the same in both groups (143). The rate of disease progression, the presence or absence of comorbid medical conditions, and physician/patient preference influence the choice of therapy in individual patients. No present data support the superiority of any particular regimen. Sequential use of single agents or combinations can be used for patients who relapse.

The use of doxorubicin-containing regimens was associated in some trials with higher response rates when compared with cyclophosphamide, methotrexate, 5-fluorouracil, or CMF-type combinations. The search for new anthracyclines with less cardiac toxicity was not entirely successful. Compared with doxorubicin 4-epidoxorubicin showed limited evidence of improved therapeutic index. Liposomal doxorubicin as a single agent yielded similar results to doxorubicin with some lesser cardiological side effects (144).

Taxanes and vinorelbine were shown to be very effective for patients with advanced breast cancer.

Their role in the treatment of advanced disease is increasingly important, alone and in combination with anthracyclines (taxanes), and 5-fluorouracil (vinorelbine). These compounds are also increasingly investigated in the adjuvant setting.

An increasing number of new taxanes are being developed in an attempt to overcome resistance to existing members of the class by possibly enhancing intracellular levels. Nanoparticle albumin-bound paclitaxel (nab-paclitaxel, abraxane) may enhance delivery to tumor tissues. The drug demonstrated a favorable safety profile and a greater efficacy than paclitaxel in a phase III trial in metastatic breast cancer.

Continuous infusions of cytotoxic drugs, such as doxorubicin and low-dose 5-fluorouracil were described to be less toxic and have a significant antitumor activity even in pretreated patients. The combination of continuous infusion 5-fluorouracil together with anthracyclines and cisplatin was found to be a very effective treatment. The combination of 5-fluorouracil with folinic acid (leucovorin) (which enhances the inhibition of fluoro-pyrimidines on thymidylate synthase) was shown to be effective even for tumors resistant to a 5-fluorouracil combination. Severe mucous toxicity should still lead to a better definition of the feasibility of this use of the drug.

Increased attention to patient's quality of life favored the development of oral chemotherapy. Capecitabine is an orally administered fluoropyrimidine carbamate recently used for the treatment of pretreated breast cancer. Capecitabine is metabolized via a three-step process to the active agent fluorouracil preferentially in malignant tissue. In patients with paclitaxel-refractory breast cancer receiving capecitabine the objective tumor response rate was about 20%. In previously untreated patients with breast cancer, the response rate was higher. Side effects were generally gastrointestinal or hematological. Other commonly reported events included hand-and-foot syndrome, fatigue, hyperbilirubinemia, dermatitis, and anorexia. Continuous oral administration of etoposide was defined as effective in inducing significant objective responses.

The term "metronomic" chemotherapy refers to frequent administration of chemotherapeutics at doses significantly below the maximum tolerated dose, with no prolonged drug-free breaks (145). Beside the cytotoxic effect, metronomic chemotherapy exerts an antiangiogenic activity (146). In two trials, the administration of oral cyclophosphamide (50 mg daily) and oral methotrexate

(2.5 mg twice daily two days per week) induced a response rate of 19% and a 32% rate of clinical benefit, and was well tolerated (147,148).

Trastuzumab (Herceptin)

Approximately 25% of breast cancers overexpress HER-2/neu. Trastuzumab (Herceptin) is a humanized monoclonal antibody that binds to the HER2/neu receptor. In patients previously treated with chemotherapy whose tumors overexpress HER-2/neu, administration of Herceptin as a single agent resulted in a response rate of 21% (149). Responses are confined to patients with HER-2 overexpression (IHC 3+) or amplification (FISH) (150). In a prospective trial, patients treated with chemotherapy (doxorubicin and cyclophosphamide or paclitaxel) plus Herceptin had an OS advantage as compared to those receiving chemotherapy alone (151). When combined with doxorubicin, Herceptin is associated with significant cardiac toxicity. Activity was shown in combination with vinorelbine, docetaxel, or cisplatin. Consequently, patients with HER-2/neu overexpressing metastatic breast cancer are candidates for treatment with the combination of Herceptin and chemotherapy.

New Agents

Lapatinib, a small molecule inhibiting tyrosine kinases associated with HER-2, has shown significant efficacy (together with capecitabine) in advanced breast cancer after failure of trastuzumab, and is being tested in the adjuvant setting.

Antibody-targeted therapy may be used to deliver cytotoxic agents specifically to antigen-expressing tumors. *Trastuzumab* linked to *DM1* (a microtubule-depolymerizing agents) displays superior activity compared with unconjugated trastuzumab while maintaining selectivity for HER-2-overexpressing tumor cells; the drug is undergoing clinical development.

Other new agents have been developed with the aim of blocking both HER-1 and HER-2 receptors. *Pertuzumab* is a recombinant humanized monoclonal antibody that binds to the HER-2 receptor, blocking heterodimerization of HER-2 with EGFR and ErbB-3 and inhibiting intracellular signaling. As a single therapy it showed a limited activity, however its combination with trastuzumab after progression on combination therapy with the latter showed an ORR of 18%.

Tanespimycin is a heat shock protein 90 inhibitor (17-AAG; KOS-953). It was administered in combination with trastuzumab in a Phase I trial showing antitumor activity in patients with HER-2+ breast cancer whose tumors have progressed during treatment with trastuzumab.

Bevacizumab, a monoclonal antibody against VEGF, has shown efficacy when combined with capecitabine and taxanes in advanced breast cancer. Combination of bevacizumab with trastuzumab as well as of Bevacizumab plus a metronomic chemotherapy has shown efficacy in metastatic disease.

Dose-Response in Metastatic Breast Cancer

High-dose chemotherapy is more effective in inducing responses, but its effect on survival is a subject of controversy. Comparative studies carried out without hemopoietic growth factors failed to show a survival advantage of this form of therapy when compared with *standard* dose cytotoxics. Although high-dose combination regimens, followed by autologous bone marrow re-infusion or peripheral blood progenitor cell support, showed a significant rate of complete remissions, many patients relapse and die of the disease. A study comparing high-dose chemotherapy with stem cell support to conventional maintenance chemotherapy in patients with metastatic disease indicates no overall or relapse-free survival benefit for patients receiving high-dose chemotherapy with stem cell support (152). Thus, the use of this modality for advanced breast cancer is still under investigation.

Combined Cytotoxics and Hormone Therapies

Combined cytotoxic drugs and endocrine therapies have theoretically an additive effect. The assumption that each might have a distinct cytocidal effect on the two target clones, and the evidence that the spectrum of their toxicities is different, represent the reasons for their combined use. The sequential administration in postmenopausal patients of endocrine therapy first, and then chemotherapy upon demonstrated resistance to endocrine agents confers an advantage, especially in patients with slow-growing tumors. Young patients with aggressive disease presentation are likely to benefit from the concomitant combination of both modalities, although this approach is not generally accepted. The current tendency is to use the modalities separately, and to reserve the combined treatment as a salvage regimen.

Secondary Treatments and Salvage Regimens

After exhaustion of initial response, most patients with advanced disease require renewed palliation. For patients who have previously received doxorubicin, this drug is useful in about 30%, and the median remission duration is about six months. Several other cytotoxics, such as taxanes (paclitaxel and docetaxel), continuous infusion of 5-fluorouracil, vinorelbine, mitomycin C, and the combination of platinum with etoposide, were all shown to have significant efficacy in providing palliation as secondary treatments.

Duration of Treatment with Chemotherapy

Although it is reasonable to continue hormone therapy until relapse, the optimal duration of chemotherapy is unknown. The optimal treatment duration for patients with responsive or stable disease has been studied by several groups. For patients who attain a complete response to initial therapy, randomized trials have shown a prolonged DFS from immediate treatment with a different chemotherapy regimen compared to observation with treatment upon relapse (153). However, neither of these studies showed an improvement in OS for patients who received immediate treatment, and, in one of these studies, survival was actually worse in the immediately treated group. Similarly, no difference in survival was noted when patients with partial response or stable disease after initial therapy were randomized to receive either a different chemotherapy versus observation (154) or a different chemotherapy regimen given at higher versus lower doses (155). The potential role for some form of maintenance cytotoxic treatment, as well as the use of an endocrine agent for such role (therapeutic attitude shared by many) is likely to be useful but remains unknown.

Table 5.13 Issues Related to the Therapy of Specific Sites of Metastatic Disease

Site (reference)	Accepted therapy	Open therapeutic research questions
Breast recurrence in the conserved breast	"Secondary" breast conservation surgery, if possible, or mastectomy.	Consider adjuvant treatment using the same criteria as for primary.
Local recurrence/Scar alone after Mastectomy	Surgery, if circumscribed. RT provides control in about half of patients. Significant response rates with systemic therapy (62–85%), which may test sensitivity to treatment.	Role of radical surgery or other techniques of local disease control. One trial demonstrated positive role of adjuvant tamoxifen in ER+ disease. Role of adjuvant CT uncertain.
Contralateral breast	Usually as a new primary.	Adjuvant systemic therapy.
Bone metastases	Systemic therapy. RT for localized pain (on average more effective than systemic therapy in providing palliation). Surgery might be considered for weight-bearing and functionally important structures.	Routine use of bisphosphonates for reducing osteolytic process and for prevention of fractures.
Brain metastases	High-dose steroids and RT. Surgery for uncertain or accessible single metastases.	Combined systemic ± RT for selected patients. High-dose CT.
Spinal cord compression	High-dose dexamethasone (given even before imaging). Radiation therapy if no bone instability or fractures. Surgery if bony instability or fracture; followed by RT.	Combination systemic therapy + RT.
Choroidal metastases	RT. Systemic therapy (improvement in 80–90%).	
Carcinomatous meningitis	Intrathecal methotrexate, thiotepa, cytosine-arabinoside, and hydrocortison. RT to symptomatic areas.	Systemic therapy.
Symptomatic malignant effusions	Drainage and instillation of tetracyclines or cytotoxics. Surgical pleurodesis (e.g., with the use of talc).	Biologicals administered locally.

Therapeutic Issues Related to Special Sites of Metastases

The treatment of metastatic disease is influenced by its anatomical spread. Data used to justify specific approaches are derived from observations and clinical experience. Table 5.13 describes the issues related to the therapy of specific sites of disease. Quality-of-life oriented end points must be considered when specific items of a palliative approach are being discussed in a multidisciplinary setting.

REFERENCES

1. Jemal A, Siegel R, Ward E et al. Cancer statistics, 2008. CA Cancer J Clin 2008; 58: 71–96.
2. Berry DA, Cronin KA, Plevritis SK et al. Effect of screening and adjuvant therapy on mortality from breast cancer. N Engl J Med 2005; 353: 1784–92.
3. Falk RT, Fears TR, Hoover RN et al. Does place of birth influence endogenous hormone levels in Asian-American women? Br J Cancer 2002; 87: 54–60.
4. Moulder S, Hortobagyi GN. Advances in the treatment of breast cancer. Clin Pharmacol Ther 2008; 83: 26–36.
5. Walsh T, King MC. Ten genes for inherited breast cancer. Cancer Cell 2007; 11: 103–5.
6. Begg CB, Haile RW, Borg A et al. Variation of breast cancer risk among BRCA1/2 carriers. JAMA 2008; 299: 194–201.
7. Shiri-Sverdlov R, Oefner P, Green L et al. Mutational analyses of BRCA1 and BRCA2 in Ashkenazi and non-Ashkenazi Jewish women with familial breast and ovarian cancer. Hum Mutat 2000; 16: 491–501.
8. Simon R, Zhang X. On the dynamics of breast tumor development in women carrying germline BRCA1 and BRCA2 mutations. Int J Cancer 2008; 122: 1916–17.
9. Frank TS, Deffenbaugh AM, Reid JE et al. Clinical characteristics of individuals with germline mutations in BRCA1 and BRCA2: analysis of 10,000 individuals. J Clin Oncol 2002; 20: 1480–90.
10. US Food and Drug Administration. Medical product safety information. http://www.fda.gov/medwatch/SAFETY/2005/safety.htm
11. Horn PL, Thompson WD. Risk of contralateral breast cancer: associations with histologic, clinical, and therapeutic factors. Cancer 1988; 62: 412–24.
12. Bernstein JL, Thompson WD, Risch N et al. Risk factors predicting the incidence of second primary breast cancer among women diagnosed with a first primary breast cancer. Am J Epidemiol 1992; 136: 925–36.
13. Trentham-Dietz A, Newcomb PA, Nichols HB et al. Breast cancer risk factors and second primary malignancies among women with breast cancer. Breast Cancer Res Treat 2007; 105: 195–207.
14. Li CI, Malone KE, Porter PL et al. Epidemiologic and molecular risk factors for contralateral breast cancer among young women. Br J Cancer 2003; 89: 513–18.
15. Marchbanks PA, McDonald JA, Wilson HG et al. Oral contraceptives and the risk of breast cancer. N Engl J Med 2002; 346: 2025–32.
16. Breast cancer and hormonal contraceptives. Collaborative reanalysis of individual data on 53,297 women with breast cancer and 100,239 women without breast cancer from 54 epidemiological studies: Collaborative Group on Hormonal Factors in Breast Cancer. Lancet 1996; 347: 1713–27.
17. Rossouw JE, Anderson GL, Prentice RL et al. Risks and benefits of estrogen plus progestin in healthy postmenopausal women: Principal results from the Women's Health Initiative randomized controlled trial. JAMA 2002; 288: 321–33.
18. Beral V. Breast cancer and hormone replacement therapy in the Million Women Study. Lancet 2003; 362: 419–27.
19. Breast cancer and hormone replacement therapy. Collaborative reanalysis of data from 51 epidemiological studies of 52,705 women with breast cancer and 108,411 women without breast cancer-Collaborative Group on Hormonal Factors in Breast Cancer. Lancet 1997; 350: 1047–59.
20. Lee SA, Ross RK, Pike MC. An overview of menopausal oestrogen-progestin hormone therapy and breast cancer risk. Br J Cancer 2005; 92: 2049–58.

21. Holmberg L, Anderson H. HABITS (Hormonal Replacement Therapy After Breast Cancer—Is It Safe?), a randomised comparison: trial stopped. Lancet 2004; 363: 453–5.

22. von Schoultz E, Rutqvist LE. Menopausal hormone therapy after breast cancer: the stockholm randomized trial. J Natl Cancer Inst 2005; 97: 533–5.

23. Powles TJ, Hickish T, Casey S et al. Hormone replacement after breast cancer. Lancet 1993; 342: 60–1.

24. DiSaia PJ, Grosen EA, Kurosaki T et al. Hormone replacement therapy in breast cancer survivors: a cohort study. Am J Obstet Gynecol 1996; 174: 1494–8.

25. O'Meara ES, Rossing MA, Daling JR et al. Hormone replacement therapy after a diagnosis of breast cancer in relation to recurrence and mortality. J Natl Cancer Inst 2001; 93: 754–62.

26. Phillips DH, Garte S. Smoking and breast cancer: is there really a link? Cancer Epidemiol Biomarkers Prev 2008; 17: 1–2.

27. Wu AH, Yu MC, Tseng C-C et al. Epidemiology of soy exposures and breast cancer risk. Br J Cancer 2008; 98: 9–14.

28. John EM, Schwartz GG, Dreon DM et al. Vitamin D and breast cancer risk: the NHANES I Epidemiologic follow-up study, 1971–1975 to 1992. National Health and Nutrition Examination Survey. Cancer Epidemiol Biomarkers Prev 1999; 8: 399–406.

29. Stevens RG, Rea MS. Light in the built environment: potential role of circadian disruption in endocrine disruption and breast cancer. Cancer Causes Control 2001; 12: 279–87.

30. Coyle YM. The effect of environment on breast cancer risk. Breast Cancer Res Treat 2004; 84: 273–88.

31. Boyle P. Global summit on mammographic screening. Ann Oncol 2003; 14: 1159–60.

32. Fonseca R, Hartmann LC, Petersen IA et al. Ductal carcinoma in situ of the breast. Ann Intern Med 1997; 127: 1013–22.

33. Hanby AM, Hughes TA. In situ and invasive lobular neoplasia of the breast. Histopathology 2008; 52: 58–66.

34. Berg JW, Hutter RV. Breast cancer. Cancer 1995; 75: 257–69.

35. Goldhirsch A, Wood WC, Gelber RD et al. Progress and promise: highlights of the international expert consensus on the primary therapy of early breast cancer 2007. Ann Oncol 2007; 18: 1133–44.

36. Veronesi U, Cascinelli N, Greco M et al. Prognosis of breast cancer patients after mastectomy and dissection of internal mammary nodes. Ann Surg 1985; 202: 702–7.

37. Pinder SE, Ellis IO, Galea MH et al. Pathological prognostic factors in breast cancer. III. Vascular invasion: relationship with recurrence and survival in a large study with long-term follow-up. Histopathology 1994; 24: 41–7.

38. Galea MH, Blamey RW, Elston CE et al. The Nottingham prognostic index in primary breast cancer. Breast Cancer Res Treat 1992; 22: 207–19.

39. Early Breast Cancer Trialists' Collaborative Group (EBCTCG). Effects of chemotherapy and hormonal therapy for early breast cancer on recurrence and 15-year survival: an overview of the randomised trials. Lancet 2005; 365: 1687–717.

40. Colleoni M, Minchella I, Mazzarol G et al. Response to primary chemotherapy in breast cancer patients with tumors not expressing estrogen and progesterone receptors. Ann Oncol 2000; 11: 1057–9.

41. van't Veer LJ, De Jong D. The microarray way to tailored cancer treatment. Nat Med 2002; 8: 13–14.

42. Bardou VJ, Arpino G, Elledge RM et al. Progesterone receptor status significantly improves outcome prediction over estrogen receptor status alone for adjuvant endocrine therapy in two large breast cancer databases. J Clin Oncol 2003; 21: 1973–9.

43. Silvestrini R, Daidone MG, Luisi A et al. Biologic and clinicopathologic factors as indicators of specific relapse types in nodenegative breast cancer. J Clin Oncol 1995; 13: 697–704.

44. Pietilainen T, Lipponen P, Aaltomee S et al. The important prognostic value of Ki-67 expression as determined by image analysis in breast cancer. J Cancer Res Clin Oncol 1996; 122: 687–92.

45. Klijn JG, Berns PM, Schmitz PI et al. The clinical significance of epidermal growth factor receptor (EGFR) in human breast cancer: a review on 5232 patients. Endocr Rev 1992; 13: 3–17.

46. Andrulis IL, Bull SB, Blackstein ME et al. neu/erbB-2 amplification identifies a poor-prognosis group of women with node-negative breast cancer. J Clin Oncol 1998; 16: 1340–9.

47. Sjögren S, Inganäs M, Lindgren A et al. Prognostic and predictive value of c-erbB-2 overexpression in primary breast cancer, alone and in combination with other prognostic markers. J Clin Oncol 1998; 16: 462–9.

48. Slamon DJ, Leyland-Jones B, Shak S et al. Use of chemotherapy plus a monoclonal antibody against HER2 for metastatic breast cancer that overexpresses HER2. N Engl J Med 2001; 344: 783–92.

49. Peyrat JP, Bonneterre J, Lubin R et al. Prognostic significance of circulating p53 antibodies in patients undergoing surgery for locoregional breast cancer. Lancet 1995; 345: 621–2.

50. Dowsett M. Improved prognosis for biomarkers in breast cancer. Lancet 1998; 351: 1753–4.

51. Porter-Jordan K, Lippman ME. Overview of the biologic markers of breast cancer. Hematol Oncol Clin North Am 1994; 8: 73–100.

52. Foekens JA, Schmitt M, van Putten LJ et al. Plasminogen activatorinhibitor-1 and prognosis in primary breast cancer. J Clin Oncol 1994; 12: 1648–58.

53. Axelsson K, Ljung B-M, Moore DH et al. Tumor angiogenesis as a prognostic assay for invasive ductal carcinoma. J Natl Cancer Inst 1995; 87: 997–1008.

54. Keyomarsi K, Tucker SL, Buchholz TA et al. Cyclin E and survival in patients with breast cancer. N Engl J Med 2002; 347: 1566–75.

55. Braun S, Pantel K, Muller P et al. Cytokeratin-positive cells in the bone marrow and survival of patients with stage I, II, or III breast cancer. N Engl J Med 2000; 342: 525–33.

56. van de Vijver MJ, He YD, van't Veer LJ et al. A gene-expression signature as a predictor of survival in breast cancer. N Engl J Med 2002; 347: 1999–2009.

57. Sotiriou C, Neo SY, McShane LM et al. Breast cancer classification and prognosis based on gene expression profiles from a population based study. Proc Natl Acad Sci USA 2003; 100: 10393–8.

58. Paik S, Shak S, Tang G et al. A multigene assay to predict recurrence of tamoxifen-treated, node-negative breast cancer. N Engl J Med 2004; 351: 2817–26.

59. Sparano JA. TAILORx. trial assigning individualized options for treatment (Rx). Clin Breast Cancer 2006; 7: 347–50.

60. Bogaerts J, Cardoso F, Buyse M et al. Gene signature evaluation as a prognostic tool: challenges in the design of the MINDACT trial. Nat Clin Pract Oncol 2006; 3: 540–51.

61. Mayer EL, Burstein HJ. Chemotherapy for metastatic breast cancer. Hematol Oncol Clin North Am 2007; 21: 257–72.

62. Sobin LH, Wittekind C. TNM Classification of Malignant Tumours. New York: UICC, Wiley-Liss, 2002.

63. Greene FL, Page DL, Fleming ID et al., eds. Breast. In: AJCC Cancer Staging Manual, 6th edn. New York: Springer, 2002: 223–40.

64. Singletary SE, Allred C, Ashley P et al. Revision of the American Joint Committee on Cancer staging system for breast cancer. J Clin Oncol 2002; 17: 3628–36.

65. Woodward WA, Strom EA, Tucker SL et al. Changes in the 2003 American Joint Committee on Cancer staging for breast cancer dramatically affect stage-specific survival. J Clin Oncol 2003; 21: 3244–8.

66. Veronesi U, Cascinelli N, Mariani L et al. Twenty-year follow-up of a randomized study comparing breast-conserving

surgery with radical mastectomy for early breast cancer. N Engl J Med 2002; 347: 1227–32.

67. Morrow M, Strom EA, Bassett LW et al. American College of Radiology; American College of Surgeons; Society of Surgical Oncology; College of American Pathology. Standard for breast conservation therapy in the management of invasive breast carcinoma. CA Cancer J Clin 2002; 52: 277–300.

68. Holli K, Saaristo R, Isola J et al. Lumpectomy with or without postoperative radiotherapy for breast cancer with favourable prognostic features: results of a randomized study. Br J Cancer 2001; 84: 164–9.

69. Veronesi U, Paganelli G, Viale G et al. A randomized comparison of sentinel-node biopsy with routine axillary dissection in breast cancer. N Engl J Med 2003; 349: 546–53.

70. Veronesi U, Paganelli G, Viale G et al. A randomized comparison of sentinel-node biopsy with routine axillary dissection in breast cancer. N Engl J Med 2003; 349: 546–53.

71. Sakorafas GH, Farley DR, Peros G. Recent advances and current controversies in the management of DCIS of the breast. Cancer Treat Rev 2008; 34: 483–97.

72. Overgaard M, Hansen PS, Overgaard J et al. Postoperative radiotherapy in high-risk premenopausal women with breast cancer who receive adjuvant chemotherapy. Danish Breast Cancer Cooperative Group 82b Trial. N Engl J Med 1997; 337: 949–55.

73. Ragaz J, Jackson SM, Le N et al. Adjuvant radiotherapy and chemotherapy in node-positive premenopausal women with breast cancer. N Engl J Med 1997; 337: 956–62.

74. Early Breast Cancer Trialists' Collaborative Group. Favourable and unfavourable effects on long-term survival of radiotherapy for early breast cancer: an overview of the randomised trials. Lancet 2000; 355: 1757–70.

75. Bartelink H. Radiotherapy to the conserved breast, chest wall, and regional nodes: is there a standard? Breast 2003; 12: 475–82.

76. Bartelink H, Horiot JC, Poortmans P et al. Recurrence rates after treatment of breast cancer with standard radiotherapy with or without additional radiation. N Engl J Med 2001; 345: 1378–87.

77. Budrukkar A. Accelerated partial breast irradiation: an advanced form of hypofractionation. J Cancer Res Ther 2008; 4: 46–7.

78. Gelber RD, Goldhirsch A. Radiotherapy to the conserved breast: Is it avoidable if the cancer is small. J Natl Cancer Inst 1994; 86: 652–4.

79. Fehlauer F, Tribius S, Holler U et al. Long-term radiation sequelae after breast-conserving therapy in women with early-stage breast cancer: an observational study using the LENT-SOMA scoring system. Int J Radiat Oncol Biol Phys 2003; 55: 651–8.

80. Chen MH, Chuang ML, Bornstein BA et al. Impact of respiratory maneuvers on cardiac volume within left-breast radiation portals. Circulation 1997; 96: 3269–72.

81. Wallgren A, Bernier J, Gelber RD et al. for the IBCSG. Timing of radiotherapy and chemotherapy following breast-conserving surgery for patients with node-positive breast cancer. Int J Radiat Oncol Biol Phys 1996; 35: 649–59.

82. Dörr W, Bertmann S, Herrmann T. Radiation induced lung reactions in breast cancer therapy. Modulating factors and consequential effects. Strahlenther Onkol 2005; 181: 567–73.

83. Burstein HJ, Winer EP. Primary care for survivors of breast cancer. N Engl J Med 2000; 343: 1086–94.

84. Loprinzi CL. It is now the age to define the appropriate follow-up of primary breast cancer patients. J Clin Oncol 1994; 12: 881–3.

85. Rosselli Del Turco M, Palli D, Cariddi A et al. Intensive diagnostic follow-up after treatment of primary breast cancer. JAMA 1994; 271: 1593–7.

86. GIVIO Investigators. Impact of follow-up testing on survival and health-related quality of life in breast cancer patients. JAMA 1994; 271: 1587–92.

87. Khatcheressian JL, Wolff AC, Smith TJ et al. American Society of Clinical Oncology 2006 Update of the Breast Cancer Follow-Up and Management Guidelines in the Adjuvant Setting. J Clin Oncol 2006; 24: 1–7.

88. Warner E, Plewes DB, Hill KA et al. Surveillance of BRCA1 and BRCA2 mutation carriers with magnetic resonance imaging, ultrasound, mammography, and clinical breast examination. JAMA 2004; 292: 1317–25.

89. Lehman CD, Gatsonis C, Kuhl CK et al. MRI evaluation of the contralateral breast in women with recently diagnosed breast cancer. N Engl J Med 2007; 356: 1295–303.

90. Shah P, Rosen MA, Stopfer J et al. Follow-up MRI screening of BRCA1/2 mutation carriers. J Clin Oncol 2008; 26: abstract 11000.

91. Keshaviah A, Dellapasqua S, Rotmensz N et al. CA15-3 and alkaline phosphatase as predictors for breast cancer recurrence: a combined analysis of seven International Breast Cancer Study Group trials. Ann Oncol 2007; 18: 701–8.

92. Bast RC Jr, Ravdin P, Hayes DF. 2000 update of recommendations for the use of tumor markers in breast and colorectal cancer: clinical practice guidelines of the American Society of Clinical Oncology. J Clin Oncol 2000; 19: 1865–78.

93. Early Breast Cancer Trialists' Collaborative Group (EBCTCG). Effects of chemotherapy and hormonal therapy for early breast cancer on recurrence and 15-year survival: an overview of the randomised trials. Lancet 2005; 365: 1687–717.

94. Fisher B, Brown AM, Dimitrov NV et al. Two months of doxorubicin-cyclophosphamide with and without interval reinduction therapy compared with 6 months of cyclophosphamide, methotrexate, and fluorouracil in positive-node breast cancer patients with tamoxifen-nonresponsive tumors: results from the National Surgical Adjuvant Breast and Bowel Project B-15. J Clin Oncol 1990; 8: 1483–96.

95. Hutchins L, Green S, Ravdin P et al. CMF versus CAF with and without tamoxifen in high risk node negative breast cancer patients and a natural history follow-up study in low-risk node-negative patients: first results of Intergroup trial INT 0102. Proc Am Soc Clin Oncol 1998; 17: 1a (abstract 1).

96. Citron ML, Berry DA, Cirrincione C et al. Randomized trial of dose-dense versus conventionally scheduled and sequential versus concurrent combination chemotherapy as postoperative adjuvant treatment of node-positive primary breast cancer: first report of Intergroup Trial C9741/Cancer and Leukemia Group B Trial 9741. J Clin Oncol 2003; 21: 1431–9.

97. Bergh J, Wiklund T, Erikstein B et al. Tailored fluorouracil, epirubicin, and cyclophosphamide compared with marrow-supported high-dose chemotherapy as adjuvant treatment for high-risk breast cancer: a randomised trial. Scandinavian Breast Group 9401 study. Lancet 2000; 356: 1384–91.

98. Nabholtz JM, Pienkowski T, Mackey J et al. Phase III trial comparing TAC (docetaxel, doxorubicin, cyclophosphamide) with FAC (5-fluorouracil, doxorubicin, cyclophosphamide) in the adjuvant treatment of node positive breast cancer (BC) patients: interim analysis of the BCIRG 001 study. Proc Am Soc Clin Oncol 2002; 21: abstract 141.

99. Goldhirsch A, Colleoni M, Coates AS et al. Adding adjuvant CMF chemotherapy to either radiotherapy or tamoxifen: are all CMFs alike? Ann Oncol 1998; 9: 489–93.

100. Colleoni M, Litman HJ, Castiglione-Gertsch M et al. Duration of adjuvant chemotherapy for breast cancer: a joint analysis of two randomised trials investigating three versus six courses of CMF. Br J Cancer 2002; 86: 1705–14.

101. The French Adjuvant Study Group. Benefit of a high-dose epirubicin regimen in adjuvant chemotherapy for node-positive breast cancer patients with poor prognostic

factors: 5-Year follow-up results of French Adjuvant Study Group 05 Randomized Trial. J Clin Oncol 2001; 19: 602–11.

102. Levine MN, Bramwell VH, Pritchard KI et al. Randomized trial of intensive cyclophosphamide, epirubicin, and fluorouracil chemotherapy compared with cyclophosphamide, methotrexate, and fluorouracil in premenopausal women with node-positive breast cancer. National Cancer Institute of Canada Clinical Trials Group. J Clin Oncol 1998; 16: 2651–8.

103. Smith RE, Bryant J, DeCillis A et al. Acute myeloid leukemia and myelodysplastic syndrome after doxorubicin-cyclophosphamide adjuvant therapy for operable breast cancer: the National Surgical Adjuvant Breast and Bowel Project Experience. J Clin Oncol 2003; 21: 1195–204.

104. Crump M, Tu D, Shepherd L et al. Risk of acute leukemia following epirubicin-based adjuvant chemotherapy: a report from the National Cancer Institute of Canada Clinical Trials Group. J Clin Oncol 2003; 21: 3066–71.

105. Henderson IC, Berry DA, Demetri GD et al. Improved outcomes from adding sequential paclitaxel but not from escalating doxorubicin dose in an adjuvant chemotherapy regimen for patients with node-positive primary breast cancer. J Clin Oncol 2003; 21: 976–83.

106. Mamounas EP, Bryant J, Lembersky BC et al. Paclitaxel (T) following doxorubicin/cyclophosphamide (AC) as adjuvant chemotherapy for node-positive breast cancer: results from NSABP B-28. Proc Am Soc Clin Oncol 2003; 22: abstract 12.

107. Citron ML, Berry DA, Cirrincione C et al. Randomized trial of dose-dense versus conventionally scheduled and sequential versus concurrent combination chemotherapy as postoperative adjuvant treatment of node-positive primary breast cancer: first report of Intergroup Trial C9741/Cancer and Leukemia Group B Trial 9741. J Clin Oncol 2003; 21: 1431–9.

108. Burnell M, Levine M, Chapman JA. A randomized trial of CEF versus dose dense EC followed by paclitaxel versus AC followed by paclitaxel in women with node positive or high risk node negative breast cancer, NCIC CTG MA.21: results of an interim analysis. 29th San Antonio Breast Cancer Symposium 2006: abstract 53.

109. Crown JP, Francis P, Di Leo A et al. Docetaxel (T) given concurrently with or sequentially to anthracycline-based (A) adjuvant therapy (adjRx) for patients (pts) with node-positive (N+) breast cancer (BrCa), in comparison with non-T adjRx: First results of the BIG 2-98 Trial at 5 years median follow-up (MFU). J Clin Oncol (2006 ASCO Annual Meeting Proceedings Part I) 2006; 24(18S): abstract LBA519.

110. Ellis PA, Barrett-Lee PJ, Bloomfield D et al. Preliminary results of the UK Taxotere as Adjuvant Chemotherapy (TACT) Trial. Breast Cancer Res Treat 2007; 106(Suppl 1): abstract 78.

111. Romond EH, Perez EA, Bryant J et al. Trastuzumab plus adjuvant chemotherapy for operable HER2-positive breast cancer. N Engl J Med 2005; 353: 1673–84.

112. Perez EA, Suman VJ, Davidson N et al. NCCTG N9831 May 2005 Update. Presented at the 2005 American Society of Clinical Oncology Annual Meeting, Orlando, FL. Available at http://www.asco.org/ac/1,1003,_12-002511-00_18-0034-00_19-005815-00_21-001,00.asp [Accessed 3 January 2006].

113. Piccart-Gebhart MJ, Procter M, Leyland-Jones B et al. Trastuzumab after adjuvant chemotherapy in HER2-positive breast cancer. N Engl J Med 2005; 353: 1659–72.

114. Smith I, Procter M, Gelber RD et al. 2-year follow-up of trastuzumab after adjuvant chemotherapy in HER2-positive breast cancer: a randomised controlled trial. Lancet 2007; 369: 29–36.

115. Slamon D, Eiermann W, Robert N et al. Phase III randomized trial comparing doxorubicin and cyclophosphamide followed by docetaxel (AC T) with doxorubicin and cyclophosphamide followed by docetaxel and trastuzumab (AC TH) with docetaxel, carboplatin and trastuzumab (TCH) in HER2 positive early breast cancer patients: BCIRG 006 study. Breast Cancer Res Treat 2005; 94(suppl 1): S5a.

116. Joensuu H, Kellokumpu-Lehtinen P-L, Bono P et al. Adjuvant docetaxel or vinorelbine with or without trastuzumab for breast cancer. N Engl J Med 2006; 354: 809–20.

117. Spielmann M, Roché H, Humblet Y et al. 3-year follow-up of trastuzumab following adjuvant chemotherapy in node positive HER2-positive breast cancer patients: results of the PACS-04 trial. 30th San Antonio Breast Cancer Symposium 2007: abstract 72.

118. Davidson NE. Ovarian ablation as adjuvant therapy for breast cancer. J Natl Cancer Inst Monogr 2001; 30: 67–71.

119. Castiglione-Gertsch M, O'Neill A, Gelber RD et al. Is the addition of adjuvant chemotherapy always necessary in node negative (N-) pre/perimenopausal breast cancer patients (pts) who receive goserelin? First results of IBCSG trial VIII. Proc Am Soc Clin Oncol 2002; 21: abstract 149.

120. Love RR, Duc NB, Havighurst TC et al. HER-2/neu overexpression and response to oophorectomy plus tamoxifen adjuvant therapy in ER-positive premenopausal women with operable breast cancer. J Clin Oncol 2003; 21: 453–7.

121. Brueggemeier RW. Aromatase inhibitors: new endocrine treatment of breast cancer. Semin Reprod Med 2004; 22: 31–43.

122. ATAC Trialists Group. Anastrozole alone or in combination with tamoxifen vs. tamoxifen alone for adjuvant treatment of postmenopausal women with early breast cancer: first results of the ATAC randomised trial. Lancet 2002; 359: 2131–9.

123. ATAC Trialists Group. Results of the ATAC (Arimidex, Tamoxifen, Alone or in Combination) trial after completion of 5 years' adjuvant treatment for breast cancer. Lancet. 2005; 365: 60–2.

124. Forbes JF, Cuzick J, Buzdar A et al. ATAC: 100 month median follow-up (FU) shows continued superior efficacy and no excess fracture risk for anastrozole (A) compared with tamoxifen (T) after treatment completion. 30th San Antonio Breast Cancer Symposium 2007: abstract 41.

125. BIG 1–98 Collaborative Group. A comparison of letrozole and tamoxifen in postmenopausal women with early breast cancer. N Engl J Med 2005; 353: 2747–57.

126. Coates AS, Keshaviah A, Thuerlimann B et al. Five years of letrozole compared with tamoxifen as initial adjuvant therapy for postmenopausal women with endocrine-responsive early breast cancer: update of study BIG 1–98. J Clin Oncol 2007; 25: 486–92.

127. Coombes RC, Hall E, Gibson LJ et al. A randomized trial of exemestane after two to three years of tamoxifen therapy in postmenopausal women with primary breast cancer. N Engl J Med 2004; 350: 1081–92.

128. Coombes RC, Kilburn LS, Snowdon CF et al. Survival and safety of exemestane vs. tamoxifen after 2–3 years' tamoxifen treatment (Intergroup Exemestane Study): a randomised controlled trial. Lancet 2007; 369: 559–70.

129. Goss PE, Ingle JN, Martino S et al. Randomized trial of letrozole following tamoxifen as extended adjuvant therapy in receptor-positive breast cancer: updated findings from NCIC CTG MA. 17. J Natl Cancer Inst 2005; 97: 1262–71.

130. Muss HB, Berry DL, Cirrincione C et al. Standard chemotherapy (CMF or AC) versus capecitabine in early-stage breast cancer (BC) patients aged 65 and older: Results of CALGB/CTSU 49907. J Clin Oncol 2008; 26: abstract 507.

131. Giordano SH, Buzdar AU, Hortobagyi GN. Breast cancer in men. Ann Intern Med 2002; 137(8): 678–87.

132. Gelber RD, Goldhirsch A, Cole BF. For the International Breast Cancer Study Group. Evaluation of effectiveness: Q-TWiST. Cancer Treat Rev 1993; 19: 73–84.

133. Therasse P, Mauriac L, Welnicka-Jaskiewicz M et al. Final results of a randomized phase III trial comparing cyclophosphamide, epirubicin, and fluorouracil with a dose-intensified epirubicin and cyclophosphamide + filgrastim as neoadjuvant treatment in locally advanced breast cancer: an EORTC-NCIC-SAKK multicenter study. J Clin Oncol 2003; 21: 843–50.

134. Harvey JM, Clark GM, Osborne CK et al. ER status by immunohistochemistry is superior to the ligand-binding assay for predicting response to adjuvant endocrine therapy in breast cancer. J Clin Oncol 1999; 17: 1474–81.

135. Pritchard KI. Endocrine therapy of advanced disease: analysis and implications of the existing data. Clin Cancer Res 2003; 9: 460S–7S.

136. Nabholtz JM, Buzdar A, Pollak M et al. Anastrozole is superior to tamoxifen as first-line therapy for advanced breast cancer in postmenopausal women: results of a North American multicenter randomized trial. Arimidex Study Group. J Clin Oncol 2000; 18: 3758–67.

137. Mouridsen H, Gershanovich M, Sun Y et al. Superior efficacy of letrozole versus tamoxifen as first-line therapy for postmenopausal women with advanced breast cancer: results of a phase III study of the International Letrozole Breast Cancer Group. J Clin Oncol 2001; 19: 2596–606.

138. Lundgren S. Progestins in breast cancer treatment. A review. Acta Oncol 1992; 31: 709–22.

139. Osborne CK, Pippen J, Jones SE et al. Double-blind, randomized trial comparing the efficacy and tolerability of fulvestrant versus anastrozole in postmenopausal women with advanced breast cancer progressing on prior endocrine therapy: results of a North American trial. J Clin Oncol 2002; 20: 3386–95.

140. Howell A, Robertson JF, Quaresma AJ et al. Fulvestrant, formerly ICI 182,780, is as effective as anastrozole in postmenopausal women with advanced breast cancer progressing after prior endocrine treatment. J Clin Oncol 2002; 20: 3396–403.

141. Minton MJ, Knight RK, Rubens RD et al. Corticosteroids for elderly patients with breast cancer. Cancer 1981; 48: 883–7.

142. Norton L. Evolving concepts in the systemic drug therapy of breast cancer. Semin Oncol 1997; 24: S10-3–S10-10.

143. Sledge GW, Neuberg D, Bernardo P et al. Phase III trial of doxorubicin, paclitaxel, and the combination of doxorubicin and paclitaxel as front-line chemotherapy for metastatic breast cancer: an intergroup trial (E1193). J Clin Oncol 2003; 21: 588–92.

144. Harris L, Batist G, Belt R et al. The TLC D-99 Study Group: Liposome-encapsulated doxorubicin compared with conventional doxorubicin in a randomized multicenter trial as first-line therapy of metastatic breast carcinoma. Cancer 2002; 94: 25–36.

145. Kerbel RS, Kamen BA. The anti-angiogenic basis of metronomic chemotherapy. Nat Rev Cancer 2004; 4: 423–36.

146. Bocci G, Nicolaou KC, Kerbel RS. Protracted low-dose effects on human endothelial cell proliferation and survival in vitro reveal a selective antiangiogenic window for various chemotherapeutic drugs. Cancer Res 2002; 62: 6938–43.

147. Colleoni M, Rocca A, Sandri MT et al. Low-dose oral methotrexate and cyclophosphamide in metastatic breast cancer: antitumor activity and correlation with vascular endothelial growth factor levels. Ann Oncol 2002; 13: 73–80.

148. Colleoni M, Orlando L, Sanna G et al. Metronomic low dose oral cyclophosphamide and methotrexate plus or minus thalidomide in metastatic breast cancer: antitumor activity and biological effects. Ann Oncol 2006; 17: 232–8.

149. Cobleigh MA, Vogel CL, Tripathy D et al. Multinational study of the efficacy and safety of humanized anti-HER2 monoclonal antibody in women who have HER2-overexpressing metastatic breast cancer that has progressed after chemotherapy for metastatic disease. J Clin Oncol 1999; 17: 2639–48.

150. Vogel CL, Cobleigh MA, Tripathy D et al. Efficacy and safety of trastuzumab as a single agent in first-line treatment of HER2-overexpressing metastatic breast cancer. J Clin Oncol 2002; 20: 719–26.

151. Slamon DJ, Leyland-Jones B, Shak S et al. Use of chemotherapy plus a monoclonal antibody against HER2 for metastatic breast cancer that overexpresses HER2. N Engl J Med 2001; 344: 783–92.

152. Stadtmauer EA, O'Neill A, Goldstein LJ et al. Conventional-dose chemotherapy compared with high-dose chemotherapy plus autologous hematopoietic stem-cell transplantation for metastatic breast cancer. Philadelphia Bone Marrow Transplant Group. N Engl J Med 2000; 342: 1069–76.

153. Coates A, Gebski V, Bishop JF et al. Improving the quality of life during chemotherapy for advanced breast cancer. A comparison of intermittent and continuous treatment strategies. New Engl J Med 1987; 317: 1490–5.

154. Muss HB, Case LD, Richards F et al. Interrupted versus continuous chemotherapy in patients with metastatic breast cancer. The Piedmont Oncology Association. N Engl J Med 1991; 325: 1342–8.

155. Falkson G, Gelman RS, Glick J et al. Metastatic breast cancer: higher versus low dose maintenance treatment when only a partial response or a no change status is obtained following doxorubicin induction treatment: an Eastern Cooperative Oncology Group study. Ann Oncol 1992; 3: 768–70.

6

Gynecological Cancer

Susana Banerjee and Martin Gore

INTRODUCTION

Gynecological cancers (ovarian, uterine, cervical, vulval, and vaginal) affect 17,000 women per year in the United Kingdom and many women still present with advanced disease with little prospect of cure. The optimal management of gynecological malignancies is increasingly complex and involves a multidisciplinary approach. There remains a significant risk of recurrence and resistance to therapy despite advances in surgical, radio, and chemotherapeutic strategies. However, over recent years, there have been improvements in our understanding of the biology of gynecological cancers and in the design of molecularly targeted therapies. This chapter summarizes the medical management of gynecological cancers and, in particular, the roles of chemotherapy and targeted agents.

OVARIAN CANCER

Epidemiology

Ovarian cancer is the second most common gynecological malignancy and the leading cause of death from a gynecological cancer. There are approximately 6000 new cases of ovarian cancer and 4500 associated deaths per year in the United Kingdom accounting for 5% of all cancer deaths. Most epithelial ovarian carcinomas (EOCs) are diagnosed in postmenopausal women and the median age at diagnosis is 63 years. Their incidence is age related with the disease being almost four times more common in the 70–74 years age group compared to 40–44 years age group. There has been little overall change in incidence and mortality rates over the past three decades but improvements in survival times and quality of life have occurred as a result of more effective surgery, chemotherapy, and a multidisciplinary approach to patient care.

Etiology

Hereditary epithelial ovarian cancer syndromes affect approximately 10% of ovarian cancer patients and as many as 90% of these cases are accounted for by *BRCA* mutations. Hereditary nonpolyposis colorectal cancer (HNPCC) can also be associated with a hereditary predisposition to ovarian cancer. Women carrying mutations of either the *BRCA1* gene (chromosome 17q) or *BRCA2* gene (chromosome 13) have a significantly higher lifetime risk of developing ovarian cancer, reported as up to 60% for *BRCA1* and 15–20% for *BRCA2*. Founder effects of *BRCA1* and *BRCA2* mutations have been identified in the Ashkenazi Jewish population where up to 2.5% of the population carry one of three genetic mutations. Nevertheless, 90% of ovarian cancers arise sporadically.

Pathology

Approximately 90% of ovarian carcinomas are epithelial in origin and develop from the surface of the ovary. The remainder arise from germ or stromal cells (see later). The ovary can also become involved by metastatic disease, especially from breast cancer or Krukenberg tumors (mucin-producing neoplastic signet-ring cells involving the ovarian stroma) from the gastrointestinal tract. The histological subtypes of ovarian cancer as defined by the World Health Organization are summarized in Table 6.1. Histological grade and type can be important prognostic factors in early-stage disease. Clear cell and mucinous types have a poorer outcome compared to other forms of epithelial ovarian cancers (1). Recent molecular evidence suggests that different histological subtypes could be considered as distinct disease entities. For example, KRAS, BRAF, and ERBB2 mutations occur in low-grade serous carcinoma but are rare in high-grade serous carcinoma.

Clinical Features

Early-stage disease often gives rise to vague, ill-defined symptoms that may be overlooked. As a result, the majority of patients present with advanced (Stage III or IV) disease. Common clinical features are abdominal distension (with ascites) and discomfort, bowel disturbance, nausea, anorexia, dyspnea (secondary to pleural effusion), and urinary tract symptoms. In view of the nature of presentation, patients are often misdiagnosed leading to delayed referral to a specialist gynecological team. Metastases often develop throughout the peritoneal cavity via transcoelomic spread of malignant cells. Common sites include all intraperitoneal (IP) surfaces, omentum, right hemi-diaphragm, para-aortic, and pelvic nodes. Hematogenous metastases are uncommon but can give rise to liver and lung metastases. The bladder and rectosigmoid may also be involved with metastases by direct extension from the ovary.

Diagnosis and Evaluation

A definitive histological diagnosis requires surgery. However, the combination of tests such as pelvic examination, transvaginal ultrasound, serum CA125, peritoneal cytology, and imaging can provide a presumptive diagnosis. A solid, irregular, fixed pelvic mass is highly suggestive of an ovarian malignancy although benign lesions such as endometriomas and tuboovarian abscesses may also give

Table 6.1 Modified WHO Classification of Ovarian Tumors

Epithelial tumors	A. Serous
	B. Mucinous
	C. Endometrioid
	D. Clear cell
	E. Brenner
	F. Mixed epithelial
	G. Undifferentiated
	H. Unclassified
Sex cord stromal tumors	A. Granulosa
	B. Sertoli-Leydig
	C. Gonadoblastoma
	D. Unclassified
Lipid cell tumors	
Germ cell tumors	A. Dysgerminoma
	B. Endodermal sinus tumor
	C. Embryonal carcinoma
	D. Polyembryona
	E. Choriocarcinoma
	F. Teratoma
	G. Mixed forms

rise to such findings. A transvaginal ultrasound scan is used to identify sonographic characteristics such as abnormal color Doppler flow suggestive of ovarian malignancy. Computerized tomography (CT) scanning is used to evaluate disease extent preoperatively and is especially useful in the assessment of retroperitoneal lymph node involvement and peritoneal disease.

Serum CA-125 is elevated (>35 U/ml) in approximately 80% of women with EOC and the sensitivity varies with stage and histological subtype. It is often high in women with serous histology but can be normal in women with mucinous cancers. CA-125 is more useful in postmenopausal women than in the premenopausal setting. A raised CA-125 is not specific for a diagnosis of ovarian cancer and it can also be increased in other malignancies such as endometrial, pancreatic, and breast cancers as well as benign conditions including endometriosis, inflammatory pelvic disease, and hepatitis. However, once ovarian cancer is confirmed in the presence of raised CA-125, this marker can be valuable as an indicator of relapsed disease, treatment response, and early treatment failure.

The potential benefit of screening is its ability to identify ovarian cancer at a more localized and curable stage, leading to reduced mortality from the disease. Screening tests under evaluation include CA-125 measurements and pelvic ultrasonography. Prospective screening trials are not yet completed, hence the impact of screening on ovarian cancer is still an open question and routine screening for ovarian cancer is not currently recommended.

Staging and Surgery

Ovarian cancer is staged surgically and is expressed according to the International Federation of Gynecologists and Obstetricians (FIGO) staging system (Table 6.2). The initial treatment of ovarian cancer is determined by the stage of disease at the time of diagnosis and therefore it is imperative that complete surgical staging is achieved to assess all likely sites of spread. A full staging laparotomy with a vertical midline incision includes a total abdominal hysterectomy (TAH), bilateral salpingo-oophorectomy (BSO), omentectomy, biopsies of suspicious areas, and peritoneal lavage or ascitic fluid sampling. Blind peritoneal, para-aortic/pelvic lymph node biopsies should be performed to exclude the possibility of microscopic Stage III disease, as up to 20% of women with apparent Stage I disease have been shown to have para-aortic lymph node involvement. Approximately 25% of women present with Stage I or II disease; the remaining 75% present with Stage III or IV ovarian cancer. Tumor stage is the most important prognostic indicator of ovarian cancer (Table 6.2).

Table 6.2 International Federation of Gynecologists and Obstetricians (FIGO) Stage Grouping for Primary Carcinoma of the Ovary and Five-Year Survival by Stage

Stage		Description	5-year survival (%)
I		Growth limited to the ovaries	
	Ia	Growth limited to one ovary; no ascites. No tumor on the external surface; capsule intact	90
	Ib	Growth limited to both ovaries; no ascites. No tumor on the external surface; capsule intact	86
	Ic	Tumor either stage Ia or Ib but with tumor on the surface of one or both ovaries, or with capsule ruptured, or with ascites present containing malignant cells or with positive peritoneal washings	83
II		Growth involving one or both ovaries with pelvic extension	
	IIa	Extension and/or metastases to the uterus and/or tubes	71
	IIb	Extension to other pelvic tissues	66
	IIc	Tumor either stage IIa or IIb but with tumor on the surface of one or both ovaries, or with capsule(s) ruptured, or with ascites present containing malignant cells or with positive peritoneal washings	71
III		Tumor involving one or both ovaries with peritoneal implants outside the pelvis and/or positive retroperitoneal or inguinal nodes or superficial liver metastases. Tumor is limited to the true pelvis but with histologicallly verified malignant extension to small bowel or omentum	
	IIIa	Tumor grossly limited to the true pelvis with negative nodes but with histologically confirmed microscopic seeding of abdominal peritoneal surfaces	47
	IIIb	Tumor of one or both ovaries with histologically confirmed implants of abdominal peritoneal surfaces, none exceeding 2 cm in diameter. Node negative	42
	IIIc	Abdominal implants greater than 2 cm in diameter and/or positive retroperitoneal or inguinal nodes	33
IV		Growth involving one or both ovaries with distant metastases. If pleural effusion is present, cytology must be positive. Parenchymal liver metastasis	19

Data from 6th Annual FIGO Report: Patients Treated 1999–2001.

The volume of residual disease postsurgery inversely correlates with survival. In addition, removal of bulky disease can improve disease-related symptoms. Optimal cytoreductive surgery ("optimum debulking") is defined as residual disease less than 1 cm in diameter. The likelihood of achieving optimal debulking depends in part on the surgeon, and gynecologists specializing in oncology should perform these procedures.

Management

The majority of ovarian cancer patients (almost all except those with low-risk Stage I tumors) require chemotherapy following initial surgery. The combination of intravenous platinum and a taxane is standard first-line therapy for women with EOC. Chemotherapy may be given either adjuvantly for early- and late-stage disease or in the neoadjuvant setting.

Adjuvant Chemotherapy for Early-Stage Ovarian Cancer

Patients with early-stage disease (Stage I or II) are initially managed with surgery. Although the prognosis for early-stage ovarian cancer is better than in advanced disease, a substantial number of women will eventually relapse and die, hence the interest in adjuvant therapy. The prognosis is not uniform among Stage I and II tumors and this is reflected in the decision regarding whom to treat. Further systemic therapy is generally not recommended for women with well-differentiated Grade I cancers (2). A worse prognosis has been associated with patients who present with one or more of the following:

Stage Ic disease
Clear cell histology
High-grade (poorly differentiated) tumors
Suboptimal surgical staging

Overall evidence suggests that there is a role for adjuvant chemotherapy in this group of patients. This issue was evaluated in two prospective randomized studies: the International Collaborative Ovarian Neoplasm (ICON-1) and the Adjuvant Treatment in Ovarian Neoplasm (ACTION) trials (3). These trials compared platinum-based adjuvant chemotherapy with observation following surgery in early-stage ovarian cancer. A combined analysis of the trials demonstrated a significant (8%) five-year survival benefit favoring the adjuvant chemotherapy group. There has been criticism of ICON-1 in relation to the lack of strict policies and checks on the completion of surgical staging. Therefore, it is possible that many patients may in fact have had advanced disease. Furthermore, subanalysis of the ACTION trial showed that this benefit may only be applicable to suboptimally staged patients suggesting that treatment of residual disease could explain the beneficial effect achieved with adjuvant chemotherapy. Results from a recent update of the ICON-1 trial favored the chemotherapy group [10 year recurrence-free survival HR = 0.70, p = 0.023; overall survival (OS) HR for death = 0.74, p = 0.066] (4). The Gynecologic Oncology Group (GOG)-157 trial addressed the issue of optimal duration of adjuvant chemotherapy.

There was no significant difference in recurrence or five-year survival with six cycles of adjuvant carboplatin/paclitaxel compared to three cycles. However, toxicity was worse with six cycles (5).

Choice of First-Line Chemotherapy Agents

Platinum agents have proven to be a critical component of the treatment of epithelial ovarian cancer. A meta-analysis of 37 randomized trials revealed a significant reduction in the risk of death (12%) that translated into an absolute 5% improvement in survival at two years (45% vs. 50%) and five years (25% vs. 30%) (p = 0.02) (6).

Carboplatin is associated with a more favorable toxicity profile compared to cisplatin having less ototoxicity, neuropathy, renal impairment, and emetogenesis. However, carboplatin causes myelosuppression that can be dose-limiting, particularly if combined with other agents. Carboplatin is now the standard platinum agent for treating ovarian carcinoma. This development is on the basis of several studies including a meta-analysis that concluded that carboplatin and cisplatin are therapeutically equivalent in women with advanced EOC (6–8).

Several randomized trials have compared cisplatin/carboplatin and paclitaxel with single agent platinum, paclitaxel, or cisplatin/cyclophosphamide. The GOG-111 trial demonstrated statistically significant improvements in the overall response rates (73% vs. 60%), progression-free survival (PFS) (18 vs. 13 months), and OS (38 vs. 24 months) in suboptimally debulked Stage III–IV patients who received cisplatin with paclitaxel compared to cisplatin with cyclophosphamide (9). A similar study (OV-10) confirmed the significant survival benefit seen with the addition of paclitaxel to cisplatin even in patients who had been optimally debulked (10). Studies were then undertaken to evaluate whether carboplatin, given the superior toxicity profile, could be substituted for cisplatin. Three randomized trials confirmed that the carboplatin–paclitaxel combination is equally effective and better tolerated than the cisplatin–paclitaxel combination (7,8,11).

The current standard first-line therapy for ovarian carcinoma is six cycles of carboplatin AUC 5-7 over one hour with paclitaxel (175 mg/m²) as a three-hour infusion every 21 days. Our practice is to administer the above regimen to patients with the high-risk features listed earlier. Chemotherapy should begin within four to six weeks of surgery. There appears to be no benefit in commencing chemotherapy any earlier (12). Despite the wide international acceptance of this regimen, several controversial issues remain which are discussed below.

In addition, a recent randomized trial from the Japanese Gynecological Oncology Group involving over 600 cases indicated superiority for first-line combination treatment in which conventional three weekly paclitaxel was replaced by a weekly paclitaxel regime (13). There was a highly significant improvement in median PFS (17 months increasing to 28 months). Confirmatory trials are therefore under discussion.

Combination vs. Single Agent Chemotherapy

It has been perceived that the platinum–paclitaxel combination is superior to single agent platinum. Two in-depth studies addressed this issue and concluded that cisplatin alone (GOG-132 trial) or single agent carboplatin (ICON-3) are as efficacious as combination therapy with paclitaxel. These findings, however, must be interpreted carefully because both trials have various shortcomings. In the GOG-132 trial (cisplatin vs. paclitaxel vs. both), half of the patients in the single arms of the trial received off-study chemotherapy prior to relapse and 85% "crossed over" by receiving the alternative drug after relapse, thereby effectively receiving sequential therapy (14). This may have obscured survival differences and led to an unintentional comparison of concurrent versus sequential therapy. Similar criticisms have been made of the ICON-3 trial (15). There was considerable heterogeneity in the study population (Stage 1c–IV) and the extent of primary surgery was not defined. Moreover, the data in this trial were not audited. Therefore, these results are not definitive and the carboplatin–paclitaxel combination remains the standard of care. However, in appropriate cases, particularly those in whom combination treatment may be poorly tolerated, single agent carboplatin is a satisfactory alternative.

Duration of Treatment, Maintenance, and High-Dose Chemotherapy

Randomized trials have failed to show the benefit of longer periods of chemotherapy in advanced EOC (e.g., five vs. eight cycles of cisplatin or carboplatin) (16). The optimum number of treatment cycles of the carboplatin–paclitaxel combination in advanced EOC has yet to be formally confirmed in a randomized setting. Conventionally, six cycles are delivered although some oncologists may administer more than six cycles, particularly when there seems to be a continuing response.

Prolonged administration of single agent chemotherapy, IP chemotherapy, and immunotherapy have been studied as maintenance therapy in ovarian cancer. So far, only one study has shown a benefit of maintenance therapy. A significant, seven-month prolongation of PFS (28 vs. 21 months, $p = 0.0023$) was achieved with 12 monthly cycles of paclitaxel compared to three monthly cycles in patients who were in remission after standard carboplatin–paclitaxel chemotherapy. However, there was no difference in the OS and neuropathy was more common with longer treatment (17). In addition, the hazard ratio for disease progression markedly increased after maintenance therapy was ceased. No survival benefit was observed in a trial (Italian After-6 protocol) that compared a shorter course of paclitaxel maintenance therapy (six cycles) with observation after six cycles of carboplatin–paclitaxel (18). Two randomized trials compared an additional four cycles of single agent topotecan after six cycles of carboplatin–paclitaxel and failed to demonstrate a benefit for maintenance therapy (19,20). The ongoing GOG-212 trial is designed to answer the question of whether taxane maintenance therapy offers a true survival benefit.

It has been proposed that drug resistance can be overcome by dose intensification. However, there has been no convincing clinical evidence to indicate that using higher doses of carboplatin improves OS. Studies of high-dose chemotherapy with stem cell transplantation as initial therapy for EOC (21) or as consolidation therapy (22) for women in remission have failed to show benefit.

Role of Other Agents

Docetaxel and paclitaxel have similar mechanisms of action but there is experimental evidence of partial noncross-resistance and a response rate of 23% was seen in a Phase II trials of docetaxel in paclitaxel-refractory Mullerian carcinoma (23). The SCOTROC study compared carboplatin–docetaxel with carboplatin–paclitaxel in previously untreated patients and found equivalent response rates and survival. The carboplatin–docetaxel combination was associated with less neurotoxicity and greater myelosuppression than carboplatin–paclitaxel (24). These findings suggest that docetaxel may be an option as a first-line agent in appropriate cases.

Liposomal doxorubicin, topotecan, gemcitabine, and epirubicin have been evaluated as first-line therapy in addition to the carboplatin and paclitaxel combination. However, the results of two Phase III trials including the GOG0182-ICON-5 did not demonstrate any benefit from the addition of a third agent (25,26).

The Role of Neoadjuvant Chemotherapy and Interval Debulking Surgery

Primary optimal debulking surgery followed by systemic chemotherapy is the conventional initial management for women with advanced ovarian carcinoma. An alternative is chemotherapy commenced prior to surgery, also known as "neoadjuvant chemotherapy." This is administered with a view to subsequent surgery or "delayed primary surgery" either in between courses or after completion of chemotherapy, depending on the degree and rate of response. This approach is applicable to patients where initial cytoreduction may not be feasible because of disease bulk and for those women that present with massive ascites, poor performance status, or significant comorbidities that may prevent aggressive surgery.

One study demonstrated a significantly greater likelihood of optimal debulking following neoadjuvant chemotherapy compared to those who had primary debulking surgery followed by adjuvant chemotherapy (95% vs. 71%) (27). Furthermore, women with extraabdominal disease who received neoadjuvant carboplatin and paclitaxel chemotherapy rather than initial debulking surgery had a significantly longer median OS compared to women who underwent initial debulking surgery (31 vs. 20 months). However, there are other data that show a negative survival effect of increasing number of chemotherapy cycles prior to interval surgery and suggest that definitive surgery should be undertaken as early in the management plan as possible (28). Preliminary findings of a randomized trial addressing the impact of neoadjuvant chemotherapy demonstrated a significantly higher optimal debulking rate, less operative blood loss, and fewer postoperative infections in patients who received neoadjuvant chemotherapy compared to initial surgery followed by chemotherapy (29). However, the differences in median OS and disease-free survival were not statistically significant. Until further results are available, initial optimal debulking is usually recommended. Currently, the optimal setting for the neoadjuvant approach is unknown and if chosen, surgical debulking should be intercalated early on during the treatment course.

Some patients undergo suboptimal debulking at primary surgery and may benefit from a further operation during chemotherapy, that is, "Interval debulking." The role of surgery in this setting remains controversial and randomized data have shown conflicting results. The results of an European Organisation for Research and Treatment of Cancer (EORTC) prospective randomized study of 278 women with ovarian cancer who had received suboptimal debulking at primary surgery support this approach. Patients were assigned surgery or no surgery after three of a total of six cycles of cyclophosphamide and cisplatin. The group that underwent a second surgical procedure demonstrated an improved two-year survival compared to the chemotherapy alone arm (56% vs. 46%) reducing the risk of death by 33% ($p = 0.008$) (30). By contrast, a GOG trial did not confirm the benefits of interval surgery. In this study, 550 suboptimally debulked patients were randomized to receive either interval debulking after three cycles or no surgery during a total of six cycles of cisplatin and paclitaxel. There was no significant difference in progression-free or OS between the two groups (31). It has been postulated that the conflicting results arise from the fact that, in contrast to patients in the EORTC trial, all the GOG trial patients underwent initial surgery by specialist gynecological-oncology teams. Therefore, interval debulking may not be useful if maximal effort at debulking has already been undertaken. Conversely, some clinicians would argue that interval debulking is a valid option in patients whose primary surgery did not achieve optimal cytoreduction.

Intraperitoneal Chemotherapy

Epithelial ovarian cancer has a unique pattern of spread and the bulk of disease tends to remain within the peritoneal cavity. This feature has led to the investigation of IP delivery of chemotherapy which allows for dose intensification while reducing systemic toxicity. However, penetration into tumor tissue is limited, and hence this approach appears best suited to patients with minimal residual disease after surgical cytoreduction. Three trials have reported a survival advantage for IP chemotherapy compared to IV administration in women with optimally cytoreduced (to <0.5 cm) Stage III epithelial ovarian cancer. The most recent trial, GOG trial 172 randomized 429 patients with optimally debulked Stage III disease between intravenous paclitaxel (135 mg/m^2 over 24 hr) followed by either intravenous cisplatin 75 mg/m^2 (control) or both IP cisplatin 100 mg/m^2 (day 2), and IP paclitaxel 60 mg/m^2 (day 8) for six cycles. IP therapy was associated with significantly improved median progression-free survival (23.8 vs. 18.3 months, $p = 0.05$) and OS (65.6 vs. 49.7 months, $p = 0.03$) although only 42% of patients in the IP group completed all six cycles because of complications (32). The interpretation of the survival data is limited for several reasons. Firstly, the control arm did not receive the current standard of care, that is, i.v. carboplatin and paclitaxel. In addition, the dose and schedule of the two drugs differ in the two arms of the study and hence the survival advantages may be as a result of higher doses of cisplatin and a higher cumulative dose of paclitaxel rather than route of administration. Furthermore, the analysis was not a true intention-to-treat analysis and given the marginal statistical differences, minor imbalances in the number of excluded patients could render the trial statistically nonsignificant. Treatment-related complications occur in up to 20% of patients and include abdominal discomfort, infection, obstruction, leakage, access problems, and bowel injury. In addition to catheter-related problems, fatigue, hematological, gastrointestinal, and neurological events were significantly higher in the IP arm of the GOG-172 trial. The use of IP chemotherapy is not universally adopted largely because of the greater toxicity associated with this approach.

Chemotherapy for Relapsed Disease

Once epithelial ovarian cancer has recurred, treatment with curative intent is no longer feasible. Several factors present at diagnosis are associated with a greater likelihood of disease relapse and include clinical stage, disease bulk, presence of ascites, age, and histology (clear cell, mucinous, poorly differentiated). Most relapsed epithelial ovarian cancers initially respond to chemotherapy but eventually the disease becomes resistant to treatment. However, the judicious use of palliative chemotherapy can improve both survival and quality of life for patients with recurrent disease.

Timing of Treatment and Surveillance. Treatment is aimed to relieve cancer-related symptoms, optimize quality of life, delay the time to symptomatic disease progression, and prolong OS. Most treatment options are associated with toxicity that could be detrimental to quality of life. An optimal window time for treatment exists and missing this opportunity may result in problematic toxicity without any palliative benefit. Biochemical and clinical surveillance to detect disease relapse is performed at regular intervals. Elevations in CA-125 may precede clinical or radiographic detection by three to six months. Recommendations for asymptomatic women with only a rising CA-125 (equivocal CT scan) are highly individualized and may include continued serial CA-125 monitoring until the development of symptoms or measurable disease, surgical reassessment, or immediate institution of systemic chemotherapy. Currently, there is no evidence to indicate that treatment of recurrent disease based on early detection of a rising CA-125 improves survival and therefore current practice in the authors' institution is to instigate chemotherapy on occurrence of disease-related symptoms or bulk (>3 cm) disease radiologically. The results of a current MRC/EORTC study that has randomized patients to receive treatment based on CA-125 alone or when clinically indicated are pending. Approximately 10–20% of patients present with normal CA-125 at diagnosis and are termed "non-secretors." This population requires close follow-up with regular scans to detect relapse prior to the development of bulky disease.

Choice of Treatment. There have been no randomized controlled trials to compare chemotherapy with best supportive care for relapsed disease and platinum-based therapy remains the preferred option for patients who have late relapse. However, several other agents have shown activity in relapsed ovarian cancer with most drugs having a response rate in the range of 10–30% for patients with a treatment-free interval of less than 12 months. The management of recurrent EOC takes into account the duration of the platinum-free interval and the response to first-line platinum therapy.

Patients can be divided into the following categories:

Platinum sensitive
Platinum-free interval of at least six months. This group has a higher chance of responding either to a rechallenge with platinum-based treatment or to other agents especially if the interval exceed two years.
Platinum resistant
Relapsed disease during or within six months from the end of first-line platinum treatment. This group is likely to have chemoresistant disease and the future chance of response to cytotoxic agents is modest.
Platinum refractory
No response or progressive disease at the end of six cycles of platinum-based chemotherapy.

Platinum-sensitive disease Many trials have concluded that second-line platinum-based therapy provides significant benefit for patients with platinum-sensitive EOC and therefore women who relapse more than six months after initial platinum treatment are usually rechallenged with platinum-based therapy. The length of platinum-free interval is highly predictive of the upper limit of the duration of disease control that can be expected with second-line cisplatin-based chemotherapy (33). The best regimen for retreatment of women with platinum-sensitive disease is not clear. Several major trials have addressed the question of whether single agent (platinum alone) or combination therapy (including platinum) should be the treatment of choice. The first randomized Phase III trial (ICON4/AGO-OVAR-2.2) assigned 802 women who relapsed with platinum-sensitive disease and a treatment-free interval of at least six months to conventional platinum-based chemotherapy or combination therapy (paclitaxel plus a platinum agent) (34). There was a significant OS benefit in favor of paclitaxel-containing combined therapy (hazard ratio, HR = 0.82), which corresponded to an absolute two-year survival benefit of 7% (57% vs. 50%), and a five-month improvement in median survival (29 vs. 24 months). The combination therapy also improved progression-free survival (HR = 0.76; one year PFS: 50% vs. 40%). A higher incidence of Grade 2–4 neurological effects (20% vs. 1%) and alopecia (86% vs. 25%) were noted with the combination therapy and a lower rate of myelosuppression in the paclitaxel-treated patients. Importantly, only 40% of patients received paclitaxel as part of the initial therapy although subset analysis did not reveal a significant difference between patients with and without prior paclitaxel exposure. Nevertheless, the major benefit numerically occurs in those women who have not previously been treated with paclitaxel. Further support for combination therapy was provided by a randomized Phase III trial (SWOG S0200) that compared liposomal doxorubicin plus carboplatin versus carboplatin alone (35). The combined therapy group had a significantly higher response rate (67% vs. 32%), median PFS (12 vs. 8 months) and median OS (26 vs. 18 months) but the results were based on accrual of only 61 of a planned 900 women, limiting the interpretation of the results. In contrast, an OS benefit was not shown for combination therapy in a Gynecologic Cancer Intergroup Phase III trial in which patients were randomly assigned to carboplatin alone (AUC 5) or carboplatin (AUC 4) plus gemcitabine (36). In fact, the trial was not powered

to show an OS difference, and the combined therapy did result in a significantly higher overall response rate (47% vs. 31%) and median PFS (8.6 vs. 5.8 months) without worsening quality of life, although hematological toxicity was worse. Taken together, these data support the superiority of combination platinum-based regimens compared to single agent platinum-based therapy alone. Some clinicians believe that single agent platinum therapy should be considered the standard of care for platinum-sensitive relapsing disease in view of the only modest survival advantages but worse toxicity of combination versus single agent therapy.

Platinum-resistant disease Many drugs have shown activity in this setting with response rates ranging from 6% to 40%. Single agent therapy is commonly chosen because although combination therapy may yield higher response rates, toxicities are greater and no OS benefit has been achieved. The most commonly used second-line agents are pegylated liposomal doxorubicin (caelyx), topotecan, and gemcitabine. The use of caelyx is associated with skin toxicity, but at a dosage of $40\,mg/m^2$ on a four weekly i.v. schedule it is generally well tolerated, with no apparent reduction in efficacy compared to the recommended dosage of $50\,mg/m^2$. Etoposide, vinorelbine, oxaliplatin, and capecitabine have also shown some activity. There is evidence of a lack of cross-resistance between topotecan and paclitaxel (37). Topotecan is associated with a high incidence of hematological toxicity which along with the inconvenient five-day intravenous schedule limits its acceptability in a palliative setting. There are data suggesting the potential for gemcitabine to modify platinum resistance and this requires further investigation. A GOG Phase II study of oral etoposide demonstrated a response rate of 32% in patients who had prior platinum and pacitaxel (38). However, hematological toxicity can be severe with etoposide as illustrated by the study above where 45% Grade 3–4 neutropenia and three treatment-related deaths were noted. Response rates of 22–30% with single agent paclitaxel in phase II and III trials of women with platinum-resistant EOC have been achieved. There is evidence for weekly paclitaxel therapy maintaining efficacy while minimizing toxicity, especially myelosuppression (39).

Endocrine therapy Although over 70% of epithelial ovarian cancers express estrogen and/or progesterone receptors (PRs), treatment with tamoxifen or LHRH agonists has shown only modest activity. A Cochrane Review of tamoxifen efficacy in relapsed ovarian cancer demonstrated an overall response rate of 9.6% and stable disease for more than four weeks in an additional 32% (40). Aromatase inhibitors have recently been investigated in Phase II trials of patients with recurrent ovarian cancer. A Phase II trial of letrozole in women with ER-positive EOC, demonstrated radiological response in 9% and disease stabilization at 12 weeks in 42% of women. A fall in CA-125 (>50%) was detected in 17% of patients. Interestingly, the CA125 response rate was highest in women who had higher estrogen receptor (ER) expression (41). The efficacy of AIs in combination with biological agents (e.g., EGFR and HER2 inhibitors) remains to be determined. Given the relatively favorable tolerability of AIs, further investigation of the role of these agents in prolonging platinum-free interval in recurrence ovarian cancer is warranted.

Surgical Resection for Relapsed Ovarian Cancer

The place of "secondary debulking" for recurrent ovarian cancer has been greatly debated. Data from mainly retrospective series show that patients in whom optimal secondary debulking is achieved have a survival advantage. Women who are offered surgical management tend to have more favorable disease characteristics and any survival benefit may be a reflection of favorable tumor biology that permits optimal debulking rather than the surgical procedure itself. The AGO-DESKTOP OVAR trial determined that good performance status, no residual disease postprimary surgery, early stage at diagnosis, and no ascites at recurrence predicted optimal resection almost 80% of the time (42). Results from Phase III trials evaluating the role of surgical management in combination with chemotherapy are eagerly awaited (LOROCSON, EORTC 55963).

Treatment of Bowel Obstruction

Bowel obstruction especially, involving the small intestine (acute or intermittent subacute), is a common problem faced by patients with end-stage ovarian cancer. Management requires a multidisciplinary approach by a team comprising palliative care specialists, surgeons, dieticians, nurses, and medical oncologists. The role of surgery as palliation for malignant bowel obstruction is well recognized, but palliative surgery is associated with a perioperative mortality of 10–15%, and 35–38% of patients do not gain any clinical benefit. It is important to identify suitable patients who are likely to benefit from chemotherapy despite a compromised performance status. Patients with newly diagnosed disease (chemotherapy-naive) and those who have relapsed after a long treatment-free interval are likely to respond to chemotherapy with symptomatic relief from bowel obstruction; otherwise, the role of chemotherapy is very limited in this situation.

Novel Therapies

Novel agents designed to target tumor cells and/or the microenvironment by exploiting specific molecular abnormalities in the tumor hold the promise of greater selectivity and lower toxicity than traditional modalities such as chemotherapy.

Angiogenesis Inhibitors. Bevacizumab, a monoclonal antibody against Vascular Endothelial Growth Factor (VEGF-A), is the first targeted agent to show significant single agent activity in ovarian carcinoma. A Phase II trial recently demonstrated a response rate and six-month PFS rate of 21% and 40%, respectively, in platinum-sensitive recurrent ovarian cancer (43). The activity of bevacizumab in ovarian cancer was confirmed in a second Phase II study in which a response rate of 16% and a 6 month PFS of 28% was observed in patients with platinum resistant disease (44). However, this trial was closed prematurely because of an unacceptable frequency of bowel perforations (11%). It seems likely that this risk can be ameliorated by avoiding the use of bevacizumab in patients with extensive bowel involvement. Two Phase III trials (GOG 218 and ICON7) of bevacizumab in combination with carboplatin–paclitaxel in front-line ovarian cancer therapy are ongoing. Bevacizumab is being evaluated in combination with anti-EGF therapy (erlotinib) and also cytotoxic

agents such as low-dose oral cyclophosphamide in Phase II trials. Other angiogenesis inhibitors are under evaluation, including oral VEGFR tyrosine kinase inhibitors such as cediranib, pazopanib, and sunitinib. Phase II data indicate a degree of efficacy for each of these and further trials involving combination and maintenance strategies (e.g., ICON-6) are underway in platinum-sensitive relapsed disease.

Poly(ADP)Ribose Polymerase (PARP) Inhibitors. Carriers of *BRCA* mutations are at risk of developing ovarian cancer (10–40% lifetime risk) and tumors arising in these individuals harbor DNA repair defects. PARP inhibitors work by generating double strand DNA breaks that require functional BRCA1 and BRCA2 proteins for efficient DNA repair. Cancers with dysfunctional *BRCA* proteins are therefore sensitive to single agent PARP inhibitor treatment. Preliminary observations from patients with *BRCA* mutations and ovarian cancer in a Phase I trial of PARP inhibition are encouraging and indicate low toxicities and promising radiological and serological clinical responses (45). Phase II trials of this drug in *BRCA* carriers with breast and/or ovarian cancer are ongoing. PARP inhibition could be more widely applicable in the treatment of sporadic ovarian cancers as BRCA dysfunction is relatively common.

Other Signaling Molecules. Preclinical evidence suggests that EGFR and HER2 are potential targets in ovarian cancer. However, results from Phase II trials of erlotinib, gefitinib (EGFR inhibitors), trastuzumab (targeting HER2), and pertuzumab (HER2 dimerization inhibitor) have all been relatively disappointing. EGFR and/or HER2 inhibitors combined with chemotherapy may further improve the efficiency of chemotherapy and final results from clinical trials addressing this are awaited. Multiple components of signaling cascades are aberrant in ovarian cancer and drugs under development that target these critical molecules include various examples of the PI3 kinase/AKT pathway (such as mTOR inhibitors), the Src pathway, and others. The folate receptor is overexpressed in >90% of ovarian cancers and MORab-003 (Morphotek Inc.), a monoclonal antibody directed against the folate receptor, is being evaluated in a Phase II trial of recurrent platinum-sensitive disease.

Immunotherapy. The host immune response is important in the clinical outcome of ovarian cancer. Immunomodulatory strategies such as monoclonal antibodies against tumor antigens and treatments against T regulatory cells are under evaluation. MAb/B43.13 (oregovomab) is a monoclonal antibody directed against CA-125, which is being studied as consolidation therapy postadjuvant treatment for ovarian cancer. Although a randomized trial of this agent versus placebo showed no alteration in time to progression, unplanned subset analysis revealed that patients who were optimally debulked and who achieved rapid serological response to chemotherapy derived increased benefit from Mab/B43.13 (46). Phase III trials looking at this specific population are in progress (IMPACT I and II). Denileukin difitox (Ontak) is a fusion protein between the diphtheria toxin and IL2 designed to downregulate T regulatory cells thereby enhancing host immunity against tumor cells. This approach is being tested in a Phase I/II trial of ovarian cancer.

Clear Cell Carcinoma of the Ovary

Clear cell carcinoma (CCC) of the ovary is a distinct histological subtype of EOC characterized by glycogen-containing clear cells and hobnail cells. CCC is associated with a high incidence of Stage I disease (especially Ic), large pelvic mass, endometriosis, thromboembolic complications, and hypercalcemia. CCC is rare in Europe and the United States (incidence 3–6%), however the incidence in Japan is more than 20%. CCC appears to be more resistant to platinum-based chemotherapy compared with serous and endometrioid subtypes of EOC and studies suggest that the survival rates are worse for patients with CCC. Primary cytoreductive surgery with maximum effort is the recommended treatment. A CCC-specific international clinical trial (GCIG/JGOG3017 trial) comparing carboplatin–paclitaxel with cisplatin–irinotecan is ongoing and aims to identify the optimal chemotherapy regimen for CCC.

Germ Cell Tumors of the Ovary
Epidemiology, Etiology, and Pathology

Ovarian germ cell tumors (OGCTs) which may be benign or malignant, arise from primordial germ cells and exhibit a spectrum of histological differentiation. Malignant germ cell tumors account for less than 5% of all ovarian malignancies. However, they represent 70% of ovarian tumors in females between 10 and 30 years of age. The etiology of malignant OGCTs is unclear but high prepregnancy body mass and use of exogenous hormones during pregnancy have been associated with higher risk. OGCTs do not appear to have a hereditary component unlike epithelial ovarian cancers.

These tumors may be divided into two main groups:

Dysgerminomas arising from primitive undifferentiated germ cells.
Nondysgerminoma-embryonal carcinoma; yolk sac tumor/endodermal sinus tumor; choriocarcinoma; teratoma.

Clinical Features

Presenting features include abdominal pain and/or distension, palpable mass, abnormal vaginal bleeding, symptoms of pregnancy (from hCG production), and, rarely, amenorrhea and precocious puberty. Patients can present with an acute abdomen due to torsion, infection, or rupture. OGCTs grow rapidly yet, in contrast to EOC, most tumors present at an early stage often confined to one ovary (Stage IA).

Diagnosis and Staging

Surgery is required for definitive histological diagnosis although abnormally high tumor markers, clinical symptoms and signs, and the radiological appearances on ultrasound make the preoperative diagnosis extremely likely.

Serum tumor markers provide highly sensitive and specific markers for the presence of certain histologic components of OGCTs. Serum AFP is generally elevated in patients with yolk sac tumor, and sometimes in embryonal carcinoma and immature teratoma. HCG is elevated in choriocarcinoma and embryonal carcinoma. Mixed germ cell tumors may contain embryonal cell, choriocarcinoma or yolk sac components and so can produce both markers.

Dysgerminomas are associated with a normal AFP. They may, however, produce lactate dehydrogenase (LDH) or small amounts of hCG.

Staging of malignant OGCTs requires surgery and is according to the International Federation of Gynecologists and Obstetricians (FIGO) staging system for epithelial ovarian cancer. Surgical staging includes total omentectomy, appendicectomy, peritoneal biopsies, and lymph node sampling. Pelvic ultrasound and CT scan are useful to assess intra-abdominal and lymph node metastases. Nodal involvement is more common with malignant OGCTs compared to EOC, and they have a greater tendency to metastasize to the liver and lung.

Management

The principles of surgical management are the same for all malignant OGCTs. Most women with malignant OGCTs are young and wish to preserve future childbearing capacity. Therefore, the current management emphasizes initial conservative surgery- unilateral salpingo-oophorectomy with preservation of the uterus and the contralateral ovary if these organs appear normal. Women who have completed childbearing undergo total abdominal hysterectomy and bilateral salpingo-oophorectomy. For patients with advanced tumors, optimal cytoreductive surgery improves outcomes. However, OGCTs are chemosensitive and so the benefits and risks of aggressive surgical cytoreductive procedures for metastatic disease must be carefully considered.

Malignant OGCTs, especially teratoma, are usually very sensitive to platinum-based chemotherapy. At least 90% of patients with early stage OGCT, and approximately 75–80% of those with advanced disease are long-term survivors. The recommended approach for both early stage and more advanced OGCTs is postoperative chemotherapy with three or four courses of bleomycin, etoposide, and cisplatin (BEP) with the exception of those with Stage I Grade 1 immature teratomas and Stage IA dysgerminomas. Despite the lack of randomized trials, several series have demonstrated that long-term survival rates with surgery followed by adjuvant BEP are in the order of 95–100% for early-stage nondysgerminomatous tumors and 75–80% for those with advanced disease at presentation. Results are even more favorable for ovarian dysgerminomas, regardless of stage at presentation. An alternative platinum-based regimen is POMBACE which aims to reduce the risk of drug resistance by alternating a relatively nonmyelosuppressive combination (cisplatin, vincristine, methotrexate, bleomycin, and folinic acid) with a more myelosuppressive triplet (actinomycin-D, cyclophosphamide, and etoposide). Trials have shown a three-year survival rate of 88%. Furthermore, this regimen appears to be effective as second-line chemotherapy for recurrent disease with 50% of patients salvaged at relapse (47).

It is important that full doses of all of the component drugs are administered at the scheduled time to ensure that the curative potential of systemic chemotherapy is not compromised. The full extent of long-term sequelae of chemotherapy on survivors are still to be determined. Most women who receive three or four courses of standard dose therapy will recover normal ovarian function, and fertility is often preserved. However, there is a risk of secondary malignancies such as leukemias following chemotherapy, in particular etoposide, which appears to be dose related. Studies are addressing prognostic factors that may permit risk stratification for future treatment choices in OGCT.

ENDOMETRIAL CANCER
Epidemiology and Etiology
Endometrial cancer is the second most common gyneco- logical malignancy in the United Kingdom. Over 6000 cases are diagnosed every year and endometrial cancer accounts for 1650 deaths annually. The incidence of endometrial cancer is rising in postmenopausal women but five-year survival rates have improved to more than 75%.

Various factors are associated with an increased risk of developing endometrial cancer. Estrogen exposure either from exogenous or endogenous sources in the absence of adequate exposure to progestins has been linked to endo- metrial cancer. Several case-control and prospective studies have shown an increased incidence of endometrial carci- noma with estrogen replacement therapy, the relative risk ranging from 3.1 to 15. The risk is related to both estrogen dose and duration of use and can be significantly reduced by the concomitant administration of progestins. Tamoxifen use is also associated with the disease. Endometrial cancer usually occurs in postmenopausal women—the median age at diagnosis is 65 years. Twenty-five percent of cases are diagnosed in premenopausal women, and 5–10% of these are in women under age 40.

Pathology
Most endometrial cancers are of epithelial origin. The histological cell types can be classified as follows:

Endometrioid adenocarcinomas (Type I)
Nonendometrioid adenocarcinomas (Type II)—papillary serous, clear cell

The most common type (80% of cases) of endometrial cancer is endometrioid adenocarcinoma. Endometrioid histology is associated with unopposed estrogen, endometrial hyper- plasia, and a younger age at diagnosis. Papillary serous and CCC account for 5–10% of cases and do not appear to be hormone related. They are highly aggressive tumors that commonly present at a more advanced stage. Mixed car- cinomas are composed of serous and endometrioid com- ponents. Rarer types include mucinous and squamous cell carcinoma.

Molecular studies show that endometrioid tumors have a different genetic profile to nonendometrioid tumors (48). Microsatellite instability and specific mutations of *PTEN*, and *K-ras* genes are more characteristic of endo- metrioid tumors, while *p53* mutations and HER2/neu overexpression predominate in nonendometrioid tumors. Endometrioid carcinomas show expression of both estrogen receptor (ER) and PR in about 90% of cases, with decreas- ing expression at higher grade. Tumors of serous histology express ER in 31% of cases and PR in 12% and CCC rarely express either receptor. In addition to cell type, three grades of differentiation are recognized: well (Grade I), moderate (Grade II), and poorly (Grade III) differentiated.

Clinical Features, Diagnosis, and Staging
The main presenting symptom is postmenopausal vaginal bleeding. However, 20% of cases occur in premenopausal women and so the signs may be subtle.

Diagnosis is confirmed on histological assessment. Tissue may be obtained by hysteroscopy with dilation and curettage (D&C) or endometrial biopsy using a Pipelle sampling device. Additional investigations include trans- vaginal ultrasound, CT, and MRI. Tumors may spread by direct extension into the myometrial wall and endocervix, lymphatic, or hematogenous routes.

Endometrial carcinoma is surgically staged according to the FIGO system (Table 6.3). Surgical staging includes hysterectomy, bilateral salpingo-oophorectomy, cytologic examination of peritoneal fluid, biopsy of any suspicious IP or retroperitoneal lesions, and retroperitoneal lymph node sampling. Synchronous primary cancers of the endo- metrium occur in 5% of cases.

Table 6.3 International Federation of Gynecologists and Obstetricians (FIGO) Stage Grouping for Endometrial Carcinoma and Five-Year Survival by Stage

Stage		Description	5-year survival (%)
I		Limited to corpus	
	Ia	Limited to endometrium	91
	Ib	Invasion of less than half of myometrium	91
	Ic	Invasion of more than half of myometrium	85
II		Involvement of the cervix	
	IIa	Glandular involvement only	83
	IIb	Cervical stromal involvement	74
III		Spread outside of uterus, confined to pelvis (excluding rectum or bladder)	
	IIIa	Involvement of uterine serosa, adnexa(e), positive peritoneal cytology	66
	IIIb	Spread to vagina	50
	IIIc	Spread to retroperitoneal nodes	57
IV		Spread to bladder, rectum, distant sites	
	IVa	Involvement of bladder and/or rectal mucosa	26
	IVb	Distant, intra-abdominal spread, inguinal nodes	20

Data from 6th Annual FIGO Report: Patients Treated 1999–2001.

Management of Early-Stage Disease

Treatment recommendations for women with endometrial cancer depend upon the estimated risk of recurrent disease, which is based upon surgical stage and tumor grade. Primary treatment is surgery comprising TAH and BSO. The role of lymphadenectomy remains controversial although it is recommended for accurate staging according to the FIGO criteria. Some clinicians believe that the morbidity associated with the procedure outweighs the benefits when the likelihood of nodal disease is very low, such as in low risk Stage I disease. Preliminary results from A Study in the Treatment of Endometrial Cancer (ASTEC) trial support this view. Women were randomly assigned to conventional surgery or conventional surgery plus lymphadenectomy; both groups had a similar three-year survival (49). Women with Grade 1 or 2 histology and Stage IA or IB endometrial cancer are considered "low-risk" for recurrence and TAH/BSO is the appropriate management. Stage IC and Grade 3 tumors (IA or IB) are of "intermediate risk." The role of adjuvant radiotherapy for intermediate-risk early-stage endometrial cancer is controversial. Prospective trials [e.g., Post Operative Radiation Therapy in Endometrial Cancer (PORTEC) and MRC ASTEC and NCIC CTG EN.5 trial] demonstrate that adjuvant radiotherapy reduces pelvic failure rates in women with early-stage endometrial cancer but there is no evidence that survival rates are improved (50). The decision whether to treat an individual patient with radiation is dependent on careful surgical staging and assessment of the benefits and risks of treatment.

The outcome of women with high-risk disease (Stage IC, Grade 3, Stage IIA and above, lymphovascular space or lower uterine segment involvement, and papillary serous or clear cell histology) is poor with surgery alone and women are offered adjuvant therapy. Recently, results from GOG 122 trial showed a survival benefit for adjuvant chemotherapy as compared to whole abdominal radiotherapy (WART) in women with Stage III–IVa disease. Three hundred and ninety six women with Stage III or IV endometrial cancer were randomly assigned to WART (30 Gy in 20 fractions, with a 15 Gy pelvic + paraaortic node boost) or postoperative chemotherapy (doxorubicin 60 mg/m^2 plus cisplatin 50 mg/m^2 every three weeks for seven courses, followed by an additional course of cisplatin). There was a statistically significant benefit for chemotherapy in terms of disease progression (stage-adjusted progression hazard ratio [HR] relative to WART 0.71), which translated into a 12% increase in five-year PFS (50% vs. 38%). There was also a significant survival benefit that favored chemotherapy (HR for death relative to WART 0.68), which translated into a 13% improvement in five-year OS (55% vs. 42 %) (51). The chemotherapy group had significantly more acute Grade 3–4 adverse events (hematological and cardiac). The best chemotherapy regimen and duration have not been defined, and toxicity may be significant. Chemotherapy regimens include carboplatin–paclitaxel and doxorubicin–cisplatin–paclitaxel.

A subset of patients may be unable to undergo TAH/BSO due to comorbid conditions or poor performance status. In these, primary radiotherapy is the treatment of choice and as external beam radiotherapy may be poorly tolerated by this group, brachytherapy may be preferable to treat disease confined to the uterus.

Management of Advanced/Recurrent Disease

Endocrine Therapy

There is a rationale for using hormone therapy in advanced or recurrent endometrial carcinoma because some tumors express estrogen and/or progesterone receptors and these are independent predictive factors for response to endocrine treatment. Hormone therapy is a particularly attractive option for the treatment of advanced endometrial cancer because it is well tolerated and lacks the usual toxicities associated with cytotoxic chemotherapy. Progestin therapy, for example, medroxyprogesterone acetate, offers a 10–20% response rate. Low-grade histology, expression of ER and/or PR and a long treatment-free interval predict a favorable response (52). Tamoxifen can be effective in women with advanced endometrial cancer in women with hormone receptor positive tumors. Whether tamoxifen is superior to a progestin for initial hormone therapy is unclear. Combinations of tamoxifen and progestins have also been studied, although none of the trials selected patients on the basis of hormone receptor expression. Randomized Phase II trials have shown response rates of 27–33% (53). Aromatase inhibitors have shown limited activity in advanced endometrial cancer.

Chemotherapy

Cytotoxic chemotherapy agents can be used alone or in combination. Doxorubicin, cisplatin, carboplatin docetaxel, and topotecan have all shown activity as monotherapy with response rates from 17% to 28%. Paclitaxel has been reported to have response rates of 27–37%. Various combination regimens that include doxorubicin and/or a platinum have been investigated. However, randomized trials have failed to show any survival benefit with combinations of doxorubicin plus either cyclophosphamide or cisplatin compared to single agent doxorubicin. These combinations are associated with toxicity in terms of myelosuppression and vomiting. Furthermore, cisplatin-containing schedules can be time consuming and inconvenient due to the hydration required and, in elderly patients, anthracycline-induced congestive cardiac failure is a concern. Trials have compared paclitaxel-based versus nonpaclitaxel-containing combination regimens and two of these suggest a survival benefit for paclitaxel-containing therapy. The GOG trial 177, randomly assigned women with Stage III/IV or recurrent endometrial cancer to doxorubicin (60 mg/m^2) plus cisplatin (50 mg/m^2), or the three drug combination of doxorubicin (45 mg/m^2 on day 1), cisplatin (50 mg/m^2 on day 1) plus paclitaxel (160 mg/m^2 over three hours on day 2) with hematopoietic colony-stimulating factor support (TAP) (54). Response rates were significantly higher with TAP (57% vs. 34%), as was median PFS (eight vs. five months) and OS (15 vs. 12 months). However, TAP was associated with more Grade 3 neuropathy and Grade 3 symptomatic heart failure. Paclitaxel plus carboplatin is an alternative less toxic combination than TAP. The GOG is currently conducting a randomized equivalency trial of TAP versus carboplatin–paclitaxel in women with advanced and recurrent endometrial cancer.

Platinum resistance or refractory disease carries a poor prognosis in endometrial cancer. Second-line single agents have low response rates (less than 10%). Paclitaxel rechallenge has been associated with 37% overall response rate and 22% in platinum-refractory patients (55).

Future Approaches

There is growing interest in targeted biological therapies for endometrial cancer management. Multiple components of signaling cascades have been identified as aberrant in endometrial cancer through the well-recognized increase in PTEN dysfunction in this disease; examples include the mammalian target of rapamycin (mTOR) which is critical for proliferation. The mTOR inhibitors have shown encouraging single agent activity in Phase II trials of advanced endometrial cancer. Their precise mechanism of action is unclear, and may involve their antiangiogenic properties. Trials of other antiangiogenic agents such as bevacizumab, sunitinib, and VEGF-Trap are currently underway. HER2, a transmembrane receptor, appears to be overexpressed in 17–50% of uterine serous papillary carcinomas. These results raise the potential for future therapeutic strategies targeting HER2 with the anti-HER2 monoclonal antibody, trastuzumab, or the orally active EGFR/HER2 tyrosine kinase inhibitor, lapatanib.

Carcinosarcoma of the Uterus

Sarcomas may also arise from the endometrium or myometrium and are associated with a poorer prognosis than endometrial carcinoma. Carcinosarcomas (malignant mixed mullerian tumors) are the most common form of uterine sarcoma and consist of both epithelial (usually papillary serous) and sarcomatous elements. These tumors are treated in a similar fashion to papillary serous and clear cell tumors. Surgery is the main form of treatment for early-stage carcinosarcoma. Few studies have addressed the effects of adjuvant therapy in individual histological subtypes of sarcoma. Nevertheless, there is evidence supporting the use of adjuvant radiotherapy and cisplatin-based chemotherapy. Several agents and combinations have shown activity in recurrent or metastatic disease and include carboplatin–paclitaxel, paclitaxel–ifosfamide, and doxorubicin–cyclophoshamide.

CARCINOMA OF THE UTERINE CERVIX
Epidemiology

Cancer of the cervix is the eleventh most common malignancy among women in the United Kingdom and the third most common gynecological malignancy accounting for 2% of female cancers. Over 3200 women are diagnosed with cervical cancer in the United Kingdom every year and around 1200 women die from this disease annually. The incidence rate is 10.6 per 100,000 and the lifetime risk of developing cervical cancer is 1 in 116. The peak incidence of cervical cancer is 40–50 years. The incidence and mortality rates of cervical cancer are falling in developed countries but there is a marked increase in the number of women with preinvasive cancer. In contrast, cervical cancer is the second most common cause of cancer-related morbidity and mortality among women in developing countries. This discrepancy is mainly due to the institution of cervical cancer screening programs which is now widespread in developed countries, but is very limited in many developing countries.

Etiology and Risk Factors

Sexual activity is the dominant risk factor for cervical neoplasia. The major factor causing these disorders is infection with the human papillomavirus (HPV). Most HPV infections occur in young women and are transient and the majority of women infected with HPV do not develop high-grade cervical lesions or cancer. High-risk HPV subtypes, such as 16 and 18, are strongly associated with high-grade lesions, persistence, and progression to invasive cancer, although they may also be associated with low-grade lesions. Cofactors in the pathogenesis of cervical cancer include immunosuppression (HIV, immunosuppressive therapy) and cigarette smoking. In contrast to squamous cell cancer of the cervix, cigarette smoking is not associated with an increased risk of adenocarcinoma of the cervix compared to nonsmokers. Herpes simplex virus (HSV), chlamydia infection, and oral contraceptive use have been implicated as cofactors that increase the risk of cervical carcinoma in women who are HPV positive; it is possibility that these factors are surrogate markers of HPV exposure rather than causal factors. It may take 15 years from initial HPV infection to development of CIN 3 and invasive cancer.

Observational evidence consistently demonstrates that introduction of cervical cytology screening programs decreases cervical cancer mortality. As compared with cytology [Papanicolaou (Pap) test], HPV testing was shown to have greater sensitivity (94.6% vs. 55.4%) but lower specificity (94.1% vs. 96.8%) for the detection of cervical intraepithelial neoplasia compared with Pap testing (56). The POBASCAM trial concluded that HPV DNA and Pap testing led to earlier detection of CIN 3 and cancerous lesions than Pap testing alone (57). Currently, Pap smear screening from age 25–65 is the U.K. recommendation.

HPV Vaccines

The introduction of targeted HPV protection with the bivalent (HPV 16/18 L1 virus-like particle vaccine) or quadrivalent vaccine (HPV 6/11/16/18 L1 VLP vaccine) is anticipated to have a significant impact on the risk for precancerous lesions and invasive cancer. Multicenter, double-blind, placebo-controlled trials for both quadrivalent (58) and bivalent (59) HPV vaccines have demonstrated efficacy in terms of incident and persistent infection and CIN. Both vaccines have an excellent safety profile.

The FUTURE II trial was a Phase III, prospective, double-blinded, placebo-controlled trial with over 12,000 women aged 15–26 years. Participants were randomly assigned to receive a three-dose regimen of quadrivalent vaccine or placebo. This study demonstrated that HPV vaccination to HPV-naive women could substantially reduce the incidence of HPV16/18-related cervical precancers and cervical cancer. Vaccine efficacy for the prevention of CIN 2 or 3, adenocarcinoma in situ, or cervical cancer related to HPV-16 or HPV-18 was 98% in the "susceptible" (HPV naive) population and 44% in an intention-to-treat population (those with or without previous infection) (60). The FUTURE I trial was a Phase III placebo-controlled trial conducted in 5455 women aged 16–24 years to assess the efficacy of quadrivalent vaccine to prevent HPV-related anogenital disease (61). Similar to FUTURE II, vaccine efficacy was 100% in preventing CIN grades 1–3 or adenocarcinoma in situ in women who were HPV naive. There was no clear evidence that vaccination altered the course of disease or infection present before administration of the first dose of vaccine in both FUTURE I and II trials. These data reinforce the use of the HPV vaccine as a prophylactic, and not as a therapeutic immunization. HPV vaccine is a major advance in the prevention of cervical cancer, but it will not replace, at least for some considerable time, the need for cervical screening.

Clinical Features, Diagnosis, and Staging

Early cervical cancer is frequently asymptomatic highlighting the importance of screening. Symptoms may include abnormal vaginal bleeding after coitus, discharge, pelvic pain, and dyspareunia. Examination findings can range from a normal appearing cervix with an isolated abnormal cervical cytology smear, to a grossly abnormal cervix that is replaced entirely with tumor. The diagnosis is confirmed with biopsies taken at colposcopy or examination under anesthetic and histological evaluation. Radiological investigations (CT or MRI scans) are undertaken to assess the urinary tract and determine the extent of disease. Staging of cervical cancer is by the FIGO system (Table 6.4).

Management

Treatment options are surgery, radiotherapy and chemotherapy and depend on factors such as the stage of disease, size of the tumor and the fitness of the patient.

The two main methods of radiotherapy delivery for cervical cancer are external photon beam radiotherapy and brachytherapy. The volume encompassed by external radiotherapy should include the lymph nodes with the primary tumor. Intrauterine brachytherapy permits the delivery of a high central dose to the primary tumor while sparing the surrounding normal tissue and can be delivered using an intracavitary approach (more commonly used) with a variety of applicators, or via an interstitial approach using needles or after loading catheters. Radiotherapy can lead to changes such as vaginal shortening, stenosis, and decreased vaginal lubrication adversely affecting overall quality of life and psychosexual well-being following treatment. Chemoradiotherapy refers to the combination of chemotherapy and radiation. The rationale for combining these modalities is that cisplatin-based chemotherapy may synergize with radiation by inhibiting the repair of radiation-induced sublethal damage and by sensitizing hypoxic cells to radiation damage. The combination of surgery and radiotherapy ideally should be avoided because of the greater risk of morbidity, particularly urological, compared to either treatment used alone.

Management of Early-Stage Disease

The treatment options for early-stage cervical cancer are surgery or chemoradiotherapy. A surgical approach (hysterectomy or trachelectomy) is generally used for younger women with stage Ia, Ib, and IIa disease in whom preservation of fertility is desired. The risk of nodal metastatic spread increases with stage. Lymphadenectomy is not performed for Stage Ia1 disease; pelvic lymphadenectomy is offered to patients with Stage IA2 or IB1; pelvic and paraaortic lymphadenectomies are undertaken in patients with IB2/IIA tumors. The main argument against a primary surgical approach is the high likelihood for multimodal therapy since the majority of women will be found to have high-risk (positive or close resection margins, positive lymph node or microscopic parametrial involvement) or intermediate-risk [tumor >4 cm, deep cervical stromal invasion (to the middle or deep one-third), lymphovascular space invasion] factors for recurrence after surgery and so postoperative adjuvant radiotherapy or chemoradiotherapy will be recommended. The benefit of chemoradiation over adjuvant radiotherapy alone was shown in a randomized trial that assigned women with high-risk, localized cervical cancer following radical hysterectomy to radiotherapy with or without four cycles of cisplatin/5-FU chemotherapy. The use of chemotherapy was associated with a significantly better four year OS (81% vs. 71%) and progression-free survival (PFS, 80% vs. 63%) (62).

Definitive primary chemoradiotherapy is an alternative option. Radical hysterectomy plus pelvic/paraaortic lymphadenectomy and definitive radiotherapy have been shown to be equally effective in Stage IB2 and IIA disease, but differ in associated morbidity and complications (63). Survival benefits of cisplatin-based chemoradiotherapy

Table 6.4 International Federation of Gynecologists and Obstetricians (FIGO) Stage Grouping for Cervical Cancer and Five-Year Survival by Stage

Stage		Description	5-year survival (%)
I Confined to the cervix	Ia	Invasive cancer identified microscopically	
	Ia1	Stromal invasion <3 mm depth and <7 mm width	98
	Ia2	Stromal invasion >3 mm and <5 mm depth and <7 mm width	95
	Ib1	Lesions <4 cm	89
	Ib2	Lesions >4 cm	76
II Extends beyond cervix, excluding lower third of vagina or pelvic wall	IIa	Extends to upper two-thirds of vagina, Not parametria	73
	IIb	Parametrail involvement, excluding pelvic side wall	66
III Pelvic sidewall involvement, lower third of vagina or causing hydronephrosis	IIIa	Lower third of vagina	40
	IIIb	Pelvic sidewall or hydronephrosis	42
IV Extension beyond true pelvis or involvement of bladder mucosa or rectum	IVa	Spread to adjacent pelvic organs	22
	IVb	Spread to distant organs	9

Data from 6th Annual FIGO report: Patients Treated 1999–2001.

compared to radiotherapy alone for locally advanced cervical cancer have been shown in randomized trials and in a meta-analysis. The meta-analysis included 4921 patients and showed a 10% OS benefit for chemoradiation compared to radiotherapy alone (64). Weekly cisplatin during radiotherapy may be a better option due to comparable efficacy and more favorable toxicity profile compared to cisplatin and 5-FU and this is currently our practice (65).

Management of Disseminated Cervical Cancer

Radiotherapy may be useful to palliate the symptoms of pelvic pain or bleeding from advanced disease. Large fraction, short course radiotherapy may also be used for local treatment of symptoms related to metastatic disease, such as alleviation of pain from skeletal metastases, or symptoms associated with brain lesions. Several single chemotherapy agents and combination regimens are active in patients with metastatic disease or recurrences that are not amenable to local therapy. Agents include cisplatin (23%), paclitaxel (17%), ifosfamide (22%), vinorelbine (15%), and topotecan (19%). Cisplatin at $50\,mg/m^2$ has been shown to give response rates of 17–38% and median OS of six to seven months. The benefit for combination chemotherapy (cisplatin–paclitaxel, cisplatin–ifosfamide, cisplatin–topotecan) as compared to single agent cisplatin has been demonstrated in randomized trials. A survival benefit was seen with the cisplatin ($50\,mg/m^2$ every three weeks) topotecan ($0.75\,mg/m^2$ days 1 to 3 every three weeks) combination. Compared to cisplatin alone, the topotecan–cisplatin group had a significantly higher response rate (27% vs. 13%), PFS (4.6 vs. 2.9 months), and median survival (9.4 vs. 6.5 months), but significantly more toxicity (70% vs. 1% grade 3 or 4 neutropenia). Despite this, the quality of life was not worse with cisplatin/topotecan compared to cisplatin (66). The combination of cisplatin–paclitaxel compared to cisplatin alone was associated with a higher response rate (36% vs. 19%), median PFS (4.8 vs. 2.8 months), and no difference in quality of life (67). Ongoing studies are exploring the role of taxanes in the treatment of cervical cancer. Currently, patients with advanced cervical cancer are offered palliative chemotherapy with either cisplatin and topotecan or cisplatin and three weekly paclitaxel.

Novel agents such as EGFR inhibitors and antiangiogenic agents are being studied in cervical cancer. A retrospective analysis of bevacizumab in combination with chemotherapy in women with heavily pretreated recurrent cervical cancer showed a clinical benefit rate of 67% (68). Results of prospective trials of bevacizumab in combination with chemotherapy and/or radiation are awaited.

CARCINOMA OF THE VAGINA

Epidemiology and Etiology

Primary cancer of the vagina is rare and comprises 0.3% of all gynecological cancers. There are 240 new cases and 100 deaths per year in the United Kingdom; the annual incidence is 1 per 100,000 women. About 90% of vaginal cancers are squamous cell carcinomas and 5% are adenocarcinomas with rarer types including melanoma and sarcoma. The most common site is the upper third of the vagina. Metastatic disease to the vagina is not uncommon and can arise from cancer of the endometrium, cervix, vulva,

ovary, breast, or rectum. The etiology of primary vaginal cancer is unknown, although vaginal intraepithelial neoplasia (VAIN) is considered to have malignant potential. The risk factors for VAIN are the same as in CIN: multiple lifetime sexual partners, early age at first intercourse, current smoker, and HPV infection. Chronic irritation (e.g., Procidentia or pessary use) may be an underlying cause. Women exposed as fetuses to diethylstilboestrol are at risk of developing clear cell adenocarcinoma of the vagina.

Clinical Features

Most cases are diagnosed at an advanced stage and present with postmenopausal or postcoital vaginal bleeding. Other manifestations include vaginal discharge, vaginal mass, urinary symptoms, and pelvic pain. Some cases are asymptomatic at diagnosis and are picked up as a result of screening for cervical cancer.

Diagnosis and Staging

Definitive diagnosis is accomplished by biopsy of the suspected lesion. Patients should be referred immediately to a gynecological oncologist. Examination under anesthesia is important and allows assessment of the bladder and rectum. Other investigations include radiology of the renal tract and CT scans of the abdomen and pelvis.

Tumors are staged clinically, based upon the above-mentioned investigations. The FIGO staging and five-year survival rates are shown in Table 6.5. Vaginal tumors may invade locally and disseminate via direct extension, lymphatic, or hematogenous routes.

Management

Treatment plans are individualized depending upon the location, size, and clinical stage of the tumor. The proximity of the bladder, urethra, and rectum to the vagina limits the administration of high-dose radiation. In addition, local anatomical constraints may not permit wide negative surgical margins without an exenterative procedure. Psychosexual issues of the patient also need to be considered.

The main treatment modality is radiotherapy. The treatment of Stage I lesions that are greater than 2 cm in diameter and patients with Stage II–IV disease is external beam radiation with or without intracavitary or interstitial brachytherapy. More superficial lesions may be treated with

Table 6.5 International Federation of Gynecologists and Obstetricians (FIGO) Stage Grouping for Vaginal Carcinoma and Five-Year Survival by Stage

Stage	Description	5-year survival (%)
I	Carcinoma limited to vaginal mucosa	78
IIa	Invasion of subvaginal tissue only	52
IIb	Parametrial involvement (not pelvic side wall)	
III	Carcinoma extends to pelvic side wall	42
IVa	Involvement of mucosa of bladder or rectum	20
IVb	Spread beyond the pelvis	13

Data from 6th Annual FIGO Report: Patients Treated 1999–2001.

brachytherapy alone. Stage I lesions in the upper vagina that are less than 2 cm in diameter may be treated with either surgery (radical hysterectomy, upper vaginectomy, and bilateral pelvic lymphadenectomy) or intracavitary radiation therapy. Lesions in the mid-to-lower vagina are typically treated with radiation therapy. Radiotherapy-related complications include rectovaginal or vesicovaginal fistulas, radiation cystitis or proctitis, rectal and vaginal strictures, and, rarely, vaginal necrosis. Radiation therapy alone is adequate treatment for Stage I and II disease. This was illustrated by a series that looked at five-year pelvic control, distant metastasis-free survival, and disease-specific survival probabilities, respectively, according to stage following radiotherapy alone: Stage I, 83%, 100%, and 92%, respectively; Stage II, 76%, 95%, and 68%, respectively; Stage III, 62%, 65%, and 44%, respectively; and Stage IV, 30%, 18%, and 13%, respectively (69). Loco-regionally advanced disease is likely to require a combined modality approach. The evidence for the use of chemotherapy is limited in squamous lesions but cisplatin-based chemoradiation has been used, as in the treatment of cervical cancer. Despite high rate of clinical response, long-term results may be disappointing. There are no large studies of chemotherapy to confirm activity in recurrent or advanced disease and so the role of chemotherapy remains unclear.

VULVAL CANCER
Epidemiology, Etiology, and Pathology

Vulval cancer accounts for 5% of all gynecological malignancies and usually occurs in postmenopausal women. Over 1000 women are diagnosed with vulval cancer every year and 380 women die from the disease annually. Vulval cancer is very rare in young women aged under 25. Rates are less than 1 per 100,000 among women aged 25–44, rising to 3 per 100,000 in those aged 45–64, and peak at 14 per 100,000 in women aged 65 and over.

Risk factors for vulval cancer include cigarette smoking, vulvlal dystrophy (e.g., lichen sclerosus), vulval (VIN) or cervical (CIN) intraepithelial neoplasia, HPV infection, immunodeficiency syndromes, and a prior history of cervical cancer. VIN and Paget's disease are likely to be precursor lesions. Approximately 9% of untreated VIN may progress to invasive disease with a latent period of progression of between one and eight years. Around 90% of vulvar malignancies are squamous cell carcinomas. Less than 5% are melanomas and the remainder are carcinomas of Bartholin's gland, other adenocarcinomas, basal cell carcinomas, verrucous carcinomas, rhabdomyosarcomas, and leiomyosarcomas. Patients with Paget's disease of the vulva (intraepithelial adenocarcinoma) and basal cell carcinoma are at increased risk of synchronous neoplasms.

Clinical Features

The most common symptom is pruritus vulvae which occurs in about two-thirds of patients. Up to half of patients also present with a vulval mass or ulcer which may be associated with bleeding or discharge. Dysuria or an enlarged lymph node in the groin are suggestive of advanced disease. Unfortunately, there can be a delay of months between the onset of symptoms and seeking medical advice and this is often confounded by delays in appropriate referral. Some patients are asymptomatic at the time of diagnosis and are most frequently found after previous treatment of CIN or cancer or the cervix or anus.

Diagnosis and Staging

The diagnosis is usually confirmed by biopsy prior to definitive treatment. Examination under anesthesia and a full thickness biopsy of the lesion and surrounding areas is important for diagnosis and delineation of the extent of the lesion. Colposcopy is sometimes indicated if preinvasive disease is also suspected. Vulval malignancies can be multifocal and therefore assessment of the cervix and vagina should also be performed. Imaging of the pelvis by CT or MRI is performed to identify the full extent of disease.

The staging of vulval cancer uses the FIGO system which is based upon pathological findings from biopsy of the vulval lesion and surgical evaluation of the lymph nodes in the groins (Table 6.6). Surgical staging is necessary because inguinofemoral lymph node status is the most important predictor of overall prognosis and clinical assessment of groin node metastases is inaccurate (false positive or false negative) in up to 30% cases. Sentinel node biopsy is under investigation as a method to avoid complete groin dissection in women with vulval malignancies, thereby potentially reducing both acute and long-term complications of lymphadenectomy. At this time, the procedure is experimental and trials are ongoing (GOG 173) to assess its efficacy in early stage vulval cancer.

Treatment of Early-Stage Disease

The main approach for early-stage vulval squamous cell carcinoma is surgery. Radical local excision without lymph node dissection is the treatment of choice in patients with

Table 6.6 International Federation of Gynecologists and Obstetricians (FIGO) Stage Grouping for Vulval Carcinoma and Five-Year Survival by Stage

Stage	Description	5-year survival (%)
I	Tumor confined to vulva or perineum with no lymph node metastases	79
Ia	Lesion 2 cm or less on vulva/perineum with stromal invasion up to 1 mm	
Ib	As in Ia except stromal invasion is >1 mm	
II	Tumor confined to vulva/perineum and more than 2 cm in greatest dimension. No lymph node metastases	59
III	Tumor of any size arising on vulva and/or perineum with adjacent spread to lower urethra or and and/or unilateral regional (inguinal and/or femoral) lymph node metastases	43
IVa	Tumor invading any of the following: upper urethra, bladder mucosa, rectal mucosa, pelvic bone, and/or bilateral regional lymph node metastases	13
IVb	Any distant metastases including pelvic lymph nodes	

Data from 6th Annual FIGO Report: Patients Treated 1999–2001.

Stage IA disease. In addition to radical local excision or modified radical vulvectomy, patients with Stage IB and II disease should also undergo inguinofemoral lymph node dissection (superficial and deep) because the risk of lymph node metastases is at least 10%. Clear surgical margins should extend at least 1 cm beyond the lesion (ideally 2 cm) to minimize the risk of a local recurrence. Retrospective series of women with resected vulval cancer have shown that adjuvant radiation therapy appears to benefit patients with two or more positive inguinal lymph nodes or positive surgical margins (70). Results are awaited of a prospective trial (GOG 145) which evaluated the role of adjuvant radiotherapy in patients with high-risk primary tumors with negative groin nodes.

Treatment of Advanced Disease

Stage III and IVa vulval squamous cell carcinoma can be resected using radical vulvectomy combined with pelvic exenteration. However, the use of stomas and reconstructive surgery is required and in view of the high morbidity of these procedures, approaches such as preoperative radiotherapy and chemoradiotherapy are often considered. Radiation-sensitizing agents such as cisplatin and 5-FU have been used in Phase II studies of chemoradiation. The role of surgery in women who achieve a complete clinical response to chemoradiotherapy is unclear. Combining chemoradiation with surgery enables more conservative surgery with a higher chance of no residual disease. However, the risk of cumulative toxicity from each procedure performed needs to be considered. Chemotherapy alone has shown limited efficacy in vulval cancer but may be considered for patients with distant metastases. The most active agents are those with substantial activity against squamous cell tumors at other sites, and include cisplatin, methotrexate, cyclophosphamide, mitomycin C, and methotrexate. EGFR tyrosine kinase inhibitors have shown promising results in small series and are likely to be investigated in future clinical trials (71).

REFERENCES

1. Hess V, A'Hern R, Nasiri N et al. Mucinous epithelial ovarian cancer: a separate entity requiring specific treatment. J Clin Oncol 2004; 22: 1040–4.
2. Young RC, Walton LA, Ellenberg SS et al. Adjuvant therapy in stage I and stage II epithelial ovarian cancer. Results of two prospective randomized trials. N Engl J Med 1990; 322: 1021–7.
3. Trimbos JB, Parmar M, Vergote I et al. International Collaborative Ovarian Neoplasm trial 1 and Adjuvant Chemo-Therapy In Ovarian Neoplasm trial: two parallel randomized phase III trials of adjuvant chemotherapy in patients with early-stage ovarian carcinoma. J Natl Cancer Inst 2003; 95: 105–12.
4. Swart AC. Long-term follow-up of women enrolled in a randomized trial of adjuvant chemotherapy for early stage ovarian cancer (ICON1). J Clin Oncol (2007 ASCO Annual Meeting Proceedings Part I) 2007; 25: 5509.
5. Bell J, Brady MF, Young RC et al. Randomized phase III trial of three versus six cycles of adjuvant carboplatin and paclitaxel in early stage epithelial ovarian carcinoma: a Gynecologic Oncology Group study. Gynecol Oncol 2006; 102: 432–9.
6. Aabo K, Adams M, Adnitt P et al. Chemotherapy in advanced ovarian cancer: four systematic meta-analyses of individual patient data from 37 randomized trials. Advanced Ovarian Cancer Trialists' Group. Br J Cancer 1998; 78: 1479–87.
7. du Bois A, Luck HJ, Meier W et al. A randomized clinical trial of cisplatin/paclitaxel versus carboplatin/paclitaxel as first-line treatment of ovarian cancer. J Natl Cancer Inst 2003; 95: 1320–9.
8. Ozols RF, Bundy BN, Greer BE et al. Phase III trial of carboplatin and paclitaxel compared with cisplatin and paclitaxel in patients with optimally resected stage III ovarian cancer: a Gynecologic Oncology Group study. J Clin Oncol 2003; 21: 3194–200.
9. McGuire WP, Hoskins WJ, Brady MF et al. Cyclophosphamide and cisplatin compared with paclitaxel and cisplatin in patients with stage III and stage IV ovarian cancer. N Engl J Med 1996; 334: 1–6.
10. Piccart MJ, Bertelsen K, James K et al. Randomized intergroup trial of cisplatin-paclitaxel versus cisplatin-cyclophosphamide in women with advanced epithelial ovarian cancer: three-year results. J Natl Cancer Inst 2000; 92: 699–708.
11. Neijt JP, Engelholm SA, Tuxen MK et al. Exploratory phase III study of paclitaxel and cisplatin versus paclitaxel and carboplatin in advanced ovarian cancer. J Clin Oncol 2000; 18: 3084–92.
12. Gadducci A, Sartori E, Landoni F et al. Relationship between time interval from primary surgery to the start of taxane-plus platinum-based chemotherapy and clinical outcome of patients with advanced epithelial ovarian cancer: results of a multicenter retrospective Italian study. J Clin Oncol 2005; 23: 751–8.
13. Isonishi S, Yasuda M, Takahashi F et al. Randomized phase III trial of conventional paclitaxel and carboplatin (c-TC) versus dose dense weekly paclitaxel and carboplatin (dd-TC) in women with advanced epithelial ovarian, fallopian tube, or primary peritoneal cancer: Japanese Gynecologic Oncology. J Clin Oncol (2008 ASCO Annual Meeting Proceedings) 2008; 26: 5506.
14. Muggia FM, Braly PS, Brady MF et al. Phase III randomized study of cisplatin versus paclitaxel versus cisplatin and paclitaxel in patients with suboptimal stage III or IV ovarian cancer: a gynecologic oncology group study. J Clin Oncol 2000; 18: 106–15.
15. International Collaborative Ovarian Neoplasm Group. Paclitaxel plus carboplatin versus standard chemotherapy with either single agent carboplatin or cyclophosphamide, doxorubicin, and cisplatin in women with ovarian cancer: the ICON3 randomised trial. Lancet 2002; 360: 505–15.
16. Lambert HE, Rustin GJ, Gregory WM et al. A randomized trial of five versus eight courses of cisplatin or carboplatin in advanced epithelial ovarian carcinoma. A North Thames Ovary Group Study. Ann Oncol 1997; 8: 327–33.
17. Markman M, Liu PY, Wilczynski S et al. Phase III randomized trial of 12 versus 3 months of maintenance paclitaxel in patients with advanced ovarian cancer after complete response to platinum and paclitaxel-based chemotherapy: a Southwest Oncology Group and Gynecologic Oncology Group trial. J Clin Oncol 2003; 21: 2460–5.
18. Conte PF, Favalli G, Gaducci A et al. Final results of After-6 protocol 1: a phase III trial of observation versus 6 courses of paclitaxel (Pac) in advanced ovarian cancer patients in complete response (CR) after platinum-paclitaxel chemotherapy (CT). J Clin Oncol (2007 ASCO Annual Meeting Proceedings Part I) 2007; 25: 5505.
19. De Placido S, Scambia G, Di Vagno G et al. Topotecan compared with no therapy after response to surgery and carboplatin/paclitaxel in patients with ovarian cancer: Multicenter Italian Trials in Ovarian Cancer (MITO-1) randomized study. J Clin Oncol 2004; 22: 2635–42.
20. Pfisterer J, Weber B, Reuss A et al. Randomized phase III trial of topotecan following carboplatin and paclitaxel in first-

line treatment of advanced ovarian cancer: a gynecologic cancer intergroup trial of the AGO-OVAR and GINECO. J Natl Cancer Inst 2006; 98: 1036–45.

21. Mobus V, Wandt H, Frickhofen N et al. Phase III trial of high-dose sequential chemotherapy with peripheral blood stem cell support compared with standard dose chemotherapy for first-line treatment of advanced ovarian cancer: intergroup trial of the AGO-Ovar/AIO and EBMT. J Clin Oncol 2007; 25: 4187–93.

22. Cure H, Battista C, Guastalla JP et al. Phase III randomized trial of high-dose chemotherapy (HDC) and peripheral blood stem cell (PBSC) support as consolidation in patients (pts) with advanced ovarian cancer (AOC): 5-year follow-up of a GINECO/FNCLCC/SFGM-TC study. J Clin Oncol [2004 ASCO Annual Meeting Proceedings (Post-Meeting Edition)] 2004; 22: 5006.

23. Verschraegen CF, Sittisomwong T, Kudelka AP et al. Docetaxel for patients with paclitaxel-resistant Mullerian carcinoma. J Clin Oncol 2000; 18: 2733–9.

24. Vasey PA, Jayson GC, Gordon A et al. Phase III randomized trial of docetaxel-carboplatin versus paclitaxel-carboplatin as first-line chemotherapy for ovarian carcinoma. J Natl Cancer Inst 2004; 96: 1682–91.

25. Bookman MA. GOG0182-ICON5: 5-arm phase III randomized trial of paclitaxel (P) and carboplatin (C) vs combinations with gemcitabine (G), PEG-lipososomal doxorubicin (D), or topotecan (T) in patients (pts) with advanced-stage epithelial ovarian (EOC) or primary peritoneal (PPC) carcinoma. J Clin Oncol (2006 ASCO Annual Meeting Proceedings Part I) 2006; 24: 5002.

26. Scarfone G, Scambia G, Raspagliesi F et al. A multicenter, randomized, phase III study comparing paclitaxel/carboplatin (PC) versus topotecan/paclitaxel/carboplatin (TPC) in patients with stage III (residual tumor >1 cm after primary surgery) and IV ovarian cancer (OC). J Clin Oncol (2006 ASCO Annual Meeting Proceedings Part I) 2006; 24: 5003.

27. Hou JY, Kelly MG, Yu H et al. Neoadjuvant chemotherapy lessens surgical morbidity in advanced ovarian cancer and leads to improved survival in stage IV disease. Gynecol Oncol 2007; 105: 211–17.

28. Bristow RE, Chi DS. Platinum-based neoadjuvant chemotherapy and interval surgical cytoreduction for advanced ovarian cancer: a meta-analysis. Gynecol Oncol 2006; 103: 1070–6.

29. Kumar L, Hariprasad R, Kumar S et al. Neoadjuvant chemotherapy (NACT) followed by interval debulking surgery versus upfront surgery followed by chemotherapy (CT) in advanced epithelial ovarian carcinoma (EOC): a prospective randomized study—Interim results. J Cli Oncol (2007 *ASCO Annual Meeting Proceedings* Part I) 2007; 25: 5531.

30. van der Burg ME, van Lent M, Buyse M et al. The effect of debulking surgery after induction chemotherapy on the prognosis in advanced epithelial ovarian cancer. Gynecological Cancer Cooperative Group of the European Organization for Research and Treatment of Cancer. N Engl J Med 1995; 332: 629–34.

31. Rose PG, Nerenstone S, Brady MF et al. Secondary surgical cytoreduction for advanced ovarian carcinoma. N Engl J Med 2004; 351: 2489–97.

32. Armstrong DK, Bundy B, Wenzel L et al. Intraperitoneal cisplatin and paclitaxel in ovarian cancer. N Engl J Med 2006; 354: 34–43.

33. Markman M, Markman J, Webster K et al. Duration of response to second-line, platinum-based chemotherapy for ovarian cancer: implications for patient management and clinical trial design. J Clin Oncol 2004; 22: 3120–5.

34. Parmar MK, Ledermann JA, Colombo N et al. Paclitaxel plus platinum-based chemotherapy versus conventional platinum-based chemotherapy in women with relapsed ovarian cancer: the ICON4/AGO-OVAR-2.2 trial. Lancet 2003; 361: 2099–106.

35. Alberts DS, Liu PY, Wilczynski SP et al. Randomized trial of pegylated liposomal doxorubicin (PLD) plus carboplatin versus carboplatin in platinum-sensitive (PS) patients with recurrent epithelial ovarian or peritoneal carcinoma after failure of initial platinum-based chemotherapy (Southwest Oncology Group Protocol S0200). Gynecol Oncol 2008; 108: 90–4.

36. Pfisterer J, Plante M, Vergote I et al. Gemcitabine plus carboplatin compared with carboplatin in patients with platinum-sensitive recurrent ovarian cancer: an intergroup trial of the AGO-OVAR, the NCIC CTG, and the EORTC GCG. J Clin Oncol 2006; 24: 4699–707.

37. Gore M, ten Bokkel Huinink W, Carmichael J et al. Clinical evidence for topotecan-paclitaxel noncross-resistance in ovarian cancer. J Clin Oncol 2001; 19: 1893–900.

38. Rose PG, Blessing JA, Mayer AR et al. Prolonged oral etoposide as second-line therapy for platinum-resistant and platinum-sensitive ovarian carcinoma: a Gynecologic Oncology Group study. J Clin Oncol 1998; 16: 405–10.

39. Markman M, Blessing J, Rubin SC et al. Phase II trial of weekly paclitaxel ($80 \, \text{mg/m}^2$) in platinum and paclitaxel-resistant ovarian and primary peritoneal cancers: a Gynecologic Oncology Group study. Gynecol Oncol 2006; 101: 436–40.

40. Williams C. Tamoxifen for relapse of ovarian cancer. Cochrane Database Syst Rev 2001; 1: CD001034.

41. Smyth JF, Gourley C, Walker G et al. Antiestrogen therapy is active in selected ovarian cancer cases: the use of letrozole in estrogen receptor-positive patients. Clin Cancer Res 2007; 13: 3617–22.

42. Harter P, Bois A, Hahmann M et al. Surgery in recurrent ovarian cancer: the Arbeitsgemeinschaft Gynaekologische Onkologie (AGO) DESKTOP OVAR trial. Ann Surg Oncol 2006; 13: 1702–10.

43. Burger RA, Sill MW, Monk BJ et al. Phase II trial of bevacizumab in persistent or recurrent epithelial ovarian cancer or primary peritoneal cancer: a Gynecologic Oncology Group Study. J Clin Oncol 2007; 25: 5165–71.

44. Cannistra SA, Matulonis UA, Penson RT et al. Phase II study of bevacizumab in patients with platinum-resistant ovarian cancer or peritoneal serous cancer. J Clin Oncol 2007; 25: 5180–6.

45. Yap T, Boss D, Fong PC et al. First in human phase I pharmacokinetic (PK) and pharmacodynamic (PD) study of KU-0059436 (Ku), a small molecule inhibitor of poly ADP-ribose polymerase (PARP) in cancer patients (p), including BRCA1/2 mutation carriers. J Clin Oncol (2007 ASCO Annual Meeting Proceedings Part I) 2007; 25: 3529.

46. Berek JS, Taylor PT, Gordon A et al. Randomized, placebo-controlled study of oregovomab for consolidation of clinical remission in patients with advanced ovarian cancer. J Clin Oncol 2004; 22: 3507–16.

47. Bower M, Fife K, Holden L et al. Chemotherapy for ovarian germ cell tumours. Eur J Cancer 1996; 32A: 593–7.

48. Hecht JL, Mutter GL. Molecular and pathologic aspects of endometrial carcinogenesis. J Clin Oncol 2006; 24: 4783–91.

49. Kitchener H. ASTEC—A Study in the Treatment of Endometrial Cancer: a randomised trial of lymphadenectomy in the treatment of endometrial cancer. 37th Annual Meeting of the Society of Gynecologic Oncologists (SGO). Gynecol Oncol 2006; 101: S21–2.

50. Creutzberg CL, van Putten WL, Koper PC et al. Surgery and postoperative radiotherapy versus surgery alone for patients with stage-1 endometrial carcinoma: multicentre randomised trial. PORTEC Study Group. Post Operative Radiation Therapy in Endometrial Carcinoma. Lancet 2000; 355: 1404–11.

51. Randall ME, Filiaci VL, Muss H et al. Randomized phase III trial of whole-abdominal irradiation versus doxorubicin and cisplatin chemotherapy in advanced endometrial carcinoma:

a Gynecologic Oncology Group Study. J Clin Oncol 2006; 24: 36–44.

52. Thigpen JT, Brady MF, Alvarez RD et al. Oral medroxyprogesterone acetate in the treatment of advanced or recurrent endometrial carcinoma: a dose-response study by the Gynecologic Oncology Group. J Clin Oncol 1999; 17: 1736–44.

53. Whitney CW, Brunetto VL, Zaino RJ et al. Phase II study of medroxyprogesterone acetate plus tamoxifen in advanced endometrial carcinoma: a Gynecologic Oncology Group study. Gynecol Oncol 2004; 92: 4–9.

54. Fleming GF, Brunetto VL, Cella D et al. Phase III trial of doxorubicin plus cisplatin with or without paclitaxel plus filgrastim in advanced endometrial carcinoma: a Gynecologic Oncology Group Study. J Clin Oncol 2004; 22: 2159–66.

55. Lissoni A, Zanetta G, Losa G et al. Phase II study of paclitaxel as salvage treatment in advanced endometrial cancer. Ann Oncol 1996; 7: 861–3.

56. Mayrand MH, Duarte-Franco E, Rodrigues I et al. Human papillomavirus DNA versus Papanicolaou screening tests for cervical cancer. N Engl J Med 2007; 357: 1579–88.

57. Bulkmans NW, Berkhof J, Rozendaal L et al. Human papillomavirus DNA testing for the detection of cervical intraepithelial neoplasia grade 3 and cancer: 5-year follow-up of a randomised controlled implementation trial. Lancet 2007; 370: 1764–72.

58. Villa LL, Costa RL, Petta CA et al. Prophylactic quadrivalent human papillomavirus (types 6, 11, 16, and 18) L1 virus-like particle vaccine in young women: a randomised double-blind placebo-controlled multicentre phase II efficacy trial. Lancet Oncol 2005; 6: 271–8.

59. Harper DM, Franco EL, Wheeler CM et al. Sustained efficacy up to 4.5 years of a bivalent L1 virus-like particle vaccine against human papillomavirus types 16 and 18: follow-up from a randomised control trial. Lancet 2006; 367: 1247–55.

60. Ault KA. Effect of prophylactic human papillomavirus L1 virus-like-particle vaccine on risk of cervical intraepithelial neoplasia grade 2, grade 3, and adenocarcinoma in situ: a combined analysis of four randomised clinical trials. Lancet 2007; 369: 1861–8.

61. Garland SM, Hernandez-Avila M, Wheeler CM et al. Quadrivalent vaccine against human papillomavirus to prevent anogenital diseases. N Engl J Med 2007; 356: 1928–43.

62. Peters WA 3rd, Liu PY, Barrett RJ 2nd et al. Concurrent chemotherapy and pelvic radiation therapy compared with pelvic radiation therapy alone as adjuvant therapy after radical surgery in high-risk early-stage cancer of the cervix. J Clin Oncol 2000; 18: 1606–13.

63. Landoni F, Maneo A, Colombo A et al. Randomised study of radical surgery versus radiotherapy for stage Ib-IIa cervical cancer. Lancet 1997; 350: 535–40.

64. Green J, Kirwan J, Tierney J et al. Concomitant chemotherapy and radiation therapy for cancer of the uterine cervix. Cochrane Database Syst Rev 2005; CD002225.

65. Kim YS, Shin SS, Nam JH et al. Prospective randomized comparison of monthly fluorouracil and cisplatin versus weekly cisplatin concurrent with pelvic radiotherapy and high-dose rate brachytherapy for locally advanced cervical cancer. Gynecol Oncol 2008; 108: 195–200.

66. Monk BJ, Huang HQ, Cella D et al. Quality of life outcomes from a randomized phase III trial of cisplatin with or without topotecan in advanced carcinoma of the cervix: a Gynecologic Oncology Group Study. J Clin Oncol 2005; 23: 4617–25.

67. Rose PG, Bundy BN, Watkins EB et al. Concurrent cisplatin-based radiotherapy and chemotherapy for locally advanced cervical cancer. N Engl J Med 1999; 340: 1144–53.

68. Wright JD, Viviano D, Powell MA et al. Bevacizumab combination therapy in heavily pretreated, recurrent cervical cancer. Gynecol Oncol 2006; 103: 489–93.

69. Tran PT, Su Z, Lee P et al. Prognostic factors for outcomes and complications for primary squamous cell carcinoma of the vagina treated with radiation. Gynecol Oncol 2007; 105: 641–9.

70. Parthasarathy A, Cheung MK, Osann K et al. The benefit of adjuvant radiation therapy in single-node-positive squamous cell vulvar carcinoma. Gynecol Oncol 2006; 103: 1095–9.

71. Olawaiye A, Lee LM, Krasner C et al. Treatment of squamous cell vulvar cancer with the anti-EGFR tyrosine kinase inhibitor Tarceva. Gynecol Oncol 2007; 106: 628–30.

7

Head and Neck Cancer

Dirk Schrijvers and Lisa Licitra

INTRODUCTION

Head and neck cancers are malignancies arising from the structures of the upper aerodigestive tract. They include cancers of the epithelium of the oral cavity, the pharynx (naso-, oro-, and hypopharynx), the larynx, nasal cavity and the paranasal sinuses (Fig. 7.1). Other types of cancers in the head and neck region are tumors of the salivary glands, thyroid, and those originating in other tissues (1).

Head and neck cancers are grouped according to the location and the histological type of the primary tumor and the extent of the disease.

The clinical manifestations of head and neck cancer affect critical parts of the human anatomy, with important repercussions on nutrition, respiration, and speech. Therefore, these tumors have an important functional and psychosocial impact on patients.

The treatment and treatment outcome of these tumors depend on the location and histology of the primary tumor, the stage of the disease, and patient-related factors.

Head and neck cancer represents about 5% of the total cancer cases. Worldwide more than 500,000 patients are diagnosed each year with head and neck cancer (1) with 100,800 people living in Europe, and almost 40,000 of European patients die from the disease (2). More men then women develop head and neck cancer; the incidence is rising (2,3) but varies greatly across Europe, especially for sites such as tongue, oral cavity, oropharynx, hypopharynx, and larynx. For these sites, cancer incidence in men is much higher in Southern Europe (France, Italy, Spain, and Switzerland) than in Central and Northern Europe.

Head and neck cancers include sites with excellent prognosis (lip, 94% five-year survival), good prognosis (larynx, 62%; salivary glands, 61%), fair prognosis (tongue, 39%; oral cavity, 45%; oropharynx, 32%; nasopharynx, 43%), and poor prognosis (hypopharynx, 25%).

The overall age-adjusted mortality rates from head and neck cancer in the European Union decreased in the period between 1992 and 2002: oral cavity and pharynx (–8%), larynx (–27%), thyroid (–23%) in men and thyroid (–28%) in women (3).

SQUAMOUS CELL CARCINOMA OF THE HEAD AND NECK
Epidemiology
In Western societies, most of the head and neck tumors are of squamous cell histology.

One-third of patients with squamous cell carcinoma of the head and neck (SCCHN) present with early stage disease and two-third have locoregional advanced disease. In less than 20%, distant metastases are found at diagnosis (1).

The most important risk factors for SCCHN are cigarette and alcohol abuse, particularly when their use is combined (4,5). These abuses may also lead to important comorbidity, including cardiovascular, pulmonary, and hepatic disease, as well as malnutrition.

Epidemiological studies show that the risk of oral cancer is five to nine times higher for smokers than for nonsmokers and this risk may increase to as much as 17 times higher for heavy smokers (80 or more cigarettes per day). In addition, if patients continue to smoke after treatment, the risk of developing a second cancer in the upper aerodigestive tract is two to six times higher than in those who stopped smoking (5). Stopping tobacco use leads to a decreasing risk over time.

Other risk factors for oral cancer are snuff or chewing tobacco and chronic use of betel nut (paan) (5). Marijuana use is also considered to be a potential risk factor (5).

Alcohol use is a major risk factor for cancers of the upper aerodigestive tract. In studies controlled for smoking, moderate-to-heavy drinkers have been shown to have a three to nine time higher risk of developing head and neck cancer (4,5).

Of even greater significance is the synergistic effect of alcohol and smoking. Patients who are both heavy smokers and drinkers have a risk of more than 100 times of normal of developing a malignancy in the head and neck region (4,5).

Infections with human papillomavirus (HPV) types 16 and 18 have been implicated in the development of cancer of the oral cavity, pharynx, and larynx (6). A meta-analysis showed that the probability of HPV detection in the oral mucosa increased with the degree of dysplasia: it was 10% (95% confidence interval, CI, 6.1–14.6) in patients with normal mucosa; 22% (95% CI 15.7–29.9) in patients with benign leukoplakia; 26.2% (95% CI 19.6–33.6) in intraepithelial neoplasia; 29.5% (95% CI 23.0–36.8) in verrucous carcinoma; and 46.5% (95% CI 37.6–55.5) in oral squamous cell carcinoma.

The probability of detection of any high-risk HPV was 2.8 times more likely than for a low-risk subtype (hazard ratio, HR, 0.24, 95% CI 0.16–0.33 and 0.09, 95% CI 0.06–0.13, respectively). Furthermore, HPV16 and HPV18 are detected in 30% of oral squamous cell carcinomas, while other high-risk types are detected in less than 1% (7).

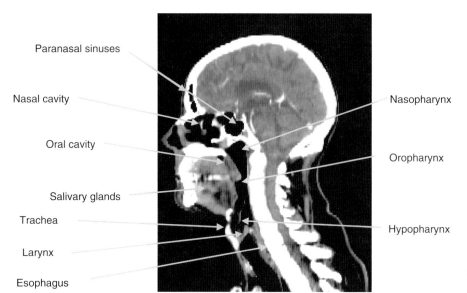

Paranasal sinuses

Nasal cavity

Oral cavity

Salivary glands

Trachea

Larynx

Esophagus

Nasopharynx

Oropharynx

Hypopharynx

Figure 7.1 Anatomy of the head and neck region.

Occupational exposure to nickel, wood, or textile fibers are risk factors for the development of sinus cancer.

Iron deficiency anemia in combination with dysphagia and esophageal webs (known as Plummer–Vinson or Paterson–Kelly syndrome) is associated with an elevated risk of carcinoma of the oral cavity and oropharynx (5).

Immunosuppression predisposes some individuals to an increased risk for oral cancer. Carcinomas of the lip have been reported in a number of kidney transplant patients receiving immunosuppressive medications, and oral carcinomas have been documented in patients with acquired immune deficiency syndrome (5).

Protective factors appear to include the consumption of fruit and vegetables.

Carcinogenesis

Carcinogenesis in patients with SCCHN is multifactorial and is a cascade of genetic events (6). There seem to be two types of important genetic events, one related to HPV and one related to the tobacco and alcohol use. However, the definite carcinogenic pathways have not yet been established.

HPV-Related Carcinogenesis

- The HPV genome encodes several early and late genes important for viral replication, transcription, and carcinogenesis (8). The early (E) open reading frames encode the E1, E2, E5, E6, and E7 proteins. Proteins E5, E6, and E7 are considered oncogenic because of their transforming and growth stimulating properties. These proteins have the ability to deregulate tumor suppressor function by binding to and abrogating the functions of the p21, p53, and pRb proteins, resulting in defects in apoptosis, DNA repair, cell cycle control, and eventually leading to cellular immortalization (Fig. 7.2). The noncoding long control region (LCR) contains binding sites for the E2 and E1 gene products, located just upstream of the P97 promoter sequence, which controls the transcription of the E6 and E7 oncogenes. There is a dose-dependent regulation of E6 and E7 expression by E2. High levels of E2 protein result in the repression of E6 and E7 expression (9). Persistent infection with high-risk HPVs is required for cancer development (10).

- Linearization and integration of the circular HPV genome into the host chromosome is a late event (i.e., in advanced precancers and the majority of invasive carcinomas). HPV integration is thought to be random throughout the host genome, with a predilection for chromosomal fragile sites; however, with respect to the viral genome, integration occurs with a break in the E1/E2 gene sequence. The disruption of the viral E2 sequence releases the HPV oncogenes from repression, resulting in overexpression of E6 and E7 and leading to the alteration of key tumor suppressor pathways (10).

- The E5 protein exerts its carcinogenic effects during the early stages of the viral infection, and this viral oncoprotein may not be required for the maintenance of the malignant phenotype. Nonetheless, the E5 protein has been shown to stimulate cell growth through the activation and upregulation of the epidermal growth factor receptor (EGFR), initiating signaling cascades leading to the overexpression of proto-oncogenes, as well as the repression of cyclin-dependent kinase inhibitor 1A (CDKN1A/p21) expression (10).

- HPV E6 protein has demonstrated growth-stimulatory abilities in conjunction with another cellular protein, E6-associated protein (E6-AP). The E6/E6-AP complex binds p53 and targets the molecule for proteosome degradation. This leads to p53 loss with inhibition of p53-mediated apoptosis and an inefficient G1/S checkpoint in cells with DNA damage, all of which contribute to defects in cell cycle regulation and, eventually, to chromosomal instability in the infected cells. The E6/E6-AP complex also prevents ubiquitination and degradation of src family tyrosine kinase, BLK, which results in

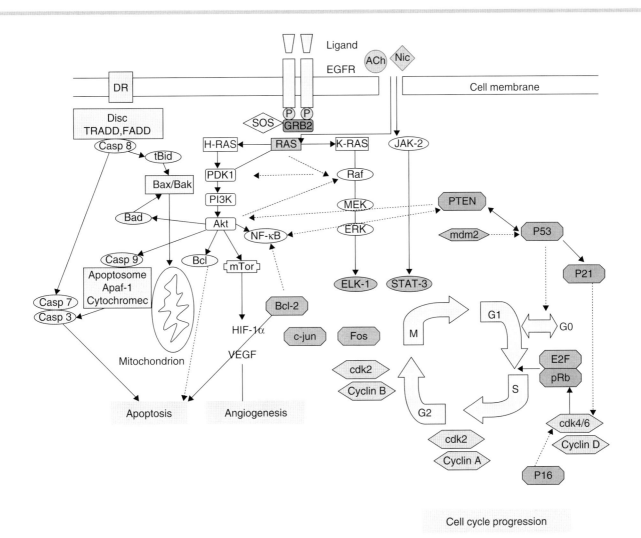

Figure 7.2 Selected pathways in head and neck cancer pathogenesis. *Abbreviations*: Ach, acetylcholine; Apaf-1, apoptotic protease activating factor; BAD, BCL2-associated agonist of cell death; BAX, BCL2-associated X protein; BCL, B-cell CLL/lymphoma; Bid, BH3 interacting domain death agonist; casp, caspase; cdk, cyclin-dependent kinase; Disc, death-inducing signaling complex; DR, death receptor; EGFR, epidermal growth factor receptor; ERK, extracellular signal-regulated kinase; FADD, Fas-associated domain; G, gap; GRB2, growth factor receptor bound protein 2; HIF, hypoxia inducible factor; JAK, Janus kinase; H-RAS, Harvey rat sarcoma; K-RAS, Kirsten rat sarcoma; M, mitosis; MEK, mitogen-activated protein/extracellular signal-regulated kinase kinase; inhibitors Nic, nicotine; mTOR, mammalian target of rapamycin; NF-κB nuclear factor of kappa B; P, phosphate; PDK1, 3-phosphoinositide-dependent protein kinase-1; pRb, retinoblastoma protein; PI3K, phosphotidylinositol 3 kinase; PTEN, phosphatase and tensin homology deleted on chromosome ten; RAF, root abundant factor; S, synthesis; STAT, signal transducer and activator of transcription; SOS, son of sevenless; TRADD, tumor necrosis factor receptor-associated death domain; VEGF, vascular endothelial growth factor; ...., inhibition; ——, activation.

stabilization of the activated form of this kinase, thereby stimulating mitosis.

- The HPV E7 protein binds and degrades the tumor suppressor protein, pRB, by ubiquitin-mediated degradation. Destabilization of pRB causes release of E2F from pRb/E2F complexes. This permits E2F, a transcriptional regulator of cell proliferation genes, to transactivate S-phase-related genes. The functional inactivation of pRB by E7 leads to overexpression of the cyclin-dependent kinase inhibitor p16INK4a. E7 also exhibits kinase activity by forming indirect complexes with cyclins A and E, which are thought to play a role in driving cellular hyperproliferation. There are several additional cellular targets of E7, such as the transcription factor JUN, TATA box-binding proteins, and the cyclin-dependent kinase inhibitors p21 and p27, which induce cell proliferation (10).

Tobacco-Related Carcinogenesis

Several mechanisms have been described in tobacco-related carcinogenesis:

- DNA adducts formation is associated with tobacco smoking (11). Molecular studies of human tumors suggest associations of p53 mutation with DNA adducts and have revealed correlations of DNA adduct levels with somatic alterations (e.g., 3p21 LOH) that are thought to occur at the very earliest stages of tobacco carcinogenesis. Changes in the tumor suppressor gene p53, located at the 17p13 chromosome have been observed in 33–76% of patients with head and neck cancer and mutations in other tumor suppressor genes (p16, p21, p27) involved in cell cycle proliferation have all been seen in patients with head and neck cancer (6).

- Nicotine and tobacco-derived nitrosamines have been shown to exhibit their pathobiologic effects also in part by activation of the nicotinic acetylcholine (ACh) receptors (nAChRs), expressed by oral keratinocytes. Activation of α7 nAChR leads to an increase of STAT-3 due to signaling through the Ras/Raf-1/MEK1/ERK or janus-activated kinase. The Ras/Raf-1/MEK1/ERK cascade culminates in upregulated expression of the gene encoding STAT-3, whereas recruitment and activation of tyrosine kinase JAK-2 phosphorylates it (Fig. 7.2) (12).
- Mutations in the retinoblastoma gene (Rb), located at 13q14 and involved in cell cycle regulation have been described in 6–74% of patients with head and neck cancer (6).
- Cyclin D, a cyclin that phophorylates Rb, leading to cell cycle progression is amplified in 12–68% of patients with head and neck cancer.
- Another important factor is the EGFR that regulates cell growth by binding to epidermal growth factor and transforming growth factor-α. This receptor is overexpressed in 43–62% of head and neck cancer patients (6).

Pathology

Several premalignant lesions have been described in patients with head and neck cancer.

Leukoplakia is a white patch or plaque that cannot be characterized clinically or pathologically as any other disease. It should be used only as a clinical term as it has no specific pathological substrate (5).

The same applies for the term erythroplakia that refers to a red patch that cannot be defined clinically or pathologically as any other condition (5).

SCCHN is subclassified according to the differentiation grade (well, moderately, and poorly differentiated) although this does not seem to be an independent prognostic factor (13,14).

Screening

Screening may lead to the detection of earlier stage cancer in asymptomatic patients and should improve treatment outcome in terms of survival.

In head and neck cancer, only the mouth is easily accessible by physical examination. The feasibility and the value of population screening by physical examination for oral cancer were tested in Sri Lanka and India. Although this screening method was feasible, the participation rate was poor (15). One important randomized controlled trial has been performed (n = 13 clusters: 191,873 participants) but there was no difference in the age-standardized oral cancer mortality rates for the screened group (16.4/100,000 person-years) and the control group (20.7/100,000 person-years). A significant 34% reduction in mortality was recorded in high-risk subjects between the intervention cohort (29.9/100,000 person-years) and the control arm (45.4/100,000) (16).

Oral exfoliative cytology is the most extensively studied screening procedure of American oral screening programs (17). Problems encountered with this screening method include a high proportion of false-negative examinations and poor voluntary participation by the highest risk individuals (heavy tobacco and alcohol users).

At the moment, there is no definitive evidence that population-based screening for head and neck cancer can reduce mortality.

However, each health professional should be aware of the problem and should try to detect head and neck cancer in an early stage. It has been shown that there may be a delay of up to 200 days between development of symptoms and diagnosis (18).

The following guidelines for oral cancer screening and mucosal lesion assessment might apply (19):

- Patient history
  - General health history and medication use
  - Oral habits and lifestyle with emphasis on tobacco use, alcohol consumption, and sexual practices
  - Symptoms of oral pain and discomfort
- Visual screening examination
  - Extra-oral examination
    Inspection of head and neck region for tenderness or swelling
    Palpation of the submandibular, neck, and supraclavicular regions for lymph nodes
    Inspection and palpation of the lips and perioral tissues
  - Intraoral examination
    Systematically inspection of all oral soft tissues with special attention to lateral and ventral aspects of the tongue, floor of the mouth, and soft palate
  - Lesion inspection
    Specific characteristics of each lesion with particular attention to size, color, texture, and outline
  - Documentation
    At each evaluation, an image of any clinically visible lesion should be obtained and kept in the patient file
- Additional visualization tools can enhance the distinction between normal tissue and the lesion and to identify satellite lesions. They are complementary to clinical examination and judgment.
  Different methods can be used:
  - Toluidine blue is a vital stain used to identify high-risk oral lesions and stained lesions have a six times higher chance of becoming cancer (20)
  - Direct fluorescence visualization which uses a cone of blue light that causes the mucosal cells to absorb light energy and emit it as visible fluorescence. Healthy oral tissue emits a pale green light, while altered tissues attenuate the passage of light and appear dark brown to black (19)
- Tissue biopsy
  - A brush biopsy may be used to perform cytology (19)
  - If a suspicious mucosal lesion persists for more than three weeks without or after an identified local irritant such as trauma, infection, or inflammation, a diagnostic biopsy is required (19).

Clinical Manifestations

The clinical presentation of head and neck cancer depends on the location of the primary tumor and the extent of the disease.

In early stage disease, the symptoms may be vague and every complaint in the head and neck region by patients with tobacco and alcohol use should be evaluated carefully.

Early symptoms of cancer of the oral cavity or pharynx include pain, ulcers that do not heal, and poorly fitting dentures.

Nasopharyngeal cancer may cause nasal obstruction, otitis media due to obstruction of the Eustachian tube, and epistaxis.

Sinusitis and nasal obstructions may be seen in cancer of the nasal cavity or paranasal sinuses.

The classical symptom of laryngeal cancer is hoarseness.

At later stage, all head and neck cancers give easily detectable signs and symptoms. They include painless swelling of lymph nodes in the neck region, pain, disfigurement, cranial neuropathies, trismus, dysphagia, bleeding, and fistulas.

Diagnosis

In patients with complaints in the head and neck region that persist for more than three weeks, a referral to a head and neck specialist is advocated (19). The definite diagnosis of head and neck cancer is made by a tissue biopsy.

Staging and Prognosis

The staging of head and neck cancers is based on the TNM (tumor, node, metastasis) classification of the International Union against Cancer (13) and the American Joint Committee on Cancer (14). It is a clinical classification. The pathological classification is similar to the clinical classification.

The T classification indicates the extent of the primary tumor. It is generally similar for the oral cavity, oropharynx, salivary gland, and thyroid cancer. T1, T2, or T3 are defined by the size of the tumor, T4a indicates that the tumor invades into the surrounding structures and is resectable, whereas T4b tumors are unresectable (13,14).

The T classification of other sites may differ in specific details because of anatomical considerations.

The N classification for cervical lymph node metastasis is uniform for all mucosal sites except for the nasopharynx. The N classification depends on the size of the lymph nodes, the number of lymph nodes involved, and the localization in the neck (unilateral/bilateral).

Regional lymph nodes are subdivided into specific anatomic subsites and grouped into seven levels (Fig. 7.3) (14):

Level I: submental, submandibular
Level II: upper jugular
Level III: midjugular
Level IV: lower jugular
Level V: posterior triangle (spinal accessory and transverse cervical) (upper, middle, and lower corresponding to the levels that define upper, middle, and lower jugular nodes)
Level VI: prelarygneal, pretracheal
Level VII: upper mediastinal
Other groups: suboccipital, retropharyngeal, parapharyngeal, buccinator (facial), preauricular, periparotid, and intraparotid.

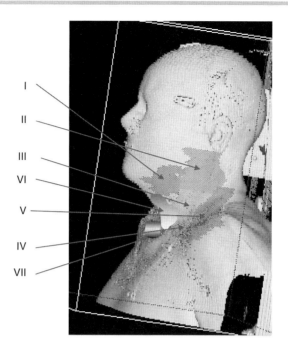

Figure 7.3 Lymph node regions in the head and neck. *See Color Plate on Page xi.*

The M classification indicates the absence (M0) or presence (M1) of distant metastasis. Metastasis are most commonly found in liver, lung, and skeleton.

Based on the TNM classification, tumors are grouped according to stage. Stage 0 indicates carcinoma in situ with no lymph node or distant metastasis; Stage I includes T1 tumors without lymph node invasion or distant metastasis; Stage II indicates T2 tumors without lymph node invasion or distant metastasis; Stage III tumors are T3N0 tumors or T1–3 tumors with N1 lymph node metastasis without distant metastasis; Stage IVA includes resectable T4a tumors and N2 lymph node metastases without distant metastasis; Stage IVB have N3 lymph node metastasis and Stage IVC includes patients with distant metastasis (13,14).

The prognosis of patients with head and neck cancer is determined by tumor location and stage. Tumors of the oral cavity, the oropharynx, and hypopharynx have a worse prognosis compared to tumors at other locations (14). Higher stage indicates a worse prognosis (14).

Prognosis seems also dependent on the carcinogenesis and patients with a HPV-related cancer have a better prognosis than those with cancer due to tobacco use (21).

Evaluation of the Patient with Head and Neck Cancer
Primary Diagnosis

The assessment of the primary tumor (T) is made by inspection, bimanual palpation, and by both indirect mirror examination and direct endoscopy.

A pan-endoscopic examination under general anesthesia with evaluation of the head and neck region, upper bronchi, and esophagus is indicated in all patients with head and neck cancer to evaluate the primary tumor and to detect second primary tumors.

Both computed tomography (CT) and magnetic resonance imaging (MRI) are highly sensitive for the detection of neoplastic invasion of the pre-epiglottic space, paraglottic space, subglottic region, and cartilage. The high negative predictive value of both CT scan and MRI allows exclusion of neoplastic cartilage invasion. The specificity of both CT scan and MRI is, however, limited and both methods may, therefore, overestimate the extent of tumor spread (22).

When comparing 18F-fluorodeoxyglucose-positron emission tomography (PET) with CT or MRI for the primary diagnosis of head and neck cancer, the sensitivity of PET ranges from 85% to 95%, compared with 67–88% for CT/MRI. The specificity of PET ranges between 80% and 100% whereas it is between 45% and 75% for CT/MRI. However, CT/MRI is needed for the anatomical visualization, and PET may be a valuable addition to these examinations.

PET can also detect some, but not all synchronous primaries that other methods failed to detect. It can also be used to detect occult primary tumors in patients with cervical lymph node metastasis (23).

The appropriate nodal (N) drainage areas are examined by careful palpation and imaging [ultrasonography (US), CT scan].

US combined with fine-needle aspiration cytology for the evaluation of lymph node metastasis in patients with head and neck cancer has a sensitivity of 89.2%; a specificity of 98.1%; and an accuracy of 94.5% and is superior to manual palpation (24).

In a meta-analysis of 32 studies (1,236 patients), PET sensitivity for identifying lymph node involvement was 79% (95% CI 72–85%) and specificity was 86% (95% CI 83–89%). For cN0 patients, sensitivity of PET was only 50% (95% CI 37–63%), whereas specificity was 87% (95% CI 76–93%). Overall, the positive likelihood ratio (LR) was 5.84 (95% CI 4.59–7.42) and the negative LR was 0.24 (95% CI 0.17–0.33) (25). In studies in which both PET and conventional diagnostic tests were performed, sensitivity and specificity of PET were 80% and 86%, respectively, and of conventional diagnostic tests were 75% and 79%, respectively. PET does not detect disease in half of the patients with metastasis and cN0 (23).

The presence of distant metastasis (M) is evaluated by chest radiography and/or CT scan of the thorax, US of the liver, and bone scintigraphy; PET can also show distant metastatic disease.

Residual/Recurrent Local Disease

Diagnosis of residual/recurrent local disease after combined modality treatment is often difficult. Patients complaining of chronic or newly developing pain should always be suspected of residual/recurrent disease. In these patients, PET has a sensitivity of at least 80% and a specificity of 90% (23). PET appears to be more accurate than CT or MRI. PET has a positive LR of 4.0 and a negative LR of 0.16 (23). A biopsy remains necessary to confirm local residual disease or local relapse.

Treatment

Patients with SCCHN may be treated by surgery, radiotherapy, and/or medication. The treatment depends on the extent of the disease and the patient's condition. Before starting a treatment, a multidisciplinary team with at least a head and neck surgeon, radiotherapist, and medical oncologist should decide on the most optimal treatment plan for the patient.

In advanced or recurrent disease, participation in an investigational protocol should be proposed to the patient.

Supportive and palliative measures should always be integrated into the treatment and care of patients with head and neck cancer.

Patients with Early Stage Disease

Patients with stage I or II disease are classified as having early stage disease. These patients may be treated with curative intent using single modality strategies (surgery or radiotherapy). With this approach 60–90% of patients will be free of disease after five years (1). There are no randomized trials comparing limited open or endoscopic surgery with radiotherapy (26). Selection of a treatment modality depends on primary tumor site, age, comorbidity, occupation, preferences and compliance, quality of life after treatment, availability of experts in each treatment modality, and a history of a previous malignancy in the head and neck region. Posttreatment voice outcomes for early glottic cancer treated by external beam radiotherapy or endoscopic laser excision provide comparable levels of voice handicap (27).

Surgery. Surgery in early stage disease will be limited and should not result in significant morbidity or long-term anatomic or functional sequels. It has the advantage of determining the microscopic extent of the disease.

Stage I–II lesions as judged by palpation of the neck are accompanied by metastatic invasion of lymph nodes in less than 30% of patients. There is a correlation between the tumor depth and lymph node metastasis and most patients with a tumor depth of more or equal to 5 mm have lymph node metastases. These patients may be candidates for elective neck dissection (28). Elective neck dissection is not indicated in other patients with small tumors and surgery may be limited to the primary tumor. A neck dissection can be postponed until recurrence without impairing the survival (29).

Radiotherapy. External beam radiotherapy is a treatment option in patients with stage I–II disease. Total doses of 65 Gray (Gy) to 70 Gy administered in daily fractions of 180–200 cGy over six to seven weeks are usual treatment schedules (30).

Radiotherapy has the advantage of sparing the anatomical structures and to include potential microscopic disease in the neck. Disadvantages are the treatment duration of six to seven weeks; acute toxicities such as mucositis, dermatitis, dysphagia, pain, and temporary loss of taste; late toxicities such as xerostomia due to decrease of the salivary gland function, fibrosis, dysphagia, or osteonecrosis.

However, in selected populations with head and neck cancer, the irradiation field may be limited by newer radiotherapy techniques (e.g., intensity-modulated radiation therapy) to a smaller portion of the head and neck region, avoiding local toxicity and fibrosis.

Brachytherapy alone or as a boost after external beam radiotherapy may be used in patients with squamous cell carcinoma of oral cavity or oropharynx with a similar outcome as external beam radiotherapy (30).

Patients with Locally Advanced Disease

Patients with stage III, IVA, and IVB cancers are classified as having locally advanced disease. Locally advanced disease may be resectable or unresectable. There is no formal definition of "resectability," and it varies significantly between disease site, disease extent, surgeon, and institution. Ideally, the determination of resectability should be made for each individual patient by the multidisciplinary team, taking into account the potential functional impact and survival benefit conferred by each treatment strategy.

- Standard treatment for patients with locally advanced resectable disease is surgery followed by radiotherapy or chemoradiation depending on negative prognostic factors and the general condition of the patient. Another possible treatment strategy is chemoradiation to preserve organ function.
- Patients with locally advanced unresectable disease are candidates for radiotherapy ± chemotherapy. The prognosis of these patients treated with radiotherapy alone remains poor with a high local relapse rate of 50–60% at two years and an overall survival of 40% at three years (1). Recurrence of locoregional disease is the most common cause of death while some patients develop distant metastases in the liver, lung, and skeleton.

Several approaches have been studied to improve treatment outcome and limit toxicity in patients with locally advanced head and neck cancer.

Radiotherapy. Tumor cell proliferation is influenced by radiotherapy. Acutely responding tumor cells have a higher alpha/beta ratio than normal tissues. An increase in total dose will therefore result in an increase in tumor kill (31).

Altered Fractionation. The impact of the fraction of the dose and the number of fractions per day has been studied extensively in patients with head and neck cancer, resulting in different fractionation schedules (acceleration, hyperfractionation). These fractionation schedules lead to an increased total dose or dose intensity with higher antitumor activity and less late damage to the normal tissue.

- In accelerated fractionation, the overall time of treatment is reduced; the total dose and the dose per fraction are either unchanged or somewhat reduced, depending on the extent of overall time reduction.
- In hyperfractionated radiotherapy, the total dose is increased; the dose per fraction is reduced and the fraction number is increased; the overall time is relatively unchanged.

In a meta-analysis of 15 trials with 6,515 patients and a median follow-up of six years, there was a benefit in locoregional control in favor of altered fractionation versus conventional radiotherapy (6·4% at five years; $p < 0·0001$), which was particularly efficient in reducing local failure,

whereas the benefit on nodal control was less pronounced. There was a significant survival benefit with altered fractionated radiotherapy, corresponding to an absolute benefit of 3.4% at five years (HR 0.92, 95% CI 0.86–0.97; $p = 0.003$). The benefit was significantly higher with hyperfractionated radiotherapy (8% at five years) than with accelerated radiotherapy (2% without total dose reduction and 1.7% with total dose reduction at five years) (32).

Altered fractionation leads to a higher acute mucosal toxicity, but does not seem to induce significantly more severe late effects compared with conventional fractionation, although late toxicity has not been systematically assessed and reported in all studies so that a moderate increase of late toxicity cannot be excluded.

Focused Radiotherapy Techniques. Intensity-modulated radiotherapy (IMRT) is a refinement of three-dimensional conformal radiotherapy (3DCRT). It uses a computerized treatment planning system along with sophisticated delivery machineries to tailor the radiation dose to the tumor target. It has the unique ability to minimize the dose delivered to normal tissues without compromising tumor coverage. As a result, side effects from high-dose radiation have decreased and patient quality of life has improved. Although no data of randomized trials are present, single institution results showed high rates of local control varying from 87% to 94% (33).

Managing Radiotherapy Side Effects. Several trials studied methods to decrease acute and late side effects of radiotherapy.

- Amifostine is a cytoprotective agent and proved to decrease acute and late side effects at the salivary glands, skin, and mucosa in patients treated with radiotherapy. It decreased the incidence of xerostomia from 56% to 34% after one year ($p = 0.002$) and from 36% to 19% after two years when given once daily at 200 mg/m² intravenously 15–30 min before each fraction of radiotherapy. It seemed also effective in patients treated with chemoradiation (34).
- Palifermin is a recombinant human keratinocyte growth factor and stimulates cellular proliferation and differentiation in mucosa throughout the alimentary tract, salivary glands, and type II pneumocytes. Randomized studies of palifermin in conjunction with concurrent chemoradiation for head and neck cancer is ongoing in the definitive treatment and adjuvant postoperative settings. These studies investigate the use of palifermin in doses of 60 µg/kg/week during and after chemoradiation (34).
- Benzydamine is a nonsteroidal anti-inflammatory drug and a potent inhibitor of tumor necrosis factor alpha. It resulted in a 30% reduction in mucosal erythema and ulceration during radiotherapy. Most of this benefit was observed once doses greater than 25 Gy had been delivered. One-third of the benzydamine patients did not develop any mucosal ulceration compared with only 18% of the placebo-treated patients ($p = 0.04$). However, although this agent was active against mucositis, data were inconclusive regarding any meaningful clinical role in treating this condition. There was no significant benefit regarding the functional sequels of mucositis (34).

• Endogenous oral flora may exacerbate the mucosal inflammatory process once the mucosal integrity is disrupted. Iseganan is a synthetic analog of protegrins that are naturally occurring peptides with a broad spectrum antimicrobial activity. In a randomized trial comparing iseganan plus standard oral care, placebo plus standard oral care and supportive oral care only, iseganan and placebo were equivalent to each other but both superior to standard oral care. Two-thirds of the patients in both arms had confluent mucositis compared with 79% in the standard oral care arm (p = 0.02). Only 2% of these last patients had no mucosal ulceration versus 9% in both the iseganan and placebo arms (p = 0.04). This show the importance of adherence to a strict regimen of oral hygiene during radiotherapy with instruction to swish and gargle at regular intervals (34).

Local treatment Combined with Medication. Local treatment with surgery or radiotherapy has been combined with medication to improve the outcome of patients with locally advanced head and neck cancer. Medication can be used for its radio-sensitizing effects or for its anticancer properties. Several sequences of medication (induction or neoadjuvant, adjuvant, alternating with radiotherapy, concomitant chemoradiation) and local treatments have been studied.

Induction Chemotherapy. Induction or neoadjuvant chemotherapy prior to local treatment has theoretical advantages. According to the Goldie and Coldman model (35) of spontaneous mutations, the fraction of drug resistant cells increases with increasing tumor size. Early treatment with chemotherapy may minimize the risk of drug resistance. Other potential advantages of induction chemotherapy are the reduction in size of the primary tumor and regional nodal disease, thereby enhancing local control by subsequent surgery or radiotherapy and facilitating surgical resection; the identification of patients with responding lesions, who can effectively be managed by surgery or radiotherapy; the identification of patients, who may benefit from additional therapy after locoregional treatment; and the treatment of occult metastatic disease.

Potential disadvantages are the delay in locoregional treatment, which could be associated with tumor regrowth and dissemination; the selection of chemotherapy and radio-resistant tumor cells; and the increase of local toxicity through subsequent surgery or radiotherapy.

Several randomized trials have examined induction chemotherapy in patients with head and neck cancer. In the older studies, only one study reported a survival benefit in a subset of patients with unresectable disease, while all others did not show an improvement in survival. Despite the high overall response rates, induction chemotherapy did not have an impact on locoregional control. However, there were less distant metastases as site of first failure. A meta-analysis of these studies could not show a survival benefit for cisplatin-based induction chemotherapy (36).

However, several studies evaluated induction chemotherapy with taxanes followed by (chemo)radiation in patients with unresectable disease (37–39). In the taxane arm the response rate, disease-free and overall survival were higher than in the nontaxane arm with acceptable toxicity. Based on these studies, taxane-based induction chemotherapy followed by (chemo)radiation has become the standard in the treatment of patients with unresectable disease.

Adjuvant Chemotherapy. Adjuvant chemotherapy is given after definitive local treatment to treat micrometastases.

Potential advantages of adjuvant chemotherapy are the immediate start of effective local treatment; the absence of a preoperative decrease of the general and nutritional status and of hematological and immunological suppression due to upfront chemotherapy; and the absence of possible interference with dose and delivery of radiotherapy due to chemotherapy-induced toxicity.

Disadvantages may be the impaired chemotherapy delivery after surgery and/or radiotherapy by alteration of the blood flow; the lack of acceptance or tolerance by the patients to any systemic treatment; the absence of immediate gratification for either patient or physician with poor patient compliance; and the overtreatment of patients, who do not benefit from a toxic treatment because of chemoresistant cell lines.

The value of adjuvant chemotherapy has been evaluated in several randomized trials and meta-analysis. No survival benefit has been demonstrated in these studies of mixed patient populations (40).

Alternating Chemotherapy and Radiotherapy. Rapidly alternating chemotherapy with radiotherapy may have theoretical advantages.

As the fraction of drug-resistant cells increases with increasing tumor size (35), rapid sequencing of different treatment modalities may minimize the risk that the tumor will become resistant. Furthermore, the repopulation after interruption of radiotherapy may be overcome by chemotherapy. Moreover, by alternating these treatments, the full therapeutic dose of chemotherapy and radiotherapy may be given with limited side effects.

Potential disadvantages are the prolongation of the locoregional treatment with the potential risk of interval regrowth, increased toxicity leading to delay of treatment or decreased dose intensity, early dissemination of disease, and increase of local toxicity of subsequent surgery.

This approach proved to be feasible and has shown to improve survival in patients with unresectable head and neck cancer (41).

Concomitant Chemoradiation. The rationale for concomitant use of medication and radiotherapy is that they each are active against cancer cells and may enhance each other's activity. They may also overcome resistant cell clones because of differences in resistance mechanisms. Resistance to chemotherapy may be because of decreased activation or increased metabolization of cytotoxic drugs, decreased uptake or increased efflux, and changed target enzymes or enzymatic activity. The activity of radiotherapy is largely independent of these mechanisms. Another advantage is that it shortens the overall treatment time compared to sequential therapy. Moreover, it may have an early effect on micrometastases in case of full dose chemotherapy and may improve locoregional control. A disadvantage is the increased local toxicity resulting in a decrease in dose of either chemotherapy or radiotherapy.

Radiotherapy with Chemotherapy. In patients with resectable disease and high-risk factors (vascular embolism, perineural disease, extracapsular nodular spread, and positive resection margins), adjuvant treatment after local resection with the combination of cisplatin (100 mg/m² d1, d22, d43) and conventional radiotherapy is standard treatment. This approach showed a positive effect on disease-free and overall survival (42).

In patients with unresectable disease, several randomized trials and meta-analyses have compared chemoradiation with radiotherapy alone. Radiotherapy combined with simultaneous 5-fluorouracil (5-FU), intravenous or intra-arterial cisplatin, carboplatin, and mitomycin C as single drug or combinations of 5-FU with one of the others resulted in a large survival advantage irrespective of the employment of radiation schedule (30).

The standard treatment in this patient population when using chemotherapy is cisplatin (100 mg/m², d1, d22, d43) in combination with conventional radiotherapy. However, this may translate in serious toxicity, decreasing the dose density of cisplatin and interruption of the radiotherapy. Other schedules of cisplatin (e.g., weekly, continuous) or other agents (e.g., carboplatin, gemcitabine) have been tested and are used in daily clinical practice.

Radiotherapy with Drugs Influencing or Benefiting of Hypoxia. Tumor hypoxia is a common phenomenon in patients with head and neck cancer and has been shown to adversely affect treatment outcome (33). It is considered an important factor contributing to radio resistance and decreasing hypoxia, and administering drugs that are cytotoxic in hypoxic conditions might improve treatment outcome.

- Increasing the oxygen delivery by increasing hemoglobin levels using erythropoiesis stimulating agents (ESAs) was tested in a randomized trial in head and neck cancer but led to a worse locoregional progression-free survival. This could be explained partially by the quadratic regression in partial oxygen pressure (pO$_2$) and hemoglobin levels: at hemoglobin levels ≤14 g/dL, increasing hemoglobin levels directly correlates with increasing pO$_2$; however, at hemoglobin above 14 g/dL, an inverse correlation is noted with lower pO$_2$ associated with increasing hemoglobin, presumably due to venostasis (30). More recently, the presence of erythropoietin (EPO) receptors in tumor cells has also been considered to be implicated with worse outcomes in patients receiving EPO (30).
- Increased vascular leakage from immature tumoral vasculatures can result in increased interstitial blood pressure, thereby worsening tumor hypoxia and impeding effective drug delivery to the tumor. Antiangiogenic agents such as bevacizumab could reverse this process but this concept has not been tested in patients with head and neck cancer. Feasibility studies showed that it was possible to combine bevacizumab with chemoradiation in patients with head and neck cancer (43).
- The combined use of the vasodilator nicotinamide and carbogen breathing is another possibility to increase pO$_2$. Accelerated radiotherapy with carbogen and nicotinamide (ARCON) can result in a three-year local control rate in excess of 80% for advanced stage T3–4 laryngeal and oropharyngeal cancers. Presently, a Phase III clinical trial testing the efficacy of ARCON in laryngeal cancers is ongoing in Europe (30).

- Tirapazamine is an agent that has a high selectivity for killing hypoxic cells. However, it has several limitations including a poor diffusion through hypoxic tissue and its requirement of less stringent hypoxia for activation that can result in normal tissue toxicity in poorly oxygenated organs. Although promising results were seen in a randomized Phase II trial with tirapazamine combined with cisplatin and radiotherapy, a Phase III trial in 861 patients with stage III or IV compared to conventional radiotherapy (70 Gy in seven weeks) concurrently with either cisplatin (100 mg/m²) on weeks 1, 4, and 7, or cisplatin (75 mg/m²) plus tirapazamine (290 mg/m²/day) on weeks 1, 4, and 7, or tirapazamine alone (160 mg/m²/day) on days 1, 3, and 5 of weeks 2 and 3 it showed no significant differences in failure-free survival, locoregional relapse rate, or overall survival. Due to toxicity resulting in radiotherapy protocol deviations, the combination of cisplatin and tirapazamine led to an increased risk of death (HR 1.56; $p < 0.0001$), any failure (HR 1.65; $p < 0.0001$), and locoregional failure (HR 1.82; $p = 0.0002$) (44).

Radiotherapy with Targeted Agents. Ionizing radiation has the potential to enhance proliferation of the surviving fraction of cells and to promote the long-term resistance to multiple cytotoxic stresses due to DNA damage and the generation of reactive oxygen species, with subsequent rapid activation of wild-type p53, ataxia telangiectasia mutated (ATM), and ATM and Rad3-related protein as well as the activation of growth factor receptors in the plasma membrane (e.g., ERBB family receptors). Receptor activation enhances the activities of RAS family transducer molecules that mediate signaling from the membrane to cause activation of multiple cytosolic signal transduction pathways (e.g., RAF-1/MAPK/ERK/PI3K pathways), which play a role in the long-term effects of cell survival and the regulation of cell growth (45). Targeted agents interact with specific steps in the cellular pathways and may block the activated pathways.

The EGFR and its ligands have been recognized as critical proteins in SCCHN and have been linked with poor outcome. Cetuximab is a human-chimeric monoclonal antibody which competitively binds to the extracellular receptor site. In a randomized trial in patients with stage III–IV locoregional advanced head and neck cancer the combination of cetuximab (intravenous loading dose of 400 mg/m² one week before starting radiotherapy, followed by a dose of 250 mg/m² weekly during radiotherapy) resulted in a higher locoregional control duration (24.4 vs. 14.9 months, HR 0.68; $p = 0.005$) and longer progression-free duration (17.1 vs. 12.4 months, HR 0.70; $p = 0.006$) and overall survival (49.0 vs. 29.3 months, HR 0.74; $p = 0.03$) compared to radiotherapy alone. With the exception of acneiform rash and infusion reactions, the incidence of Grade 3 or greater toxic effects did not differ significantly between the two groups (46).

Radiotherapy with Radio-Sensitizers. Several antimetabolites (e.g., 5-FU, hydroxyurea, gemcitabine) have been shown to have radio-sensitizing properties in vitro. They target DNA replication by inhibition of the biosynthesis of deoxyribonucleotides for DNA replication (thymidylate synthase inhibitors, such as 5-FU, and ribonucleotide reductase inhibitors, such as hydroxyurea), or by becoming substrates for DNA polymerases (nucleoside/nucleobase analogs, such as gemcitabine). Some of the antimetabolite radio-sensitizers have more than one of these actions (47).

Several trials have studied the addition of these drugs to radiotherapy as radio-sensitizers in patients with locally advanced resectable and unresectable head and neck cancer. The doses of these drugs are lower than when used as cytotoxic agents (e.g., gemcitabine). In phase I–II studies the combination of these drugs was feasible, but their value should be confirmed in randomized trials.

Patients with Recurrent and/or Metastatic Disease

Patients with locoregional recurrent disease after failure of surgery or radiotherapy alone may be salvaged by further surgery and/or radiotherapy.

Reirradiation in combination with chemotherapy for salvage following failure of radiotherapy has resulted in long-term survival in a small number of patients. It may be considered for small recurrences after radiation therapy, especially in patients who refuse or are not candidates for surgery. This approach has been studied by several groups combining radiotherapy with several chemotherapy schedules including hydroxyurea-5-FU-cisplatin. These treatments are tolerable and long-term disease-free survival has been reported. However, careful patient selection is required because of the relatively high incidence of treatment-related morbidity (48).

In patients with unresectable locally recurrent disease that is not amenable for reirradiation or with metastatic disease, the median survival is six months with 20% of patients being alive at one year. There is no clear indication that the use of chemotherapy has changed these statistics. A study by the European Organization for Research and Treatment of Cancer failed to answer the question whether weekly methotrexate plus best supportive care was superior to best supportive care alone due to insufficient accrual.

However, patients with local recurrent disease or distant metastases may be treated with chemotherapy in a palliative setting to alleviate symptoms. Chemotherapy may induce responses in 10–40% of patients, depending on the pretreatment. However, responses normally last only for three to six months (1).

The most active agents and their response rates are listed in Table 7.1. These data are cumulative data and response rates in different studies differed widely due

to patient-related (performance status, prior treatment) and tumor-related factors (extent and site of disease) in addition to treatment-related factors.

Single Agent Treatment. Response rates of 20% or more have been reported in nonrandomized studies for single agent intravenous methotrexate, cisplatin, 5-FU, bleomycin, anthracyclines, docetaxel and paclitaxel, topotecan, vinorelbine, and gemcitabine. In randomized studies, these response rates decrease and there are no randomized trials of single agents to suggest a superiority of any drug over standard-dosed methotrexate.

A cisplatin-containing gel may be directly injected into the tumor and this technique was tested in a small Phase III trial in which 87 patients were randomly assigned to either cisplatin ($n = 62$) or placebo gel for six weekly intra-tumoral injections in an eight-week period. The response rate was 34% in the cisplatin arm versus 0% in the placebo arm ($p < 0.001$). More patients treated with cisplatin gel achieved palliative benefit than did those treated with placebo gel (37% vs. 12%; $p = 0.036$). The most frequent side effects were local pain and local cutaneous reactions, which resolved over 3–12 weeks. Renal and hematologic toxicities were rare (49).

Targeted agents have also been tested as first-line treatment in patients with recurrent/metastatic head and neck cancer.

Erlotinib is an oral tyrosine-kinase inhibitor that was administered in an oral dose of 150 mg/day to 115 patients with advanced recurrent and/or metastatic squamous cell cancer of the head and neck. The overall objective response rate was 4.3% (95% CI 1.4–9.9%) and disease stabilization was obtained in 38.3% for a median duration of 16.1 weeks. The median progression-free survival was 9.6 weeks (95% CI 8.1–12.1 weeks) and the median overall survival 6 months (95% CI 4.8–7.0 months). Subgroup analyses revealed a significant difference in overall survival favoring patients who developed at least grade 2 skin rashes versus those who did not ($p = 0.045$). Rash and diarrhea were the most common drug-related toxicities, encountered in 79% and 37% of patients, respectively (50).

The prognosis for patients progressing after first-line treatment is particularly poor. In these patients, the alternative therapeutic options are discouraging and the response rates are generally less than 5%. Single agent cetuximab was tested alone in 103 patients who progressed after platinum-based chemotherapy. There was a response rate of 13% and a disease control rate (complete response/partial response/stable disease) of 46% with a median time to progression of 70 days. These results show that cetuximab is active as a single agent in this group of patients whose prognosis is particularly dismal (51).

Combination Therapy. Several combination schedules have been tested in patients with head and neck cancer. The standard combination schedule of intravenous cisplatin (100 mg/m²/day, d1) with continuous 5-FU (1000 mg/m²/day, d1–d4) every three weeks can induce response rates of 40% in first-line treatment (1). Combination chemotherapy does give higher response rates compared to single agent methotrexate but at the cost of increased toxicity and with no gain in survival in patients with recurrent and/or metastatic disease (52).

Table 7.1 Activity of Single Agents in Recurrent and/or Metastatic Squamous Cell Cancer of the Head and Neck

Agent	Number of patients	Response rate (%)
Methotrexate	998	31
5-fluorouracil	118	15
Bleomycin	347	21
Cisplatin	288	28
Paclitaxel	67	33
Docetaxel	146	29

Newer drugs have been used to replace one of the drugs in the standard cisplatin and 5-FU combination. In a Phase III study, 218 patients with locally advanced, recurrent, or metastatic disease were randomly assigned to standard cisplatin-5-FU or cisplatin 75 mg/m² and paclitaxel 175 mg/m² every three weeks until progression or a minimum of six cycles with complete response or stable disease. There was no significant difference in overall survival (8.7 vs. 8.1 months) or response rate (27% vs. 26%). Toxicity was similar between groups and most frequently myelosuppression with thrombocytopenia and anemia, nausea and vomiting, and stomatitis were reported (52).

The Eastern Cooperative Oncology Group carried out a Phase III trial where 117 patients with recurrent/metastatic SCCHN were randomly assigned to receive cisplatin 100 mg/m² every four weeks, with weekly cetuximab or placebo. There was a higher response rate in the cetuximab arm than in the placebo arm (26% vs. 10%; $p = 0.03$) but no difference in progression-free or overall survival (53).

Erlotinib was also combined with cisplatin in patients with recurrent or metastatic SCCHN and a daily oral dose of erlotinib 100 mg could be combined with intravenous cisplatin 75 mg/m² every 21 days. The response rate in 45 patients treated at this dose was 21% (95% CI 10–36%), and disease stabilization was achieved in 21 patients (49%, 95% CI 33–65%). Median progression-free survival was 3.3 months (95% CI 2.7–4.8 months) and median overall survival 7.9 months (95% CI 5.6–9.5). Subgroup analysis suggested that patients who developed higher grade skin rashes during Cycle 1 had better survival outcomes ($p = 0.034$) (54).

Cetuximab (400 mg/m² followed by 250 mg/m²/week) was added to a platinum-based combination (cisplatin 100 mg/m² or carboplatin area under the curve 5 mg/ml/min) plus 5-FU (1000 mg/m²/d for 4 days) every 3 weeks for a maximum of 6 cycles in a randomized study in 442 patients with untreated recurrent or metastatic SCCHN. In the group of patients treated with the cetuximab combination there was a prolonged median progression-free survival time (3.3 vs. 5.6 months, HR 0.54; p<0.001), an increased response rate (20 vs. 36%; p<0.001) and better median overall survival (7.4 vs. 10.1 months; HR 0.80; 95% CI 0.64 to 0.99; p=0.04) (73).

Cetuximab has also been combined with cisplatin as second-line treatment after platinum-based chemotherapy. Overall response rates ranged from 10% to 13% and disease control rates from 46% to 56%. The median time to disease progression was between 2.2 and 2.8 months, and the median overall survival between 5.2 and 6.1 months. Cetuximab did not increase the toxicities associated with chemotherapy (51).

At the moment, single agent methotrexate (40 mg/m²/week and escalated depending on tolerance) still remains the standard in patients with recurrent/metastatic disease, although the cisplatin/5-FU combination may induce higher responses. The addition of cetuximab to a platinum-5-FU combination increases overall survival and might be considered as first-line treatment in patients with a good condition.

Supportive Care

Patients who undergo treatment for head and neck cancers often suffer from acute or late reactions to therapy.

Acute toxicity ranges from mild complains such as gastrointestinal disturbances (nausea, vomiting, dysphagia) or pain to life-threatening complication such as severe mucositis leading to weight loss and necessitating enteral or total parenteral nutrition or hematologic toxicity (neutropenic fever). Late toxicity is mutilation from surgery, xerostomia, fibrosis or osteonecrosis because of radiotherapy, permanent tube feeding, or speech impairment (55). Therefore, head and neck cancer patients are in need of intense supportive care during and after therapy. Following surgical neck dissection and external beam radiation they need rehabilitation and they should be taken care for by a multidisciplinary team for support, revalidation, and rehabilitation (56).

Chemoprevention

Most patients with Stage I and Stage II disease may be treated successfully. However, failure remains common and is manifested by local recurrences or second primary cancers. These second primary tumors occur in other sites within the head and neck region, in the esophagus, or the lung. They are consequences of field cancerization of the upper aerodigestive tract due to chronic exposure to tobacco and alcohol.

The prevalence of a concomitant second primary tumor lays around 14%. The expected incidence of second primaries varies by initial cancer site and by tobacco use and is estimated to be 4% each year (57). Prevention of second cancers is therefore of great clinical relevance.

Several randomized trials of β-carotene and retinoids have reported significant chemopreventive efficacy in oral precancerous lesions (58). Retinoids have also been evaluated as chemopreventive agents in head and neck cancer, with one trial reporting significant benefit with regard to second primary tumors but two others showing no benefit. β-carotene did not prevent second head and neck cancers (58).

New compounds are tested in chemoprevention trials in head and neck cancer such as curcumin analogs, green tea extracts, and agents such as selenium, polyphenols of pomegranate juice, Bowman–Birk inhibitor from soybeans, and others. The National Cancer Institute has funded a series of large individual or multi-investigator studies looking at combinations of celecoxib, a selective COX-2 inhibitor with erlotinib on the basis of extensive clinical data suggesting efficacy in head and neck cancer cell lines and xenografts (58).

At this moment, there is no indication to use these interventions in the secondary prevention of head and neck cancer outside a clinical trial. Most important is to advice patients to quit smoking and limit alcohol intake in combination with healthy nutrition.

Follow up

Patients with head and neck cancer have a high incidence of second malignancies but there are no evidence-based guidelines for follow up (59).

Hypothyroidism is seen in 15–45% of patients treated for head and neck cancer with radiotherapy (60). Therefore, a control of the thyroid function is indicated every six months after radiotherapy.

NASOPHARYNGEAL CANCER

Introduction

Nasopharyngeal cancer is clearly a distinct tumor entity among head and neck cancers. It has a specific geographical distribution, epidemiology, clinical expression, and response to treatment.

Epidemiology

In Europe, it represents a rare disease with an annual incidence of less than 1 per 100,000. The incidence is higher in the Mediterranean countries of Europe (Greece, former Yugoslavia, Italy, France, Spain), whereas it is endemic in the Far East (1).

It is related to the Epstein–Barr virus (EBV) infection (61).

Pathology

Nasopharyngeal cancer is classified according to the World Health Organization (62) in different categories including nonkeratinizing carcinoma, keratinizing squamous cell carcinoma, and basaloid squamous cell carcinoma. The keratinizing squamous cell carcinoma is the most frequent type in the Western countries whereas the nonkeratinizing (undifferentiated) form is more frequently seen in the Far East (1).

Staging and Prognosis

Nasopharyngeal cancer has its own TNM classification system (13,14) both for the primary tumor site (which is not based on tumor dimensions) and for nodal extension (Table 7.2).

The distribution and the prognostic impact of regional lymph node spread is different from those of other head and neck mucosal cancers justifying a different N classification.

Undifferentiated nasopharyngeal cancer has a high propensity to distant failure, which may occur in up to 30% of patients whose disease is controlled locally and in 40% of patients with locoregional failure (61).

Evaluation of a Patient with Nasopharyngeal Cancer

Diagnosis is made by a biopsy during a pan-endoscopic evaluation under anesthesia. Staging of the disease should include an MRI of the head and neck region, which seems to be superior to CT scan.

A total body radiological evaluation, along with a bone scan, is highly recommended mainly in patients with undifferentiated nasopharyngeal cancer. All these examinations can be replaced by a PET scan.

EBV integration in tumor cells is useful to prove the disease while serum levels of EBV-DNA are useful to determine prognosis and during follow-up.

Regular follow up after treatment completion is suggested for early detection of locoregional relapse that may be still curable.

Treatment

Before starting treatment, a multidisciplinary team with a head and neck surgeon, a radiotherapist, and a medical

Table 7.2 TNM Definitions of Nasopharyngeal Cancer

Primary tumor (T)
- TX: Primary tumor cannot be assessed
- T0: No evidence of primary tumor
- Tis: Carcinoma in situ
- T1: Tumor confined to the nasopharynx
- T2: Tumor extends to soft tissues
  - T2a: Tumor extends to the oropharynx and/or nasal cavity without parapharyngeal extension[a]
  - T2b: Any tumor with parapharyngeal extension[a]
- T3: Tumor invades bony structures and/or paranasal sinuses
- T4: Tumor with intracranial extension and/or involvement of cranial nerves, infratemporal fossa, hypopharynx, orbit, or masticator space

Parapharyngeal extension denotes posterolateral infiltration of tumor beyond the pharyngobasilar fascia

Regional lymph nodes (N)
- NX: Regional lymph nodes cannot be assessed
- N0: No regional lymph node metastasis
- N1: Unilateral metastasis in lymph node(s), 6 cm or less in greatest dimension, above the supraclavicular fossa[a]
- N2: Bilateral metastasis in lymph node(s), 6 cm or less in greatest dimension, above the supraclavicular fossa[a]
- N3: Metastasis in a lymph node(s)[a] >6 cm and/or to supraclavicular fossa
  - N3a: Greater than 6 cm in dimension
  - N3b: Extension to the supraclavicular fossa[b]

Distant metastasis (M)
- MX: Distant metastasis cannot be assessed
- M0: No distant metastasis
- M1: Distant metastasis

AJCC stage groupings of nasopharyngeal cancer

Stage	T	N	M
Stage 0	Tis	N0	M0
Stage I	T1	N0	M0
Stage IIA	T2a	N0	M0
Stage IIB	T1-T2a-b	N1	M0
	T2b	N0	M0
Stage III	T1	N2	M0
	T2a-b	N2	M0
	T3	N1-2	M0
Stage IVA	T4	N0-2	M0
Stage IVB	Any T	N3	M0
Stage IVC	Any T	Any N	M1

[a]Midline nodes are considered ipsilateral nodes.
[b]Supraclavicular zone or fossa is relevant to the staging of nasopharyngeal carcinoma and is the triangular region originally described by Ho. It is defined by three points: (1) the superior margin of the sternal end of the clavicle, (2) the superior margin of the lateral end of the clavicle, (3) the point where the neck meets the shoulder. Note that this would include caudal portions of levels IV and V. All cases with lymph nodes (whole or part) in the fossa are considered N3b.
Source: From Ref. 14.

oncologist should decide on the most optimal treatment plan for the patient.

Unlike other head and neck cancers, surgery plays a minor role in the treatment of nasopharyngeal cancer whereas radiotherapy is the main treatment modality. All histotypes but in particular the nonkeratinizing type are particularly sensitive to radiotherapy and chemotherapy.

Treatment is delivered according to tumor stage. Early stage tumors are treated with radiotherapy alone while concomitant chemoradiation is the standard treatment for advanced stage III and IV nasopharyngeal cancer. Modern radiotherapy including IMRT together with concomitant chemotherapy has significantly improved patient's outcome, so that today the majority of patients with nasopharyngeal cancer can be cured. The role of induction chemotherapy is still debated and is marginal as compared to concomitant chemotherapy that has to be delivered during radiotherapy (61,63).

Nasopharyngeal cancer is sensitive to cisplatin-based regimens. Cisplatin alone is the treatment of choice when radiotherapy is given concomitantly.

Induction chemotherapy usually combining cisplatin, 5-FU, and epirubicin with or without bleomycin and more recently with taxanes is feasible (63).

Locoregional recurrent disease might be cured with reirradiation or salvage surgery in selected patients; in most patients palliative platinum-based polychemotherapy is the treatment of choice. Response rates are not negligible and a good disease control can be achieved. Painful bone metastases should be irradiated.

THYROID CANCER

Introduction

Although thyroid cancer is an uncommon cancer, it is the most common malignancy of the endocrine system (64). Most thyroid cancers (95%) are differentiated cancers deriving from the follicular epithelial cells and are either papillary or follicular thyroid carcinomas. Another 5% are medullary carcinomas and 1% is of anaplastic histology.

When managed adequately, the vast majority of patients with thyroid cancer can be cured.

After treatment, local or regional recurrences develop in up to 30% of patients and distant metastases in up to 20%. The recurrence rate increases in time and cumulative 40-year recurrence rates are about 35% (65). Overall 8–10% of patients with a diagnosis of thyroid cancer die of their disease.

Epidemiology

Thyroid cancer accounts for 1% of all new cancers and affects women more commonly than men. It occurs primarily in young and middle aged adults, rarely in children. The mean age is the mid-40s to mid-50s for the papillary type, 50s for the follicular and medullary type, and 60s for the less common undifferentiated (anaplastic) type. Standardized incidence rates per 100,000 population vary in different parts of the world from 0.8 to 5.0 in men and 1.9 to 19.4 in women. The incidence of this malignancy has been increasing over the last decade.

Risk factors for thyroid cancer are radiation exposure during childhood, endemic goiter, lymphocytic thyroiditis, family or personal history of thyroid nodules, Cowden's syndrome, familial adenomatosis polyposis, and familial thyroid cancer.

Carcinogenesis

Several defects in tumor suppressor genes and oncogenes have been described in patients with thyroid cancer.

- The activation of RET proto-oncogene due to several mechanism (gain-of-function mutations or chromosomal rearrangements) plays a causative role in the pathogenesis of a large proportion of papillary cancer. Also among the hereditary and sporadic forms of medullary cancer, germ-line activating point mutations of the RET proto-oncogene are observed.
- The activation of B-Raf is another genetic alteration involved in thyroid cancer pathogenesis. The B-Raf V600E mutation is the most common genetic change in papillary cancer, B-Raf mutation is also present in up to 24% of anaplastic carcinomas arisen in association with papillary cancer.
- Oncogenic *ras* mutations occur rarely, in about 10% of patients, mostly in the follicular variant.
- Elevated levels of vascular endothelial growth factor (VEGF) have been found in thyroid tumor tissue compared to normal thyroid, and it could be hypothesized that other pathways, such as VEGFR- and EGFR-dependent signaling, also participate in tumor growth and development.
- Anaplastic cancer expresses along with TP53 mutations and also other targets such as beta-catenine, cyclin E and cyclin D1, and EGFR. No EGFR mutations or gene amplifications were found in a little series of anaplastic carcinoma, while high polisomy was detected by fluorescence in situ hybridization (FISH) in 61% of patients.

Clinical significance of these observations is still unknown, although these targets could be considered for biological therapies (66).

Pathology

The most recent WHO 2004 pathologic classification is reported in Table 7.3.

Screening

Patients with medullary cancer, whether familial or sporadic, should be tested for RET mutations. If they are positive, family members should also be tested.

Family members who are gene carriers should undergo specific close monitoring or prophylactic thyroidectomy at an early age depending on mutation type.

Clinical Manifestations

Thyroid cancer commonly presents as a solitary or multinodular swelling in the neck. It may give rise to hoarseness or stridor and swelling of the cervical lymph nodes.

In case of distant metastasis, there may be pain due to bone metastases.

Table 7.3 Pathology of Thyroid Cancer

- Papillary carcinoma
  - Papillary/follicular carcinoma
- Follicular carcinoma
  - Hurthle cell carcinoma
- Medullary carcinoma
- Anaplastic carcinoma
  - Small cell carcinoma
  - Giant cell carcinoma

Medullary carcinoma usually presents as a hard thyroidal mass and is often accompanied by blood vessel invasion. Metastasis to regional lymph nodes are found in about 50% of patients. It occurs in two forms: a sporadic and familial form. In the sporadic form, the tumor is usually unilateral. In the familial form, the tumor is almost always bilateral and may be associated with benign or malignant tumors of other endocrine organs, commonly referred to as the multiple endocrine neoplasia syndromes (MEN 2A or MEN 2B). In these syndromes, there is an association with pheochromocytoma of the adrenal gland and parathyroid hyperplasia.

Staging and Prognosis

The staging of thyroid cancers is based on the TNM classification of the International Union against Cancer (13) and the American Joint Committee on Cancer (14) (Table 7.4). It is a clinical classification. The pathological classification is similar to the clinical classification.

- The T classification indicates the extent of the primary tumor. It is based on the size of the tumor, whereas T4 indicates that the tumor extends beyond the thyroid capsule (14).
- The N classification for cervical lymph node metastasis is based on the localization of the lymph nodes in the neck (unilateral/bilateral).
- The M classification indicates the absence (M0) or presence (M1) of distant metastasis. Metastases are most often found in liver, lung, and skeleton.

Based on the TNM classification, histology, and age thyroid cancers are grouped according to stage (Table 7.4).

Several risk scoring systems have been proposed. Three of these which are the most frequently used are AGES (based on age, grade, extent, size); AMES (based on age, size, extent, distant metastasis); and MACIS (based on age, size, local invasion, completeness of resection, distant metastasis). The prognostic significance of lymph node status remains controversial (13). All these systems have shortcomings such as histotype variants and genetic profile.

Evaluation of a Patient with Thyroid Cancer

The assessment of the primary tumor is by inspection and bimanual palpation of the thyroid and the neck. A neck ultrasound and a fine needle biopsy will give the diagnosis.

In addition to the clinical examination, calcitonine (medullary carcinoma), a thyroid function test, thyroid antibodies, and thyroglobulin should be determined (67).

Additional tests particularly in patients with large neck masses are inspection of the function of the vocal cords, and a CT scan without Iodine (I)-containing contrast or MRI of the thyroid and neck region.

Distant metastasis can be detected by chest radiography and ^{123}I or Technetium scintigraphy.

Treatment

Before treatment, a multidisciplinary team with a head and neck surgeon, a radiotherapist, an endocrinologist, a pathologist, and a medical oncologist should decide on the most optimal treatment plan for the patient.

All patients with a differentiated thyroid cancer should be treated by surgery (65,68). A thyroidectomy and

Table 7.4 TNM Classification of Thyroid Cancer

Primary tumor (T)
All categories may be subdivided into (a) solitary tumor or (b) multifocal tumor (the largest determines the classification).
- TX: Primary tumor cannot be assessed
- T0: No evidence of primary tumor
- T1: Tumor 2 cm or less in greatest dimension limited to the thyroid
- T2: Tumor more than 2 cm but not more than 4 cm in greatest dimension limited to the thyroid
- T3: Tumor more than 4 cm in greatest dimension limited to the thyroid or any tumor with minimal extrathyroid extension (e.g., extension to sternothyroid muscle or perithyroid soft tissues)
- T4a: Tumor extends beyond the thyroid capsule and invades any of the following: subcutaneous soft tissue, larynx, trachea, oesophagus, recurrent laryngeal nerve
- T4b: Tumor invades prevertebral fascia, mediastinal vessels, or encases carotid artery (any size) extends beyond the thyroid capsule

Regional lymph nodes (N)
- NX: Regional lymph nodes cannot be assessed
- N0: No regional lymph node metastasis
- N1: Regional lymph node metastasis
  - N1a: Metastasis in level IV (pretracheal and paratracheal, including pretracheal and Delphian lymph nodes)
  - N1b: Metastasis in other unilateral, bilateral, or contralateral cervical or upper/superior mediastinal lymph nodes

Distant metastases (M)
- MX: Distant metastasis cannot be assessed
- M0: No distant metastasis
- M1: Distant metastasis

Stage grouping
Papillary or follicular under 45 years

Stage I	Any T	Any N	M0
Stage II	Any T	Any N	M1

Papillary or follicular 45 years and older and medullary

Stage I	T1	N0	M0
Stage II	T2	N0	M0
Stage III	T3	N0	M0
	T1-3	N1a	M0
Stage IVA	T1-3	N1b	M0
	T4a	N0,1	M0
Stage IVB	T4b	Any N	M0
Stage IVC	Any T	Any N	M1

Anaplastic/undifferentiated (all cases are stage IV)

Stage IVA	T4a	Any N	M0
Stage IVB	T4b	Any N	M0
Stage IVC	Any T	Any N	M1

Source: From Ref. 14.

a lymph node dissection of Level VI should be performed. In case of suspicious lymph nodes at other levels, a frozen section examination has to be done, and in case of tumor invasion, lymph node dissection of levels II, III, and IV should be performed. Postoperative radiotherapy in poorly differentiated cancers with poor prognostic features such as T extension and presence of nodal involvement has been advocated (68).

Papillary Carcinoma and Follicular Carcinoma

In patients with tumors smaller than 1 cm and no lymph node involvement, a lobectomy and thyroid stimulating hormone (TSH) suppression therapy is sufficient.

In high-risk patients (documented persistent or at high risk of persistent or recurrent disease), a total thyroidectomy followed by ^{131}I ablation and long-term TSH suppression therapy is indicated (67).

In all other patients (low-risk group) radio-ablation is still controversial.

Radio-ablation with ^{131}I will be started three to four weeks after surgery without thyroid substitution therapy. TSH should at that moment be higher than 30 mu/L. In case tri-iodothyronine was started postoperatively, it should be stopped for two weeks before radio-ablation.

Long-term TSH suppression is with thyroxine. The dose of thyroxine should gradually be increased until TSH levels are below 0.1 mu/L.

Medullary Carcinoma

The primary treatment is a total thyroidectomy and lymph node dissection. Adjuvant radiotherapy is not given, but radiotherapy may be used for local control in patients with inoperable or recurrent disease. Targeted radiotherapy with somatostatin analogs or ^{131}I-meta-iodobenzylguanidine (MIBG) has a very limited value. Chemotherapy based on dacarbazine either alone or in combination has been associated with tumor reduction in approximately 30% of patients.

Anaplastic Carcinoma

This is a very aggressive tumor with a median survival of less than six months. Surgery is indicated to maintain an open airway and is followed by external radiotherapy with or without chemotherapy. Some authors claim that chemoradiation followed by surgery gives a better result.

Many patients may present with unresectable neck masses; in this situation chemoradiation with cisplatin represents the standard treatment.

In patients with metastatic disease, chemotherapy may be used for palliation. Doxorubicin, paclitaxel, and cisplatin have some activity in these patients (69).

Recurrent Disease

For recurrent disease in the thyroid bed or cervical lymph nodes of papillary and follicular carcinoma, surgery in combination with radio-ablation is the treatment of choice.

Metastatic disease should be treated with radio-ablation. Painful bone metastases may be treated with external beam radiotherapy.

In radio-iodine-resistant tumors chemotherapy is not effective although some responses have been reported with doxorubicin (less than 20%). Some authors reported promising results in patients with poorly differentiated thyroid cancer treated with chemotherapy preceded by TSH stimulation (68).

Targeted therapy with tyrosine kinase inhibitors has been recently proven to be of some interest in radio-iodine-resistant and medullary cancer (66). Promising drugs are axitinib, sorafenib, vandetanib, motesanib, and sunitinib (68). Also, thalidomide has shown some activity (68).

Follow up

Patients with thyroid cancer should be followed for early detection of recurrence and for efficacy of TSH suppression. Patients are seen every three months during the first two years, then every six months during the third year and then once yearly. Medullary cancer should be followed with serum calcitonin and carcino-embryonic antigen (CEA).

SALIVARY GLAND TUMORS

Introduction

Salivary glands contribute to less than 1% of head and neck cancers. The most common salivary gland cancers are localized in the major glands (parotid, submandibular, and sublingual). Carcinomas of the minor salivary glands originate from submucosal glands located in the upper aerodigestive tract and are most commonly localized in the soft palate (19%), followed by the paranasal sinuses/nasal cavity (17%), and the tongue (14%) (70).

Epidemiology

Salivary gland tumors are more frequent in Europe and North America compared to Asia and Africa. They are more common in men than in women with an incidence ratio of 1.3:1 (70).

Risk factors for salivary gland cancer include exposure to radiation and tobacco use (70).

Carcinogenesis

Genetic abnormalities in salivary glands cancers include trisomy 8, loss of genetic material (Y chromosome), and loss of heterogeneity in 6q21–23.3 and 6q27 (71). These chromosomal abnormalities may reflect inactivation of tumor suppressor genes. Specific histological tumor types are also associated with specific abnormalities: adenoid cystic carcinoma has a translocation [t(6;9)(q21–24;p13–23)] as well as mucoepidermoid carcinoma [t(11;19)(q14–21;p12–13)] (71).

Among several biological alterations molecular analysis has shown Her-2 and EGFR amplification/overexpression particularly in malignant tumors originating from excretory duct, such as salivary duct cancer and adenocarcinoma. Also, androgen receptors have been found to be overexpressed mainly in the same histotypes.

Kit was shown to be overexpressed mainly in adenoid cystic carcinoma while VEGFR overexpression has been seen in mucoepidermoid cancer and adenoid cystic carcinoma (71).

Pathology

The most recent pathologic classification for salivary gland cancer is that of the World Health Organization (62) reported in Table 7.5.

Clinical Manifestations

Every painless swelling of a major salivary gland without signs of inflammation is suspicious. More than 80% of the tumors in the parotid are benign while more than 50% of those arising in the submandibular or sublingual glands are malignant.

Clinical indicators suggesting a malignant salivary gland tumor are rapid growth, pain, facial nerve involvement, and cervical adenopathy. Facial nerve palsy may be a sign of a locally infiltrating parotid cancer. Another symptom is parapharyngeal or palatal fullness. Trismus, skin ulceration, and fistulae may be present in advanced stages.

Table 7.5 Malignant Tumors of the Salivary Glands

- Low-grade malignancies:
    - Acinic cell tumors
    - Mucoepidermoid carcinoma (grades I or II)
- High-grade malignancies:
    - Mucoepidermoid carcinoma (Grade III)
    - Adenocarcinoma, poorly differentiated carcinoma, anaplastic carcinoma
    - Squamous cell carcinoma
    - Malignant mixed tumors
    - Adenoid cystic carcinoma

Minor salivary gland tumors may cause a painless submucosal swelling or a mass with a small ulcer. If the nasopharynx or the nasal cavity is infiltrated, facial pain, nasal obstruction, or bleeding may occur. A tumor in the larynx or trachea can cause hoarseness, voice changes, or dyspnea.

Staging and Prognosis

The staging of salivary gland cancers is based on the TNM of the International Union against Cancer (13) and American Joint Committee on Cancer (14) (Table 7.6). It is a clinical classification. The pathological classification is similar to the clinical classification.

Tumor stage, histology, and grade are independent prognostic factors for survival (88). The prognosis of adenoid cystic carcinoma depends on perineural invasion, positive margins, and solid histological features (72).

Distant metastases occur in approximately 30% of patients. In adenoid cystic carcinoma it may reach 50%.

Evaluation of the Patient with Salivary Gland Cancer

Physical examination is the most important diagnostic tool.

Ultrasonography of the affected salivary glands has a high sensitivity and is excellent to differentiate intra- from extraglandular lesions.

CT scan or MRI may be useful for a surgical planning, especially in patients with larger tumors and those arising in deep structures and/or involving them.

Fine needle aspiration is used for diagnosis and has an accuracy from 87% to 96% (70). Open biopsy of parotid or submandibular mass is not recommended because of the risk of seeding. In the presence of small masses in minor salivary glands (palate, tongue) a biopsy is preferable to direct excision, unless resection is possible with adequate margins.

CT scan is useful in the presence of deep infiltrating tumors, high-grade tumors with occult cervical metastases, and in patients with minor salivary gland tumors. The advantages of MRI include multiplanar imaging, elimination of dental artifacts, and the ability to distinguish between a tumor and obstructed secretions.

A CT scan of the chest is useful for excluding the presence of distant lung metastasis.

Treatment

Before treatment, a multidisciplinary team with a head and neck surgeon, a radiotherapist, and a medical oncologist should decide on the most optimal treatment plan for the patient.

Table 7.6 TNM Classification of Salivary Gland Tumors

Primary tumor (T)
- TX: Primary tumor cannot be assessed
- T0: No evidence of primary tumor
- T1: Tumor 2 cm or less in greatest dimension without extraparenchymal extension
- T2: Tumor more than 2 cm but not more than 4 cm in greatest dimension without extraparenchymal extension
- T3: Tumor more than 4 cm and/or extraparenchymal extension
- T4a: Tumor invades skin, mandible, ear cancal, and/or facial nerve
- T4b: Tumor invades base of skull and/or pterygoid plates and/or encases carotid artery

Regional lymph nodes (N)
- NX: Regional lymph nodes cannot be assessed
- N0: No regional lymph node metastasis
- N1: Metastasis in a single ipsilateral lymph node, 3 cm or less in greatest dimension
- N2: Metastasis in a single ipsilateral lymph node, more than 3 cm but not more than 6 cm in greatest dimension, or in multiple ipsilateral lymph nodes, none more than 6 cm in greatest dimension, or in bilateral or contralateral lymph nodes, none more than 6 cm in greatest dimension
    - N2a: Metastasis in a single ipsilateral lymph node more than 3 cm but not more than 6 cm in greatest dimension
    - N2b: Metastasis in multiple ipsilateral lymph nodes, none more than 6 cm in greatest dimension
    - N2c: Metastasis in bilateral or contralateral lymph nodes, none more than 6 cm in greatest dimension
- N3: Metastasis in a lymph node more than 6 cm in greatest dimension

Distant metastasis (M)
- MX: Distant metastasis cannot be assessed
- M0: No distant metastasis
- M1: Distant metastasis

AJCC stage groupings

Stage I	T1	N0	M0
Stage II	T2	N0	M0
Stage III	T3	N0	M0
	T1-3	N1	M0
Stage IVA	T4a	N0-1	M0
	T1-4a	N2	M0
Stage IVB	T4b	Any N	M0
	Any T	N3	M0
Stage IVC	Any T	Any N	M1

Source: From Ref. 14.

Surgery is the treatment of choice for resectable major and minor salivary glands tumors.

A prophylactic neck dissection is not routinely recommended since lymph node metastases occur in only 15% of patients. However, since lymph node metastases occur more frequently in high-grade tumors or in tumors larger than 4 cm, elective lymph node dissection of levels I, II, and III and of levels II, III, IV, and V is recommended for submaxillary-sublingual and parotid gland tumors, respectively.

Primary radiotherapy may be used in patients with unresectable disease or those who refuse surgery. Adjuvant radiotherapy may be used in both major and minor salivary gland tumors in case of undifferentiated and high-grade tumors; in case of extensive nodal involvement; or after capsular rupture. It is not indicated in patients with adenoid cystic carcinoma.

Chemotherapy may be used for palliation. Response rates to polychemotherapy vary widely due to the different chemosensitivity of the different histotypes. The response rate is 30% in recurrent and/or metastatic disease.

The most studied regimen is the combination of cyclophosphamide, doxorubicin, and cisplatin (CAP). Since there are no randomized trials, it is not known whether combination chemotherapy has any advantage over single agent treatment (70). Therefore, a standard regimen is still lacking.

In most patients with an indolent course, a conservative attitude should be strongly considered.

Based on the presence of several cellular targets a number of targeted drugs have been employed. Results obtained both with gefitinib, cetuximab, and lapatinib are not impressive. No objective response was recorded, although disease stabilizations (35% with lapatinib and 43% with cetuximab) lasting more than six months were observed. These observations may depend on the behavior of adenoid cystic carcinoma (histology mainly included in the studies), for which a cytostatic activity of the drugs themselves is difficult to prove.

REFERENCES

1. Vokes EE, Cohen EE, Grandis JR. Introduction: head and neck cancer. Semin Oncol 2008; 35: 196–7.
2. Sant M, Aareleid T, Berrino F et al. EUROCARE-3: survival of cancer patients diagnosed 1990-94--results and commentary. Ann Oncol 2003; 14(Suppl 5): v61–118.
3. Bosetti C, Bertuccio P, Levi F et al. Cancer mortality in the European Union, 1970–2003, with a joinpoint analysis. Ann Oncol 2008; 19: 631–40.
4. Decker J, Goldstein J. Current concepts in otolaryngology. Risk factors in head and neck cancer. N Engl J Med 1982; 306: 1151–5.
5. Neville BW, Day TA. Oral cancer and precancerous lesions. CA Cancer J Clin 2002; 52: 195–215.
6. Gleich LL, Salamone FN. Molecular genetics of head and neck cancer. Cancer Control 2002; 9: 369–78.
7. Ragin CC, Modugno F, Gollin SM. The epidemiology and risk factors of head and neck cancer: a focus on human papillomavirus. J Dent Res 2007; 86: 104–14.
8. Hoory T, Monie A, Gravitt P et al. Molecular epidemiology of human papillomavirus. J Formos Med Assoc 2008; 107: 198–217.
9. Steger G, Corbach S. Dose-dependent regulation of the early promoter of human papillomavirus type 18 by the viral E2 protein. J Virol 1997; 71: 50–8.
10. Stanley MA, Pett MR, Coleman N. HPV: from infection to cancer. Biochem Soc Trans 2007; 35: 1456–60.
11. Wiencke JK. DNA adduct burden and tobacco carcinogenesis. Oncogene 2002; 21: 7376–91.
12. Arredondo J, Chernyavsky AI, Jolkovsky DL et al. Receptor-mediated tobacco toxicity: cooperation of the Ras/Raf-1/MEK1/ERK and JAK-2/STAT-3 pathways downstream of alpha7 nicotinic receptor in oral keratinocytes. FASEB J 2006; 20: 2093–101.
13. International Union against Cancer. In: Sobin LH, Wittekind Ch, eds. TNM Classification of Malignant Tumors, 6th edn. New York: Wiley-Liss, 2002.
14. American Joint Committee on Cancer. In: Greene FL, Page DL, Fleming ID et al., eds. AJCC Cancer Staging Handbook, 6th edn. New York: Springer, 2002.
15. Warnakulasuriya KA, Nanayakkara BG. Reproducibility of an oral cancer and precancer detection program using a primary health care model in Sri Lanka. Cancer Detect Prev 1991; 15: 331–4.
16. Ramadas K, Sankaranarayanan R, Jacob BJ et al. Interim results from a cluster randomized controlled oral cancer screening trial in Kerala, India. Oral Oncol 2003; 39: 580–8.
17. Prout MN, Sidari JN, Witzburg RA et al. Head and neck cancer screening among 4611 tobacco users older than forty years. Otolaryngol Head Neck Surg 1997; 116: 201–8.
18. Abdo EN, Garrocho Ade A, Barbosa AA et al. Time elapsed between the first symptoms, diagnosis and treatment of oral cancer patients in Belo Horizonte, Brazil. Med Oral Patol Oral Cir Bucal 2007; 12: 469–73.
19. British Columbia Oral Cancer Prevention Program, BC Cancer Agency; College of Dental Surgeons of British Columbia. Guideline for the early detection of oral cancer in British Columbia 2008. J Can Dent Assoc 2008; 74: 245.
20. Chen YW, Lin JS, Wu CH et al. Application of in vivo stain of methylene blue as a diagnostic aid in the early detection and screening of oral squamous cell carcinoma and precancer lesions. J Chin Med Assoc 2007; 70: 497–503.
21. Dahlstrand H, Näsman A, Romanitan M et al. Human papillomavirus accounts both for increased incidence and better prognosis in tonsillar cancer. Anticancer Res 2008; 28: 1133–8.
22. Becker M. Diagnosis and staging of laryngeal tumors with CT and MRI. Radiologe 1998; 38: 93–100.
23. Facey K, Bradbury I, Laking G et al. Overview of the clinical effectiveness of positron emission tomography imaging in selected cancers. Health Technol Assess 2007; 11: iii–iv, xi–267.
24. Knappe M, Louw M, Gregor RT. Ultrasonography-guided fine-needle aspiration for the assessment of cervical metastases. Arch Otolaryngol Head Neck Surg 2000; 126: 1091–6.
25. Kyzas PA, Evangelou E, Denaxa-Kyza D et al. 18F-fluorodeoxyglucose positron emission tomography to evaluate cervical node metastases in patients with head and neck squamous cell carcinoma: a meta-analysis. J Natl Cancer Inst 2008; 100: 712–20.
26. Dey P, Arnold D, Wight R et al. Radiotherapy versus open surgery versus endolaryngeal surgery (with or without laser) for early laryngeal squamous cell cancer. Cochrane Database Syst Rev 2002; CD002027.
27. Cohen SM, Garrett CG, Dupont WD et al. Voice-related quality of life in T1 glottic cancer: irradiation versus endoscopic excision. Ann Otol Rhinol Laryngol 2006; 115: 581–6.
28. Kane SV, Gupta M, Kakade AC et al. Depth of invasion is the most significant histological predictor of subclinical cervical lymph node metastasis in early squamous carcinomas of the oral cavity. Eur J Surg Oncol 2006; 32: 795–803.
29. Brazilian Head and Neck Cancer Study Group. End results of a prospective trial on elective lateral neck dissection vs type III modified radical neck dissection in the management of supraglottic and transglottic carcinomas. Head Neck 1999; 21: 694–702.
30. Corvò R. Evidence-based radiation oncology in head and neck squamous cell carcinoma. Radiother Oncol 2007; 85: 156–70.
31. Williams M, Denekamp J, Fowler J. A review of alpha/beta ratios for experimental tumors: implications for clinical studies of altered fractionation. Int J Radiat Oncol Biol Phys 1985; 11: 87–96.
32. Bourhis J, Overgaard J, Audry H et al. Hyperfractionated or accelerated radiotherapy in head and neck cancer: a meta-analysis. Lancet 2006; 368: 843–54.
33. Lee NY, Le QT. New developments in radiation therapy for head and neck cancer: intensity-modulated radiation therapy and hypoxia targeting. Semin Oncol 2008; 35: 236–50.
34. Brizel DM. Pharmacologic approaches to radiation protection. J Clin Oncol 2007; 25: 4084–9.

35. Goldie JH, Coldman AJ. A mathematic model for relating the drug sensitivity of tumors to their spontaneous mutation rate. Cancer Treat Rep 1979; 63: 1727–33.

36. Specenier PM, Vermorken JB. Neoadjuvant chemotherapy in head and neck cancer: should it be revisited? Cancer Lett 2007; 256: 166–77.

37. Hitt R, López-Pousa A, Martínez-Trufero J et al. Phase III study comparing cisplatin plus fluorouracil to paclitaxel, cisplatin, and fluorouracil induction chemotherapy followed by chemoradiotherapy in locally advanced head and neck cancer. J Clin Oncol 2005; 23: 8636–45.

38. Vermorken JB, Remenar E, van Herpen C et al. Cisplatin, fluorouracil, and docetaxel in unresectable head and neck cancer. N Engl J Med 2007; 357: 1695–704.

39. Posner MR, Hershock DM, Blajman CR et al. Cisplatin and fluorouracil alone or with docetaxel in head and neck cancer. N Engl J Med 2007; 357: 1705–15.

40. Pignon JP, Bourhis J, Domenge C et al. Chemotherapy added to locoregional treatment for head and neck squamous-cell carcinoma: three meta-analyses of updated individual data. MACH-NC Collaborative Group. Meta-Analysis of Chemotherapy on Head and Neck Cancer. Lancet 2000; 355: 949–55.

41. Merlano M. Alternating chemotherapy and radiotherapy in locally advanced head and neck cancer: an alternative? Oncologist 2006; 11: 146–51.

42. Bernier J, Vermorken JB, Koch WM. Adjuvant therapy in patients with resected poor-risk head and neck cancer. J Clin Oncol 2006; 24: 2629–35.

43. Seiwert TY, Haraf DJ, Cohen EE et al. Phase I study of bevacizumab added to fluorouracil- and hydroxyurea-based concomitant chemoradiotherapy for poor-prognosis head and neck cancer. J Clin Oncol 2008; 26: 1732–41.

44. Rischin D, Peters L, O'Sullivan B et al. Phase III study of tirapazamine, cisplatin and radiation versus cisplatin and radiation for advanced squamous cell carcinoma of the head and neck. J Clin Oncol 2008; 26: S1010.

45. Valerie K, Yacoub A, Hagan MP et al. Radiation-induced cell signaling: inside-out and outside-in. Mol Cancer Ther 2007; 6: 789–801.

46. Bonner JA, Harari PM, Giralt J et al. Radiotherapy plus cetuximab for squamous-cell carcinoma of the head and neck. N Engl J Med 2006; 354: 567–78.

47. Shewach DS, Lawrence TS. Antimetabolite radiosensitizers. J Clin Oncol 2007; 25: 4043–50.

48. Langendijk JA, Bourhis J. Reirradiation in squamous cell head and neck cancer: recent developments and future directions. Curr Opin Oncol 2007; 19: 202–9.

49. Castro DJ, Sridhar KS, Garewal HS et al. Intratumoral cisplatin/epinephrine gel in advanced head and neck cancer: a multicenter, randomized, double-blind, phase III study in North America. Head Neck 2003; 25: 717–31.

50. Soulieres D, Senzer NN, Vokes EE et al. Multicenter phase II study of erlotinib, an oral epidermal growth factor receptor tyrosine kinase inhibitor, in patients with recurrent or metastatic squamous cell cancer of the head and neck. J Clin Oncol 2004; 22: 77–85.

51. Vermorken JB, Herbst RS, Leon X et al. Overview of the efficacy of cetuximab in recurrent and/or metastatic squamous cell carcinoma of the head and neck in patients who previously failed platinum-based therapies. Cancer 2008; 112: 2710–19.

52. Gibson MK, Li Y, Murphy B et al. Randomized phase III evaluation of cisplatin plus fluorouracil versus cisplatin plus paclitaxel in advanced head and neck cancer (E1395): an intergroup trial of the Eastern Cooperative Oncology Group. J Clin Oncol 2005; 23: 3562–7.

53. Burtness B, Goldwasser MA, Flood W et al. Eastern Cooperative Oncology Group. Phase III randomized trial of cisplatin plus placebo compared with cisplatin plus cetuximab in metastatic/recurrent head and neck cancer: an Eastern Cooperative Oncology Group study. J Clin Oncol 2005; 23: 8646–54.

54. Siu LL, Soulieres D, Chen EX et al. Phase I/II trial of erlotinib and cisplatin in patients with recurrent or metastatic squamous cell carcinoma of the head and neck: a Princess Margaret Hospital phase II consortium and National Cancer Institute of Canada Clinical Trials Group Study. J Clin Oncol 2007; 25: 2178–83.

55. Kaanders JH, Hordijk GJ, Dutch Cooperative Head and Neck Oncology Group. Carcinoma of the larynx: the Dutch national guideline for diagnostics, treatment, supportive care and rehabilitation. Radiother Oncol 2002; 63: 299–307.

56. Cheville AL. Cancer rehabilitation. Semin Oncol 2005; 32: 219–24.

57. Haughey BH, Gates GA, Arfken CL et al. Meta-analysis of second malignant tumors in head and neck cancer: the case for an endoscopic screening protocol. Ann Otol Rhinol Laryngol 1992; 101: 105–12.

58. Khuri FR, Shin DM. Head and neck cancer chemoprevention gets a shot in the arm. J Clin Oncol 2008; 26: 345–7.

59. de Visscher AV, Manni JJ. Routine long-term follow-up in patients treated with curative intent for squamous cell carcinoma of the larynx, pharynx, and oral cavity. Does it make sense? Arch Otolaryngol Head Neck Surg 1994; 120: 934–9.

60. Tell R, Sjodin H, Lundell G et al. Hypothyroidism after external radiotherapy for head and neck cancer. Int J Radiat Oncol Biol Phys 1997; 39: 303–8.

61. Licitra L, Bernier J, Bossi P et al. Cancer of nasopharynx. www.startoncology.net

62. Barnes L, Eveson JW, Reichart P et al., eds. WHO classification of tumours. Pathology and Genetics of Head and Neck Tumours. Lyon: IARC Press, 2005.

63. Baujat B, Audry H, Bourhis J et al. Chemotherapy as an adjunct to radiotherapy in locally advanced nasopharyngeal carcinoma. Cochrane Database Syst Rev 2006; CD004329.

64. DeLellis R, Lloyd R, Heintz PU et al., eds. World Health Organization. Classification of Tumours. Pathology and Genetics. Tumours of Endocrine Organs. Lyon: IARC Press, 2004.

65. Sherman S. Thyroid carcinoma. Lancet 2003; 361: 501–11.

66. Bossi P, Locati L, Licitra L. Biological agents in head and neck cancer. Expert Rev Anticancer Ther 2007; 7: 1643–50.

67. Pacini F, Schlumberger M, Dralle H et al. European consensus for the management of patients with differentiated thyroid carcinoma of the follicular epithelium. Eur J Endocrinol 2006; 154: 787–803.

68. Brown RL. Standard and emerging therapeutic approaches for thyroid malignancies. Semin Oncol 2008; 35: 298–308.

69. Pudney D, Lau H, Ruether JD et al. Clinical experience of the multimodality management of anaplastic thyroid cancer and literature review. Thyroid 2007; 17: 1243–50.

70. Licitra L, Bruzzi P, Bernier J et al. Major and minor salivary glands tumors. http//www.startoncology.net

71. Seifert G, Sobin LH. The World Health Organization's Histological Classification of Salivary Gland Tumors. A commentary on the second edition. Cancer 1992; 70: 379–85.

72. Spiro RH, Huvos AG. Stage means more than grade in adenoid cystic carcinoma. Am J Surg 1992; 164: 623–8.

73. Vermorken JB, Mesia R, Rivera F, et al. Platinum-based chemotherapy plus cetuximab in head and neck cancer. N Engl J Med 2008; 359: 1116–27.

8

Primary Malignant Tumors of the Lung and Pleura

Heine H. Hansen and Helle Pappot

The continuous increase in the incidence of lung cancer, which is now the most frequent cancer type in men in most European countries and rapidly increasing in women, makes the understanding of the etiology, prevention, and treatment of this disease more important than ever. Although the key etiological factor, smoking with its many carcinogens, has been known for years, the long lag between exposure and the clinical symptoms of the tumor has hampered the initiation of preventive programs in this disease. In addition, reducing tobacco consumption has major economic and political ramifications. In spite of the increasing knowledge of the biology of the disease and the development of new active cytostatic drugs and targeted therapies against lung cancer, the long-term survival rate remains low, implying that the treatment of lung cancer will continue to be a major therapeutic challenge for many years to come. Data from the Eurocare database imply that there are fairly large variations in survival within Europe, and that despite improvements in both the diagnosis and treatment, the overall prognosis for patients with nonsmall cell lung cancer (NSCLC) has hardly improved over time. In contrast, the introduction and improvement of chemotherapy since the 1970s have given rise to an improvement in survival in small cell lung cancer (SCLC) (1). In the most recent update of the Eurocare study, including data from 83 cancer registries on 2.7 million cancer patients, the five-year survival for all lung cancer patients has increased from 9.2% in 1990–1994 to 10.2% in 1995–1999 (2) and 10.9% in 2000–2002 (3).

EPIDEMIOLOGY AND ETIOLOGY
Incidence and Mortality
The incidence of lung cancer has increased rapidly during the last four decades and lung cancer is now the most common cancer in the world according to the most recent studies. It has been estimated that approximately 1.35 million throughout the world were diagnosed with lung cancer in year 2002, corresponding to 18% of all cancers in the more developed regions of the world and 16% in the rest of the world (4). The estimated number of lung cancer deaths in 2003 was 1.18 million—more than for any other type of cancer (5). The frequency seems to be leveling off in men in some countries but it continues to rise in other countries and in women. The mortality trends for men and for women vary considerably in the world, including the European countries; the trend since the 1980s of a decreasing incidence of lung cancer among men and an increasing incidence among women observed in northern Europe

seems to occur later in southern and eastern Europe (Fig. 8.1), most probably as a result of more recent changes in smoking habits among women in the latter countries (6). Among women, the peak in incidence was not reached in the 1990s. If this pattern continues, a dramatic increase is to be expected among women in southern and eastern Europe and in other parts of the world, such as countries in Asia, North Africa, and South America within the next two decades. In addition, the proportion of adenocarcinoma has been increasing over time and is expected to continue rising—the most likely explanation being the shift to low-tar filter cigarettes, which allow deep inhalations of the smoke into the periphery of the lung. A second complementary hypothesis suggests that smoking low-tar cigarettes may increase the risk for adenocarcinoma because of the higher nitrate content of these cigarettes. In contrast, the incidence of more centrally located histological tumor types (squamous cell carcinoma and small cell carcinoma) is decreasing.

Risk Factors and Prevention
It is well established that the dominant risk factor for lung cancer is cigarette smoking, causing 90% of all lung cancers in the developed world. It is estimated that giving up smoking at 60 years of age reduces the lifetime risk of lung cancer by 40%, giving up at 50, 40, and 30 years of age reduces the risk by 60%, 80%, and 90%, respectively. The risk increases with the number of cigarettes smoked daily, the duration of smoking, young age at onset of smoking, degree of inhalation, the tar and nicotine content, and the use of unfiltered cigarettes. Also other types of smoking, including passive smoking, and occupational exposures to carcinogenic agents such as asbestos fibers, arsenic compounds, alkylating agents, chromium compounds, mustard gas, nickel compounds, ionizing radiation, soots, tars, and some mineral oils, are associated with the risk of developing lung cancer. A multiplicative, synergistic interaction has been observed for asbestos, ionizing radiation, and arsenic compounds in combination with tobacco smoking, in such a way that the combined exposure is associated with a lung cancer risk that far exceeds that expected from the separate exposure to each of the agents. In many European countries, the risk of pleural mesothelioma will continue to increase among males and also among women but at a much lower level. The delayed period effect of the asbestos regulation by the late 1970s in many countries will probably have its greatest effects in the mesothelioma rates around 2010.

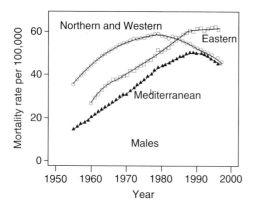
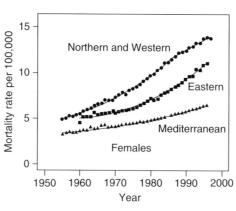

Figure 8.1 Estimated incidence and mortality of cancer of the lung. *Source*: From Ref. 6.

As the association between certain definite factors, as mentioned above, and lung cancer is well established, prevention by eliminating risk factors seems obvious, and, fortunately, preventive activities are being established in many countries and recently also with increasing, but modest, governmental support. However, there is still a major need for public information, especially for young people, about this manmade disease that was almost unknown about a century ago.

EARLY DETECTION AND SCREENING

The major problem in the treatment of lung cancer has been that patients at the time of exhibiting symptoms, and thus diagnosis, usually have had advanced stage disease. This has encouraged researchers to set up screening programs to detect the disease in more localized stages. Screening programs using chest radiographs and sputum cytology have been disappointing, as these tests not were able to decrease mortality from lung cancer (7). New technology have since emerged giving hope to better screening modalities, and recent studies using spiral CT screening in combination with sputum cytology seem to detect more early stage lung cancers than previous screening tools. It is still controversial whether spiral CT screening can decrease lung cancer mortality (8,9) and a number of randomized studies are ongoing in the United States, Europe, and Japan with data on disease-specific mortality (10). Apart from imaging, also molecular markers are being investigated as screening tools. Especially in high-risk populations, lung cancer molecular diagnostics, including chemoprevention, could become an important part of future screening methodologies (11). When the best screening tool has been identified, other issues remain to be elucidated, such as health-economic calculations and identification of the optimal screening population, before screening programs can become part of the healthcare standard prevention program, such as screening for breast cancer and cervical cancer.

LUNG CANCER BIOLOGY AND ITS APPLICATION TO CLINICAL PRACTICE
Histogenesis, DNA Damage, and Genetic Alterations
All normal cells in the tracheobronchial tree originate from differentiation of an epithelial pluripotent stem cell, which probably is also responsible for the development of lung tumors, expressing various phenotypes. If DNA damage occurs in the lung epithelium, for example, as a result of carcinogens, it is of great importance that repair takes place in order to avoid malignant transformation of the cell. It is conceivable that certain individuals may be genetically predisposed to lung cancer, for example, by the manner in which DNA damage is repaired and carcinogens are activated or inactivated. There is increasing evidence to indicate that many cancers arise via a multistep process in which multiple genetic alterations occur affecting the control of cell differentiation, cell division, and growth. Examples of such genetic alterations in lung cancers are loss of chromosomal material, for example, deletion of material from chromosome region 3p21; mutations of tumor-suppressor genes, such as p53, and mutations or changes in the levels of expression of proto-oncogenes, for example, RAS, NEU, JUN, MYC, and c-ERB-B2 (12). The frequency of genetic alterations differs among the various types of lung cancer, and these changes are most likely not only important for tumorigenesis but also for tumor growth and spread. Other processes seem to be activated by for example, p53 mutations, which influence apoptosis, induce insensitivity to antigrowth signals, and leads to genomic instability predisposing to other alterations. In addition, considerable "crosstalk" between components of the different systems mentioned above, is observed (12). The prognostic impact of some of these genetic factors has been studied clinically by genomic and proteomic assays, showing prognostic impact in subgroups of operated NSCLC. However, these findings have not been used clinically. It has been demonstrated that molecular markers (13) may predict patient benefit from chemotherapy (ERCC1, RRM1, p27(kip1), p53 expression) or targeted therapy (different EGFr forms). Direct genetic therapy as an approach in lung cancer therapy still seems difficult, as it is well established that not only lung cancer, but malignant diseases in general arise after numerous molecular changes, many of which are interrelated.

Growth Factors, Angiogenesis, and Proteolytic Enzymes
A number of peptides have been identified in human lung cancer cell lines. Insulin-like growth factor (IGF), epidermal

growth factor (EGF), vascular epidermal growth factor (VEGF), and transforming growth factor (TGF) are examples of growth factors acting in lung cancer by binding to specific receptors, and thereby influencing both tumor growth and angiogenesis. Experimental in vitro studies have shown that blocking of the receptors EGFr and VEGFr inhibit the growth of lung cancer cell lines, and drugs acting directly against the receptors, as antibodies, or inhibiting the receptor tyrosine kinase have been developed. These compounds have been tested in clinical trials, and have in combination with chemotherapy shown poorer results than expected, probably because of antagonism (14).

Also several enzymes and peptide hormones are produced and released by lung cancer cells. A great number of these substances are consistently produced by SCLCs and less often by the other major histological types. With regard to the expression of genetic alterations and growth factors there is considerable overlap of properties supporting the concept of a common origin for all lung cancers, but differing with respect to biological qualities. SCLCs are particularly well known for the ectopic production of hormones. Serum from such patients often shows elevated levels of, for example, hormones such as calcitonin, adrenocorticotrophic hormone (ACTH), antidiuretic hormone, and neuron-specific enolase (NSE), oxytocin resulting in various paraneoplastic syndromes see later. In SCLC cell lines drugs inhibiting the proteasome, farnesyltransferase, and Bcl2 have been tested and are now moving into clinical studies (15).

HISTOPATHOLOGY OF MALIGNANT TUMORS OF THE LUNG AND PLEURA

As mentioned, bronchogenic carcinoma apparently originates as a single malignant clone, but rapid cell proliferation and mutations result in the creation of heterogeneous tumors with many subpopulations. This heterogeneity is microscopically reflected by the presence of various histological types, indicating differentiation in more than one direction, even in the same patient.

More than 95% of bronchial tumors can be classified into four major cell types: squamous cell carcinoma (WHO I), small cell carcinoma (WHO II), adenocarcinoma (WHO III), and large cell carcinoma (WHO IV) (Table 8.1). The remaining 5% include mesotheliomas and carcinoids. Table 8.1 shows the most recent classification published by the WHO in collaboration with the International Academy of Pathology and International Association for the Study of Lung Cancer (IASLC) and it shows the morphologic codes of the International Classification for Oncology and the systematized Nomenclature of Medicine (16). The relative frequency of each type varies among different series and different countries. This variation may not only be based on geographical differences, but may also reflect variations in the histopathological classification applied. The frequency of small cell carcinoma seems rather constant (15–25%), whereas the variations in frequency for WHO I, III, and IV are somewhat greater with a steady increase in adenocarcinoma over the last two decades. For practical and therapeutic purposes the last three types are commonly referred to as NSCLC. The diagnosis of lung cancer is usually carried out on the basis of histopathological biopsy

material obtained at bronchoscopy, mediastinoscopy, lung biopsy, and the like. In some cases it may be difficult to obtain material for histopathological evaluation and the diagnosis is then based on the less precise cytological material. The WHO classification is based on light microscopic criteria using common staining procedures. Results of electron microscopy and immunohistochemistry are usually not included as diagnostic criteria in the classification, but they may in some cases clarify the diagnosis.

Squamous cell carcinoma is associated with squamous metaplasia and carcinoma in situ in its earliest form and with further growth the tumor invades the basement membrane and extends into the bronchial lumen. The tumor is histologically composed of sheets of epithelial cells being well or poorly differentiated with the most well-differentiated cells demonstrating keratin pearls, whereas the more poorly differentiated ones have positive keratin staining.

Small cell carcinoma is characterized by diffuse growth or solid nests of small cells with oval to spindle nuclei, finely granular nuclei, inconspicuous nucleoli, thin nuclear membrane, scanty faintly stained, or very finely granular and ill-defined cell borders. Cancer cells are smaller than lymphocytes. Mitotic figures are frequently seen, often 60 to 70 per high power field. A variant combined small cell carcinoma is defined as small cell carcinoma combined with nonsmall cell elements, such as adenocarcinoma, squamous cell- or large cell carcinoma. Using immunohistochemistry SCLCs can often be distinguished from NSCLCs by a more frequent expression of neuroendocrine differentiation markers, such as, for example, NSE, chromogranin, and the like. The presence of these markers is, however, not diagnostic for SCLCs.

Adenocarcinomas form glands and produce mucin. Within adenocarcinomas, bronchoalveolar carcinoma is pathologically different, showing growth along alveolar septa and little if any desmoplastic or glandular change. Adenocarcinomas may stain positively for carcinoembryonic antigen (CEA) and keratin.

Large cell carcinoma is the less frequent type of lung cancer (<15%); large cell, undifferentiated carcinomas usually have sheets of highly atypical cells with focal necrosis without keratinization or gland formation, and, occasionally the presence of multinucleated "giant cells."

Carcinoid tumors, which are seen more rarely, are believed to arise from enterochromaffin cells and are able to secrete a variety of components. Histologically, it is difficult to distinguish between benign and malignant tumors. The tumors are composed of monotonous sheets of small, round cells with uniform nuclei and cytoplasm. Another rare tumor is mesothelioma, which arises from pleura. There are three histological variants, the epithelial form characterized by tubular, papillary, solid, or vacuolated cells is the most frequently occurring type (60%), whereas the sarcomatoid and mixed forms are less common.

The histopathological classification constitutes a significant, independent prognostic factor, with a relatively better prognosis being obtained for squamous cell carcinoma. Among the adenocarcinomas, the bronchioloalveolar carcinoma has a better prognosis than the other subtypes with special biologic features (17), and for both squamous cell carcinoma and adenocarcinoma the outcome for the

Table 8.1   Histological Classification of Lung and Pleural Tumors

1   Epithelial tumors
   1.3   Malignant
      1.3.1   Squamous cell carcinoma Variants
         1.3.1.1   Papillary
         1.3.1.2   Clear cell
         1.3.1.3   Small cell
         1.3.1.4   Basaloid
      1.3.2   Small cell carcinoma Variant
         1.3.2.1   Combined
      1.3.3   Adenocarcinoma
         1.3.3.1   Acinar
         1.3.3.2   Papillary
         1.3.3.3   Bronchioloalveolar carcinoma
            1.3.3.3.1   Nonmucinous
            1.3.3.3.2   Mucinous
            1.3.3.3.3   Mixed mucinous and nonmucinous or indeterminate cell type
         1.3.3.4   Solid adenocarcinoma with mucin
         1.3.3.5   Adenocarcinoma with mixed subtypes
         1.3.3.6   Variants
            1.3.3.6.1   Well-differentiated fetal adenocarcinoma
            1.3.3.6.2   Mucinous ("colloid") adenocarcinoma
            1.3.3.6.3   Mucinous cystadenocarcinom
            1.3.3.6.4   Signet-ring adenocarcinoma
            1.3.3.6.5   Clear cell adenocarcinoma
      1.3.4   Large cell carcinoma Variants
         1.3.4.1   Large cell neuroendocrine carcinoma
            1.3.4.1.1   Combined large cell neuroendocrine carcinoma
         1.3.4.2   Basaloid carcinoma
         1.3.4.3   Lymphoepithelioma-like carcinoma
         1.3.4.4   Clear cell carcinoma
         1.3.4.5   Large cell carcinoma with rhabdoid phenotype
      1.3.5   Adenosquamous carcinoma
      1.3.6   Carcinomas with pleomorphic, sarcomatoid, or sarcomatous elements
         1.3.6.1   Carcinomas with spindle and/or giant cells
            1.3.6.1.1   Pleomorphic carcinoma
            1.3.6.1.2   Spindle cell carcinoma
            1.3.6.1.3   Giant cell carcinoma
         1.3.6.2   Carcinosarcoma
         1.3.6.3   Pulmonary blastoma
         1.3.6.4   Others
      1.3.7   Carcinoid tumor
         1.3.7.1   Typical carcinoid
         1.3.7.2   Atypical carcinois
      1.3.8   Carcinomas of salivary gland type
         1.3.8.1   Mucoepidermoid carcinoma
         1.3.8.2   Adenoid cystic carcinoma
         1.3.8.3   Others
      1.3.9   Unclassified carcinoma

well-differentiated tumors is better than for the poorly differentiated tumors.

CLINICAL PRESENTATIONS AND SYMPTOMS
Locoregional and Metastatic Manifestations

The signs and symptoms manifested by the lung cancer patient depend on the location of the tumor, its locoregional spread, the effect of metastatic growth, and possibly paraneoplastic syndromes, which are more frequent in lung cancer than in any other type of cancer. Ten to fifteen per cent of lung cancers are detected incidentally in the asymptomatic state on a chest radiograph, including screening. These tumors are usually small and therefore associated with a higher rate of resectability and a better five-year survival rate than symptomatic tumors.

The most frequently presenting signs and symptoms for NSCLC and SCLC patients are given in Table 8.2 (18). The local symptoms include cough, hemoptysis, dyspnea, and chest pain, with the development of cough or a change in the character of a preexisting cough being the most common symptom. Dyspnea is a frequent symptom, which may be caused by pleural effusion, diaphragmatic paralysis resulting from phrenic nerve involvement, obstructive pneumonitis or lymphangitic metastases. In addition, lung cancer patients often have coexistent chronic obstructive pulmonary disease that contributes to their dyspnea. Chest pain may be present in patients with tumors invading the

Table 8.2 Presenting Signs and Symptoms in 1024 Patients with Lung Cancer (Based on Data from Ref. 18)

Symptoms	Percentage of patients with	
	NSCLC	SCLC
Cough	45	49
Dyspnea	37	53
Hemoptysis	33	30
Chest pain	27	48
Anorexia	22	37
Fatigue	22	37
Weight loss (>10% body weight)	16	21
Wheeze	10	23
Bone pain	10	13
Hoarseness	7	21
Dysphagia	3	9
Asymptomatic	15	5

Table 8.3 Paraneoplastic Syndromes Associated with Bronchogenic Carcinoma

Endocrine	Musculoskeletal and cutaneous
Cushing's syndrome	Hypertrophic osteoarthropathy
Inappropriate ADH secretion	Clubbing
Hypercalcemia	Dermatomyositis
Carcinoid syndrome	Acanthosis nigricans
Gynecomastia	Pruritus
Hyperglycemia	Urticaria
Hypoglycemia	Erythema multiforme
Galactorrhea	Hyperpigmentation
Growth hormone excess	**Hematological**
Secretion of thyroid-stimulating	Hemolytic anemia
hormone	Red cell aplasia
Calcitonin secretion	Polycythemia
Neuromuscular	Thrombocytosis
Polymyositis	Eosinophilia
Myasthenic syndrome	Leukoerythroblastic reaction
Sensorimotor neuropathy	including thrombocytopenia
Encephalopathy	**Others**
Myelopathy	Nephrotic syndrome
Psychosis	Hyperuricemia
Dementia	Amyloidosis
Cardiovascular	
Superficial thrombophlebitis	
Arterial thrombosis	
Marantic endocarditis	

pleura or chest wall. Hoarseness and dysphagia can occur as results of vocal cord paralysis by pressure on the left recurrent laryngeal nerve in the mediastinum, and through compression of the esophagus by mediastinal lymphadenopathy or direct invasion of primary tumor in esophagus, respectively. Anorexia, fatigue, and weight loss are less specific but frequently occurring symptoms, often associated with metastatic spread. Two frequent clinical syndromes associated with lung cancer are related to the local effects of the tumor: superior vena cava syndrome (SVCS) and Pancoast's syndrome (or superior sulcus tumors). The SVCS consists of edema of the face and upper extremities, along with dilated superficial veins in the neck, arms, and thorax. This is most frequently observed in SCLC and it may be caused either by direct invasion of the superior vena cava or by compression from mediastinal metastases. Pancoast's syndrome is caused by a tumor in the apex of the lung, which may also involve the first and second ribs, vertebral column, spinal cord, and brachial plexus. As a result of involvement of the cervical sympathetic nerves, Horner's syndrome may also be present in patients with Pancoast's syndrome. Pancoast's tumors are often squamous cell carcinomas and adenocarcinomas, rarely, small cell carcinoma.

Frequently, evidence of extrathoracic metastases is seen at the time of diagnosis. Lymph node enlargement in the supraclavicular and cervical regions may be initial findings. Bone pain is also a common presenting symptom, caused by osseous metastases. The spine, pelvis, femur, ribs, and skull are the most frequently involved regions, but any bone may be affected. If hepatomegaly occurs as a presenting symptom it is most likely that the patient has SCLC. In 10–15% of lung cancer patients, evidence of metastases to the central nervous system is the initial manifestation, including cerebral and cerebellar metastases, again mostly observed in SCLC.

Paraneoplastic Syndromes

Paraneoplastic syndromes are often specific entities caused by remote, nonmetastatic effects of the tumor. They may be present in 10–20% of all lung cancer patients (Table 8.3) and are most commonly observed in SCLC.

Ectopic ACTH production may produce Cushing's syndrome, while inappropriate secretion of antidiuretic hormone (the Eaton–Lambert syndrome) may cause severe hyponatremia. Hypercalcemia is usually caused by osseous metastases or by ectopic secretion of parathyroid-like hormone, an osteolytic substance or prostaglandin; hypercalcemia is often observed in NSCLC and rarely in SCLC in spite of the high frequency of bone marrow metastases in SCLC. Less frequent endocrine syndromes include carcinoid syndrome, gynecomastia, and hypoglycemia.

A neurological paraneoplastic syndrome associated with SCLC is the myasthenic syndrome (Eaton–Lambert syndrome). Rarely, ataxia caused by cerebellar degeneration or cerebral atrophy may be a presenting symptom.

Several musculoskeletal and cutaneous manifestations are also occasionally seen, including digital clubbing, hypertrophic pulmonary osteoarthropathy, polymyositis, acanthosis nigricans, and dermatomyositis.

The most common hematological abnormalities include anemia of chronic disease, whereas thrombocytopenia is often a sign of bone marrow metastases in SCLC.

DIAGNOSIS AND STAGING OF LUNG CANCER
Detection of Primary Tumor and Locoregional Spread

To verify a suspicion of lung cancer a chest radiograph is generally the first procedure following the clinical examination. Tumors must be at least 1 cm in greatest diameter to be detectable by chest radiography. A chest radiograph is best at detecting peripherally located cancers, which are most likely to be large cell carcinomas and adenocarcinomas, whereas centrally located or hilar lesions are more likely to be small cell carcinomas or squamous cell carcinomas. Chest radiography also allows evaluation of the anatomical extent of the tumor, including mediastinal metastases, chest wall involvement, metastases to the ribs, tracheal compression, pleural effusion, and atelectasis, whereas computed tomography (CT) is especially valuable in defining more accurately multiple nodules, multiple intrapulmonary lesions, mediastinal lymphadenopathy, and chest wall or mediastinal invasion. More recently, endobronchial ultrasonography (EBUS) with transbronchial needle aspiration and, especially, 18F-fluorodeoxyglucose (FDG) positron emission tomography (18FDG-PET) with or without a CT have emerged as important procedures in the workup of patients with (suspected) lung cancer. This is so especially in the evaluation of the mediastinum, including lymph node involvement (19) and the procedure is now recommended by the European Society of Thoracic Surgeons, American College of Chest Physicians, and European Society of Medical Oncology (20–22).

Also in the evaluation of mediastinal response, PET-CT evaluation is superior to repeat mediastinoscopy with sensitivity, specificity, and accuracy of PET-CT being 77%, 92%, and 83%, respectively, whereas those for repeat mediastinoscopy were 29%, 100%, and 60%, respectively. Sensitivity ($p < 0.0001$) and accuracy ($p = 0.012$) were thus significantly better for PET-CT compared with mediastinoscopy (23).

When a tumor has been visualized on a chest radiograph or by CT, a biopsy is essential for obtaining the right diagnosis. The introduction of the flexible fiber optic bronchoscope has enabled the diagnosis of lung cancer to be made by a procedure that albeit invasive, is fast, safe, and performed under local anesthesia. Using the flexible scope the endobronchial distance that may be visualized has been extended to include third and fourth order bronchi. If lung lesions are visible, the rate of positive diagnoses from bronchial brushings and biopsy is up to 90%, the success rate depending on the size of the tumor. Small cell carcinoma has a tendency to cause submucosal invasion, so a deep biopsy should be performed, and this is also necessary in areas with swollen mucosa without visible tumor.

To obtain material from intrapulmonary lesions and mediastinal lymph nodes, transbronchial biopsy aspiration, sometimes ultrasound guided, should be carried out using special needles. If diagnostic material cannot be obtained by bronchoscopy, other procedures should be applied, such as transthoracic needle aspiration or thoracoscopy with biopsy, or thoracocentesis if pleural effusion is present. Mediastinoscopy or mediastinotomy are important techniques to assess superior mediastinal lymph nodes; more recently developed methods include video-assisted thoracoscopy. In selected cases thoracotomy may be needed before the diagnosis of lung cancer can be established.

Detection of Distant Metastases

Systemic manifestations of lung cancer are present in more than 50% of cases at diagnosis, so once the diagnosis of lung cancer is made, and before therapy is chosen, an evaluation of the extent of the disease is required. Most patients undergo chest radiography, CT of the chest and abdomen, and/or ultrasonography to detect mediastinal lymph node enlargement or unsuspected pulmonary, liver, or adrenal metastases. As metastases to liver, bone, and brain are the most frequent distant metastatic sites in lung cancer, with varying frequency dependent on histological types, procedures to detect these metastases are usually applied in lung cancer patients.

Biochemical variables, such as transaminases, bilirubin, alkaline phosphatase, and coagulation factors are used to detect liver (and bone) metastases, but the specificity of these is low, and other noninvasive diagnostic imaging procedures may be more helpful. Liver metastases can be detected with either ultrasonography with biopsy or CT, with the last having a greater potential of revealing abnormalities located in the adrenals, pancreatic region, and retroperitoneal lymph nodes.

When lung cancer affects the bones, two organs may be involved: the bone marrow or the osseous tissue, clinically characterized by either hemopoietic changes such as thrombocytopenia and/or bone pain. The bone marrow can often be evaluated by aspiration and biopsy from the iliac crest—routine procedures in small cell carcinoma. Bone radiography is too insensitive to be used for screening, but may be relevant when specific bone pain is present. Bone scans are rarely used anymore, but have been replaced by magnetic resonance imaging (MRI) as the best procedure to detect malignant bone lesions.

Central nervous system (CNS) metastases can often be revealed by a thorough clinical neurological examination, lumbar puncture with cytological evaluation of the cerebrospinal fluid and supplemented by myelography, CT, and MRI, depending on the clinical signs and symptoms. The recommended routine staging investigations are depicted in Table 8.4.

Staging Systems

The TNM classification is the most commonly used staging system: T indicates the localization and size of the primary tumor including possible local invasion; N is the degree of nodal involvement; and M is the presence of distant metastases (24). The TNM descriptors are outlined in Table 8.5. Applying the TNM classification, patients with lung cancer can be staged into various groups, as indicated in Table 8.5; the stages can be subdivided into five categories depending on the origin of the information on which the staging is performed. *Clinical diagnostic staging* (cTNM), permits the incorporation of information from all investigations performed before treatment; *surgical evaluative staging* (sTNM), is based on information from thoracotomy; *pathological staging* (pTNM), is possible if resection is undertaken and a detailed histological assessment is available, whereas *retreatment staging* (rTNM), may include additional investigations obtained if further treatment has become necessary. *Autopsy staging* (aTNM), is based on postmortem findings. The lung cancer stages include: occult carcinoma, Stage 0, Stage I, Stage II, Stage IIIa and b, and Stage IV defined according to the latest revision of the International System for Staging of Lung Cancer (24,25):

- *Occult stage*: TXN0M0. An occult carcinoma with bronchopulmonary secretions containing malignant cells but without other evidence of tumor, metastases to the regional lymph nodes or distant metastases.
- *Stage 0*: TisN0M0. Carcinoma in situ.
- *Stage I*: T1N0M0, T2N0M0. A tumor that can be classified as T1 with no metastases, or T2 without any metastases

Table 8.4 Recommended Staging Procedures for Patients with Lung Cancer—Clinical Practice

Procedure	Local treatment modality under consideration	
	No	Yes
General procedures		
Patient history	+	+
Physical examination		
Blood counts	+	+
Serum biochemistry		
Cytological or histological documentation	+	+
Procedures for local disease		
Chest radiograph	+	+
Chest computed tomography	–	+
Fiber bronchoscopy	–	+
Mediastinoscopy	–	+[a]
Endoesophageal ultrasound (EUS)		
Endobronchial ultrasonography (EBUS)	–	+[a]
Positron emission tomography (PET)		
18-FDG-PET	–	+[a]
Cytology of effusion	–	+
Cytology of supraclavicular node	–	+[b]
Procedures for distant disease		
Bone		
Bone scan	–	+[e]
Bone radiographs	–	+[c,e]
MR scan	–	+[c,e]
Liver and retroperitoneal organs		
Ultrasonography or abdominal computed tomography with fine-needle aspiration/biopsy	–	+[e]
Bone marrow: aspirate and biopsy	–	+[d]
Brain: computed tomography or MR-scan	–	+[f]

[a]Only if needed by surgeon for preoperative work-up.
[b]If the findings are doubtful and the establishment of a positive finding affects the treatment.
[c]Only of areas of increased uptake on bone scan.
[d]Only in small cell carcinoma.
[e]Only if either serum biochemistry is abnormal or patient has clinical symptoms.
[f]Only if clinical symptoms are present.

Table 8.5 Stage Grouping of TNM Subsets[a]

Stage	TNM Subset
0	Carcinoma in situ
IA	T1N0M0
IB	T2N0M0
IIA	T1N1M0
IIB	T2N1M0
	T3N0M0
IIIA	T3N1M0
	T1N2M0
	T2N2M0
	T3N2M0
IIIB	T4N0M0
	T4N1M0
	T4N2M0
	T1N3M0
	T2N3M0
	T3N3M0
	T4N3M0
IV	Any T Any N M1

[a]Staging is not relevant for occult carcinoma, designated TXN0M0

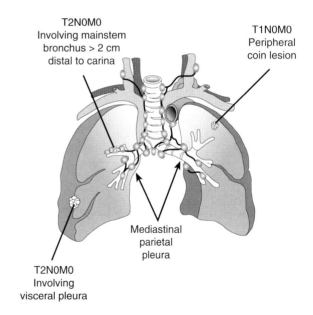

Stage I
No lymph node involvement

T2N0M0
Involving mainstem bronchus > 2 cm distal to carina

T1N0M0
Peripheral coin lesion

Mediastinal parietal pleura

T2N0M0
Involving visceral pleura

Figure 8.2 Stage I disease. *Source*: From Ref. 74.

to nodes or distant organs. TXN1M0 is theoretically possible but clinically difficult to make. If such a diagnosis occurs, it would be included in this stage (Fig. 8.2).
- *Stage IIa*: T1N1M0. A tumor classified as T1 with metastases to the lymph nodes in the peribronchial ipsilateral hilar region only (Fig. 8.3).
- *Stage IIb*: T2N1M0, T3N0M0. A tumor classified as either T2 or T3 with metastases to the lymph nodes in the peribronchial or ipsilateral hilar region only (Fig. 8.4).
- *Stage IIIa*: T3N1M0, T1N2M0, T2N2M0, T3N2M0. Any tumor with ipsilateral mediastinal lymph nodes only or T3 tumor without contralateral mediastinal, scalene, supraclavicular or distant metastases (Fig. 8.5).
- *Stage IIIb*: T4N0M0, T4N1M0, T4N2M0, T1N3M0, T2N3M0, T3N3M0, T4N3M0. Any tumor with contralateral, mediastinal, scalene, or supraclavicular lymph nodes or any T4 tumor without spread beyond the thorax (Fig. 8.6)
- *Stage IV*: Any tumor with distant metastases.

The TNM subsets and the stage grouping are outlined in Table 8.5. The staging of lung cancer by the TNM staging system is also referred to as the New International Staging System (ISS) because American, Japanese, and European cancer committees have agreed in 1986 on this worldwide staging system, and it is now used extensively. The most recent revision took place in 1997 (24) and was based on a relatively small surgically treated cohort of 5319 patients treated in the United States. Therefore, the International Association for the Study of Lung Cancer

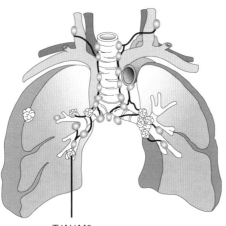

Stage IIA
Intrapulmonary and/or hilar nodes involved
Tumor <3 cm

T1N1M0
<3 cm involving
ipsilateral peribronchial and/or
ipsilateral hilar lymph nodes

Figure 8.3   Stage IIA disease.

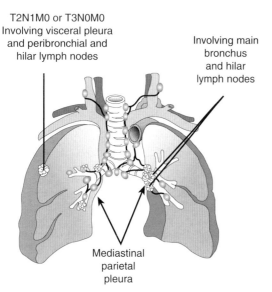

Stage IIB
Intrapulmonary and/or hilar nodes involved
Tumor >3 cm

T2N1M0 or T3N0M0
Involving visceral pleura
and peribronchial and
hilar lymph nodes

Involving main
bronchus
and hilar
lymph nodes

Mediastinal
parietal
pleura

Figure 8.4   Stage IIB.

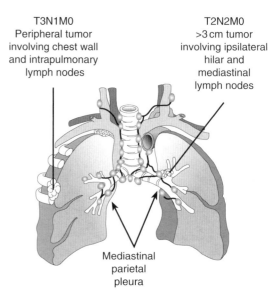

Stage IIIA

T3N1M0
Peripheral tumor
involving chest wall
and intrapulmonary
lymph nodes

T2N2M0
>3 cm tumor
involving ipsilateral
hilar and
mediastinal
lymph nodes

Mediastinal
parietal
pleura

Figure 8.5   Stage IIIA disease.

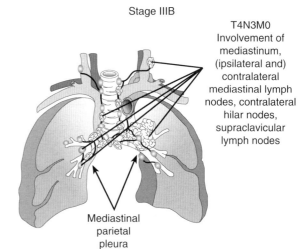

Stage IIIB

T4N3M0
Involvement of
mediastinum,
(ipsilateral and)
contralateral
mediastinal lymph
nodes, contralateral
hilar nodes,
supraclavicular
lymph nodes

Mediastinal
parietal
pleura

Figure 8.6   Stage IIIB disease. *Source*: From Ref. 74.

(IASLC) has initiated a global (including entries from Europe, North America, Asia, and Australia) retrospective dataset covering patients treated for primary lung cancer from 1990 to 2000. Recent reports of the IASLC Lung Cancer Staging Project provide proposals of the TNM descriptors in the seventh edition of the TNM classification system. This TNM staging system is scheduled to be pub-

lished after approval by the UICC and AJCC in 2009. Unlike the current sixth edition of the TNM classification, which was internally validated only, data in the IASLC database were subjected to internal validation using a larger data set and external validation using the Surveillance Epidemiology and End Results Cancer Registry. The IASLC project has been summarized recently, including presentation of the new proposed staging system (24).

The lung cancer stages are quite accurate in predicting overall survival in lung cancer patients (Fig. 8.7), and despite the emergence of biochemical and genetic markers as prognostic indicators, stage together with histological type is still the strongest predictive parameter.

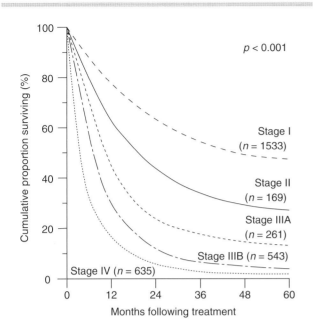

Figure 8.7 Cumulative proportion of patients surviving five years by clinical stage of disease (1986 classification). *Source:* From Ref. 74.

TREATMENT

The management of lung cancer should primarily be based on the histopathological type, secondarily on the stage. NSCLC represents one treatment group and SCLC another. Accordingly, the treatment will be described separately. Less common lung tumors include neuroendocrine tumors including carcinoids and pleural malignancies, such as mesothelioma.

Nonsmall Cell Lung Cancer

Surgery

The primary curative treatment for NSCLC is surgery. In stages I and II a complete surgical resection is almost always possible. Before surgery is performed, evaluation of the pulmonary function is necessary to estimate the maximum tolerated extent of pulmonary resection. The extent of the resection should preferably be planned in advance, even though final selection of the operative procedures must take place at the time of operation. The procedure of choice is the one that encompasses all existing tumor tissue and provides maximum conservation of the lung tissue, as determined by the location and degree of tumor involvement, including sampling of all mediastinal nodal stations or complete lymph node dissection. Segmental resection will be selected for patients with small, peripheral tumors (<2 cm in diameter), with no evidence of extension or metastases (T1N0M0). Lobectomy is performed for patients with a centrally located tumor mass within the lobe, and an adequate tumor-free margin is required for this type of resection. There may be lymph node extension or metastases that are limited to intrapulmonary or immediate hilar lymphatic drainage which can be totally encompassed by "en bloc dissection." Pneumonectomy is the procedure of choice for patients having

more extensive disease, with tumors extending to the orifice of the lobar bronchus and tumors originating within or extending to the main stem bronchus, with involvement of more than one lobe. Within recent years, video-assisted thoracic surgery is gaining ground being less traumatic. The therapeutic role of mediastinal lymph node dissection is at present uncertain (26).

Adjuvant Therapy in Resectable Stage I, II, and IIIa

As more than two-thirds of all resected patients relapse, great attention has been given to adjuvant treatment, such as postoperative radiation therapy and adjuvant chemotherapy, and numerous randomized studies have also been undertaken. The rationale for applying postoperative chemotherapy is to achieve reduction of circulating tumor cells and eradication of subclinical metastases not recognized at surgery. Various cytotoxic agents and combinations have been used as postoperative adjuvant chemotherapy in randomized prospective studies, but with disappointing results and until recently without major survival benefit, as demonstrated in a meta-analysis performed in 1995 (27). Data from 14 randomized trials, both published and unpublished, including 4357 patients were analyzed. Five trials employed alkylating agents and six had cisplatin-based regimens. Tegafur or UFT were administered in the remaining three trials. Alkylating agents were detrimental. The hazard ratio estimate of 1.15 ($p = 0.005$) favored surgery alone. This 15% increase in the risk of death translated into an absolute decrease in survival of 4% at two years and 5% at five years. Cisplatin-based chemotherapy was beneficial; the absolute improvements were 3% at two years and 5% at five years ($p = 0.08$). The trials employing Tegafur and UFT were found to have a hazard ratio of 0.89 ($p = 0.30$) in favor of chemotherapy. Based on these results, postoperative chemotherapy was not routinely adopted in 1995, but the results constituted the rationale for a new generation of randomized trials with cisplatin-based regimens performed in Europe, United States, and Japan.

The results of some of these trials have been published and a meta-analysis including five of these cisplatin-based chemotherapy trials with 4584 patients have been performed. The analysis demonstrated a hazard ration of 0.89 (95% CI 0.82–0.96, $p = 0.004$), which translates into a survival benefit of 5.3% ± 1.6% at five years by adjuvant chemotherapy for the total group. Cisplatin and vinorelbine was the most widely used chemotherapy protocols. Based on these data, cisplatin-based adjuvant chemotherapy is recommended in Stages II and IIIA whereas it is optional in Stage IB (28).

With respect to postoperative radiotherapy after complete resection, it does decrease the rate of local recurrences, but has no significant impact on survival, probably because distant metastases are common regardless of the control of intrathoracic disease (29). The topic remains controversial—especially after the Post-Operative Radiation Trial's (PORT) group concluded in a meta-analysis that postoperative radiotherapy in patients with stages I and II may be associated with a detrimental effect (30). The main criticism of the PORT analysis is the failure to consider the way in which radiotherapy is administered, including the use of Cobalt 60 irradiations.

Preoperative and Postoperative Therapies in Potentially Resectable Stage IIIa

In NSCLC patients with Stage III disease other than T3 lesions, the extent of disease usually prohibits surgical resection. Therefore, investigations have been initiated in which different types of preoperative chemotherapy or radiotherapy, either alone or in combination, has been applied to minimize the extent of tumor before surgery, thereby increasing the possibility of radical resection. Some studies have shown encouraging results with regard to downstaging using chemotherapy and/or radiotherapy, but the final impact on survival still awaits the results of larger, randomized studies.

Combined Modality Therapy in Unresectable Stage III

As the effects of radiotherapy and chemotherapy used alone have been modest, the combination of these has been explored extensively in nonresectable and locoregional NSCLC (31,32). The efficacy of concurrent chemoradiation has been confirmed in several meta-analyses of randomized trials, showing combined modality therapy to be superior to radiation alone, and it is now considered the standard of care for the treatment of locally advanced NSCLC. What still remains to be clarified are the optimal volume, dose, schedule, and fractionation of radiotherapy, issues which are currently under investigation in multinational trials, including identification of the best chemotherapy regimen.

Chemotherapy for Stage IIIb (Malignant Pleural Effusion) and Stage IV

NSCLC is one of the most chemoresistant solid tumors with a response rate of 15–25% for single agents (Table 8.6), usually of three to five months' duration. However, when combining two or three of the most active drugs, the response rates increase to 30–50%, mainly due to new more active and less toxic cytotoxic agents, such as taxanes, vinorelbine, and gemcitabine (33). Examples of commonly used combination chemotherapy as first-line treatment are

given in Table 8.7. No one regimen has been demonstrated to be superior in the first-line treatment for patients with advanced NSCLC. At present, it is generally accepted that platinum-based chemotherapy should be standard first-line treatment to advanced NSCLC patients in good performance status, as documented median survival benefit of two to four months is achieved and symptom relief is documented to occur in 40–60% of all patients. Chemotherapy is usually administered for no more than four to six cycles in patients with Stage IV NSCLC. Until recently, none of the two-drug combinations applied had demonstrated any major differences in activity among the various histologic types of NSCLC. Very recently, however, a large study comparing cisplatin plus gemcitabine with cisplatin plus permetrexed in chemotherapy-naïve patients with advanced NSCLC, including 1735 patients, has shed new light on this question (34). Patients were not randomly assigned according to histology, but in a prespecified subset analysis of the 847 patients with adenocarcinomas there was an improved survival for the cisplatin plus pemetrexed arm compared to the cisplatin plus gemcitabine arm (12.6 vs. 10.9 months, respectively; hazard ratio 0.84; 95% CL 0.71–0.99, $p = 0.03$). In contrast, in patients with squamous cell carcinoma ($N = 473$), survival analysis favored the cisplatin plus gemcitabin arm compared with cisplatin plus premetrexed (10.8 months vs. 9.4 months, respectively; hazard ratio 1.23; 95% CL 1.00–1.51, $p = 0.05$). The authors propose a molecular rationale for these results based on the observation that premetrexed inhibits thynidylate synthetase (TS). Baseline of TS gene is significantly higher in squamous cell carcinoma than in adenocarcinoma and preclinical data suggest that there is a reduced activity of premetrexed with a high expression of TS. Further studies are obviously needed to elucidate these results, including analysis for various biomarkers.

Table 8.6 Most Frequently Chosen Active Agents for Inclusion in Combination Chemotherapy in Nonsmall Cell Lung Cancer

Alkylating agents
   Cis-platinum
   Carboplatin
   Ifosfamide
Antimitotic agentse
   Docetaxel (Taxotere®)
   Paclitaxel (Taxol®)
   Vinblastine (Velbe®)
   Vinorelbine (Navelbine®)
Antimetabolites
   Gemcitabine (Gemzar®)
   Pemetrexed (Alimta®)
Topoisomerase inhibitors
   Etoposide
   Mitomycin
   Irinotecan (Camptho®)

Table 8.7 Commonly Used Regimens in NSCLC[a]

Regimen	Doses and schedule
Cisplatin	75–80 mg/m² day 1
Paclitaxel	135 mg/m²/24 day 1 every 21 days; or 175 mg/m²/3 hr day 1
Carboplatin	AUC = 6 day 1
Paclitaxel	225 mg/m² day 1 every 21 days
Cisplatin	100 mg/m² day 1
Vinorelbine	25 mg/m²/wk every 28 days
Cisplatin	100 mg/m² day 1
Gemcitabine	1,000 mg/m²/wk every 28 days
Carboplatin	AUC = 6 day 1
Gemcitabine	1000 mg/m² day 1 and 8
Cisplatin	75 mg/m² day 1
Doxetaxel	75 mg/m² day 1 every 21 days
Gemcitabine	1100 mg/m² day 1 and 8
Docetaxel	100 mg/m² day 8 every 21 days
Paclitaxel	200 mg/m² day 1
Gemcitabine	1000 mg/m² day 1 and 8 every 21 days
Cisplatin	75 mg/m² day 1 every 3 wks
Pemetrexed	500 mg/m² day 1 every 3 wks

[a]Modified after Socinski MA, Morris DE, Masters GA et al. Chemotherapeutic management of stage IV non-small cell lung cancer. Hest 2003; 123: 226S–43S. (Ref. 32).
Abbreviation: AUC, area under the concentration curve.

With respect to the elderly patients having advanced lung cancer, treatment tends to be complicated by their comorbid conditions. However, studies have shown that the "fit" elderly are likely to benefit as much from chemotherapy as their younger counterparts (35). The response rate, toxicity, and survival in fit elderly NSCLC patients receiving combination chemotherapy, including platinum-containing regimens, appear to be similar to those in younger patients.

In a disease with poor survival it is important also to focus on the palliative effect of therapy, including quality-of-life parameters (and costs), and these parameters are being increasingly included, not only in the evaluation of clinical trials, but also in the day-to-day management of newly diagnosed patient with advanced NSCLC.

Second-line chemotherapy to NSCLC has become a new treatment option, as single-agent therapy with docetaxel in doses of 75mg/m^2 i.v. q. 3 weeks in patients not previously treated with this drug has shown both quality-of-life benefit and slight improvement in the overall survival in randomized trials when compared to best supportive care in patients with advanced NSCLC with a performance status of 0 to 2 (36). Among the newer cytostatic agents, pemetrexed (Alimta) has been shown to be noninferior to docetaxel, with a more favorable toxicity profile (37). Noteworthy is also that one of the new vincaalkaloids, vinflunine, has shown equivalent activity when compared with docetaxel as second-line treatment in a study with 557 patients with NSCLC (38).

Radiotherapy

As the vast majority of NSCLC patients present with tumors too advanced for surgery, other treatment options are necessary. Radiotherapy has an important palliative effect in controlling troublesome symptoms caused by local tumor effects or metastases, whereas the curative role is less clear, but it appears that a small, highly selected group may be cured by radical radiotherapy, using three-dimensional (3-D) conformal or stereotactic radio surgery, thereby achieving a five-year survival rate of up to 40% (39). The latter group includes otherwise operable patients in whom medical contraindication to surgery exists or in patients refusing surgery. Intended curative radiotherapy should cover a treatment volume including the primary tumor, hilar, and mediastinal lymph node areas, with a margin allowing for the microscopic extension of tumor. Various dose and fractionation schedules are used, including hyperfractionation with treatment given twice daily at total doses ranging from 5500 to 6500 Gy, yielding better results. In the pivotal study by Saunders et al (40). 563 patients were randomly allocated in a 3:2 ratio to either conventional radiotherapy (30 fractions of 2 Gy to a total dose of 60 Gy in six weeks) or continuous hyperfractionated accelerated radiotherapy (CHART) which uses 36 small fractions of 1.5 Gy given three times per day, to give 54 Gy in only 12 consecutive days. Overall, there was a 24% reduction in the relative risk of death, which is equivalent to an absolute improvement in two-year survival of 9% from 20% to 29% (95% CI 0.63–0.92). Subgroup analyses suggest that the largest benefit occurred in patients with squamous cell carcinoma.

Randomized studies of newer fractionation schedules with or without chemotherapy are exploring higher than 60 Gy conventionally fractionated doses in carefully selected patients.

Palliative radiotherapy, for example, 20 Gy in five fractions, can be used for relief of symptoms, such as hemoptysis, dyspnea caused by bronchial obstruction, dysphagia caused by mediastinal lymph node compression, superior vena caval obstruction, and local pain caused by chest wall or rib involvement (41). Also, extrathoracic manifestations of NSCLC may benefit from palliative radiotherapy. Palliative radiotherapy is also applied for brain metastases in combination with corticosteroids, usually resulting in a short-lasting effect of two to three months, with reduction of intracranial pressure and edema. In patients with compression of the spinal cord, radiotherapy is also indicated after surgical decompression. Pain caused by bone metastases can also be relieved by palliative radiotherapy and usually single fractions, for example, 8 Gy, may be sufficient.

Biologic Therapy

Much hope has been given to new biologic agents against NSCLC (42,43) including:

a. Receptor-targeted therapy
b. Signal transduction—cell cycle inhibitors
c. Angiogenetic inhibitors
d. Gene therapy
e. Vaccines

Many of these agents are now in clinical development with most experience having been obtained with the oral, small-molecule epidermal growth factor receptor tyrosine kinase inhibitors gefitinib (Iressa®) and erlotinib (Tarceva®), and the angiogenetic inhibitor bevacizumab (Avastin®) (42,43). As a single agent, gefitinib resulted in response rates of 12–18% and symptom improvement in 40–43% lasting from a few weeks to several months at a dosage level of 250 or 500 mg p.o. daily. All patients had failed one or more previous chemotherapy regimens. Highest activity was observed among patients with adenocarcinoma, especially alveolar cell carcinoma and among females. Response has also been seen in patients with CNS metastases including some patients who had progressed after having received brain irradiation (44). Most frequent adverse toxicity was generally mild, and included rash, pruritus, and dry skin. Gefitinib has also been investigated with two-drug chemotherapy in two large randomized double-blind placebo controlled Phase III trials, each enrolling more than 1000 previously untreated advanced NSCLC patients. There were no significant differences in response rates, time to progression, or survival between the gefitinib alone or placebo arm of either trial. The reasons for the negative results are unclear (45,46). The results obtained with erlotinib are mainly similar to the experience with gefitinib, and erlotinib is now recommended and registered for second- and third-line therapy in Stage IV NSCLC as a single agent. Several studies are also ongoing exploring various EGFR-inhibitors as first-line therapy in certain subsets of patients with advanced NSCLC (47). Among these, preliminary data by Pirker et al. have demonstrated a median survival advantage (11.3 months vs. 10 months, hazard ratio 0.87, 95% CI 0.762–0.996, $p < 0.044$) in favor of a combination of cisplatin, vinorelbine plus cetuximab

(Erbitux) compared with cisplatin and vinorelbine in a study with 1125 patients with advanced NSCLC, expressing EGFR, including an increase in response rate from 26% to 29% ($p = 0.05$) (48). Much effort has been exerted to identify the patients expected to benefit from this targeted therapy, but a golden standard aiming at this has not yet been obtained (13). Several studies including recent large randomized trials indicate that EGFR mutations and high copy number are predictive of response to erlotonib and that EGFR FISH is the strongest prognostic marker and a significant predictive marker of differential survival benefit from erlotinib (49). As in other cancers the effect of the inhibitor of angiogenesis, bevacizumab, has been studied in combination with chemotherapy and based on an improvement in overall survival of two months when given in combination with first-line chemotherapy to Stage IV non-squamous NSCLC, the drug has been approved in both the United States and Europe. The adverse events in non-squamous NSCLC have been modest, but the drug has caused lethal hemorrhagic adverse events in squamous cancers preventing the use of the drug in this subgroup (50).

The effect of other biologic agents interacting with the EGFR or EGFR pathway and other growth factors is at the moment being investigated further.

Small Cell Lung Cancer

Updated clinical guidelines have recently been presented by both European and North American Organizations (7–10,51–53).

Chemotherapy

The disseminated nature of SCLC, displaying a high frequency of metastases at the time of diagnosis combined with a high sensitivity to cytostatic agents, has led to the use of chemotherapy as the primary treatment of choice in all its stages.

The most effective agents are listed in Table 8.8. The most commonly used combinations include a platinum compound together with the podophyllotoxins, usually etoposide. Combinations including vincristine, cyclophosphamide/ifosfamide, or doxorubicin are also highly active. Examples of frequently used treatment schedules are listed in Table 8.9. In a trial by Sundstrøm et al. (54) including 436 eligible patients with limited (214) and extensive

Table 8.8 Agents Used in SCLC. Most Frequently Chosen Agents for Inclusion in Combination Regimens for SCLC

Alkylating agents
  Cisplatin
  Carboplatin
  Ifosfamide
  Cyclophosphamide
Antimitotic agents
  Vincristine
  Paclitaxel (Taxol®)
Topoisomerase inhibitors
  Etoposide
  Irinotecan (Camptho®)
  Topotecan (Hycamtin®)
  Doxorubicin

Table 8.9 Commonly Used Regimens in Small Cell Carcinoma

Regimen	Dosage and schedule
PE	
Cisplatin	25 mg/m² i.v. on days 1–3 or 60–80 mg/m² i.v. on day 1
Etoposide	100 mg/m² i.v. on days 1–3 or 115 mg/m² i.v. days 3–5
CE	
Carboplatin	AUC 6 day 1 i.v.
Etoposide	100–120 mg/m² day 1–3 q. 3 wks
ICE	
Ifosfamide	5000 mg/m² day 1+
Carboplatin	300–400 mg/m² day 1
Etoposide	100–120 mg/m² day 1–3 + mesna 500 mg/m² day 1 and 3000 mg day 2.
CAV	
Cyclophosphamide	1000 mg/m² i.v. on day 1 q 3 wks
Adriamycin	45 mg/m² i.v. on day 1 q 3 wks
Vincristine	1.4 mg/m² i.v. on day 1
CAVE	
Cyclophosphamide	1000 mg/m² i.v. on day 1
Adriamycin	50 mg/m² i.v. on day 1
Vincristine	1.5 mg/m² i.v. on day 1
Etoposide	60 mg/m² i.v. on days 1–5

disease (222), a combination of etoposide and cisplatin was shown to be superior to a three-drug combination of cyclophosphamide, epirubicin, and vincristine. For all patients the two and five-year survival rates in the EP arm (14% and 5%) were significantly higher compared with the EP arm (6%) ($p = 0.0004$). Patients with limited disease received thoracic radiotherapy concurrently with chemotherapy cycle 3, and those achieving complete remission during the treatment period also received prophylactic cranial irradiation. In a recently published Japanese study (55), which included only patients with extensive disease, survival rates with a combination of irinotecan plus cisplatin were superior to those with etoposide and cisplatin with one-year survival being 56% versus 34%. A confirmatory trial in the United States failed to confirm the encouraging data, which may be related to a change in the treatment schedule causing more toxicity in the U.S. study (56). Among the other new compounds, topotecan appears to be the most promising, with studies indicating that oral topotecan is as effective as intravenous etoposide in combination with cisplatin (57).

Scheduling of drugs as well as the actual combination used is of great importance. Thus, etoposide is more effective when given as a five-day course than when the same dose is given over 24 hours (58).

For both limited (stages I–III) and extensive (Stage IV) disease the response rates achieved are over 80%. Complete response, with no clinical or histopathological evidence of malignant disease, is initially obtained in 30–40% of patients with limited disease and 15–20% of patients with extensive disease. The primary problem in managing this disease is that the median survival for patients with limited disease is only about 14–16 months and usually 8–10 months for extensive disease, whereas long-term survival (beyond five years) is 10–15% and 3–5%, respectively, for the two stages. One should be aware that survival results vary according to selection criteria, and more representative results from large national studies are less encouraging (1,59). With respect to the duration of treatment needed to produce optimal results, a period of six months corresponding to six cycles of chemotherapy is currently an acceptable standard. In patients presenting with poor prognostic factors such as performance status 3 to 4, involvement of the liver and bone marrow and/or severe comorbid diseases, the initial dose of chemotherapy should be reduced, and careful monitoring is recommended over the first weeks.

Within recent years, new approaches to chemotherapy have been undertaken to improve treatment results. The intensity of chemotherapy can also be increased, particularly as consolidation treatment by the use of autologous bone marrow infusion, and by peripheral blood stem cells; several randomized trials have been performed, but most of the data published so far have not resulted in clinically significant superiority compared to standard therapy. Noteworthy is that in a single study, more intensive treatment with four drugs instead of two drugs resulted in improved one-year survival (40% vs. 27%), but with more severe hematologic toxicity (60).

Other treatment approaches include scheduling of drugs based on cell kinetic observations or the use of anticoagulants, such as warfarin and antiangionetic agents such as thalidomide, but the results are inconclusive. Another attempt to improve chemotherapy is alternating combination chemotherapy using different noncross-resistant combinations, because resistant clones of SCLC cells, which develop either at the time of diagnosis or during chemotherapy, are thought to be the reason for treatment failure in most patients. Again, the impact on survival is modest. The use of biological response modifiers, such as interferons as maintenance therapy, has also been tested, but again with disappointing results. Granulocyte colony-stimulating factor (CSF) and granulocyte–macrophage CSF, given to counter the hematological effects of combination chemotherapy, lessen the severity of neutropenic episodes, but they do not significantly appear to influence survival in spite of the increased doses of chemotherapy.

When patients relapse, and most do within the first two years, the results of second-line treatment with combination chemotherapy are usually disappointing. Using noncross-resistant regimens at multifocal relapse, a response rate of 20–25% is obtained with a median duration of survival of three to four months. If there is a longer chemotherapy-free interval of >3 months before relapse, the same drug combination that initially produced a response may be repeated with a response rate of up to 50%, but again the effect is rather short lasting. In a recent study the use of topotecan 1.0mg/m^2 i.v. daily × 5 was as effective as a three-drug combination of cyclofosfamide, adriamycin, and vincristine (CAV) given i.v (61). It has also been demonstrated that addition of oral topotecan to best supportive care (BSC) significantly increased overall survival and resulted in better symptom control. In the study with 141 patients with relapsed SCLC the median survival times were 25.9 weeks versus 13.9 weeks in topotecan + BSC and BSC alone, respectively ($p = 0.01$) (62). If the patient has a local relapse and has not received irradiation previously,

the latter should be the treatment of choice. In addition, expandable metal stents and endobronchial laser beam therapy are also valuable tools in patients with obstructive intrathoracic tumor components.

Radiotherapy

Among the different types of lung cancer, SCLC is by far the most radiosensitive. Three decades ago radiotherapy was the main mode of therapy for this disease, but the recognition that SCLC disseminates early and widely has changed the role of radiotherapy. A small but statistically definite benefit of a 5% improvement in three-year survival based on meta-analysis can be seen in patients with limited disease when thoracic irradiation is added to combination chemotherapy (63). Limited disease is defined as a tumor that can be encompassed in a single radiation port. Limited disease is thus confined to one hemithorax with regional lymph node metastases, including lobar, ipsilateral supraclavicular mediastinal, and/or contralateral lobar nodes. Chest irradiation also significantly decreases the rate of local recurrence, and a dose-response relationship exists for up to 45–50 Gy with conventional 2-Gy daily fractions. The exact timing of irradiation is uncertain when given in relation to chemotherapy, but probably irradiation given concurrently with the first two courses is the most optimal. With respect to hyperfractionation, the results from two randomized trials (64,65) have been published. One of these included 147 patients and showed statistically significant superiority of 10 twice-daily irradiation sessions compared with daily irradiation, with five-year survival rates of 26% and 16%, respectively (64). A similar effect was not observed in the other study (65), possibly because radiotherapy was started after three cycles of chemotherapy and given as a split-course rather than continuously starting on day 1 with cycle 1, as applied in the study of Turrisi et al (64).

Because of the high propensity of SCLC to metastasize early to the brain, elective (prophylactic) cranial irradiation for SCLC has been applied for many years, especially in patients achieving a complete response. In all 10–15% of these patients will develop brain metastases. Cranial irradiation reduces brain metastases significantly and it also increases the time before brain metastases become symptomatic in patients having obtained a complete response to induction therapy. Furthermore, in several meta-analyses, prophylactic cranial irradiation (PCI) has been demonstrated to have a statistically significant impact on survival in patients with limited disease who achieve a complete remission. Three-year survival with PCI was 20.7% versus 15.3% without PCI (66). Very recently, a study by the EORTC has also shown prolongation of survival (6.7 months vs. 5.4 months, $p = 0.0033$) when PCI was added within five weeks of completion of chemotherapy in a randomized trial including 286 patients with extensive SCLC (67). The optimal dose and timing of radiotherapy are again uncertain; usually the total dose does not exceed 30 Gy, given in fractions of 2.5 Gy daily.

In SCLC patients presenting with CNS metastases, complete responses shown on brain CT and neurological improvement after induction might be achieved by chemotherapy alone, because brain metastases respond as frequently as metastatic SCLC disease at other sites.

Surgery

The very few SCLC patients who present with T_{1-2}, N_{0-1} disease are candidates for surgical treatment. As a result of the disseminated nature of this type of lung cancer, postoperative chemotherapy is indicated for a period of 6 months in these patients and prophylactic cranial irradiation may be considered.

Follow-up

Although the impact of routine radiologic follow-up of asymptomatic patients is not clearly defined in the literature, follow-up should be considered. For patients who achieve long-term survival, monitoring for development of a second primary cancer may be considered. Smoking cessation is recommended.

Neuroendocrine Tumors, including
Pulmonary Carcinoids

In contrast to small cell carcinoma, the other neuroendocrine tumors originating in the lung are on the rise, according to data published by Skuladottir et al. (59) Surgery is the only potentially curative therapy in patients with carcinoids. Radiotherapy can be used to treat symptomatic metastases, but has no place in the primary treatment of this disease entity. Also, the application of chemotherapy is in general disappointing, but combination chemotherapy with platinum and etoposide sometimes yields worthwhile long-lasting responses in patients with aggressive pulmonary neuroendocrine tumors, including carcinoids (68).

Management of Other Malignant Tumors of the Lung and Pleura
Mesothelioma

Malignant pleural mesothelioma (MPM) is an aggressive and locally invasive malignant tumor of the pleura arising from the mesothelial cells lining the pleura. MPM is usually associated with a history of chronic asbestos exposure and the incidence of this disease is increasing throughout the world. The incidence is expected to peak within the next 10–15 years.

The initial clinical presentation is usually progressive dyspnea and/or chest wall pain caused by pleural effusion with chest wall invasion. Weight loss, cough, and fatigue are also common symptoms.

A diagnosis of MPM is usually conducted on the basis of chest x-ray, CT-scan of the thorax combined with MRI of the chest and also PET with the latter ones being applied if potentially curative surgery is being considered for the patient.

A diagnosis of MPM may be based on pleural fluid cytology in 20–30% of the patients and in the remaining by a needle biopsy of one of the pleural masses, either CT-guided or using video-assisted thoracoscopy (VATS).

In addition to standard histology, special immunohistochemical stains should be applied to reach a reliable diagnosis, thereby distinguishing MPM from adenocarcinoma with staining for calretinin and vimentin being typical for MPM cure lacking in adenocarcinoma of the lung. Recently, a new serum marker called soluble mesothelin-related protein (SMRP) has been observed to occur in 80–90% of all patients with MPM, and mesothelin expression in <50% of the MPM malignant cells has been demonstrated to be a significant negative prognostic factor (69).

The treatment is dependent on the stage with the most commonly accepted staging system being the International Mesothelioma Staging System (IMIG) (Table 8.10).

The prognosis for patients with MPM is usually poor with median survival of 6–12 months and cures occur only in the subset of patients presenting with Stage I and II in performance ECOC 0-1 undergoing extrapleural pneumonectomy with resection of the diaphragm.

Two-year survival rates in this group of patients vary in recent studies from 20% to 45% (70,71). With respect to radiotherapy, mesothelioma is rather resistant and radical irradiation with 40–50Gy to the entire pleural space and the mediastinum followed by boost irradiation up to 55–70Gy to areas of gross disease are being used, but is

Table 8.10   Staging of Mesotheliomas

Stage	Tumor	Lymph nodes	Metastases
Stage Ia	Limited to the ipsilateral parietal pleura, including the mediastinal and diaphragmatic pleurae	None detectable N_0	None M_0
Stage Ib T_{1b},N_0,M_0	Ipsilateral parietal pleura, including the mediastinal and diaphragmatic pleurae	None detectable N_0	None M_0
Stage II T_2,N_0,M_0	Each ipsilateral pleural surface	N_0	M_0
Stage III Any T_3 Any N_1 or N_2 M_0	Locally advanced, technically unresectable tumor (each ipsilateral pleural surface)	Metastases in ipsilateral bronchopulmonary or hilar lymph nodes. or Metastases in subcarinal or ipsilateral mediastinal lymph nodes, including ipsilateral internal mammary lymph nodes	No distant metastases
Stage IV Any T_4 Any N_3 Any M_1	Locally advanced, technically unresectable tumor (each ipsilateral pleural surface)	Metastases in contralateral mediastinal, contralateral internal mammary, and ipsilateral or contralateral supraclavicular lymph nodes.	Distant metastases present

difficult to apply without significant toxicity. Radiocolloids, such as ^{198}Au or ^{32}P, have also been given into the pleural cavity but with disappointing results. With respect to chemotherapy the response rates to both single agent and combination chemotherapy have been low (<20%). In a study, including a total of 448 patients, the use of pemetrexed (Alimta), an antifolate with multiple mechanisms of action, given together with cisplatin resulted in significant improvement of both survival and quality of life compared with cisplatin alone, with response rates of 40% compared to 16.7% for cisplatin alone, and median overall survival of 12.1 months versus 9.3 months; also improvement of lung function and subjective quality of life were noted (72). Also the combination of cisplatin and raltitrexed has been demonstrated to be superior to cisplatin in patients with MPM in a randomized trial with 250 patients based on both response rates (24% vs. 14%) and median survival (11.1 vs. 8.8 months) (73).

Ongoing studies are exploring the effect of combination chemotherapy given as an adjunct to extrapleural pneumonectomy and/or radiotherapy, including intensity-modulated radiation therapy (IMRI) as part of multimodality treatment with chemotherapy being given both pre- and postoperatively. Overall, there is an increasing tendency to apply trimodality therapy using this approach based on the results of a series of Phase II trials in both the United States and Europe (70,71).

With respect to targeted therapies, a variety of biological agents have been explored or are undergoing evaluation in MPM patients, but the results of studies testing EGFR tyrasine kinase inhibitors (gefitinib and erlotinib) have shown limited or no activity, and so have trials with imatinib mesylate.

REFERENCES

1. Janssen-Heijnen MLG, Coebergh J-WW. Trends in incidence and prognosis of their histological subtypes of lung cancer in North America, Australia, New Zealand and Europe. Lung Cancer 2001; 31: 123–7.
2. Berrino F, De Angelis R, Rosso S et al., the EUROCARE-4 Working group. Survival for eight major cancers and all cancers combined for European adults diagnosed in 1995–99: results of the EUROCARE-4 study. Lancet Oncol 2007; 8: 773–83.
3. Verdecchia A, Francisci S, Brenner H et al., the EUROCARE-4 Working Group. Recent cancer survival in Europe: a 2000–02 period analysis of EUROCARE-4 data. Lancet Oncol 2007; 8: 784–96.
4. The GLOBOCAN 2002 database. http://www-dep.iarc.fr/globocan/database.htm
5. Youlden DR, Cramb SM, Baade PD. The international epidemiology of lung cancer. Geographical distribution and secular trends. J Thorac Oncol 2008; 3: 819–31.
6. Borràs JM, Fernandez E, Gonzalez JR et al. Lung cancer mortality in European regions (1955-1997). Ann Oncol 2003; 14: 159–61.
7. Fontana RS, Sanderson DR, Woolner LB et al. Lung cancer screening: the Mayo program. J Occup Environ Med 1996; 28: 746–50.
8. Henschke CI. CT screening for lung cancer is justified. Nat Clin Pract Oncol 2007; 4: 440–1.
9. Gleeson FV. Screening for lung cancer with spiral CT is not justified. Nat Clin Pract Oncol 2007; 4: 442–3.
10. Yau G, Lock M, Rodrigues G. Systematic review of baseline low-dose CT lung cancer screening. Lung Cancer 2007; 58: 161–70.
11. Conrad DH, Goyette J, Thomas PS. Proteomics as a method for early detection of cancer: a review of proteomics, exhaled breath condensate and lung cancer screening. J Gen Intern Med 2007; 23: 78–84.
12. Herbst RS, Haymach JV, Lippman SC. Lung Cancer. N Engl J Med 2008; 359: 1367–80.
13. Dziadzinsko R, Hirsch FR. Advances in genomic and proteomic studies of non-small-cell lung cancer: clinical and translational research perspective. Clin Lung Cancer 2008: Mar; 9: 78–84.
14. Bunn PA Jr, Thatcher N. Systemic treatment for advanced (stage IIIb/IV) non-small cell lung cancer: more treatment options; more things to consider. Conclusion. Oncologist 2008; 13(suppl 1): 37–46.
15. Fischer B, Arcaro A. Current status of clinical trials for small cell lung cancer. Rev Recent Clin Trials 2008, 3: 40–61.
16. Travis WD, Brambilla E, Müller-Hermelink HK et al., eds. WHO Classification: Pathology and Genetics of Tumours of the Lung, Pleura, Thymus and Heart. Lyon: IARC Press, 2004: 10.
17. Raz DJ, Rosell R, Jablons DM. Current concepts on bronchioloalveolar carcinoma biology. Clin Cancer Res 2006; 12: 3698–704.
18. Hawson G, Firouz-Abadi A, Ford CA et al. Primary lung cancer: characterisation and survival of 1024 patients treated in a single institution. Med J Aust 1990; 152: 230–4.
19. Ung YC, Maziak DE, Vanderveen JA et al. 18Fluorodeoxyglucose positron emission tomography in the diagnosis and staging of lung cancer: a systematic review. J Natl Cancer Inst 2007; 99: 1753–67.
20. De Leyn P, Lardinois D, Van Schil PE et al. ESTS guidelines for preoperative lymph node staging for non-small cell lung cancer. Eur J Cardiothorac Surg 2007; 32: 1–8
21. Silvestri GA, Could MK, Margolis ML et al. Noninvasive staging of non-smal cell lung cancer: ACCP evidenced-based clinical practice guidelines (2nd edition). Chest 2007; 132: 178S–201S.
22. ESMO Guidelines Working Group. Non-small-cell lung cancer: ESMO Clinical Recommendations for diagnosis, treatment and follow-up. Ann Oncol 2007; 18(Suppl 2): ii30–1.
23. De Leyn P, Stroobants S, De Wever W et al. Prospective comparative study of integrated positron emission tomography-computed tomography scan compared with remediastinoscopy in the assessment of residual mediastinal lymph node disease after induction chemotherapy for mediastinoscopy-proven stage IIIA-N2 non-small-cell lung cancer: a Leuven Lung Cancer Group Study. J Clin Oncol 2006; 24: 3333–9.
24. Mountain CF. Revisions in the international system for staging lung cancer. Chest 1997; 111: 1710–17.
25. Kloover JS, van Klaveren RJ. Staging, staging procedures and prognostic factors. In: Hansen HH ed. Lung Cancer Therapy Annual 6. London: Informa HealthCare, 2008: 57–90.
26. Keller SM. Complete mediastinal lymph node dissection—does it make a difference? Lung Cancer 2002; 36: 7–8.
27. Non-Small Cell Lung Cancer Collaborative Group, Chemotherapy in non-small cell lung cancer: a meta-analysis using updated data on individual patients from 52 randomised clinical trials. BMJ 1995; 311: 899–909.
28. Pignon J, Tribodet H, Scagliotti G et al. Lung Adjuvant Cisplatin Evaluation (LACE): A pooled analysis of five randomized clinical trials including 4,584 patients. J Clin Oncol 2006; 24: 366s (abstract 7008).
29. Arriagada R, Le Pechoux C, Pignon JP. Resected non-small cell lung cancer: Need for adjuvant lymph-node treatment? From hope to reality. Lung Cancer 2003; 42(Suppl 1): S57–64.

30. PORT Meta-analysis Trialist Group. Postoperative radiotherapy in non-small-cell lung cancer: systematic review and meta-analysis of individual patients data from nine randomised controlled trials. Lancet 1998; 352: 257.

31. Govindan R, Bogart J, Vokes EE. Locally advanced non-small cell lung cancer: the past, present, and future. J Thorac Oncol 2008; 3: 917–28.

32. Auperin A, Le Pechoux C, Pignon JP et al. Concomitant radio-chemotherapy based on platin compounds in patients with locally advanced non-small cell lung cancer (NSCLC): a meta-analysis of individual data from 1764 patients. Ann Oncol 2006; 17: 473–83.

33. Molina JR, Adjei AA, Jett JR. Advances in chemotherapy of non-small cell lung cancer. Chest 2006; 130: 1211–19.

34. Scagliotti GV, Parikh P, von Pawel J et al. Phase III study comparing cisplatin plus gemcitabine with cisplatin plus pemetrexed in chemotherapy-naive patients with advanced-stage non-small-cell lung cancer. J Clin Oncol 2008; 26: 3543–51.

35. Weinmann M, Jeremic B, Toomes H et al. Treatment of lung cancer in the elderly. Part I: non-small cell lung cancer. Lung Cancer 2003; 39: 233–54.

36. Shepherd FA, Dancey J, Ramlau R et al. Prospective randomized trial of docetaxel versus best supportive care in patients with non-small cell lung cancer previously treated with platinum-based chemotherapy. J Clin Oncol 2000; 18: 2095–103.

37. Hanna N, Shepherd FA, Fossella FV et al. Randomized phase III trial of pemetrexed versus docetaxel in patients with non-small-cell lung cancer previously treated with chemotherapy. J Clin Oncol 2004; 22: 1589–97.

38. Douillard JY, Coudert B, Gridelli C et al. Phase III study of i.v. vinflunine (VFL) versus i.v. docetaxel (DTX) in patients with advanced or metastatic non-small cell lung cancer (NSCLC) previously treated with a platinum-containing regimen. Eur J Cancer Suppl 2007; 5: 358.

39. Onishi H, Shirato H, Nagata Y et al. Hypofractionated stereotactic radiotherapy (HypoFXSRT) for stage I non-small cell lung cancer: updated results of 257 patients in a Japanese multi-institutional study. J Thorac Oncol 2007; 2(Suppl 3): S94–100.

40. Saunders M, Dische S, Barrett A et al. Continuous hyperfractionated accelerated radiotherapy (CHART) versus conventional radiotherapy in non-small-cell lung cancer: a randomised multicentre trial. CHART Steering Committee. Lancet 1997; 350: 161–5.

41. Kramer GW, Wanders SL, Noordijk EM et al. Results of the Dutch National study of the palliative effect of irradiation using two different treatment schemes for non-small-cell lung cancer. J Clin Oncol 2005; 23: 2962–70.

42. Kelly K, Huang C. Biological agents in non-small cell lung cancer: a review of recent advances and clinical results with a focus on epidermal growth factor receptor and vascular endothelial growth factor. J Thorac Oncol 2008; 3: 664–73.

43. Pirker R, Minar W, Filipits M. Integrating EGFR targeted therapies into platinum-based chemotherapy regimens for newly diagnosed non-small cell lung cancer. Clin Lung Cancer, 2008; 9: S109–115.

44. Cappuzzo F, Ardizzoni A, Soto-Parra H et al. Epidermal growth factor receptor targeted therapy by ZC 1839 (Iressa) in patients with brain metastases from non-small cell lung cancer (NSCLC). Lung Cancer 2003; 41: 227–31.

45. Giaccone G, Herbst RS, Manegold C et al. Gefitinib in combination with gemcitabine and cisplatin in advanced non-small-cell lung cancer: a phase III trial—INTACT 1. J Clin Oncol 2004; 22: 777–84.

46. Herbst RS, Giaccone G, Schiller JH et al. Gefitinib in combination with paclitaxel and carboplatin in advanced non-small-cell lung cancer: a phase III trial—INTACT 2. J Clin Oncol 2004; 22: 785–94.

47. Fong T, Morgensztern D, Govindan R. EGFR inhibitors as first-line therapy in advanced non-small cell lung cancer. J Thorac Oncol 2008; 3: 303–10.

48. Pirker R, Szczesna A, von Pawel J et al. FLEX: a randomized, multicenter, phase III study of cetuximab in combination with cisplatin/vinorelbine (CV) versus CV alone in the first-line treatment of patients with advanced non-small cell lung cancer (NSCLC). 2008 ASCO Annual Meeting Proceedings. J Clin Oncol 2008; 26: 6s (abstract 3).

49. Zhu C-Q, Santos GdC, Ding K et al. Role of KRAS and EGFR as biomarkers of response to erotinib in National Cancer Institute of Canada Clinical Trials Group Study BR.21. J Clin Oncol 2008; 26: 4268–75.

50. Cohen MH, Gootenberg J, Keegan P et al. FDA Drug Approval Summary: Bevacizumab (Avastin®) plus carboplatin and paclitaxel as first-line treatment of advanced/metastatic recurrent nonsquamous non-small cell lung cancer. Oncologist 2007; 12: 713–18.

51. ESMO Guidelines Working Group. Small-cell lung cancer: ESMO Clinical Recommendations for diagnosis, treatment and follow-up. Ann Oncol 2007; 18(Suppl 2): ii32–3.

52. Samson DJ, Sidenfeld J, Simon GR et al. Evidence for management of small cell lung cancer: ACCP evidence-based clinical practice guidelines (2nd edition). Chest 2007; 132: 314S–23S.

53. National Comprehensive Cancer Network. Clinical Practice Guidelines in Oncology™. Small Cell Lung Cancer v.1.2008. http://www.nccn.org/professionals/physician_gls/pdf/sclc.pdf2008

54. Sundstrøm S, Bremnes RM, Kaasa S et al. Cisplatin and etoposide (EP-regimen is superior to cyclophosphamide, epirubicin, and vincristine (CEV-regimen) in small cell lung cancer: results from a randomized phase III trial with 5-year follow-up. Eur J Cancer 2001; 37(Suppl 6): S153 (abstract 556).

55. Noda K, Nistriwaki Y, Kawahara M et al. Irinotecan plus cisplatin compared with etoposide plus cisplatin for extensive small cell lung cancer. N Engl J Med 2002; 346: 85–91.

56. Natale RB, Lara PN, Chansky K et al. SO124: A randomized phase III trial comparing irinotecan/cisplatin (IP) with etoposide/cisplatin (EP) in patients with previously untreated extensive stage small cell lung cancer (E-SCLC). J Clin Oncol 2008; 26: 400s (abstract 7512).

57. Eckardt JR, von Pawel J, Pujol JL et al. Phase III study of oral compared with intravenous topotecan as second-line therapy in small-cell lung cancer. J Clin Oncol 2007; 25: 2086–92.

58. Souhami RL, Spiro SG, Rudd RM et al. Five-day oral etoposide treatment for advanced small-cell lung cancer: randomized comparison with intravenous chemotherapy. J Natl Cancer Inst 1997; 89: 577–80.

59. Skuladottir H, Hirsch FR, Hansen HH et al. Pulmonary neuroendocrine tumors: Incidence and prognosis of histological subtypes. A population-based study in Denmark. Lung Cancer 2002; 37: 127–35.

60. Pujol JL, Daurès JP, Rivière A et al. Etoposide plus cisplatin with or without the combination of 4'-epidoxorubicin plus c yclophosphamide in treatment of extensive small-cell lung cancer: a French Federation of Cancer Institutes Multicenter Phase III randomized study. J Natl Cancer Inst 2001; 93: 300–8.

61. von Pawel J, Schiller JH, Shepherd FA et al. Topotecan vs cyclophosphamide, doxorubicin, and vincristine for the treatment of recurrent small-cell lung cancer. J Clin Oncol 1999; 7: 658–67.

62. O'Brien ME, Ciuleanu TE, Tsekov H et al. Phase III trial comparing supportive care alone with supportive care with oral topotecan in patients with relapsed small-cell lung cancer. J Clin Oncol 2006; 24: 5441–7.

63. Pignon JP, Arriagada R, Ihde DC et al. A meta-analyses of thoracic radiotherapy for small cell lung cancer. New Eng J Med 1992; 327: 1618–24.

64. Turrisi AT, Kim K, Blum R et al. Twice daily compared with once daily radiotherapy in limited small cell lung cancer treated concurrently with cisplatin and etoposide. N Engl J Med 1999; 340: 265–71.

65. Schild SE, Bonner JA, Shanahan TG et al. Long-term results of a phase III trial comparing once-daily radiotherapy with twice-daily radiotherapy in limited-stage small-cell lung cancer. Int J Radiat Oncol Biol Phys 2004; 59: 943–51.

66. Cochrane Collaboration Consumer. Prophylactic cranial irradiation improves survival rate of patients with small-cell lung cancer in complete remission. An update on: "Cranial irradiation for preventing brain metastases of small cell lung cancer in patients in complete remission" (Cochrane Review). In: The Cochrane Library, 2, 2001. Oxford: Update Software.

67. Slotman B, Faivre-Finn C, Kramer G et al. Prophylactic cranial irradiation in extensive small-cell lung cancer. N Engl J Med 2007; 357: 664–72.

68. Gustafsson BI, Kidd M, Chan A. Bronchopulmonary neuroendocrine tumors. Cancer 2008; 113: 5–21.

69. Roe OD, Creaney J, Lundgren S et al. Mesothelin-related predictive and prognostic factors in malignant mesothelioma: A nested case-control study. Lung Cancer 2008; 61: 235–43.

70. Baas P. Optimising survival in malignant mesothelioma. Lung Cancer 2007; 57(Suppl 2): S24–9.

71. Tsiouris A, Walesby RK. Malignant pleural mesothelioma: current concepts in treatment. Nat Clin Pract Oncol 2007; 4: 344–52.

72. Vogelzang NJ, Rusthoven JJ, Symanowski J et al. Phase III study of pemetrexed in combination with cisplatin versus cisplatin alone in patients with malignant pleural mesothelioma. J Clin Oncol 2003; 21: 2636–44.

73. van Meerbeeck JP, Gaafar R, Manegold C et al. Randomized phase III study of cisplatin with or without reltitrexed in proteins with malignant pleural mesothelioma: an Intergroup study of the Europen Organisation for Research and Treatment of Cancer Lung Cancer Group and the National Cancer Institute of Canada. J Clin Oncol 2005; 23: 6881–8.

74. Mountain CF. A new international staging system for lung cancers. Chest 1986; 89: 225S–33S.

9

Gastrointestinal Cancer

Rachel Wong, Ian Chau, and David Cunningham

Gastrointestinal (GI) cancers are the most common cancers in Europe and the United States and represent a major public health problem worldwide. Recent advances have increased the complexity of the management of GI cancer and many GI cancers now require a multimodality approach to treatment. The multidisciplinary team—comprising of medical, radiation, and surgical oncologists, radiologists, nuclear medicine physicians, gastroenterologists, pathologists, specialist nurses, and pharmacists—has therefore become imperative when determining optimal management. For medical oncologists, considerable progress has been made not only in refining the delivery of chemotherapy, but also in establishing a role for molecular targeted therapies in the treatment of many GI malignancies. Treatment paradigms, of course, continue to evolve, facilitated by participation in clinical trials that should be encouraged. This chapter summarizes current oncological practice in the treatment of GI cancers.

ESOPHAGEAL AND GASTRIC CANCERS
Esophageal Cancer

The histological profile of esophageal cancer has changed over the past few decades. Squamous cell carcinoma (SCC) is no longer the predominant histological subtype. Worldwide, the incidence of esophageal cancer is increasing. Western countries in particular have seen a significant rise in the incidence of esophageal adenocarcinoma. The long-term outcome for esophageal cancer remains poor mainly as a result of distal relapse or advanced disease at presentation. Five-year survival is less than 20% (1).

Epidemiology and Presentation

Squamous cell carcinoma is strongly associated with alcohol consumption and smoking (2). Furthermore, these tumors tend to occur in the middle and upper thirds of the esophagus. In contrast, esophageal adenocarcinoma, which typically involves the distal esophagus, is associated with gastroesophageal reflux and the development Barrett's metaplasia. The risk of developing invasive adenocarcinoma in Barrett's metaplasia is approximately 0.5% per year (3). The role of surveillance endoscopy in patients with Barrett's metaplasia remains unclear. Symptoms often present only in the later stages of disease and include dysphagia, odynophagia, regurgitation of food or fluids, retrosternal discomfort/burning, anorexia, and weight loss.

Staging

The median survival of patients with esophageal cancer is strongly correlated with stage at diagnosis. Careful selection of patients suitable for an aggressive approach to management is vital. Initial staging investigations performed on patients with esophageal cancer may include computed tomography (CT) of chest and abdomen, endoscopic ultrasound (EUS), positron emission tomography (PET), laparoscopy, and thoracoscopy.

EUS is a key tool for locoregional staging although it is not without its limitations. A recent meta-analysis reported the sensitivity and specificity for detecting regional lymph nodes at 0.80 and 0.70 respectively and 0.85 (sensitivity) and 0.96 (specificity) for coeliac nodes (4). Understaging may occur if the ultrasound is unable to traverse the tumor, as neither the entire tumor nor the coeliac axis nodes can be visualized. Furthermore, accuracy of TNM classification is lower after neoadjuvant therapy due to the inability to differentiate between fibrosis, inflammation, or residual tumor. The sensitivity of CT and PET to detect regional lymph nodes is lower (0.50 and 0.57) although specificity is higher (0.83 and 0.85) (4). CT and PET are useful modes to detect distant metastases, and the use of combined CT-PET, providing both anatomical and functional information, is increasing. The rate of detection of occult distal metastases in patients with esophageal cancer by FDG-PET have been reported to be as high as 20% (4).

It remains unclear whether the optimal management of adenocarcinomas arising at the gastroesophageal junction (GOJ) should follow an esophageal or gastric treatment paradigm. A consensus conference has defined GOJ tumors as those with their centers arising within 5cm proximal and distal of the anatomical cardia and further classifies GOJ tumors into three different types as outlined in Table 9.1 (5). The management of GOJ tumors is discussed with the management of gastric cancers.

Treatment Strategies
Localized Esophageal Cancer

There is no current standard treatment approach for localized esophageal cancer. Treatment options range from surgery alone or definitive chemoradiation (CRT) to the neoadjuvant approaches combining induction chemotherapy with surgery, chemotherapy followed by CRT and CRT with surgery. There is a paucity of studies supporting the use of postoperative adjuvant chemotherapy or CRT.

Table 9.1 Siewert's Classification of Gastroesophageal Junction Adenocarcinoma (5)

Type I Distal esophageal adenocarcinoma, usually arising from an area with specialized intestinal metaplasia of the esophagus (i.e., Barrett's esophagus) and which may infiltrate the gastroesophageal junction from above
Type II True carcinoma of the cardia arising from the cardiac epithelium or short segments with intestinal metaplasia at the gastroesophageal junction; this entity is also often referred to as "junctional carcinoma"
Type III Subcardial gastric carcinoma which infiltrates the gastroesophageal junction and distal esophagus from below

Surgery. Surgical resection of esophageal primary tumors remains the treatment of choice for the majority of patients with localized esophageal cancer. Although improved patient selection and refinement of surgical techniques has reduced perioperative mortality, with surgery alone, five-year survival rates are only approximately 35% (6). Multimodality therapy improves outcome; however, no international consensus on treatment approach has been reached.

Preoperative Radiotherapy. The updated systematic review of preoperative radiotherapy in esophageal cancer confirmed that any impact of preoperative radiotherapy is modest (absolute improvement in survival of around 3–4%) (7). The lack of new randomized controlled trials (RCTs) comparing surgery to preoperative radiotherapy and surgery reflects the acceptance of chemoradiation as a superior treatment modality to radiation alone.

Neoadjuvant Chemotherapy. The two largest RCTs evaluating neoadjuvant cisplatin and 5-FU in patients with resectable or esophageal SCC or adenocarcinoma produced conflicting results. The U.S. Intergroup-0113 study randomized 467 patients to surgery alone or three cycles of chemotherapy (cisplatin 100 mg/m^2, days 1, 29, and 58, and 5-FU, 1000 mg/m^2 by continuous infusion, days 1 to 5 of each cycle) (8). Responders and those with stable disease could receive a further two cycles of chemotherapy postoperatively with a lower dose of cisplatin (75 mg/m^2). No significant difference in median survival was detected.

In contrast, the larger U.K. MRC OE02 study randomized 802 patients to surgery alone or two three-weekly cycles of chemotherapy (cisplatin 80 mg/m^2 day 1 and 5-FU, 1000 mg/m^2 by continuous infusion days 1 to 4) (9). Nine percent of patients in each group also received preoperative radiotherapy. Overall survival (OS) was significantly better in the group receiving chemotherapy (hazard ratio 0.79; 95% CI 0.67–0.93; $p = 0.004$) as was two-year survival (43% vs. 34%). A further U.K. MRC trial (MAGIC) and the French FNLCC/FFCD trial (see section on "Gastric and Gastroesophageal Junction Cancers") both included patients with lower esophageal and GOJ adenocarcinomas and resulted in improved OS from the addition of perioperative chemotherapy (10,11).

It has been postulated that the lack of survival benefit seen in the Intergroup study may be due to a combination of treatment-related toxicity and a delay to definitive surgery in patients not responding to neoadjuvant chemotherapy.

A recent meta-analysis of eight RCTs ($n = 1724$) found the hazard ratio (HR) for all cause mortality for neoadjuvant chemotherapy was 0.90 (0.81–1.00; $p = 0.05$), corresponding to a two-year absolute survival benefit of 7%. Chemotherapy did not have a significant effect on all cause mortality for patients with SCC (HR 0.88; $p = 0.12$), however a significant benefit in esophageal adenocarcinoma was found (HR 0.78; $p = 0.014$) (12).

Preoperative Chemoradiation. Several RCTs evaluating neoadjuvant CRT have been conducted. The HR for all-cause mortality in a meta-analysis of 10 RCTs comparing neoadjuvant chemoradiotherapy to surgery alone ($n = 1209$) for preoperative CRT compared to surgery alone was 0.81 (95% CI 0.70–0.93; $p = 0.002$), corresponding to a 13% absolute difference in survival at two years (12).

Direct comparison of these two preoperative approaches has not occurred. A randomized phase III trial comparing preoperative chemotherapy followed by surgery to preoperative chemotherapy followed by CRT followed by surgery closed early due to poor accrual, but reported a trend toward improved survival in the CRT arm, albeit with higher perioperative morbidity (13).

Definitive Radiation or Chemoradiation Versus Surgery. A review of 19 randomized trials evaluating CRT versus radiation for localized osophageal cancer, reported that as definitive treatment, CRT alone results in superior disease control rates (local and distant) and survival compared to radiation alone (14). Ten of these trials included patients with SCC only, whereas the remaining nine included both SCC and esophageal adenocarcinomas.

Although surgery results in better locoregional control rates compared to chemoradiation followed by surgery, survival outcomes are similar. The French trial FFCD 9102 treated 444 patients with potentially resectable T3, N0-1, M0 esophageal SCC (90%) or adenocarcinoma (10%) with induction chemoradiation. Responders ($n = 259$) were then randomized to further chemoradiotherapy or surgery. Median survival for patients randomized to surgery was 17.7 months compared to 19.3 months for those who continued CRT. The trial reached its primary end point of noninferiority for two-year survival ($p = 0.03$) (15). Toxicity was higher with the combined modality emphasizing the importance of careful patient selection. For selected patients with SCC, chemoradiation alone is a viable treatment option, with surgery reserved for patients with residual or recurrent local disease.

Adjuvant Treatment. There is currently no evidence to support the routine use of postoperative CRT, RT, or chemotherapy post esophagectomy. Adjuvant RT may improve local control rates, but not survival and is associated with increased toxicity. The postoperative management of GOJ adenocarcinomas is discussed in the section on "Gastric and Gastroesophageal Junction Cancers."

Advanced Disease
Palliative treatment options for patients with locally advanced inoperable or metastatic esophageal carcinoma can range from local treatments (e.g., CRT, RT alone, endoluminal stenting) to systemic chemotherapy. There is currently no gold standard chemotherapy regimen for

advanced esophageal cancer. Chemotherapeutic options for advanced esophageal cancer are discussed in the section on "Gastric and Gastroesophageal Junction Cancers."

Gastric and Gastroesophageal Junction Cancers

Gastric cancer is the fourth most common cancer worldwide and is a leading cause of cancer-related death. The incidence of gastric cancer varies widely according to geographic location. Despite recent advances in the management of localized disease, five-year survival remains poor in most parts of the world (20%) with the exclusion of Japan where five-year survival is approximately 60% (16).

Epidemiology

Approximately 90% of gastric cancers are adenocarcinomas, with lymphoma, sarcoma, and other rare histological types comprising the remaining 10%. This section will focus solely on the management of gastric and GOJ adenocarcinoma. Anatomically, gastric adenocarcinoma can be subdivided into distal (noncardia) or proximal (cardia) tumors. Worldwide, noncardia gastric cancers are the predominant subtype.

Risk factors for the development of noncardia gastric cancer include *Helicobacter pylori* infection, diets rich in preserved foods and low in fresh fruits and vegetables, low socioeconomic class, and smoking. Improved sanitation leading to decreased incidence of *H. pylori*, increased availability of fresh fruit and vegetables, and decreasing consumption of preserved foods are thought to be the main factors resulting in the decreased incidence of noncardia gastric cancer in developed countries. On the other hand, the incidence of cardia gastric adenocarcinomas have increased or remained constant in developed countries. Risk factors include male gender, Caucasian racial background, obesity, smoking, and gastroesophageal reflux (16).

Mass screening programmes have been instituted in countries such as Japan, where there is a particularly high incidence of the disease, resulting in a high rate of diagnosis in the early stage of the disease and improved mortality rates; however this approach currently does not have sufficient evidence to support worldwide usage (16).

Treatment Strategies

Gastric adenocarcinoma has a propensity for early dissemination and the majority of patients present with advanced disease, except in countries where screening programmes exist. For patients presenting with early stage disease, surgery is the standard of care, especially in Stage I and Stage II disease. A number of perioperative and adjuvant strategies have been investigated to improve outcomes from surgery alone. For patients of good performance status who present with advanced disease, palliative chemotherapy improves survival and quality of life compared to best supportive care (BSC).

Treatment of Early Stage Gastric and Gastroesophageal Cancer

Surgery. At a minimum, staging of patients with early stage disease includes endoscopy and CT chest, abdomen, and pelvis. Endoscopic ultrasound can provide further information regarding local (T and N) staging and

PET may be useful to detect occult metastases, but may miss peritoneal disease and is often not readily available. Diagnostic laparoscopy is essential in patients being considered for curative surgery and can identify occult metastases in 23% to 37% of patients and thus spare patients from noncurative laparotomy (17).

The extent of resection to be performed remains controversial. D1 resection involves dissection of perigastric lymph nodes whereas D2-4 dissection involves more extensive en-bloc resection of lymph nodes outside the perigastric area. The two largest randomized prospective trials comparing D1 and D2 resections were conducted in Holland and the United Kingdom. There was no difference in recurrence rates or five-year survival rates in either trial, and increased hospital morbidity and perioperative mortality in patients undergoing D2 gastric resections (18).

Adjuvant Chemotherapy. Several meta-analyses have been published suggesting that there is a small benefit associated with adjuvant chemotherapy; however the majority of trials conducted have been small, and the chemotherapy regimens used have varied widely. More favorable results have been reported in Asian studies compared with Western trials, but differences in tumor location, prevalence of early stages, extent of preoperative staging evaluation, and type of surgery must also be taken into account.

S1 is an oral combination of tegafur, a prodrug of fluorouracil, and 5-chloro-2,4-dihydropyrimidine and potassium oxonate. The recently published Adjuvant Chemotherapy Trial of TS-1 for Gastric Cancer (ACTS-GC) randomized 1059 patients with stage II/III gastric cancer to S-1 monotherapy versus surgery alone after curative D2 gastrectomy. Three-year OS was 80.1% in the S-1 group and 70.1% in the surgery only group (HR for death 0.68; 95% CI 0.52–0.87; $p = 0.0024$) (19). Whether or not these results can be translated to a non-Japanese patient population remains to be seen.

Perioperative Chemotherapy. The U.K. Medical Research Council Adjuvant Gastric Infusional Chemotherapy (MAGIC) Trial randomized 503 patients with operable gastroesophageal cancer to perioperative chemotherapy with epirubicin, cisplatin, and fluorouracil (ECF) with three cycles before and after surgery, or to surgery alone. Perioperative chemotherapy resulted in tumor downstaging, and a significant improvement in OS from 23% to 36% (HR for death 0.75; 95% CI 0.60–0.93; $p = 0.009$) and progression-free survival (HR for progression 0.66; 95% CI 0.53–0.81; $p < 0.001$) (10). There was no difference in the rates of operative complications or mortality between the two arms.

A smaller French study using perioperative cisplatin and 5-FU also reported improved disease-free survival (DFS)(HR 0.65; 95% CI 0.48–0.89) and OS (HR for death 0.69; 95% CI 0.50–0.95; $p = 0.02$), thus confirming the benefits of this multimodality approach (11).

Neoadjuvant administration of chemotherapy allows early treatment of micrometastatic disease and results in tumor downstaging. Recovery from major gastrointestinal surgery may often preclude the use of postoperative treatment. Concerns that tumor progression may occur during neoadjuvant chemotherapy or that operative morbidity may be increased by this approach have not been substantiated. Perioperative chemotherapy is now the standard of care in Europe for potentially resectable gastric and gastroesophageal junction tumors.

Adjuvant Chemoradiation. The U.S. Intergroup 0116 trial evaluated the combination of radiotherapy plus 5-FU/leucovorin (LV) in resected gastric cancer versus surgery alone. A significant OS benefit was observed in the chemoradiation arm (median OS: 36 vs. 27 months; $p = 0.005$) alongside significantly increased local control rates (30 vs. 19 months; $p = 0.001$) (20). The majority of patients had D0 or D1 resections (54% and 36%, respectively). Based on the results of this study, postoperative chemoradiation became the standard of care in the United States for patients undergoing surgery for gastric cancer.

Treatment of Advanced Gastric and Gastroesophageal Junction Cancers

Although radiotherapy, endoscopic stenting, and even surgery may have a role in the treatment of advanced gastric cancer in a minority of patients presenting with inoperable disease (depending on symptomatology), systemic chemotherapy is the main mode of treatment available . Four RCTs have demonstrated that chemotherapy is superior to BSC for OS (increase in median survival from 3–4 months to 7–10 months) and also reported improvements in quality of life (21).

Many agents including 5-fluorouracil (5-FU), doxorubicin, mitomycin C, cisplatin, S1, taxanes, and irinotecan have demonstrated single agent activity with response rates around 20% to 30%. It is, however, recognized that combination chemotherapy is superior to single agent chemotherapy. Despite this, there is no international consensus on which chemotherapy regimen should be used first-line. Table 9.2 outlines some of the key and recent Phase III RCTs in advanced gastric cancer. Across much of Europe, ECF has been the most commonly used regimen since it was demonstrated to have superior efficacy compared to FAMTX, which had been the reference regimen in the 1990s. In this study, ECF had a higher response rate and OS compared to FAMTX (45% vs. 21%; 8.9 vs. 5.7 months at 1 year respectively) (22). Cisplatin/5-FU (CF) has also been commonly used. Phase III RCTs directly comparing ECF to CF have not been conducted. A recent meta-analysis has demonstrated three-drug regimens containing 5-FU, anthracyclines, and cisplatin to be superior to two-drug regimens containing either cisplatin/5-FU or anthracycline/5-FU in terms of OS (23).

Two recent Phase III RCTs have demonstrated that oral capecitabine can replace infused 5-FU in the treatment of advanced gastric cancer without compromising efficacy. REAL-2 randomized 1002 patients in a 2×2 factorial design to show noninferiority in OS for both capecitabine compared to infused 5-FU and oxaliplatin compared to cisplatin (24). The HR for death was 0.86 (95% CI 0.80–0.99) for the capecitabine regimens compared to the 5-FU regimens. The

Table 9.2 Selected Phase III Studies in Advanced Gastric Cancer Comparing Chemotherapy Regimens

Author (Ref.)	Treatment arms	Number of patients	Overall survival		p Value for overall survival
			Median (months)	1 year (%)	
Webb et al. (22)	FAMTX	130	6.1	22	0.0005
Waters et al. (155)	ECF	126	8.7	37	
Ross et al. (156)	MCF	285	8.7	32.7	0.315
	ECF	289	9.4	40.2	
Dank et al. (157)	Irinotecan/5-FU/folinic acid	170	9.0	NR	0.53
	Cisplatin/5FU	163	8.7	NR	
Van Cutsem et al. (27)	DCF	221	9.2	40	0.02
	5-FU/cisplatin	224	8.6	32	
Kang et al. (25)	5-FU/cisplatin	156	9.5	NR	0.27
	Capecitabine/cisplatin	160	10.5	NR	
Boku et al. (30)	5-FU	234	10.8	44.0	
	Irinotecan/cisplatin	236	12.3	52.5	0.055 (5-FU vs. irinotecan/cisplatin)
	S1	234	11.4	47.9	0.034 (5-FU vs. S1)
Koizumi et al. (31)	S1/cisplatin	148	13.0	54.1	0.04
	S1	150	11.0	46.7	
Cunningham et al. (24)	ECF	263	9.9	37.7	0.61 (ECF vs. EOF)
	EOF	245	9.3	40.4	0.39 (ECF vs. ECX)
	ECX	250	9.9	40.8	0.02 (ECF vs. EOX)
	EOX	244	11.2	46.8	
Al-Batran et al. (26)	5-FU/leucovorin/oxaliplatin	112	10.7	45	NS
	5-FU/leucovorin/cisplatin	106	8.8	40	
Imamura et al. (32)	S1/irinotecan	164	12.8	52.0	0.23
	S1	162	10.5	44.9	
Ajani et al. (154)	S1/cisplatin	521	8.6	NR	0.1983
	5-FU/cisplatin	508	7.9	NR	

Abbreviations: DCF, docetaxel/cisplatin/5-FU; ECF, epirubicin/cisplatin/5-FU; ECX, epirubicin/cisplatin/capecitabine; EOF, epirubicin/oxaliplatin/5-FU; EOX, epirubicin/oxaliplatin/capecitabine; FAMTX, 5-FU/doxorubicin/methotrexate; MCF, mitomycin/cisplatin/5-FU; NS, not significant.

ML17032 study compared capecitabine/cisplatin with cisplatin/5-FU, again with noninferiority as the primary end point (25). Again the primary end point of noninferiority was met (HR 0.81). The results of these two trials confirmed that capecitabine can be used as a substitute for infused 5-FU, thus avoiding the inconvenience and potential complications of central venous catheters.

REAL-2 also demonstrated noninferiority of oxaliplatin compared to cisplatin. In the secondary analysis, EOX had longer OS compared to ECF (HR for death 0.80; 95% CI; 0.66–0.97; $p = 0.02$) as well as a more favorable toxicity profile (24). A smaller study of 220 patients randomized to infused 5-FU plus LV and oxaliplatin (FLO) or infused 5-FU plus LV and cisplatin (FLP) reported reduced toxicity and a trend toward improved progression-free survival (PFS) with the combination of FLO compared to FLP. An unplanned subgroup analysis of patients aged >65 noted that treatment with FLO resulted in significant improvements in RR, TTF, and PFS as well as improved OS (13.9 vs. 7.2 months) for this age group (26).

The ECF regimen can therefore be modified to EOX by substituting capecitabine for infused 5-FU and oxaliplatin for cisplatin, resulting in a combination at least as efficacious as ECF and with a more convenient mode of administration and an acceptable toxicity profile. EOX is currently being used as the reference regimen in the U.K. REAL-3 trial, which is evaluating first-line use of EOX with or without the EGFR-inhibitor panitumumab.

V325 was a Phase II/III study evaluating the role of docetaxel in combination with cisplatin in untreated advanced gastric cancer. In the Phase II study, docetaxel in combination with cisplatin and infused 5-FU (DCF) resulted in a higher over all response rate (ORR) than docetaxel in combination with cisplatin (43% vs. 26%) and was therefore selected as the experimental arm for the Phase III study which randomized 445 patients to DCF or the doublet CF. A modest, but significant improvement in OS (9.2 vs. 8.6 months; $p = 0.020$) was seen with the addition of docetaxel (27). This, however, occurred at the cost of significantly more toxicity, including febrile neutropenia. Furthermore, the study population was younger and fitter than the average patient with advanced gastric cancer, with a median age of 55 years and Karnofsky performance status of 80% to 100% in the majority of patients prior to commencing treatment.

Nevertheless, docetaxel clearly has activity in combination with CF combinations. Phase III RCTs directly comparing DCF to ECF have not yet been conducted, so neither regimen has proven to be superior to the other. A Phase II Swiss trial compared DCF to ECF and reported a much higher rate of complicated neutropenia (41% vs. 18%) (28). Alternative docetaxel dosing regimens have been evaluated in Phase II trials with improved toxicity profiles and similar efficacy, but require further evaluation in Phase III trials (29).

In Japan, S1 is commonly used first-line in advanced gastric cancer. A three-arm RCT comparing 5-FU to S1 and irinotecan plus cisplatin met its primary end point of noninferiority for OS of S1 compared to 5-FU. The response rate for single agent S1 was 28% and median survival was 10.2 months (30). The SPIRITS trial evaluated the addition of cisplatin to S1. Three hundred and five patients were randomized to S1 or S1 plus cisplatin, with a primary end point of OS. The combination of S1 and cisplatin was significantly better than S1-alone in terms of OS (13.0 vs. 11.0 months HR for death 0.77; 95% CI 0.61–0.98; $p = 0.04$) and PFS (6.0 vs. 4.0 months) (31). The combination of irinotecan and S1 compared to S1 alone has also been investigated in the Phase III IRI-S trial reported at GI ASCO 2008. Although the combination treatment arm had a higher response rate (41.5% vs. 26.9%; $p = 0.035$), no statistically significant difference in OS has been observed to date (32). Outside Japan, (mainly USA, Europe and South America), the multinational First-Line Advanced Gastric Cancer Study (FLAGS) randomized patients to fluorouracil/platinum or S1/platinum and failed to demonstrate superior survival with the S1 combination (154).

Several Phase II trials have investigated irinotecan in combination with cisplatin (IC) or LV and 5-FU (ILF and FOLFIRI). In the Phase II part of V-306, ILF was superior to IC in terms of OS, TTP, and RR and was therefore selected as the experimental treatment for the Phase III component of the study. The Phase III study comparing ILF to CF found a nonsignificant trend toward improved TTP (5.0 vs. 4.2 months) and no difference in OS between the two arms (21).

Despite chemosensitivity to many first-line therapeutic regimens, the duration of benefit derived by patients remains limited to months. There is no current standard second-line chemotherapy option for patients with advanced gastric or GOJ tumors. Chemotherapy regimens demonstrating activity in Phase II trials include irinotecan in combination with cisplatin or fluoropyrimidines, FOLFOX, docetaxel alone or in combination with oxaliplatin, and paclitaxel alone or in combination with platinum agents (21).

Key Points

- In esophageal cancer, the addition of neoadjuvant chemotherapy or CRT results in superior outcomes to surgery alone (Fig. 9.1)
- CRT alone may be a treatment option for patients with early stage esophageal SCC or esophageal adenocarcinoma deemed not suitable for resection (Fig. 9.1)
- Perioperative chemotherapy for GOJ and gastric adenocarcinoma results in superior disease-free and overall survival and is now considered the standard of care in Europe. Adjuvant CRT is an alternative treatment option and is the current standard in North America (Fig. 9.1)
- Palliative chemotherapy prolongs survival and improves quality of life and should be offered to patients with adequate performance status

---

PANCREATIC CANCER

Cancer of the exocrine pancreas is the one of the commonest causes of cancer-related death in the Western world. Due to the universally poor outcome of pancreatic cancer, incidence and mortality rates are similar. Five-year survival rates are dismal, and rarely exceed 5% (33).

Epidemiology

The incidence of pancreatic cancer increases with age with the highest incidence in the seventh and eighth decades of life. A clear association with smoking has been identified in several studies and a recent meta-analysis reported a 75%

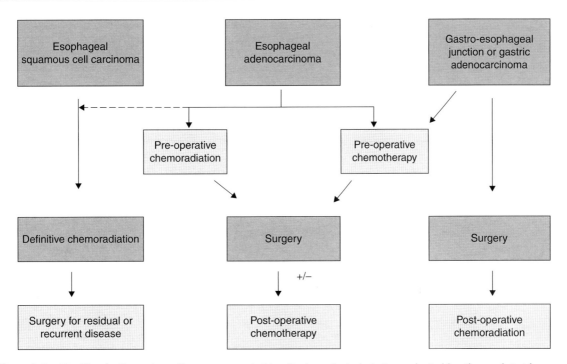

Figure 9.1 Algorithm for the perioperative management of localized esophageal, gastroesophageal junction, and gastric cancer.

increased risk in developing pancreatic cancer in smokers compared to nonsmokers (34). Other potential risk factors include chronic pancreatitis and diabetes mellitus.

Diagnosis and Staging

Common presenting symptoms include abdominal pain, weight loss, and obstructive jaundice. Confirmation of the diagnosis is based on radiological and histological appearance.

Accurate staging of pancreatic cancer is vital to plan appropriate management and avoid unnecessary morbidity. Commonly used imaging modalities for the diagnosis and staging of pancreatic cancer include abdominal ultrasound, CT, and EUS. In experienced hands, EUS has approximately 95% sensitivity for detecting pancreatic cancer and is particularly useful in determining the characteristics of small lesions (33). Furthermore, EUS-FNA can provide histological confirmation of diagnosis in patients deemed unresectable, or with potentially resectable lesions of uncertain etiology. Despite conclusive evidence, many clinicians will choose to avoid percutaneous biopsy of resectable lesions due to a theoretical risk of needle track and intraperitoneal seeding (33).

Further staging information may be acquired via staging laparoscopy and additional imaging modalities including endoscopic retrograde cholangiopancreatography (ERCP), which has the added advantage of enabling therapeutic management of obstructive jaundice; MRI; magnetic resonance cholangiopancreatography (MRCP); and PET with or without CT.

Although cancer associated antigen 19-9 (CA 19-9) is frequently elevated in pancreatic cancer, both sensitivity and specificity are low. Elevated levels can occur in benign disorders as well as in other malignancies. CA 19-9 level is not recommended as a screening test, although it may be useful to monitor response to treatment in locally advanced or unresectable pancreatic cancer or to prompt further investigations to detect recurrence in patients who have undergone primary resection.

Treatment Strategies

Treatment of Resectable Pancreatic Cancer

Approximately 10% to 15% of patients will proceed to potentially curative pancreatic surgery; however median survival for these patients is still limited to 11 to 20 months and five-year survival rates from surgery alone is less than 25% (33). Both adjuvant chemoradiation and chemotherapy have been evaluated as potential strategies to improve surgical outcome. Results of selected trials are represented in Table 9.3.

Adjuvant Chemoradiation. The GITSG trial comparing bolus 5-FU plus split course radiation followed by two years of 5-FU to observation was the first RCT demonstrating the benefit of adjuvant therapy (35). The study closed early due to poor accrual; however due to a statistically significant improvement in survival, adjuvant CRT was adopted as standard therapy in the United States. This approach has not been incorporated into routine practice in Europe as two subsequent European studies (EORTC and ESPAC-1) failed to find a statistically significant advantage in favor of adjuvant CRT. In fact ESPAC-1 found a trend toward worse survival with the addition of CRT (HR for death 1.28; 95% CI 0.99–1.66; $p = 0.05$) (36). A subsequent meta-analysis did not find a significant effect on risk of death with adjuvant CRT and subgroup analysis favored

Table 9.3 Selected Phase III Randomized Controlled Trials of Adjuvant Therapy in Pancreatic Cancer

Study/author (Ref.)	Treatment	Number of patients	Overall survival (months)	p Value
Adjuvant chemoradiotherapy				
GITSG (35)	Bolus 5-FU + RT followed by maintenance 5-FU for 2 years	21	21	0.035
	Observation	22	11	
EORTC (158)	5-FU CI + RT	110	24.5	0.208
	Observation	108	19	
ESPAC 1 (36)	Bolus 5-FU/LV + RT	145	15.9	0.05
	No chemoradiation	147	14.8	
Adjuvant chemotherapy				
ESPAC 1 (36)	5-FU/LV	147	20.1	0.009
	No chemotherapy	142	15.5	
Kosuge et al. (39)	Cisplatin/5-FU	45	12.5	NS
	Observation	44	15.8	
CONKO-001(38)[a]	Gemcitabine	179	22.8	0.005
	Observation	175	20.2	
RTOG 97-04 (40)	CRT + gemcitabine	221	18	NS
	CRT + 5-FU	230	16	
	Pancreatic head tumors			
	CRT + gemcitabine	187	20.5	0.09
	CRT + 5-FU	201	16.9	
Kosuge et al. (39)[b]	Gemcitabine	60	22.31	0.29
	Observation	58	18.36	

[a]DFS 13.3 versus 6.9 months, *p* <0.001. DFS was the primary end point for CONKO-001.
[b]DFS 11.44 versus 4.97 months, *p* = 0.01.
Abbreviations: 5-FU, 5-Fluorouracil; CI, continuous infusion; CRT, chemoradiation; LV, leucovorin; NS, not significant; RT, radiation.

adjuvant CRT in patients with positive resection margins, although the confidence intervals crossed unity (37).

The definitive role of CRT as adjuvant treatment for pancreatic cancer remains uncertain. The ESPAC-1, GITSG, and EORTC studies administered CRT that is probably inferior to modern regimens which utilize infused 5-FU and single course radiation. Furthermore, in the GITSG trial patients received maintenance 5-FU in addition to CRT, and it is impossible to determine which component of treatment is responsible for the observed effect. Prospective RCTs comparing modern CRT regimens to nonradiation-containing regimens have not been conducted. Whether gemcitabine and/or other systemic agents will succeed 5-FU in chemoradiation regimens also remains to be seen.

Adjuvant Chemotherapy. A number of studies have evaluated the role of single agent and combination adjuvant chemotherapy. The ESPAC-1 reported a statistically significant OS advantage for adjuvant bolus 5-FU/LV and this treatment regimen has been compared to adjuvant gemcitabine in the ESPAC-3 trial which completed accrual for pancreatic cancer in December 2006.

The CONKO-001 study evaluated six months of gemcitabine versus observation. This study met its primary end point of a significant improvement in DFS (13.3 vs. 6.9 months; *p* < 0.001) and also demonstrated an OS benefit (22.8 vs. 20.2 months; *p* = 0.005) translating into an estimated five-year survival of 21% versus 9.0% (38). Kosuge et al. also recently reported a significant improvement in DFS for three months of adjuvant gemcitabine compared to observation (11.44 vs. 4.97 months; *p* = 0.01) but not OS (22.3 vs. 18.4 months) (39).

The RTOG 9704 trial compared gemcitabine to 5-FU when given both pre- and post-CRT (infused 5-FU and single course radiation) (40). There was no significant difference in OS or DFS for all patients. A nonsignificant trend toward improved survival was noted for patients with pancreatic head tumors.

In the 2005 meta-analyses of adjuvant therapy for pancreatic cancer adjuvant chemotherapy resulted in a 25% reduction in the risk of death (HR = 0.75; *p* = 0.001) and this improvement was maintained with the inclusion of the CONKO-001 data (24% reduction in the risk of death) (37,41). Adjuvant chemotherapy with 5-FU or gemcitabine confers significant improvements in disease-free and/or OS. The results of ESPAC-3 are awaited to determine the best agent to use in this setting.

Treatment of Locally Advanced Pancreatic Cancer

The optimal management of patients with locally advanced pancreatic cancer is yet to be determined. A 2007 meta-analysis of combined radiation/combined modality therapy for locally advanced pancreatic cancer found a survival advantage for chemoradiation compared to radiation alone but not for chemoradiation followed by chemotherapy (42). A RCT comparing gemcitabine chemotherapy to cisplatin-5FU based chemoradiation followed by maintenance gemcitabine chemotherapy stopped prematurely after a significant OS advantage was found for upfront gemcitabine compared to combined modality therapy (13 vs. 8.6 months, *p* = 0.03) (43). In contrast, the E4201 trial reported a modest OS improvement for gemcitabine-based chemoradiation compared to gemcitabine alone (11.0 vs. 9.2 months; HR 0.574; *p* = 0.034) (44). These results must be interpreted with caution however, since the trial closed early after recruiting only 74 out of a planned 316 patients due to poor accrual.

Furthermore, there was no difference in RR or PFS between the two treatment arms and more grade 3/4 toxicity in the chemoradiation arm.

A newer approach currently under evaluation is the administration of initial chemotherapy followed by CRT in the absence of disease progression. Attempts to refine chemoradiation regimens are also ongoing. The role of neoadjuvant therapy in an attempt to downstage unresectable tumors remains unknown and should be limited to the context of clinical trials.

Treatment of Metastatic Pancreatic Cancer

The majority of patients with pancreatic cancer present with advanced (inoperable or metastatic) disease. Prognosis is extremely poor with a median survival, if untreated, in the order of three to four months. The aims of treatment are tumor control, to improve symptoms and to maintain and improve quality of life (QOL).

The benefits of palliative chemotherapy in addition to BSC have been demonstrated in a number of studies. In a 2007 meta-analysis, chemotherapy resulted in a 36% improvement in survival compared with BSC (HR = 0.64; 95% CI 0.42–0.98) (45).

Single agent gemcitabine has been the accepted standard of care for advanced pancreatic cancer after it was demonstrated to have superior survival and clinical benefit to 5-FU in a single RCT (46). Gemcitabine (1000 mg/m^2 over 30 minutes weekly × 7 followed by one week's rest, and then weekly × 3 every 4 weeks) was superior to 5-FU (600 mg/m^2 weekly) in terms of clinical benefit response (23.8% compared with 4.8% $p = 0.0022$) and median survival (5.65 and 4.41 months, $p = 0.0025$). Approaches to improving the efficacy of gemcitabine have included utilizing fixed dose regimens (FDR) as well as combining gemcitabine with other systemic agents.

Gemcitabine requires initial phosphorylation by deoxycytidine kinase to gemcitabine monophosphate, and subsequent phosphorylation to gemcitabine diphosphate and gemcitabine triphosphate, the active form of the drug (47). Deoxycytidine kinase has saturable kinetics and it has been demonstrated that infusing gemcitabine at 10 mg/m^2/min achieves steady state plasma levels of 20 μmol/L thereby maximizing the rate of formation of gemcitabine triphosphate. Despite initial promising results from Phase II studies, the three-arm Phase III E6201 study failed to reach its primary end point of a 33% or more difference in survival using either FDR gemcitabine or FDR gemcitabine with oxaliplatin compared to standard gemcitabine therapy (48).

Gemcitabine has been combined with several other chemotherapy agents including fluoropyrimidines (5-FU and capecitabine), platinum agents (oxaliplatin and cisplatin), docetaxel, topoisomerase inhibitors (irinotecan and exatecan), and pemetrexed. Results have been largely disappointing, with few regimens resulting in significant improvements in OS. Gemcitabine combined with cisplatin, epirubicin, and 5-FU resulted in statistically significant higher OS compared to gemcitabine alone (5.4 vs. 3.3 months; $p = 0.0033$), however the median OS for each arm was less than the expected median OS for gemcitabine alone (49). This regimen also resulted in significantly higher rates of hematological toxicity. Although gemcitabine combined with oxaliplatin (Gemox) does not appear to improve OS (9.1 vs. 7.1 months;

$p = 0.04$), the significant improvement in RR (26.8% vs. 17.3%; $p = 0.04$), DFS (5.8 vs. 3.7 months; $p = 0.04$), and clinical benefit (38.2% vs. 26.9%; $p = 0.03$) compared to gemcitabine alone indicated that the Gemox regimen represents an active and reasonable treatment option for advanced pancreatic cancer, albeit at the cost of greater hematological, GI, and neurological toxicity (50).

Two Phase III RCTs comparing gemcitabine alone or combined with capecitabine (GemCap) have been conducted in Europe. Updated results from the U.K. NCRI (National Cancer Research Institute) GemCap study report statistically significant improvements in RR (19.4% vs. 12.4%) and PFS (HR 0.78; $p = 0.004$) and a trend toward improved OS (7.1 vs. 6.2 months, HR 0.86; $p = 0.08$) with a good toxicity profile (51). The second study did not find a significant difference in OS, RR, or PFS between the two arms (52). A post hoc analysis, however, found a significant prolongation in OS (10.1 vs. 7.1 months, $p = 0.014$) for patients with KPS 90-100. There was an excess of early disease-related deaths amongst poor PS patients in the GemCap arm, which may account for the lack of significant difference for all patients between the treatment arms. Meta-analysis of the three RCTs comparing GemCap with gemcitabine alone (total 935 patients) indicates a significant OS advantage for combination chemotherapy (HR 0.85; 95% CI 0.76–0.99) with no significant heterogeneity.

Targeted Therapies. The efficacy of molecular targeted agents in combination with gemcitabine has also been investigated. Randomized phase III studies have been conducted comparing gemcitabine to gemcitabine combined with marimastat, tipifarnib, erlotinib, cetuximab, and bevacizumab. Results are summarized in Table 9.4.

In the NCIC CTG PA.3 study, erlotinib combined with gemcitabine conferred a small, albeit statistically significant, OS benefit compared to gemcitabine alone (6.24 vs. 5.91 months, HR 0.82, $p = 0.038$) (53). Although many would argue that the actual clinical benefit of this combination is minimal, on the basis of this single RCT, erlotinib was approved for use combined with gemcitabine in the first-line setting. Preliminary results of two Phase III studies presented at ASCO 2007 comparing gemcitabine to gemcitabine/bevacizumab, and gemcitabine/cetuximab have not demonstrated a significant improvement in OS, PFS, or RR.

AVITA, a double blind, placebo controlled study of gemcitabine and erlotinib with or without bevacizumab also failed to result in an improvement in OS (6.0 vs. 7.1 months with the addition of bevacizumab, HR 0.89; $p = 0.2087$) although a small improvement in median PFS was observed (3.6 vs. 4.6 months, HR 0.73; $p = 0.0002$) (54).

Second-Line Chemotherapy. There is no standard second-line treatment for advanced pancreatic cancer. Several regimens have been evaluated including 5-FU/LV, irinotecan, rubitecan, paclitaxel, gemcitabine plus oxaliplatin, oxaliplatin plus fluoropyrimidines, capecitabine plus erlotinib, and raltitrexed plus oxaliplatin/or irinotecan; however few randomized Phase III studies have been completed.

CONKO 003 initially compared BSC to oxaliplatin/5-FU/LV (OFF regimen) in patients who had progressed after first-line gemcitabine therapy. Results after recruiting 46 patients reported a significant improvement in median OS for OFF (4.8 vs. 2.3 months, $p = 0.0077$) (55). The trial

Table 9.4   Selected Phase III Randomized Controlled Trials of Gemcitabine and Targeted Therapies in Metastatic Pancreatic Cancer

Study/author (Ref.)	Treatment arms	DFS/PFS median (months)	p Value	Median survival (months)	p Value	Response rate (%)
Moore et al. (159)	Gemcitabine/marimastat	1.68	0.001	3.74	<0.001	<1
	Gemcitabine	3.5		6.59		5
Van Cutsem et al. (160)	Gemcitabine/tipifarnib	3.73	0.72	6.43	0.75	6
	Gemcitabine	3.63		6.06		8
NCIC CTG PA.3 (53)	Gemcitabine/erlotinib	3.75	0.004	6.24	0.038	48.9
	Gemcitabine	3.55		5.91		41.2
SWOG S0205 (161)	Gemcitabine/cetuximab	3.5	0.058	6.4	0.14	12
	Gemcitabine	3.0		5.9		14
CALGB 80303 (162)	Gemcitabine/bevacizumab	4.9	0.99	5.8	0.78	11
	Gemcitabine	4.7		6.1		10
AVITA (54)	Gemcitabine/erlotinib	4.6	0.0002	7.1	0.2087	13.5
	Gemcitabine/erlotinib/ bevacizumab	3.6		6.0		8.6

Abbreviation: DFS/PFS, disease free survival/progression free survival.

was subsequently modified to use 5-FU/LV as the control arm. Compared to 5-FU/LV, OFF resulted in a significant improvement in both PFS (13 vs. 9 weeks; $p = 0.012$) and OS (26 vs. 13 weeks; $p = 0.014$) (56). OFF therefore represents a regimen with clinically significant activity for patients who have progressed after first-line gemcitabine.

Other Treatment Options. Palliative stenting, bypass surgery, radiotherapy, nerve plexus blocks, and intrathecal infusions may also provide symptomatic relief in selected patients.

Key Points

- For patients with resected pancreatic cancer, adjuvant chemotherapy with 5-FU is the current European standard of care with gemcitabine emerging as a potential alternative
- The definitive role of adjuvant chemoradiation remains uncertain amongst European oncologists. In North America, adjuvant chemoradiation is the standard postoperative approach
- Palliative chemotherapy results in improved survival and quality of life
- Erlotinib combined with gemcitabine confers a superior, although modest OS improvement compared to gemcitabine monotherapy
- The combination of capecitabine with gemcitabine is well tolerated and results in improved PFS and response rate compared to gemcitabine monotherapy. In addition, a meta-analysis demonstrates a significant improvement in OS for the combination therapy
- The combination of oxaliplatin with gemcitabine results in improved PFS, radiological and clinical response rates compared to gemcitabine monotherapy, but may be less well tolerated
- Oxaliplatin/5-FU/LV is an active second-line treatment regimen after failure of gemcitabine therapy

---

HEPATOBILIARY CANCERS
Hepatocellular Carcinoma
Epidemiology
Although hepatocellular carcinoma (HCC) can occur in patients without known risk factors, the majority of cases are associated with hepatitis B virus (HBV), hepatitis C virus (HCV), alcoholic liver disease, and cirrhosis of any cause. The combination of HBV and HCV increases the risk of developing HCC.

The incidence of HCC is rising and it is the third most common cause of cancer-related death worldwide. The prognosis is poor because of high rates of recurrence, late stage presentation, and limited treatment options. Five-year survival is around 5% and OS for patients diagnosed with unresectable disease is around six months. Although there is no evidence of survival benefit with early diagnosis, many groups now advocate six monthly surveillance ultrasound and alpha-fetoprotein (AFP) in patients at high risk of developing the disease (57).

Diagnosis and Staging
Diagnosis can often be made without biopsy by the combination of liver imaging (CT scan and MRI) and serum markers (AFP). CT of the thorax is also required to complete staging.

Treatment Strategies
Treatment of Localized Operable Disease
Surgery. For a selected minority of patients presenting with early stage disease, surgical resection or liver transplantation (LT) may be viable and potentially curative treatment options. Factors influencing suitability for surgical resection include adequate liver function (Child-Pugh classification A), anatomic location, size, and number of lesions. Although no RCTs comparing outcomes of resection to transplantation have been conducted, LT may result in superior outcomes in terms of both recurrence and survival and with careful patient selection, five-year survival for LT can exceed 70% (58). Surgical resection along with transarterial chemoembolization (TACE) and radiofrequency ablation (RFA) can be used as bridging treatments while awaiting a suitable donor liver.

Local Therapies. Local ablative techniques using percutaneous ethanol injection or thermal ablation (RFA or microwave therapy) results in complete destruction in 90% of small lesions (≤3 cm). Recent RCTs suggest thermal ablation to be superior to percutaneous ethanol injection for both recurrence and survival (59).

Adjuvant Therapy. There is no standard adjuvant treatment for HCC postresection and reports from studies are often contradictory. In a meta-analysis of preoperative or postoperative transarterial chemotherapy, systemic chemotherapy, or a combination of systemic and transarterial chemotherapy, only postoperative transarterial chemotherapy was likely to improve survival and decrease recurrence risk (60). Adjuvant interferon (IFN-α) has been evaluated in a number of RCTs which have reported improved local recurrence and/or survival rates. However, this treatment is often poorly tolerated and current evidence is not sufficient to warrant routine use of adjuvant IFN-α (59). Retinoids following resection or local ablation were associated with a significant lower incidence of recurrence in a randomized control trial (RCT) compared with placebo (27% vs. 45%) and are undergoing further evaluation (59).

Treatment of Inoperable Disease
Arterial embolization techniques, particularly with chemotherapy (TACE) has been the main treatment option for patients with advanced HCC. A recent review confirmed that while TACE improves survival for patients with advanced HCC and is the most preferred embolization prodecure, there is no evidence that TACE has a survival advantage compared to transarterial embolization alone (61). This question is currently being evaluated in the U.K. NCRN TACE trial.

The discovery of hormonal receptors on HCC lines has not led to further therapeutic options. A meta-analysis of tamoxifen in HCC found no effect on median survival or tumor response rate (62). Several chemotherapeutic agents including doxorubicin, fluoropyrimidines, cisplatin, etoposide, epirubicin, oxaliplatin, gemcitabine, and irinotecan have been investigated either as single agents or in combination. Results have been disappointing with response rates of less than 20% and little (if any) impact on survival, often at the cost of significant toxicity (59).

Sorafenib, a multitargeted orally active small molecule tyrosine kinase inhibitor (TKI) has emerged as the new reference standard treatment option for advanced HCC. The Phase III SHARP trial randomized 602 patients with untreated, advanced HCC to sorafenib 400 mg twice daily or placebo. Treatment with sorafenib resulted in a 44% improvement in OS compared to placebo (median survival 10.7 vs. 7.9 months; HR 0.69; $p = 0.0077$) as well as improved time to progression (5.5 vs. 2.8 months; $p = 0.000007$). Disease control rate was also improved (43% vs. 32%), although actual overall response rates were low (2.3%) (63).

Biliary Tract Cancers
Cancers of the gallbladder and cholangiocarcinomas are rare and are generally associated with a poor prognosis. Cholangiocarcinomas are subclassified according to anatomical site intrahepatic (10%), perihilar (50–60%), and distal/extrahepatic (20–30%) (64).

Epidemiology
Identified risk factors for biliary cancers include chronic cholelithiasis, primary sclerosing cholangitis, choledochal cysts, Caroli's disease, bile duct adenomas, smoking, thorotrast exposure, HCV infection, parasitic biliary infestation, and chronic typhoid carrier state (64).

Treatment Strategies
Treatment of Localized Biliary Tract Cancers
The only potentially curative treatment is surgery, however few patients present with disease amenable to complete resection. Radical/extended cholecystectomy is recommended in patients with localized gallbladder cancers with the exception of T1a tumors, who have five-year survival over 85% with simple cholecystectomy alone (65). Patients with intrahepatic lesions require partial hepatectomy whereas distal lesions require pancreatoduodenectomy. Negative tumor margins and the absence of lymph node involvement are known predictors of five-year survival which is in the order of 20% to 40%.

Although adjuvant CRT or chemotherapy may confer a survival benefit or improve local control rates because of the rarity of the disease, there are few RCT trials to allow definite conclusions to be drawn. Adjuvant therapy remains the subject of ongoing trials.

Treatment of Advanced Disease
For patients of good performance status, palliative treatment options include chemotherapy, radiation, and photodynamic therapy (PDT). Biliary drainage, preferably by endoscopic stenting can provide good symptomatic relief. Metallic stents are preferable to plastic stents in patients with a prognosis longer than six months (64). PDT as an alternative or in addition to stenting has been evaluated in two RCTs and was found to result in superior OS; 630 versus 210 days for PDT compared to BSC ($p = 0.0109$) and 493 versus 98 days for PDT plus stent compared to stent alone ($p = 0.001$) (66).

Chemotherapy appears to confer benefits for both quality of life and survival over BSC, although improvements in OS are modest. Several agents have been evaluated including fluoropyrimidines, anthracyclines, gemcitabine, platinum agents, docetaxel, and irinotecan; however, few randomized Phase III trials have been conducted. A 2007-pooled analysis of 104 published trials concluded that gemcitabine combined with platinum agents was the most active regimen (67). ABC-02 is an ongoing U.K. NCRI randomized Phase III trial directly comparing gemcitabine to gemcitabine/cisplatin in advanced biliary cancers.

Key Points

Hepatocellular carcinoma

- Hepatic resection and liver transplantation are potentially curative treatment options for selected patients with localized HCC
- There is no standard adjuvant treatment for HCC
- Transarterial chemoembolization improves survival in patients with inoperable HCC
- Sorafenib improves OS and TTP in patients with advanced HCC and has emerged as the new reference treatment option

Biliary tract cancer

- Surgery is the primary treatment modality for localized disease
- The role of adjuvant treatment is currently being evaluated
- There is no standard chemotherapy regimen for advanced biliary tract cancer Active enrolment into clinical trials is essential to establish best practice

NEUROENDOCRINE TUMORS AND CANCER OF THE SMALL BOWEL

Gastroenteropancreatic Neuroendocrine Tumors

Gastroenteropancreatic neuroendocrine tumors are a rare entity, accounting for approximately 2% of all GI tumors. The incidence of carcinoid tumors has been rising and is now around 2.5 to 5 cases per 100,000 (68).

Over 90% of neuroendocrine tumors (NETs) arise in the gastrointestinal tract. Other sites of presentation include the bronchus and gonads, although they can arise in almost any organ. Neuroendocrine tumors s are traditionally classified according to their embryological site of origin (Foregut–Bronchi, stomach, pancreas, gallbladder, duodenum; midgut–jejunum, ileum, appendix, right colon; hindgut–left colon, rectum). However, this mode of classification has largely been replaced by the WHO classification of gastroenteropancreatic endocrine tumors, which classifies according to predicted clinical behavior depending on histopathologic features. Carcinoid tumors, arising from enterochromaffin cells, account for the majority of all NETS and most frequently occur in the gastrointestinal tract.

A recently published study of patients in England and Wales reported five-year survival rates of 45.9% and 56.5% for all NETs and well-differentiated NETs respectively (69).

Diagnosis and Staging

Symptoms relating to NETs vary widely from no symptomatology, to symptoms relating to anatomical location (abdominal pain, mechanical obstruction, bleeding) or relating to secretion of neuroamines and peptides including 5-hydroxytryptophan (5HT), gastrin, insulin, glucagons, somatostatin, histamine, and vasoactive intestinal peptide (VIP). Of note a significant proportion of pancreatic NETs are nonfunctioning (40%) (68).

Carcinoid syndrome occurs in approximately 10% of patients with carcinoid tumors, and is characterized by the triad of facial flushing, secretory diarrhea, and bronchospasm. Patients with carcinoid syndrome may also develop cardiac fibrosis, predominantly resulting in right sided valvular heart disease.

Staging Investigations. A combination of conventional imaging modalities (CT and MRI) and nuclear medicine scans, in particular somatostatin receptor scintigraphy (SRS) is often required to assess the full extent of NETs. Eighty percent of carcinoid tumors have type 2 somatostatin receptors and can thus be localized by scintigraphy with radio-labelled octreotide. The SRS can also provide useful information regarding likely response to somatostatin analogues.

Biochemical markers play an important role in the diagnosis, monitoring, and management of NETs. Chromogranin A levels are often elevated, even in nonfunctioning tumors. For carcinoid tumors, the serotonin breakdown product 5-hydroxyindolacetic acids (5HIAA) can be measured by 24-hour urine collection. Other serum markers (gastrin, insulin, glucagon, somatostatin, histamine, VIP) relating to functioning tumors may be elevated and will often result in distinct clinical syndromes.

Accurate histopathological classification of NETs is essential since characteristics such as degree of differentiation, mitoses per high power field, and proliferation index (Ki-67) are predictive for tumor grade and prognosis.

Treatment Strategies

Surgery. Surgery is the treatment of choice for the minority of patients presenting with localized resectable disease and offers the only chance of cure. Patients presenting with incidental carcinoid of the appendix at appendicectomy less than <2 cm, involving the tip and with no mesoappendiceal invasion are usually cured by appendicectomy alone. The European Neuroendocrine Tumor Society consensus guidelines recommend performing a right hemicolectomy for appendiceal carcinoid tumors if the following features are present: tumor >2 cm; deep mesoappendiceal invasion, and/or positive margins (70). The presence of other histological features associated with aggressive behavior such as high mitotic index or high Ki67, angio- or neural invasion, or tumor location at the base of the appendix may also be indications for more extensive surgery.

For patients with advanced disease cytoreductive surgery to reduce tumor burden (ideally by 90%) and therefore reduce hormone secretion may provide palliation of symptoms. Several, albeit small, retrospective studies have cited the benefits of hepatic cytoreduction with most studies reporting improved symptomatology in more than 90% of patients and five-year survival rates of 41% to 92% (71). Furthermore, reducing the tumor burden may prolong or restore the effectiveness of anti-secretory therapies, to which most tumors eventually become refractory.

Chemoembolization/RFA. For patients deemed not suitable for surgical cytoreduction, interventional radiological techniques such as chemoembolization or embolization alone may provide effective palliation of symptoms by reducing hepatic artery bloodflow and causing tumor necrosis. Chemoembolization or embolization involves catheterization of the hepatic artery and injection of chemotherapy, gel foam powder, or microspherical particles. Radiofrequency ablation is also used alone or in combination with either surgery or embolization techniques.

Chemotherapy. There are few large prospective randomized trials evaluating the role of chemotherapy in NETs. Many published trials are small, retrospective and/or include biochemical responses in the overall response rate. The highest response rates to systemic chemotherapy agents are generally seen in poorly differentiated, anaplastic NETS where the combination of cisplatin and etoposide has produced response rates around 70% (72). Pancreatic NETS, which tend to be well to moderately differentiated, are more likely to respond to streptozocin-based chemotherapy than other NETS. Streptozocin, in combination with doxorubicin, 5-FU, or both, produces higher response rates than streptozocin alone. Actual radiological response rates to streptozocin-combinations are between 6% and 40% (73). For patients who have progressed on standard chemotherapy, a small case series has reported tumor response or stabilization in all six evaluable patients with the combination of temozolamide and capecitabine (74).

Somatostatin Analogues and Interferon. For patients with symptomatic metastatic NETs, antisecretory treatment with the somatostatin analogues octreotide or lanreotide can markedly reduce the circulating amounts of bioactive amines and control symptoms. Clinical response rates are in the order of 75%, although objective tumor response rates are low (5%) (68).

Alpha-interferon has been demonstrated to have antitumor activity in a number of studies with clinical response rates of 40% to 70%, biochemical response rates of up to 50%, and objective tumor response rates of 10% to 15% (75).

Although a potential additive effect of somatostatin analogues and alpha-interferon has been demonstrated, a recently published review of the literature found a lack of statistically significant evidence favoring the upfront use of the combination and increased toxicity, particularly when higher doses of alpha-interferon were used (75).

Radioisotopes. Targeted radionuclide therapy is a treatment option for patients and can achieve good symptomatic responses and tumor stabilization rates. Agents used include ^{131}I-MIBG and, for patients with positive ^{111}In-octreotide and ^{111}In-lanreotide SRS scans, ^{90}Y-octreotide and ^{90}Y-lanreotide respectively. Approximately 15% to 20% of patients may achieve an objective response to ^{90}Y-octreotide or ^{90}Y-lanreotide, although the majority generally achieve tumor stabilization (72). Myelosuppression is the main side effect experienced. Renal failure can occur with ^{90}Y-octreotide due to tubular reuptake of peptide analogues. Ensuring adequate renal function prior to treatment and pretreatment with amino acids has been shown to minimize this risk.

Molecular Targeted Therapies. The overexpression in NETs of growth factors, including VEGF and downstream signaling molecules, platelet derived growth factor and insulin-like growth factor receptor 1, has generated interest in the antitumor effects of targeted therapies alone or in combination with somatostatin analogues. Of these agents, the angiogenesis inhibitors—bevacizumab and the small molecule tyrosine kinase inhibitors sunitinib, sorafenib, and valatinib—and the mTOR protein kinase inhibitors—temsirolimus and everolimus—appear the most promising, although actual radiological response rates in Phase II trials are less than 20% (68).

Small Bowel Cancer

Small bowel tumors are rare, accounting for 2% of all GI malignancies (1). The main histological subtypes are adenocarcinoma and carcinoid (discussed previously), comprising 45% and 29% of small bowel tumors respectively. Carcinomas occur most commonly in the duodenum, whereas carcinoids occur more commonly in the distal small bowel. Presenting symptoms of adenocarcinomas of the small bowel may relate to local effects (bleeding, obstruction, pain) or, more frequently, metastatic disease.

Surgery is the only curative option for patients with localized disease and can result in median survival of

20 months and five-year survival of 26% (76). Due to the rarity of the disease, there are no RCTs regarding systemic treatment of small bowel tumors. In practice, most oncologists will treat duodenal tumors in a similar fashion to gastric cancers, whereas more distal small bowel tumors are treated with colorectal cancer protocols. Small, retrospective case series provide some support for the use of 5-FU either alone or in combination with other cytotoxics in the metastatic setting. Combinations of 5-FU and platinum can produce response rates around 20% and irinotecan may have efficacy as second-line therapy (77).

Key Points

- Surgery offers potentially curative treatment for NETs, but is only feasible in a minority of patients
- Several treatment modalities including chemoembolization/RFA, chemotherapy, somatostatin analogues, targeted radionuclide therapy, and surgery to reduce tumor burden are aimed at achieving symptom control
- Small bowel tumors are rare and surgery again is the primary curative treatment
- Systemic chemotherapy can be offered to patients with distant metastases, however the evidence is based on retrospective case series or extrapolation from gastric and colorectal cancer trials

---

COLORECTAL CANCER

Colorectal cancer (CRC) is the most common gastrointestinal malignancy and the third most common cancer worldwide with over one million new cases diagnosed annually. Although significant progress has been made in the treatment of colorectal cancer over the past few decades, each year over 500,000 patients will still die from the disease (16).

Epidemiology

The step-wise mutations that occur as normal colonic epithelium develops increasing levels of dysplasia and finally transforms to invasive carcinoma are well described (the adenoma-carcinoma sequence). Both environmental and genetic factors influence the risk of developing CRC.

A family history of CRC is a major risk factor for developing CRC. The presence of a single first degree relative with CRC almost doubles an individual's risk of developing the disease. Autosomal dominant genetic disorders such as familial adenomatous polyposis (FAP) and hereditary nonpolyposis colon cancer (HNPCC or Lynch syndrome) are associated with a very high risk of developing the disease. However, inherited mutations in the APC gene, responsible for FAP, and mutations associated with HNPCC (e.g., hMLH1, hMSH2) only account for 3% to 5% of cases (78). Inflammatory bowel disease also increases the risk of developing malignancy. Epidemiological studies have identified environmental risk factors including diet, alcohol intake, smoking, and physical activity (79). Aspirin, nonsteroidal anti-inflammatory agents (including COX-2 inhibitors), and hormone replacement therapy are potential chemopreventative agents, but routine use is not recommended due to the associated toxicity of these agents and uncertainty regarding cost-effectiveness, dosage, and duration of therapy (80).

Individuals considered at high risk of developing CRC should undergo regular screening/surveillance colonoscopies. This includes patients with an inherited predisposition toward CRC (e.g., FAP or HNPCC), patients with a personal history of adenomatous polyps, CRC, or inflammatory bowel disease, and individuals with a family history of two or more first degree relatives with CRC, or one first degree relative diagnosed at a young age. Increasingly, throughout the European Union and elsewhere, mass screening programmes, mainly utilizing fecal occult blood tests and flexible sigmoidoscopy, are being introduced for individuals considered at average or slightly above average risk for developing CRC.

Diagnosis and Staging

The presenting symptoms of CRC vary widely and may include weight loss, symptomatic anaemia, abdominal pain, constipation or diarrhea, per rectum bleeding, bowel obstruction, or perforation. Many patients with CRC remain asymptomatic until their disease is at an advanced stage. With screening programs and increased public awareness, patients with asymptomatic disease may be diagnosed at an earlier stage, thereby increasing the chance of cure. For colorectal cancer, the minimum baseline diagnostic work-up should include histological confirmation, total colonoscopy, and CT CAP. Assessment of patients with rectal cancer requires additional imaging in the form of MRI of the pelvis or endorectal ultrasound. Equivocal lesions seen on CT may also require further evaluation with MRI of the liver and/or PET.

Accurate staging to predict prognosis of colorectal cancer is essential and requires a combination of imaging, histopathological review, and good quality surgery. The long-term outcome of localized resected colon cancer is intimately related to lymph node status. It is therefore imperative that careful attention is paid to the number of lymph nodes harvested during surgery as well as the number of lymph nodes involved when considering if adjuvant therapy should be recommended. It is recommended that a minimum of 12 nodes should be examined if true node negativity is to be declared (81).

For rectal cancer, circumferential resection margin (CRM) involvement, defined as tumor ≤1 mm from the resection margin, is an important prognostic factor. Even with the advent of total mesorectal excision (TME) and preoperative CRT, the power of the CRM to predict for local recurrence and survival remains high (82). Increasing T (T1-2, T3, T4) and N (N0, N1, N2) stage had a negative impact on prognosis in a pooled analysis of five North American trials (83). In this analysis, three distinct groups of at risk patients were identified according to T and N status; intermediate risk (T1-2/N1, T3/N0), moderately high (T1-2/N2, T3/N1, T4/N0), and high (T3/N2, T4/N1, T4/N2). Additionally, for T3 tumors, depth of penetration into the muscularis propria, particularly if tumor extends more than 5 to 6 mm beyond the muscularis propria is associated with a higher locoregional recurrence rate and a poorer five-year survival rate (84). All these factors must be taken into account when selecting patients for more aggressive combined modality therapy.

Accurate local staging of primary rectal cancer is therefore of utmost importance and further information can be obtained by additional imaging with pelvic MRI, endorectal ultrasound, or both. Pretreatment MRI assessment of rectal tumors is particularly favored in Europe. The multinational MERCURY study demonstrated that MRI can accurately stage extramural spread and that tumor within 1 mm of the mesorectal fascia on MRI strongly predicts for CRM involvement (85). Endorectal ultrasound is most useful to measure depth of tumor invasion in early stage T1 and T2 rectal cancers, but is limited in its ability to assess bulky tumors growing into the mesorectum and nodal disease.

Treatment Strategies for Localized Colon Cancer

Although the majority of patients present with localized colon cancer amenable to curative surgery, a significant proportion will develop recurrent disease. Adjuvant chemotherapy is aimed at the eradication of micrometastatic disease and therefore the prevention of recurrent disease. Selected patients with very early tumors may be candidates for local excision via polypectomy, but specimens require careful histological examination to determine depth of invasion and confirm clear margins and exclude the need for more extensive resection.

Adjuvant Therapy for Colon Cancer

Since the late 1980s, the results of several large randomized trials have demonstrated a clear indication for adjuvant therapy in resected Stage III colon cancer. Initial adjuvant chemotherapy regimens have evolved over time. Current trials are evaluating the potential role of bevacizumab in the treatment of adjuvant colon cancer. A further development has been the recognition of three-year DFS as an appropriate end point for adjuvant CRC trials, after a pooled analysis of 18 RCTs demonstrated high correlation between three-year DFS and five-year OS (86).

Intravenous (IV) Fluoropyrimidines. After the initial demonstration of both improved DFS and OS for patients with Stage III colon cancer with adjuvant chemotherapy, FU/levimasole became the standard of care in the United States, and the reference arm for many randomized clinical trials. Subsequent RCTs evaluating bolus 5-FU regimens addressed questions such as duration of treatment; modulation of 5FU with levimasole, LV or both; and the role of high versus low dose LV (81). Collectively, these trials defined six months of bolus 5-FU/LV as the standard adjuvant regimen for colon cancer in many countries.

Adjuvant trials comparing infused and bolus 5-FU regimens have consistently reported less toxicity with the infused regimens with similar relapse-free and OS (81). Infused 5-FU regimens are therefore a reasonable substitute for bolus 5-FU regimens and have been used as the reference treatment arm in subsequent European RCTs.

Oral Fluoropyrimidines. The X-ACT trial was a noninferiority study comparing oral capecitabine to bolus 5-FU/LV (Mayo regimen) (87). Almost 2000 patients were recruited, with 1004 patients randomized to oral capecitabine. The primary end point—equivalence in DFS was met (HR 0.87; 95% CI 0.75–1.00; $p < 0.001$ for noninferiority). Significantly less diarrhea, nausea or vomiting, stomatitis, and neutropenia occurred with capecitabine, although higher rates of hand-foot-syndrome and hyperbilirubinae-mia were observed. On the basis of this trial, the adjuvant use of oral capecitabine for CRC was approved in the United States, Europe, and elsewhere.

Oral UFT (combined uracil/tegafur) in combination with LV has also been shown to have similar efficacy to bolus 5-FU. In the NSABP C06 trial, there was no differ-ence in five-year DFS or OS for UFT/LV compared to 5-FU/LV. Health-related QOL data was similar, although patients reported oral UFT/LV as a more convenient mode of delivery than IV 5-FU/LV (88). Despite this, UFT has not been approved for use in the United States, but is available elsewhere, including Europe.

Combination Regimens. Success with the addition of oxaliplatin and irinotecan in the metastatic CRC setting has led to evaluation of these drugs in the adjuvant setting (Table 9.5). Ongoing RCTs are also evaluating the impact of the addition of targeted agents to adjuvant chemotherapy.

The MOSAIC (Multicenter International Study of Oxaliplatin/5-Fluorouracil/Leucovorin in the Adjuvant Treatment of Colon Cancer) trial investigated the addition of oxaliplatin (85 mg/m^2 day 1) to infused 5-FU/LV (De Gramont regimen). Initial results reported a 23% reduc-tion in the risk of relapse with the addition of oxaliplatin ($p = 0.002$) (89). On the basis of these results oxaliplatin was approved for the adjuvant treatment of Stage III CRC by several drug regulatory authorities. Updated results from the MOSAIC trial presented at ASCO 2007 con-firmed the significant improvement in five-year DFS for all patients, a significant benefit in OS for Stage III patients (HR 0.80; $p = 0.029$) and a trend toward improved OS for all patients (HR 0.85; $p = 0.057$) (90). A second study conducted in North America, NSABP C07, evaluated the addition of the same dose of oxaliplatin (weeks 1, 3, and 5) to the Roswell Park bolus 5-FU/LV regimen. Again a statistically significant improvement in DFS was observed (19% risk reduction in favor of the oxaliplatin-containing regimen; $p = 0.002$) as well as a trend toward improved OS survival (HR 0.85; $p = 0.06$) (91). However, much higher rates of grade 3/4 GI toxicity occurred in both

arms compared to the regimens used in the MOSAIC trial.

Both trials reported a significant increase in grade 3/4 neuropathy with the addition of oxaliplatin, although the rates of persisting severe neuropathy decreased to 1.1% after 12 months of follow-up and 0.6% 12 months after randomization for the MOSAIC and NSABP C07 trials respectively. Grade 3/4 neutropenia, nausea, vomiting, and diarrhea were also increased with the addition of oxaliplatin compared to fluoropyrimidine-therapy alone. Although severe oxaliplatin-related neuropathy improves with time, patients can develop permanent residual neu-ropathy and must therefore be carefully monitored for development of neurotoxicity while on therapy. Dose reductions or omissions should occur as determined by severity of symptoms.

Efficacy results from a RCT comparing oxaliplatin in combination with capecitabine (XELOX or Capox—a regimen used with increasing frequency in the metastatic CRC setting) to bolus 5-FU/LV are not yet available, how-ever the planned safety analysis has indicated a manage-able toxicity profile in the adjuvant setting (92). Further information regarding the efficacy of this regimen is also expected from a number of other ongoing adjuvant trials.

Adjuvant CRC trials designed to investigate the effi-cacy of irinotecan have failed to demonstrate a benefit for the addition of irinotecan to 5-FU/LV. The CALGB C89803 trial randomized 1264 patients to irinotecan plus 5-FU/LV (Roswell Park regimen) or 5-FU/LV alone. No difference in DFS or OS was seen, however toxicities and treatment-related mortality were much higher in the irinotecan-treatment arm (93). The PETACC-3 and FNCLCC Accord02/FFCD9802 studies compared the more tolerable FOLFIRI regimen to the De Gramont infused 5-FU regimen, the latter trial in patients considered to have high-risk Stage III disease. Again, neither trial demonstrated a benefit for the addition of irinotecan to fluoropyrimidines for the adjuvant treatment of CRC (81).

The optimal postoperative management of Stage II colon cancer has been less clear largely due to the majority of studies being small and underpowered. Recently,

Table 9.5 Selected Phase III Randomized Controlled Trials of Adjuvant Combination Chemotherapy for Colon Cancer

Study/author (Ref.)	Treatment arms	Number of patients	HR DFS (95% CI)	*p* value	HR death (95% CI)	*p* value
Fluoropyrimidine + oxaliplatin						
MOSAIC (80,90)	Oxaliplatin/infused 5-FU/LV	1123	0.77[a] (0.65–0.91)	0.002	0.85 (0.71–1.01)[c]	0.057
	Infused 5-FU/LV	1123	0.80[b] (0.68–0.93)	0.003	0.80 (0.66–0.98)[d]	0.029
NSABP C07 (91)	Oxaliplatin/bolus 5-FU/LV	1200	0.81 (0.70–0.93)	0.002	0.85 (0.72–1.01)	0.06
	Bolus 5-FU/LV	1209				
Fluoropyrimidine + irinotecan						
CALGB C89803 (93)	Irinotecan/5-FU/LV	629	No difference	0.85	No difference	0.74
	5-FU/LV	635				
PETACC-3 (163)	Irinotecan/infused 5-FU/LV	1044	0.89[a] (0.77–1.11)	0.091	NR	
	Infused 5-FU/LV	1050				
Accord 02/FFCD 9802 (164)	Irinotecan/infused 5-FU/LV	200	1.19 (0.90–1.59)	0.22	1.06 (0.79–1.42)	0.68
	Infused 5-FU/LV	200				

[a]3 year DFS all patients.
[b]5 year DFS all patients.
[c]All patients.
[d]Stage III patients only.
Abbreviations: 5-FU/LV, 5-fluorouracil/leucovorin; DFS, disease free survival; HR, hazard ratio; NR, not reported.

however, the randomized Phase III QUASAR study (which included 2963 patients with Stage II CRC) confirmed that 5-FU-based adjuvant treatment confers a reduction in risk of recurrence and a 3.6% absolute improvement in survival for patients with uncertain indications for adjuvant chemotherapy (94). At ASCO 2008, an analysis of patients according to tumor mismatch repair (MMR) status demonstrated a lack of response to 5-FU based chemotherapy in patients with Stage II MMR deficient tumors. In fact, patients with Stage II MMR deficient tumors treated with 5-FU chemotherapy had a worse OS compared to untreated patients (HR 3.15; 95% CI 1.07–9.29; $p = 0.03$) (95). The role of oxaliplatin-containing regimens in these patients remains unknown.

The risk-benefit profile must therefore be carefully taken into account when discussing the role of adjuvant chemotherapy with patients with Stage II colon cancer, and immunohistochemistry for MMR proteins or testing for microsatellite instability (MSI) should be considered. The presence of the following adverse prognostic factors, presentation with intestinal obstruction/perforation, T4 tumors, poorly differentiated tumors, presence of extramural venous or lymphatic invasion or perineural invasion, is considered to indicate a high risk of relapse and, providing there are no medical contraindications, adjuvant chemotherapy should be offered. These high-risk patients may also derive further benefit from a combination oxaliplatin-fluoropyrimidine regimen (90).

Treatment Strategies for Localized Rectal Cancer

Optimizing the treatment of localized rectal cancer is a prime example of the importance of a multidisciplinary approach to management. Accurate staging of the primary tumor using MRI or endorectal ultrasound (discussed previously) is essential. Curative treatment generally requires surgery, however local recurrence (LR) rates with conventional resection are 25% to 40%. Only the earliest stage of tumors can be effectively managed with surgery alone. Several treatment approaches have therefore been developed, aimed at reducing both the risk of LR and distal metastases.

Surgery. Although selected very early tumors (e.g., T1N0) may be appropriate for local procedures such as transanal endoscopic microdissection, the majority of tumors require more extensive surgical excision. Recurrence rates with TME, defined as a sharp dissection under clear vision with the excision of the rectum and mesorectum within the mesorectal fascia, have consistently been reported as <10%. Although no RCTs currently compare conventional surgery to TME, due to the reported lower rates of recurrence and superior survival, TME has been adopted as the standard surgical procedure in several European countries.

Preoperative and Postoperative Radiotherapy. Preoperative short course RT administered as 5 Gy daily for five days improves LR rates compared to both conventional surgery and TME. The Swedish Rectal Cancer Trial randomized patients to short course RT and conventional surgery or conventional surgery alone. Five-year LR rates decreased from 27% to 11% ($p < 0.001$) and overall five-year survival improved from 48% to 58% ($p = 0.004$) with the addition

of RT to surgery (96). The Dutch Colorectal Cancer Group (CKVO 95-04 trial) compared the same RT regimen and TME to TME alone. Again five-year LR rates were improved (5.6% vs. 10.9%; $p < 0.001$) in the RT arm. However, there was no difference in five-year OS (64.2% vs. 63.5%; $p = 0.902$) (97). The recently published results of the MRC CR07 study also reported a significant improvement in three-year LR rates (4.4% vs. 10.6%) and three-year DFS (78% vs. 72%) for preoperative RT and surgery compared to surgery followed by postoperative CRT only if the CRM was positive. There was no difference in OS between the groups (98).

The 2007 Cochrane review of preoperative radiotherapy and curative surgery for the management of localized rectal carcinoma analyzed 19 trials comparing preoperative RT to surgery alone (99). Both LR and OS were improved by the addition of preoperative RT, although the actual improvement in OS was marginal (HR for death 0.93; 95% CI 0.87–1.00).

Single modality postoperative RT is not recommended. The Colorectal Cancer Collaborative Group's 2001 meta-analysis found similar reductions in the risk of recurrence for preoperative and postoperative RT, however preoperative RT was more dose efficient than postoperative RT (100). A RCT directly comparing short course preoperative RT and prolonged postoperative RT reported better LR rates with the preoperative RT approach (13% vs. 22%, $p = 0.02$) (101). Furthermore, the NCCTG 79-47-51 study reported both a survival advantage and reduced LR rates with postoperative CRT compared to postoperative RT, making combined therapy the preferred approach (102).

Preoperative and Postoperative Chemoradiotherapy. Until recently, postoperative 5-FU-based CRT was the standard of care in the United States for stage II and III rectal cancers. Postoperative CRT was superior to RT alone in the NCCTG trial, and the GITSG 7175 trial demonstrated a significant advantage for adjuvant CRT over surgery alone for both LR rates (33% vs. 55%, $p = 0.005$) and survival ($p = 0.01$) (103). The NSABP R-01 study did not evaluate postoperative CRT, but results indicated that compared to surgery alone, adjuvant chemotherapy was superior for DFS and adjuvant RT was superior for LR rates (104). The combined results of these trials led to the NIH consensus conference recommendation of postoperative CRT as standard therapy. A subsequent study determined that 5-FU delivered as a protracted venous infusion was superior to bolus 5-FU in terms of time to relapse ($p = 0.01$) and survival ($p = 0.005$), and that there was no additional benefit with the addition of semustine (105).

Increasingly, the approach for patients with locally advanced rectal cancer is moving toward the use of preoperative CRT. Neoadjuvant CRT has several potential benefits. In addition to the synergistic effect of chemotherapy combined with RT, micrometastatic disease is treated early and tumor downstaging may allow increased rates of sphincter-preserving surgery. The disadvantage is overtreatment of patients with early pathological stage or occult metastases.

At least three RCTs have addressed the question of preoperative versus postoperative CRT. Both the NSABP R-03 and INT-0147 trials closed prematurely due to poor accrual. Over 800 patients were recruited to the German

CAO/ARO/AIO-94 study, which reported improved local control rates (6% vs. 13%, p = 0.006) and reduced acute (27% vs. 47%, p = 0.01) and long-term (14% vs. 24%, p = 0.01) toxicity with the preoperative approach (106). More patients were able to have sphincter-preserving surgery following preoperative CRT. No difference in OS or DFS was seen between the two approaches. This trial prompted the move in the United States from postoperative to preoperative CRT. Due to a more convenient mode of administration, capecitabine is often substituted for infused 5-FU. The ongoing NSABP R-04 trial is designed to evaluate noninferiority of capecitabine and RT to infused 5-FU and RT, as well as the efficacy of adding oxaliplatin to fluoropyrimidine-based CRT.

Preoperative Radiotherapy or Preoperative Chemoradiation. Trials comparing preoperative CRT and preoperative RT have also been conducted. Two European studies, the FFCD 9203 and the EORTC 22921 evaluated the addition of 5-FU to long course preoperative RT (45 Gy in 25 fractions) in patients with T3-4 rectal cancers (107,108). Total mesorectal excision was the recommended surgery (from 1999 onward for EORTC 22921) although compliance was variable. Patients in the FFCD 9203 study also received postoperative chemotherapy, whereas patients within the EORTC 22921 study had a second randomization to postoperative chemotherapy or observation. Adding chemotherapy to long-course RT resulted in pathological downstaging and improved LR rates, but no difference in OS. In the EORTC study, LR rates were improved by the addition of chemotherapy whether it was administered preoperatively (with RT) or as adjuvant therapy. A small Polish study randomized patients to preoperative short-course RT (5 Gy in 5 fractions) or CRT (50.4 Gy in 28 fractions, bolus 5-FU/LV) followed by TME. Combined therapy resulted in higher rates of pathological downstaging, but also higher rates of early toxicity and no difference in survival or LR rates (109).

It therefore remains uncertain if preoperative short-course RT or preoperative long-course CRT should be the preferred approach. When interpreting these results, consideration should also be given to the degree of quality control on multiple levels, including accuracy of initial staging, delivery of treatment (particularly TME quality), and histopathology reporting. Due to the increased rates of pathological downstaging, many European centers would elect to administer preoperative CRT to patients T3-4N0-2 tumors if the CRM is threatened or involved.

Adjuvant Chemotherapy. Fluoropyrimidine-based adjuvant chemotherapy is commonly given in both stage II and III rectal cancer. Limitations of preoperative staging techniques and the histological downstaging that follows preoperative therapy means that the current challenge is accurately predicting risk of relapse and who will benefit from adjuvant chemotherapy. Adjuvant chemotherapy is superior to surgery alone (104).

The EORTC 22921 study reported trends toward improved PFS and OS with the addition of adjuvant chemotherapy to preoperative RT or CRT; however these results were not statistically significant (108). The QUASAR trial included 948 patients with rectal cancer and allowed adjunctive RT, but not CRT. The relative risk of recurrence with fluoropyrimidine-chemotherapy compared to observation for patients with primary rectal tumors was 0.68 (p = 0.004) and the relative risk of death was 0.77 (p = 0.05) (94).

The evidence supporting fluoropyrimidines-based adjuvant chemotherapy in rectal cancer is therefore increasing. Regimens commonly used include bolus 5-FU/LV, infused 5-FU, and oral capecitabine. Extrapolating from colon cancer trials, oxaliplatin-containing regimens are also used. Prospective RCTs have not yet demonstrated definitively the benefits of adjuvant chemotherapy following neoadjuvant CRT.

Follow-up

Patients who have completed curative treatment for colorectal cancer should be followed up for the development of recurrent disease and require lifelong surveillance for the development of adenomatous polyps and second colorectal primary tumors. For patients at higher risk of recurrence deemed appropriate for intervention, the current ASCO guidelines recommend history and examination every three to six months for the first three years and every six months during years 4 and 5, CEA every three months for at least the first three years, and annual CT chest, abdomen, and pelvis (rectal cancer) for three years after primary therapy. Colonoscopy is recommended at three years postoperative treatment and, if normal, every five years thereafter. Routine CXR, full blood count, or liver function tests are not recommended (110).

The current ESMO guidelines suggest follow-up for colon cancer comprising of history and examination; CEA every three to six months for three years and every 6–12 months in years 4 and 5 after surgery if initially elevated, liver ultrasound every six months for three years and after four and five years, and colonoscopy after one year and thereafter every three to five years. Annual CT chest and abdomen for three years can be considered in patients who are at higher risk for recurrence. Chest X-ray has a low sensitivity but can be considered every year for five years (111).

Treatment Strategies for Advanced Colorectal Cancer

Despite improved surgical techniques, adjuvant and neoadjuvant treatment strategies, and the introduction of national screening programs, a significant proportion of patients will still develop or present with advanced CRC. The past decade has seen substantial developments in the treatment of metastatic colorectal cancer (mCRC). Active chemotherapeutic agents include IV and oral fluoropyrimidines, oxaliplatin, irinotecan, and raltitrexed. Molecular targeted agents also have an established role in the treatment of mCRC, although the high cost associated with these agents prohibits routine use in many countries. Recent RCTs have reported median OS in excess of 20 months with the use of active chemotherapy agents with and without targeted agents. For a small number of patients with limited metastatic disease, curative resection of liver or lung metastases may be possible. Evaluation of strategies to improve outcomes for patients with potentially curable metastatic disease is ongoing.

Chemotherapy for Advanced Colorectal Cancer

For patients with advanced CRC and adequate PS, systemic chemotherapy can confer both symptomatic and survival advantages. Although combination regimens are most frequently used first-line, RCTs comparing initial combination to sequential chemotherapy have, perhaps surprisingly, not demonstrated a significant difference in OS with combination therapy (112).

Fluoropyrimidines. Fluoropyrimidines have long been regarded as the backbone of treatment in mCRC. Bolus IV 5-FU on its own produces RR around 10%. The addition of LV to 5-FU results in improved RR and OS, and for many years bolus 5-FU/LV regimens were considered standard therapy (113). The main toxicities associated with bolus 5-FU/LV are gastrointestinal and hematological, along with hand-foot syndrome. Subsequently, due to improved toxicity profiles and superior efficacy, infused 5-FU/LV regimens have largely replaced bolus regimens both in practice and in clinical trials, although the need for central venous catheters and their associated potential complications must not be disregarded (114).

With this in mind, the oral fluoropyrimidines capecitabine and UFT provide convenient alternatives to infused 5-FU. Compared to bolus 5-FU, capecitabine has been shown to have at least equivalent time to disease progression (TTP) and OS in two large RCTs (115). Different toxicity profiles were also observed, with significantly less grade 3/4 stomatitis, neutropenia, and febrile neutropenia/sepsis, but increased hand-foot syndrome and hyperbilirubinaemia with capecitabine. In the mCRC setting, UFT plus LV has been compared to 5-FU in two Phase III studies and also resulted in similar efficacy and an improved safety profile (115). In contrast to capecitabine, UFT resulted in less hand-foot syndrome (frequency 2%) compared to 5-FU (116). UFT is not approved for the treatment of mCRC in the United States.

Raltitrexed. Raltitrexed is a folate analogue that directly inhibits thymidylate synthase. Four RCTs comparing raltitrexed (3 mg/m² every three weeks) to bolus IV or infused 5-FU/LV have been conducted, three of which demonstrated equivalent efficacy (117). The main side effects are neutropenia and diarrhea. Due to 50% of the drug being renally excreted unchanged, close monitoring of renal function is essential to prevent undue toxicity. Raltitrexed can be used as an alternative to fluoropyrimidines in patients who are intolerant of fluoropyrimidines due to dihydropyrimidine dehydrogenase deficiency, or fluoropyrimidine-induced coronary artery spasm. Raltitrexed is not licensed for use in the United States.

Irinotecan. Single agent irinotecan was adopted as standard second-line therapy based on the results of two RCTs which demonstrated significantly improved OS for irinotecan compared to BSC (9.2 vs. 6.5 months, $p = 0.0001$) and infused 5-FU (10.8 vs. 8.5 months, $p = 0.035$) (118,119). When added to fluoropyrimidines in the first-line setting, irinotecan results in superior survival. A European study compared irinotecan with infused 5-FU/LV to infused 5-FU/LV and resulted in improved RR (49% vs. 31%, $p < 0.001$), TTP (6.7 vs. 4.4 months, $p < 0.001$), and OS (17.4 vs. 14.1 months, $p = 0.031$) with a manageable toxicity profile.

A North American study assigned patients to irinotecan/5-FU/LV (IFL), 5-FU/LV, or irinotecan alone (120). Compared to 5-FU/LV, IFL resulted in significantly improved OS (14.8 vs. 12.6 months, $p = 0.04$), PFS (7.0 vs. 4.3 months, $p = 0.004$), and RR (50% vs. 29%, $p < 0.001$). Irinotecan monotherapy had similar efficacy to 5-FU/LV. Further information regarding the optimal irinotecan-fluoropyrimidine combination has been gained from the BICC-C trial. This study initially randomized patients to FOLFIRI, modified IFL (mIFL), or irinotecan plus oral capecitabine (CapeIRI) and then to either celecoxib or placebo (121). Compared to mIFL, FOLFIRI was superior for PFS (7.6 vs. 5.9 months, $p = 0.004$) and there was a trend toward improved OS (23.1 vs. 17.6 months, $p = 0.09$). CapeIRI was associated with increased toxicity; namely severe vomiting, diarrhea, and dehydration, and inferior PFS and OS compared to FOLFIRI. This arm was discontinued when the protocol was modified to include bevacizumab.

FOLFIRI has emerged as the preferred irinotecan-fluoropyrimidine regimen based on efficacy and toxicity profile. The main toxicities associated with irinotecan are: delayed onset diarrhea, which can be severe and life threatening, neutropenia, nausea, vomiting, asthenia, acute cholinergic syndrome, and alopecia.

Oxaliplatin. Oxaliplatin in combination with infused 5-FU/LV (FOLFOX) is an accepted treatment regimen in both the first- and second-line setting. Initial Phase III studies reported improved PFS compared to infused 5-FU/LV (9.0 vs. 6.2 months, $p = 0.0003$) and bolus 5-FU/LV (7.8 vs. 5.3 months, $p = 0.0001$) as well as significantly improved response rates when used first-line (122,123). Although OS was not significantly improved in either trial, this was attributed to a significant proportion of patients assigned to 5-FU/LV receiving oxaliplatin-chemotherapy after progression. An OS benefit for the first-line use of FOLFOX was demonstrated in the U.S. Intergroup 9741 study, leading to adoption of FOLFOX as standard first-line therapy for mCRC. In the final design of this study, patients were assigned to IFL, FOLFOX, or a combination of irinotecan and oxaliplatin (IROX). FOLFOX was significantly superior to IFL in terms of TTP (HR 0.74, $p = 0.0014$), RR (45% vs. 31%, $p = 0.002$) and OS (HR 0.66, $p = 0.0001$) (124). IFL also resulted in significantly higher rates of GI toxicity, febrile neutropenia, and dehydration than FOLFOX. Comparison of FOLFOX to IROX is discussed below. Second-line FOLFOX after failure of an irinotecan-containing regimen is also superior to infused 5-FU/LV in terms of RR, TTP, and relief of tumor-related symptoms (125).

Unlike CapeIRI, capecitabine combined with oxaliplatin is a well-tolerated regimen with at least similar efficacy to FOLFOX. The largest trial comparing XELOX to FOLFOX, the NO16966 trial, met its primary end point of noninferiority for XELOX versus FOLFOX for PFS (HR 1.04; 95% CI 0.93–1.16) (126).

Both FOLFOX and Capox are acceptable treatment options for the treatment of mCRC. Specific oxaliplatin-related toxicities are cold-induced dysaesthesia and cumulative peripheral sensory neuropathy which is the dose-limiting toxicity.

Irinotecan, Oxaliplatin, or Both? With both oxaliplatin and irinotecan available for use in mCRC, questions then arose regarding the optimal sequencing of effective regimens and the potential role of oxaliplatin combined with irinotecan. A GERCOR study was designed to specifically address the issue of FOLFIRI-FOLFOX sequencing. Patients were randomized to FOLFIRI then FOLFOX6, or the reverse (127). Median TTP was similar (8.5 vs. 8.0 months, $p = 0.26$) as were initial response rates (56% vs. 54%). Although second-line FOLFIRI resulted in a lower response rate compared to second-line FOLFOX (4% vs. 15%), there was no significant difference in OS (21.5 vs. 21.6 months, $p = 0.99$). A second Italian study, comparing first-line FOLFOX to FOLFIRI also reported no difference in ORR, TTP, or OS (128). Similar numbers of patients in each group received second-line therapy.

Updated results from the U.S. Intergroup 9741 trial have confirmed that IROX is not superior to FOLFOX in terms of TTP (HR 1.39, $p < 0.0001$), RR (36% vs. 43%, $p = 0.002$), or OS (1.34, $p = 0.0001$) (129). Two published RCTs have compared the combination of oxaliplatin, irinotecan, and 5-FU (FOLFOXIRI) with FOLFIRI with conflicting results. The first study, conducted by the Hellenic Oncology Research Group failed to detect a significant difference in OS (21.5 vs. 19.5 months, $p = 0.337$), RR (43% vs. 33.6%, $p = 0.17$), or TTP (8.4 vs. 6.9 months, $p = 0.17$) (130). On the other hand, the second study conducted by the Gruppo Oncologico Nord Ovest reported significantly improved OS (22.6 vs. 16.7 months, $p = 0.0006$), RR (66% vs. 41%, $p = 0.033$), or TTP (9.8 vs. 6.9 months, $p = 0.032$) (131). The differing results may be explained, in part by differing dosing schedules and the enrolment of a younger and fitter patient population in the second study. On the basis of the available data, however, FOLFOXIRI cannot be accepted as standard first-line therapy, although may be an option for younger patients of good PS.

Molecularly Targeted Agents and Advanced Colorectal Cancer

Recent years have seen the emergence of several biological agents in the treatment of gastrointestinal and other malignancies. In advanced colorectal cancer, RCTs have demonstrated that the vascular endothelial growth factor (VEGF) receptor monoclonal antibody, bevacizumab, and the epidermal growth factor receptor (EGFR) inhibitors, cetuximab and panitumumab, have efficacy. The optimal setting for the use of these agents, however, remains uncertain and treatment paradigms continue to evolve. Furthermore, due to the high cost associated with these drugs and the often modest clinical benefit, for many countries, incorporation of these drugs into routine practice is not feasible from a health-economic point of view.

Bevacizumab. Since angiogenesis is a requirement for tumor growth, invasion, and metastasis, there has been much interest in the development of antiangiogenic drugs. Bevacizumab, an IgG1 recombinant monoclonal antibody, binds and inactivates all isoforms of VEGF to inhibit angiogenesis and has activity in CRC in both the first- and second-line settings (Table 9.6). The main toxicities associated with bevacizumab are hypertension, proteinuria, bleeding, and impaired wound healing and, more rarely, arterial thrombosis and gastrointestinal perforation.

The Hurwitz study randomized 813 patients to irinotecan and bolus 5-FU/LV (IFL); plus bevacizumab (5 mg/kg fortnightly) or placebo (132). The primary end point of the study was met, with a significant improvement in OS from 15.6 to 20.3 months with the addition of bevacizumab (HR 0.66, $p < 0.001$). This study was commenced prior to the routine use of oxaliplatin for mCRC, consequently only 25% of all patients received subsequent oxaliplatin. The rate of any second-line therapy was similar between the two arms. Progression-free survival improved from a median of 6.2 to 10.6 months, ORR from 34.8% to 44.8%, and median duration of response from 7.1 to 10.4 months. A combined analysis of three RCTs evaluating 5-FU/LV in combination with bevacizumab or placebo also reported improved response rate (34.1% vs. 24.5%), PFS (HR 0.63, $p \leq 0.0001$), and OS (HR 0.74, $p = 0.008$) with the addition of bevacizumab (133). On the basis of these results,

Table 9.6 Selected Randomized Studies of Bevacizumab in Metastatic Colorectal Cancer

Study/author (Ref.)	Treatment arms	Number of patients	HR DFS	*p* Value	HR death	*p* Value
First line						
Hurwitz et al. (132)	IFL + bevacizumab	411	0.054	<0.001	0.66	<0.001
	IFL + placebo	402				
Kabbinavar (165)	5-FU/LV + bev 5 mg/kg	35	0.46	0.005	0.63	0.137
	5-FU/LV + bev 10 mg/kg	33	0.66	0.217	1.17	0.582
	5-FU/LV + placebo	36				
Kabbinavar et al. (166)	5-FU/LV + bevacizumab	104	0.50	0.0002	0.79	0.16
	5-FU/LV + placebo	105				
BICC-C (121, 134)	IFL + bevacizumab	60	NS	0.28	1.79	0.037
	FOLFIRI + bevacizumab	57				
NO16966 (136)	XELOX/FOLFOX + bev	699	0.83	0.0023	0.89	0.077
	XELOX/FOLFOX	701				
Second line						
E3200 (137)	FOLFOX4 + bevacizumab	286	0.61	0.0001[a]	0.75	0.0011[a]
	FOLFOX4	296				
	Bevacizumab[b]	243				

[a]FOLFOX4 + bevacizumab versus FOLFOX4.
[b]Bevacizumab-alone arm closed early after an interim safety analysis suggested inferior survival.
Abbreviations: 5-FU/LV, 5-fluorouracil/leucovorin; bev, bevacizumab; DFS, disease-free survival; FOLFIRI, 5-fluorouracil/leucovorin/irinorecan; FOLFOX, 5-fluorouracil/leucovorin/oxaliplatin; HR, hazard ratio; IFL, Irinotecan/5-fluorouracil/leucovorin; NS, not significant; XELOX, capecitabine/oxaliplatin.

bevacizumab in combination with fluoropyrimidine-based chemotherapy (5-FU/LV or 5-FU/LV/irinotecan) was approved for use in first-line mCRC by the U.S. FDA in April 2004, and the European Commission in 2005. Following the FDA approval of bevacizumab in April 2004, the aforementioned BICC-C study was modified to include a randomization of 117 patients to FOLFIRI and bevacizumab or modified IFL and bevacizumab. With a median follow-up of 34.4 months, FOLFIRI/bevacizumab had superior OS compared to IFL/bevacizumab (HR 1.79, p = 0.037) (134). FOLFIRI/bevacizumab should therefore be used in preference to IFL/bevacizumab.

Bevacizumab has also been evaluated in the first-line (TREE2 and NO16966) and second-line (E3200) settings in combination with oxaliplatin/fluoropyrimidine chemotherapy. TREE2 reported nonsignificant trends toward improved RR, TTP, and OS with the addition of bevacizumab to oxaliplatin in combination with bolus, infused, or oral fluoropyrimidines (135). NO16966 randomized 1400 patients to XELOX or FOLFOX alone or in combination with bevacizumab. A significant improvement in PFS (the primary end point) was observed (8.0 vs. 9.4 months, HR 0.93, p = 0.0023), but not OS (HR 0.89, p = 0.077) (136). An interesting observation from this study is the equivalent median duration of treatment in both the bevacizumab and placebo arms despite differing PFS, suggesting that patients were not treated with bevacizumab until progressive disease. This led the authors to conclude that patients may need to be treated with bevacizumab until progression to derive the maximum benefit. The E3200 study randomized 829 patients to FOLFOX4, FOLFOX4/bevacizumab, or bevacizumab alone (137). The bevacizumab-alone arm was discontinued after an interim analysis suggested inferiority compared to the chemotherapy-containing arms. The addition of bevacizumab to FOLFOX4 chemotherapy resulted in statistically significant improvements in OS (12.9 vs. 10.8 months), PFS (7.3 vs. 4.7 months), and RR (22.7% vs. 8.6%) and led to FDA approval for use of bevacizumab in second-line treatment of mCRC.

Cetuximab and Panitumumab. The EGFR is involved in the pathogenesis of many malignancies and is correlated with poorer outcome. The rate of EGFR expression in CRC is around 70% (138). EGFR inhibitors such as cetuximab and panitumumab act by binding to the extracellular domain of EGFR, thus preventing phosphorylation and activation of intracellular downstream signal transduction pathways. Several trials have demonstrated the efficacy of these agents (Table 9.7). The most commonly observed toxicities associated with EGFR inhibitors are skin toxicity, typically an acneiform rash, and hypomagnesemia.

The BOND study established the role of cetuximab in patients with irinotecan-refractory mCRC (139). Three hundred and twenty nine patients were randomly assigned in a 2:1 fashion to cetuximab in combination with an irinotecan based regimen or cetuximab alone. Cross-over to the combination treatment arm at progression was permitted. The primary end point, ORR was met and was significantly superior for the combination treatment arm (22.9% vs. 10.8%, p = 0.007), demonstrating that cetuximab has the ability to overcome irinotecan-resistance. Time to progression was also in favor of combination therapy (4.1 vs. 1.5 months, p < 0.001) and there was a trend toward an OS advantage (8.6 vs. 6.9 months, p = 0.48). Subsequent trials have also resulted in a significant PFS for cetuximab + irinotecan compared to irinotecan-alone in patients who have failed oxaliplatin chemotherapy (EPIC) and cetuximab compared to BSC alone in chemotherapy refractory patients (CO.17) (140,141). Furthermore, the CO.17 study, unlike BOND and EPIC did not permit crossover and also resulted in a statistically significant improvement in OS (HR 0.77; p = 0.0005).

Little data is currently available regarding the efficacy of cetuximab in combination with oxaliplatin-fluoropyrimidine therapy. EXPLORE was a randomized Phase III trial designed to evaluate FOLFOX versus FOLFOX-cetuximab in patients previously treated with irinotecan, that closed early after recruiting only 102 patients out of a planned 1100 patients (142). In the first-line setting, Phase II studies

Table 9.7 Randomized Studies of Cetuximab and Panitumumab in Metastatic Colorectal Cancer

Study/author (Ref.)	Treatment arms	Number of patients	Median DFS	HR DFS (p value)	Median OS	HR death (p value)
First line						
CRYSTAL (143)	FOLFIRI + cetuximab	599	8.9 mo	0.851	19.9 mo	0.93
	FOLFIRI	599	8.0 mo	(0.0479)	18.6 mo	(0.31)
Second or subsequent line						
BOND (139)	Irinotecan + cetuximab	218	4.1 mo	0.54	8.6 mo	NS
	Cetuximab	111	1.5 mo	(<0.001)	6.9 mo	
CO.17 (140)	Cetuximab Best supportive care	287	1.9 mo	0.68	6.1 mo	0.77
		285	1.8 mo	(<0.001)	4.6 mo	(0.005)
EPIC (141)	Irinotecan + cetuximab	648	4.0 mo	0.692	10.7 mo	0.975
	Irinotecan	650	2.6 mo	(≤0.0001)	10.0 mo	(0.71)
EXPLORE (142)	FOLFOX + cetuximab	50	4.4 mo	NS	NR	
	FOLFOX	52	4.1 mo			
Van Cutsem et al. (144)	Panitumumab Best supportive care	231	8.0 wk	0.54	~6 mo	NS
		232	7.3 wk	(<0.0001)	~6 mo	

Abbreviations: DFS, disease-free survival; FOLFIRI, 5-fluorouracil/leucovorin/irinorecan; FOLFOX, 5-fluorouracil/leucovorin/oxaliplatin; HR, hazard ratio; NR, not reported; NS, not significant; OS, overall survival.

have demonstrated efficacy of the combination of FOLFOX and cetuximab and the ongoing U.K. Phase III COIN study will provide further efficacy data regarding this regimen.

In the first-line setting, the CRYSTAL trial met its primary end point of PFS, with improved PFS for FOLFIRI-cetuximab compared to FOLFIRI alone (8.9 vs. 8.0 months, HR 0.851, $p = 0.0479$) (143). ORR also significantly favored the cetuximab-containing arm (46.9% vs. 38.7%, $p = 0.0038$) and a higher percentage of patients receiving cetuximab proceeded to surgery with curative intent (6.0% vs. 1.5%) and achieved R0 resection (4.3% vs. 1.5%, $p = 0.0034$). There was no significant difference in OS. K-ras mutation analysis of 540 of the 1198 patients recruited demonstrated that the PFS benefit associated with the addition of cetuximab was limited to patients with wild-type K-ras (HR 0.68, $p = 0.017$) as opposed to mutated K-ras (HR 1.07, $p = 0.47$) (143).

In a RCT of chemotherapy refractory patients, panitumumab had superior PFS compared to BSC alone (HR 0.54, $p < 0.0001$) (144). Although statistically significant, the actual improvement in PFS was from 7.3 to 8.0 weeks. A significant OS benefit was not observed in this study; however, crossover to the active treatment arm at progression was allowed, a phenomenon that may have obscured any potential OS advantage. As in the CRYSTAL study, response to panitumumab was limited to patients with wild-type K-ras, with no patient with mutant K-ras responding to panitumumab (145). Furthermore, patients with wild-type K-ras fared better than mutant K-ras (HR death 0.67) regardless of treatment, suggesting that K-ras is both a prognostic and predictive factor for this group of patients. The FDA approved panitumumab for use in chemorefractory mCRC in September 2006. In Europe, conditional marketing authorization was granted for use of panitumumab in EGFR expressing mCRC with nonmutated (wild-type) KRAS after failure of standard chemotherapy regimens.

Future Directions for Targeted Therapies. Several other targeted agents including sunitinib, pazopanib, cetiranib, and aflibercept are in the early phases of development. Other agents such as vatalanib and the tyrosine kinase inhibitors gefitinib and erlotinib alone or in combination with chemotherapy have so far yielded disappointing results.

For the targeted agents with confirmed efficacy, efforts are now focused on defining the optimal setting in which to administer these agents, identification of predictive factors and better selection of patients more likely to respond to therapy, optimization of dosing regimens, and the role of dual targeted therapy. Initial excitement regarding dual targeted therapy has been dampened by recent clinical trials. The combination of panitumumab and bevacizumab with either oxaliplatin or irinotecan-based chemotherapy was found to be detrimental in the interim analysis of the PACCE trial, leading to early closure of the trial (146). BOND-2 also closed early due to poor recruitment, but did not report any unexpected toxicity in the 83 patients from the addition of bevacizumab to either randomized to cetuximab and bevacizumab or irinotecan and, cetuximab and bevacizumab (147). However, in the Dutch CAIRO II study, the addition of cetuximab to the combination of Capox-bevacizumab resulted in increased toxicity and worse PFS (HR 1.21, $p = 0.01$) compared to Capox-bevacizumab, although OS was similar (19.4 m vs. 20.3 m, $p = 0.16$) (148).

Management of Potentially Resectable Metastatic Disease

Patients with mCRC limited to the liver (and less frequently the lung) may be candidates for potentially curative resection. Appropriate selection of surgical candidates requires consideration of the patient's clinical state and the likelihood of achieving a successful R0 resection. For patients with liver metastases, conservation of adequate residual liver parenchyma is also important. Careful review of imaging modalities including CT, PET, and MRI allows exclusion of extrahepatic (or pulmonary) disease and clarification of the size, number, and distribution of metastases, as well as the relationship of metastatic lesions to vascular structures. A small percentage of patients with initially unresectable metastases may be sufficiently downstaged by systemic therapy to become candidates for potential resection and early data suggest that the rates of "conversion" may be increased by the addition of targeted agents to chemotherapy.

Surgical resection of liver metastases results in five-year survival rates around 35% (149). Although adjuvant chemotherapy is frequently administered, actual supporting data from RCTs is limited. To date, no study has demonstrated an OS benefit although a significant improvement in relapse-free survival was observed in the published Intergroup study which evaluated adjuvant intra-arterial floxuridine and IV-infused 5-FU chemotherapy (four-year

---

Key Points

- Adjuvant oxaliplatin-fluoropyrimidine therapy chemotherapy should be routinely offered to fit patients with Stage III colon cancer. For those not suitable for oxaliplatin therapy, oral capecitabine (or IV-infused 5-FU) is a reasonable option
- Oral capecitabine is at least equivalent to intravenous 5-FU in the adjuvant and metastatic settings
- For patients with Stage II colon cancer, fluoropyrimidine chemotherapy offers a small clinical benefit and should be considered in patients considered at high-risk of relapse. Mismatch repair status should be determined by either immunohistochemistry or MSI, since Stage II patients with deficient MMR tumors do not appear to benefit from adjuvant 5-FU alone
- Surgery (ideally TME) is the primary curative treatment modality for rectal cancer
- For locally advanced rectal tumors, preoperative short course radiation or long-course chemoradiation results in improved LR rates
- Palliative systemic chemotherapy is beneficial for patients of adequate performance status. Exposure to the active agents oxaliplatin, irinotecan, and fluoropyrimides correlates with longer median OS
- The targeted agents bevacizumab, cetuximab, and panitumumab can result in improved response rates and PFS. Bevacizumab in the first- and second-line setting can prolong OS. Cetuximab can improve OS in chemorefractory patients, can reverse irinotecan resistance, and is more efficacious in combination with irinotecan
- Emerging data indicates that in mCRC, K-ras mutations confer resistance to EGFR monoclonal antibodies. K-ras analysis should be performed if considering treatment with cetuximab or panitumumab
- Selected patients with metastatic disease confined to the liver and/or lung may be candidates for potentially curative resection

recurrence free rate 25.2% vs. 45.7%, $p = 0.04$) (150). The EORTC 40983 (EPOC) trial employed a different approach, randomizing patients to perioperative FOLFOX chemotherapy (six cycles pre- and six cycles postoperatively) or surgery alone (149). Three year PFS improved for both the eligible and resected patient populations with the addition of perioperative chemotherapy (HR 0.77, $p = 0.041$, and HR 0.73, $p = 0.025$, respectively). For all randomized patients, three-year PFS improved from 28.1% to 35.4% (HR 0.79, $p = 0.058$), corresponding to a 7.3% absolute improvement in PFS. Overall survival data from this trial is awaited.

ANAL CANCER

Squamous cell carcinoma of the anus is uncommon with an estimated 4650 new cases in the United States for 2007 (1).

Epidemiology
The incidence of anal cancer is increasing, most likely due to the rising prevalence of exposure to risk factors such as cigarette smoking, anal intercourse, HPV infection, and multiple lifetime sexual partners (151). Oncogenic human papillomavirus infection types (e.g., type 16) are frequently detected.

Treatment Strategies
Treatment of Localized Anal Cancer
Combined chemoradiation using 5-FU and mitomycin C is the standard of care, with surgery reserved for residual or recurrent disease after chemoradiation.

Two randomized studies demonstrated superiority of chemoradiation over radiotherapy alone with regards to local control rates, although neither resulted in an OS benefit. A third study demonstrated that incorporating mitomycin C into 5-FU-radiation regimens improved both colostomy-free and disease-free rates (152). The RTOG 98-11 trial comparing standard chemoradiation to two cycles of induction cisplatin/5-FU followed by cisplatin/5-FU-based chemoradiation reported a higher rate of colostomies in the experimental arm and no difference in DFS or OS (153). Current randomized Phase III studies are evaluating substitution of cisplatin for mitomycin C, the role of adjuvant chemotherapy and alternative radiation schedules.

Treatment of Metastatic Disease
Less than 20% of patients with anal cancer will develop distal metastases. There is no standard treatment although several agents have been evaluated. Cisplatin in combination with 5-FU is a commonly used regimen with relatively high response rates in nonrandomized trials, however median survival for these patients remains limited to 9 to 12 months (152).

Key Points

- Definitive chemoradiation with mitomycin C and 5-FU is standard of care
- Surgery is usually reserved as salvage therapy
- There is no standard treatment regimen for metastatic disease

REFERENCES

1. Jemal A, Siegel R, Ward E et al. Cancer statistics, 2007. CA Cancer J Clin 2007; 57: 43–66.
2. Thun MJ, Peto R, Lopez AD et al. Alcohol consumption and mortality among middle-aged and elderly U.S. adults. N Engl J Med 1997; 337: 1705–14.
3. Sharma P, Falk GW, Weston AP et al. Dysplasia and cancer in a large multicenter cohort of patients with Barrett's esophagus. Clin Gastroenterol Hepatol 2006; 4: 566–72.
4. van Vliet EP, Heijenbrok-Kal MH, Hunink MG et al. Staging investigations for oesophageal cancer: a meta-analysis. Br J Cancer 2008; 98: 547–57.
5. Siewert JR, Stein HJ. Classification of adenocarcinoma of the oesophagogastric junction. Br J Surg 1998; 85: 1457–9.
6. Omloo JM, Lagarde SM, Hulscher JB et al. Extended transthoracic resection compared with limited transhiatal resection for adenocarcinoma of the mid/distal esophagus: five-year survival of a randomized clinical trial. Ann Surg 2007; 246: 992–1000, discussion-1.
7. Arnott SJ, Duncan W, Gignoux M et al. Preoperative radiotherapy for esophageal carcinoma. Cochrane Database Syst Rev 2005; CD001799.
8. Kelsen DP, Ginsberg R, Pajak TF et al. Chemotherapy followed by surgery compared with surgery alone for localized esophageal cancer. N Engl J Med 1998; 339: 1979–84.
9. Medical Research Council Oesophageal Cancer Working Group. Surgical resection with or without preoperative chemotherapy in oesophageal cancer: a randomised controlled trial. Lancet 2002; 359: 1727–33.
10. Cunningham D, Allum WH, Stenning SP et al. Perioperative chemotherapy versus surgery alone for resectable gastroesophageal cancer. N Engl J Med 2006; 355: 11–20.
11. Boige V, Pignon J, Saint-Aubert B et al. Final results of a randomized trial comparing preoperative 5-fluorouracil (F)/cisplatin (P) to surgery alone in adenocarcinoma of stomach and lower esophagus (ASLE): FNLCC ACCORD07-FFCD 9703 trial. J Clin Oncol (Meeting Abstracts) 2007; 25(18 Suppl): 4510.
12. Gebski V, Burmeister B, Smithers BM et al. Survival benefits from neoadjuvant chemoradiotherapy or chemotherapy in oesophageal carcinoma: a meta-analysis. Lancet Oncol 2007; 8: 226–34.
13. Stahl M, Walz MK, Stuschke M et al. Preoperative chemotherapy (CTX) versus preoperative chemoradiotherapy (CRTX) in locally advanced esophagogastric adenocarcinomas: First results of a randomized phase III trial. J Clin Oncol (Meeting Abstracts) 2007; 25(18 Suppl): 4511.
14. Wong R, Malthaner R. Combined chemotherapy and radiotherapy (without surgery) compared with radiotherapy alone in localized carcinoma of the esophagus. Cochrane Database Syst Rev 2006; CD002092.
15. Bedenne L, Michel P, Bouche O et al. Chemoradiation followed by surgery compared with chemoradiation alone in squamous cancer of the esophagus: FFCD 9102. J Clin Oncol 2007; 25: 1160–8.
16. Kamangar F, Dores GM, Anderson WF. Patterns of cancer incidence, mortality, and prevalence across five continents: defining priorities to reduce cancer disparities in different geographic regions of the World. J Clin Oncol 2006; 24: 2137–50.
17. Abdalla EK, Pisters PW. Staging and preoperative evaluation of upper gastrointestinal malignancies. Semin Oncol 2004; 31: 513–29.
18. van de Velde CJ. Resection for gastric cancer in the community. Semin Oncol 2005; 32(6 Suppl 9): S90–S93.
19. Sakuramoto S, Sasako M, Yamaguchi T et al. Adjuvant chemotherapy for gastric cancer with S-1, an oral fluoropyrimidine. N Engl J Med 2007; 357: 1810–20.

20. Macdonald JS, Smalley SR, Benedetti J et al. Chemoradiotherapy after surgery compared with surgery alone for adenocarcinoma of the stomach or gastroesophageal junction. N Engl J Med 2001; 345: 725–30.

21. Rivera F, Vega-Villegas ME, Lopez-Brea MF. Chemotherapy of advanced gastric cancer. Cancer Treat Rev 2007; 33: 315–24.

22. Webb A, Cunningham D, Scarffe JH et al. Randomized trial comparing epirubicin, cisplatin, and fluorouracil versus fluorouracil, doxorubicin, and methotrexate in advanced esophagogastric cancer. J Clin Oncol 1997; 15: 261–7.

23. Wagner AD, Grothe W, Haerting J et al. Combination chemotherapies in advanced gastric cancer: an updated systematic review and meta-analysis. J Clin Oncol (Meeting Abstracts) 2007; 25(18 Suppl): 4555.

24. Cunningham D, Starling N, Rao S et al. Capecitabine and oxaliplatin for advanced esophagogastric cancer. N Engl J Med 2008; 358: 36–46.

25. Kang YK, Kang WK, Shin DB et al. Capecitabine/cisplatin versus 5-fluorouracil/cisplatin as first-line therapy in patients with advanced gastric cancer: a randomised phase III non-inferiority trial. Ann Oncol 2009; 20: 666–73.

26. Al-Batran S-E, Hartmann JT, Probst S et al. Phase III Trial in metastatic gastroesophageal adenocarcinoma with fluorouracil, leucovorin plus either oxaliplatin or cisplatin: a study of the arbeitsgemeinschaft internistische onkologie. J Clin Oncol 2008; 26: 1435–42.

27. Van Cutsem E, Moiseyenko VM, Tjulandin S et al. Phase III study of docetaxel and cisplatin plus fluorouracil compared with cisplatin and fluorouracil as first-line therapy for advanced gastric cancer: a report of the V325 study group. J Clin Oncol 2006; 24: 4991–7.

28. Roth AD, Fazio N, Stupp R et al. Docetaxel, cisplatin, and fluorouracil; docetaxel and cisplatin; and epirubicin, cisplatin, and fluorouracil as systemic treatment for advanced gastric carcinoma: a randomized phase II trial of the Swiss Group for Clinical Cancer Research. J Clin Oncol 2007; 25: 3217–23.

29. Tebbutt N, Sourjina T, Strickland A et al. ATTAX: randomised phase II study evaluating weekly docetaxel-based chemotherapy combinations in advanced esophago-gastric cancer, final results of an AGITG trial. J Clin Oncol (Meeting Abstracts) 2007; 25(18 Suppl): 4528.

30. Boku N, Yamamoto S, Shirao K et al. Randomized phase III study of 5-fluorouracil (5-FU) alone versus combination of irinotecan and cisplatin (CP) versus S-1 alone in advanced gastric cancer (JCOG9912). J Clin Oncol (Meeting Abstracts) 2007; 25(18 Suppl): LBA4513.

31. Koizumi W, Narahara H, Hara T et al. S-1 plus cisplatin versus S-1 alone for first-line treatment of advanced gastric cancer (SPIRITS trial): a phase III trial. Lancet Oncol 2008; 9: 215–21.

32. Imamura H, Iishi H, Tsuburaya A et al. Randomized phase III study of irinotecan plus S-1 (IRIS) versus S-1 alone as first-line treatment for advanced gastric cancer (GC0301/TOP-002). In: ASCO Gastrointestinal Cancers Symposium, Orlando, Florida, 2008.

33. Alexakis N, Halloran C, Raraty M et al. Current standards of surgery for pancreatic cancer. Br J Surg 2004; 91: 1410–27.

34. Iodice S, Gandini S, Maisonneuve P et al. Tobacco and the risk of pancreatic cancer: a review and meta-analysis. Langenbecks Arch Surg 2008; 393: 535–45.

35. Kalser MH, Ellenberg SS. Pancreatic cancer. Adjuvant combined radiation and chemotherapy following curative resection. Arch Surg 1985; 120: 899–903.

36. Neoptolemos JP, Stocken DD, Friess H et al. A randomized trial of chemoradiotherapy and chemotherapy after resection of pancreatic cancer. N Engl J Med 2004; 350: 1200–10.

37. Stocken DD, Buchler MW, Dervenis C et al. Meta-analysis of randomised adjuvant therapy trials for pancreatic cancer. Br J Cancer 2005; 92: 1372–81.

38. Neuhaus P, Riess H, Post S et al. Deutsche Krebsgesellschaft (CAO/AIO). CONKO-001: final results of the randomized, prospective, multicenter phase III trial of adjuvant chemotherapy with gemcitabine versus observation in patients with resected pancreatic cancer (PC). J Clin Oncol 2008; 26(May 20 Suppl): abstract LBA 4504.

39. Kosuge T, Ueno H, Matsuyama Y et al. A randomized phase III study comparing gemcitabine monotherapy with observation in patients with resected pancreatic cancer. Eur J Cancer Supplements 2007; 5: 260.

40. Regine WF, Winter KA, Abrams RA et al. Fluorouracil vs gemcitabine chemotherapy before and after fluorouracil-based chemoradiation following resection of pancreatic adenocarcinoma: a randomized controlled trial. JAMA 2008; 299: 1019–26.

41. Ghaneh P, Smith R, Tudor-Smith C et al. Neoadjuvant and adjuvant strategies for pancreatic cancer. Eur J Surg Oncol 2008; 34: 297–305.

42. Sultana A, Tudur Smith C, Cunningham D et al. Systematic review, including meta-analyses, on the management of locally advanced pancreatic cancer using radiation/combined modality therapy. Br J Cancer 2007; 96: 1183–90.

43. Chauffert B, Mornex F, Bonnetain F et al. Phase III trial comparing intensive induction chemoradiotherapy (60 Gy, infusional 5-FU and intermittent cisplatin) followed by maintenance gemcitabine with gemcitabine alone for locally advanced unresectable pancreatic cancer. Definitive results of the 2000-01 FFCD/SFRO study. Ann Oncol 2008; 19: 1592–9.

44. Loehrer PJ, Powell ME, Cardenes HR et al. Eastern Cooperative Oncology Group. A randomized phase III study of gemcitabine in combination with radiation therapy versus gemcitabine alone in patients with localized, unresectable pancreatic cancer: E4201. J Clin Oncol 2008; 26(May 20 Suppl): abstract 4506.

45. Sultana A, Smith CT, Cunningham D et al. Meta-analyses of chemotherapy for locally advanced and metastatic pancreatic cancer. J Clin Oncol 2007; 25: 2607–15.

46. Burris HA 3rd, Moore MJ, Andersen J et al. Improvements in survival and clinical benefit with gemcitabine as first-line therapy for patients with advanced pancreas cancer: a randomized trial. J Clin Oncol 1997; 15: 2403–13.

47. Tempero M, Plunkett W, Ruiz Van Haperen V et al. Randomized phase II comparison of dose-intense gemcitabine: thirty-minute infusion and fixed dose rate infusion in patients with pancreatic adenocarcinoma. J Clin Oncol 2003; 21: 3402–8.

48. Poplin E, Levy DE, Berlin J et al. Phase III trial of gemcitabine (30-minute infusion) versus gemcitabine [fixed-dose-rate infusion (FDR)] versus gemcitabine + oxaliplatin (GEMOX) in patients with advanced pancreatic cancer (E6201). J Clin Oncol (Meeting Abstracts) 2006; 24(18 Suppl): LBA4004.

49. Reni M, Cordio S, Milandri C et al. Gemcitabine versus cisplatin, epirubicin, fluorouracil, and gemcitabine in advanced pancreatic cancer: a randomised controlled multicentre phase III trial. Lancet Oncol 2005; 6: 369–76.

50. Louvet C, Labianca R, Hammel P et al. Gemcitabine in combination with oxaliplatin compared with gemcitabine alone in locally advanced or metastatic pancreatic cancer: results of a GERCOR and GISCAD phase III trial. J Clin Oncol 2005; 23: 3509–16.

51. Cunningham D, Chau I, Stocken C et al. Phase III randomised comparison of gemcitabine (GEM) versus

gemcitabine plus capecitabine (GEM-CAP) in patients with advanced pancreatic cancer. Eur J Cancer Supplements 2005; 3: abstract PS11.

52. Herrmann R, Bodoky G, Ruhstaller T et al. Gemcitabine plus capecitabine compared with gemcitabine alone in advanced pancreatic cancer: a randomized, multicenter, phase III trial of the Swiss Group for Clinical Cancer Research and the Central European Cooperative Oncology Group. J Clin Oncol 2007; 25: 2212–17.

53. Moore MJ, Goldstein D, Hamm J et al. Erlotinib plus gemcitabine compared with gemcitabine alone in patients with advanced pancreatic cancer: a phase III trial of the National Cancer Institute of Canada Clinical Trials Group. J Clin Oncol 2007; 25: 1960–6.

54. Vervenne W, Bennouna J, Humblet Y et al. A randomized, double-blind, placebo (P) controlled, multicenter phase III trial to evaluate the efficacy and safety of adding bevacizumab (B) to erlotinib (E) and gemcitabine (G) in patients (pts) with metastatic pancreatic cancer. J Clin Oncol 2008; 26(May 20 Suppl): abstract 4507.

55. Riess H, Pelzer U, Stieler J et al. A randomized second line trial in patients with gemcitabine refractory advanced pancreatic cancer—CONKO 003. J Clin Oncol (Meeting Abstracts) 2007; 25(18 Suppl): 4517.

56. Pelzer U, Kubica K, Stieler J et al. A randomized trial in patients with gemcitabine refractory pancreatic cancer. Final results of the CONKO 003 study. J Clin Oncol 2008; 26(May 20 Suppl): abstract 4508.

57. Ryder SD. Guidelines for the diagnosis and treatment of hepatocellular carcinoma (HCC) in adults. Gut 2003; 52(Suppl 3): iii1–8.

58. Baccarani U, Isola M, Adani GL et al. Superiority of transplantation versus resection for the treatment of small hepatocellular carcinoma. Transpl Int 2008; 21: 247–54.

59. Rougier P, Mitry E, Barbare JC et al. Hepatocellular carcinoma (HCC): an update. Semin Oncol 2007; 34(2 Suppl 1): S12–S20.

60. Mathurin P, Raynard B, Dharancy S et al. Meta-analysis: evaluation of adjuvant therapy after curative liver resection for hepatocellular carcinoma. Aliment Pharmacol Ther 2003; 17: 1247–61.

61. Marelli L, Stigliano R, Triantos C et al. Transarterial therapy for hepatocellular carcinoma: which technique is more effective? A systematic review of cohort and randomized studies. Cardiovasc Intervent Radiol 2007; 30: 6–25.

62. Nowak AK, Stockler MR, Chow PK et al. Use of tamoxifen in advanced-stage hepatocellular carcinoma. A systematic review. Cancer 2005; 103: 1408–14.

63. Llovet JM, Ricci S, Mazzaferro V et al. Sorafenib in advanced hepatocellular carcinoma. N Engl J Med 2008; 359: 378–90.

64. Malhi H, Gores GJ. Cholangiocarcinoma: modern advances in understanding a deadly old disease. J Hepatol 2006; 45: 856–67.

65. Mekeel KL, Hemming AW. Surgical management of gallbladder carcinoma: a review. J Gastrointest Surg 2007; 11: 1188–93.

66. Ortner MA, Dorta G. Technology insight: photodynamic therapy for cholangiocarcinoma. Nat Clin Pract Gastroenterol Hepatol 2006; 3: 459–67.

67. Eckel F, Schmid RM. Chemotherapy in advanced biliary tract carcinoma: a pooled analysis of clinical trials. Br J Cancer 2007; 96: 896–902.

68. Modlin IM, Oberg K, Chung DC et al. Gastroenteropancreatic neuroendocrine tumours. Lancet Oncol 2008; 9: 61–72.

69. Lepage C, Rachet B, Coleman MP. Survival from malignant digestive endocrine tumors in England and Wales: a population-based study. Gastroenterology 2007; 132: 899–904.

70. Plockinger U, Couvelard A, Falconi M et al. Consensus guidelines for the management of patients with digestive neuroendocrine tumours: well-differentiated tumour/carcinoma of the appendix and goblet cell carcinoma. Neuroendocrinology 2008; 87: 20–30.

71. Wright BE, Lee CC, Bilchik AJ. Hepatic cytoreductive surgery for neuroendocrine cancer. Surgical Oncol Clin N Am 2007; 16: 627–37.

72. Ramage JK, Davies AH, Ardill J et al. Guidelines for the management of gastroenteropancreatic neuroendocrine (including carcinoid) tumours. Gut 2005; 54(Suppl 4): iv1–16.

73. Kouvaraki MA, Ajani JA, Hoff P et al. Fluorouracil, doxorubicin, and streptozocin in the treatment of patients with locally advanced and metastatic pancreatic endocrine carcinomas. J Clin Oncol 2004; 22: 4762–71.

74. Fine RL, Fogelman DR, Schreibman SM. Effective treatment of neuroendocrine tumors with temozolomide and capecitabine. J Clin Oncol (Meeting Abstracts) 2005; 23(16 Suppl): 4216.

75. Fazio N, de Braud F, Delle Fave G et al. Interferon-alpha and somatostatin analog in patients with gastroenteropancreatic neuroendocrine carcinoma: single agent or combination? Ann Oncol 2007; 18: 13–19.

76. Dabaja BS, Suki D, Pro B et al. Adenocarcinoma of the small bowel: presentation, prognostic factors, and outcome of 217 patients. Cancer 2004; 101: 518–26.

77. Locher C, Malka D, Boige V et al. Combination chemotherapy in advanced small bowel adenocarcinoma. Oncology 2005; 69: 290–4.

78. Jo WS, Chung DC. Genetics of hereditary colorectal cancer. Semin Oncol 2005; 32: 11–23.

79. Lieberman DA, Prindiville S, Weiss DG et al. Risk factors for advanced colonic neoplasia and hyperplastic polyps in asymptomatic individuals. JAMA 2003; 290: 2959–67.

80. Chlebowski RT, Wactawski-Wende J, Ritenbaugh C et al. Estrogen plus progestin and colorectal cancer in postmenopausal women. N Engl J Med 2004; 350: 991–1004.

81. Chau I, Cunningham D. Adjuvant therapy in colon cancer—what, when and how? Ann Oncol 2006; 17: 1347–59.

82. Nagtegaal ID, Quirke P. What is the role for the circumferential margin in the modern treatment of rectal cancer? J Clin Oncol 2008; 26: 303–12.

83. Gunderson LL, Sargent DJ, Tepper JE et al. Impact of T and N stage and treatment on survival and relapse in adjuvant rectal cancer: a pooled analysis. J Clin Oncol 2004; 22: 1785–96.

84. Miyoshi M, Ueno H, Hashiguchi Y et al. Extent of mesorectal tumor invasion as a prognostic factor after curative surgery for T3 rectal cancer patients. Ann Surg 2006; 243: 492–8.

85. MERCURY Study Group. Diagnostic accuracy of preoperative magnetic resonance imaging in predicting curative resection of rectal cancer: prospective observational study. BMJ 2006; 333: 779.

86. Sargent DJ, Wieand HS, Haller DG et al. Disease-free survival versus overall survival as a primary end point for adjuvant colon cancer studies: individual patient data from 20,898 patients on 18 randomized trials. J Clin Oncol 2005; 23: 8664–70.

87. Twelves C, Wong A, Nowacki MP et al. Capecitabine as adjuvant treatment for stage III colon cancer. N Engl J Med 2005; 352: 2696–704.

88. Kopec JA, Yothers G, Ganz PA et al. Quality of life in operable colon cancer patients receiving oral compared with intravenous chemotherapy: results from National Surgical Adjuvant Breast and Bowel Project Trial C-06. J Clin Oncol 2007; 25: 424–30.

89. Andre T, Boni C, Mounedji-Boudiaf L et al. Oxaliplatin, fluorouracil, and leucovorin as adjuvant treatment for colon cancer. N Engl J Med 2004; 350: 2343–51.

90. de Gramont A, Boni C, Navarro M et al. Oxaliplatin/5FU/LV in adjuvant colon cancer: updated efficacy results of the MOSAIC trial, including survival, with a median follow-up of six years. J Clin Oncol (Meeting Abstracts) 2007; 25(18 Suppl): 4007.

91. Wolmark N, Wieand S, Kuebler PJ et al. A phase III trial comparing FULV to FULV + oxaliplatin in stage II or III carcinoma of the colon: survival results of NSABP Protocol C-07. J Clin Oncol 2008; 26(May 20 Suppl): abstract LBA 4005.

92. Schmoll H-J, Cartwright T, Tabernero J et al. Phase III trial of capecitabine plus oxaliplatin as adjuvant therapy for stage III colon cancer: a planned safety analysis in 1,864 patients. J Clin Oncol 2007; 25: 102–9.

93. Saltz LB, Niedzwiecki D, Hollis D et al. Irinotecan fluorouracil plus leucovorin is not superior to fluorouracil plus leucovorin alone as adjuvant treatment for stage III colon cancer: results of CALGB 89803. J Clin Oncol 2007; 25: 3456–61.

94. Quasar Collaborative Group, Gray R, Barnwell J et al. Adjuvant chemotherapy versus observation in patients with colorectal cancer: a randomised study. Lancet 2007; 370: 2020–9.

95. de Gramont A. for the Adjuvant Colon Cancer End points (ACCENT) Group. Association between 3-year (yr) disease free survival (DFS) and overall survival (OS) delayed with improved survival after recurrence (rec) in patients receiving cytotoxic adjuvant therapy for colon cancer: findings from the 20,800 patient (pt) ACCENT dataset. J Clin Oncol 2008; 26(May 20 Suppl): abstract 4007.

96. Improved survival with preoperative radiotherapy in resectable rectal cancer. Swedish Rectal Cancer Trial. N Engl J Med 1997; 336: 980–7.

97. Peeters KC, Marijnen CA, Nagtegaal ID et al. The TME trial after a median follow-up of 6 years: increased local control but no survival benefit in irradiated patients with resectable rectal carcinoma. Ann Surg 2007; 246: 693–701.

98. Sebag-Montefiore D, Stephens RJ, Steele R, et al. Preoperative radiotherapy versus selective postoperative chemoradiotherapy in patients with rectal cancer (MRC CR07 and NCIC-CTG C016): a multicentre, randomised trial. Lancet 2009; 373: 811–20.

99. Wong RK, Tandan V, De Silva S et al. Pre-operative radiotherapy and curative surgery for the management of localized rectal carcinoma. Cochrane Database Syst Rev 2007; CD002102.

100. Colorectal Cancer Collaborative Group. Adjuvant radiotherapy for rectal cancer: a systematic overview of 8,507 patients from 22 randomised trials. Lancet 2001; 358: 1291–304.

101. Frykholm GJ, Glimelius B, Pahlman L. Preoperative or postoperative irradiation in adenocarcinoma of the rectum: final treatment results of a randomized trial and an evaluation of late secondary effects. Dis Colon Rectum 1993; 36: 564–72.

102. Krook JE, Moertel CG, Gunderson LL et al. Effective surgical adjuvant therapy for high-risk rectal carcinoma. N Engl J Med 1991; 324: 709–15.

103. Douglass HO Jr, Moertel CG, Mayer RJ et al. Survival after postoperative combination treatment of rectal cancer. N Engl J Med 1986; 315: 1294–5.

104. Fisher B, Wolmark N, Rockette H et al. Postoperative adjuvant chemotherapy or radiation therapy for rectal cancer: results from NSABP protocol R-01. J Natl Cancer Inst 1988; 80: 21–9.

105. O'Connell MJ, Martenson JA, Wieand HS et al. Improving adjuvant therapy for rectal cancer by combining protracted-infusion fluorouracil with radiation therapy after curative surgery. N Engl J Med 1994; 331: 502–7.

106. Sauer R, Becker H, Hohenberger W et al. Preoperative versus postoperative chemoradiotherapy for rectal cancer. N Engl J Med 2004; 351: 1731–40.

107. Gerard J-P, Conroy T, Bonnetain F et al. Preoperative radiotherapy with or without concurrent fluorouracil and leucovorin in T3-4 rectal cancers: results of FFCD 9203. J Clin Oncol 2006; 24: 4620–5.

108. Bosset JF, Collette L, Calais G et al. Chemotherapy with preoperative radiotherapy in rectal cancer. N Engl J Med 2006; 355: 1114–23.

109. Bujko K, Nowacki MP, Nasierowska-Guttmejer A et al. Long-term results of a randomized trial comparing preoperative short-course radiotherapy with preoperative conventionally fractionated chemoradiation for rectal cancer. Br J Surg 2006; 93: 1215–23.

110. Desch CE, Benson AB III, Somerfield MR et al. colorectal cancer surveillance: 2005 Update of an American Society of Clinical Oncology practice guideline. J Clin Oncol 2005; 23: 8512–19.

111. Van Cutsem EJ, Oliveira J. Colon cancer: ESMO clinical recommendations for diagnosis, adjuvant treatment and follow-up. Ann Oncol 2008; 19(Suppl 2): ii29–30.

112. Schmoll H-J, Sargent D. Single agent fluorouracil for first-line treatment of advanced colorectal cancer as standard? Lancet 2007; 370: 105–7.

113. Thirion P, Michiels S, Pignon JP et al. Modulation of fluorouracil by leucovorin in patients with advanced colorectal cancer: an updated meta-analysis. J Clin Oncol 2004; 22: 3766–75.

114. de Gramont A, Bosset JF, Milan C et al. Randomized trial comparing monthly low-dose leucovorin and fluorouracil bolus with bimonthly high-dose leucovorin and fluorouracil bolus plus continuous infusion for advanced colorectal cancer: a French intergroup study. J Clin Oncol 1997; 15: 808–15.

115. Mayer RJ. Oral versus intravenous fluoropyrimidines for advanced colorectal cancer: By either route, it's all the same. J Clin Oncol 2001; 19: 4093–6.

116. Douillard JY, Hoff PM, Skillings JR et al. Multicenter phase III study of uracil/tegafur and oral leucovorin versus fluorouracil and leucovorin in patients with previously untreated metastatic colorectal cancer. J Clin Oncol 2002; 20: 3605–16.

117. Cunningham D, Zalcberg J, Maroun J et al. Efficacy, tolerability and management of raltitrexed (Tomudex) monotherapy in patients with advanced colorectal cancer. a review of phase II/III trials. Eur J Cancer 2002; 38: 478–86.

118. Cunningham D, Pyrhonen S, James RD et al. Randomised trial of irinotecan plus supportive care versus supportive care alone after fluorouracil failure for patients with metastatic colorectal cancer. Lancet 1998; 352: 1413–18.

119. Rougier P, Van Cutsem E, Bajetta E et al. Randomised trial of irinotecan versus fluorouracil by continuous infusion after fluorouracil failure in patients with metastatic colorectal cancer. Lancet 1998; 352: 1407–12.

120. Saltz LB, Cox JV, Blanke C et al. Irinotecan plus fluorouracil and leucovorin for metastatic colorectal cancer. Irinotecan Study Group. N Engl J Med 2000; 343: 905–14.

121. Fuchs CS, Marshall J, Mitchell E et al. Randomized, controlled trial of irinotecan plus infusional, bolus, or oral fluoropyrimidines in first-line treatment of metastatic colorectal cancer: Results from the BICC-C study. J Clin Oncol 2007; 25: 4779–86.

122. de Gramont A, Figer A, Seymour M et al. Leucovorin and fluorouracil with or without oxaliplatin as first-line treatment in advanced colorectal cancer. J Clin Oncol 2000; 18: 2938–47.

123. Grothey A, Deschler B, Kroening H et al. Phase III study of bolus 5-fluorouracil (5-FU)/folinic acid (FA) (Mayo) vs weekly high-dose 24h 5-FU infusion/FA + oxaliplatin in

advanced colorectal cancer. Proc Am Soc Clin Oncol 2002; 21: 129a.

124. Goldberg RM, Sargent DJ, Morton RF et al. A Randomized controlled trial of fluorouracil plus leucovorin, irinotecan, and oxaliplatin combinations in patients with previously untreated metastatic colorectal cancer. J Clin Oncol 2004; 22: 23–30.

125. Rothenberg ML, Oza AM, Bigelow RH et al. Superiority of oxaliplatin and fluorouracil-leucovorin compared with either therapy alone in patients with progressive colorectal cancer after irinotecan and fluorouracil-leucovorin: interim results of a phase III trial. J Clin Oncol 2003; 21: 2059–69.

126. Cassidy J, Clarke S, Diaz-Rubio E et al. Randomized phase iii study of capecitabine plus oxaliplatin compared with fluorouracil/folinic acid plus oxaliplatin as first-line therapy for metastatic colorectal cancer. J Clin Oncol 2008; 26: 2006–12.

127. Tournigand C, Andre T, Achille E et al. FOLFIRI followed by FOLFOX6 or the reverse sequence in advanced colorectal cancer: a randomized GERCOR study. J Clin Oncol 2004; 22: 229–37.

128. Colucci G, Gebbia V, Paoletti G et al. Phase III randomized trial of FOLFIRI versus FOLFOX4 in the treatment of advanced colorectal cancer: a multicenter study of the Gruppo Oncologico Dell'Italia Meridionale. J Clin Oncol 2005; 23: 4866–75.

129. Ashley AC, Sargent DJ, Alberts SR et al. Updated efficacy and toxicity analysis of irinotecan and oxaliplatin (IROX): intergroup trial N9741 in first-line treatment of metastatic colorectal cancer. Cancer 2007; 110: 670–7.

130. Souglakos J, Androulakis N, Syrigos K et al. FOLFOXIRI (folinic acid, 5-fluorouracil, oxaliplatin and irinotecan) vs FOLFIRI (folinic acid, 5-fluorouracil and irinotecan) as first-line treatment in metastatic colorectal cancer (MCC): a multicentre randomised phase III trial from the Hellenic Oncology Research Group (HORG). Br J Cancer 2006; 94: 798–805.

131. Falcone A, Ricci S, Brunetti I et al. Phase III trial of infusional fluorouracil, leucovorin, oxaliplatin, and irinotecan (FOLFOXIRI) compared with infusional fluorouracil, leucovorin, and irinotecan (FOLFIRI) as first-line treatment for metastatic colorectal cancer: the Gruppo Oncologico Nord Ovest. J Clin Oncol 2007; 25: 1670–6.

132. Hurwitz H, Fehrenbacher L, Novotny W et al. Bevacizumab plus irinotecan, fluorouracil, and leucovorin for metastatic colorectal cancer. N Engl J Med 2004; 350: 2335–42.

133. Kabbinavar FF, Hambleton J, Mass RD et al. Combined analysis of efficacy: the addition of bevacizumab to fluorouracil/leucovorin improves survival for patients with metastatic colorectal cancer. J Clin Oncol 2005; 23: 3706–12.

134. Fuchs CS, Marshall J, Barrueco J. Randomized, controlled trial of irinotecan plus infusional, bolus, or oral fluoropyrimidines in first-line treatment of metastatic colorectal cancer: updated results from the BICC-C study. J Clin Oncol 2008; 26: 689–90.

135. Hochster HS, Hart LL, Ramanathan RK et al. Safety and efficacy of oxaliplatin/fluoropyrimidine regimens with or without bevacizumab as first-line treatment of metastatic colorectal cancer (mCRC): Final analysis of the TREE-Study. J Clin Oncol (Meeting Abstracts) 2006; 24(18 Suppl): 3510.

136. Saltz LB, Clarke S, Diaz-Rubio E et al. Bevacizumab in combination with oxaliplatin-based chemotherapy as first-line therapy in metastatic colorectal cancer: a randomized phase III study. J Clin Oncol 2008; 26: 2013–19.

137. Giantonio BJ, Catalano PJ, Meropol NJ et al. Bevacizumab in combination with oxaliplatin, fluorouracil, and leucovorin (FOLFOX4) for previously treated metastatic colorectal cancer: results from the Eastern Cooperative Oncology Group Study E3200. J Clin Oncol 2007; 25: 1539–44.

138. Porebska I, Harlozinska A, Bojarowski T. Expression of the tyrosine kinase activity growth factor receptors (EGFR, ERB B2, ERB B3) in colorectal adenocarcinomas and adenomas. Tumour Biol 2000; 21: 105–15.

139. Cunningham D, Humblet Y, Siena S et al. Cetuximab monotherapy and cetuximab plus irinotecan in irinotecan-refractory metastatic colorectal cancer. N Engl J Med 2004; 351: 337–45.

140. Jonker DJ, O'Callaghan CJ, Karapetis CS et al. Cetuximab for the treatment of colorectal cancer. N Engl J Med 2007; 357: 2040–8.

141. Sobrero AF, Maurel J, Fehrenbacher L et al. EPIC: Phase III trial of cetuximab plus irinotecan after fluoropyrimidine and oxaliplatin failure in patients with metastatic colorectal cancer. J Clin Oncol 2008; 26: 2311-19.

142. Polikoff J, Mitchell EP, Badarinath S et al. Cetuximab plus FOLFOX for colorectal cancer (EXPLORE): preliminary efficacy analysis of a randomized phase III trial. J Clin Oncol (Meeting Abstracts) 2005; 23(16 Suppl): 3574.

143. Van Cutsem E, Kohne C-H, Hitre E, et al. Cetuximab and Chemotherapy as Initial Treatment for Metastatic Colorectal Cancer. N Engl J Med 2009; 360: 1408–17.

144. Van Cutsem E, Peeters M, Siena S et al. Open-label phase III trial of panitumumab plus best supportive care compared with best supportive care alone in patients with chemotherapy-refractory metastatic colorectal cancer. J Clin Oncol 2007; 25: 1658–64.

145. Amado RG, Wolf M, Peeters M et al. Wild-type KRAS is required for panitumumab efficacy in patients with metastatic colorectal cancer. J Clin Oncol 2008: JCO 2007; 14: 7116.

146. Hecht JR, Mitchell E, Chidiac T, et al. A randomized phase IIIB trial of chemotherapy, bevacizumab, and panitumumab compared with chemotherapy and bevacizumab alone for metastatic colorectal cancer. J Clin Oncol 2009; 27: 672–80.

147. Saltz LB, Lenz HJ, Kindler HL et al. Randomized phase II trial of cetuximab, bevacizumab, and irinotecan compared with cetuximab and bevacizumab alone in irinotecan-refractory colorectal cancer: the BOND-2 study. J Clin Oncol 2007; 25: 4557–61.

148. Tol J, Koopman M, Cats A, et al. Chemotherapy, bevacizumab, and cetuximab in metastatic colorectal cancer. N Engl J Med 2009; 360: 563–72.

149. Nordlinger B, Sorbye H, Glimelius B et al. Perioperative chemotherapy with FOLFOX4 and surgery versus surgery alone for resectable liver metastases from colorectal cancer (EORTC Intergroup trial 40983): a randomised controlled trial. Lancet 2008; 371: 1007–16.

150. Kemeny MM, Adak S, Gray B et al. Combined-modality treatment for resectable metastatic colorectal carcinoma to the liver: surgical resection of hepatic metastases in combination with continuous infusion of chemotherapy—an intergroup study. J Clin Oncol 2002; 20: 1499–505.

151. Daling JR, Madeleine MM, Johnson LG et al. Human papillomavirus, smoking, and sexual practices in the etiology of anal cancer. Cancer 2004; 101: 270–80.

152. Cummings BJ. Current management of anal canal cancer. Semin Oncol 2005; 32(6 Suppl 9): S123–S128.

153. Ajani JA, Winter KA, Gunderson LL et al. Fluorouracil, mitomycin, and radiotherapy vs fluorouracil, cisplatin, and radiotherapy for carcinoma of the anal canal: a randomized controlled trial. JAMA 2008; 299: 1914–21.

154. Ajani JA, Rodriguez G, Bodoky G et al. Multicenter phase III comparison of cisplatin/S-1 (CS) with cisplatin/5-FU (CF) as first-line therapy in patients with advanced gastric cancer (FLAGS). Abstr 8. In 2009 Gastrointestinal Cancers Symposium.

155. Waters JS, Norman A, Cunningham D, et al. Long-term survival after epirubicin, cisplatin and fluorouracil for gastric cancer: results of a randomized trial. Br J Cancer 1999; 80: 269–72.

156. Ross P, Nicolson M, Cunningham D, et al. Prospective randomized trial comparing mitomycin, cisplatin, and protracted venous-infusion fluorouracil (PVI 5-FU) with epirubicin, cisplatin, and PVI 5-FU in advanced esophagogastric cancer. J Clin Oncol 2002; 20: 1996–2004.

157. Dank M, Zaluski J, Barone C, et al. Randomized phase 3 trial of irinotecan (CPT-11) + 5FU/folinic acid (FA) vs CDDP + 5FU in 1st-line advanced gastric cancer patients. J Clin Oncol (Meeting Abstracts) 2005; 23: 4003.

158. Klinkenbijl JH, Jeekel J, Sahmoud T, et al. Adjuvant radiotherapy and 5-fluorouracil after curative resection of cancer of the pancreas and periampullary region: phase III trial of the EORTC gastrointestinal tract cancer cooperative group. Ann Surg 1999; 230: 776–82.

159. Moore MJ, Hamm J, Dancey J, et al. Comparison of gemcitabine versus the matrix metalloproteinase inhibitor BAY 12-9566 in patients with advanced or metastatic adenocarcinoma of the pancreas: a phase III trial of the National Cancer Institute of Canada Clinical Trials Group. J Clin Oncol 2003; 21: 3296–302.

160. Van Cutsem E, van de Velde H, Karasek P, et al. Phase III trial of gemcitabine plus tipifarnib compared with gemcitabine plus placebo in advanced pancreatic cancer. J Clin Oncol 2004; 22: 1430–8.

161. Philip PA, Benedetti J, Fenoglio-Preiser C, et al. Phase III study of gemcitabine [G] plus cetuximab [C] versus gemcitabine in patients [pts] with locally advanced or metastatic pancreatic adenocarcinoma [PC]: SWOG S0205 study. J Clin Oncol (Meeting Abstracts) 2007; 25: LBA4509.

162. Kindler HL, Niedzwiecki D, Hollis D, et al. A double-blind, placebo-controlled, randomized phase III trial of gemcitabine (G) plus bevacizumab (B) versus gemcitabine plus placebo (P) in patients (pts) with advanced pancreatic cancer (PC): A preliminary analysis of Cancer and Leukemia Group B (CALGB. J Clin Oncol (Meeting Abstracts) 2007; 25: 4508.

163. Van Cutsem E, Labianca R, Hossfeld D et al. Randomized phase III trial comparing infused irinotecan/5-fluorouracil (5-FU)/folinic acid (IF) versus 5-FU/FA (F) in stage III colon cancer patients (pts). (PETACC 3). J Clin Oncol (Meeting Abstracts) 2005; 23: LBA8.

164. Ychou M, Raoul JL, Douillard JY, et al. A phase III randomised trial of LV5FU2 + irinotecan versus LV5FU2 alone in adjuvant high-risk colon cancer (FNCLCC Accord02/FFCD9802). Ann Oncol 2009; 20: 674–80.

165. Kabbinavar F, Hurwitz HI, Fehrenbacher L, et al. Phase II, randomized trial comparing bevacizumab plus fluorouracil (FU)/leucovorin (LV) with FU/LV alone in patients with metastatic colorectal cancer. J Clin Oncol 2003; 21: 60–5.

166. Kabbinavar FF, Schulz J, McCleod M, et al. Addition of bevacizumab to bolus fluorouracil and leucovorin in first-line metastatic colorectal cancer: results of a randomized phase II trial. J Clin Oncol 2005; 23: 3697–705.

10

Cancers of the Genitourinary Tract

Ronald de Wit and Cora N. Sternberg

CANCER OF THE PROSTATE

Prostate cancer is the most common cancer (excluding skin cancer) in men and the second leading cause of death from cancer, exceeded only by lung cancer. It primarily affects men over the age of 70 years.

In all, 89% of men diagnosed with prostate cancer will survive at least five years and 63% will survive at least 10 years. Substantial controversy exists about the advisability and effectiveness of screening, the most appropriate staging evaluations, and the optimal management of patients with all stages of prostate cancer. For metastatic disease, hormonal androgen deprivation therapy has been the mainstay of treatment for many years. Uncertainty exists about optimal therapy and timing. For patients who have become refractory to androgen ablation, chemotherapy was recently recognized to prolong survival.

Staging

The International Union Against Cancer (UICC) 1997 tumor, node, metastasis (TNM) staging classification is generally used for prostate cancer. Measurement of serum prostate-specific antigen (PSA) is useful both in diagnosis and in staging.

Pathology

Over 90% of prostate cancers are adenocarcinomas. Other histologic variants include small cell carcinoma, transitional, and squamous cell carcinomas. Although several pathologic grading systems for adenocarcinoma of the prostate have been developed, the Gleason grading system, based on the glandular pattern of the tumor, has gained most acceptance (Table 10.1). Both the predominant and the second most prevalent architectural patterns are identified and assigned a grade from 1 (the most differentiated) to 5 (undifferentiated). Because both patterns are influential in predicting prognosis, the Gleason score is obtained by adding the sum of the primary and the secondary grades.

Localized Prostate Cancer

Due to the increasing use of screening and PSA, 60% of all prostate cancers are discovered while they are still confined to the prostate. The five-year relative survival rate for localized prostate cancer in the United States approaches 100%. Management options include radiation therapy (RT), radical surgery, and conservative management. The ideal approach for every individual patient remains unclear, as prospective comparative data are limited. Few trials have been conducted or are in progress that may shed new light on existing controversies (1,2).

The majority of men receiving radical treatment will survive 10 years following optimal RT or radical prostatectomy. RT is often selected for patients with coexisting medical problems that would preclude major surgery. Patients treated by RT tend to be older and have higher grade, higher stage tumors, and higher PSA levels. The younger, healthier men with smaller, localized tumors more often undergo surgery. The strategy of initial conservative management and delayed hormone therapy is an alternative for elderly patients with Grade 1 or 2 minimal volume tumors (2).

After RT, local control is maintained in 92% of Stage T1 and 75% of Stage T2 tumors, with an overall survival of 82% and 55% at 5 and 10 years, respectively. Biopsies of the prostate may reveal viable cancer cells in up to 90% of patients, however, at five years. Sexual impotence is observed in 14% to 46% of patients after RT and in 7% to 13% after interstitial implantation. New techniques using three-dimensional conformal external beam RT and intensity modulated radiation therapy (IMRT) may permit delivery of a higher dose within the tumor and minimal dose to the surrounding tissue, decreasing both acute and late toxicity (3).

Additional (adjuvant) hormonal androgen deprivation therapy, when started simultaneously with RT, may improve local control and survival in patients with locally advanced prostate cancer (4). An European Organisation for Research and Treatment of Cancer (EORTC) comparative trial of external beam RT versus RT plus three years of goserelin (an agonist analogue of gonadotropin-releasing hormone) has shown a survival benefit at five years. When the use of six months versus three years was evaluated, patients who underwent three years of hormonal therapy had an advantage in terms of biochemical progression-free survival (PFS) (5).

Radical prostatectomy entails the removal of seminal vesicles and ampullae of the vas as well as the prostate with its capsule. Modifications in the surgical technique have led to improved continence and potency rates (2,3). Excluding patients with positive seminal vesicles or lymph nodes, the five-year actuarial PFS is 87% for patients with negative margins, 60% for those with focally positive margins, and 35% for those with extensive positive margins (6). Several studies have shown that additional RT for patients with pT3 prostate carcinoma improves biochemical failure-free survival, especially in patients with positive surgical margins (7). A report on long-term follow-up in a study from the South West Oncology Group (SWOG) of immediate

Table 10.1 Gleason Grading System for Adenocarcinoma of the Prostate

Score 1	Lobular masses, uniform small glands, no invasion
Score 2	Lobular masses, irregular glands, "broad front" invasion, ± cribriform pattern
Score 3	Irregular glands, infiltrative invasion, cribriform pattern, papillary pattern
Score 4	Sheets of large cells with pale cytoplasm, infiltrative invasion, ± glands (like renal cell carcinoma)
Score 5	Sheets of anaplastic cells, ± foci of glands (like small cell carcinoma)

RT versus observation in PT3 prostate cancer recently demonstrated an overall survival benefit, 47% versus 37%.

Advanced Disease

Approximately 30% to 35% of patients with prostate cancer will present with regional or metastatic tumors, whereas an additional 25% will develop metastases in the course of the disease. Metastases predominantly occur in the bone. In patients presenting with metastatic disease and those treated with androgen deprivation therapy, the median survival is 2.5 years.

Hormone-Naive Disease

The mainstay of therapy is androgen deprivation, which is palliative rather than curative. Hormonal therapy can produce objective tumor regression in soft tissue sites in more than 80% of cases, normalization of PSA in 70%, and an improvement in the bone scan in 30% to 50% of cases. Despite the initially highly active androgen deprivation therapy, eventually 90% of patients will die within three years. Surgical castration (bilateral orchiectomy) has been the gold standard of androgen deprivation therapy for many years. Luteinizing hormone releasing hormone (LHRH) agonists result in continuous stimulation of pituitary receptors for LHRH, paradoxically resulting in decreased secretion of LH and follicle-stimulating hormone (FSH). Testosterone production by the testis is then turned off achieving serum levels of testosterone similar to those obtained by orchiectomy. Antiandrogens interfere with testosterone binding to the androgen receptor (AR).

The decision to use an LHRH analogue or to perform orchiectomy as the initial hormone treatment for advanced prostate cancer is based on the preferences of the patient and the physician. LHRH agonists may cause an initial increase in testosterone levels. In patients with widespread metastatic disease, this can cause dangerous clinical sequela and can be circumvented by concurrent administration of antiandrogens during the initial weeks of therapy. Direct LHRH antagonists are also being developed and may circumvent this flare phenomenon as these agents directly inhibit the release of LH and FSH.

Combined androgen blockade (CAB) was conceived as a means of blocking the adrenal androgens. It has been evaluated by many investigators in patients with metastatic prostate cancer with contradictory results. Although three studies demonstrated a positive effect with CAB, numerous trials have failed to demonstrate any benefit to CAB. A meta-analysis including 27 published randomized trials showed no survival benefit at two years.

The antiandrogens are generally divided into steroidal and nonsteroidal compounds. The nonsteroidal antiandrogens (flutamide, nilufamide, and biculatamide) are the most frequently used agents. These agents are thought to be therapeutically equivalent, with clinical differences primarily related to adverse-effect profiles and half-lives. Of note, the antiandrogens alone do not result in castrate levels of testosterone and are generally not considered sufficient treatment for use in overt metastatic disease. The advantage to using these agents alone, though, is the potential for preserving sexual potency, and for this reason, these agents are used as initial therapy in patients with biochemical (PSA) failure after local treatment. The timing of treatment of patients with evidence of biochemical failure remains controversial (8).

Hormone-Refractory Prostate Cancer

Hormone-refractory prostate cancer (HRPC) is defined as a progressive disease despite serum castration levels of the testosterone. The development of hormonal resistance predictably occurs after androgen deprivation. HRPC reflects a heterogeneous patient population. Formerly, HRPC consisted of symptomatic patients with impaired performance status. Now, due to intensive PSA-guided follow-up, patients may have HRPC without having extensive macroscopic disease. The knowledge that tumor has escaped preliminary hormonal control (rising PSA) is disturbing to most patients and further therapies are usually requested (8). This term is gradually being replaced by the term castration-resistant prostate cancer (CRPC), as patients may still respond to hormonal maneuvers after failing initial hormonal therapy.

The median time to progression following androgen deprivation therapy is 18 months. Median survival of patients with HRPC in older studies was approximately 12 months. Due to stage migration, this is no longer entirely realistic and different categories of patients must be taken into account in the interpretation of the results of trials in HRPC and individual patient management. An American study recently developed a prognostic model, based on lactic dehydrogenase (LDH), PSA, alkaline phosphatase, Gleason sum, ECOG performance status, hemoglobin, and presence of visceral metastases, that discriminated between four risk groups, the worst group having a median survival duration of 7.5 months and the best group surviving a median of 27 months.

In addition, interpretation of trials in advanced prostate cancer has been confounded by the lack of measurable disease. Bone is the dominant site of metastases in 90% of patients with metastatic prostatic cancer. For this reason, objectively measurable criteria for response evaluation are lacking in a majority of patients. In many patients, bone pain and decreased performance status are predominant and relief from these symptoms is as important as the prolongation of survival. Use of surrogate end points, such as reduction in PSA or improvement in pain, has been used to evaluate new therapies. Although the value of PSA decline as a measure of therapeutic benefit has not been definitively established, recent studies have indicated that a >30% decrease in PSA at three months is the best surrogate measure for survival (9,10) associated with prolonged survival. New guidelines have been developed for the conduct of clinical trials based upon some of these considerations (11).

Second-Line Hormonal Therapy

Second-line hormonal treatment may exert its effects by diminishing circulating adrenal androgens causing tumor regression by suppressing any remaining hormone-dependent prostatic cancer cells. A variety of hormonal therapies, including both nonsteroidal and steroidal antiandrogens, have been used as second-line therapy with modest results. Measurable disease regression is rare and responses are of brief duration. An alternative agent that blocks the adrenal production of testosterone by CYP17 blockade is ketoconazole. However, ketoconazole is a rather weak CYP17 inhibitor, and a much more potent agent with this target is abiraterone. Recent data indicate that this agent is well tolerated and highly efficacious in HRPC. Randomized studies are planned incorporating the addition of dexamethasone to augment the effect of the drug.

An interesting and clinically meaningful observation is the "antiandrogen withdrawal syndrome." Up to 40% of patients failing CAB will respond when the antiandrogen is discontinued. This paradoxical response was first documented with flutamide withdrawal, but was subsequently shown to occur with other nonsteroidal antiandrogens such as bicalutamide and nilutamide. Long-term androgen ablation with antiandrogens may lead to increased expression and activity and mutation of ARs. This may explain why discontinuation of the antiandrogen may lead to a decrease in PSA. It should be pointed out that no second-line hormonal manipulation has been proven to have led to an increase in survival.

Chemotherapy

Clinical results of chemotherapy in HRPC have been disappointing for many years. The objective response rate to chemotherapy in a total of 26 studies conducted between 1987 and 1991 was only 8.7% (95% CI 6.4–9.0%). In those years, clinical investigators were reluctant to treat asymptomatic patients, especially if the disease could not be evaluated using standard measurability criteria. Consequently, the majority of patients enrolled in studies had widespread disease that had already caused impaired performance status, which had an additional negative impact on the effectiveness of any type of systemic treatment.

With the recognition that PSA levels were correlated with survival and could serve as a surrogate end point for evaluable disease, and the development of "palliative measurement scales" by Canadian investigators (pain, analgesic consumption, performance status, and quality of life, QOL), prospective clinical studies were designed to enroll hormone-refractory patients earlier in the course of their disease.

Using these parameters, a randomized study in Canada and a study in the United States showed mitoxantrone plus prednisone or hydrocorticone to be beneficial. Although there was no measurable improvement in survival, the mitoxantrone–prednisone combination was accepted standard treatment for HRPC.

In the same time frame, proof-of-concept trials were being conducted using the taxanes. Several docetaxel-based regimens were investigated: a three-weekly (q3w) regimen, a weekly (q1w) regimen (due to the assumption that this regimen would be better tolerated in an elderly population), and combinations of docetaxel and estramustine. Promising objective response rates and median survival prompted the initiation of two large randomized Phase III studies, TAX 327 and SWOG 99-16, that were designed to test for a survival benefit (12,13).

TAX 327 was a three-arm study in which 1006 patients were randomized to receive either q3w docetaxel (75 mg/m²) plus low-dose prednisone (10 mg daily), docetaxel q1w (30 mg/m² for five of six weeks) plus prednisone, or mitoxantrone (12 mg/m² q3w) plus prednisone (12). The treatment duration was 30 weeks in all three arms. Patients who received the docetaxel q3w regimen had significantly longer survival and higher PSA and pain response rates compared with those who received mitoxantrone. The median survival was 18.9 months in the q3w docetaxel arm compared with 16.5 months in the mitoxantrone arm; a 2.4-month survival benefit that corresponded to a 24% reduction in the risk of death [hazard ratio (HR) of death 0.76 (95% CI 0.62–0.92)]. The docetaxel q1w regimen showed a trend toward survival benefit compared with mitoxantrone, but this did not reach statistical significance. A significantly greater proportion of patients who were treated with q3w docetaxel experienced a reduction in pain (35% vs. 22%, $p = 0.01$), a ≥50% reduction in PSA (45% vs. 32%, $p < 0.001$), and an improvement in QOL (22% vs. 13%, $p = 0.009$) compared with patients who received mitoxantrone. Grade 3/4 toxicity was infrequent other than neutropenia (32%), but the incidence of febrile neutropenia during the entire course of chemotherapy was, at most, 3%.

An updated survival analysis from the TAX 327 study showed that the significant improvement in survival associated with the q3w docetaxel regimen compared with the mitoxantrone regimen was sustained at three years (19.2 vs. 16.3 months, HR 0.79, $p = 0.004$) (14). The updated analysis also confirmed previous findings that the survival benefit associated with q3w docetaxel is relevant in all investigated subgroups; the HR for overall survival favored docetaxel regardless of age (<68 years, ≥68 years) and pain versus no pain, and for those with baseline PSA above and below the median value of 115 ng/ml.

The SWOG 99-16 study was designed on the premise that the combination of two cytotoxic agents, docetaxel with estramustine, would have a greater efficacy than the combination of one cytotoxic agent with a steroid (13). As such, SWOG 99-16 was a head-to-head comparison of docetaxel (60 mg/m², day, q3w) plus estramustine (280 mg, TID, days 1–5, q3w) with mitoxantrone (12 mg/m², day 1, q3w) plus prednisone (10 mg daily). The patient characteristics were quite similar to those of the TAX 327 study, as were the survival outcomes; patients who received the docetaxel plus estramustine regimen experienced a significant improvement in overall survival of 1.9 months compared with those who received mitoxantrone plus prednisone (17.5 vs. 15.6 months, $p = 0.02$).

The addition of estramustine to docetaxel, though, was associated with a significant increase in grade 3–5 gastrointestinal and cardiovascular toxicity compared with mitoxantrone plus prednisone. The most frequent cardiovascular toxicities were thrombosis and pulmonary embolism that were attributed to the estrogenic effects of estramustine.

The results of these two studies clearly demonstrate that chemotherapy is an effective approach for patients with metastatic HRPC. Three-weekly docetaxel with low-dose prednisone was associated with the most favorable outcomes; q1w docetaxel was possibly inferior in terms of efficacy and did not appear to be better tolerated than q3w administration in terms of nonhematological toxicities. The use of estramustine combined with docetaxel was associated with increased toxicity and did not appear to have improved efficacy compared with the q3w docetaxel plus prednisone regimen. As such, the docetaxel q3w plus low-dose prednisone is now considered the standard treatment for patients with metastatic HRPC (15).

The TAX 327 and SWOG 99-16 results were the first demonstration of a survival advantage for chemotherapy with docetaxel in patients with metastatic HRPC. Some physicians interpret these data with caution, and indeed it is often asked whether a 2.5-month increase in survival is enough to warrant the use of chemotherapy in an elderly patient population. Although in isolation this may appear to be a reasonable argument, it is important to consider two key facts about these results that are not immediately apparent. First, the increase in overall survival gained by the use of q3w docetaxel was not a 2.5-month increase compared with no therapy, but it was in fact, a 2.5-month increase over the benefit provided by the comparator arm, which also comprised effective chemotherapy (i.e., mitoxantrone), which was considered the standard of care. Second, in both trials, up to 40% of patients who were randomized to the mitoxantrone arm of the study crossed over to receive docetaxel after failure on mitoxantrone therapy. These patients were not excluded from the survival analysis. Despite the confounding effect of second-line treatment using the more effective therapy, the survival benefit associated with the q3w docetaxel regimen remained significant (16).

Many physicians support the notion that chemotherapy should be deferred until the disease becomes symptomatic in order to delay the exposure of patients to the potential side effects of chemotherapy. Although this may be a suitable approach in some patients with indolent disease, there are many patients in whom further disease progression and the development of symptoms is more imminent and for whom the start of chemotherapy should not be postponed. A secondary analysis of the Tax 327 cohort evidenced that pretreatment PSA and PSA doubling time (PSADT) were both independent predictors of survival (17). Also, patients with a short PSADT (<55 days) had a lower chance of survival compared with patients who had a more indolent PSADT. A multivariate analysis was conducted that also incorporated these PSA kinetics. It was found that well-established prognostic factors such as the presence or absence of pain, performance status, the number of metastatic sites (three or more), presence of liver metastases, baseline hemoglobin and alkaline phosphatase, and type of progressions at baseline (measurable soft tissue disease or bone scan progression vs. PSA only or nonmeasurable disease progression) all had independent prognostic importance for survival. Also, the baseline PSA concentration remained highly statistically significant ($p < 0.001$). PSADT remained borderline statistical significant in the multivariate model (17).

The consideration of prognostic parameters for survival is extremely informative and could facilitate treatment decisions. Nomograms are useful tools in this setting and one such item has been constructed using the above multivariate factors for survival from the TAX 327 results (17). Through assessment of a number of factors including PSA concentration, PSADT, pain at baseline, the presence of new metastatic sites, alkaline phosphatase, and hemoglobin, a patient's disease status can be assigned points that can be translated into one-, two-, and five-year probabilities of survival for that patient. The use of nomograms could facilitate the tailoring of therapy to suit the pattern of disease on an individual basis. Those patients who have no actual symptoms, but are more likely to develop symptoms in the near future because of bone scan progression and/or unfavorable PSA kinetics should be considered as candidates for docetaxel chemotherapy (Table 10.2).

Secondary analyses using the TAX 327 and SWOG 99-16 databases have also revealed that both PSA decline and pain response are only modest surrogate measures for benefit and survival, especially during the first three months of chemotherapy (16). As both PSA and pain may increase during the initial cycles of chemotherapy before the start to decrease, these early changes may best be ignored unless there is clinically compelling evidence of disease progression (11,16).

It is important to note that the docetaxel Phase 3 data were obtained in patients with documented metastatic disease. Therefore, these results cannot be extrapolated to earlier disease in patients with rising PSA without evidence of metastases.

As it is assumed that in the setting of HRPC some clones of the tumor spread may have retained their sensitively to hormonal manipulations, patients with HRPC are usually kept on androgen ablation therapy, even during cytotoxic treatment.

Radiation Therapy

Bone pain is often a debilitating component of metastatic prostate cancer. Single 8 Gy fractions are convenient both for administration and for pain relief (18). The β-emitting radioisotope [89]Strontium is an alternative means of palliating bone pain but may cause prolonged myelosuppression, which may prevent the use of chemotherapeutic options.

Table 10.2 Treatment Algorithm for Hormone-Refractory Prostate Cancer

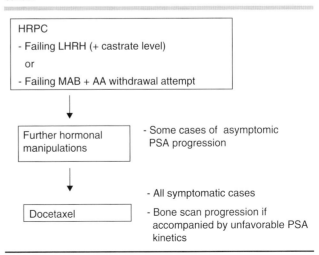

Bisphosphonates

Bisphosphonates are primarily known for their ability to inhibit osteoclast-mediated bone resorption and are widely used to delay skeletal complications in patients with breast cancer and multiple myeloma. Conventional bisphosphonates failed to show objective benefit in patients with prostate cancer and (mostly) osteoblastic bone lesions. New generation bisphosphonates, however, have shown to be more potent osteoblast mediators. Zoledronic acid significantly reduced the proportion of patients who experienced skeletal complications and extended the time to first skeletal complications. Other promising agents to prevent skeletal-related events include monoclonal antibodies to RANK-ligand (densumab).

New Developments

Increased insight into the biology of prostate cancer has led to new developments in immunotherapy, dendritic cell therapy, and gene vaccination therapy (19). Molecular targeted small molecule therapy and monoclonal antibodies that target signaling cascades in tumor growth have been identified, and antiangiogenesis agents such as bevacizumab and VEGF-TRAP are being evaluated in combination with docetaxel in large Phase IIII clinical trials. So too are endothelin A antagonists (atrasentan A and ZD 4504) under evaluation in combination with docetaxel or prior to docetaxel in clinical trials. Novel chemotherapeutic agents that work at different points in the cell cycle are other options for preclinical and clinical development. Also, a number of trials are in progress to investigate docetaxel chemotherapy earlier in the course of the disease, that is, in the neoadjuvant setting or noncastrate metastatic disease.

Abiraterone acetate is an emerging agent that inhibits 17 α-hydroxylase and C17,20-lyase, and has been demonstrated to decrease serum androgen to undetectable levels. It has been studied both in patients with metastatic HRPC who have progressed on docetaxel and in patients who have not received chemotherapy (20). A Phase III trial is comparing placebo-prednisolone with abiraterone-prednisolone in patients progressing after docetaxel.

Prostate cancer continues to rely on AR signaling, which remains a target of hormonal therapy. Modifications of the AR via mutations, amplification, phosphorylation, and changes in AR cofactors are implicated in the activation of AR signaling. The development of new strategies and drugs that can abrogate AR signaling may result in benefits. MDV 3100 is a small molecule that blocks nuclear translocation of AR, DNA binding without agonist activity when AR is overexpressed. Ongoing trials are evaluating BMS-641988 and MDV3100, which are novel and potent AR antagonists.

CANCER OF THE BLADDER

Bladder cancer is the fifth most common cancer in men and the seventh in women, The male to female occurrence is three to one. Smoking is a significant risk factor. It is primarily a disease of the elderly, with 80% of cases in the 50 to 79 years age group.

In cases involving regional spread or distant spread, five-year survival rates are 49% and 6%, respectively. When bladder cancer is found at a localized superficial stage, the five-year survival rate is 94%. Seventy-five percent of all bladder cancers are superficial at presentation, limited to the mucosa, submucosa, or lamina propria. Recurrence rates after initial treatment are 50% to 80%, with progression to muscle-invading tumor in 10% to 25%. For superficial disease, prevention of recurrence and progression are the primary issues. In muscle-invading bladder cancers, there is a 50% risk of distant metastases.

Pathology

In the Western world, the majority of bladder carcinomas are transitional cell carcinoma (TCC), whereas squamous cell carcinoma and adenocarcinomas account for 5% and 2%, respectively. Squamous cell carcinomas are often associated with chronic irritation or infection. The distinct variants of squamous cell carcinomas, with diverse etiologies and biology, are beyond the scope of this chapter.

Clinical Presentation

The diagnosis can be elusive as bladder cancer can mimic urinary tract infection or prostatitis. In an adult, especially over 50 years of age, with asymptomatic hematuria or irritative voiding symptoms, this diagnosis should be considered.

Staging

Evaluation of a patient with potentially muscle invasive bladder cancer should include computerized axial tomography (CT scan) or nuclear magnetic resonance (NMR) to evaluate the lymph nodes and stratified transurethral resection of the bladder (TURB) of the bladder.

Superficial Bladder Cancer

Superficial bladder cancers are usually low grade. They rarely become invasive, but locally recur in approximately 50% of patients within 6 to 12 months. The risk of progression is related to grade and stage of the cancer. The rate of progression for Grade I is approximately 2%, 11% for Grade II, and 45% for Grade III; approximately 4% with Ta progress, compared with 30% of patients with T1 tumors.

Carcinoma in situ (CIS) is a flat, nonpapillary, noninvasive, anaplastic epithelium closely resembling high-grade TCC. The association of CIS with low-stage, low-grade tumors has been linked with increased risk of subsequent progression and muscle invasion.

Treatment of Superficial Bladder Cancer

Intravesical therapy provides close proximity of the drug with the tumor, thus avoiding the toxicity of systemic therapy. No therapy is recommended for patients with low risk for recurrence, that is, patients with solitary Stage Ta, grade 1–2 TCC. For patients at intermediate risk, those with infrequent recurrence of grade 1–2, Stage Ta tumor, no treatment may be required. For those who require therapy, BCG (Bacillus Calmette Guerin) is used in the United States, although urologists in Europe use either BCG or intravesical chemotherapy, mostly mitomycin. Patients at high risk of disease progression should be treated with intravesical BCG. High-risk patients are defined as those with CIS, Grade 3 TCC, Stage 1 TCC, or positive postresection urinary cytology. BCG is the most effective intravesical agent for the prevention of recurrence and progression of bladder cancer (21).

Muscle-Invasive Bladder Cancer

Although radical cystectomy has been the treatment of choice for patients with muscle-invading tumors in the United States, RT has been a standard alternative therapeutic option in Europe and Canada. Predictors for relapse after cystectomy include the depth of invasion, the involvement of adjacent viscera (perivesicular fat, vascular invasion, prostate, vagina), and the presence of nodal metastases. Recurrence is related to stage and nodal status. High-grade, high-stage (pT3–4) tumors are frequently (40–60%) found to have lymph node involvement (pN+) at the time of radical cystectomy. Current selected studies indicate a 15% to 20% five-year survival after cystectomy in patients with nodal metastases. With direct invasion into the adjacent viscera, cure is obtained in less than 10%. Other known prognostic factors include histology, grade, presence or absence of ureteral obstruction, and the extent of surgical resection.

Surgery

Radical cystectomy implies the removal of the bladder and pelvic lymph nodes, and in male patients the prostate and the seminal vesicles. In the female patient, radical cystectomy means the removal of the bladder, female urethra, and pelvic lymph nodes. It also involves the removal of the uterus, fallopian tubes, and ovaries, and a variable amount of the upper vagina. This surgery is associated with considerable morbidity and mutilation and requires adaptation of lifestyle. It is only offered to patients in good medical condition.

Several techniques of bladder substitution have been described, which recently have also included female patients. The patient's enhanced self-image following continent urinary diversion is the major advantage of this type of surgery.

Neoadjuvant Chemotherapy

Following cystectomy for muscle invasive bladder carcinoma, up to 50% of patients may develop metastases. This most often occurs within two years. Most patients relapse in distant sites; only one-third of patients relapse in the pelvis alone. Response rates of 40% to 70% with combination chemotherapy regimens have led to investigation of their use for locally invasive disease in combination with conventional modalities of treatment, either as neoadjuvant or classic adjuvant therapy.

There have been many single arm, nonrandomized pilot studies that have established the feasibility and safety of administering neoadjuvant chemotherapy. The overall response rates of 60% to 70% with CR rates in the 30% range have been frequently reported. These trials have demonstrated that neoadjuvant chemotherapy can produce tumor "downstaging."

The International EORTC/MRC trial of chemotherapy prior to cystectomy or radiotherapy versus cystectomy or radiotherapy is the largest trial of neoadjuvant chemotherapy. The trial enrolled 976 patients. In this trial, first published in the *Lancet*, a 15% reduction in the risk of death, which translated into a three-year survival difference of 5.5% (50% in the no chemotherapy arm) was observed. Looking at the HR of 0.85 (95% CI 0.71–1.02), this difference was not statistically significant. The median length of follow-up for patients alive was four years. These results have been updated to 7.4 years (22). With more events, the data have just reached statistical significance (HR = 0.85; 95% CI 0.72–1.00; $p = 0.048$) in favor of patients treated with CMV chemotherapy. The five-year survival rate was 44% versus 50%, and the seven-year survival rate was 37% versus 43%. Hence, the 2002 results provide longer follow-up, but no real change in absolute benefit.

Also, a SWOG Intergroup trial reported the benefits of three cycles of neoadjuvant M-VAC chemotherapy prior to cystectomy versus cystectomy alone (23). This trial evaluated 307 patients and reported a difference in median survival in favor of M-VAC chemotherapy. According to an intent-to-treat analysis, the authors reported that median survival was 46 months for the cystectomy patients as compared to 47.7 months in M-VAC-treated patients. Five-year survival was 42.1% for cystectomy alone versus 57.2% for M-VAC-treated patients. In view of limited sample size, these results reached only borderline statistical significance, $p = 0.06$.

These results show a trend in favor of neoadjuvant chemotherapy. In a recent meta-analysis including data from 2688 patients from 10 available randomized trials, the use of combination chemotherapy showed a 5% absolute benefit at five years (24). It is important to emphasize that the survival benefit by optimal surgery, that is, radical cystectomy plus extensive pelvic lymphadenectomy is greater than the modest benefit provided by neoadjuvant chemotherapy. The approach of neoadjuvant chemotherapy is therefore only a justifiable approach if followed by radical surgery including state-of-the-art lymphadenectomy.

Neoadjuvant Chemotherapy and Bladder Preservation

As orthotopic bladder substitution has become available, many urologists prefer early definitive therapy with this ideal form of continent urinary diversion. Bladder preservation is a second option, also used in the treatment of other solid tumors.

Following neoadjuvant chemotherapy, or radiochemotherapy, bladder preservation may be possible in highly selected cases. Pathologically complete responses in the cystectomy specimen (pT0) were obtained in 38% of M-VAC-treated patients in the SWOG trial. Likewise, the pT0 rate in patients in the EORTC/MRC trial who underwent surgery was 33% for patients who had CMV chemotherapy, as compared to 12% for those who had TURB and cystectomy alone without chemotherapy. Bladder sparing in selected patients on the basis of response to neoadjuvant chemotherapy is a feasible approach that must be confirmed in prospective randomized trials (25).

Adjuvant Chemotherapy

The principal advantage of adjuvant chemotherapy over the neoadjuvant approach is that the cystectomy specimen is immediately available for pathologic evaluation. Prognostic factors for relapse and/or metastases can be determined. Patients can then be selected to receive chemotherapy who may benefit most. As the cystectomy is performed immediately, there is no delay in definitive treatment.

The disadvantage to adjuvant chemotherapy is the delay in giving systemic therapy for occult metastases whereas treatment for the primary tumor is emphasized. In addition, it is difficult to administer the chemotherapy shortly after a cystectomy.

There have been few randomized trials evaluating adjuvant chemotherapy. The trials have been difficult to interpret because of problems such as small sample size and early closure. Some trials have suggested that there may be a benefit for adjuvant chemotherapy, whereas others have shown differing results (26). The EORTC attempted to enlist 660 patients in a study of adjuvant chemotherapy. This study evaluating four cycles of immediate chemotherapy (Gemcitabine/Cisplatin, MVAC, or HD-MVAC) versus therapy at the time of relapse in high-risk patients with pT3–pT4 or node positive disease was unfortunately closed to accrual after only 298 patients were entered.

Metastatic Disease

Following the recognition in the 1980s of the chemosensitivity of urothelial cell cancer, with Phase II studies demonstrating the activity of cisplatin, methotrexate, adriamycin, vinblastine in advanced and/or metastatic disease, the next step to the development of effective therapy was to combine the most effective agents known at that time into two-, three-, and four-drug combinations.

In 1985, investigators from Memorial Sloan Kettering Cancer Center (MSKCC) reported on a four-drug regimen that was built by combining the two active two-drug regimen studies at MSKCC, cisplatin plus doxorubicin and methotrexate plus vinblastine (M-VAC). The initial study on 24 patients gave an overall response rate of 71%.

With increasing experience, the overall worldwide response rate became slightly lower, ranging from 40% to 57%, but the median survival of 12 to 13 months was maintained. Subsequent randomized Phase III trials demonstrated the superiority of M-VAC compared to single agent cisplatin, and to CISCA (cisplatin/cyclophosphamide/adriamycin), in terms of both response rates and overall survival (27).

Unfortunately M-VAC therapy is associated with significant morbidity. The median age of patients presenting with metastatic urothelial cell cancer is 70 years, and because of smoking as an associated risk factor, many patients have pulmonary and/or cardiovascular diseases. In addition, many patients have impaired renal function that hampers the safe administration of cisplatin-based chemotherapy. Previous studies have also shown that impaired performance status, weight loss, high alkaline phosphate, and visceral metastases are adversely related with response to chemotherapy. In a report on 199 patients treated with M-VAC at MSKCC, investigators were able to identify performance status and the presence of visceral metastases as

the two most important independent prognostic factors that had an impact on median survival. Median survival times for patients who had zero, one, or two risk factors were 33, 13.4, and 9.3 months, respectively ($p = 0.0001$).

Even in patients who are still in good clinical condition, M-VAC causes clinically significant myelosuppression, with up to a 25% incidence of granulocytopenic fever at any time during the course of M-VAC therapy, and a 3% drug-related mortality.

The EORTC conducted a randomized Phase III trial comparing classical M-VAC to a schedule-intensified regimen every two weeks, using G-CSF support during all cycles (28). There were differences in complete response rate, PFS, and survival at two years in favor of the escalated M-VAC schedule. However, this did not translate into an improved median survival, which was 14.5 months on escalated M-VAC versus 14.1 months on classic M-VAC. Consequently, escalated M-VAC therapy remains an investigational approach.

In view of the toxicity associated with M-VAC, particularly in patients with impaired renal function, carboplatin has been substituted for cisplatin in various combinations. Single-agent activity of carboplatin derived from pooled data from seven Phase II studies is 12% (range 6–21%), appears inferior to that obtained with cisplatin. The combination of carboplatin with methotrexate and vinblastine (Carbo-MV) has shown response rates of 30% to 40% and a median survival of 8 to 10 months, and again these results appear inferior to those obtained with M-VAC (27).

New Active Agents and Combinations

In the past decade, with new agents becoming available, substantial single agent activity has been demonstrated for the antifolate piritrexim, the multitargeted antifolate (MTA), the taxanes paclitaxel and docetaxel, and gemcitabine (27,29). Responses in Phase II trials with piritrexim and Phase II trials with either paclitaxel or docetaxel in patients not previously treated with chemotherapy ranged from 25% to 40%. In patients who have previously been treated with cisplatin-based chemotherapy though, these agents appear considerably less effective. Initial Phase II studies of two-drug combinations of docetaxel, or paclitaxel, with cisplatin, have shown activity in untreated patients, with response rates that are in the same range as those obtained with M-VAC, but to date there are no comparative data. Several studies have tested the combination of paclitaxel with carboplatin, but again, in view of reported median survival figures as low as 8.5 to 9.5 months, there is concern as to whether carboplatin should be substituted for cisplatin in those patients who are potentially fit to tolerate a cisplatin-based regimen.

Gemcitabine is an antimetabolite. Interestingly, the overall 27% response rate appears not to be influenced by previous cisplatin-based chemotherapy, suggesting that there is no complete cross-resistance between these agents. Three Phase II studies of the GC (gemcitabine and cisplatin) combination have demonstrated the feasibility of the two-drug combination and have produced response rates similar to that obtained with M-VAC (27,29).

A large multinational Phase III trial comparing GC with M-VAC was conducted (30). The study was designed to detect a four-month improvement in the median survival with GC. A total of 405 patients were entered. With a median follow-up of 19 months, overall survival was found to be similar on both arms, GC 13.8 months, M-VAC 14.8 months (HR 1.04; 95% CI 0.82–1.32, $p = 0.75$), as were time to progressive disease (7.4 months on both arms) and overall response (GC, 49%; MVAC, 46%). Fewer patients on GC, compared with M-VAC patients, had neutropenic fever (2% vs. 14%), neutropenic sepsis (1% vs. 12%), and grade 3/4 mucositis (1% vs. 22%).

Although the study failed to detect a significant difference in survival, which was the primary end point, the favorable risk–benefit ratio has led many investigators to consider GC as first-line therapy for advanced urothelial cancer. This can be justified by the easier administration of GC, its lower toxicity, fewer hospitalizations related to sepsis and mucositis, and use of fewer medical resources. GC can be considered a valuable alternative for the vast majority of patients with metastatic bladder cancer in whom GC may achieve a similar clinical response to M-VAC, but with the benefit of fewer adverse effects (27).

Investigators in Spain have conducted Phase I/II trials of the triplet combination of paclitaxel, cisplatin, gemcitabine in a total of 61 patients. The studies gave an overall response rate of 78% and a median survival time for the Phase I and the Phase II part of the study of 24 and 16 months, respectively. An international trial, led by the EORTC, recently investigated this triplet combination in a Phase III randomized trial versus the cisplatin, gemcitabine study. The study accrued 627 patients from 2001 to 2004. The initial trial results showed a higher overall response rate and slightly better survival in the triplet arm (15.7 vs. 12.8 months), but in view of the trial design to test for a four-month survival benefit, this did not reach statistical significance (HR 0.86; 95% CI 0.72–1.03; $p = 0.12$) (31).

Improved understanding of the molecular biology of urothelial malignancies may enable us to define the role of new prognostic indices, which can direct appropriate therapeutic options. There is a strong scientific and clinical rationale to combine new molecular targeted agents with chemotherapy combinations in the treatment of locally advanced or metastatic TCC of the bladder. Several strategies including EGFR and VEGFR inhibition are now being initiated, combining chemotherapy with these new compounds.

CANCER OF THE KIDNEY

Renal cell carcinoma (RCC) accounts for 3% of adult malignancies, with a male to female ratio of 2:1. It is most commonly seen between the ages of 50 and 70 years. During the early 1990s, studies demonstrated that the Von Hippel–Lindau (VHL) tumor suppressor gene was inactivated in a majority of patients with sporadic clear cell renal carcinomas through mutation or methylation (32). Functional VHL encodes a protein that targets hypoxia inducible factor (HIF) for degradation. Inactivation of VHL leads to upregulation of HIF-1H, and as a result, it leads to transcription of multiple genes involved in tumorigenesis including vascular endothelial growth factor (VEGF), platelet-derived growth factor (PDGF), and fibroblast growth factor (FGF). Subsequent studies demonstrated that the protein mTOR (mammalian target of rapamycin) also plays an important

role in promoting the translation of HIF-1H mRNA (33). Based on this work, several novel targets emerged for anticancer therapy in renal carcinoma.

Patients with localized tumors can usually be cured by surgery. However, one-third of patients present with metastatic disease and another 30% to 40% will eventually develop distant metastases. These patients have a median survival that was 12 months, with 5% to 10% five-year survival. This may be changing because of earlier diagnosis and novel therapies that have reached the clinic.

Clinical Presentation

There appears to have been an increase in the proportion of patients diagnosed with RCC at an earlier stage; this has led to an improvement in five-year survival. Both trends are likely because of improvements in diagnostic capabilities. The classic triad of hematuria, abdominal mass, and costovertebral pain nowadays occurs in a small percentage of patients. At least one of these symptoms, most commonly hematuria, may be present in up to 50% of patients. Other symptoms include weakness, weight loss (28%), anemia (21%), and fever (7%). Paraneoplastic syndromes may occur in up to 25% of patients. These include Cushing's syndrome, polycythemia (3%), hypercalcemia (3%), and hepatic dysfunction (7%).

Pathology

The most prevalent form of sporadic RCC is clear cell carcinoma that occurs in 75% of patients with renal carcinoma. It is 15% who develop papillary ca, of whom 5% is Type 1 and 10% is Type 2. cMET pertains to type 1 (thus 5%) FH and cMYC to type 2 (thus 10%). Other types of RCC include chromophobe (5%) and oncocytoma (5%) (34). Whereas most RCCs are of proximal tubular epithelial origin, less common subtypes, including collecting duct carcinomas, chromophobe cell carcinoma, and papillary cystadenocarcinoma, probably arise from distal parts of the nephron. Distinctions as to histologic subtype of RCC are fundamental (35).

Better survival is reported for tumors confined to the kidney, with five-year survival rates from 80% to >90% following radical nephrectomy for T1-2 tumors (36). The grade of the primary tumor and size are important prognostic variables that may impact upon survival. The presence of lymph node metastases has a significant adverse effect on survival, with reports of 10% to 25% five-year survival.

The incidence of positive nodes depends on tumor stage. Positive nodes are found in 5% to 10% of tumors confined to the renal capsule, in 30% of tumors extending through the renal capsule, and in 50% with distant metastases.

Surgery

There has been an overall increase in the frequency in which surgery is utilized as the primary treatment for RCC. Partial nephrectomy rather than total nephrectomy can be considered in patients with Stage I RCC, a solitary kidney, or in bilateral kidney cancer (36). Radical nephrectomy is indicated for tumors that are locally advanced or large tumors that have not invaded adjacent organs. A large randomized study has shown that lymphadenectomy did not increase survival in patients with negative nodes on CT scan.

Tumors with penetration of the perirenal fat, positive margins, or regional nodal metastases are at higher risk for local and distant recurrence. Neither adjuvant RT nor adjuvant systemic therapy has an established role (37).

Metastatic Disease

Prognostic Factors

Several independent prognostic factors are associated with survival in patients with metastatic disease, metastatic RCC (mRCC). At MSKCC, a prognostic model was made based on five variables that predicted a short survival: low KPS, high LDH, low Hb, high corrected serum calcium, and time from initial RCC diagnosis to treatment of <1 year. Patients were assigned to three risk groups: those with 0 risk factors (favorable risk), those with 1–2 (intermediate risk), and those with ≥3 (poor risk). Median survival in the favorable risk group was 30 months, intermediate risk group was 14 months, and poor risk group was 5 months (38).

Investigators at the Cleveland Clinic have added the number of metastatic sites to this model and French investigators favor a more simplified model that includes only PS and the number of metastatic sites.

Surgery

Surgery is appropriate in select patients with solitary or a small number of metastatic lesions. This usually indicates patients with pulmonary lesions and a good performance status. Five-year survivals ranging from 25% to 35% have been reported. Spontaneous regressions following nephrectomy have been reported in 1% to 4% of patients, primarily those with minimal pulmonary metastases. Most have not been histologically documented. Nephrectomy on this basis is not justified. Two large randomized trials have shown that radical nephrectomy before interferon (IFN)-based immunotherapy delays time to progression and improves survival of patients with mRCC who present with good performance status, compared to IFN-based therapy alone (39,40).

Chemotherapy

The results of chemotherapy in the treatment of RCC are consistently disappointing. In a review of 83 trials of 63 single agents and 20 combinations in 4093 patients with advanced disease, only 6% responded (35). It is likely that multiple mechanisms of drug resistance are involved in the intrinsic resistance of RCC to chemotherapeutic agents. The only single agents with some efficacy are the fluorinated pyrimidines fluorouracil (5-FU), capecitabine, floxuridine (FUDR), and gemcitabine (41).

Interferon (IFN)

Since successful treatment of RCC by IFN was described in 1983, IFN has become the most widely accepted treatment for metastatic RCC. IFNs are natural glycoproteins with antiviral, antiproliferative, and immunomodulatory properties. IFN-α appears to be the most active in the treatment of RCC, with IFN-β and IFN-γ being less useful. IFN-α has

a response rate (RR) of approximately 15%. An intermediate dose is probably best, consisting of approximately 9 million IU subcutaneously three times weekly. Principal side effects include flu-like symptoms such as fever, myalgia, and asthenia. Occasionally, confusion, depression, liver dysfunction, and myelosuppression may occur. Toxicity leads to dose reduction or discontinuation in 20% to 40% of patients. Patient selection is important, with up to a 30% RR in selected patients with a good PS and pulmonary metastases. IFN has less activity in bone, liver, and brain metastases.

Immunotherapy for RCC was submitted to a systematic Cochrane database literature review comparing both IFN-α and high dose interleukin-2 (HD-IL-2) to other options. Forty-two studies involving 4216 patients were eligible in terms of response and 26 studies reported survival outcome (3089 patients). This analysis concluded that IFN-α provided a modest survival benefit compared to other commonly used treatments and could be considered for the control arm of trials with other systemic agents. IL-2 was not validated in controlled randomized studies.

Interleukin-2 (IL-2)

IL-2 is a cytokine secreted by activated T lymphocytes, which in addition to producing IL-2 also increase the expression of high affinity IL-2 receptors. The mechanism of action of IL-2 is the induction and activation of T lymphocytes and natural killer cells, and the secondary release of cytokines such as IFN-gamma, tumor necrosis factor, granulocyte-macrophage colony stimulating factor, IL-1, and IL-6, which in turn stimulate the activity of other cells in the immune system, such as the monocyte-macrophage lineage (42).

High dose IL-2 at a dose of 600,000 or 720,000 IU/kg as an i.v. bolus in 15 minutes every 8 hours was the only approved therapy for metastatic RCC in the United States. This approval was based on results in 255 patients in 7 clinical trials, with 12 complete (5%) and 24 partial (9%) responses. The overall median duration of response was 20 months when approved, and in an update was 84+ months and not yet reached (NYR) at >5 years follow-up (35). Toxicity included a vascular leak syndrome characterized by a generalized increase in capillary permeability, fluid accumulation, and hypotension. As a result of this toxicity, high-dose IL-2 is infrequently used and should be used in patients who express CA-IX (43). A review of phase I and II trials in over 1400 patients treated with combinations of IFN or IL-2 have revealed response rates of 20% to 21%, with CR in 3% to 5%.

Novel Single Agents in Advanced Renal Carcinoma

Multiple novel agents have been approved for use in RCC or are under review by regulatory agencies based on the results of well-conducted Phase III trials completed over the past five years.

Bevacizumab. Bevacizumab is a monoclonal antibody that binds and neutralizes VEGF-A. In a "proof of concept" trial by Yang, 166 patients with mRCC (refractory to IL-2) were randomized to bevacizumab at two different dose levels (10 mg/kg every two weeks or 3 mg/kg every two weeks) versus placebo (44). The objective response rate and the time to disease progression were the primary end points. The trial was stopped early after an interim analysis demonstrated a doubling in the time to disease progression in the 10 mg/kg bevacizumab treated group compared with placebo. There was no significant difference in survival among the three groups in this small hypothesis generating Phase II trial.

Two randomized Phase III trials (CALGB-90206 and the European AVOREN study) subsequently compared IFN-α plus bevacizumab to IFN-α alone as first-line treatment in mRCC. The AVOREN trial randomized 649 patients to IFN-α (9 million IU subcutaneously three times weekly) plus bevacizumab (10 mg/kg every two weeks) or IFN-α plus placebo (45). Although the primary end point of the trial was overall survival, the study was unblinded after a preplanned final analysis of PFS demonstrated a significant improvement. Patents were encouraged to cross over to the bevacizumab arm. At the time of unblinding, the duration of PFS was significantly longer in the combination arm than in the IFN arm (10.2 vs. 5.4 months; HR 0.63; 95% CI 0.52–0.75; $p = 0.0001$). The most common side effects in the bevacizumab group were fatigue and asthenia. Based on these data, bevacizumab plus IFN-α has already been approved in Europe.

CALGB 90206 utilized a similar (although not placebo-controlled) design and identical dosing regimen as the AVOREN trial (46). In a preliminary report after 732 patients were enrolled, the median time to progression was 8.5 months for patients receiving bevacizumab plus IFN-α compared to 5.2 months with IFN-α monotherapy (HR 0.71; 95% CI 0.61–0.83; $p < 0.0001$). Toxicity was greater in the bevacizumab plus IFN-α arm, including Grade 3 hypertension (9% vs. 0%), anorexia (17% vs. 8%), fatigue (35% vs. 28%), and proteinuria (13% vs. 0%).

Sunitinib. Sunitinib is an orally bioavailable potent inhibitor of multiple receptor tyrosine kinases (tyrosine kinase inhibitor, TKI) including VEGFR types 1–3 and PDGF. Two Phase II trials explored the activity of sunitinib in mRCC patients who had progressed on prior cytokines (47,48). In both trials, sunitinib was given at a dose of 50 mg orally daily for four weeks followed by two weeks rest. In a pooled analysis of both trials including 186 patients, the RR was 34% (95% CI 25–44%) with a median PFS of 8.3 months. Adverse events associated with sunitinib included fatigue, diarrhea, neutropenia, elevation of lipase, anemia, hand-foot syndrome, and thyroid function abnormalities. Given the activity in cytokine refractory patients, sunitinib is approved for the treatment of mRCC.

A randomized Phase III trial subsequently compared sunitinib with IFN-α in untreated patients with advanced clear cell RCC (49). Sunitinib revealed a significant improvement in PFS compared with IFN-α (11 vs. 5 months; HR 0.415; $p < 0.000001$). Patients treated with sunitinib also reported better QOL. All risk groups appeared to benefit. Based on these results, sunitinib has become a standard first-line treatment for patients with mRCC. Updated results presented at ASCO 2008 demonstrated an improvement in survival with sunitinib compared with IFN-α, despite cross-over with a HR of 0.82 (95% CI 0.67–1.001; $p = 0.051$) (50).

Sorafenib. Sorafenib is another potent orally bioavailable multitargeted TKI with activity against Raf, VEGFR2,

PDGFR, Flt3, and c-KIT. A novel trial design was initially used to explore the activity of sorafenib in mRCC (51). In this randomized discontinuation trial, patients were treated with sorafenib 400 mg orally twice daily for an initial treatment period. After restaging, patients achieving an objective response continued treatment, those who progressed were taken off study, and those with stable disease were randomized to sorafenib versus placebo. The last group, enriched for patients with a uniform natural history, provided a statistically sound assessment of the potential cytostatic nature of sorafenib. Of the 202 patients enrolled, 73 patients achieved an objective response whereas 65 patients had stable disease at 12 weeks and were randomized to continue sorafenib versus placebo. At 24 weeks, 50% of the sorafenib-treated patients were progression free versus 18% of the placebo-treated patients ($p = 0.0077$). Adverse events associated with sorafenib included fatigue, hand-foot syndrome, diarrhea, and hypertension.

Based on the promising results of this trial, a randomized Phase III trial compared sorafenib to placebo as second-line therapy (after cytokines or chemotherapy) in patients with good and intermediate risk clear cell advanced RCC (52). The TARGET trial enrolled 905 patients. After a planned interim analysis, the median PFS was 5.5 months in the sorafenib group and 2.8 months in the placebo arm (HR = 0.44; 95% CI 0.35–0.55; $p < 0.01$). Sorafenib is approved for the treatment of advanced RCC.

A randomized Phase II trial of sorafenib versus IFN-α as first-line therapy has been completed (53). The primary end point was PFS and the study did include an option of dose escalation to sorafenib 600 mg twice daily at the time of progression or cross-over from IFN-α to sorafenib at progression. The median PFS was 5.7 months (95% CI 5.0–7.4 months) versus 5.6 months (95% CI 3.7–7.4 months) for sorafenib versus IFN-α. This trial unfortunately enrolled patients with very poor prognostic features and may not have been a fair test of sorafenib as first-line therapy. There has been a suggestion of a potential benefit from sorafenib dose escalation in other trials.

Temsirolimus. Temsirolimus is an inhibitor of mTOR. In a randomized Phase II trial, three dose levels of weekly temsirolimus (25, 75, and 250 mg given i.v.) were evaluated in patients with cytokine-refractory RCC (54). Temsirolimus resulted in an objective RR of 7% (1 CR), a minor response rate of 26% and median survival of 15 months. The most frequent adverse events were skin toxicity (maculopapular rash), mucositis, asthenia, nausea, hyperglycemia, hyperphosphatemia, and hypertriglyceridemia. Neither toxicity nor efficacy was associated with the dose level of temsirolimus. A retrospective analysis compared actual outcomes based on MSKCC risk grouping and suggested that patients with poor risk disease benefited the most from temsirolimus.

After this subgroup analysis, a Phase III study compared temsirolimus versus IFN-α versus the combination in 626 patients with modified MSKCC poor-risk prognostic features (55). Treatment with single-agent temsirolimus was associated with a survival benefit compared to IFN-α alone (10.9 vs. 7.3 months; HR 0.73; $p < 0.007$), whereas the combination regimen was not superior to IFN-α (8.4 months; HR 0.95; $p = 0.69$). Patients with nonclear cell cancer also appeared to benefit. Temsirolimus is approved for the treatment of advanced RCC. An ongoing Phase III trial is comparing temsirolimus with sorafenib in patients with disease progression after first-line treatment with sunitinib. Another trial is planned comparing bevacizumab combined with either IFN-α or temsirolimus.

Everolimus. With the widespread use of the multitargeted TKIs as first-line therapy for mRCC, the optimal management of patients progressing on these agents has remained unclear. To prospectively evaluate the efficacy of an mTOR inhibitor in patients with clear cell RCC progressing on sunitinib, sorafenib, and/or bevacizumab, a Phase III trial of the oral mTOR inhibitor everolimus (RAD-001) versus placebo was completed. In February 2008, the study was stopped after interim analysis demonstrated a significantly better PFS in patients who received everolimus. These data were presented at ASCO in 2008; 410 patients were enrolled and treatment was associated with a significant improvement in PFS compared with placebo, the primary end point of the trial (4.0 vs. 1.9 months; HR 0.30; 95% CI 0.22–0.40; $p < 0.001$) (56). Additionally, all risk groups appeared to benefit.

Other New Agents

There are a multitude of other new agents with novel mechanisms of action for patients with RCC including perifosine, axitinib, and pazopanib.

Axitinib. Axitinib is a slightly more selective multitargeted TKI than sorafenib or sunitinib with predominant activity against VEGFR-1, VEGFR-2, and VEGFR-3. A Phase II study explored the activity of axitinib in patients with cytokine refractory RCC (57). There were two complete and 21 partial responses for an overall response rate (RRe) of 44.2% (95% CI 30.5–58.7). The median time to progression was 15.7 months, and the median overall survival was 29.9 months. The most common treatment-related adverse events included diarrhea, hypertension, fatigue, nausea, and hoarseness. Axitinib is currently being compared with sorafenib in a randomized Phase III trial in patients with mRCC who have progressed on prior treatment with sunitinib.

Pazopanib. Pazopanib is an orally administered multitargeted inhibitor of the VEGF receptors, PDGFR-α, PDGFR-β, and c-kit. To explore the activity of pazopanib in patients with mRCC, a multinational randomized discontinuation Phase II trial was performed (58). Patients received pazopanib 800 mg orally daily for 12 weeks. Responding patients continued treatment, progressing patients were discontinued from treatment, and those patients with stable disease were randomized 1:1 to continue pazopanib versus placebo. Two hundred and twenty-five patients were enrolled. Due to significant activity with this agent, with an objective RR of 40% and stable disease rate of 42% at week 12, an independent monitoring committee recommended discontinuing the randomized portion of the trial. The most common treatment-related adverse events included transaminase elevation, diarrhea, fatigue, and nausea.

A multicenter international Phase III study evaluating pazopanib in patients with locally advanced or metastatic RCC who are untreated or have failed prior cytokine treatment has completed accrual, and results from this trial are awaited. Another Phase III head-to-head trial is planned comparing pazopanib to sunitinib in previously untreated patients with mRCC.

Novel Combinations in Advanced Renal Carcinoma

The optimal strategies for combining targeted therapies are the subject of ongoing research and current approaches have focused on both inhibiting different receptor tyrosine kinases with diverse functions such as the combination of sunitinib and erlotinib inhibiting at different points upstream and downstream in the same pathway such as the combination of bevacizumab and sunitinib. Virtually every combination of available agents has been evaluated or is planned for study. In an effort to determine the benefit of combination therapy, ECOG 2804 trial (also known as BEST for Bevacizumab, Sorafenib, Temsirolimus) is randomizing 240 untreated patients with advanced RCC either bevacizumab monotherapy or combination therapy with bevacizumab plus sorafenib versus bevacizumab plus temsirolimus versus temsirolimus plus sorafenib. The primary end point of this trial is PFS.

Based on a better understanding of the pathogenesis of advanced RCC, the past decade has brought a host of advances rapidly translated from the bench to the bedside. Several new classes of agents have been approved for the treatment of mRCC with additional molecules demonstrating exciting activity in current Phase II trials. Over the next several years, the optimal sequence and/or combination of these agents will be a major focus of clinical research. Early efforts at combination therapy have shown some promise, but the ability to combine "noncytotoxic" therapies, with often varying and cumulative toxicities, has proven challenging. Additional safety and efficacy data of combination therapy is needed before these regimens become a part of the rapidly expanding armamentarium for renal carcinoma.

Studies evaluating targeted agents in high-risk patients in the adjuvant postoperative setting are underway and include the MRC led and EORTC SORCE trial of adjuvant sorafenib one versus three years versus placebo, the U.S. led ASSURE trial of sunitinib versus sorafenib versus placebo for one year, and the pharmaceutical industry sponsored STAR trial of adjuvant of sunitinib versus placebo.

There is a strong rationale for targeting angiogenesis and multiple pathways in patients with advanced RCC. Novel targeted agents have demonstrated an increase in PFS in first and second line and an increase in survival in poor risk therapy naive patients and in first-line patients treated with sunitinib.

They are better tolerated than cytokines, but there is toxicity associated with these agents. The effect of the novel targets in the neoadjuvant setting on the primary tumor and whether or not nephrectomy is still required in metastatic patients is under evaluation.

CANCER OF THE TESTIS

Although testis cancer accounts for only 1% of tumors in males, with an incidence of 3 per 100,000 men per year, it is the most common malignancy in men from age 15 to

35 years. Remarkable progress has been achieved in the past 20 years, rendering testicular cancer one of the most curable solid tumors. Better understanding of prognostic risk factors, radiologic techniques, the availability of serum markers, effective multidrug chemotherapy regimens, and ramifications in surgical approaches have led to considerable improvements. In the early 1970s, less than 10% of patients with distant metastases survived; today cure is obtained in 70% to 90% of patients with metastatic disease.

Epidemiology and Etiology

There has been a steady increase in the incidence of testicular cancer (59). The highest incidence of testis cancer is in white males from the United States, Scandinavia, and Western Europe. A white male has a 1 in 500 chance of developing testicular cancer. The peak incidence of nonseminomatous germ cell tumor (NSGCT) is between the ages of 20 and 40. Pure seminomas and combined tumors (seminoma plus NSGCT) typically occur a decade later.

About 10% of patients with testicular cancer have a prior history of cryptorchism. The relative risk of developing testis cancer in patients with maldescent is 8.8. Orchidopexy prior to age 10 seems to reduce the risk. Of note, 5% to 10% of patients with a history of cryptorchism develop testis cancer in the contralateral normal testis. This may represent carcinoma in situ (CIS) or hormonal dysfunction. Dysgenetic gonads or almost any condition associated with abnormal gonadal development, including those related to sex chromosomal abnormalities, have been associated with an increased incidence of testicular tumors.

Patients with testis cancer are at increased risk of developing a metachronous testicular cancer on the contralateral side, with a risk 25 times higher than that of the normal age-matched population.

The unusual cytogenetic abnormality of an isochrome of the short arm of chromosome 12, (12p) is found in the majority of testis cancers and in CIS cells. This occurs more frequently in nonseminoma (81%) than in seminoma (30%) (59).

Clinical Presentation

Most patients with testis cancer present with a testicular primary, the remainder present with metastatic disease, such as a neck mass, respiratory symptoms, abdominal, or back pain. The characteristic finding on exam is a tumor that is solid and usually not nodular. About 10% to 15% may present with pain, which may lead to a mistaken diagnosis of epididymo-orchitis. Gynecomastia is sometimes seen, related to increased serum levels of human chorionic gonadotrophin (HCG). A sonogram of the testis is a rapid method for distinguishing hydrocele or epididymitis from testis cancer.

Histologic diagnosis is confirmed by inguinal orchiectomy. The testis is removed intact. The dense membrane of the tunica albuginea tends to limit local spread of tumor. Local recurrence is exceptionally rare. NSGCT is often associated with the presence in the serum of tumor marker products, i.e, alphafetoprotein (AFP) and the beta subunit of HCG in the serum as tumor marker products. The half-life of HCG, following surgery for removal of the primary tumor or metastases, or following the initiation of chemotherapy is 24 to 36 hours. The half-life of AFP is five to seven days. During the first two weeks after the start of chemotherapy, however, the pattern in the decline of AFP and HCG is unpredictable and may even transiently increase. The mechanism of this so-called surge phenomenon is not known. Initially it was assumed that such transient increase was due to the huge release of these glycoproteins from necrotic cells, but there is one report that, at least for AFP, a surge is an adverse prognostic sign. Also, the prognostic importance of speed of decline of HCG and AFP has been investigated by a number of groups. Although prolonged half-lives of both HCG and AFP were reported as adverse prognostic features, this could not be confirmed by others and to date has remained a controversial issue (60).

Pathology

More than 95% of testicular cancer is of germ cell origin and approximately 50% are NSGCT and 50% are seminoma. Germinal elements are responsible for 93% of testis cancers, with 38% representing pure histological types and 62% mixed types. Sex-cord stromal tumors arising from Sertoli or Leydig cells account for 4% to 6% of testis cancers; metastases from these occur only rarely.

Recent interest in CIS as the premalignant phase of NSGCT has been stimulated by investigators in Denmark who performed testicular biopsies on the contralateral testis of 500 patients with testis cancer. Of 27 who were found to have CIS, progression to invasive cancer was 50% within five years. There is controversy, however, if biopsy of the contralateral testis is necessary in all patients and most investigators do not proceed with such biopsy routinely (61).

Staging

In a patient with suspected diagnosis of testis cancer, serum AFP and HCG levels are obtained and radiological examinations include CT scan of the chest, abdomen, and pelvis. Patients with central nervous system symptoms or those with multiple pulmonary metastases or very high levels of HCG (>20,000 IU, which is typically seen in patients with predominantly choriocarcinoma elements) are investigated by either a CT or NMR scan of the brain.

The American Joint Committee on Cancer (AJCC) and the UICC have provided a new universal staging system for all stages of disease. Stage I can now be divided into tumors with or without lymphatic/vascular invasion and those with persistently elevated AFP or B-HCG in the absence of clinical or radiologic evidence of disease. Stage II includes retroperitoneal disease without distant metastases, with or without increased markers. Stage III disease includes only distant metastases or elevated marker levels.

Many investigators in Europe use the Royal Marsden Hospital Classification as it easily categorizes extent and sites of disease; stages II and III reflect retroperitoneal and mediastinal nodal disease, A-D reflects size of the metastases, and Stage IV indicates visceral metastases.

In addition, multiple classifications have attempted to categorize patients into risk groups, regarding treatment outcome following cisplatin-based combination chemotherapy. Most of these classifications incorporated both the bulk and site of the metastatic tumor load, as well as concentrations of AFP, HCG, and LDH in the serum, but minor and major differences between categories were rendering it impossible to compare trial results.

An international consensus classification was defined after an international group of investigators analyzed prognostic factors in 5202 patients with NSGCT and 660 with advanced seminoma treated with cisplatin-based chemotherapy (62). This classification divides patients into three clinical groups. Definitions of good, intermediate, and poor prognosis are found in Table 10.3. For reasons of simplicity of the model, both NSGCT and seminoma are included.

There is separation of mediastinal from nonmediastinal primary (i.e., testis, retroperitoneal, or unknown) primary sites. Nonpulmonary visceral disease such as liver, bone, brain, and skin are included as adverse features. There is heavy reliance on tumor marker estimations (AFP, HCG, and LDH), which are the only factors to distinguish good and intermediate risk patients. The proportion of patients falling into each category is as follows: good 60% of all patients, intermediate 26%, and poor 14% of patients. Survival at five years for good risk patients is 90%, 78% for intermediate risk, and 48% for poor risk patients. This classification represents an important advance in the interpretation of trial results and provides a means for international collaboration. Ninety percent of patients with metastatic seminoma is in the good prognosis group, although there is controversy if seminoma patients with very high levels of LDH may be considered good risk (63).

Treatment for Clinical Stage I NSGCT

The definitive procedure for pathologic diagnosis and local treatment is removal of the testis by an inguinal approach. Clinical Stage I is defined as tumor confined to the testis with no clinical or radiological evidence of metastatic spread and with normal (or normalized) serum markers.

Modern radiological techniques and serum markers, coupled with the experience that metastatic disease from earlier occult spread can be effectively treated has led to various ways of managing clinical Stage I disease. Current options include retroperitoneal lymph node dissection (RPLND), surveillance, and chemotherapy (64). In the United States, the standard approach to patients with clinical Stage I has been RPLND. Those in favor of RPLND note that up to 30% of patients who are clinical Stage I are found to be pathologic Stage II at RPLND, and the operation itself can be curative. RPLND is the most reliable method for staging purposes. The most important disadvantage of RPLND has been induction of retrograde ejaculation caused by autonomic nerve dissection in the region of the aortic bifurcation. Modifying the technique has reduced the morbidity and incidence of ejaculatory dysfunction. After right-sided RPLND, retrograde ejaculation occurs rarely. Following left-sided RPLND, problems may arise in up to one-third of patients. These techniques are time consuming and require considerable experience.

With survival rates of more than 95%, emphasis has been on reducing the toxicity of therapy, while maintaining high curability. Surveillance alone following orchiectomy has become increasingly popular. The strategy is based upon thorough clinical assessment after orchiectomy and early detection of metastases, with regular tumor marker estimations, chest x-rays, and CT scans of the chest/abdomen and pelvis during the first two years (64).

Table 10.3 Testis Cancer Classification by the International Germ Cell Cancer Collaborative Group

Good prognosis

Nonseminoma	*Good markers
Testis/retroperitoneal primary AND	AFP <1000 ng/ml AND
Good markers* AND	HCG <1000 ng/ml (<5000 IU/l)
No nonpulmonary visceral mets	AND LDH <1.5 × N
	(N = upper limit of normal)
Seminoma	
Any primary site AND	
Any markers AND	
No nonpulmonary visceral mets	

Intermediate prognosis

Nonseminoma	*Intermediate markers
Testis/retroperitoneal primary AND	AFP 1000–10,000 ng/ml OR
Intermediate markers* AND	HCG 1000–10,000 ng/ml
No nonpulmonary visceral mets	(5000–50,000 IU/l) OR
	LDH 1.5–10 × N
Seminoma	
Any primary site AND	
Any markers AND	
Nonpulmonary visceral mets[a]	

Poor prognosis

Nonseminoma	*Poor markers
Mediastinal primary site or testis/	AFP >10,000 ng/ml OR
retroperitoneal with either:	HCG >10,000 ng/ml
Nonpulmonary visceral mets[a]	(>50,000 IU/l) OR
OR Poor markers*	LDH >10 × N

*,[a]Nonpulmonary visceral disease refers to liver, bone, brain, and skin.

Results of numerous surveillance studies conducted throughout the world are now available. Of 1771 patients culled from the literature in such programs, the median follow-up is 54 months, with a range from 3 to 144 months. In all, 28% (500 patients) relapsed and 54% of the relapses were in the retroperitoneal lymph nodes. The median time to relapse in most series is six months (0–58 months) after orchiectomy. Patients who relapsed were generally treated by chemotherapy. The overall survival (98%) is comparable to that seen in surgical series. Presence of vascular (either blood vessel or lymphatic vessel) invasion indicates a higher risk of recurrence after orchiectomy alone. Patients with evidence of vascular invasion in the primary tumor have a 40% risk of harboring occult metastatic spread; for those patients who have no vessel invasion, the risk is 15% to 20%. A "wait-and-see" policy, if conducted properly, is clearly an alternative option in patients at low risk for relapse, that is, in those with no vascular invasion. Patient compliance is essential, and this method of careful observation has been widely accepted, particularly in Europe, as an alternative option to RPLND (64).

Although a wait-and-see policy is also a viable option in patients having vascular invasion, and studies have indicated that patients may prefer such policy as long as the relapse risk does not exceed 50%, several centers in Europe proceed with adjuvant chemotherapy in these patients. This mostly consists of two cycles of chemotherapy and may be better accepted than initial RPLND or the alternative option of three cycles of chemotherapy and possible RPLND at the time of relapse. Chemotherapy studies in clinical Stage I have shown that two cycles of BEP appear to be sufficient treatment to prevent recurrence of metastatic disease in more than 95% of the patients (65,66). To date, there have been no randomized trials of adjuvant chemotherapy against RPLND to test for therapeutical equivalence or patient preferences. However, there is increasing concern with the cardiovascular morbidity in testis cancer survivors following cisplatin-based chemotherapy (67–69). The most recent and extensive data indicate a two-fold excess acute myocardial infarction rate because of cardiovascular disease. Also, there is accumulating evidence of an increased incidence of second solid malignancies in testis cancer survivors after chemotherapy (69,70). In light of these concerns, the use of even two cycles of adjuvant chemotherapy in over 50% of patients who do not need any chemotherapy is becoming debatable (64).

Treatment for Clinical Stage II NSGCT

Clinical Stage II is defined as metastatic disease limited to the retroperitoneal lymph nodes. With regard to disease management, in the United States, RPLND remains an option in Stage II A (0–2 cm) and Stage IIB (2–5 cm) nodal disease, with two courses of additional chemotherapy if macroscopic nodal involvement is found, whereas in Europe initial chemotherapy for patients with clinical Stage II disease has become the standard approach (71) in the hope of avoiding surgery altogether. Postchemotherapy surgery is then reserved to those patients who have postchemotherapy and residual radiographic abnormalities. Recent reports though, that up to a third of patients deemed radiological Stage II upon lymph node dissection were found pathological Stage I (72), as well as high rates of postchemotherapy surgery to resect residual mature teratoma, following chemotherapy for Stage II A, B disease, may shift the pendulum back to primary definitive surgery, especially in patients with Stage II A disease and/or those who do not have elevated serum tumor markers (73).

Chemotherapy in Metastatic Disease

Good Prognosis Metastatic Disease

For patients with good prognosis disease, the main goal is to continue to achieve good results with the least amount of toxicity. A number of randomized trials in Europe and in the United States have been conducted with this purpose. Using the gold standard regimen of four cycles of cisplatin, etoposide, bleomycin (BEP) as a framework (74), modifications have included the deletion of bleomycin (to reduce the risk of pulmonary fibrosis and sometimes fatal pneumonitis), the substitution of carboplatin for cisplatin, and to reduce the chemotherapy by one cycle (3 BEP). The standard BEP regimen comprises of cisplatin at $20 \, mg/m^2$, days 1–5 ($100 \, mg/m^2$ per cycle); etoposide is given at $100 \, mg/m^2$, days 1–5 ($500 \, mg/m^2$ per cycle); and bleomycin is given at $30 \, mg/week$. The regimen is scheduled every three weeks.

Two studies have investigated three cycles versus four cycles (74). The largest study that was conducted by the EORTC and MRC was designed to show therapeutical equivalence and enrolled 812 patients (75). PFS (90% on 3 BEP, 89% on 4 cycles) and survival were similar. The study also investigated in a 2×2 factorial design whether the chemotherapy could be delivered over three days (using

the same total dose of the chemotherapy per cycle), instead of the usual five days. Also, this comparison showed therapeutical equivalence. However, in those patients receiving four cycles over three days, more ototoxicity was reported. Hence, the three-day regimen can be considered for patients for whom three cycles is sufficient therapy. For those patients scheduled to receive four cycles, the standard five-day regimen is advised.

Several studies have demonstrated that bleomycin cannot be deleted from regimens that were used in the 1980s, and that may be considered suboptimal therapy today; cisplatin, vinblastine, bleomycin (PVB) and four cycles of $BE_{360}P$, (comprising of a reduced dose of etoposide of $360 \, mg/m^2$ per cycle) (74).

It is likely that bleomycin can be omitted from four cycles of $BE_{500}P$ in good prognosis disease. Long-term follow-up data from 289 patients, treated at MSKCC with four $E_{500}P$ and who could be reclassified good prognosis according to the international consensus criteria have shown PFS in 93% of patients, which is similar to PFS obtained in the above EORTC/MRC study, indicates therapeutical identical results for 4 EP and 3 BEP (76). A study that was recently reported on a direct comparison of 3 BEP versus 4 EP was underpowered to provide a more definitive answer (77). To date, available data suggest that if there are reasons for concern against the use of bleomycin (sportsmen on one hand and existing pulmonary comorbidity/cigarette smoking/age above 40 on the other hand), four cycles of $E_{500}P$ is a valid alternative treatment option (78).

A study conducted by EORTC and MRC that showed a significant inferior treatment outcome in patients receiving carboplatin-based chemotherapy (CEB vs. BEP) conclusively terminated the use of carboplatin in patients with metastatic germ cell cancer.

Postchemotherapy Surgery

Postchemotherapy RPLND should be performed in patients with residual radiographic abnormalities and normal serum markers after chemotherapy for nonseminoma. The presence of elevated markers is usually, but not always, considered a contraindication to adjunctive surgery after chemotherapy, as in selected cases, patients may be rendered disease-free by such surgery. At surgery, necrotic debris or fibrosis is found in 40% to 50% of specimens, mature teratoma in 40%, and viable germ cell tumor in the remaining 10% to 20%. PET scanning in the evaluation of postchemotherapy masses has shown conflicting data and remains investigational.

Viable tumor found at surgery is associated with an adverse prognosis despite complete resection. Mature teratoma should be removed as it may grow and become unresectable. In due course, there is also the risk of possible malignant transformation to immature teratoma or nongerm cell malignancies, including sarcoma or adenocarcinoma, which may not satisfactorily respond to chemotherapy.

Treatment of Patients in Specialized Centers

Differences in chemotherapy dose and schedule adherence by oncologists working in specialized centers, as well as the precise radiological recognition of postchemotherapy residuals and appropriate resection of such residuals, are important factors that are associated with a significant better treatment outcome of patients treated by physicians who have obtained the routines and skills in the management of germ cell cancer patients (79).

Intermediate and Poor Prognosis (IGCCCG)

For patients with intermediate or poor-risk NSGCT, the potential cure rate is lower. Studies have addressed alternating chemotherapy, increasing the dose and schedule intensity of cisplatin, using upfront ifosfamide (VIP) and various combinations of these approaches (74). As yet, there is no evidence from randomized studies of improved results compared to treatment with four cycles of standard BEP. Research efforts must focus upon this group of patients with intermediate and poor prognosis. The approach that is currently investigated in a randomized study in Europe is the incorporation of paclitaxel (Taxol) in the standard BEP regimen (T-BEP). The alternative approach of dose-intensified VIP chemotherapy plus autologous progenitor cell support that was recently being studied in Europe as upfront therapy in patients presenting with poor prognosis disease was stopped in light of a study report from investigators in the United States that did not show a survival benefit by using two cycles of BEP followed by two cycles of high dose chemotherapy, versus conventionally dosed BEP alone (80).

Salvage Chemotherapy

In the salvage setting, approximately 40% to 50% may attain disease-free status, but long-term PFS has been reported as 20% to 25% or less, although the outlook may recently be improving. An incomplete response to first-line treatment is a poor prognostic factor. It is important to note that pre- or postchemotherapy debulking surgery is a key element of successful salvage therapy, particularly for localized disease (81).

For more than a decade, ifosfamide-based chemotherapy was considered standard first-line salvage therapy. Vinblastine, ifosfamide, and cisplatin (VeIP) was able to achieve a CR in 56 patients (45%) with 29 (23%) alive and continuously disease-free at 27 months. New agents such as paclitaxel have been shown to have activity in relapsed NSGCT, and paclitaxel, ifosfamide, and cisplatin (TIP) regimens have recently been assessed as alternative first-line salvage regimens (82). Other new active agents that may be considered for use in the salvage setting are gemcitabine and oxaliplatin.

High-dose chemotherapy with autologous peripheral blood progenitor cell support has been investigated as salvage treatment for patients who failed first- or second-line chemotherapy (83,84). Data from Europe and the United States on 283 patients revealed a prognostic classification based on four independent variables: remission status prior to high-dose therapy, primary mediastinal NSGCT, sensitivity to cisplatin, and HCG >1000 U/l. Patients who are deemed "relapsed good risk" may be salvaged successfully with conventional dose chemotherapy comprising one or two new agents such as TIP, or with reinduction conventional dose chemotherapy followed by one single cycle of high-dose therapy. Patients who are in the "relapsed poor risk" category have a dismal prognosis (5% PFS), unless repetitive (2–3) cycles of high-dose therapy are being utilized (85,86). Hence, in relapsed poor risk disease,

dose intensification may appear a more favorable approach than incorporating new agents in conventional dose regimens.

Side Effects of Therapy

Apart from acute side effects of chemotherapy, including cisplatin-induced emesis, alopecia, and a modest risk of mucositis and neutropenic complications, BEP chemotherapy is usually well tolerated. Most of the patients return to ordinary daily life within a few months after the completion of therapy. Some patients complain of prolonged fatigue that may be because of chemotherapy or anxiety over the possibility of a disease relapse (which may recur especially during the first 1–2 years after treatment). In addition, patients may develop sensory neuropathy, ototoxicity, and/or Raynaud's phenomenon. These symptoms frequently diminish within one year. The risk of bleomycin-induced acute and late severe pulmonas toxicity and death, especially with the use of 3 BEP (cumulative dose of bleomycin 270 mg), has become rare. Even when the 360 mg total dose is administered (4 BEP), bleomycin-related death had decreased to less than 1% of patients. In addition, although pulmonary function tests during or shortly after the completion of four BEP cycles reveals abnormalities in approximately 25% of patients, clinical sequelae are infrequent and these changes have shown to be mostly reversible within one to two years, especially in nonsmokers. In the 1980s, anecdotal observations of perioperative pulmonary complications have been attributed to bleomycin-induced pneumonitis (BIP), elicited by high inspired oxygen fractions during surgery. Today, such pulmonary symptoms would be categorized as the multifactorial adult respiratory distress syndrome, and the paradigm of avoiding high inspired oxygen fractions forever after previous bleomycin exposure has been largely abandoned (87).

One of the most disturbing long-term effects identified is the increased risk for cardiovascular morbidity in testis cancer survivors who have received chemotherapy (67–69). Several risk factors have been identified, including hypertension, hypercholesterolemia, microalbuminuria, hormonal alterations, as well as an increased body mass index and decreased physical activity. As many of these factors can be notably improved by changes in lifestyle habits, patients should be encouraged to resume physical activity after completion of treatment (88).

Men with testicular cancer are at elevated risk for second neoplasms. Treatment for testicular cancer may be associated with secondary solid tumors attributed both to chemotherapy and to RT (69,70). Secondary leukemias have also been associated with chemotherapy.

Although spermatogenesis does recover in the majority of patients who have normal sperm counts before chemotherapy, a compensated insufficiency of the function of Leydig cells may be observed up to 60 months after therapy.

Seminoma

Seminoma occurs most frequently in the fourth decade of life. Approximately, 75% of patients with seminoma present with Stage I disease.

Stages I and IIA, IIB

Survival rates of >90% have been reported for patients with clinical Stage I and low Stage II (<5 cm), with orchiectomy followed by RT to the retroperitoneal and ipsilateral pelvic lymph nodes. Seminoma is radiosensitive and relapses rarely occur within the radiation field. Local control is achieved in 92% to 98% of patients (89). The majority of relapsing patients are successfully salvaged with chemotherapy, with an overall survival of >95%.

In the past, 35 Gy was traditionally used. Today, in most centers, 25 Gy are given. The MRC conducted a randomized study in 478 men with Stage I (T1–T3) seminoma to evaluate the optimal field size of adjuvant abdominal RT. Conventional "dog leg" RT (para-aortic lymph nodes and ipsilateral iliac lymph nodes) was compared to reduced field RT to the para-aortic lymph nodes alone. The dose in both arms was 30 Gy in three weeks. At a median follow-up of 36 months, the recurrence rate was 4% with equal numbers of relapses in both arms. Toxicity was less in the reduced field arm. In patients with undisturbed lymph node drainage, adjuvant RT confined to the para-aortic nodes is recommended as a standard treatment approach.

Surveillance for Stage I Seminoma

In the United Kingdom, Scandinavia, and Canada, investigators have questioned whether RT is necessary in all patients. The concern is that the majority of patients are overtreated with RT and there has also been a preoccupation over the increased number of second cancers in patients 15 to 20 years after RT (69,70,90). Surveillance has, therefore, been explored as an alternative, but it has not been adopted in the same way as for nonseminomatous germ cell cancer (NSGCT), partly because of the lack of serum tumor markers, as well as recurrences occurring more frequently beyond two years, as compared with NSGCT. It has also been more difficult to identify consistently useful prognostic factors for Stage I seminoma; the main risk factors appear to be size of the primary tumor and the presence or absence of rate testis invasion and to a lesser extent the presence or absence of vascular invasion.

The main advantage of surveillance is that >80% of patients can be spared overtreatment. The main disadvantage is the need for long-term follow-up that is expensive and stressful to the patient. Good patient compliance, mandatory to an observation policy, is often difficult on a long-term basis (64).

To date, in view of the recognized risk of late toxicity, there may be an increasing role for surveillance in Stage I seminoma, especially in patients with small tumors (less than 4 cm) and no rate testis invasion (59).

Adjuvant Carboplatin for Stage I Seminoma

The MRC and EORTC investigated one cycle of carboplatin with adjuvant RT in a study involving 1477 clinical Stage I seminoma patients. The relapse-free survival rates at three and five years were similar, 95% on carboplatin, and 96% on RT (64 and updated report presented at ASCO 2008). As most relapses in the carboplatin group occurred below the diaphragm and hence an identical strict radiological follow-up is mandatory as when opting for surveillance, many investigators today still prefer RT for high-risk seminoma and surveillance for low-risk patients.

Stages ≥IIC Metastatic Seminoma

RT has an unacceptably high failure rate of 40% to 80% in bulky Stage II (>5 cm) seminoma. For these patients and all seminoma patients who present with Stage III nodal or visceral metastasis, cisplatin-based chemotherapy is highly effective. BEP is the standard regimen, but bleomycin needs to be used cautiously in older patients. In elderly patients the alternative option is four cycles of EP.

In patients with advanced seminoma, 90% of patients still fall into the good risk category and the remaining 10% are intermediate prognosis (Table 10.3). They are never in the poor prognosis group.

Controversy exists as to the best strategy for patients who present with bulky seminoma and have persistent radiographic abnormalities on CT scan after cisplatin-based chemotherapy. Seminoma differs from NSGCT in that residual teratoma is rare and RPLND is usually technically demanding due to extensive fibrosis in response to chemotherapy. The majority of residual lesions may shrink in time, and a policy of observation, with intervention if resolution does not occur, has been adopted in many centers. If the abnormality is >3 cm, options include surgery or continued observation. The use of a postchemotherapy PET scan may also help to discriminate between fibrotic remains and viable tumor.

CONCLUSIONS

Significant improvements have been made during the past few decades with respect to the understanding and treatment in all four major genitourinary cancers. Chemotherapy has become a feasible option in CRPC. More effective and less toxic chemotherapy regimens have been developed in bladder cancer. There have been significant advances and approval of novel targeted agents in renal cell cancer, and testis cancer has become a model for a curable solid cancer.

REFERENCES

1. Holmberg L, Bill-Axelson A, Helgesen F et al. A randomized trial comparing radical prostatectomy with watchful waiting in early prostate cancer. N Engl J Med 2002; 347: 781–9.
2. Linton KD, Hamdy FC. Early diagnosis and surgical management of prostate cancer. Cancer Treat Rev 2003; 29: 151–60.
3. Parker CC, Dearnaley DP. Radical radiotherapy for prostate cancer. Cancer Treat Rev 2003; 29: 161–9.
4. Bolla M, van Tienhoven G, de Reijke THM et al. and EORTC Radiation Oncology and Genitourinary Tract Cancer Groups. Concomitant and adjuvant androgen deprivation (ADT) with external beam irradiation (RT) for locally advanced prostate cancer: 6 months versus 3 years ADT – Results of the randomized EORTC Phase III trial 22961. Proc Annu Meet Am Soc Clin Oncol 2007; 25: 238s.
5. D'Amico AV, Denham JW, Bolla M et al. Short- vs long-term androgen suppression plus external beam radiation therapy and survival in men of advanced age with node-negative high-risk adenocarcinoma of the prostate. Cancer 2007; 109: 2004–10.
6. Epstein JI, Pizov G, Walsh PC. Correlation of pathologic findings with progression after radical retropubic prostatectomy. Cancer 1993; 71: 3582–93.
7. van der Kwast TH, Bolla M, Van Poppel H et al. Identification of patients with prostate cancer who benefit from immediate

postoperative radiotherapy: EORTC 22911. J Clin Oncol 2007; 25: 4178–86.

8. Dreicer R. Controversies in the systemic management of patients with evidence of biochemical failure following radical prostatectomy. Cancer Treat Rev 2002; 28: 189–94.

9. Petrylak DP, Ankerst DP, Jiang CS et al. Evaluation of prostate-specific antigen declines for surrogacy in patients treated on SWOG 99-16. J Natl Cancer Inst 2006; 98: 516–21.

10. Armstrong AJ, Garrett Mayer E, Ou Yang YC et al. Prostate-specific antigen and pain surrogacy analysis in metastatic hormone-refractory prostate cancer. J Clin Oncol 2007; 25: 3965–70.

11. Scher HI, Halabi S, Tannock I et al. Design and endpoints of clinical trials for patients with progressive prostate cancer and castrate levels of testosterone: recommendations of the Prostate Cancer Clinical Trials Working Group (PCWG2). J Clin Oncol 2008; 26: 1148–59.

12. Tannock IF, de Wit R, Berry WR et al. Docetaxel plus prednisone or mitoxantrone plus prednisone for advanced prostate cancer. N Engl J Med 2004; 351: 1502–12.

13. Petrylak DP, Tangen CM, Hussain MH et al. Docetaxel and estramustine compared with mitoxantrone and prednisone for advanced refractory prostate cancer. N Engl J Med 2004; 351: 1513–20.

14. Berthold DR, Pond GR, Soban F et al. Docetaxel plus prednisone or mitoxantrone plus prednisone for advanced prostate cancer: updated survival in the TAX 327 study. J Clin Oncol 2008; 26: 242–5.

15. de Wit R. Shifting paradigms in prostate cancer: docetaxel plus low-dose prednisone — finally an effective chemotherapy. Eur J Cancer 2005; 41: 502–7.

16. Berthold DR, Pond GR, Roessner M et al. Treatment of hormone-refractory prostate cancer with docetaxel or mitoxantrone: relationships between PSA, pain and quality of life response and survival in the Tax-327 Study. Clin Cancer Res 2008; 14: 2763–7.

17. Armstrong AJ, Garrett-Mayer ES, Yang YC et al. A contemporary prognostic nomogram for men with hormone-refractory metastatic prostate cancer: a TAX327 study analysis. Clin Cancer Res 2007; 13: 6396–403.

18. van den Hout WB, van der Linden YM, Steenland E et al. Single- versus multiple-fraction radiotherapy in patients with painful bone metastases: cost-utility analysis based on a randomized trial. J Natl Cancer Inst 2003; 95: 222–9.

19. Nelson GW, De Marzo AM, Isaacs WB. Mechanisms of disease: prostate cancer. N Engl J Med 2004; 349: 366–81.

20. Attard G, Reid AH, Yap TA et al. Phase I clinical trial of a selective inhibitor of CYP17, abiraterone acetate, confirms that castration-resistant prostate cancer commonly remains hormone driven. J Clin Oncol 2008; 26: 4563–71.

21. Oosterlinck W, Lobel B, Jakse G et al. European association of urology guidelines on bladder cancer. Eur Urol 2002; 41: 105–12.

22. Hall, R. R. Updated results of a randomised controlled trial of neoadjuvant cisplatin (C), methotrexate (M) and vinblastine (V) chemotherapy for muscle-invasive bladder cancer. Intl Collaboration of Trialists of the MRC Advanced Bladder Cancer Group. Proc Annu Meet Am Soc Clin Oncol 2002; 21: 178a.

23. Grossman HB, Natale RB, Tangen CM et al. Neoadjuvant chemotherapy plus cystectomy compared with cystectomy alone for locally advanced bladder cancer. N Engl J Med 2003; 349: 859–66.

24. Advanced Bladder Cancer Meta-analysis Collaboration. Neo-adjuvant chemotherapy in invasive bladder cancer: a systematic review and meta-analysis. Lancet 2003; 361: 1927–34.

25. Sternberg CN, Pansadoro V, Calabrò F et al. Can patient selection for bladder preservation be based on response to chemotherapy? Cancer 2003; 97: 1644–52.

26. Stockle M, Meyenburg W, Wellek S. Adjuvant polychemotherapy of nonorgan-confined bladder cancer after radical cystectomy revisited: long term results of a controlled prospective study and further clinical experience. J Urol 1995; 153: 47–52.

27. de Wit R, Bellmunt J. Chemotherapy in metastatic urothelial cancer. Am J Cancer 2002; 1: 23–31.

28. Sternberg CN, de Mulder PHM, Schornagel JH et al. Randomized phase III trial of high dose intensity methotrexate, vinblastine, doxorubicin, and cisplatin (MVAC) chemotherapy and recombinant human granulocyte colony-stimulating factor versus classic MVAC in advanced urothelial tract tumors: European Organization for Research and Treatment of Cancer. Protocol No. 30924. J Clin Oncol 2001; 19: 2638–46.

29. Sternberg CN, Vogelzang NJ. Gemcitabine, paclitaxel, pemetrexed and other newer agents in urothelial and kidney cancers. Crit Rev Oncol Hematol 2003; 46(Suppl): S105–15.

30. von der Maase H, Hansen SW, Roberts JT et al. Gemcitabine and cisplatin versus methotrexate, vinblastine, doxorubicin, and cisplatin in advanced or metastatic bladder cancer: results of a large, randomized, multinational, multicenter, phase III study. J Clin Oncol 2000; 18: 3068–77.

31. Bellmunt J, von der Maase H, Mead GM et al. Randomized phase III study comparing paclitaxel/cisplatin/gemcitabine and gemcitabine/cisplatin in patients with locally advanced or metastatic urothelial cancer without prior systemic therapy: EORTC 30987/intergroup study. Proc Annu Meet Am Soc Clin Oncol 2007; 25: 242s.

32. Kim WY, Kaelin WG. Role of VHL gene mutation in human cancer. J Clin Oncol 2004; 22: 4991–5004.

33. Hanna SC, Heathcote SA, Kim WY. mTOR pathway in renal cell carcinoma. Expert Rev Anticancer Ther 2008; 8: 283–92.

34. Linehan WM, Vasselli J, Srinivasan R et al. Genetic basis of cancer of the kidney: disease-specific approaches to therapy. Clin Cancer Res 2004; 10: 6282S–6289S.

35. Vaishampayan U. A review of current and future treatment options in renal cancer. Am J Cancer 2003; 2: 201–10.

36. Novick AC. Current surgical approaches, nephron-sparing surgery and the role of surgery in the integrated immunologic approach to renal cell carcinoma. Semin Oncol 1995; 22: 29–33.

37. Glaspy JA. Therapeutic options in the management of renal cell carcinoma. Semin Oncol 2002; 29: 41–6.

38. Motzer RJ, Bacik J, Murphy BA et al. Interferon-alfa as a comparative treatment for clinical trials of new therapies against advanced renal cell carcinoma. J Clin Oncol 2002; 20: 289–96.

39. Mickisch GH, Garin A, Van Poppel H et al. and European Organisation for Research and Treatment of Cancer (EORTC) Genitourinary Group. Radical nephrectomy plus interferon-alfa-based immunotherapy compared with interferon alfa alone in metastatic renal-cell carcinoma: a randomised trial. Lancet 2001; 358: 966–70.

40. Flanigan RC, Salmon SE, Blumenstein BA et al. Nephrectomy followed by interferon alfa-2b compared with interferon alfa-2b alone for metastatic renal-cell cancer. N Engl J Med 2001; 345: 1655–9.

41. Mertens WC, Eisenhauer EA, Moore M et al. Gemcitabine in advanced renal cell carcinoma. A phase II study of the national cancer Institute of Canada Clinical Trials Group. Ann Oncol 1993; 4: 331–2.

42. Margolin KA. Interleukin-2 in the treatment of renal cancer. Semin Oncol 2000; 27: 194–203.

43. Sandlund J, Oosterwijk E, Grankvist K et al. Prognostic impact of carbonic anhydrase IX expression in human renal cell carcinoma. BJU Int 2007; 100: 556–60.

44. Yang JC, Haworth L, Sherry RM et al. A randomized trial of bevacizumab, an anti-vascular endothelial growth factor antibody, for metastatic renal cancer. N Engl J Med 2003; 349: 427–34.

45. Escudier B, Pluzanska A, Koralewski P et al. Bevacizumab plus interferon alfa-2a for treatment of metastatic renal cell carcinoma: a randomised, double-blind phase III trial. Lancet 2007; 370: 2103–11.

46. Rini B, Halabi S, Rosenberg JE et al. CALGB 90206: a phase III trial of bevacizumab plus interferon-alpha versus interferon-alpha monotherapy in metastatic renal cell carcinoma. Genitourinary Cancer Symposium San Francisco, CA, 2008.

47. Motzer RJ, Michaelson MD, Redman BG et al. Activity of SU11248, a multitargeted inhibitor of vascular endothelial growth factor receptor and platelet-derived growth factor receptor, in patients with metastatic renal cell carcinoma. J Clin Oncol 2006; 24: 16–24.

48. Motzer RJ, Rini BI, Bukowski RM et al. Sunitinib in patients with metastatic renal cell carcinoma. JAMA 2006; 295: 2516–24.

49. Motzer RJ, Hutson TE, Tomczak P et al. Sunitinib versus interferon alfa in metastatic renal-cell carcinoma. N Engl J Med 2007; 356: 115–24.

50. Figlin R, Hutson TE, Tomczak P et al. Overall survival with sunitinib versus interferon-alfa as first-line treatment of metastatic renal cell carcinoma. Proc Annu Meet Am Soc Clin Oncol 2008; 26: abstract 5024.

51. Ratain MJ, Eisen T, Stadler WM et al. Phase II placebo-controlled randomized discontinuation trial of sorafenib in patients with metastatic renal cell carcinoma. J Clin Oncol 2006; 24: 2505–12.

52. Escudier B, Eisen T, Stadler WM et al. Sorafenib in advanced clear-cell renal-cell carcinoma. N Engl J Med 2007; 356: 125–34.

53. Szczylik C, Demkow T, Staehler M et al. Randomized phase II trial of first-line treatment with sorafenib versus interferon in patients with advanced renal cell carcinoma: final results. Proc Annu Meet Am Soc Clin Oncol 2007; 25: abstract 5025.

54. Atkins MB, Hidalgo M, Stadler WM et al. Randomized phase II study of multiple dose levels of CCI-779, a novel mammalian target of rapamycin kinase inhibitor, in patients with advanced refractory renal cell carcinoma. J Clin Oncol 2004; 22: 909–18.

55. Hudes G, Carducci M, Tomczak P et al. Temsirolimus, interferon alfa, or both for advanced renal-cell carcinoma. N Engl J Med 2007; 356: 2271–81.

56. Motzer R, Escudier B, Oudard S et al. Efficacy of Everolimus in advanced renal cell carcinoma: a double-blind, randomised, placebo-controlled phase III trial. Lancet 2008; 372: 449–56.

57. Rixe O, Bukowski RM, Michaelson MD et al. Axitinib treatment in patients with cytokine-refractory metastatic renal-cell cancer: a phase II study. Lancet Oncol 2007; 8: 975–84.

58. Hutson TE, Davis ID, Machiels JP et al. Pazopanib (GW786034) is active in metastatic renal cell carcinoma (RCC): interim results of a phase II randomized discontinuation trial (RDT). Proc Annu Meet Am Soc Clin Oncol 2007; 25: 242s.

59. Jones RH, Vasey PA. New directions in testicular cancer; molecular determinants of oncogenesis and treatment success. Eur J Cancer 2003; 39: 147–56.

60. Toner GC. Early identification of therapeutic failure in non-seminomatous germ cell tumors by assessing serum tumor marker decline during chemotherapy: still not ready for routine clinical use. J Clin Oncol 2004; 19: 3842–5.

61. Herr HW. Is biopsy of the contralateral testis necessary in patients with germ cell tumors? J Urol 1997; 158: 1331–4.

62. International Germ Cell Cancer Collaborative Group. International germ cell consensus classification: a prognostic factor based staging system for metastatic germ cell cancers. J Clin Oncol 1997; 15: 594–603.

63. Fossa SD, Oliver RTH, Stenning SP et al. Prognostic factors for patients with advanced seminoma treated with platinum-based chemotherapy. Eur J Cancer 1997; 33: 1380–7.

64. de Wit R, Fizazi K. Controversies in the management of clinical stage I testis cancer. J Clin Oncol 2006; 24: 5482–92.

65. Klepp O, Dahl O, Flodgren P et al. Risk-adapted treatment of clinical stage 1 non-seminoma testis cancer. Eur J Cancer 1997; 33: 1038–44.

66. Horwich A, Cullen MH, Stenning SP. Primary chemotherapy after orchidectomy for stage I and II nonseminoma. Semin Oncol 1998; 25: 154–9.

67. Huddart RA, Norman A, Shahidi M et al. Cardiovascular disease as a long-term complication of treatment for testicular cancer. J Clin Oncol 2003; 21: 1513–23.

68. Van den Belt-Dusebout AW, Nuver J, de Wit R et al. Long-term risk of cardiovascular disease in 5-year survivors of testicular cancer. J Clin Oncol 2006; 24: 467–75.

69. Van den Belt-Dusebout AW, de Wit R, Gietema JA et al. Treatment-specific risks of second malignancies and cardiovascular disease in 5-year survivors of testicular cancer. J Clin Oncol 2007; 25: 4270–378.

70. Travis LB, Fossa DS, Schonfeld SJ et al. Second cancers among 40,576 cancer patients: focus on long-term survivors. J Natl Cancer Inst 2005; 97: 1354–65.

71. Culine S, Theodore C, Court BH et al. Evaluation of primary standard cisplatin-based chemotherapy for clinical stage II non-seminomatous germ cell tumours of the testis. Br J Urol 1997; 79: 258–62.

72. Stephenson AJ, Bosl GJ, Motzer RJ et al. Non-randomized comparison of primary chemotherapy and retroperitoneal lymph node dissection for clinical stage II A and II B non-seminomatous germ cell testicular cancer. J Clin Oncol 2007; 25: 5597–602.

73. de Wit R. Optimal management of retroperitoneal metastatic nonseminomatous testicular cancer; towards better selection between scalpel and needle. J Clin Oncol 2007; 25: 5550–2.

74. de Wit R. Treatment of disseminated non-seminomatous testicular cancer: the european experience. Semin Surg Oncol 1999; 17: 250–6.

75. de Wit R, Roberts JT, Wilkinson P et al. Equivalence of three or four cycles of bleomycin, etopposide, and cisplatin chemotherapy and of a 3- or 5-day schedule in good-prognosis germ cell cancer: a randomized study of the European Organization for Research and Treatment of Cancer Genitourinary Tract Cancer Cooperative Group and the Medical Research Council. J Clin Oncol 2001; 19: 1629–40.

76. Kondagunta GV, Bacik J, Bajorin DF et al. Etoposide and cisplatin chemotherapy for metastatic good-risk germ cell tumors. J Clin Oncol 2005; 23: 9290–4.

77. Culine S, Kerbrat P, Kramar A et al. Refining the optimal chemotherapy regimen for good-risk metastatic nonseminomatous germ-cell tumors: a randomized trial of the Genito-Urinary Group of the French Federation of Cancer Centers (GETUG T93BP). Ann Oncol 2007; 18: 917–24.

78. de Wit R. Refining the optimal chemotherapy regimen in good prognosis germ cell cancer; interpretation of the current body of knowledge. J Clin Oncol 2007; 25: 4346–9.

79. Collette L, Sylvester RJ, Stenning SP et al. Impact of the treatment institution on survival of patients with "poor-prognostic" metastatic nonseminoma. J Natl Cancer Inst 1999; 91: 839–46.

80. Motzer RJ, NIchols CJ, Margolin KA et al. Phase III randomized trial of conventional-dose chemotherapy with or without high-dose chemotherapy and autologous hematopoietic stem-cell rescue as first-line treatment for patients with poor prognosis metastatic germ cell tumors. J Clin Oncol 2007; 25: 239–40.

81. Fizazi K, Tjulandin S, Salvioni R et al. Viable malignant cells after primary chemotherapy for disseminated nonseminomatous germ cell tumors: prognostic factors and role of post-surgery chemotherapy—results from an international study group. J Clin Oncol 2001; 19: 2647–57.

82. Kondagunta GV, Bacik J, Donadio A et al. Combination of paclitaxel, ifosfamide, and cisplatin is an effective second-line

therapy for patients with relapsed testicular germ cell tumors. J Clin Oncol 2005; 23: 6549–55.

83. Rick O, Kollmannsberger C, Beyer J et al. Current aspects of high-dose chemotherapy in germ-cell tumors. Crit Rev Oncol Hematol 2003; 47: 237–48.

84. Bokemeyer C, Harstrick A, Beyer J et al. The use of dose-intensified chemotherapy in the treatment of metastatic non-seminomatous testicular germ cell tumours. German Testicular Cancer Study Group. Semin Oncol 1998; 25(2 Suppl 4): 24–32.

85. Motzer RJ, Mazumdar M, Sheinfeld J et al. Sequential dose-intensive paclitaxel, ifosfamide, carboplatin, and etoposide salvage therapy for germ cell tumor patients. J Clin Oncol 2000; 18: 1173–80.

86. Bhatia S, Abonour R, Porcu P et al. High-dose chemotherapy as initial salvage chemotherapy in patients with relapsed testicular cancer. J Clin Oncol 2000; 18: 3346–51.

87. de Wit R, Sleijfer S, Kaye SB et al. Bleomycin and scuba diving; where is the harm? Lancet Oncol 2007; 8: 954–5.

88. Meinardi MT, Gietema JA, Graaf van der WTA et al. Cardiovascular morbidity in long-term survivors of metastatic testicular cancer. J Clin Oncol 2000; 18: 1725–32.

89. Schultz HP, von der Maase H, Rorth M et al. Testicular seminoma in Denmark 1976–1980. Acta Radiol Oncol 1984; 23: 263–9.

90. Zagars GK, Ballo MT, Lee AK et al. Mortality after cure of testicular seminoma. J Clin Oncol 2004; 22: 640–7.

11

Sarcomas

Jean-Yves Blay and Isabelle Ray-Coquard

Soft tissue sarcomas (STS) represent a group of rare tumors, accounting for less than 2% of all adult malignancies and 10% to 15% of children malignancies. They constitute a heterogeneous group of rare tumors arising from the resident cells of connective tissues (1). The overall yearly incidence of sarcoma from all sites is not well known, but has likely been underestimated and probably ranges between 5 and 7 new cases/100,000/year (2).

In adults, 50% of the patients will relapse into their disease. A careful clinical management by a multidisciplinary team of experienced cancer specialists is crucial in these diseases. Patient survival is dependent on the quality of care provided, at any stage of patient management, from diagnosis to treatment. This chapter describes the major diagnostic features and the natural history of sarcomas, summarizes strategies for the clinical management of the disease, and describes ongoing development in the systemic treatments of this disease.

HISTOPATHOLOGY OF SOFT TISSUE SARCOMAS

STSs are a heterogeneous group of diseases with distinct histological, cytological, and molecular features. Tumors originate from mesodermal or, more rarely, ectodermal tissues and are classified histologically according to the soft tissue cell that they resemble: in leiomyosarcomas, for instance, cells have cytological and phenotypical characteristics also observed in smooth muscle cells. At macroscopic examination, STS generally present as tan-white masses with a fish-flesh appearance with frequent focal hemorrhage and necrosis, the two features considered relevant for prognosis.

The histological classification of sarcomas has been revisited recently (3). Each type may be divided into several subtypes depending on genetic abnormalities and large differences in disease history. Well-differentiated liposarcomas, for instance, are slow-growing, localized tumors that may acquire additional genetic alteration and become dedifferentiated; conversely, myxoid and round cell liposarcomas are associated with aggressive local and metastatic behavior and have a completely different set of genetic alterations; finally, pleomorphic liposarcoma represents a third subtype of liposarcoma with an even more aggressive clinical presentation and a third different set of genetic alterations. Some of the major histological subtypes described in the previous large series, such as malignant fibrous histiocytomas (MFHs), have been redistributed into other subtypes following the identification of phenotypic

differences revealed by immunohistochemical analysis or molecular markers specific for different histological subtypes. Other histopathological or molecular entities will likely be identified through the ongoing development of novel molecular biology techniques (4,5).

Despite the increasing knowledge of the molecular alteration of these tumors, prognosis is still based on a simple histological grading of the tumor. Among several grading systems available, the most widely accepted is the classification initially proposed by the Sarcoma Group of the French Federation of Cancer Centers now used in the WHO classification (6,7). Tumors are classified according to three parameters: the mitotic index, the presence of necrosis, and cell differentiation. This classification has demonstrated prognostic value for predicting the risk of local relapse, metastatic spread or death, with five-year survival rates of 95%, 75%, and 45% in patients with grade 1, 2, or 3 tumors, respectively (6).

MOLECULAR BIOLOGY OF SARCOMAS

There is a wide variety of DNA alterations observed in sarcoma. These tumors can be classified into distinct molecular and pathological entities: six molecular subgroups of connective tissue tumors may be distinguished as of now, keeping in mind that this is a rapidly evolving classification (4,5,8–18):

1. Sarcomas with specific translocations generating fusion gene whose protein products modulate transcription or may act as growth factors (e.g., EWS/Fli1 in Ewing family of tumors, PDGF-col1a1 in DFSP). These translocations give rise to fusion genes whose protein products often exert transcriptional regulatory activity. These translocations are specific for nosological entities and were identified initially by cytogenetic approaches (4,5,8,9). Now they can be identified using polymerase chain reaction (PCR) or fluorescence in situ hybridization (FISH) for diagnostic purposes. The most frequent translocations are described in Table 11.1.
2. Sarcomas with mutated activated kinases (e.g., KIT in gastrointestinal stromal tumor, GIST). These alterations affect genes coding for cytokines or cytokine tyrosine kinase receptors. GISTs, for instance, are characterized by frequent mutations of *KIT*, the gene encoding for the stem cell factor receptor, or platelet-derived growth factor receptor alpha (PDGFRA) whose activated protein products play an important role in the oncogenic process of these tumors (10–12).

Table 11.1 Translocations in Sarcomas

Tumor	Translocation	Fusion gene	Incidence (%)
Ewing/PNET	t(11;22)(q24;q12)	EWS-FLI1	85
	t(21;22)(q22;q12)	EWS-ERG	10
	t(7;22)(p22;q12)	EWS-ETV1	Rare
	t(17;22)(q12;q12)	EWS-E1AF	Rare
	t(2;22)(q33;q12)	EWS-FEV	Rare
DSRCT[a]	t(11;22)(p13;q12)	EWS-WT1	95
Myxoid liposarcoma	t(12;16)(q13;p11)	TLS-CHOP	95
	t(12;22)(q13;q12)	EWS-CHOP	5
Extraskeletal myxoid chondrosarcoma	t(9;22)(q22;q12)	EWS-CHN	75
Clear cell sarcoma	t(12;22)(q13;q12)	EWS-ATF1	Unknown
Synovialosarcoma	t(X;18)(p11.23;q11)	SYT-SSX1	65
	t(X;18)(p11.21;q11)	SYT-SSX2	35
Alveolar	t(2;13)(q35;q14)	PAX3-FKHR	75
Rhabdomyosarcoma	t(1;13)(p36;q14)	PAX7-FKHR	10
Dermatofibrosarcoma protuberans	t(17;22)(q22;q13)	COL1A1-PDGFB	Unknown
Congenital fibrosarcoma	t(12;15)(p13;q25)	ETV6-NTRK3	Unknown

[a]Desmoplastic small round cell tumor.

3. Sarcomas with deletion of tumor suppressor genes such as NF1 in sarcomas associated with Recklinghausen disease or rhabdoid tumors (INI1) (13,14).
4. Sarcomas with simple genetic alterations [mdm2/cdk4 amplification in well differentiated/dedifferentiated (WD/DD) liposarcomas] (15,16).
5. Sarcomas with gross genetic alterations, including amplifications and deletion of large chromosome segments (e.g., leiomyosarcomas) (17). These alterations frequently involve the *Rb* gene.
6. Closely linked to sarcoma are connective tissue tumors with locoregional spreading behavior with alterations of the intercellular adhesion pathways, for example, aggressive fibromatosis with APC alterations—in Gardner's syndrome—or beta catenin mutations (18).

EPIDEMIOLOGY OF SOFT TISSUE SARCOMAS

STSs are known to be a collection of rare diseases, but altogether, these rare tumors are not that infrequent. Overall, the incidence of soft tissue, bone, and visceral sarcomas is probably close to 6/100,000/year. However, this is the overall incidence of all 50+ subtypes, and for some subtypes the incidence may be as low as 1/1,000,000/year (2).

The etiology of these diseases is not known for most patients (1). Several predisposing genetic abnormalities have been identified, such as constitutional mutations of the genes *Rb* (hereditary retinoblastoma), *p53* (Li–Fraumeni syndrome), *APC* (Gardner syndrome), *NF1* (neurofibromatosis), *WRN* (Werner syndrome), or *c-kit* (familial GIST).

Exposure to ionizing radiation is a well-established extrinsic risk factor for the disease. Sarcomas often develop at the site of radiation. This holds true independent of the part of the body that is affected, although most studies have investigated sarcomas developing after breast cancer treatment, mainly osteosarcomas, angiosarcomas, and MFH. Chronic lymphedema (Stewart–Treves syndrome) has also been identified as a major risk factor, just as exposure to toxic substances such as some herbicides and food preservatives (phenoxyacetic acids and chlorophenols), thorotrast or vinyl chloride has been shown to increase the risk of developing sarcoma. Finally, retrospective studies frequently mention a history of previous injuries as a possible triggering factor for the disease, though no clear causative link has yet been demonstrated.

CLINICAL PRESENTATION OF SOFT TISSUE SARCOMAS

A sarcoma should be suspected in any patient presenting with a superficial or deep tumor of unidentified histological type, larger than 5 cm, arising in the soft tissues. More than 70% of STS are larger than 5 cm at initial diagnosis (6). The diagnostic procedure of sarcoma, including specific imaging and biopsy by an expert surgeon or radiologist should be considered in this case, ideally following a multidisciplinary consultation (19,20).

STS can occur at any age, in any part of the body. However, histological type varies with age: synovial sarcomas, rhabdomyosarcomas, and Ewing's sarcomas are more likely to occur in young adults, whereas MFH and leiomyosarcomas are more frequent in the elderly, and liposarcomas are generally diagnosed in patients between the ages of 40 and 50. These ranges are only meant as a rough guide, and any STS subtype may arise at virtually any age.

The sites most frequently involved are the lower (40%) and upper (15%) extremities, the abdomen and retroperitoneum (15%), the viscera (uterus, gastrointestinal track, lung, kidney, etc.) (20%), the thorax (5%), and the head and neck (5%).

Disease progression is first local with invasion of neighboring structures and possible dissemination to adjacent tissue compartments (fascia, skin, organ, cortical bone, vessels, nerves, etc.). Tumors are rarely metastatic at initial diagnosis and 80% to 90% of tumors are discovered in the localized phase. Distant spread of malignant cells occurs through the bloodstream to other organs; this occurs in 50% of the patients principally to the lung (the most common metastatic site for extraabdominal tumors), less frequently to the liver or bones. Intraabdominal or retroperitoneal sarcomas are generally associated with local and regional relapses, with metastases developing in the abdomen, the peritoneal cavity, or the liver. Metastases to the soft tissues or the brain also occur in patients with end-stage disease or with specific histological subtypes of STS. In all cases, nodal involvement is rare.

MORPHOLOGICAL ASSESSMENT AND INITIAL BIOPSY

Morphological assessment is performed to evaluate disease extension, notably to identify a possible extension of the tumor to the vascular system or to the adjacent bone structures and organs. Morphological imaging may also guide in determining the tumor type and in making treatment decisions.

Precise histological examination of a tumor specimen is required to confirm the diagnosis before treatment is initiated. For all soft tissue tumors of unknown etiology larger than 5 cm, it is essential to have a careful review of the biopsy tissue performed by an experienced pathologist. If performed by a surgeon, the biopsy should always be obtained by the surgeon who will eventually remove the tumor. A small incision, oriented parallel to the long axis of the extremity, is required so that the biopsy trajectory and scar are encompassed by the subsequent definitive resection of the tumor. After histopathological examination, samples are processed and stored for molecular analysis. In collaboration with the clinicians involved in the surgical management of the patients, skilled imaging specialists should obtain tissue biopsies for histopathological examination and diagnosis of malignancy (19–22). For GISTs, preoperative biopsy is not uniformly recommended in consensus guidelines (23).

Morphological assessment includes computed tomography (CT) scan and magnetic resonance imaging (MRI). MRI is the technique of choice for limb localizations, whereas CT scan examination is preferred for tumors arising in the abdomen or the chest. Preoperative staging is based on thoracic CT scan, and for some subtypes (GIST, abdominal, and pelvic sarcomas), abdominal and pelvic CT scan. Other investigations may be required according to the specific clinical signs and symptoms of each patient.

Unfortunately, in most European countries, the majority of patients is not treated according to these guidelines and are referred to expert centers following the initial locoregional treatment. A retrospective study suggested a detrimental impact on patient survival in case of noncompliance to clinical practice guidelines and treatment outside networks or expert centers (20).

STAGING AND PROGNOSTIC FACTORS FOR SOFT TISSUE SARCOMAS

Clinicopathological staging of the tumor is essential for determining the most effective treatment strategy. The classification systems most frequently used are based on the size (T1 < 5 cm, T2 > 5 cm) and histological grade (1–3) of the tumor and also differentiate between superficial (above the superficial fascia) and deep lesions (6,7). The risks of local recurrence, metastatic relapse, or disease-related death depend on several factors, including the type and location of the tumor and patient clinical management (1,6,7).

Young age, female gender, low histological grade, and Stage 1 tumors are associated with good prognosis and low invasiveness, whereas the prognosis for patients with high-grade (Grade 3) Stage 2 tumors, positive (R1 or R2) resection margins, local relapses, or aggressive histological subtypes (leiomyosarcoma, neurosarcoma, or synovial sarcoma) is generally poor.

TREATMENT OF SOFT TISSUE SARCOMAS

STSs are heterogeneous diseases that require multidisciplinary clinical management combining surgery, radiation oncology, and chemotherapy, based on accurate radiological and histological diagnosis.

Surgery

Surgical excision of the primary tumor is the treatment of choice for patients with a soft tissue or visceral sarcoma diagnosed on initial biopsy (1,19,21). It should be the first treatment option when conservative resection is both feasible in agreement with clinical practice guidelines, that is, en bloc, macro- and microscopically complete surgical excision of the gross tumor encompassing the biopsy scar (this defines an R0 resection). The persistence of microscopic residual disease (R1 resection) is associated with a higher risk of relapse, and re-resection should be considered when technically feasible. Patients with macroscopically incomplete surgery will all relapse and secondary surgical excision of residual disease is therefore mandatory unless the medical condition of the patients makes it unfeasible.

Microscopically complete resection (R0) can be difficult at some sites (sarcomas of the retroperitoneum, for instance). Multidisciplinary team collaboration is therefore essential at all stages of the surgical process (biopsy, initial surgery, secondary resection). Most experienced teams perform systematic secondary surgery when the above criteria are not met.

For sarcomas of the extremities, an adequate surgery may require amputation, a complete resection of the tumor bed or wide local excision with negative tissue margins. The optimal extent of these resection margins is currently debated. The procedure most frequently used is conservative limb-sparing local surgery; amputation is less frequently proposed in recent years following the publication of the results of a randomized trial showing similar outcome in patients treated with amputation versus conservative surgery and radiotherapy (24). In the case of a tumor with a locoregional extent that would not allow for any conservative treatment, neoadjuvant chemotherapy may be proposed by experienced teams after a careful consideration of the operability of the patients; in some patients, this strategy may aid in proposing a conservative treatment if sufficient shrinkage of the tumor can be obtained (25). Combination with hyperthermia has been reported to improve local tumor control in a single randomized trial reported by Issels et al. at ASCO 2007 (26). This technique is however available only in a limited number of centers in some countries (26).

Amputation is still considered in cases of local relapse following an optimal locoregional treatment. However, in some European centers, isolated limb perfusion with tumor necrosis factor (TNF) is used as a rescue treatment, as it has been demonstrated to induce tumor shrinkage enabling complete resection of the relapsing tumor without amputation in up to 70% of the cases (27,28).

Radiation Therapy

This is the second option for the local treatment of STS. Radiation therapy alone at the classical 60 Gy dose per 2 Gy fractions is insufficient to achieve local control of the disease. It is generally used in combination with conservative surgery for patients with R0 or R1 tumors, notably lesions with microscopically positive margins or residual disease (R1) for which secondary resection is not feasible. Several randomized trials have shown that radiation therapy, either brachytherapy or external beam radiotherapy, improves local tumor control (29–31). The total radiation dose is usually between 50 and 60 Gy, given in 1.8- to 2-Gy daily fractions delivered to a target volume encompassing the tumor and safety margins. A randomized trial of preoperative radiotherapy versus postoperative radiotherapy showed no significant difference in tumor control, but a significantly higher early toxicity in the preoperative arm, with however a higher rate of late complications in the postoperative arm (31).

Patients with macroscopically positive margins (R2) must undergo secondary resection to achieve R0 or R1 before receiving radiation therapy. If not feasible, radiation therapy may be given with a palliative intent in this setting. Proton beam therapy and carbon ion therapy have been reported to yield encouraging results in these clinical situations. In a study reported on 57 patients, Kamada et al. reported an overall local control rate of 73% at three years, with three-year overall survival (OS) rates 82% and 46%, respectively (32).

Chemotherapy

In 2000, three drugs were considered to have a proven efficacy against STS: doxorubicin, ifosfamide, and dacarbazine (DTIC). Still in 2008, most first-line regimens contain doxorubicin either used as a single agent (A) at an optimal dose of 75 mg/m^2 or a combination of doxorubicin and ifosfamide (AI) possibly associated with dacarbazine (MAID). Higher response rates are obtained with combined chemotherapy regimens, but Phase III comparative studies have not demonstrated any survival benefit of the combination of drugs over single-agent doxorubicin (33).

Four types of approaches are used in patients with STS: adjuvant or neoadjuvant chemotherapy, isolated limb perfusion, and chemotherapy for metastatic disease.

Adjuvant Chemotherapy

Sixteen randomized Phase III trials have evaluated the benefit of postoperative adjuvant chemotherapy to prevent local relapse in high-risk STS patients with localized disease. Because STS is a rare disease, most trials have involved relatively small patient populations. In a majority of cases, a reduction of the risk of local recurrence has been observed among patients receiving adjuvant chemotherapy. Some other studies have shown a lower risk of metastatic progression, whereas only few have reported improved survival. A meta-analysis of all published studies has confirmed a

significant reduction of the risk of relapse, either local or metastatic, but with a nonsignificant reduction of the risk of death (–4%) (34). A more recent trial from the Italian Sarcoma Group showed a significant improvement in OS for patients with high-risk sarcoma of the extremities receiving adjuvant chemotherapy with ifosfamide (35), but the OS benefit was not sustained with additional follow-up. Individual variations in the risk of relapse, respect of dose intensity, variable dosing of drugs, as well as other, yet unknown, factors may account for these discrepancies. In 2007, the largest adjuvant trial of chemotherapy with doxorubicin and ifosfamide in STS performed with the EORTC STBSG presented at ASCO 2007 and 2008 meetings failed to demonstrate a significant survival benefit for adjuvant chemotherapy (36).

Therefore, with the exception of Ewing's sarcoma of the soft parts (see under "Ewing family of tumors") and alveolar or embryonal rhabdomyosarcomas of the soft tissues, adjuvant chemotherapy cannot be considered a standard option for patients with STS and treatment must be tailored to the needs of each individual patient (13).

Neoadjuvant Chemotherapy

As mentioned above, neoadjuvant chemotherapy is used prior to surgery to control microscopic residual disease and shrink the size of the tumor in order to allow complete "oncological" surgical resection (R0, or at least R1). This strategy is used for the treatment of "locally advanced" tumors. The chemotherapy regimens most commonly used in the neoadjuvant setting are combinations of drugs because of the superior response rates observed in several of the randomized trials (33). The exact benefit of this strategy and in particular the percentage of patients achieving conservative tumor resection with this strategy has however not been prospectively addressed. Again, a multidisciplinary approach is advised for these patients. Finally it should be noted that the only randomized trial comparing neoadjuvant chemotherapy followed by surgery versus surgery only, which was reported by the EORTC STBSG failed to demonstrate a significant tumor control rate or survival advantage (37).

Isolated Limb Perfusion with TNF and Melphalan

The technique previously mentioned in the surgery section combines surgery and drug treatment. Tumor necrosis factor, a cytokine able to disrupt tumor neovascularization and the cytotoxic drug melphalan are delivered directly into the limb after temporary isolation of its vasculature to spare the rest of the body from the side effects of treatment. Surgical resection of the residual tumor mass is performed after two or three months. This treatment strategy achieves effective local control of the disease and makes limb-sparing surgery possible for patients with local relapse or locally advanced tumors of the extremities (27,28).

Chemotherapy for Metastatic Disease: Individualization in Progress

Since 2000, treatment of advanced sarcoma has undergone major changes. In the setting of advanced disease, chemotherapy with a doxorubicin-based regimen is the treatment of choice for most histological subtypes, although response rates are in most series in the 25% to 35% range with doxorubin and ifosfamide combinations, with median progression-free survival (PFS) and OS of 6 and 12 months, respectively (38). These features have shown little or no improvement over the past 20 years and most regimens have been considered too toxic, while in most cases failing to show a survival advantage over single agent doxorubicin. Of note, regardless of the regimen, a small proportion of patients with advanced disease will be long-term survivors; the proportion reaches 20% for patients achieving CR, but ranges from 3% to 4% of patients with PR and SD as best response to first line treatment (39). Advanced sarcoma should therefore be considered as a potentially curable disease, even though the proportion of cured patients still remains very low in 2008.

There is therefore room for improvement in advanced STSs, and most innovative treatments for sarcomas are currently developed for metastatic disease. Emerging drugs for the treatment of sarcomas can be divided into two large groups of agents: cytotoxic agents (i.e., chemotherapy) and molecular targeted agents (i.e., targeted therapies).

New Cytotoxic Agents in Sarcomas

Different cytotoxic agents have now shown activity in sarcomas, including taxanes, trabectedin, and other agents still under evaluation.

The taxanes, docetaxel, and paclitaxel enhance microtubule assembly and inhibit the depolymerization of tubulin when given at high doses in vitro; they act through disruption of microtubule dynamics at therapeutic doses in vivo. The activities of docetaxel and gemcitabine remain limited as single agents in the treatment of sarcomas. However, docetaxel when combined with gemcitabine has shown high activity (18.4% objective response rate in STS and up to 53% in leiomyosarcoma) in first- and second-line chemotherapy with a rather favorable toxicity profile (40). A randomized Phase II study demonstrated improved PFS with G + D as compared to G, with an original Bayesian statistical methodology (41). Of note this is the first ever published randomized trial showing improvement in OS in advanced sarcoma. At ASCO 2008, however, a small randomized study by the French sarcoma group, including only patients with leiomyosarcomas and comparing the same two options, failed to confirm the advantage of G + D over G, possibly because of limited power of the study (42). Interestingly, in the rare subset of angiosarcomas, paclitaxel has been reported to induce remarkable activity in retrospective studies, in particular in lesions of the head and neck and the scalp, a disease considered generally as chemo resistant after failure of doxorubicin (43,44).

Trabectedin (ecteinascidin 743, ET-743), is a marine-derived compound that binds covalently to the DNA minor groove, blocking G2/M progression, inducing p53 independent apoptosis, and blocking transcription of inducible genes. The recommended dose is 1.5 mg/m² as a 24-hour continuous infusion. Several Phase II trials assessing the efficacy and toxicity of ET-743 in patients with advanced STS failing first-line chemotherapy have been published (45–47): all trials have shown rather low response rates (4%, 8%, and 8%, respectively), but a high rate of prolonged stable disease (six months PFS = 24%, 29%, and more than 20%, respectively). Toxicities in these trials were mainly

hepatic and hematological and they were mild with less than 10% febrile neutropenia, no febrile neutropenia in the American trial, about 20% grade 3–4 thrombocytopenia, and 40% to 50% of patients experiencing AST and/or ALT elevation. ET-743 has therefore an interesting activity in advanced sarcoma with a manageable toxicity profile. Preliminary results of a randomized Phase II trial, STS201, comparing ET743 1.5 mg/m²/day 24 CI every 21 days versus 0.58 mg/m² as a three-hour weekly infusion three weeks out of four, showed an improvement in PFS and a trend for OS benefit with the three-weekly schedule (47). ET-743 may be particularly efficient for the treatment of some molecular subtypes of sarcomas, in particular myxoid liposarcomas (46).

Brostallicin is a new cytotoxic agent that binds to the DNA minor groove with specificity for TA rich sequences. Phase II of brostallicin has recently been published (48) showing promising activity of this compound in STS. In non-GIST STS (*n* = 43) (patients failing first-line chemotherapy), two PRs were seen (ORR = 5%) and six months PFS was 22%. Based on these results, a randomized EORTC Phase II study of brostallicin versus doxorubicin as first-line chemotherapy in patients with advanced or metastatic STSs was initiated and completed in 2008.

Molecular Targeted Agents: Successes and Failures of Rationally Based Approaches

The development of specific agents in histotypes has been guided by the known molecular biology of these tumors. Not unexpectedly, the identification of a driver—or consistent—molecular alteration in a specific histotype has been more efficient to identify active treatment than the sole expression of a specific marker.

Dermatofibrosarcoma Protuberans (DFSP)

DFSP is a rare skin neoplasm with essentially a locally malignant behavior (9). Its molecular hallmark is a translocation juxtaposing the *col1A1* gene with the *PDGFA* gene, resulting in a fusion protein overproduced in tumor cells with autocrine growth activities (9). Several retrospective and prospective studies based on the inhibitory activities of imatinib on PDGFRA have reported on a significant antitumor effect of imatinib in the disease in both localized and locally advanced disease and metastatic diseases (49). Two Phase II trials have been completed within EORTC (62027) and SARC, and the drug is already registered in many countries for this rare indication in which no agent has previously demonstrated any efficacy.

Imatinib in Pigmented Villonodular Synovitis-Tenosynovial Giant Cell Tumor

Pigmented villonodular synovitis (PVNS), also known as tenosynovial giant cell tumor (TGCT), is a rare pathological entity affecting the synovium in young adults. Initially considered as an inflammatory reactive process, recent observations have shown that this disease may actually be a neoplastic process with specific genetic alterations and rare metastases (50). Indeed, a specific t(1;2) translocation, involving the collagen *6A3* gene (on 2q35) and the *M-CSF* (a.k.a CSF1) gene (on 1p13), is present in a fraction of tumor cells in PVNS/TGCT. This fusion gene expressed by a fraction of the cells encodes for a fusion protein that attracts nonneoplastic cells expressing M-CSFR, through a paracrine—"landscape"—effect. PVNS/TGCT is generally treated by surgery alone. However, relapses may occur and reexcision may be needed with possible important functional impairment. In addition to its inhibitory activity on bcr-abl, KIT, and PDGFRA, imatinib has recently been reported to block M-CSFR activation at therapeutic concentration (50). These observations prompted us to evaluate imatinib in a patient with recurrent and symptomatic PVNS/TGCT following surgery: a complete remission was observed in this patient, and additional studies are required to confirm its antitumor activity (50).

HER1 in Sarcomas

Both gene expression profile analysis and tissue microarrays have shown that several sarcoma histotypes, in particular synovial sarcomas and malignant peripheral nerve sheath tumors (MPNSTs), express high levels of EGFR. Two Phase II studies testing EGFR tyrosine kinase inhibitors in advanced STS, gefitinib, in synovial sarcoma, and erlotinib in MPNST, respectively, were reported and both showed no efficacy of the investigational drug in these settings (51). This is a good example of a model where the expression of the target does not imply a role in tumor progression.

Hormonal Manipulation of Endometrial Stromal Sarcomas

Estrogen and progesterone receptors are observed in a subset of uterine sarcoma, the low-grade endometrial stromal sarcomas (52). These sarcomas are characterized by frequent hormone receptor expression and a t(7;17) translocation. In several retrospective analysis of patients with advanced ESS treated with aromatase inhibitors (AIs) (anastrozole and letrozole), long-lasting responses were reported (52).

IGF1R in Ewing's Sarcomas and Other Sarcomas

Ewing's sarcomas are characterized by fusion genes that encode for transcription factors regulating a number of genes; among these the IGFBP3 gene has been found downregulated by the fusion protein. IGFBP3 regulates the IGF1/IGF1R pathway by interacting with IGF1, and the recombinant IGFBP3 inhibits the proliferation of ES cells and promote apoptosis in Ewing's sarcoma cell lines (8). With this strong biological rationale, phase I and II trials of IGF1R Ab are underway, and preliminary results suggest 40% to 50% rates of tumor control in patients with refractory diseases in very preliminary results (53). Despite its rarity (incidence <3/1,000,000/year) several clinical trials have been initiated with IGF1R antibodies in this tumor.

RANK Ligand Antibody in Giant Cell Tumor of the Bone

Giant cell tumor of the bone is a rare primary neoplastic lesion of the bone, most often with a locoregional behavior but occasionally causing metastases. Giant cell growth is promoted by a complex interaction between the reactive cell environment and the tumor cells, though a RANKL/RANK paracrine pathway. Very limited agents have antitumor activity in this disease. In a trial reported at ASCO 2008, denosumab, an anti-RANKL Ab showed impressive antitumor activity, promoting metabolic response, bone reconstruction, and reduction of the number of size of the metastasis in 85% of patients in a small cohort of patients (54).

Imatinib in Chordoma

Chordoma cells express PDGFR at the cell surface in an activated phosphorylated form (55). Imatinib was tested in this disease and was found capable of inducing prolonged stabilization in some patients (55). A clinical trial exploring a combination with cytotoxic (CDDP) is underway.

Molecular Targeted Agents: Empirical Approaches

Although a growing numbers of sarcomas exhibit molecular alterations on proteins whose function can be modulated, the majority of subsets still has not yet a druggable "driver" molecular alteration. In these cases, targeting a biological pathway shared by different histotypes can still be a proposed strategy. Trials exploring inhibitors of mTOR, of VEGFR, and modulators of heat shock proteins can be grouped within such an empirical approach.

Estrogens Antagonists and Imatinib in Desmoids Tumors

Desmoids tumors are infiltrating tumors composed of fibroblasts and myofibroblasts, which have a significant potential for local and locoregional relapses but which most often do not metastasize (56). Until recently, their biology was largely unknown and developments of agents have therefore followed empiric approaches or were guided by low levels of evidence. These tumors exhibit characteristic molecular alterations on the beta catenin and APC pathway: beta catenin mutations (18). Initially considered as a low-grade sarcoma, a significant proportion of these tumors may have a very prolonged indolent course, or even spontaneous regression, resulting in very heterogeneous treatment strategies in the literature. However, a proportion of these tumors will progress and ultimately may lead to patient death, in particular for tumors of the trunk (56). Several systemic treatments have a reported antitumor activity in this disease: NSAIDS, antiestrogens, low dose or standard dose cytotoxics, and more recently, imatinib (56), which has demonstrated antitumor activity in this disease with 15% response rates and a one-year PFS of 40% and 65% in the two reported trials (57). The biological mechanisms of the antitumor activity of imatinib in this disease remain unknown.

Inhibitors of mTOR

The mammalian target of rapamycin (mTOR) is a serine-theronine kinase playing a central role in several pathways involved in cancer progression, including functions such as survival, metabolism, proliferations, translation, ribosome biogenesis, and autophagy. Three inhibitors of mTOR are currently in clinical development: CCI-779 (temsirolimus), RAD-001 (everolimus), and AP23573-deforolimus

(Ariad Pharmaceuticals, Los Angeles, California). The most documented for the treatment of sarcomas is deforolimus with the initial results of a large Phase II trial being reported in 2006 by Chawla et al. (ASCO abstract) and completed this year by a phase study or an oral formulation of the same agent (58). In the initial trial with an IV formulation, the ORR was only 2.5% (5/193 evaluable patients), but clinical benefit (i.e., CR + PR + SD by RECIST criteria for more than four months) was observed for 54 patients (28%), confirming again (as for trabectedin) that objective response is probably not the most relevant end point to identify efficient drugs in sarcomas. This molecule is now under evaluation in a Phase 3 trial testing maintenance following response or stable disease in first to third line of treatment.

Agents Targeting Angiogenesis

Most of the currently available treatments targeting angiogenesis block VEGF (bevacizumab, VEGF-trap) or the VEGF receptors (tyrosine kinase inhibitors sunitinib, sorafenib). Several antiangiogenic agents have been reported to induce limited response rates but prolonged stabilizations beyond the reported rate of "active agents" reported in the EORTC database (59). Bevacizumab, a humanized monoclonal antibody to human VEGF, was combined in a Phase II trial with doxorubicin in chemotherapy-naïve patients with advanced sarcoma (59). Objective response rate was only 12%, close or similar to the usual doxorubicin single agent response rate, and toxicity was found substantial since 6 of 17 patients experienced grade ≥2 cardiac toxicity.

Several small molecule tyrosine kinase inhibitors targeting angiogenesis are currently in clinical development, some of them in patients with advanced STS. A Phase II trial with VEGFR tyrosine kinase inhibitor GW786034 (pazopanib) has completed accrual in patients with advanced STS, stratified for histological subtypes (leiomyosarcoma, liposarcomas, synovial sarcomas, and others). Antitumor activity was observed with a median PFS beyond that of active agents according to the EORTC model (60) for all subtypes but liposarcomas, with responses in synovial sarcomas and leiomyosarcomas and four months PFS >40% for all subgroups but LPS; some patients are still experiencing prolonged PFS 30+ months after initiation of the treatment (60). Similar encouraging results have been reported with sorafenib and sunitinib in similar Phase II trials enrolling patients in different strata according to histotypes.

GIST AND TYROSINE KINASE INHIBITORS: A MODEL OF TARGETED CHEMOTHERAPY FOR SOLID TUMORS

GIST is the most frequent sarcoma of the GI tract. These tumors that derive from the precursors of the interstitial cells of Cajal may occur anywhere in the GI tract, but most often from the stomach and small intestine (12). Their incidence is estimated to be approximately 1.5/100,000/year (61). Approximately 95% of GISTs are CD117/KIT positive in immunohistochemistry (IHC). In 1998, Hirota et al. identified an activating mutation in the *KIT* gene, which encodes for the stem cell factor (SCF) receptor (10), and it is now recognized that 75% to 80% of GIST harbor a mutation of

the *KIT* gene (12). These mutations are located mainly to exons 11 and 9 (close to 2/3 and 10% respectively), mutations of exons 13, 14, and 17 being infrequent (0.5–1% respectively) (12). More recently, a subset of GIST with no KIT mutations was found to be driven by an activating mutation in the gene encoding for PDGFRA (11). These are present in 5% to 7% of advanced GIST, but may be more frequent in localized forms, and are mutually exclusive with KIT mutations, leaving approximately 12% to 15% of GIST with no identified mutation. The latter are observed particularly in pediatric forms, NF1, and Carney-associated forms. Mutations of KIT and PDGFR have been found in biopsies of early stage GIST, and more recently in the incidental forms found in 30% of normal individuals in autopsy series (12).

In 2008, surgery remains the only potentially curative treatment for patients with localized GIST (21): optimal surgery of a primary GIST requests complete excision of the tumor without rupture in order to avoid seeding of tumor cells, usually in the peritoneal cavity. Several prognostic factors have been identified in patients with localized GIST, two of them are the basis for the most common prognostic classification: the size of the primary tumor and the mitotic rate assessed per 50 high power fields. More recently, the primary tumor site and possibly the nature of mutations have also been found to influence the outcome of these patients and will likely soon be integrated for treatment decision purposes (62–64). In 2009, adjuvant imatinib was approved by US and EU health autorities for GIST with a substantial risk of relapse.

Conversely, in advanced disease, surgery has no established role yet, even though short-term remissions can be observed following complete resection of metastases (21,61,65). In advanced stages, imatinib mesylate (IM) 400 mg/day is therefore the standard upfront treatment (66–69). The median time to progression under imatinib therapy is two years, with 5% of patients exhibiting primary resistance whereas the majority of patients will be developing secondary resistance, either early within one year or later (66–69). At progression, imatinib 800 mg/day enables transient tumor control in 30% to 35% of the patients with a median PFS of four months (70). Following the report of the meta-analysis of the two randomized studies comparing imatinib 400 mg/day to 800 mg/day, the dose of imatinib 800 mg/day is now recognized to induce a longer PFS than 400 mg/day in patients with exon 9 mutation, and this dose is now recommended as the standard first-line treatment in the ESMO 2008 guideline (21,23,71). Treatment interruption in advanced setting associated with a median PFS of 6 months as demonstrated in the BFR14 trial, in which imatinib interruption was randomized vs continuation at 1 year and 3 years (69). Even though most patients responded again upon treatment reintroduction, the impact of treatment interruption on OS remains unknown. In 2006, sunitinib malate was approved for patients failing imatinib therapy because of toxicity or disease progression (72). These treatments enable tumor control, that is, CR-PR or SD in 8% and 60% of patients, respectively, in imatinib-resistant patients. Median PFS with sunitinib after imatinib failure is close to six months (72). Other agents targeting KIT and PDGFRA have shown very promising results, such as nilotinib, which was developed as a second-line therapy for IM-resistant chronic myeloid leukemia (CML) and seems to show a high efficiency in GISTs failing imatinib therapy, combined with a favorable toxicity profile (49,50). A phase I/II trial reported a CR/PR/SD rate of 65% with a median TTP of 23 weeks in imatinib- and sunitinib-resistant patients; a Phase III trial of nilotinib in imatinib (IM)-resistant GIST has recently completed accrual.

The role of imatinib in the adjuvant setting is currently under active investigation in four trials in Europe, United States, and Japan comparing one year adjuvant imatinib 400 mg/day versus placebo (ACOSOG-Z9001), two years adjuvant imatinib 400 mg/day versus no treatment (EORTC 62024), one year adjuvant imatinib 400 mg/day versus three years (SSG/AIO), one year adjuvant imatinib 400 mg/day versus six months (Japanese trial). These trials investigate the role of imatinib versus placebo after complete excision in patients classified as having a larger than 3 cm tumor (ACOSOG) and in patients with GIST of the intermediate to high risk of relapse (EORTC, SSG/AIO, Japanese group). In the latter group, the long-term risk of relapse is in the range of 60% to 70%. The preliminary results of the ACOSOG trial presented at ASCO 2007 (73) showed a dramatic reduction of the risk of relapse; whether adjuvant imatinib prevents or delays relapse is unknown; the impact of adjuvant treatment on the response to imatinib at the time of metastatic relapse is neither known. Conversely, the identification of groups of patients with a >85% risk of relapse (60) prompts the discussion of a more prolonged (five years, lifelong?) treatment with imatinib in the adjuvant setting, given the results of the BFR14 trial.

BONE SARCOMAS

Bone sarcomas include a wide variety of histological subtypes and are 10-fold less frequent than STSs. Osteogenic sarcomas and Ewing's sarcomas (Ewing family of tumors, EFTs) are the most frequent histotypes, followed by chondrosarcomas (74–77). Osteogenic sarcoma have an overall incidence of two to three new cases/1,000,000/year and occur mostly between the ages of 10 and 30. They occur most often in the metaphysis of a long bones, in the lower femur or upper tibia; iliac bone, vertebrae, or craniofacial bones lesions are observed most often in older adults patients (76). EFT of the bone is the not only the second most common primary malignant bone cancer in children and adolescents, but it is also seen in adults up to 70. In all, 20% of patients have EFT of the pelvic bones, 50% show extremity tumors; 20% originate from soft tissues, in particular in adults. Chondrosarcomas represent the third group of malignant bone tumors and are observed most often in adults.

Diagnosis

Bone tumors are revealed most often by pain and swelling, with bone radiographs showing highly suspect osteolytic lesions, sometimes with extraosseous bone formation. At this stage, referral to an expert center is highly advised. The primary tumor must be evaluated by plain radiographs in two planes. Magnetic resonance imaging (MRI) for long bones with CT scans for axial and craniofacial lesions should be performed before biopsy when the diagnosis is suspected. The whole involved bone as well as

the adjacent joints must be analyzed on the MRI and/or CT scan.

Biopsy is mandatory for definitive diagnosis and should be performed only after a multidisciplinary assessment of the lesion, with the pathologist, the surgeon, and the radiologist. Inappropriate biopsies reduce the possibilities for limb salvage and cure. By definition, the malignant cell population of an osteogenic sarcoma produces osteoïd tissue. In more than 80% of the cases, osteogenic sarcoma are high-grade malignancies; different histological subtypes are distinguished (osteoblastic, chondroblastic, and fibroblastic) but these are currently managed similarly. Conversely, low-grade osteosarcomas, in particular periosteal, parosteal, or intramedullary low-grade osteosarcomas, have a distinct prognosis and are generally treated without systemic treatment (76). EFTs are small, blue round-cell tumors, expressing CD99 (MIC2)-positive, and all are high-grade malignancies. All EFTs, from bone or from the soft tissues and organs, share a common gene rearrangement involving the EWS gene on chromosome 22. In most cases, a reciprocal translocation t(11;22)(q24;q12) is found, but t(21;22)(q22;q12) and others may also occur (78).

Systemic staging should include chest X-rays, a CT scan of the thorax, abdomen, and pelvis and a radionuclide bone scan; in case of secondary bone lesions, X-rays, MRI, or CT scans of affected areas are recommended. In EFTs, bone marrow aspirates and biopsies taken at sites distant from the primary tumor are recommended.

There are no specific tumor markers for bone sarcoma [alkaline phosphatase (AP) and LDH are nonspecific]. A biological evaluation of liver and renal function, blood cell count, evaluation of LVEF using either radionuclide ventriculography or echocardiography is standard practice. Collection and storage of sperm before the initiation of treatment is recommended for male patients of reproductive age.

Treatment
Osteogenic Sarcomas

Patients with osteogenic sarcoma should be treated in specialized centers where therapy is usually given within prospective multi-institutional trials. Curative treatment for high-grade osteogenic sarcoma consists of surgery and chemotherapy.

Two randomized trials have demonstrated that adjuvant and/or neoadjuvant systemic chemotherapy of high-grade osteosarcoma increases disease-free survival probabilities from only 10% to 20% to more than 50% (76,77). Adjuvant or neoadjuvant chemotherapy have been reported to be similarly effective, in a small size randomized trial (79,80), as well as in the different large prospective trials reported to date (78,81,82). The goal of surgery is the complete removal of the tumor (including the biopsy tract) with the aim to preserve limb function. Radiotherapy has a limited role and is generally reserved for inoperable situations and for specific sites such as the craniofacial sites, which are generally associated with a higher risk of locoregional relapses (83).

Active cytotoxic agents in osteogenic sarcomas include doxorubicin, cisplatin, ifosfamide, and high-dose methotrexate with leucovorin rescue for children and adolescents (79–85). The optimal combination is currently investigated in multicentric trials. Dose intensification of dose dense regimens with hematopoietic growth factors have so far failed to improve survival (82). Recently, muramyl tripeptide (MTPPE) added to chemotherapy was found to yield an improved OS in a single randomized trial (86). Histological response to preoperative chemotherapy is a major prognostic information, along with proximal extremity or axial tumor site, large tumor volume, elevated serum ALP or LDH, and foremost detectable primary metastases (85). It is however not demonstrated whether altering postoperative chemotherapy in poor responders improves outcomes. Low-grade central and parosteal osteogenic sarcoma are treated by surgery only. Importantly, the conclusions obtained from multidisciplinary treatment principles were generated in children and young adults with high-grade central osteogenic sarcoma. The applicability of these observations for extraosseous osteogenic sarcoma is unknown and these are often managed like STSs without adjuvant or neoadjuvant chemotherapy if the primary tumor is deemed resectable. In this case, adjuvant radiotherapy may be proposed. Similarly, the role of chemotherapy has not been defined for craniofacial osteosarcoma.

A curative approach should also be undertaken for primary metastatic osteogenic sarcoma as for localized disease; surgical removal of all metastatic lesions must however be performed. Twenty percent of all patients with osteogenic sarcoma with lung metastasis and close to 30% of those who achieve a complete surgical remission become long-term survivors (87). The prognosis is much less favorable for patients with bone metastasis. In the case of recurrence, the prognosis is poor with long-term survival under 20%. Patients with recurrent osteogenic sarcoma to the lung with completely potentially resectable disease should be considered as curable, and complete removal of all metastases should be attempted whenever possible. There is no standard regimen for the treatment of relapsing osteosarcoma, even though the addition of chemotherapy was associated with an improved outcome in some studies (88).

Ewing Family of Tumors

In EFT, multidisciplinary treatments including combination chemotherapy and surgery and/or radiotherapy also represent the standard of care (78). The ongoing clinical trials include most often six cycles of initial chemotherapy after biopsy, followed by local therapy and another six to eight cycles of chemotherapy usually applied at three-week intervals. The most active agents are cyclophosphamide, ifosfamide, vincristine, dactinomycin, and etoposide. Most regimens include four or more of these agents, with at least one alkylating agent (78,89–91). Recently a dose dense regimen given at two weeks intervals was reported to improve OS. Following neoadjuvant treatment, complete surgery, where feasible, is regarded as the best modality for achieving local control. Radiotherapy should be applied if radical surgery is impossible, and in the adjuvant setting if complete histological response is not achieved. Radiotherapy is applied at doses of 40 to 45 Gy for microscopic residues and 50 to 60 Gy for macroscopic disease with 1.8 to 2 Gy fractions (92).

Patients with metastatic EFT receive the same treatment as for localized disease with appropriate local treatment of metastases, with surgery and/or radiotherapy (78). Two groups of patients should be distinguished: those with lung only metastases and those with bone or bone marrow metastases, with a much worse prognosis. The EuroEwing trial is currently assessing the value of more intensive, high-dose chemotherapy approaches, followed by autologous stem cell rescue in the first group of patients. Patients with bone or bone marrow metastases are deemed incurable (93). Chemotherapy regimens in relapsing EFT are not standardized and are commonly based on topoisomerase inhibitors (topotecan or irinotecan) (94). As mentioned above, several trials are also investigating the role of anti-IGF1R antibody treatment in second or more line settings with encouraging preliminary results.

CONCLUSIONS

Sarcomas represent a family of cancers with heterogeneous histological and molecular patterns. Multidisciplinary management, in particular proper diagnostic procedures, surgery by an expert physician, and adequate systemic treatments are essential from the very first steps of the management of patients. Advances in the molecular characterization of these tumors have led to the introduction of effective targeted treatment strategies, as shown in GIST using imatinib. Other examples of targeted treatment on driver mutations in connective tissue tumors are now being developed.

REFERENCES

1. Clark MA, Fisher C, Judson I et al. Soft-tissue sarcomas in adults. N Engl J Med 2005; 353: 701–11.
2. Toro JR, Travis LB, Wu HJ et al. Incidence patterns of soft tissue sarcomas, regardless of primary site, in the surveillance, epidemiology and end results program, 1978–2001: An analysis of 26,758 cases. Int J Cancer 2006; 119: 2922–30.
3. Fletcher CD. The evolving classification of soft tissue tumours: an update based on the new WHO classification. Histopathology 2006; 48: 3–12.
4. Helman LJ, Meltzer P. Mechanisms of sarcoma development. Nat Rev Cancer 2003; 3: 685–94.
5. Mitelman F, Johansson B, Mertens F. The impact of translocations and gene fusions on cancer causation. Nat Rev Cancer 2007; 7: 233–45.
6. Coindre JM, Terrier P, Bui NB et al. Prognostic factors in adult patients with locally controlled soft tissue sarcoma. A study of 546 patients from the French Federation of Cancer Centers Sarcoma Group. J Clin Oncol 1996; 14: 869–77.
7. Coindre JM, Terrier P, Guillou L et al. Predictive value of grade for metastasis development in the main histologic types of adult soft tissue sarcomas: a study of 1240 patients from the French Federation of Cancer Centers Sarcoma Group. Cancer 2001; 91: 1914–26.
8. Prieur A, Tirode F, Cohen P et al. EWS/FLI-1 silencing and gene profiling of Ewing cells reveal downstream oncogenic pathways and a crucial role for repression of insulin-like growth factor binding protein 3. Mol Cell Biol 2004; 24: 7275–83.
9. McArthur G. Dermatofibrosarcoma protuberans: recent clinical progress. Ann Surg Oncol 2007; 14: 2876–86.
10. Hirota S, Isozaki K, Moriyama Y et al. Gain-of-function mutations of c-kit in human gastrointestinal stromal tumors. Science 1998; 279: 577–80.

11. Heinrich MC, Corless CL, Duensing A et al. PDGFRA activating mutations in gastrointestinal stromal tumors. Science 2003; 299: 708–10.

12. Corless CL, Fletcher JA, Heinrich MC. Biology of gastrointestinal stromal tumors. J Clin Oncol 2004; 22: 3813–25.

13. Biegel JA, Rousseau-Merck MF, Fiette L et al. Chromosome mechanisms and INI1 inactivation in human and mouse rhabdoid tumors. Cancer Genet Cytogenet 2005; 157: 127–33.

14. Korf BR. Diagnosis and management of neurofibromatosis type 1. Curr Neurol Neurosci Rep 2001; 1: 162–7.

15. Sirvent N, Coindre JM, Maire G et al. Detection of MDM2-CDK4 amplification by fluorescence in situ hybridization in 200 paraffin-embedded tumor samples: utility in diagnosing adipocytic lesions and comparison with immunohistochemistry and real-time PCR. Am J Surg Pathol 2007; 31: 1476–89.

16. Italiano A, Cardot N, Dupré F et al. Gains and complex rearrangements of the 12q13-15 chromosomal region in ordinary lipomas: the "missing link" between lipomas and liposarcomas? Int J Cancer 2007; 121: 308–15.

17. Idbaih A, Coindre JM, Derré J et al. Myxoid malignant fibrous histiocytoma and pleomorphic liposarcoma share very similar genomic imbalances. Lab Invest 2005; 85: 176–81.

18. Kotiligam D, Lazar AJ, Pollock RE et al. Desmoid tumor: a disease opportune for molecular insights. Histol Histopathol 2008; 23: 117–26.

19. Casali PG, Jost L, Sleijfer S et al. ESMO Guidelines Working Group. Soft tissue sarcomas: ESMO clinical recommendations for diagnosis, treatment and follow-up. Ann Oncol 2008; 19(Suppl 2): ii89–93.

20. Ray-Coquard I, Thiesse P, Ranchere-Vince D et al. Conformity to clinical practice guidelines, multidisciplinary management and outcome of treatment for soft tissue sarcomas. Ann Oncol 2004; 15: 307–15.

21. Casali PG, Jost L, Reichardt P et al. ESMO Guidelines Working Group. Gastrointestinal stromal tumors: ESMO clinical recommendations for diagnosis, treatment and follow-up. Ann Oncol 2008; 19(Suppl 2): ii35–8.

22. Ray-Coquard I, Ranchere-Vince D, Thiesse P et al. Evaluation of core needle biopsy as a substitute to open biopsy in the diagnosis of soft-tissue masses. Eur J Cancer 2003; 39: 2021–5.

23. Demetri GD, Benjamin RS, Blanke CD et al. NCCN Task Force. NCCN Task Force report: management of patients with gastrointestinal stromal tumor (GIST)—update of the NCCN clinical practice guidelines. J Natl Compr Canc Netw 2007; 5(Suppl 2): S1–29, quiz S30.

24. Yang JC, Rosenberg SA. Surgery for adult patients with soft tissue sarcomas. Semin Oncol 1989; 16: 289–96.

25. Hohenberger P, Wysocki WM. Neoadjuvant treatment of locally advanced soft tissue sarcoma of the limbs: which treatment to choose? Oncologist 2008; 13: 175–86.

26. Issels RD, Lindner LH, Wust P et al. Regional hyperthermia (RHT) improves response and survival when combined with systemic chemotherapy in the management of locally advanced, high grade soft tissue sarcomas (STS) of the extremities, the body wall and the abdomen: a phase III randomised pros. J Clin Oncol (ASCO Annual Meeting Proceedings Part I) 2007; 25(18S June 20 Suppl): 10009.

27. Grünhagen DJ, de Wilt JH, ten Hagen TL et al. Technology insight: utility of TNF-alpha-based isolated limb perfusion to avoid amputation of irresectable tumors of the extremities. Nat Clin Pract Oncol 2006; 3: 94–103.

28. Bonvalot S, Laplanche A, Lejeune F et al. Limb salvage with isolated perfusion for soft tissue sarcoma: could less TNF-alpha be better? Ann Oncol 2005; 16: 1061–8.

29. Pisters PW, Harrison LB, Woodruff JM et al. A prospective randomized trial of adjuvant brachytherapy in the management of low-grade soft tissue sarcomas of the extremity and superficial trunk. J Clin Oncol 1994; 12: 1150–5.

30. Yang JC, Chang AE, Baker AR et al. Randomized prospective study of the benefit of adjuvant radiation therapy in the treatment of soft tissue sarcomas of the extremity. J Clin Oncol 1998; 16: 197–203.

31. O'Sullivan B, Davis AM, Turcotte R et al. Preoperative versus postoperative radiotherapy in soft-tissue sarcoma of the limbs: a randomised trial. Lancet 2002; 359: 2235–41.

32. Kamada T, Tsujii H, Tsuji H et al. Working Group for the Bone and Soft Tissue Sarcomas. Efficacy and safety of carbon ion radiotherapy in bone and soft tissue sarcomas. J Clin Oncol 2002; 20: 4466–71.

33. Bramwell VH, Anderson D, Charette ML. Doxorubicin-based chemotherapy for the palliative treatment of adult patients with locally advanced or metastatic soft-tissue sarcoma: a meta-analysis and clinical practice guideline. Sarcoma 2000; 4: 103–12.

34. Sarcoma Meta-analysis Collaboration. Adjuvant chemotherapy for localize resectable soft-tissue sarcoma of adults: meta-analysis of individual data. Lancet 1997; 350: 1647–54.

35. Frustaci S, Gherlinzoni F, De PA et al. Adjuvant chemotherapy for adult soft tissue sarcomas of the extremities and girdles: results of the Italian randomized cooperative trial. J Clin Oncol 2001; 19: 1238–47.

36. Woll PJ, van Glabbeke M, Hohenberger P et al. Adjuvant chemotherapy with doxorubicin and ifosfamide in resected soft tissue sarcoma: interim analysis of a randomized phase III trial. Proc Am Soc Clin Oncol 2007: abstract 10008.

37. Gortzak E, Azzarelli A, Buesa J et al. E.O.R.T.C. Soft Tissue Bone Sarcoma Group and the National Cancer Institute of Canada Clinical Trials Group/Canadian Sarcoma Group. A randomised phase II study on neo-adjuvant chemotherapy for "high-risk" adult soft-tissue sarcoma. Eur J Cancer 2001; 37: 1096–103.

38. Van Glabekke M, van Oosterom AT, Oosterhuis JW et al. Prognostic factors for the outcome of chemotherapy in advanced soft tissue sarcoma: an analysis of 2,185 patients treated with anthracycline-containing first-line regimens—a European Organization for Research and Treatment of Cancer Soft Tissue and Bone Sarcoma Group Study. J Clin Oncol 1999; 17: 150–7.

39. Blay JY, van Glabbeke M, Verweij J et al. Advanced soft-tissue sarcoma: a disease that is potentially curable for a subset of patients treated with chemotherapy. Eur J Cancer 2003; 39: 64–9.

40. Bay JO, Ray-Coquard I, Fayette J et al. Docetaxel and gemcitabine combination in 133 advanced soft-tissue sarcomas: a retrospective analysis. Int J Cancer 2006; 119: 706–11.

41. Maki RG, Wathen JK, Patel SR et al. Randomized phase II study of gemcitabine and docetaxel compared with gemcitabine alone in patients with metastatic soft tissue sarcomas: results of sarcoma alliance for research through collaboration study 002. J Clin Oncol 2007; 25: 2755–63.

42. Duffaud F, Bui BN, Penel N et al. A FNCLCC French Sarcoma Group—GETO multicenter randomized phase II study of gemcitabine (G) versus gemcitabine and docetaxel (G+D) in patients with metastatic or relapsed leiomyosarcoma (LMS). Clin Oncol 2008; 26(May 20 suppl): abstract 10511.

43. Fata F, O'Reilly E, Ilson D et al. Paclitaxel in the treatment of patients with angiosarcoma of the scalp or face. Cancer 1999; 86: 2034–7.

44. Penel N et al. Weekly paclitaxel for metastatic or unresectable angiosarcoma. Results of a FNCLCC—French Sarcoma Group Phase II trial, the ANGIOTAX Study. J Clin Oncol 2008; 26: 5269–74.

45. Le Cesne A, Blay JY, Judson I et al. Phase II study of ET-743 in advanced soft tissue sarcomas: a European Organisation for the Research and Treatment of Cancer (EORTC) Soft Tissue

and Bone Sarcoma Group Trial. J Clin Oncol 2005; 23: 576–84.

46. Grosso F, Jones RL, Demetri GD et al. Efficacy of trabectedin (ecteinascidin-743) in advanced pretreated myxoid liposarcomas: a retrospective study. Lancet 2007; 8: 595–602.

47. Samuels BL, Rushing D, Chawla SP et al. Randomized phase II study of trabectedin (ET-743) given by two different dosing schedules in patients (pts) with leiomyosarcomas (LMS) or liposarcomas (LPS) refractory to conventional doxorubicin and ifosfamide chemotherapy. J Clin Oncol (ASCO Meeting Abstracts) 2004; 22: 9000.

48. Leahy M, Ray-Coquard I, Verweij J et al. Brostallicin, an agent with potential activity in metastatic soft tissue sarcoma: a phase II study from the EORTC soft tissue and bone sarcoma group. Eur J Cancer 2007; 43: 308–15.

49. Maki RG, Awan RA, Dixon RH et al. Differential sensitivity to imatinib of 2 patients with metastatic sarcoma arising from dermatofibrosarcoma protuberans. Int J Cancer 2002; 100: 623–6.

50. Blay JY, El Sayadi H, Thiesse P et al. Complete response to imatinib in relapsing pigmented villonodular synovitis/tenosynovial giant cell tumor (PVNS/TGCT). Ann Oncol 2008; 19: 821–2.

51. Blay J, Le Cesne A, Whelan J et al. Gefitinib in second line treatment of metastatic or locally advanced synovial sarcoma expressing HER1: a phase II trial of EORTC Soft Tissue and Bone Sarcoma Group. J Clin Oncol (2006 ASCO Annual Meeting Proceedings Part I) 2006; 24(18S June 20 Suppl): 9517.

52. Pink D, Lindner T, Mrozek A et al. Harm or benefit of hormonal treatment in metastatic low-grade endometrial stromal sarcoma: single center experience with 10 cases and review of the literature. Gynecol Oncol 2006; 101: 464–9.

53. Hidalgo M, Tirado Gomez M, Lewis N et al. A phase I study of MK-0646, a humanized monoclonal antibody against the insulin-like growth factor receptor type 1 (IGF1R) in advanced solid tumor patients in a q2 wk schedule. J Clin Oncol 2008; 26(May 20 suppl): abstract 3520.

54. Thomas D, Chawla SP, Skubitz K et al. Denosumab treatment of giant cell tumor of bone: Interim analysis of an open-label phase II study. J Clin Oncol 2008; 26(May 20 suppl): abstract 10500.

55. Casali PG, Stacchiotti S, Sangalli C et al. Chordoma. Curr Opin Oncol 2007; 19: 367–70.

56. Janinis J, Patriki M, Vini L et al. The pharmacological treatment of aggressive fibromatosis: a systematic review. Ann Oncol 2003; 14: 181–90.

57. Heinrich MC, McArthur GA, Demetri GD et al. Clinical and molecular studies of the effect of imatinib on advanced aggressive fibromatosis (desmoid tumor). J Clin Oncol 2006; 24: 1195–203.

58. Sabatini DM. mTOR and cancer: insights into a complex relationship. Nat Rev Cancer 2006; 6: 729–34.

59. D'Adamo DR, Anderson SE, Albritton K et al. Phase II study of doxorubicin and bevacizumab for patients with metastatic soft-tissue sarcomas. J Clin Oncol 2005; 23: 7135–42.

60. Sleijfer S, le Cesne A, Scurr M et al. Phase II study of pazopanib (GW786034) in patients (pts) with relapsed or refractory soft tissue sarcoma (STS): EORTC 62043. J Clin Oncol 2007; 25: 552s, abstract 10031.

61. Nilsson B, Bumming P, Meis-Kindblom JM et al. Gastrointestinal stromal tumors: the incidence, prevalence, clinical course, and prognostication in the preimatinib mesylate era—a population-based study in western Sweden. Cancer 2005; 103: 821–9.

62. Blay JY, Bonvalot S, Casali P et al. Consensus meeting for the management of gastrointestinal stromal tumors. Report of the GIST consensus conference of 20-21 March 2004, under the auspices of ESMO. Ann Oncol 2005; 16: 566–78.

63. Fletcher CD, Berman JJ, Corless C et al. Diagnosis of gastrointestinal stromal tumors: a consensus approach. Hum Pathol 2002; 33: 459–65.

64. Miettinen M, Lasota J. Gastrointestinal stromal tumors: pathology and prognosis at different sites. Semin Diagn Pathol 2006; 23: 70–83.

65. Raut CP, Posner M, Desai J et al. Surgical management of advanced gastrointestinal stromal tumors after treatment with targeted systemic therapy using kinase inhibitors. J Clin Oncol 2006; 24: 2325–31.

66. Demetri GD, von MM, Blanke CD et al. Efficacy and safety of imatinib mesylate in advanced gastrointestinal stromal tumors. N Engl J Med 2002; 347: 472–80.

67. Verweij J, Casali PG, Zalcberg J et al. Progression-free survival in gastrointestinal stromal tumours with high-dose imatinib: randomised trial. Lancet 2004; 364: 1127–34.

68. Blanke CD, Rankin C, Demetri GD et al. Phase III randomized, intergroup trial assessing imatinib mesylate at two dose levels in patients with unresectable or metastatic gastrointestinal stromal tumors expressing the kit receptor tyrosine kinase: S0033. Clin Oncol 2008; 26: 626–32.

69. Blay JY, Le Cesne A, Ray-Coquard I et al. Prospective multicentric randomized phase III study of imatinib in patients with advanced gastrointestinal stromal tumors comparing interruption versus continuation of treatment beyond 1 year: the French Sarcoma Group. J Clin Oncol 2007; 25: 1107–13.

70. Zalcberg JR, Verweij J, Casali PG et al. Outcome of patients with advanced gastro-intestinal stromal tumours crossing over to a daily imatinib dose of 800 mg after progression on 400 mg. Eur J Cancer 2005; 41: 1751–7.

71. Debiec-Rychter M, Dumez H, Judson I et al. Use of c-KIT/PDGFRA mutational analysis to predict the clinical response to imatinib in 575 patients with advanced gastrointestinal stromal tumours entered on phase I and II studies of the EORTC Soft Tissue and Bone Sarcoma Group. Eur J Cancer 2004; 40: 689–95.

72. Demetri GD, van Oosterom AT, Garrett CR et al. Efficacy and safety of sunitinib in patients with advanced gastrointestinal stromal tumour after failure of imatinib: a randomised controlled trial. Lancet 2006; 368: 1329–38.

73. DeMatteo R, Owzar K, Maki R et al. the American College of Surgeons Oncology Group (ACOSOG) Intergroup Adjuvant GIST Study Team. Adjuvant imatinib mesylate after resection of localised, primary gastrointestinal stromal tumour: a randomised, double-blind, placebo-controlled trial. Lancet 2009; 373: 1097–104.

74. Arndt CA, Crist WM. Common musculoskeletal tumors of childhood and adolescence. N Engl J Med 1999; 341: 342–52.

75. Fletcher CDM, Unni KK, Mertens F, eds. WHO Classification of Tumours. Pathology and Genetics of Tumours of Soft Tissue and Bone. Lyon: IARC Press, 2002.

76. Link MP, Goorin AM, Miser AW et al. The effect of adjuvant chemotherapy on relapse-free survival in patients with osteosarcoma of the extremity. N Engl J Med 1986; 314: 1600–6.

77. Eilber F, Giuliano A, Eckardt J et al. Adjuvant chemotherapy for osteosarcoma: a randomized prospective trial. J Clin Oncol 1987; 5: 21–6.

78. Bernstein M, Kovar H, Paulussen M et al. Ewing's sarcoma family of tumors: current management. Oncologist 2006; 11: 503–19.

79. Goorin AM, Schwartzentruber DJ, Devidas M et al. Presurgical chemotherapy compared with immediate surgery and adjuvant chemotherapy for nonmetastatic osteosarcoma: Pediatric Oncology Group Study POG-8651. J Clin Oncol 2003; 21: 1574–80.

80. Bramwell VH, Burgers M, Sneath R et al. A comparison of two short intensive adjuvant chemotherapy regimens in operable osteosarcoma of limbs in children and young adults: the first study of the European Osteosarcoma Intergroup. J Clin Oncol 1992; 10: 1579–91.

81. Souhami RL, Craft AW, Van der Eijken JW et al. Randomised trial of two regimens of chemotherapy in operable

osteosarcoma: a study of the European Osteosarcoma Intergroup. Lancet 1997; 350: 911–17.

82. Lewis IJ, Nooij MA, Whelan J et al. Improvement in histologic response but not survival in osteosarcoma patients treated with intensified chemotherapy: a randomized phase III trial of the European Osteosarcoma Intergroup. J Natl Cancer Inst 2007; 99: 112–28.

83. Carrle D, Bielack SS. Current strategies of chemotherapy in osteosarcoma. Int Orthop 2006; 30: 445–51.

84. Grimer RJ, Cannon SR, Taminiau AM et al. Osteosarcoma over the age of forty. Eur J Cancer 2003; 39: 157–63.

85. Bielack SS, Kempf-Bielack B, Delling G et al. Prognostic factors in high-grade osteosarcoma of the extremities or trunk: an analysis of 1,702 patients treated on neoadjuvant cooperative osteosarcoma study group protocols. J Clin Oncol 2002; 20: 776–90.

86. Meyers PA, Schwartz CL, Krailo MD et al. Osteosarcoma: the addition of muramyl tripeptide to chemotherapy improves overall survival—a report from the Children's Oncology Group. J Clin Oncol 2008; 26: 633–8.

87. Ferrari S, Briccoli A, Mercuri M et al. Post-relapse survival in osteosarcoma of the extremities: prognostic factors for long-term survival. J Clin Oncol 2003; 21: 710–15.

88. Kempf-Bielack B, Bielack SS, Jürgens H et al. Osteosarcoma relapse after combined modality therapy: an analysis of unselected patients in the Cooperative Osteosarcoma Study Group (COSS). J Clin Oncol 2005; 23: 559–68.

89. Nesbit ME Jr, Gehan EA, Burgert EO et al. Multimodal therapy for the management of primary, nonmetastatic Ewing's sarcoma of bone: a long-term follow-up of the First Intergroup study. J Clin Oncol 1990; 8: 1664–74.

90. Burgert EO Jr, Nesbit ME, Garnsey LA et al. Multimodal therapy for the management of nonpelvic, localized Ewing's sarcoma of bone: intergroup study IESS-II. J Clin Oncol 1990; 8: 1514–24.

91. Grier HE, Krailo MD, Tarbell NJ et al. Addition of ifosfamide and etoposide to standard chemotherapy for Ewing's sarcoma and primitive neuroectodermal tumor of bone. N Engl J Med 2003; 348: 694–701.

92. Schuck A, Ahrens S, Paulussen M et al. Local therapy in localized Ewing tumors: results of 1058 patients treated in the CESS 81, CESS 86, and EICESS 92 trials. Int J Radiat Oncol Biol Phys 2003; 55: 168–77.

93. Paulussen M, Ahrens S, Craft AW. Ewing's tumors with primary lung metastases. Survival analysis of 114 (European Intergroup) Cooperative Ewing's Sarcoma Study patients. J Clin Oncol 1998; 16: 3044–52.

94. Wagner LM, McAllister N, Goldsby RE et al. Temozolomide and intravenous irinotecan for treatment of advanced Ewing Sarcoma. Pediatr Blood Cancer 2007; 48: 132–9.

12

Leukemias

Guido Marcucci, Meir Wetzler, John C. Byrd, Krzysztof Mrózek, and Clara D. Bloomfield

Leukemias are malignant hematopoietic disorders characterized by increased proliferation, extended survival, and/or disruption of differentiation of hematopoietic progenitors that result in clonal expansion of leukemic cells in the bone marrow, blood, or other tissues. The most common types of leukemia are acute myeloid leukemia (AML), acute lymphoblastic leukemia (ALL), chronic myelogenous leukemia (CML), and chronic lymphocytic leukemia (CLL), which differ with regard to the incidence, clinical presentation, disease course, and prognosis, as well as the underlying biology and cytogenetic and molecular genetic alterations (1–4).

INCIDENCE AND ETIOLOGY

The incidence and median age of patients at diagnosis of the four major leukemia types in the United States are presented in Table 12.1 (5). Although AML, CML, and CLL are predominantly adult diseases, with median age at presentation >65 years, most patients with ALL are children and adolescents, with median age at diagnosis of 13 years and 61% of the patients being diagnosed under the age of 20. For all leukemia types, the age-adjusted incidence is higher in men than in women, with the greatest difference in CLL (5.6 vs. 2.8/100,000/year) and the smallest in ALL (1.8 vs. 1.4/100,000/year). With the exception of ALL, the incidence of leukemias increases with age.

The etiology of leukemia is unknown in most cases. Risk factors for developing leukemia include heredity, radiation, chemical exposure, and chemotherapeutic drugs. The risk of developing acute leukemia (both ALL and AML) is increased in patients with constitutional chromosome aneuploidies such as +21 in Down and XXY in Klinefelter syndromes, and inherited diseases with excessive chromatin fragility, e.g., Bloom syndrome and ataxia telangiectasia, as well as neurofibromatosis and Schwachman–Diamond syndrome. Syndromes associated with particular types of leukemia include Fanconi anemia and Kostmann syndrome associated with AML and Langerhans cell histiocytosis with ALL (6). Germline mutations of the CEBPA and RUNX1 genes have also been shown to predispose the development of AML (7).

Large case–control studies showed that the risk ratio for first-degree relatives of CLL patients to have CLL was higher than for that for most other cancers (8). Approximately 8% to 10% of CLL patients have a first- or second-degree relative with CLL (9), and relatives of patients with CLL also seem to have a higher frequency of other lymphoproliferative disorders and auto-immune diseases (10,11). Patients with familial CLL do not seem to be genetically or clinically different from individuals with sporadic CLL. To date, only a single germline mutation in the DAPK gene has been convincingly shown to be related to familial predisposition in a single CLL family (12).

Exposure to chemicals including benzene, petroleum products, herbicides, pesticides, and tobacco smoking is associated with the risk of developing AML (13,14), whereas CLL is recognized as a service-related illness among Vietnam War veterans who were exposed to Agent Orange. Notably, the most common source of benzene exposure is cigarette smoking; smoking has been associated with 1.2 to 2.3 times increase in the incidence of AML (1,14).

Up to 10% of patients exposed to chemotherapy eventually develop therapy-associated AML (15). Alkylating agent–associated leukemias occur on average four to six years after exposure and present commonly with monosomies or deletions of the long arms of chromosomes 5 or 7. Topoisomerase II inhibitor–associated leukemias occur one to three years after exposure, and affected individuals often harbor balanced translocations, frequently involving band 11q23/MLL.

Warfare or occupational exposure to ionizing radiation predisposes to AML and ALL; CLL is the only leukemia type whose incidence is not increased following exposure to radiation. The risk of developing AML after therapeutic radiation may increase following exposure to alkylating agents (16,17).

ACUTE MYELOID LEUKEMIA

AML is currently categorized according to the World Health Organization classification, which uses the cutoff of ≥20% blasts for diagnosis (18). In this classification (Table 12.2), AMLs with certain recurrent cytogenetic aberrations are recognized as distinct subsets. In patients with t(8;21)(q22;q22), inv(16)(p13q22) or t(16;16)(p13;q22), or t(15;17)(q22;q12), the diagnosis of AML is made even with <20% marrow blasts. Characteristic morphologic findings such as the association of t(15;17) with increased promyeloblasts and inv(16)/t(16;16) with dysplastic eosinophils facilitate the recognition of these entities. In the recently updated 2008 classification, AMLs with certain submicroscopic genetic aberrations (i.e., CEBPA or NPM1 mutations) have been recognized as new provisional entities (Table 12.2). Other AMLs are grouped based on myelodysplasia-related changes, receipt of prior chemotherapy or radiotherapy, and the

Table 12.1 The Incidence and Median Patient Age at Diagnosis of the Four Major Leukemia Categories in the United States in 2001–2005

Type of leukemia	Median age at diagnosis (years)	Incidence[a] (M/F)	Estimated number of cases in 2008 (M/F)
AML	67	3.6 (4.5/2.9)	13,290 (7200/6090)
ALL	13	1.6 (1.8/1.4)	5,430 (3220/2210)
CML	66	1.5 (1.9/1.1)	4,830 (2,800/2,030)
CLL	72	4.0 (5.6/2.8)	15,110 (8750/6360)

[a]Age-adjusted incidence rate per 100,000 men and women per year.
Abbreviations: M, males; F, females.
Source: From Ref. 5.

Table 12.2 World Health Organization Classification of AML

AML with recurrent genetic abnormalities
  AML with t(8;21)(q22;q22); *RUNX1-RUNX1T1*
  AML with inv(16)(pl3.1q22) or t(16;16)(p13.1;q22); *CBFB-MYH11*
  Acute promyelocytic leukemia with t(15;17)(q22;q12); *PML-RARA*
  AML with t(9;11)(p22;q23); *MLLT3-MLL*
  AML with t(6;9)(p23;q34); *DEK-NUP214*
  AML with inv(3)(q21q26.2) or t(3;3)(q21;q26.2); *RPN1-EVI1*
  AML (megakaryoblastic) with t(1;22)(p13;q13); *RBM15-MKL1*
  AML with mutated NPM1
  AML with mutated CEBPA
AML with myelodysplasia-related changes
Therapy-related myeloid neoplasms
AML not otherwise specified
  AML with minimal differentiation
  AML without maturation
  AML with maturation
  Acute myelomonocytic leukemia
  Acute monoblastic and monocytic leukemia
  Acute erythroid leukemia
  Acute megakaryoblastic leukemia
  Acute basophilic leukemia
  Acute panmyelosis with myelofibrosis
Myeloid sarcoma
Myeloid proliferations related to Down syndrome
  Transient abnormal myelopoiesis
  Myeloid leukemia associated with Down syndrome

Source: From Ref. 18.

presence of myeloid sarcomas or Down syndrome. On the basis of clinical history, AML with multilineage dysplasia is subdivided into specific types with or without prior myelodysplastic syndromes (MDS). The remaining cases are classified based on morphology as AML not otherwise specified (18).

Clinical Presentation
Symptoms

At diagnosis, nearly half the patients report fatigue or weakness, anorexia, and weight loss. Patients often present with fever with or without an identifiable infection and symptoms or signs of abnormal hemostasis (bleeding, easy bruising) due to neutropenia and thrombocytopenia, respectively, from abnormal hematopoiesis. On occasion, bone pain, cough, headache, or diaphoresis may be present at diagnosis. Patients may rarely have symptomatic mass lesions located in the soft tissues, cranial or spinal dura, or other

organs. These masses, called myeloid sarcoma or chloroma, represent tumor growth of leukemic cells, and may present with or without marrow involvement. Although the initial approach to these manifestations may include local radiation therapy, systemic chemotherapy is required because most patients with myeloid sarcoma and no evidence of leukemia eventually develop marrow and blood involvement. This rare presentation is more common in patients with t(8;21).

Physical Findings

On physical examination, fever, splenomegaly, hepatomegaly, lymphadenopathy, sternal tenderness, and evidence of infection and hemorrhage are often found. Significant gastrointestinal bleeding and intrapulmonary and/or intracranial hemorrhages can occur because of disseminated intravascular coagulation, which most often associates with acute promyelocytic leukemia (APL), monocytic AML, or extreme degrees of leukocytosis. Infiltration of the gingivae, skin, soft tissues, or the meninges with leukemic blasts at diagnosis is characteristic of the monocytic subtypes and those with chromosomal abnormalities involving 11q23/*MLL*.

Hematologic Findings

AML is usually suspected from the study of the blood smear and confirmed with the examination of a marrow aspirate, which shows hypercellularity in most cases. Blast immunophenotyping shows surface antigens associated with myeloid differentiation (e.g., CD33, CD13). Laboratory evaluation often reveals normochromic normocytic anemia due to erythropoiesis failure or active bleeding because of concurrent thrombocytopenia. The median leukocyte count at presentation is about 15,000/μl. Between 25% and 40% of patients have counts <5000/μl, and 20% have counts >100,000/μl. Fewer than 5% have no detectable leukemic cells in the blood. Neutrophils, if present, may be functionally impaired and therefore fever should be treated aggressively with broad-spectrum antibacterial and antifungal drugs. Patients with high numbers of circulating blasts may abruptly develop signs of leukostasis (headache, confusion, and dyspnea), which requires immediate intervention with leukophoresis, cytoreductive chemotherapy, and eventually radiation therapy for central nervous system involvement. Thrombocytopenia is a common finding at diagnosis. Because quantitative and qualitative platelet dysfunction and/or concurrent infections may increase the likelihood of bleeding, platelet transfusions may be justified even with only moderately decreased platelet counts.

In about 50% of patients, serum uric acid levels were increased at presentation and can be worsened by the initiation of chemotherapy due to tumor lysis and may rapidly lead to uric acid nephropathy and renal failure. Therefore, presenting AML patients are usually given prophylaxis with allopurinol and hydration. Rasburicase (recombinant uric oxidase enzyme) may be used in patients allergic to allopurinol or unable to tolerate oral therapies or for the treatment of uric acid nephropathy. Finally, the presence in high concentrations of lysozyme, usually associated with monocytic differentiation, may lead to renal tubular dysfunction.

Prognostic Factors

To achieve long survival and/or cure, treated AML patients must achieve complete remission (19). Complete remission is defined as <5% blasts in the marrow, a blood neutrophil count ≥1000/μl, and a platelet count ≥100,000/μl following induction chemotherapy. Circulating blasts should be absent. Rare blasts detectable in blood during marrow regeneration should disappear on successive studies. Extramedullary leukemia should not be present.

Failure to achieve complete remission may be due to treatment-related toxicity and death or resistance to treatment. Many factors influence the likelihood of entering complete remission and remission duration. Older age is associated with a poorer prognosis likely because of its influence on the patient's ability to survive induction therapy, because of chronic and intercurrent co-morbid conditions, or because of chemoresistance mediated by multidrug resistance 1 efflux pump expression (20). Other factors that confer higher risk of resistance to therapy such as prior chemotherapy for an unrelated cancer, antecedent hematopoietic disorders, and/or presence of poor-risk cytogenetic abnormalities are also relatively common in older patients. Regardless of age, performance status and hyperleukocytosis (>100,000/μl) influence independently the ability to survive induction therapy and response to treatment (21).

Structural and numerical chromosome aberrations have been identified as one of the most important factors that influence the outcome of AML patients (Table 12.3) (22). Based on the presence or absence of recurrent chromosome aberrations, AML patients are assigned to a favorable, intermediate, or poor cytogenetic risk group. In cytogenetically normal patients (40–45% of the entire AML population) who lack any chromosome aberrations, submicroscopic genetic alterations should be used to refine outcome prediction (Table 12.4) (23). Internal tandem duplications (ITDs) within the juxtamembrane domain of the *FLT3* gene are detectable in 28% to 33% of the cytogenetically normal AML patients and predict poor outcome, especially if the *FLT3*-ITD/*FLT3*-wild-type allelic ratio is high (24). In addition to *FLT3*-ITD, *FLT3* point mutations have been discovered, but their prognostic significance remains unclear. Mutations of the *NPM1* gene are the most frequent in cytogenetically normal AML patients, reported in 46% to 62% (25). The presence of *NPM1* mutations is associated with a significantly improved outcome, especially in the absence of *FLT3*-ITD (26). Other less-frequent genetic abnormalities in cytogenetically normal AML patients have also been associated with better outcome, e.g., *CEBPA* mutations, or adverse outcome, e.g., the partial tandem duplication of the *MLL* gene (*MLL*-PTD), *WT1* mutations, and overexpression of the *BAALC*, *ERG*, or *MN1* genes (27–34).

Submicroscopic markers can also refine prognostication in patients with specific, prognostic chromosome aberrations. In the favorable subset of AML patients with t(8;21) or inv(16)/t(16;16) (collectively referred to as core-binding factor AML), mutations in the *KIT* gene have been shown to adversely affect the clinical outcome (33).

Treatment

Induction Therapy

Treatment of newly diagnosed AML patients is usually divided into two phases, induction and postremission management. Once induction treatment is completed and complete remission obtained, further consolidation therapy must be used to prolong survival and achieve cure. The initial induction chemotherapy and subsequent postremission treatment approaches are often chosen based on the patient's age and other clinical and genetic prognostic factors.

Standard induction chemotherapy regimens for patients younger than 60 years, without a history of antecedent hematologic diseases such as MDS or treatment-related AML, include a combination of cytarabine (cytosine arabinoside) and an anthracycline (21). Cytarabine at a dose of 100 to 200 mg/m²/day is usually administered as a continuous intravenous infusion for seven days. Attempts to escalate the dose of cytarabine during induction therapy resulted in higher mortality and did not translate to better complete remission rates. Anthracyclines (e.g., daunorubicin or idarubicin) are given intravenously on days 1 to 3 (the 7 and 3 regimen). Although several studies have been conducted to assess which of the anthracyclines may confer higher probability of disease response, this remains controversial (1). The addition of etoposide may improve remission duration.

After induction chemotherapy, the marrow is examined to determine the response. Approximately 70% of adults younger than 60 years with de novo AML achieve complete remission. The remaining patients fail to achieve complete remission because of death from treatment-related complications or resistant disease. Patients younger than 70 years who fail to attain complete remission after induction treatment should be considered for salvage regimens, which include high-dose cytarabine or novel therapeutic agents, although some patients could be considered

Table 12.3 Cytogenetic Risk Groups in AML

Cytogenetic risk group	Chromosome aberration
Favorable	t(8;21); inv(16)/t(16;16); t(15;17)
Intermediate	Normal karyotype; –Y, del(7q), del(9q), t(9;11); del(11q), isolated +8, +11, +21, del(20q)
Adverse	Complex karyotype; inv(3)/t(3;3); –7 t(6;9); t(6;11); t(11;19)(q23;p13.3); –5; del(5q)

Table 12.4 Molecular Prognostic Markers in Cytogentically Normal AML

Marker	Marker location	Prognostic impact
NPM1 mutations	5q35	Favorable
CEBPA mutation	19q13.1	Favorable
FLT3-ITD	13q12	Adverse
FLT3-TKD	13q12	Adverse
WT1 mutations	11p13	Adverse
MLL-PTD	11q23	Adverse
BAALC overexpression	8q22.3	Adverse
ERG overexpression	21q22.3	Adverse
MN1 overexpression	22q12.1	Adverse

Abbreviations: ITD, internal tandem duplication; TKD, point mutation of tyrosine kinase domain; PTD, partial tandem duplication.

immediately for an allogeneic stem-cell transplantation if an appropriate donor exists, especially if no circulating blasts are observed.

Supportive care of AML patients through a prolonged period of granulocytopenia and thrombocytopenia is critical to the success of therapy. AML clinical trials involving the use of recombinant hematopoietic growth factors have shown reduced median time to neutrophil recovery but no significant improvement in the outcome (34,35). The use of growth factors as supportive care for AML patients is therefore controversial, and, outside clinical trials, they should be administered according to published guidelines (36).

Multilumen right atrial catheters should be used in AML patients for administering intravenous medications, fluid, and transfusions, as well as for drawing blood. Platelet transfusions should be given to maintain a platelet count >10,000/μl to 20,000/μl. In febrile patients and during episodes of active bleeding or disseminated intravascular coagulation, it may be necessary to keep platelet counts at higher levels. Red blood cell transfusions should be administered to keep the hemoglobin level >8g/dl. Higher levels of hemoglobin should be targeted for patients with heavy bleeding, disseminated intravascular coagulation, or known history of cardiovascular disease. All blood products should be leukodepleted by filtration and irradiated to prevent serious side effects such as alloimmunization, fever, and transfusion-associated graft-versus-host disease. Cytomegalovirus-negative blood should be used in cytomegalovirus-seronegative patients who are potential candidates for allogeneic stem-cell transplantation.

Complications due to infections remain the major cause of morbidity and death during the treatment of AML. Prophylactic systemic administration of antibiotics may be considered based on institutional epidemiologic data. Prophylaxis to prevent oral candidiasis and herpetic infection (in herpes simplex virus antibody titer-positive patients) is recommended. Fever should be aggressively treated with early initiation of empirical broad-spectrum antibacterial and antifungal antibiotics (37).

Postremission Therapy

Induction of a first longlasting complete remission is critical to long-term disease-free survival of AML patients. However, without further therapy, virtually all patients experience relapse. Approaches to postremission therapy in AML are often based on age and other prognostic factors (38). For younger patients, most studies include intensive chemotherapy and autologous or allogeneic stem-cell transplantation.

High-dose cytarabine is more effective than standard-dose cytarabine based on the Cancer and Leukemia Group B (CALGB) experience (39). Multiple courses of high-dose cytarabine appear particularly effective in patients with core-binding factor AML and those with cytogenetically normal AML (40–43).

Allogeneic and autologous stem-cell transplantations in first complete remission have been studied extensively in younger patients with no major organ dysfunction. Allogeneic stem-cell transplantation reduces the risk of relapse, but a more favorable impact on survival when compared with chemotherapy or autologous stem-cell transplantation

remains to be demonstrated (44–46). This is likely due to the relatively high toxicity arising from the treatment associated with allogeneic stem-cell transplantation, which may offset the benefit from reduced risk of relapse derived from this procedure. In contrast, in patients treated with autologous stem-cell transplantation, the toxicity is significantly lower, but the relapse rate is higher than in patients treated with allogeneic stem-cell transplantation. In cytogenetically normal AML with high-risk molecular features such as *FLT3*-ITD, the optimal postinduction therapy is controversial, although recent results suggest an increased survival for patients treated with allogeneic stem-cell transplantation in first complete remission (47,48). No such advantage has been clearly reported when transplantation is used for core-binding factor AML in first complete remission. Prognostic factors may help select patients with high-risk disease for whom allogeneic stem-cell transplantation may represent the most effective approach.

Treatment of Acute Promyelocytic Leukemia

The identification of the fusion gene *PML/RARA*, created as a result of t(15;17) or rare cryptic chromosome rearrangements, is the molecular hallmark of APL (49,50). Recognition of APL is important because this is a highly curable disease. Although APL is responsive to cytarabine and daunorubicin, only about 10% of patients treated with these drugs die because of disseminated intravascular coagulation induced by the release of granule components by apoptotic leukemic cells. The outcome of APL patients has improved with the introduction of all-*trans*-retinoic acid, an oral drug that induces the differentiation of leukemic cells bearing the *PML/RARA* fusion gene. However, when treating APL patients with all-*trans*-retinoic acid, the physician should be aware of a treatment-related complication called retinoic acid syndrome, which is characterized by increasing leukocyte counts, fever, dyspnea, chest pain, pulmonary infiltrates, pleural and pericardial effusions, and hypoxia. This condition is effectively treated by glucocorticoids and/or chemotherapy and supportive measures.

All-*trans*-retinoic acid plus concurrent anthracycline-based chemotherapy is a standard treatment for APL (50). Addition of cytarabine to the induction therapy remains controversial. Up to 90% of APL patients achieve complete remission, and the goal of the subsequent consolidation therapy is to maintain a molecular remission for a long term. This is usually achieved with consolidation with all-*trans*-retinoic acid and anthracycline. Recently, the benefit of including two cycles of arsenic trioxide during the first complete remission has been reported by CALGB (51). There is evidence that patients with APL may benefit from the maintenance therapy with all-*trans*-retinoic acid with or without chemotherapy, but additional data remain to be collected to verify whether this approach is beneficial for all or only for distinct subsets of patients (52,53). Given the high cure rates of APL patients, current efforts are aimed at identifying those patient subsets that can achieve cure with a substantial decrease in the chemotherapy and those at a greatest risk of relapse that may benefit from innovative and more aggressive approaches (54).

The detection of minimal residual disease during complete remission by RT-PCR of *PML/RARA* transcript has been shown to predict relapses. Sequential RT-PCR monitoring of *PML/RARA* is now considered standard for postremission monitoring of APL (55). Patients with disease refractory to all-*trans*-retinoic acid or those in molecular or clinical relapse should be treated with arsenic trioxide that produces meaningful responses in up to 85% of the cases (56). Thereafter, patients showing clinical response should be considered for autologous stem-cell transplantation, if complete molecular remission was achieved, or for allogeneic stem-cell transplantation, if *PML/RARA* can still be detected.

Treatment of Relapsed AML

Once relapse occurs following initial treatment, patients are rarely treated further with standard-dose chemotherapy. The factors most predictive of response in relapsed patients are duration of previous complete remission and number of previous salvage regimens received. Patients eligible for allogeneic stem-cell transplantation should receive transplants expeditiously in the first relapse or second complete remission. The outcome of patients who received allogeneic stem-cell transplantation in second complete remission is likely better than the outcome of those transplanted in first relapse (57). Nonetheless, allogeneic stem-cell transplantation may be a better choice than chemotherapy in patients in first relapse with refractory disease or those with complete remission that has lasted less than 6 to 12 months (58). For this group of patients, the complete remission rate following salvage chemotherapy is only 10% to 20%. The long-term disease-free survival of relapsed patients eventually treated with allogeneic stem-cell transplantation is approximately 40%.

For patients older than 60 years, for whom clinical trials are not available, gemtuzumab ozogamicin (Mylotarg™), a humanized anti-CD33 antibody linked to calicheamicin, is a therapeutic alternative (59). The overall complete remission rate in response to this therapy is ~30% but is quite limited in patients who relapse early (<6 months) or have refractory disease.

Novel Approaches and Future Directions

Progress made in understanding the pathophysiology of AML has allowed the development of novel molecularly targeted strategies (Table 12.5) (59). Aberrant tyrosine kinase activity has been shown to play an important role in the pathogenesis of AML. Mutations of the *FLT3* gene that encodes a tyrosine kinase receptor have been shown to be suitable targets for tyrosine kinase inhibitors. Current studies are investigating the combination of tyrosine kinase inhibitors with induction and/or consolidation regimens in previously untreated AML patients or with salvage regimens in refractory or relapsed AML patients. Treatments with tyrosine kinase inhibitors are also being explored in core-binding factor AML harboring *KIT* mutations.

Other emerging investigational therapies include agents targeting aberrant epigenetic changes in AML blasts (59). Epigenetic silencing of structurally normal genes by aberrant DNA methylation and/or histone deacetylation has been described in AML. In contrast to genetic deletions causing irreversible loss of gene function, epigenetic gene silencing induced by DNA methylation and/or histone deacetylation can be reversed via pharmacologic inhibition

Table 12.5 Selected New Agents under Study for the Treatment of Adults with AML

Class of drugs	Examples of agents in class
Tyrosine kinase inhibitors	PKC412, MLN518, SU11248, CHIR-258, Imatinib (STI571, Gleevec), dasatinib, AMN107
Demethylating agents	Decitabine, 5-azacytidine
Histone deacetylase inhibitors	Suberoylanilide hydroxamic acid (SAHA), MS275, LBH589, Valproic Acid
Heavy metals	Arsenic trioxide, Antimony
Multidrug resistance 1 modulators	Cyclosporine, LY335979, Valspodar
Farnesyl transferase inhibitors	R115777, SCH66336
HSP-90 antagonists	17-allylaminogeldanamycin (17-AAG), DMAG, or derivatives
Cell cycle inhibitors	Flavopiridol, CYC202 (R-Roscovitine), SNS-032
Nucleoside analogs	Clofarabine, Troxacitabine
Humanized antibodies	Anti-CD33 (SGN33), anti-DR4, anti-DR5, anti-KIR
Toxin-conjugated antibodies	Gemtuzumab ozogamicin
Radiolabeled antibodies	Yttrium-90-labeled human M195

of DNA methyltransferases and histone deacetylases, respectively. Hypomethylating agents currently used in the clinic include 5-azacytidine and decitabine (collectively called azanucleosides), both approved by the U.S. Food and Drug Administration for use in MDS. Treatment with azanucleoside alone or in combination with histone deacetylase inhibitors represents a rational approach to AML therapy.

In addition, other classes of agents being tested in AML include the farnesyltransferase inhibitor tipifarnib (R115777, Zarnestra), the alkylating agent cloretazine (VNP40101M), the nucleoside analog clofarabine, and the proteasome inhibitor bortezomib. All these compounds have shown encouraging results in high-risk patients (older and/or refractory/relapsed AML).

In contrast, targeting the multidrug resistance 1 efflux pump activity with inhibitors (e.g., Valspodar) has not been successful, except for the addition of cyclosporine to daunorubicin and high-dose cytarabine, which seemingly improved the outcome (60). Inhibition of the *BCL2* anti-apoptotic activity that mediates chemoresistance in AML may be a promising strategy, but it remains to be validated in clinical trials.

ACUTE LYMPHOBLASTIC LEUKEMIA

Acute lymphoblastic leukemia, a clonal malignant disease of the immature lymphoid hematopoietic progenitors that can arise in the marrow, thymus, lymph nodes, or spleen, is presently categorized according to the World Health Organization classification, which uses morphology, immunophenotype, and, increasingly, genetic and cytogenetic findings. In contrast to AML, there is no agreed-upon lower limit for the blast percentage required for ALL diagnosis; many treatment protocols use 25% of blast as the cutoff for diagnosis, and, in general, ALL diagnosis should be avoided when there are <20% of blasts (18). The recently updated 2008 World Health Organization classification includes now several B-lineage ALL (B-ALL), but not T-lineage ALL (T-ALL), categories recognized as separate entities based on the presence of specific chromosome/molecular abnormalities (Table 12.6) (18).

Pathophysiology

The theories about the origin of the leukemia-initiating cell in ALL vary. Some relate it to an already committed B- or T-lineage cell (61–63), whereas others propose that, in at least some ALL subtypes, the leukemic blasts may arise from a more phenotypically primitive hematopoietic stem cell (64–67).

Secondary ALL, defined as ALL following another malignancy, irrespective of whether patients received prior therapy, is a rare entity characterized by increased frequency of 11q23/*MLL* aberrations in all age groups, increased frequency of *BCR-ABL*-positive disease in pediatric patients and its decreased frequency in older patients (68). As in secondary AML, the outcome continues to be extremely poor.

Clinical Presentation

Symptoms

The symptoms are not significantly different from those of patients with AML. Patients may present with fever, pallor, complaints of palpitations due to anemia and/or infection, spontaneous bleeding, and fatigue.

Physical Findings

Findings on physical examination range from fever, petechiae/ecchymoses, hepatomegaly, splenomegaly, and peripheral lymphadenopathy. Involvement of central nervous system is detected in approximately 10% of the cases and is more prevalent in T-ALL.

Hematologic Findings

White blood cell (WBC) counts $\geq 30 \times 10^9/l$ occur in approximately 25% to 63% of the patients; T-ALL tends to present with higher WBC counts. Platelet counts $\geq 50 \times 10^9/l$ occur in approximately 50% of the patients. Hemoglobin $<10\,g/dl$ can be found in approximately 70%, and elevated lactate dehydrogenase in 40% to 59% of patients.

Morphological, cytochemical, immunophenotypic, genetic, and molecular characteristic are described in Table 12.7. The leukemic blasts may resemble hematogones, the normal lymphoid progenitors. Morphologic distinction between hematogones and residual ALL cells is difficult. However, hematogones display the continuum of B-cell markers, whereas the leukemic blasts overexpress or underexpress specific markers. Further, ALL with myeloid markers can be relatively easily distinguished from its normal counterpart because hematogones are devoid of myeloid markers. Finally, some ALL cases contain several populations of blasts from one or more lineages. Leukemia of ambiguous lineage is a new entity defined by the World Health Organization (18). It includes biphenotypic leukemia, describing a single blast population expressing antigens from more than one lineage, and bilineage leukemia, describing separate population of blasts from more than one lineage. The two most common examples are leukemias with t(9;22) and 11q23/*MLL* translocations.

Table 12.6 World Health Organization Classification of ALL

Precursor lymphoid neoplasms
   B lymphoblastic leukemia/lymphoma
      B lymphoblastic leukemia/lymphoma, NOS
      B lymphoblastic leukemia/lymphoma with recurrent genetic abnormalities
      B lymphoblastic leukemia/lymphoma with t(9;22)(q34;q11.2); *BCR-ABL1*
      B lymphoblastic leukemia/lymphoma with t(v;11q23); *MLL* rearranged
      B lymphoblastic leukemia/lymphoma with t(12;21)(p13;q22); *TEL-AML1 (ETV6-RUNX1)*
      B lymphoblastic leukemia/lymphoma with hyperdiploidy
      B lymphoblastic leukemia/lymphoma with hypodiploidy (hypodiploid ALL)
      B lymphoblastic leukemia/lymphoma with t(5;14)(q31;q32); *IL3-IGH*
      B lymphoblastic leukaemia/lymphoma with t(1;19)(q23;p13.3); *E2A-PBX1*; *(TCF3-PBX1)*
   T lymphoblastic leukemia/lymphoma

Mature B-cell neoplasms
   Burkitt lymphoma

Source: From Ref. 18.

Prognostic Factors

Common prognostic factors (high risk denoted in parentheses) in ALL include age at diagnosis (>60 years of age), performance status (poor), WBC at diagnosis ($>30 \times 10^9/l$ in B-ALL; $>100 \times 10^9/l$ in T-ALL), immunophenotype (B-cell), multidrug resistance (expression of multidrug resistance proteins), and lactate dehydrogenase (high level, which is also associated with central nervous system disease). Persistence of normal residual hematopoiesis and intense leukemic cell mitotic activity are associated with favorable outcome. In addition to the pretreatment variables, lack of cytoreduction and absence of complete remission correlate with adverse prognosis in ALL.

Recurring chromosome abnormalities divide ALL into unfavorable, intermediate and favorable groups based on the probability of continuous complete remission or disease-free survival (Table 12.8). Cytogenetic and molecular analyses at diagnosis can assist in developing risk-adapted therapeutic strategies and in devising new treatment modalities by unraveling of the molecular basis of the disease. The Philadelphia chromosome, i.e., t(9;22)(q34;q11.2), is the most common aberration in adult B-ALL being detected in 11% to 34% of patients, with an increased prevalence in those >60 years. The translocation results in the head-to-tail fusion of variable numbers of 5′ exons of the *BCR* gene, mapped to 22q11.2, with exon 2 of the *ABL* gene, located at 9q34, which creates the chimeric gene *BCR/ABL*. There are two main variants of *BCR/ABL* that encode two types of fusion proteins: the p190[BCR/ABL] harboring the first exon of *BCR* and the p210[BCR/ABL] containing *BCR* exon 13 or exon 14. They are almost equally distributed among ALL cases. Interestingly, deletion of the *IKZF1* gene has been recently found in most *BCR/ABL*-positive ALL patients (69). Adult Philadelphia chromosome-positive (referred to thereafter as Philadelphia-positive) ALL patients are usually considered for allogeneic stem-cell transplantation or investigational therapies, as they are not cured with chemotherapy alone.

Table 12.7 Characteristics of Adult ALL

Characteristics	B-ALL	T-ALL	Ph+ ALL	Burkitt leukemia
Blast morphology	Blasts range from homogenous small cells with high nuclear-to-cytoplasmic ratio and inconspicuous nucleoli to more pleomorphic cells that are often larger in size, have a lower nuclear-to-cytoplasmic ratio and prominent nucleoli			Medium-sized homogenous cells with dispersed chromatin, multiple nucleoli, and a moderate amount of deep blue cytoplasm with clearly defined vacuoles
Bone marrow morphology	Hypercellular with almost complete replacement of the normal bone marrow with the leukemic blasts; increased reticulin deposits can be found in up to 70% of B-cell precursor-ALL			"Starry sky" appearance: tinted body macrophages (the stars) scattered among sheets of dark blue blasts (the sky)
Cytochemistry				
MPO	Negative	Negative	Negative	Negative
TdT	Positive	Positive	Positive	Negative
PAS	"Block" positivity	"Block" positivity	"Block" positivity	
AP	Negative	Positive	Negative	Negative
Oil red O	Negative	Negative	Negative	Positive
Ki-67	Variable	Variable	Variable	>99% positive
Immunophenotype				
CD19	Positive	Negative	Positive	Positive
CyCD79a	Positive	Negative in 90% of cases	Positive	Positive
CyCD22	Positive	Negative	Positive	Positive
CD10	Positive[a]	May be positive	Positive	Positive
PAX5[b]	Positive	Negative	Positive	Positive
SIg	Negative[c]	Negative	Negative	Positive
CD1a	Negative	Positive	Negative	Negative
CyCD3	Negative	Positive	Negative	Negative
CD4/8	Negative	Positive	Negative	Negative
Cytogenetics	Translocations involving 11q23/*MLL* gene; 4q21/*AFF1* is the most common 11q23/*MLL* partner	del(9p); loss of *CDKN2A* in about 30% of cases	t(9;22)(q34;q11.2)	t(8;14)(q24;q32) t(2;8)(p12;q24) t(8;22)(q24;q11)
Molecular				
Clonal DJ rearrangement	Positive	Positive in 20% of cases	Positive	Positive
T-cell receptor gene rearrangements	Positive (up to 70%)	Positive	Positive	Negative
NOTCH1	Negative	Activating mutations in the extracellular domain and/or C-terminal PEST domain of *NOTCH1*	Negative	Negative
HOX11 (TLX1)	Negative	Positive in 30% of cases	Negative	Negative
HOX11L2 (TLX3)	Negative	Positive in 10–15% of cases	Negative	Negative
MYC translocation	Negative	Negative	Negative	Positive

[a]Except those with t(v;11q23); MLL rearranged.
[b]Also positive in AML with t(8;21).
[c]Can be present but provided that other morphologic and cytogenetics are consistent with B-lineage ALL.
Abbreviations: AFF1, gene from chromosome 4 fused with the *MLL* gene; AP, acid phosphatase; CD, Cluster designation; CDKN2A, cyclin-dependent kinase inhibitor 2A; Cy, cytoplasmic; *MLL*, myeloid/lymphoid or mixed-lineage leukemia gene; MPO, myeloperoxidase; PAS, periodic acid-Schiff; PAX5, paired box 5; Sig, surface immunoglobulins; TdT, terminal deoxynucleotide transferase.

Translocations involving 11q23/*MLL* involve many different fusion partners. In some cases, these partners encode transcriptional trans-activators [e.g., t(4;11)(q21;q23), t(9;11)(p22;q23), and t(11;19)(q23;p13.3)] (70). The most common *MLL* partner in adults is the *AFF1* (*AF4*) gene at 4q21; t(4;11)/*MLL*/*AFF1* confers adverse prognosis.

Progress has been made in molecular characterization of ALL. The transcription factor *PAX5* was found to be inactivated in B-ALL by deletion or point mutation (71). The *PAX5* gene, located at 9p13.2, is also involved in translocations, e.g., t(7;9)(q11;p13) resulting in the PAX5-ENL protein shown to inhibit the function of the wild-type

PAX5 (72). Although other molecular aberrations are being discovered, their prognostic significance remains to be explored.

Similarly, in T-ALL, the expression of certain oncogenes has been closely linked to the developmental arrest at particular stages of normal thymocyte development (70,73,74). For example, activating somatic mutations in *NOTCH1* were found in approximately 50% of T-ALL cases. The mutations target different areas within *NOTCH1*, leading to increased signaling. The NOTCH1 protein, either normal or aberrant, is cleaved by the γ-secretase complex, leading to its translocation to the nucleus, where it induces

Table 12.8 Cytogenetic Risk Groups in ALL

Risk group	Cytogenetic abnormality
Favorable	del(12p) or t(12p)
	t(14)(q11-q13)
	Hyperdiploid
Intermediate	None (normal karyotype)
	+21
	del(9p) or t(9p)
	del(6q)
Unfavorable	t(9;22)(q34;q11.2)
	−7
	+8 t(4;11)(q21;q23)
	Hypodiploid
	t(1;19)(q23;p13)

the transcription of *NOTCH1*-target genes. Current clinical trials evaluate the role of γ-secretase inhibitors in T-ALL. Lack of *HOX11* expression (75), and high *ERG* and *BAALC* expression (76) are predictive of adverse outcome in T-ALL.

The presence of minimal residual disease after treatment is associated with poor outcome. Molecular analysis and flow cytometry are the mainstay techniques to detect minimal residual disease (77). Detection of clonotypic *TCR* and *IGH* gene rearrangements was used initially. Later, tumor-specific RNA was used to detect fusion gene transcripts (e.g., *BCR/ABL*, *MLL/AFF1*) or aberrantly expressed genes (e.g., *FLT3*, *WT1*). Flow cytometry is another method to detect minimal residual disease in ALL. Flow cytometry can identify one abnormal cell in 10^4 to 10^5 cells. Of note, clonal evolution may cause the disappearance of one or more antigens detected at diagnosis. Taking into consideration the aforementioned caveats, absence of minimal residual disease revealed by either molecular techniques or quantitative flow cytometry at the end of induction therapy was associated with better clinical outcome in some adult ALL studies (77,78).

Treatment

Different treatment approaches are outlined in Table 12.9. Overall, the outcome in either B- and T-ALL with any of

these approaches results in approximately 30% to 40% five-year survival (79). The main achievements in the last few years, are the inclusion of imatinib mesylate (Gleevec®) in Philadelphia-positive ALL, the approval of nelarabine (Arranon®) for T-ALL, the use of pediatric regimens to treat ALL in adolescents and young adults, and the inclusion of anti-CD20 antibody in the Burkitt leukemia armamentarium; these are discussed in detail below.

Imatinib Mesylate

Imatinib is described fully in the section on "Chronic Myelogenous Leukemia." Imatinib alone was not sufficient to induce prolonged remission in Philadelphia-positive ALL patients. Therefore, several groups studied its combination with chemotherapy, either sequentially (aiming to reduce toxicities) or concurrently (80–90). Overall, the results demonstrate a significant improvement over chemotherapy-alone approaches; although the follow-up is relatively short (the longest is three years).

The mechanisms of resistance to imatinib are delineated in the section on "Chronic Myelogenous Leukemia." Unique to Philadelphia-positive ALL is that kinase domain mutations may precede imatinib-based therapy and give rise to relapse in patients with *de novo* Philadelphia-positive ALL (91). These data suggest that, in contrast to CML, mutational analysis could be considered at diagnosis in Philadelphia-positive ALL and treatment could be tailored accordingly.

In CML, decreased intracellular imatinib concentrations are addressed by intensifying the therapy with higher (up to 800 mg/day) imatinib doses. This approach is not useful in treating Philadelphia-positive ALL as the recommended dose is already at its maximum. As discussed in the section "Chronic Myelogenous Leukemia," the novel BCR/ABL kinase inhibitors are more potent than imatinib and can overcome this mechanism of resistance.

Alternative signaling pathways have been implicated in resistance to imatinib. Specifically, the Src family kinase members, Lyn, Hck, and Fgr, have been shown elevated in the hematopoietic cells of mice with Philadelphia-positive ALL and required for the induction of Philadelphia-positive

Table 12.9 Treatment of Adult ALL

B-ALL and T-ALL	Ph+ ALL	Burkitt
BFM-like regimen Induction with VCR, PRED, daunorubicin, and L-ASP; Early intensification with CTX, ARA-C, 6-MP, VCR; CNS prophylaxis with intrathecal MTX with either cranial irradiation or high dose MTX and ARA-C; Late intensification with doxorubicin, VCR, DEXA, CTX, 6-TG, and ARA-C; Maintenance with VCR, PRED, 6-MP, and MTX to complete 24 months	Addition of imatinib to any of the approaches described for B-lineage diseases	CTX, VCR, doxorubicin, high-dose MTX, and intrathecal therapy alternating with ifosfamide, VP-16, high-dose ARA-C and intrathecal therapy
Hyper-CVAD regimen Alternating courses of CTX, VCR, doxorubicin, and DEXA with MTX and high dose ARA-C; CNS prophylaxis includes intrathecal chemotherapy; Maintenance with VCR, PRED, 6-MP, and MTX to complete 24 months		
New treatment aspects: anti-CD20 antibody (for B-ALL), nelarabine (for T-ALL), different regimens for adolescents and young adults	New treatment aspects: new tyrosine kinase inhibitors	New treatment aspects: anti-CD20 antibody

Abbreviations: ARA-C, cytosine arabinoside; BFM, Berlin-Frankfurt-Munster; CTX, cyclophosphamide; DEXA, dexamethasone; L-ASP, L-asparaginase; MTX, methotrexate; PRED, prednisone; VCR, vincristine; VP-16, etoposide.

ALL (92). Dasatinib (Sprycel®) and bosutinib (SKI-606) target the Src family kinase members (see section "Chronic Myelogenous Leukemia"). Another pathway involved in imatinib resistance in Philadelphia-positive ALL is stromal support. Although the BCR/ABL kinase continued to be inhibited by imatinib, leukemia cells have been shown to proliferate in the presence of stromal support (93). These data suggest that the stroma selects imatinib resistant BCR/ABL cells that are less dependent on the kinase activity; interrupting the interaction between the lymphoblasts and the stroma may be of benefit in Philadelphia-positive ALL.

Dasatinib for Philadelphia-positive ALL

Dasatinib was tested in imatinib-resistant and naive Ph+ ALL patients. Dasatinib as a single agent was indeed shown to induce rapid hematologic and cytogenetic responses in adult Ph+ ALL patients with resistance or intolerance to imatinib (94). With a minimum follow-up of eight months, complete hematologic responses were achieved by 31% and complete cytogenetic responses by 58% of the patients. The lower rate of hematologic responses compared with cytogenetic responses stems from the cytopenias associated with dasatinib.

Dasatinib and prednisone were recently studied as a front-line therapy in the induction of newly diagnosed Philadelphia-positive ALL (95). All patients achieved complete remission by day 22 and only one patient relapsed. In addition, preliminary results of the combination of dasatinib with hyper-CVAD were shown to induce complete remission in 93% of patients and cytogenetic responses in all but one patient.

Nilotinib for Philadelphia-positive ALL

Nilotinib (Tasigna®) (described in the section "Chronic Myelogenous Leukemia") was tested in imatinib-resistant Philadelphia-positive ALL patients. As monotherapy, nilotinib had promising activity in imatinib-resistant disease (96). Trials combining nilotinib with chemotherapy for Philadelphia-positive ALL are forthcoming.

New Drugs for Philadelphia-positive ALL

Bosutinib (discussed in the section "Chronic Myelogenous Leukemia") is currently undergoing clinical trials in patients with CML and Philadelphia-positive ALL who have failed treatment with imatinib, dasatinib, and/or nilotinib. The results will be available in the near future.

Nelarabine for T-ALL

Nelarabine is a new purine analog shown to have significant activity in T-ALL patients whose disease has not responded to or has relapsed following treatment with at least two chemotherapy regimens (97). In the adult clinical trial, the rate of complete remission was 31% and the overall response rate was 41%. The principal toxicity was grade 3 or 4 neutropenia (37% of patients) and thrombocytopenia (26% of patients). Nelarabine is now going to be studied in newly diagnosed T-ALL.

Treating Adolescents and Young Adults

Adolescents and young adults represent a challenging group for both pediatric and adult oncologists. Several groups recently evaluated the outcome of patients aged 16 to 21 years based on their treatment on adult or pediatric protocols (Fig. 12.1) (98). Despite an assortment of treatment approaches among the different groups, the results of these retrospective analyses consistently demonstrated that adolescents and young adults treated on pediatric protocols had a significantly better five-year survival than those treated on adult protocols. Several reasons were suggested for these differences including more intensive use of nonmyelosuppressive agents (e.g., steroids, L-asparaginase, vincristine), earlier central nervous system prophylaxis, and longer maintenance in the pediatric protocols. Moreover, protocol adherence/compliance, by both treating physicians and patients, was raised as a contributing factor to outcome differences. Therefore, several groups have started offering pediatric regimens to adolescents and young adults in a prospective manner. Preliminary results from two European studies (99,100), employing pediatric regimens for adolescents and young adults up to age 30, are very encouraging.

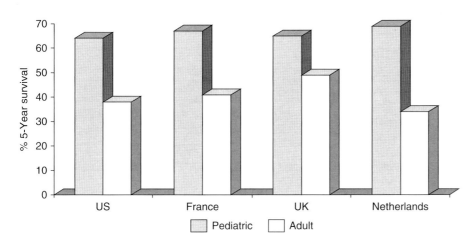

Figure 12.1 Five-year survival of adolescents and young adults with ALL treated on pediatric or adult protocols.

Treatment of Burkitt Disease

Burkitt leukemia is a subtype of ALL whose hallmark is the t(8;14)(q24;q32) and its variants, t(2;8)(p12;q24) and t(8;22)(q24;q11). As a result of t(8;14), the *MYC* gene at 8q24, is juxtaposed to the enhancer elements of the *IGH* gene at 14q32. In the variant translocations, one of the immunoglobulin light chain genes, mapped to 2p12 (*IGK*) or 22q11 (*IGL*), is translocated to a telomeric region of *MYC* (101). Consequently, *MYC* is activated and expressed at high levels. Because the product of the *MYC* gene, a DNA binding protein, is implicated in the regulation of other critical genes, its constitutive production results in uncontrolled proliferation of cells with one of the translocations.

The treatment of adult Burkitt disease underwent a significant improvement when pediatric regimens, including repetitive cycles of fractionated alkylating agents and aggressive central nervous system therapy, were employed (79). Since Burkitt disease is characterized by strong CD20 expression, two groups (102,103) successfully included the anti-CD20 antibody, rituximab (Rituxan®), in their treatment regimens. In addition to the favorable outcome in these patients, concerns about increased infectious complications, due to the use of rituximab, were dismissed by these trials.

Allogeneic Stem-Cell Transplantation

Allogeneic stem-cell transplantation continues to represent an effective treatment approach for adult ALL. We currently recommend an allogeneic stem-cell transplantation for all ALL patients unless enrolled onto a specific clinical trial, e.g., Philadelphia-positive ALL, where autologous transplantation is also an option. Most data suggest that the inclusion of total body irradiation in the preparatory regimen results in better outcome (104). However, graft-versus-leukemia does not seem to be as potent in ALL as in other diseases. Therefore, employing reduced-intensity preparatory regimens for the elderly, those with poor performance status or co-morbidities, presents a challenge.

Future Directions

Pegylated asparaginase (Oncospar®) decreases the immunogenicity of the enzyme, thus reducing the risk of hypersensitivity reactions. Another advantage of pegylated asparaginase is its long half-life. Its use in adult ALL patients has been lagging behind when compared with its use in pediatric ALL patients, because of lack of pharmacokinetic and pharmacodynamic data in adults. However, two recent publications may change this trend. Specifically, the recent demonstration of the safety of intravenous pegylated asparaginase during remission induction in adult ALL with favorable pharmacodynamics and decreased hypersensitivity reactions (105) suggests that this route will replace other routes of administration. Further, the finding that effective asparagine depletion with pegylated asparaginase resulted in improved outcome in adult ALL (106) suggests that monitoring for asparagine depletion will become part of the treatment approach in these patients.

Finally, clofarabine (Clolar®) is a novel deoxyadenosine analog with clinical activity in refractory and relapsed pediatric ALL patients. Its role in combination with other drugs in relapsed/refractory adult ALL patients is being investigated (107,108). Upon completion of optimal dose and combination identification, clofarabine will be tested as a front-line agent in adult ALL.

CHRONIC MYELOGENOUS LEUKEMIA

CML is a myeloproliferative disorder defined by the presence of the *BCR/ABL* chimeric gene, a product of a reciprocal t(9;22) occurring in a hematopoietic stem cell (3). *BCR/ABL* plays a central role in the development of CML. It is transcribed into a hybrid *BCR/ABL* mRNA in which exon 1 of *ABL* is replaced by variable numbers of 5' *BCR* exons. The BCR/ABL fusion proteins, p210$^{BCR/ABL}$, contain NH$_2$-terminal domains of BCR from exon one up to either exon 13 or exon 14 fused to exon two of ABL. A rare breakpoint, occurring at exon 19 of *BCR*, yields a fusion protein of 230 kDa.

The mechanism(s) by which p210$^{BCR/ABL}$ promotes the transition from the benign to the fully malignant state is still unclear. The attachment of the *BCR* sequences to *ABL* results in three critical functional changes: (1) the ABL protein becomes constitutively active as a tyrosine kinase enzyme, subsequently activating downstream kinases that prevent apoptosis; (2) the DNA-protein-binding activity of ABL is attenuated; and (3) the binding of ABL to cytoskeletal actin microfilaments is enhanced. The BCR/ABL proteins can transform hematopoietic progenitor cells in vitro; reconstituting lethally irradiated mice with marrow cells infected with retrovirus carrying the gene encoding the p210$^{BCR/ABL}$ leads to the development of a myeloproliferative syndrome resembling CML in 50% of mice.

Clinical Presentation
Symptoms

CML in approximately half of the patients is diagnosed during routine health screening; the others may present with fatigue, malaise, and weight loss or have symptoms resulting from splenic enlargement. Occasionally, patients present with leukostatic manifestations. Patients with p23-$^{BCR/ABL}$-positive CML have had a more indolent course, at least in the pre-imatinib era.

Progression of CML is associated with worsening symptoms. Unexplained fever, significant weight loss, increasing dose requirement of the drugs controlling the disease, bone and joint pain, bleeding, thrombosis, and infections suggest transformation into accelerated or blastic phases. Less than 10% to 15% of newly diagnosed patients present with accelerated disease or with de novo blastic phase CML.

Physical Findings

Minimal to moderate splenomegaly is the most common physical finding in CML patients; mild hepatomegaly is found occasionally. Lymphadenopathy and myeloid sarcomas are unusual.

Hematologic Findings

Elevated WBC counts, with different levels of myeloid maturation, are found in CML patients at diagnosis. Usually <5% circulating blasts are noted. Platelet counts are usually elevated, and a mild degree of normochromic normocytic anemia may be present. Phagocytic functions are preserved at diagnosis and remain normal during the chronic phase.

The marrow cellularity is increased at diagnosis, with a greatly altered myeloid to erythroid ratio. The marrow blast percentage is generally normal or slightly elevated. Marrow or blood basophilia, eosinophilia, and monocytosis may be present. Collagen fibrosis in the marrow is unusual at presentation, but significant degrees of reticulin stain–measured fibrosis are noted in about half of the patients.

Accelerated phase of CML is defined by the development of increasing degrees of anemia unaccounted for by bleeding or chemotherapy; clonal cytogenetic evolution; blood or marrow blasts between 10% and 19%, blood or marrow basophils ≥20%, or platelet count <100,000/μl. *Blast phase* is diagnosed when blood or marrow blasts are ≥20% or when an extramedullary blast proliferation occurs. In approximately 70% of patients, blast cells are of myeloid lineage and may include neutrophilic, monocytic, eosinophilic, basophilic, megakaryocytic, or erythroid blasts or any combination thereof. Lymphoblasts are found in 20% to 30% of patients (18).

Cytogenetic and Molecular Findings

The cytogenetic hallmark of CML is the t(9;22)(q34;q11.2). Some patients have *variant translocations* that involve one to three chromosomes in addition to chromosomes 9 and 22. However, the molecular consequences of *variant translocations* appear similar to those resulting from the typical t(9;22), i.e., the creation of *BCR/ABL*. For CML diagnosis, each patient should have evidence of the translocation from cytogenetics, fluorescence in situ hybridization (FISH), and/or molecular analysis.

In the pre-imatinib era, CML was likely to transform from the chronic phase to accelerated and blastic phases. The events associated with this transition included chromosomal instability of the malignant clone, and heterogeneous alterations in such genes as *TP53*, *RAS*, *PP2A*, and *MYC*. Sporadic reports have documented progressive de novo DNA methylation at the *BCR/ABL* locus and hypomethylation of the *LINE-1* retrotransposon promoter. Further, large deletions adjacent to the translocation breakpoint on the derivative chromosome 9 have been associated with shorter survival, even in the post-imatinib era. Finally, CML that develops resistance to imatinib by any of the mechanisms listed below is at increased risk to progress to accelerated phase/blast crisis. In summary, multiple pathways to disease transformation exist, but the exact timing and relevance of each remain unclear.

Prognostic Factors

Several prognostic models identifying different risk groups in CML have been developed. These staging systems were derived from multivariable analyses of prognostic factors. The *Sokal index* was developed based on chemotherapy-treated patients, and the *Hasford system* was developed on interferon α-treated patients (3). Preliminary results suggest that both the Sokal and Hasford systems are applicable to imatinib-treated patients.

Treatment

The therapy of CML is rapidly undergoing evolution because we have a targeted treatment option (imatinib) with outstanding outcome. The role of stem-cell transplantation is clearly diminishing in CML.

The current treatment goal in CML is to achieve prolonged, non-neoplastic, nonclonal hematopoiesis, with eradication of any residual cells containing the *BCR/ABL* transcript. However, complete cytogenetic remission and major molecular response (≥3 log reduction in *BCR/ABL* transcript) at 18 months were associated with estimated survival, without progression, of 100% at five years (109). Therefore, the need to achieve complete eradication of any residual cells may change in the upcoming years.

Imatinib Mesylate

Imatinib functions through competitive inhibition at the adenosine triphosphate binding site of the ABL kinase in the inactive conformation, which leads to inhibition of tyrosine phosphorylation of proteins involved in BCR/ABL signal transduction. It shows a high degree of specificity for BCR/ABL, the receptor for platelet-derived growth factor and KIT tyrosine kinases. Imatinib does not affect the hematopoietic progenitor cells (110).

In newly diagnosed CML, a recent randomized phase III study of imatinib (400 mg/day) versus interferon-α and cytarabine revealed an estimated complete hematologic remission rate of 98% at 60 months in imatinib-treated patients (109). Data on interferon-α–treated patients were not presented since most of the patients crossed over to the imatinib arm. The estimated complete cytogenetic remission rate at 60 months was 87% in imatinib-treated patients. Major molecular response was shown in 58% at 12 months and 80% of patients at four years. At 60 months, the estimated event-free survival was 83%; 93% of patients did not progress to the accelerated or blastic phase.

Based on these unsurpassed results, specific milestones have been developed for chronic-phase CML patients (Table 12.10) (111,112). For example, chronic-phase CML patients who do not achieve any cytogenetic remission following six months of treatment with imatinib are unlikely to achieve major molecular response in the future and therefore should be offered other treatment approaches.

Progression to accelerated/blastic phases of the disease decreased gradually to <1% during the fourth and fifth years, and no patient who achieved cytogenetic complete remission during the first year of imatinib treatment progressed to the accelerated/blastic phases of the disease.

Imatinib is administered orally and has an acceptable toxicity profile. The main side effects are fluid retention, nausea, muscle cramps, diarrhea, and skin rashes. The management of these side effects is usually supportive. Myelosuppression is the most common hematologic side effect. Myelosuppression, while rare, may require blood, platelet and/or growth factor support. Doses of <300 mg/day seem ineffective and may lead to development of resistance. To our current knowledge, imatinib needs to be administered for life.

Four mechanisms of resistance to imatinib have been described to date. These are (1) gene amplification, (2) mutations at the kinase site, (3) decreased intracellular imatinib levels, and (4) alternative signaling pathways functionally compensating for the imatinib-sensitive mechanisms (113). All four mechanisms are being targeted in clinical trials. Another common mechanism of imatinib failure is

Table 12.10 CML Milestones Based on Imatinib Treatment

Time	National comprehensive cancer network (NCCN)	European leukemia net (ELN)	
		Failure	Suboptimal response
3 Months	CHR	No hematologic response	<CHR
6 Months	Any cytogenetic response	<CHR, no cytogenetic response	<PCyR
12 Months	PCyR	<PCyR	<CCyR
18 Months	CCyR	<CCyR	<MMR
Anytime	Loss of previously achieved hematologic, cytogenetic or molecular response	Loss of CHR Loss of CCyR Mutation	Additional chromosome abnormalities in Ph+ cells Loss of MMR Mutation

Abbreviations: CCyR, complete cytogenetic response (0 Ph+ cells); CHR, complete hematologic response; MMR, major molecular response (≥3 log reduction in *BCR/ABL* message); PCyR, partial cytogenetic response (<35% Ph+ cells).

patient compliance (114). Data suggest that up to 25% of patients are noncompliant (compliance was defined as medication possession ratio = apparent mg taken vs. mg prescribed) (115).

BCR/ABL gene amplification and decreased intracellular imatinib concentrations are addressed by intensifying the therapy with higher (up to 800 mg/day) imatinib doses. Early intensification of imatinib dose in newly diagnosed CML patients led to improved major molecular response when compared to historical controls treated with 400 mg/day. However, a randomized study comparing 400 to 800 mg/day in newly diagnosed CML patients did not find any difference in achieving major molecular response except in the subset of patients with the highest risk for disease progression (116).

Mutations at the kinase domain are being targeted by novel tyrosine kinase inhibitors that have a different conformation than imatinib, demonstrating activity against most imatinib-resistant mutations. Nilotinib, like imatinib, binds to the kinase domain in the inactive conformation (117). Dasatinib binds to the kinase domain in the open conformation and also inhibits the SRC family of kinases, addressing the last mechanism of resistance (118). Both are oral agents with toxicity profiles similar to imatinib with small, albeit significant, differences. Specifically, both agents are associated with more pronounced myelosuppression than imatinib. Nilotinib was associated with sudden death in six of approximately 550 CML patients. A suspected relationship to nilotinib was reported in two of these cases. Dasatinib was shown to cause pleural effusion in 22% of the patients, with 7% developing grade 3 to 4 toxicity. Finally, the current tyrosine kinase inhibitors are ineffective against some mutations (e.g., T315I); several clinical trials target these mutations, e.g., homoharringtonine (Omacetaxine®).

The approval of these new agents has changed the treatment algorithm of CML (111,112). For example, patients who do not achieve any cytogenetic remission at six months with imatinib will now be offered dasatinib, nilotinib, clinical trial with novel agents, or stem-cell transplantation. Interferon-α will be offered only if all other options, including clinical trials, have failed.

The encouraging results with imatinib have led clinicians to offer it as a first-line therapy for newly diagnosed CML patients, including those who otherwise would have benefited from transplantation (e.g., young patients with a sibling matched donor). Several groups have shown that prior exposure to imatinib does not affect transplantation

outcome negatively. However, delaying transplantation for high-risk (Sokal/Hasford criteria) patients, who fail to achieve the treatment milestones (Table 12.10), may result in worse outcome.

Chemotherapy
Initial management of patients with chemotherapy is currently reserved for rapid lowering of WBC counts, reduction of symptoms, and reversal of symptomatic splenomegaly. Hydroxyurea, a ribonucleotide reductase inhibitor, induces rapid disease control. The initial dose is 1 to 4 g/day; the dose should be halved with each 50% reduction of the WBC. Unfortunately, cytogenetic remissions with hydroxyurea are uncommon.

Allogeneic Stem-Cell Transplantation
Allogeneic stem-cell transplantation is the only proven curative option for CML patients. However, it is complicated by early mortality owing to the transplantation procedure. Outcome of stem-cell transplantation depends on multiple factors, including (1) the patient (e.g., age and phase of disease); (2) the type of donor [e.g., syngeneic (monozygotic twins) or HLA-compatible allogeneic, related or unrelated]; (3) the preparative regimen (myeloblative or reduced intensity); (4) graft-versus-host disease; and (5) post–stem-cell transplantation treatment. Allogeneic stem-cell transplantation is reserved nowadays only for CML patients whose disease has developed resistance to imatinib (119).

Future Directions
Attempts to discontinue imatinib treatment have failed because of disease recurrence. Thus, future directions concentrate on the eradication of the hematopoietic progenitor cells initiating the disease to allow discontinuation of imatinib (109). In addition, several studies concentrate on the advanced stages of the disease. For example, abrogation of DNA methylation with decitabine has shown clinical activity in the advanced stages of CML (120). Inhibition of RAS with a farnesyl transferase inhibitor that blocks its insertion into the membrane may have antitumor activity in CML on the basis of early clinical trials (121,122). A clinical trial with a vaccine targeting the BCR/ABL e14a2 sequences with two adjuvants (CMLVAX100) showed improved cytogenetic responses in imatinib-resistant patients (123). Pre-clinical studies have also shown that therapeutic

induction of PP2A may have promise against imatinib-resistant CML (124).

CHRONIC LYMPHOCYTIC LEUKEMIA

CLL represents a common mature B-cell clonal disease (125–131), characterized by monoclonal circulating lymphocytes ($\geq 5 \times 10^9$/l) and/or infiltration of bone marrow and other hematopoietic organs (lymph nodes and spleen). CLL is subdivided prognostically based upon IgV$_H$ mutational status (132,133). However, in addition to the prognostic significance, IgV$_H$ mutational status may identify subtypes with distinct mechanisms of leukemogenesis. Differences in B-cell receptor signaling exist between these subtypes, with IgV$_H$ unmutated patients having enhanced signaling. A role of disordered apoptosis in CLL has been suggested. Studies have also demonstrated that clonal lymphocytes have constitutive activation of several anti-apoptotic transcription factors including NF-κB, NFAT, and STAT3. The source of activation of these different transcription factors is not completely defined but may in part be due to autocrine and paracrine networks involving BAFF, APRIL, VEGF, IL4, and CD40. CLL cells are also maintained through contact with stromal cells (marrow and dendritic) and nurse-like cells through a complex interface of adhesion molecules and stromal survival factors. Exposure to these factors promotes up-regulation of anti-apoptotic proteins such as BCL2, MCL1, and survival signaling pathways involving NF-κB, PI3-kinase, and ERK that promote survival of CLL cells. The importance of the in vivo environment to CLL survival is supported by the increased apoptosis, which occurs when CLL cells are cultured in vitro.

Diagnosis and Presentation
Symptoms
CLL patients often present with no symptoms, although a small proportion of patients have symptoms related to marrow replacement (fatigue, dyspnea, or petechiae secondary to anemia and thrombocytopenia), lymphadenopathy or hepatosplenomegaly, autoimmune complications (hemolytic anemia or idiopathic thrombocytopenic purpura), or B-symptoms (fevers, night sweats, and weight loss).

Hematologic Findings
In addition to blood and marrow lymphocytosis, a few abnormal laboratory findings are commonly observed in CLL. Neutropenia, anemia, and thrombocytopenia can develop as a consequence of marrow infiltration or therapy administered to eliminate the leukemia. A positive direct antiglobulin test (DAT), or Coomb's, test consistent with the diagnosis of autoimmune antibodies directed at red cells is observed in approximately 10% to 25% of CLL patients sometime during the course of the disease (134). A subset of these patients will develop symptomatic hemolytic anemia as a consequence of antibody-mediated red cell destruction. Similarly, autoimmune thrombocytopenia or neutropenia may be present, although marrow replacement or chemotherapy side effects are much more common causes and should be excluded. Pure red cell aplasia can sometimes be observed and presents with isolated anemia

and absence of red cell precursor cells. Hypogammaglobulinemia is common and becomes more frequent and marked as the disease progresses. In contrast, hypercalcemia and markedly elevated lactate dehydrogenase is not common in CLL and suggests Richter's transformation, which represents change of CLL to diffuse large cell lymphoma. This generally occurs after patients have been treated for their CLL (135,136). Richter's transformation is generally associated with a very poor outcome, and investigational therapies and/or stem-cell transplantation should be considered (135,136).

The diagnosis of CLL relies on immunophenotypic confirmation, and flow cytometry should therefore be performed on all patients at diagnosis. CLL cells have a relatively consistent immunophenotype, which differentiates CLL from other indolent B-cell malignancies. CLL cells express a variety of B-cell markers, including dim surface immunoglobulins (sIg), CD19, dim CD20, and CD23, as well as the pan T-cell marker CD5. Kappa or lambda immunoglobulin light chain restriction is always present, establishing the presence of a clonal B-cell population, although sIg expression may be so weak that light chain restriction may be difficult to determine. In contrast, presence of CD10, FMC7, or CD79b (all typically absent on CLL cells) or bright expression of CD11c, CD20, or CD25 (all typically dim on CLL cells) suggests an alternative low-grade B-cell lymphoproliferative malignancy. Expression of CD5 without CD23 suggests mantle cell lymphoma, and FISH for t(11;14)(q13;q32) should be performed to exclude this diagnosis.

Staging and Prognostic Factors
Until recently, the staging of CLL in patients has been done using the Rai or Binet system. Both systems discriminate CLL stages by the sites of disease and degree of cytopenias induced by leukemia marrow replacement. The Rai staging system is shown in Table 12.11 (137). For early-stage patients (Rai low and intermediate stage), a relatively large range of time to developing symptoms exists. The lack of survival advantage with early treatment, the observation that some patients will never require therapy, and the varied natural history of the disease have driven research efforts in CLL to identify specific biologic or clinical factors that predict time to progression. Features other than the Rai or Binet systems used in daily practice include plasma/serum assays of thymidine kinase activity and beta-2-microglobulin,

Table 12.11 Rai Staging System of CLL (137)

Rai stage at diagnosis	Percent of patients never requiring CLL therapy	Expected survival in months from initial diagnosis
0 Lymphocytosis >5 × 10⁹/l only	59	150
1 Lymph node (LN) enlargement	21	101
2 Spleen/liver (S/L) enlargement ± LN	23	71
3 Anemia with hemoglobin <11 g/dl ± LN or S/L	5	19
4 Thrombocytopenia <100 × 10¹²/l ± LN or S/L	0	19

whose higher levels portend rapid disease progression and short survival.

Cytogenetic abnormalities have been proven prognostic in CLL. Conventional metaphase cytogenetics identifies chromosomal aberrations in only 20% to 50% of cases. Interphase FISH of known abnormalities is therefore required to adequately assess genetic findings in CLL and distinguish genetic subtypes of the disease, given the absence of CLL cell proliferation without mitogen stimulation. Cytogenetic abnormalities in CLL are different from those observed in other types of leukemia. They are mostly deletions; balanced translocations are rare. The largest study of interphase FISH detected abnormalities in >80% of patients (138). The del(13)(q14) is by far the most common cytogenetic abnormality, followed by trisomy 12, del(11) (q22.3), del(17)(p13.1), and del(6)(q22.3). Patients with del(11)(q22.3) and del(17)(p13.1) generally have accelerated disease progression and poor survival (138).

Döhner and colleagues (138) constructed a hierarchical model consisting of five genetic subgroups on the basis of regression analysis of CLL patients studied by FISH. Patients with a del(17p) had the shortest median survival (32 months) and treatment-free interval (nine months), whereas patients with del(11q) followed closely with 79 months and 13 months, respectively (138). The favorable del(13)(q14) group had a long median treatment-free interval (92 months) and survival (133 months), whereas the group without detectable chromosomal anomalies and patients with trisomy 12 was included in an intermediate group, with median survivals of 111 and 114 months, and treatment-free intervals of 33 and 49 months, respectively. Based on this pivotal study, CLL patients are prioritized in a hierarchical order [del(17)(p13)>del(11)(q22-q23)>trisomy 12>no aberration>del(13)(q14)] (138). Interestingly, patients with high-risk interphase cytogenetic abnormalities or complex abnormalities usually have IgV$_H$ unmutated CLL (139). The impact of high-risk interphase cytogenetics relative to disease progression, outside of its association with IgV$_H$ unmutated CLL, is unknown.

IgV$_H$ mutational status of the CLL clone is an important prognostic factor (131,132). Approximately 60% of CLL patients have cells with mutated IgV$_H$ genes (<98% sequence identity with germline), whereas the remaining patients have cells exhibiting unmutated IgV$_H$ (≥98% identity with germline). The prognostic significance of the absence of IgV$_H$ gene mutations is substantial, with all studies uniformly showing an inferior survival and high predisposition to requiring early treatment (132,133,140–143). Although other biomarkers have been suggested as surrogate markers to IgV$_H$ gene mutational status, including ZAP-70, CD38, these are either not reproducible or not uniformly predictive of IgV$_H$ gene mutational status.

Despite the usefulness of these clinical and laboratory tests to predict the natural history of CLL, no study to date has demonstrated that earlier treatment will alter the natural history of patients even in the higher-risk groups. Therefore, at present, staging and predictive biomarkers should be used only to provide patients with information relative to the expected course of their disease, but these should never be used to initiate therapy in patients with asymptomatic disease and no indication for treatment. A detailed discussion of how these tests will be used with the patient should occur, and the option of not performing them should be provided. In a subset of patients, significant anxiety can be produced by identifying high-risk features for which intervention remains only observation. Table 12.12 provides the typical evaluation provided by our group when seeing a newly diagnosed CLL patient.

Treatment

Initial Treatment

Treatment of CLL is not initiated until symptoms develop based upon several studies that failed to show an improvement in overall survival when early therapeutic intervention with chlorambucil therapy was administered to asymptomatic patients (144). The National Cancer Institute–sponsored Working Group on CLL established guidelines for the initiation of treatment and were recently updated (145); a modified version is provided in Table 12.13. A useful paradigm for clinical practice is to institute treatment in CLL only for cytopenias or directly referable symptoms. When treatment is necessary, treatment options have expanded with the introduction of several new agents. In addition, several retrospective (146–150) and prospective trials (151,152) have recently demonstrated that some of the same prognostic features that predict the time to progression and need for therapy may also predict treatment outcome (Fig. 12.2).

Table 12.12 Evaluation of CLL Patients at Diagnosis

History
B-symptom and fatigue assessment
Infectious history assessment
Occupational assessment for chemical exposure
Familial history of CLL and lymphoproliferative disorders
Preventive interventions for infections and secondary cancers

Physical exam

Laboratory assessment
Complete blood count with differential
Morphology assessment of lymphocytes
Chemistry, LFT enzymes, lactate dehydrogenase
Flow cytometry assessment to confirm immunophenotype of CLL
Serum immunoglobulins
Serum β_2M levels
Interphase cytogenetics for del(17)(p13.1), del(11)(q22.3), del(13) (q14), del(6)(q21), trisomy 12
IgV$_H$ mutational analysis
Stimulated metaphase karyotype (if available)

Selected tests under certain circumstances
Direct antiglobulin test (DAT), haptoglobin, riticulocyte count if anemia present
CT scan if unexplained abdominal pain or enlargement present
PET scan and/or biopsy if large nodal mass present
Bone marrow aspirate and biopsy if cytopenias present
Familial counseling if first degree relative with CLL

Teaching
Varicella zoster Identification Instruction
Skin cancer Identification
Disease education [Leukemia and Lymphoma Society, CLL Topics, Association of Cancer Online Resources (ACOR)]

Table 12.13 Modified Indications for Treatment of CLL (145)

Grade 2 or greater fatigue limiting life activities

B-symptoms persisting for 2 weeks or greater

Lymph nodes greater than 10 cm or progressively enlarging lymph nodes causing symptoms

Spleen or liver with progressive enlargement or causing symptoms

Anemia (hemoglobin <11 g/dl) referable to CLL

Thrombocytopenia (platelets <100 $\times$ 10^{12}/l) referable to CLL

Autoimmune hemolytic anemia or idiopathic thrombocytopenic purpura poorly responsive to traditional therapy

WBC >300 $\times$ 10^9/l on two occasions two weeks apart if no alternative co-morbid diseases increase morbidity of treatment

Severe paraneoplastic process (insect hypersensitivity, vasculitis, myositis, etc.) related to CLL not responsive to traditional therapies

Although CLL therapy for many years consisted of chlorambucil or other alkylating agents, several randomized trials have demonstrated that monotherapy with fludarabine (153), bendamustine (154), or alemtuzumab (155) is superior to this approach as indicated by improved response rates and remission duration. However, toxicities (cytopenias, infection, infusion toxicity) are often more frequent with these newer approaches as well. Given the more extended experience with the purine analogs for over two decades, combination-based approaches have been built upon them. Fludarabine was combined with cyclophosphamide (fludarabine/cyclophosphamide) in three randomized phase III studies of younger CLL patients, and all three demonstrated improved response and progression-free survival (156–158). The benefit of this combination was greatest in patients younger than 65 years. In addition, although del(11)(q22.3) patients had inferior outcome with fludarabine-based regimens, the addition of cyclophosphamide appears to abrogate this (158). If confirmed, this would suggest that del(11)(q22.3) patients would benefit the most from fludarabine/cyclophosphamide.

Rituximab was introduced for CLL in the late 1990s and had only modest activity as monotherapy in relapsed patients. However, when given in combination with fludarabine (159,160) or fludarabine/cyclophosphamide (FCR) (161), significant responses and extended remissions were observed. Studies with both fludarabine and fludarabine/cyclophosphamide have demonstrated that patients with del(17)(p13.1) do not respond well and that patients with IgV_H unmutated disease have shorter remission durations.

The humanized monoclonal antibody alemtuzumab is directed against the surface antigen CD52. The broad expression CD52 on normal lymphocytes and monocytes is predictive of the increased neutropenia, lymphopenia, and infectious complications, which have been observed with alemtuzumab therapy. Although clinical activity has been observed with alemtuzumab, its use will likely be limited by the significant toxicity and associated immune suppression.

Bendamustine is the most recently approved agent for CLL treatment. Although chemical properties of bendamustine suggest it acts as an alkylating agent, preclinical work demonstrates it has a novel mechanism of action (162). A recent randomized study comparing bendamustine to chlorambucil demonstrated bendamustine's superiority with respect to response and progression-free survival (154). The U.S. Food and Drug Administration has approved bendamustine for use in initial and salvage treatment of CLL. However, the role of bendamustine related to high-risk interphase cytogenetics and IgV_H unmutated disease and the potential long-term risks of secondary leukemia remain to be defined.

Treatment of Relapsed CLL

The approach to reinitiating therapy for CLL patients who relapsed after initial therapy is similar to that applied for initial therapy assessment. Patients need not receive therapy at the first sign of relapse. Rather, they should have an indication for treatment, as discussed above. Patients should have repeat interphase FISH analysis of the blood

---

Clinical trial is always first choice

Young patient (<70) with good performance status

- Del(17)(p13.1)-FCR or trial followed by non-myeloablative allogeneic stem cell transplant
- Del(11)(q22.3)-FCR
- Other genetic features-FR

Older patient (>70) with good performance status

- Del(17)(p13.1)-alemtuzumab
- Del(11)(q22.3)-PCR
- Other genetic features FR or PCR, bendamustine

Older patient (>70) with poor performance status

- Rituximab or chlorambucil

Figure 12.2 Treatment approach for symptomatic previously untreated CLL at the Ohio State University, Columbus, Ohio.

or marrow aspirate, because they may have acquired additional cytogenetic abnormalities such as the del(17)(p13.1). A marrow analysis should be performed if cytopenias are present to confirm that CLL is the cause and exclude other potential causes, including transformed lymphoma, prolonged marrow toxicity from prior therapy, or development of treatment-related myelodysplasia. For relapsing patients aged 70 years or older, re-treatment with the same therapy or with an alternative antibody or investigational agent can be considered. In general, for a patient younger than 70 years who has experienced a good remission with initial therapy (>12 months), an FCR regimen (161), preferably in combination with an investigational agent, is suggested. If a complete remission is obtained in patients without a del(17)(p13.1), our approach at this point is to observe. If a del(17)(p13.1) is present or a complete remission is not obtained, we generally consider a nonmyeloablative stem-cell transplantation.

For relapsing patients 70 years or older, we do not administer FCR regimen due to concerns of increasing toxicity. Any patient who does not attain complete remission following second therapy or who harbors del(17)(p13.1) at the time of relapse should be considered as a candidate for a reduced intensity allogeneic stem-cell transplantation. Although transplantation is associated with more initial treatment-related mortality, the long-term benefit of stem-cell transplantation for high-risk genomic CLL makes it an attractive option for these patients. Specifically, extended disease-free intervals and plateau in relapse frequency have been observed in CLL with both full and reduced-intensity transplantation for CLL. Given the older age of most CLL patients, reduced-intensity transplantations are becoming more acceptable. In contrast, autologous stem-cell transplantation does not offer the graft-versus-leukemia effect of a reduced-intensity allogeneic stem-cell transplantation and is associated with a continuous risk of relapse from CLL over time. Autologous stem-cell transplantation is therefore not generally used.

Future Directions of CLL Therapy

There are currently multiple investigational agents in phase I, II, and III testing for relapsed CLL. Agents such as lenalidomide, flavopiridol, and ofatumumab have demonstrated single agent clinical activity, and are currently in phase III registration studies for potential approval for use in relapsed and refractory CLL patients. Other agents such as lumiliximab and genasense have very modest clinical activity but appear to augment the effectiveness of chemotherapy or chemoimmunotherapy. Phase III combination studies with these agents and chemotherapy or chemoimmunotherapy are either underway or completed.

Many other therapeutic agents are currently in early phase I/II clinical trials for CLL or will be entering the clinic within the next year. Therapeutic antibodies or small modular immune pharmaceuticals (SMIP™) targeting surface antigens including CD40, HLA-DR, CD19, CD20, CD37, CD74, and CD200 are under development. Additionally, therapeutic agents targeting signal transduction pathways (HSP-90 inhibitors, AKT inhibitors, PI3K-δ inhibitors, syk inhibitors, PKC-δ inhibitors, and PP2A activating agents) are in early clinical development. Finally, agents targeting epigenetic events (histone deacetylase inhibitors,

hypomethylating agents), micro-RNA directed therapy, or innate immune activation (CpG oligonucleotides or IL21) have promising preclinical data to support their ongoing early clinical investigation (163,164).

Conclusions

The understanding of the biology and treatment of CLL has significantly improved over the past two decades. With these advances has come the identification of new biomarkers that can predict early disease progression, poor response to therapy, and inferior survival. Concurrent with these developments, new therapies have also emerged that are increasing the proportion of CLL patients going into complete remission and having prolonged treatment-free intervals. Understanding the impact of these new prognostic features and treatment approaches will be essential to assuring optimal management of CLL patients.

ACKNOWLEDGMENTS

This study was supported in part by National Cancer Institute, Bethesda, Maryland (MD) grants CA16058 and R01CA102031, PO1 CA110496, The Leukemia and Lymphoma Foundation, The D Warren Brown Foundation, and The Coleman Leukemia Research Foundation.

REFERENCES

1. Estey E, Döhner H. Acute myeloid leukaemia. Lancet 2006; 368: 1894–907.
2. Pui CH, Robison LL, Look AT. Acute lymphoblastic leukaemia. Lancet 2008; 371: 1030–43.
3. Hehlmann R, Hochhaus A, Baccarani M. Chronic myeloid leukaemia. Lancet 2007; 370: 342–50.
4. Dighiero G, Hamblin TJ. Chronic lymphocytic leukaemia. Lancet 2008; 371: 1017–29.
5. Ries LAG, Melbert D, Krapcho M et al., eds. SEER Cancer Statistics Review, 1975–2004, National Cancer Institute. Bethesda, MD. http://seer.cancer.gov/csr/1975_2004/, based on November 2007 SEER data submission, posted to the SEER web site, 2008.
6. Sandler DP, Ross JA. Epidemiology of acute leukemia in children and adults. Semin Oncol 1997; 24: 3–16.
7. Owen C, Barnett M, Fitzgibbon J. Familial myelodysplasia and acute myeloid leukaemia—a review. Br J Haematol 2008; 140: 123–32.
8. Goldgar DE, Easton DF, Cannon-Albright LA et al. Systematic population-based assessment of cancer risk in first-degree relatives of cancer probands. J Natl Cancer Inst 1994; 86: 1600–8.
9. Yuille MR, Matutes E, Marossy A et al. Familial chronic lymphocytic leukaemia: a survey and review of published studies. Br J Haematol 2000; 109: 794–9.
10. Conley CL, Misiti J, Laster AJ. Genetic factors predisposing to chronic lymphocytic leukemia and to autoimmune disease. Medicine (Baltimore) 1980; 59: 323–34.
11. Cuttner J. Increased incidence of hematologic malignances in first-degree relatives of patients with chronic lymphocytic leukemia. Cancer Invest 1992; 10: 103–9.
12. Raval A, Tanner SM, Byrd JC et al. Downregulation of death-associated protein kinase 1 (DAPK1) in chronic lymphocytic leukemia. Cell 2007; 129: 879–90.
13. Travis LB, Li C-Y, Zhang Z-N et al. Hematopoietic malignancies and related disorders among benzene-exposed workers in China. Leuk Lymphoma 1994; 14: 91–102.

14. Kane EV, Roman E, Cartwright R et al. Tobacco and the risk of acute leukaemia in adults. Br J Cancer 1999; 81: 1228–33.

15. Smith SM, Le Beau MM, Huo D et al. Clinical-cytogenetic associations in 306 patients with therapy-related myelodysplasia or myeloid leukemia: the University of Chicago series. Blood 2003; 102: 43–52.

16. Nakanishi M, Tanaka K, Shintani T et al. Chromosomal instability in acute myelocytic leukemia and myelodysplastic syndrome in patients among atomic bomb survivors. J Radiat Res (Tokyo) 1999; 40: 159–67.

17. von Mühlendahl KE. Chernobyl fallout, nuclear plants and leukaemia: review of recent literature. Eur J Pediatr 1998; 157: 602–4.

18. Swerdlow SH, Campo E, Harris NL et al., eds. World Health Organization Classification of Tumours of Haematopoietic and Lymphoid Tissues. Lyon: IARC Press, 2008.

19. Cheson BD, Bennett JM, Kopecky KJ et al. Revised recommendations of the International Working Group for diagnosis, standardization of response criteria, treatment outcomes, and reporting standards for therapeutic trials in acute myeloid leukemia. J Clin Oncol 2003; 21: 4642–9.

20. Estey E. Acute myeloid leukemia and myelodysplastic syndromes in older patients. J Clin Oncol 2007; 25: 1908–15.

21. Stone RM, O'Donnell MR, Sekeres MA. Acute myeloid leukemia. Hematology Am Soc Hematol Educ Program 2004: 98–117.

22. Mrózek K, Bloomfield CD. Chromosome aberrations, gene mutations and expression changes, and prognosis in adult acute myeloid leukemia. Hematology Am Soc Hematol Educ Program 2006: 169–77.

23. Mrózek K, Marcucci G, Paschka P et al. Clinical relevance of mutations and gene-expression changes in adult acute myeloid leukemia with normal cytogenetics: are we ready for a prognostically prioritized molecular classification? Blood 2007; 109: 431–48.

24. Thiede C, Steudel C, Mohr B et al. Analysis of FLT3-activating mutations in 979 patients with acute myelogenous leukemia: association with FAB subtypes and identification of subgroups with poor prognosis. Blood 2002; 99: 4326–35.

25. Gale RE, Green C, Allen C et al. The impact of FLT3 internal tandem duplication mutant level, number, size, and interaction with NPM1 mutations in a large cohort of young adult patients with acute myeloid leukemia. Blood 2008; 111: 2776–84.

26. Döhner K, Schlenk RF, Habdank M et al. Mutant nucleophosmin (NPM1) predicts favorable prognosis in younger adults with acute myeloid leukemia and normal cytogenetics: interaction with other gene mutations. Blood 2005; 106: 3740–6.

27. Fröhling S, Schlenk RF, Stolze I et al. CEBPA mutations in younger adults with acute myeloid leukemia and normal cytogenetics: prognostic relevance and analysis of cooperating mutations. J Clin Oncol 2004; 22: 624–33.

28. Whitman SP, Ruppert AS, Marcucci G et al. Long-term disease-free survivors with cytogenetically normal acute myeloid leukemia and MLL partial tandem duplication: a Cancer and Leukemia Group B study. Blood 2007; 109: 5164–7.

29. Paschka P, Marcucci G, Ruppert AS et al. Wilms' tumor 1 gene mutations independently predict poor outcome in adults with cytogenetically normal acute myeloid leukemia: a Cancer and Leukemia Group B study. J Clin Oncol 2008; 26: 4595–602.

30. Baldus CD, Tanner SM, Ruppert AS et al. BAALC expression predicts clinical outcome of de novo acute myeloid leukemia patients with normal cytogenetics: a Cancer and Leukemia Group B study. Blood 2003; 102: 1613–18.

31. Marcucci G, Maharry K, Whitman SP et al. High expression levels of the ETS-related gene, ERG, predict adverse outcome and improve molecular risk-based classification of cytogenetically normal acute myeloid leukemia: a Cancer and Leukemia Group B study. J Clin Oncol 2007; 25: 3337–43.

32. Heuser M, Beutel G, Krauter J et al. High meningioma 1 (MN1) expression as a predictor for poor outcome in acute myeloid leukemia with normal cytogenetics. Blood 2006; 108: 3898–905.

33. Paschka P, Marcucci G, Ruppert AS et al. Adverse prognostic significance of KIT mutations in adult acute myeloid leukemia with inv(16) and t(8;21): a Cancer and Leukemia Group B study. J Clin Oncol 2006; 24: 3904–11.

34. Löwenberg B, van Putten W, Theobald M et al. Effect of priming with granulocyte colony-stimulating factor on the outcome of chemotherapy for acute myeloid leukemia. N Engl J Med 2003; 349: 743–52.

35. Amadori S, Suciu S, Jehn U et al. Use of glycosylated recombinant human G-CSF (lenograstim) during and/or after induction chemotherapy in patients 61 years of age and older with acute myeloid leukemia: final results of AML-13, a randomized phase III study. Blood 2005; 106: 27–34.

36. Smith TJ, Khatcheressian J, Lyman GH et al. 2006 update of recommendations for the use of white blood cell growth factors: an evidence-based clinical practice guideline. J Clin Oncol 2006; 24: 3187–205.

37. Segal BH, Freifeld AG, Baden LR et al. Prevention and treatment of cancer-related infections. J Natl Compr Canc Netw 2008; 6: 122–74.

38. Rowe JM. Consolidation therapy: what should be the standard of care? Best Pract Res Clin Haematol 2008; 21: 53–60.

39. Mayer R, Davis R, Schiffer C et al. Intensive postremission chemotherapy in adults with acute myeloid leukemia. N Engl J Med 1994; 331: 896–903.

40. Bloomfield CD, Lawrence D, Byrd JC et al. Frequency of prolonged remission duration after high-dose cytarabine intensification in acute myeloid leukemia varies by cytogenetic subtype. Cancer Res 1998; 58: 4173–9.

41. Byrd JC, Dodge RK, Carroll A et al. Patients with t(8;21) (q22;q22) and acute myeloid leukemia have superior failure-free and overall survival when repetitive cycles of high-dose cytarabine are administered. J Clin Oncol 1999; 17: 3767–75.

42. Byrd JC, Ruppert AS, Mrózek K et al. Repetitive cycles of high-dose cytarabine benefit patients with acute myeloid leukemia and inv(16)(p13q22) or t(16;16)(p13;q22): results from CALGB 8461. J Clin Oncol 2004; 22: 1087–94.

43. Farag SS, Ruppert AS, Mrózek K et al. Outcome of induction and postremission therapy in younger adults with acute myeloid leukemia with normal karyotype: a Cancer and Leukemia Group B study. J Clin Oncol 2005; 23: 482–93.

44. Cassileth PA, Harrington DP, Appelbaum FR et al. Chemotherapy compared with autologous or allogeneic bone marrow transplantation in the management of acute myeloid leukemia in first remission. N Engl J Med 1998; 339: 1649–56.

45. Suciu S, Mandelli F, de Witte T et al. EORTC and GIMEMA Leukemia Groups. Allogeneic compared with autologous stem cell transplantation in the treatment of patients younger than 46 years with acute myeloid leukemia (AML) in first complete remission (CR1): an intention-to-treat analysis of the EORTC/GIMEMA AML-10 trial. Blood 2003; 102: 1232–40.

46. Harousseau J-L, Cahn J-Y, Pignon B et al. Comparison of autologous bone marrow transplantation and intensive chemotherapy as postremission therapy in adult acute myeloid leukemia. Blood 1997; 90: 2978–86.

47. Gale R, Hills R, Kottaridis PD et al. No evidence that FLT3 status should be considered as an indicator for transplantation in acute myeloid leukemia (AML): an analysis of 1135 patients, excluding promyelocytic leukemia, from the UK MRC AML10 and 12 trials. Blood 2005; 106: 3658–65.

48. Schlenk RF, Döhner K, Krauter J et al. Mutations and treatment outcome in cytogenetically normal acute myeloid leukemia. N Engl J Med 2008; 358: 1909–18.

49. Wang ZY, Chen Z. Acute promyelocytic leukemia: from highly fatal to highly curable. Blood 2008; 111: 2505–15.

50. Sanz MA. Treatment of acute promyelocytic leukemia. Hematology Am Soc Hematol Educ Program 2006: 147–55.

51. Powell BL, Moser B, Stock W et al. Arsenic trioxide consolidation improves event-free and overall survival among patients with newly diagnosed acute promyelocytic leukemia: North American intergroup protocol c9710. Ann Hematol 2008; 87(Suppl 1): S77–S78.

52. Bourgeois E, Chevret S, Sanz M et al. Long-term follow-up of APL treated with ATRA and chemotherapy (CT) including incidence of late relapses and overall toxicity. Blood 2003; 102: 140a–1a.

53. Sanz MA, Martin G, González M et al. Risk-adapted treatment of acute promyelocytic leukemia with all-*trans*-retinoic acid and anthracycline monochemotherapy: a multicenter study by the PETHEMA group. Blood 2004; 103: 1237–43.

54. Estey E, Garcia-Manero G, Ferrajoli A et al. Use of all-*trans* retinoic acid plus arsenic trioxide as an alternative to chemotherapy in untreated acute promyelocytic leukemia. Blood 2006; 107: 3469–73.

55. Lo-Coco F, Ammatuna E. Front line clinical trials and minimal residual disease monitoring in acute promyelocytic leukemia. Curr Top Microbiol Immunol 2007; 313: 145–56.

56. Tallman MS. Treatment of relapsed or refractory acute promyelocytic leukemia. Best Pract Res Clin Haematol 2007; 20: 57–65.

57. Breems DA, Van Putten WLJ, Huijgens PC et al. Prognostic index for adult patients with acute myeloid leukemia in first relapse. J Clin Oncol 2005; 23: 1969–78.

58. Wong R, Shajahan M, Wang X et al. Prognostic factors for outcomes of patients with refractory or relapsed acute myelogenous leukemia or myelodysplastic syndromes undergoing allogeneic progenitor cell transplantation. Biol Blood Marrow Transplant 2005; 11: 108–14.

59. Blum W, Marcucci G. New approaches in acute myeloid leukemia. Best Pract Res Clin Haematol 2008; 21: 29–41.

60. List AF, Spier C, Greer J et al. Phase I/II trial of cyclosporine as a chemotherapy-resistance modifier in acute leukemia. J Clin Oncol 1993; 11: 1652–60.

61. Russell NH. Biology of acute leukaemia. Lancet 1997; 349: 118–22.

62. Castor A, Nilsson L, Åstrand-Grundström I et al. Distinct patterns of hematopoietic stem cell involvement in acute lymphoblastic leukemia. Nat Med 2005; 11: 630–7.

63. Kong Y, Yoshida S, Saito Y et al. CD34+CD38+CD19+ as well as CD34+CD38–CD19+ cells are leukemia-initiating cells with self-renewal capacity in human B-precursor ALL. Leukemia 2008; 22: 1207–13.

64. Quijano CA, Moore D II, Arthur D et al. Cytogenetically aberrant cells are present in the CD34+CD33–38–19– marrow compartment in children with acute lymphoblastic leukemia. Leukemia 1997; 11: 1508–15.

65. Cox CV, Evely RS, Oakhill A et al. Characterization of acute lymphoblastic leukemia progenitor cells. Blood 2004; 104: 2919–25.

66. Cox CV, Martin HM, Kearns PR et al. Characterization of a progenitor cell population in childhood T-cell acute lymphoblastic leukemia. Blood 2007; 109: 674–82.

67. le Viseur C, Hotfilder M, Bomken S et al. In childhood acute lymphoblastic leukemia, blasts at different stages of immunophenotypic maturation have stem cell properties. Cancer Cell 2008; 14: 47–58.

68. Shivakumar R, Tan W, Wilding GE et al. Biologic features and treatment outcome of secondary acute lymphoblastic leukemia–a review of 101 cases. Ann Oncol 2008; 19: 1634–8.

69. Mullighan CG, Miller CB, Radtke I et al. *BCR-ABL1* lymphoblastic leukaemia is characterized by the deletion of Ikaros. Nature 2008; 453: 110–14.

70. O'Neil J, Look AT. Mechanisms of transcription factor deregulation in lymphoid cell transformation. Oncogene 2007; 26: 6838–49.

71. Mullighan CG, Goorha S, Radtke I et al. Genome-wide analysis of genetic alterations in acute lymphoblastic leukaemia. Nature 2007; 446: 758–64.

72. Bousquet M, Broccardo C, Quelen C et al. A novel PAX5-ELN fusion protein identified in B-cell acute lymphoblastic leukemia acts as a dominant negative on wild-type PAX5. Blood 2007; 109: 3417–23.

73. Graux C, Cools J, Michaux L et al. Cytogenetics and molecular genetics of T-cell acute lymphoblastic leukemia: from thymocyte to lymphoblast. Leukemia 2006; 20: 1496–510.

74. Aifantis I, Raetz E, Buonamici S. Molecular pathogenesis of T-cell leukaemia and lymphoma. Nat Rev Immunol 2008; 8: 380–90.

75. Baak U, Gökbuget N, Orawa H et al. Thymic adult T-cell acute lymphoblastic leukemia stratified in standard- and high-risk group by aberrant HOX11L2 expression: experience of the German multicenter ALL study group. Leukemia 2008; 22: 1154–60.

76. Baldus CD, Martus P, Burmeister T et al. Low *ERG* and *BAALC* expression identifies a new subgroup of adult acute T-lymphoblastic leukemia with a highly favorable outcome. J Clin Oncol 2007; 25: 3739–45.

77. Szczepański T. Why and how to quantify minimal residual disease in acute lymphoblastic leukemia? Leukemia 2007; 21: 622–6.

78. Brüggemann M, Raff T, Flohr T et al. Clinical significance of minimal residual disease quantification in adult patients with standard-risk acute lymphoblastic leukemia. Blood 2006; 107: 1116–23.

79. Larson S, Stock W. Progress in the treatment of adults with acute lymphoblastic leukemia. Curr Opin Hematol 2008; 15: 400–7.

80. Schultz KR, Bowman WP, Slayton W et al. Improved early event free survival (EFS) in children with Philadelphia chromosome-positive (Ph+) acute lymphoblastic leukemia (ALL) with intensive imatinib in combination with high dose chemotherapy: Children's Oncology Group (COG) study AALL0031. Blood 2007; 110: 9a.

81. Thomas DA, Kantarjian HM, Ravandi F et al. Long-term follow-up after frontline therapy with hyper-CVAD and imatinib mesylate regimen in adults with Philadelphia (Ph) positive acute lymphocytic leukemia (ALL). Blood 2007; 110: 10a.

82. Potenza L, Luppi M, Riva G et al. Efficacy of imatinib mesylate as maintenance therapy in adults with acute lymphoblastic leukemia in first complete remission. Haematologica 2005; 90: 1275–7.

83. de Labarthe A, Rousselot P, Huguet-Rigal F et al. Imatinib combined with induction or consolidation chemotherapy in patients with de novo Philadelphia chromosome-positive acute lymphoblastic leukemia: results of the GRAAPH-2003 study. Blood 2007; 109: 1408–13.

84. Wetzler M, Stock W, Donohue KA et al. Autologous stem cell transplantation (SCT) following sequential chemotherapy and imatinib for adults with newly diagnosed Philadelphia chromosome positive acute lymphoblastic leukemia (Ph+ ALL)—CALGB study 10001. Blood 2007; 110: 843a.

85. Yanada M, Takeuchi J, Sugiura I et al. High complete remission rate and promising outcome by combination of imatinib and chemotherapy for newly diagnosed *BCR-ABL*-positive acute lymphoblastic leukemia: a phase II study by the Japan Adult Leukemia Study Group. J Clin Oncol 2006; 24: 460–6.

86. Wassmann B, Pfeifer H, Goekbuget N et al. Alternating versus concurrent schedules of imatinib and chemotherapy as front-line therapy for Philadelphia-positive acute lymphoblastic leukemia (Ph⁺ ALL). Blood 2006; 108: 1469–77.

87. Lee K-H, Lee J-H, Choi S-J et al. Clinical effect of imatinib added to intensive combination chemotherapy for newly diagnosed Philadelphia chromosome-positive acute lymphoblastic leukemia. Leukemia 2005; 19: 1509–16.

88. Delannoy A, Delabesse E, Lhéritier V et al. Imatinib and methylprednisolone alternated with chemotherapy improve the outcome of elderly patients with Philadelphia-positive acute lymphoblastic leukemia: results of the GRAALL AFR09 study. Leukemia 2006; 20: 1526–32.

89. Ottmann OG, Wassmann B, Pfeifer H et al. Imatinib compared with chemotherapy as front-line treatment of elderly patients with Philadelphia chromosome-positive acute lymphoblastic leukemia (Ph⁺ ALL). Cancer 2007; 109: 2068–76.

90. Vignetti M, Fazi P, Cimino G et al. Imatinib plus steroids induces complete remissions and prolonged survival in elderly Philadelphia chromosome-positive patients with acute lymphoblastic leukemia without additional chemotherapy: results of the Gruppo Italiano Malattie Ematologiche dell'Adulto (GIMEMA) LAL0201-B protocol. Blood 2007; 109: 3676–8.

91. Pfeifer H, Wassmann B, Pavlova A et al. Kinase domain mutations of BCR-ABL frequently precede imatinib-based therapy and give rise to relapse in patients with de novo Philadelphia-positive acute lymphoblastic leukemia (Ph⁺ ALL). Blood 2007; 110: 727–34.

92. Hu Y, Liu Y, Pelletier S et al. Requirement of Src kinases Lyn, Hck and Fgr for *BCR-ABL1*-induced B-lymphoblastic leukemia but not chronic myeloid leukemia. Nat Genet 2004; 36: 453–61.

93. Mishra S, Zhang B, Cunnick JM et al. Resistance to imatinib of bcr/abl p190 lymphoblastic leukemia cells. Cancer Res 2006; 66: 5387–93.

94. Ottmann O, Dombret H, Martinelli G et al. Dasatinib induces rapid hematologic and cytogenetic responses in adult patients with Philadelphia chromosome-positive acute lymphoblastic leukemia with resistance or intolerance to imatinib: interim results of a phase 2 study. Blood 2007; 110: 2309–15.

95. Foa R, Vignetti M, Vitale A et al. Dasatinib as front-line monotherapy for the induction treatment of adult and elderly Ph+ acute lymphoblastic leukemia (ALL) patients: interim analysis of the GIMEMA prospective study LAL1205. Blood 2007; 110: 10a.

96. Ottman OG, Larson RA, Kantarjian HM et al. Nilotininb in patients (pts) with refractory/relapsed Philadelphia chromosome-positive acute lymphoblastic leukemia (Ph⁺ ALL) who are resistant or intolerant to imatinib. Blood 2007; 110: 828a.

97. Cohen MH, Johnson JR, Justice R et al. FDA drug approval summary: nelarabine (Arranon®) for the treatment of T-cell lymphoblastic leukemia/lymphoma. Oncologist 2008; 13: 709–14.

98. Sallan SE. Myths and lessons from the adult/pediatric interface in acute lymphoblastic leukemia. Hematology Am Soc Hematol Educ Program 2006: 128–32.

99. Ribera J-M, Oriol A, Sanz M-A et al. Comparison of the results of the treatment of adolescents and young adults with standard-risk acute lymphoblastic leukemia with the Programa Español de Tratamiento en Hematología pediatric-based protocol ALL-96. J Clin Oncol 2008; 26: 1843–9.

100. Usvasalo A, Räty R, Knuutila S et al. Acute lymphoblastic leukemia in adolescents and young adults in Finland. Haematologica 2008; 93: 1161–8.

101. Ferry JA. Burkitt's lymphoma: clinicopathologic features and differential diagnosis. Oncologist 2006; 11: 375–83.

102. Thomas DA, Faderl S, O'Brien S et al. Chemoimmunotherapy with hyper-CVAD plus rituximab for the treatment of adult Burkitt and Burkitt-type lymphoma or acute lymphoblastic leukemia. Cancer 2006; 106: 1569–80.

103. Oriol A, Ribera J-M, Bergua J et al. High-dose chemotherapy and immunotherapy in adult Burkitt lymphoma: comparison of results in human immunodeficiency virus-infected and noninfected patients. Cancer 2008; 113: 117–25.

104. Stein A, Forman SJ. Allogeneic transplantation for ALL in adults. Bone Marrow Transplant 2008; 41: 439–46.

105. Douer D, Yampolsky H, Cohen LJ et al. Pharmacodynamics and safety of intravenous pegaspargase during remission induction in adults aged 55 years or younger with newly diagnosed acute lymphoblastic leukemia. Blood 2007; 109: 2744–50.

106. Wetzler M, Sanford BL, Kurtzberg J et al. Effective asparagine depletion with pegylated asparaginase results in improved outcomes in adult acute lymphoblastic leukemia: Cancer and Leukemia Group B study 9511. Blood 2007; 109: 4164–7.

107. Faderl S, Gandhi V, O'Brien S et al. Results of a phase 1-2 study of clofarabine in combination with cytarabine (ara-C) in relapsed and refractory acute leukemias. Blood 2005; 105: 940–7.

108. Karp JE, Ricklis RM, Balakrishnan K et al. A phase 1 clinical-laboratory study of clofarabine followed by cyclophosphamide for adults with refractory acute leukemias. Blood 2007; 110: 1762–9.

109. Druker BJ, Guilhot F, O'Brien SG et al. Five-year follow-up of patients receiving imatinib for chronic myeloid leukemia. N Engl J Med 2006; 355: 2408–17.

110. Savona M, Talpaz M. Getting to the stem of chronic myeloid leukaemia. Nat Rev Cancer 2008; 8: 341–50.

111. Baccarani M, Saglio G, Goldman J et al. Evolving concepts in the management of chronic myeloid leukemia: recommendations from an expert panel on behalf of the European LeukemiaNet. Blood 2006; 108: 1809–20.

112. O'Brien S, Berman E, Bhalla K et al. Chronic myelogenous leukemia. J Natl Compr Canc Netw 2007; 5: 474–96.

113. Apperley JF. Part I: mechanisms of resistance to imatinib in chronic myeloid leukaemia. Lancet Oncol 2007; 8: 1018–29.

114. Giles FJ, DeAngelo DJ, Baccarani M et al. Optimizing outcomes for patients with advanced disease in chronic myelogenous leukemia. Semin Oncol 2008; 35(Suppl 1): S1–S17.

115. Tsang J, Rudychev I, Pescatore SL. Prescription compliance and persistency in chronic myelogenous leukemia (CML) and gastrointestinal stromal tumor (GIST) patients (pts) on imatinib (IM). J Clin Oncol 2006; 24(Suppl): 330s.

116. Cortes J, Baccarani M, Guilhot F et al. First report of the TOPS study: a randomized phase III trial of 400 mg vs 800 mg imatinib in patients with newly diagnosed, previously untreated CML in chronic phase using molecular endpoints. Haematologica 2008; 93(Suppl 1): 160.

117. le Coutre P, Ottmann OG, Giles F et al. Nilotinib (formerly AMN107), a highly selective BCR-ABL tyrosine kinase inhibitor, is active in patients with imatinib-resistant or -intolerant accelerated-phase chronic myelogenous leukemia. Blood 2008; 111: 1834–9.

118. Hochhaus A, Baccarani M, Deininger M et al. Dasatinib induces durable cytogenetic responses in patients with chronic myelogenous leukemia in chronic phase with resistance or intolerance to imatinib. Leukemia 2008; 22: 1200–6.

119. Schiffer CA. BCR-ABL tyrosine kinase inhibitors for chronic myelogenous leukemia. N Engl J Med 2007; 357: 258–65.

120. Oki Y, Kantarjian HM, Gharibyan V et al. Phase II study of low-dose decitabine in combination with imatinib mesylate in patients with accelerated or myeloid blastic phase of chronic myelogenous leukemia. Cancer 2007; 109: 899–906.

121. Cortes J, Quintás-Cardama A, Garcia-Manero G et al. Phase 1 study of tipifarnib in combination with imatinib for

patients with chronic myelogenous leukemia in chronic phase after imatinib failure. Cancer 2007; 110: 2000–6.

122. Cortes J, Jabbour E, Daley GQ et al. Phase 1 study of lonafarnib (SCH 66336) and imatinib mesylate in patients with chronic myeloid leukemia who have failed prior single-agent therapy with imatinib. Cancer 2007; 110: 1295–302.

123. Bocchia M, Gentili S, Abruzzese E et al. Effect of a p210 multipeptide vaccine associated with imatinib or interferon in patients with chronic myeloid leukaemia and persistent residual disease: a multicentre observational trial. Lancet 2005; 365: 657–62.

124. Neviani P, Santhanam R, Oaks JJ et al. FTY720, a new alternative for treating blast crisis chronic myelogenous leukemia and Philadelphia chromosome-positive acute lymphocytic leukemia. J Clin Invest 2007; 117: 2408–21.

125. Danilov AV, Danilova OV, Klein AK et al. Molecular pathogenesis of chronic lymphocytic leukemia. Curr Mol Med 2006; 6: 665–75.

126. Seiler T, Döhner H, Stilgenbauer S. Risk stratification in chronic lymphocytic leukemia. Semin Oncol 2006; 33: 186–94.

127. Shanafelt TD, Kay NE. The clinical and biologic importance of neovascularization and angiogenic signaling pathways in chronic lymphocytic leukemia. Semin Oncol 2006; 33: 174–85.

128. Calin GA, Croce CM. Genomics of chronic lymphocytic leukemia microRNAs as new players with clinical significance. Semin Oncol 2006; 33: 167–73.

129. Raval A, Byrd JC, Plass C. Epigenetics in chronic lymphocytic leukemia. Semin Oncol 2006; 33: 157–66.

130. Ghia P, Caligaris-Cappio F. The origin of B-cell chronic lymphocytic leukemia. Semin Oncol 2006; 33: 150–6.

131. Klein U, Tu Y, Stolovitzky GA et al. Gene expression profiling of B cell chronic lymphocytic leukemia reveals a homogeneous phenotype related to memory B cells. J Exp Med 2001; 194: 1625–38.

132. Damle RN, Wasil T, Fais F et al. Ig V gene mutation status and CD38 expression as novel prognostic indicators in chronic lymphocytic leukemia. Blood 1999; 94: 1840–7.

133. Hamblin TJ, Davis Z, Gardiner A et al. Unmutated Ig V_H genes are associated with a more aggressive form of chronic lymphocytic leukemia. Blood 1999; 94: 1848–54.

134. Diehl LF, Ketchum LH. Autoimmune disease and chronic lymphocytic leukemia: autoimmune hemolytic anemia, pure red cell aplasia, and autoimmune thrombocytopenia. Semin Oncol 1998; 25: 80–97.

135. Tsimberidou AM, Keating MJ. Richter syndrome: biology, incidence, and therapeutic strategies. Cancer 2005; 103: 216–28.

136. Tsimberidou AM, Keating MJ. Richter's transformation in chronic lymphocytic leukemia. Semin Oncol 2006; 33: 250–6.

137. Rai KR, Sawitsky A, Cronkite EP et al. Clinical staging of chronic lymphocytic leukemia. Blood 1975; 46: 219–34.

138. Döhner H, Stilgenbauer S, Benner A et al. Genomic aberrations and survival in chronic lymphocytic leukemia. N Engl J Med 2000; 343: 1910–16.

139. Kröber A, Seiler T, Benner A et al. V_H mutation status, CD38 expression level, genomic aberrations, and survival in chronic lymphocytic leukemia. Blood 2002; 100: 1410–16.

140. Hamblin TJ, Orchard JA, Ibbotson RE et al. CD38 expression and immunoglobulin variable region mutations are independent prognostic variables in chronic lymphocytic leukemia, but CD38 expression may vary during the course of the disease. Blood 2002; 99: 1023–9.

141. Matrai Z, Lin K, Dennis M et al. CD38 expression and Ig V_H gene mutation in B-cell chronic lymphocytic leukemia. Blood 2001; 97: 1902–3.

142. Lin K, Sherrington PD, Dennis M et al. Relationship between p53 dysfunction, CD38 expression, and IgV_H mutation in chronic lymphocytic leukemia. Blood 2002; 100: 1404–9.

143. Jelinek DF, Tschumper RC, Geyer SM et al. Analysis of clonal B-cell CD38 and immunoglobulin variable region sequence status in relation to clinical outcome for B-chronic lymphocytic leukaemia. Br J Haematol 2001; 115: 854–61.

144. CLL Trialists' Collaborative Group. Chemotherapeutic options in chronic lymphocytic leukemia: a meta-analysis of the randomized trials. J Natl Cancer Inst 1999; 91: 861–8.

145. Hallek M, Cheson BD, Catovsky D et al. Guidelines for the diagnosis and treatment of chronic lymphocytic leukemia: a report from the International Workshop on Chronic Lymphocytic Leukemia (IWCLL) updating the National Cancer Institute-Working Group (NCI-WG) 1996 guidelines. Blood 2008; 111: 5446–56.

146. Byrd JC, Gribben JG, Peterson BL et al. Select high-risk genetic features predict earlier progression following chemoimmunotherapy with fludarabine and rituximab in chronic lymphocytic leukemia: justification for risk-adapted therapy. J Clin Oncol 2006; 24: 437–43.

147. Döhner H, Fischer K, Bentz M et al. p53 gene deletion predicts for poor survival and non-response to therapy with purine analogs in chronic B-cell leukemias. Blood 1995; 85: 1580–9.

148. Chevallier P, Penther D, Avet-Loiseau H et al. CD38 expression and secondary 17p deletion are important prognostic factors in chronic lymphocytic leukaemia. Br J Haematol 2002; 116: 142–50.

149. el Rouby S, Thomas A, Costin D et al. p53 gene mutation in B-cell chronic lymphocytic leukemia is associated with drug resistance and is independent of MDR1/MDR3 gene expression. Blood 1993; 82: 3452–9.

150. Lozanski G, Heerema NA, Flinn IW et al. Alemtuzumab is an effective therapy for chronic lymphocytic leukemia with p53 mutations and deletions. Blood 2004; 103: 3278–81.

151. Grever MR, Lucas DM, Dewald GW et al. Comprehensive assessment of genetic and molecular features predicting outcome in patients with chronic lymphocytic leukemia: results from the US Intergroup Phase III Trial E2997. J Clin Oncol 2007; 25: 799–804.

152. Eichhorst BF, Busch R, Hopfinger G et al. Fludarabine plus cyclophosphamide versus fludarabine alone in first-line therapy of younger patients with chronic lymphocytic leukemia. Blood 2006; 107: 885–91.

153. Rai KR, Peterson BL, Appelbaum FR et al. Fludarabine compared with chlorambucil as primary therapy for chronic lymphocytic leukemia. N Engl J Med 2000; 343: 1750–7.

154. Knauf WU, Lissichkov T, Aldaoud A et al. Bendamustine versus chlorambucil in treatment-naive patients with B-cell chronic lymphocytic leukemia (B-CLL): results of an international phase III study. Blood 2007; 110: 609a.

155. Hillmen P, Skotnicki AB, Robak T et al. Alemtuzumab compared with chlorambucil as first-line therapy for chronic lymphocytic leukemia. J Clin Oncol 2007; 25: 5616–23.

156. Eichhorst BF, Busch R, Hopfinger G et al. Fludarabine plus cyclophosphamide versus fludarabine alone in first-line therapy of younger patients with chronic lymphocytic leukemia. Blood 2006; 107: 885–91.

157. Flinn IW, Neuberg DS, Grever MR et al. Phase III trial of fludarabine plus cyclophosphamide compared with fludarabine for patients with previously untreated chronic lymphocytic leukemia: US Intergroup Trial E2997. J Clin Oncol 2007; 25: 793–8.

158. Catovsky D, Richards S, Matutes E et al. Assessment of fludarabine plus cyclophosphamide for patients with chronic lymphocytic leukaemia (the LRF CLL4 Trial): a randomised controlled trial. Lancet 2007; 370: 230–9.

159. Byrd JC, Peterson BL, Morrison VA et al. Randomized phase 2 study of fludarabine with concurrent versus sequential treatment with rituximab in symptomatic, untreated patients with B-cell chronic lymphocytic leukemia: results from Cancer and Leukemia Group B 9712 (CALGB 9712). Blood 2003; 101: 6–14.

160. Byrd JC, Rai K, Peterson BL et al. Addition of rituximab to fludarabine may prolong progression-free survival and overall survival in patients with previously untreated chronic lymphocytic leukemia: an updated retrospective comparative analysis of CALGB 9712 and CALGB 9011. Blood 2005; 105: 49–53.

161. Wierda W, O'Brien S, Wen S et al. Chemoimmunotherapy with fludarabine, cyclophosphamide, and rituximab for relapsed and refractory chronic lymphocytic leukemia. J Clin Oncol 2005; 23: 4070–8.

162. Leoni LM, Bailey B, Reifert J et al. Bendamustine (Treanda) displays a distinct pattern of cytotoxicity and unique mechanistic features compared with other alkylating agents. Clin Cancer Res 2008; 14: 309–17.

163. Grever MR, Lucas DM, Johnson AJ et al. Novel agents and strategies for treatment of p53-defective chronic lymphocytic leukemia. Best Pract Res Clin Haematol 2007; 20: 545–56.

164. Wierda WG. Current and investigational therapies for patients with CLL. Hematology Am Soc Hematol Educ Program 2006: 285–94.

13

Non-Hodgkin's Lymphomas

Jean-François Larouche and Bertrand Coiffier

Non-Hodgkin's lymphomas (NHLs) are a heterogeneous group of cancers arising from B or T lymphocytes, also rarely from NK cells. This heterogeneity results from the numerous histological entities, the lymphoma's location in nodal or extranodal sites, its capacity to remain localized or to disseminate throughout the body, and the patients' age and associated diseases. The prognostic implications related to these variables must be known before therapeutic options are proposed. Because of the multiplicity of lymphoma entities and of the possible lymphoma manifestations, it is difficult to accurately predict the outcome of therapy in individual patients. Defining subgroups among large numbers of patients with histologically similar lymphomas and similar clinical manifestations is, however, likely to lead to the identification of meaningful prognostic indicators.

Over the past 15 years, new information from research has led to the recognition of new entities, definition of better prognostic parameters, and determination of standard treatments. This evolution has enabled the development of a risk-adapted therapy based on lymphoma cell characteristics, spread of the tumor, and the patient's response to this tumor. The main aim of lymphoma treatment should be to provide cure or, at least for patients older than 70 years, a long-term, disease-free survival.

EPIDEMIOLOGY

The incidence of lymphoma is steadily increasing worldwide for the past 30 years. Age-adjusted incidence rates among 100,000 people in the United States were 11.1, 16.7, and 20.4 in 1975, 1987, and 2004, respectively. Lymphoma is the sixth most common cancer in the United States (1). European studies show similar result.

Among elderly people, this increase may be explained by age-related immunodeficiency. The relative importance of the human immunodeficiency virus (HIV) in this increase is probably minor, because in Europe, only 1% of all lymphomas occur in patients with acquired immune deficiency syndrome (AIDS). Other viruses such as Epstein-Barr virus (EBV), hepatitis C virus (HCV), human T-cell lymphoma/leukemia virus (HTLV-I), and human herpes virus (HHV-8) certainly have a role in causing lymphoma, but the different steps from viral infection to lymphoma's development are unknown and factors other than viral infection may have a role. In other entities, stimulation by bacteria such as *Helicobacter pylori* or *Borrelia burgdorferi* has been recognized as the initial trigger. However, an increased incidence of

these pathogens has not been observed, and therefore, their role in the increased incidence of lymphoma remains uncertain.

Exposure to environmental agents such as herbicides or hair dyes has recently been identified as a risk factor for development of lymphoma, but the overall contribution of such agents still needs to be defined. Immunosuppression as in solid organ or bone marrow transplantation is a well-established risk factor for NHL. Also, NHL is found to be associated with autoimmune disorders such as rheumatoid arthritis, Sjögren's syndrome, Hashimoto thyroiditis, and systemic lupus. However, immunosuppression for organ transplantation or autoimmune disorders cannot explain the rise in NHL incidence.

On the other hand, the outcome of lymphoma treatment improved from the 1990s to the early 21st century. American data showed an increase in the 10-year relative survival from 39.4% to 56.3% in all age groups and all subtypes of NHL (2).

CLINICAL PRESENTATION AND STAGING

A patient is suspected of having a NHL in three clinical situations: 1) the presence of one or several lymph nodes that grow more or less rapidly, 2) an extranodal tumor that has either a typical aspect such as lymphomatous skin lesions, a typical localization (e.g., conjunctiva), or that looks like any solid tumor, or 3) systemic manifestations such as fever, weight loss, or severe fatigue. In any case, a definitive diagnosis of lymphoma requires the full characterization of the tumor. A substantial tissue specimen must be obtained to establish the diagnosis by pathological examination including immunophenotyping and the presence of CD20 or CD3 antigen qualifying the lymphoma as B-cell or T-cell proliferation. Additional analyses of fresh cells or cryopreserved specimens may be useful for obtaining or confirming the diagnosis in difficult cases and for establishing biological and molecular prognostic factors: immunoglobulin or T-cell receptor (TCR) gene rearrangement, chromosomal abnormalities, oncogene expressions, and proliferation-associated parameters. Whenever possible, and in any questionable case, the diagnosis should be confirmed by one or several pathologists experienced in lymphoid malignancies.

Clinical and laboratory investigations should be performed as soon as possible. The presence or absence of constitutional symptoms should be noted: fever >38°C, night sweats, and/or unintentional weight loss of greater than 10% of body weight over six months. After assessing the patient's general condition (performance status, PS) and possible underlying diseases, care should be taken to look for nodal and extranodal dissemination by detailed clinical examination and computed tomography (CT) scan of the abdomen and thorax. Specialized evaluation of the gastrointestinal tract is indicated in patients with gastrointestinal symptoms. Tumor burden should be evaluated to aid in assessing prognosis and to determine therapeutic efficacy. Bone marrow biopsy is mandatory to assess marrow infiltration. Although leptomeningeal infiltration is found at diagnosis in 5% or fewer of the patients with aggressive presentation, we recommend a systematic evaluation of cerebrospinal fluid in all clinically aggressive lymphomas because of the adverse prognosis of such involvement and the specificity of the treatment required. In addition to routine laboratory examinations (complete blood count, uric acid level, assessment of heart, kidney, and liver functions), serum lactate dehydrogenase (LDH) and serum β2-microglobulin levels should be determined to complete the prognostic staging. HIV serology should be performed in all patients because of the specificity of management in these patients. We also recommend hepatitis B and C serology, as it can influence the management (3,4). Other tests may be done on a research basis but have yet to prove their clinical interest (5).

Positron emission tomography (PET) is a noninvasive metabolic imaging that uses a radiopharmaceutical to target a physiologic process. The most widely used agent is 8-fluoro-deoxyglucose (FDG), which is an analog of glucose. PET shows high sensitivity and specificity in the evaluation of most lymphomas. Some subtype as diffuse large B-cell lymphoma, follicular lymphoma, and mantle cell lymphoma, are considered more FDG avid than others (marginal zone lymphoma, small lymphocytic lymphoma, and T-cell lymphoma). Sensitivity and specificity of PET scan for initial staging are around 80% to 90%. PET in initial staging is currently not standard because it alters the stage and therapy in only a minority of patients (6). However, pre-therapy PET is strongly encouraged because it helps in the interpretation of post-therapy PET. The clearest role of PET is response assessment at the conclusion of therapy, especially for lymphoma with a curative potential. Use of PET for monitoring response to therapy is under study in clinical trials (7). The combination of PET with CT scan as a single modality (PET/CT) represents a major advance in the field of lymphoma imaging, the results of which is better than that of both tests separately.

PROGNOSTIC PARAMETERS AND PROGNOSTIC INDEX

Independently of lymphoma entity, various clinical and biological features have been identified and associated with response to treatment and survival. Features most frequently associated with the ability to achieve complete remission and long-term survival reflect tumor's growth and invasive potential, patient's response to tumor, or patient's ability to tolerate intensive therapy (8,9).

Parameters Associated with High Tumor Burden

A large tumor mass has long been recognized as a significant adverse parameter even though the assessment

methods vary from one study to another. Parameters associated with large tumor mass and a poorer outcome are high number of nodal sites, high number of extranodal sites, certain specific locations, large tumor diameter, disseminated stage, high serum LDH level, and high β2-microglobulin level.

Ann Arbor Stage

Stage was originally described for Hodgkin's disease but was subsequently applied to NHL as well. However, the Ann Arbor stage was described for what is essentially a nodal disease and is somewhat difficult to apply to NHL because of the extranodal primary localizations and the weak correlation between extranodal involvement and outcome in some lymphoma subtypes. Stage, however, is related to outcome, and stage I patients have a longer survival than do stage IV patients. Moreover, disseminated stage seems to be the only parameter associated with a high risk of late relapse.

Number of Extranodal Sites

The number of lymphoma localizations depends on specialized examinations used to detect them (i.e., computed tomography, PET scan, endoscopy, serous fluid examinations, and biological examinations). Presence of more than one extranodal site has been associated with poor prognosis and has proved to be one of the strongest prognostic factors in aggressive lymphomas and follicular lymphomas.

Largest Diameter of the Tumor

A poor outcome has been associated with larger tumors, but the cutoff varies from 5 to 10 cm, depending on the study. Large tumors are thought to be associated with an increased risk of developing aggressive cell clones, but this adverse risk factor often does not persist in multiparametric analyses (10).

Specific Extranodal Localizations

Lymphoma cells may appear in any organ or lymph node. Although some of these extranodal sites are associated with a poorer outcome in retrospective studies, multiparametric analyses have always shown that poorer outcome was a function of the number of extranodal sites rather than secondary to a specific location (10).

Patients with bone marrow involvement have a poorer outcome. Bone marrow involvement is present in more than 70% of patients with follicular lymphoma (FL), small lymphocytic lymphoma (SLL), or mantle cell lymphoma (MCL), but these tumors may not modify the prognosis. However, bone marrow involvement in patients with Burkitt lymphoma (BL) or lymphoblastic lymphoma (LL) has a considerably worse prognosis. Only 20% to 25% of patients with diffuse large B-cell lymphoma (DLBCL) have bone marrow involvement at the time of diagnosis, but these patients have poorer responses to therapy and shorter survival than those without bone marrow involvement. For DLBCL patients, bone marrow infiltration was subdivided into infiltration by large cells, similar to those seen in lymph nodes, and by small cells. Patients with

DLBCL and bone marrow infiltration with small cells have a higher risk of relapse but a longer survival than patients with large cell involvement.

Gastrointestinal involvement is the most common extranodal site, but its prognostic significance as well as its optimal therapy are still matters of debate. This reflects the presence among these localizations of different lymphoma entities, mostly MALT lymphoma and DLBCL, but also BL or MCL. In fact, treatment of these extranodal locations should not be based on specific location but on the lymphoma histology.

CNS lymphomas occur in four different subgroups of patients: those with meningeal localization, those with a spinal extradural involvement with cord compression, those with primary DLBCL of cerebral parenchyma, and lymphoma in immunocompromised patients, especially HIV-positive patients. We consider all these presentations as poor prognosis.

Lactic Dehydrogenase

LDH above normal levels has been identified as the major prognostic factor in lymphoma patients in almost all published prognostic analyses (10). Moreover, the higher the LDH level, the poorer is the outcome.

β2-Microglobulin Level

Adverse prognosis associated with a high β2-microglobulin serum level in lymphoma was recognized years ago, but this parameter has not been widely used. The putative importance of the β2-microglobulin level has been recognized and applied to prognostic analyses in several centers (11), and, like LDH level, it predicts the risk of relapse for patients. However, few physicians consider it in clinical practice, and this parameter is not really use except in follicular lymphoma (12).

Parameters Associated with Patient Response to the Tumor

These parameters include B symptoms, performance status, serum albumin, and hemoglobin levels. They probably reflect the same phenomenon, cytokine secretion by either neoplastic cells or the patient's immune cells in response to the tumor. Earlier studies focused on B symptoms; the more recent ones, such as the International Prognostic Index, have focused on performance status, whereas statisticians tend to prefer either serum albumin or hemoglobin levels because these two parameters are more reproducible and less affected by other independent parameters such as transient infection (9).

Parameters Associated with Patient Ability to Tolerate Treatment

Outcome for patients may be different, depending on comorbidities not related to lymphoma and on their age at time of diagnosis. In a Southwest Oncology Group study, older patients had worse outcomes because they responded less well to treatment and relapsed more often. This poorer outcome was related to a decrease in chemotherapy dose intensity. In other studies, more elderly patients died during initial courses of treatment, whereas

Table 13.1   Definition of "Elderly" Patients According to Different Standards

Standard	Definition	Elderly
Biologic age	Decrease in physiologic reserve which decrease capacity to respond adequately to stress	Unknown
Renal function	Decline of glomerular filtration and tubular secretion rates <50%	>70
Hormonal status	Menopause in women	>50–55
Treatment	Capacity to tolerate allogeneic marrow transplantation	>50
Treatment	Capacity to tolerate autologous stem cell transplantation	>60–65
Prognosis	Modification of survival curves in International Prognostic Index	>60–65

those who completed chemotherapy and responded did not have higher relapse rate. Elderly patients are more likely to develop complications after chemotherapy because of their age and the possible existence of comorbidities. The cutoff age for old patients with DLBCL is between 60 and 65 years (10). However, if tolerance to treatment decreases with age, it is not perfectly correlated to the numeric age but rather with biologic age as defined in Table 13.1.

Prognostic Index

A number of investigators have used the subset of clinical features that retained independent significance in multivariate analysis of their patients to develop prognostic factor models predictive of an individual patient's risk of shortened survival. Although the specific clinical features used in the prognostic factor models differ, each model incorporates features that reflect the volume of disease and extent of tumor involvement at diagnosis, confirming the primary importance of these factors (13).

In 1990, there was a consensus that an international classification system based on clinically relevant prognostic factors in DLBCL should be developed (10). This International Prognostic Index (IPI) is based on age, tumor stage, serum LDH level, performance status, and number of extranodal disease sites. IPI renders possible to identify four risk groups corresponding to the number of adverse parameters. In young patients, an age-adjusted IPI based on tumor stage, serum LDH level, and performance status identified four risk groups. In both models, the increased risk of death was the result of both a lower rate of complete responses and a higher rate of relapses. The IPI may also be effectively applied to patients presenting with lymphoma subtypes other than DLBCL (14). Other indexes developed for follicular lymphoma include the Follicular Lymphoma International Prognostic Index (FLIPI), mantle cell lymphoma, or peripheral T-cell lymphoma, but currently these have not been proven clearly superior to IPI (15). IPI and age-adjusted IPI were proven to be significantly more accurate than Ann Arbor classification in predicting long-term survival. Today, one of these indexes should be used in the design of therapeutic trials and in the selection of appropriate therapeutic approaches for individual patients.

New Prognostic Parameters

The IPI incorporates in its definition only surrogate markers of profound alterations in cellular biology of tumor cells. Since its description, and in the future, biological or genetic alterations have been, and will be, described that may replace all or some of the classical parameters. These putative parameters include gene alterations of cell-cycle regulator proteins (p53, p27, cyclin D), apoptotic proteins (survivin, bcl-2), cytokines (TNF, IL-6, IL-10), adhesion molecules (CD44, ICAM-1), and angiogenic peptides (VEGF) (16). Currently, bcl-2 protein expression is one of the best biological parameters associated with outcome (17). Gene microarray analysis is a promising tool to characterize genetic abnormalities related to lymphoma and this microenvironment in the function of prognosis (18–20). Finally, proteomic analysis has the potential to reveal new biomarkers of prognostic significance (21).

HISTOLOGICAL CLASSIFICATIONS OF NHL

Many histological classifications have been proposed, with the Rappaport classification (1956), the Kiel classification and the Working Formulation for Clinical Usage (1982) being the most frequently used. Based on morphological, immunological, and genetic characterization of the tumor, the Revised European–American Classification for lymphoid neoplasms (REAL classification) has been proposed by the International Lymphoma Study Group. This classification has evolved to the World Health Organization (WHO) classification, which is the classification commonly used nowadays (Table 13.2). A complete histological description may be found in the original description (22).

The incidence of each type of lymphoma may vary from country to country and center to center according to referral policy. Figure 13.1 shows the frequency observed among patients treated during nine years in Lyon (Centre Hospitalier Lyon-Sud) and in an international review in eight centers around the world (23,24). The frequency is not different from that observed in Europe or North America. In Japan and other Eastern countries, some entities such as peripheral T-cell lymphomas (PTCLs) and adult T-cell lymphoma/leukemia (ATL) are more frequently observed, whereas others such as follicular lymphoma (FL) are rare.

Indolent lymphomas have a propensity for increasing their histological aggressiveness as they recur. This may be translated as transformation into a proliferation of large cells from low-grade lymphoma, such as in FL, marginal zone lymphoma (MZL), small lymphocytic lymphoma (SLL), or lymphoplasmacytic lymphoma (LPL). This transformation is often associated with a large mass, a decrease in the performance status, a high LDH level, and additional genetic abnormalities. These abnormalities occur in key steps regulating cell cycle, proliferation, and apoptosis (CDKN2A, CKKN2B, c-myc, TP53, bcl-2, etc.). This leads to disease refractoriness to treatment and poor outcome.

Mature B-cell Lymphomas (Table 13.2)
Small Lymphocytic Lymphoma

Small lymphocytic lymphoma (SLL) represents the lymphoma counterpart of chronic lymphocytic leukemia (CLL),

Table 13.2 World Heath Organization (WHO) Classification of Lymphoid Tumors[a]

B cell neoplasms
  Precursor B-cell neoplasm
    Precursor B-cell lymphoblastic *leukemia*/lymphoma
  Mature B-cell neoplasms
    Chronic lymphocytic leukemia(CLL)/small lymphocytic lymphoma (SLL)
    B cell prolymphocytic leukemia
    Lymphoplasmacytic lymphoma (LPL)/Waldenström macroglobulinemia
    Splenic marginal zone lymphoma
    Hairy cell leukemia
    Plasma cell neoplasms: plasma cell myeloma, plasmacytoma, monoclonal immunoglobulin deposition diseases, heavy-chain diseases
    Extranodal marginal zone B-cell lymphoma (MALT lymphoma)
    Nodal marginal zone B-cell lymphoma
    Follicular lymphoma (FL)
    Mantle cell lymphoma (MCL)
    Diffuse large B-cell lymphomas (DLBCL)
      Subtypes
        Mediastinal large B-cell lymphoma
        Intravascular large B-cell lymphoma
        Primary effusion lymphoma
    Burkitt Lymphoma/leukemia (BL)

T cell neoplasms
  Precursor T-cell neoplasm
    Precursor T-cell lymphoblastic *leukemia*/lymphoma (LL)
  Mature T-cell and NK cell neoplasms
    T-cell prolymphocytic leukemia
    T-cell large granular lymphocyte leukemia
    Aggressive NK cell leukemia
    Adult T-cell leukemia/lymphoma
    Extranodal NK/T cell lymphoma, nasal type
    Enteropathy-type T-cell lymphoma
    Hepatosplenic T-cell lymphoma
    Subcutaneous panniculitis-like T-cell lymphoma
    Blastic NK cell lymphoma
    Mycosis fungoides/Sézary syndrome (CTCL)
    Primary cutaneous CD30-positive T-cell lymphoproliferative disorders: primary cutaneous anaplasic large cell lymphoma, lymphomatoid papulosis, borderline lesions
    Angioimmunoblastic T-cell lymphoma
    Peripheral T-cell lymphomas (PTCL), unspecified
    Systemic anaplastic large cell lymphoma (ALCL)

Hodgkin's lymphoma (Hodgkin's disease)
  Nodular lymphocyte predominance Hodgkin's lymphoma
  Classical Hodgkin's lymphoma
    Nodular sclerosis Hodgkin's lymphoma
    Mixed cellularity Hodgkin's lymphoma
    Lymphocyte-rich classic Hodgkin's lymphoma
    Lymphocyte depleted Hodgkin's lymphoma

[a]Clinical entities in italics will be discussed in other chapters of this book.

which is about three to seven times more frequent than SLL (25). SLL is what remains of the small lymphocytic subtype of the Working Formulation after the now well-defined subtypes, mantle cell lymphoma (MCL) and marginal zone lymphoma (MZL), have been dropped. It represents 4% to 5% of lymphomas. Lymph node involvement is characteristics. There is usually effacement of lymph node architecture. The infiltrate consists predominantly of small lymphocytes, which appear slightly larger than a normal lymphocyte with a slightly more abundant

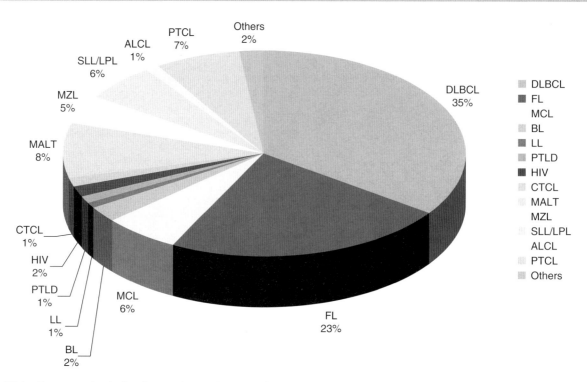

Figure 13.1 Frequency of major lymphoma subtypes observed in Centre Hospitalier Lyon-Sud (Lyon, France) among 3267 patients referred between 1990 and 2007. Acute and chronic lymphocytic leukemias and plasma cell disorders are not included. *Abbreviations*: ALCL, systemic anaplastic large cell lymphoma; BL, Burkitt lymphoma/leukemia; CTCL, mycosis fungoides/Sézary syndrome; DLBCL, diffuse large B-cell lymphomas; FL, follicular lymphoma; HIV, human immunodeficiency virus-related lymphomas; LL, precursor T-cell lymphoblastic *leukemia*/lymphoma; LPL, lymphoplasmacytic lymphoma; MALT, extranodal marginal zone B-cell lymphoma; MCL, mantle cell lymphoma; MZL, marginal zone lymphoma; PTCL, peripheral T-cell lymphomas; PTLD, post-transplantation lymphomas; SLL, small lymphocytic lymphoma.

basophilic cytoplasm and clumped chromatin. There are also some large lymphoid cells (prolymphocytes and paraimmunoblasts), which are grouped together in pseudofollicles. Few mitoses are also seen. Tumor cells express B cell-associated antigens and are CD5⁺, CD19⁺, CD23⁺, CD20 (weak), CD43⁺, FMC7⁻, CD10⁻, CD79a⁺, surface IgM or IgM and IgD (weak), and cyclin D1⁻.

SLLs are heterogeneous in their clinical picture, response to treatment and outcome, and may comprise several entities. SLLs are characterized as mentioned earlier by nodal involvement. Patients are usually asymptomatic, and the diagnosis is made following the discovery of enlarged lymph nodes. General symptoms (fever, night sweats, or weight loss) are infrequent. A high proportion of SLL presents infiltration of blood and bone marrow. By definition, infiltration of the blood must be minimal, less than 5000 lymphocytes/μL; otherwise, the condition becomes CLL. Extranodal infiltration is possible but unusual. A small M component may be found in some patients. Anemia or thrombocytopenia can be found, either from bone marrow involvement or by autoimmune phenomenon. Blood abnormalities related to autoimmunity seem to have a better prognosis (26). Hypogammaglobulinemia may be observed, especially with advanced disease, and can be related to infectious complications.

A number of parameters with prognostic significance have been discovered in the past as clinical stage (Binet or Rai) and bone marrow infiltration pattern. In the past decade, new analysis became available in clinical practice: CD38 expression, ZAP-70, IgV$_H$ mutational status, and cytogenetics (27). Most of them have been evaluated in CLL, but recent data suggest that SLLs have less cytogenetic abnormalities, more CD38 expression, and more mutated immunoglobulin variable heavy-chain region gene status than CLL (25). Patients with del11q represent a subgroup characterized clinically by extensive lymphadenopathy.

Few prospective trials have been designed specifically for patients with SLL, and the best therapeutic approach is not known. Actual therapies are based on CLL, as it is considered the same disease. Response to treatment and survival look similar (25). Overall median survival for patients with SLL/CLL is around 10 years but range from 2 to 20 years. Asymptomatic patients with low tumor burden disseminated disease can be followed with no treatment, as delay in therapy does not have impact on survival. Usual indications for treatment include disease related-symptoms, symptomatic cytopenia, progressive disease, and repeated infections. For many years, the treatment for most patients was single-agent chemotherapy (chlorambucil or cyclophosphamide) or a multidrug regimen with or without doxorubicin (cyclophosphamide + vincristine + prednisone ± doxorubicin). However, very few patients reached complete remission, but most responded to treatment, and they had

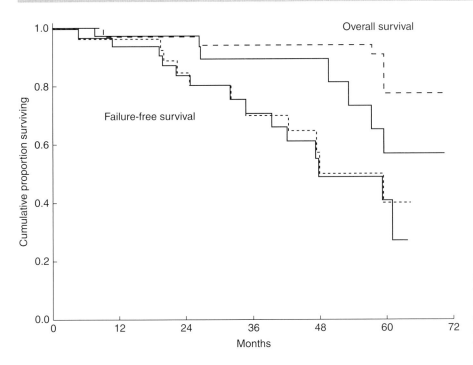

Figure 13.2 Overall survival and failure-free survival of 34 patients with mantle cell lymphoma treated with combination chemotherapy and rituximab followed by high-dose therapy and autologous stem cell transplant. *Source:* From Ref. 69.

a median time to failure (TTF) of two to five years. Introduction of purine analogs such as fludarabine showed improve overall response rate, complete response rate, and progression-free survival with no significant improvement in overall survival. Combination of fludarabine with cyclophosphamide (FC) showed improved results when compared with single-agent treatment. Addition of rituximab to FC improved results compared with FC, at least in CLL (phase III study results not yet published). Another antibody directed against CD52, alemtuzumab, showed clinical activity in CLL but has been least effective in patients with adenopathy, especially the large ones. New promising agents include lenalidomide and ofatumumab (fully humanized anti-CD20). More intensive therapy with total body irradiation and autologous stem cell transplantation (ASCT) or allogeneic stem cell transplantation may be proposed for young patients with histological transformation and for relapsing patients, but their role has not yet been defined.

Marginal Zone Lymphomas

Marginal zone lymphomas (MZL) regroup tumors that have recently been recognized, such as extranodal marginal zone B-cell lymphoma of mucosa associated lymphoid tissue (MALT lymphoma), splenic marginal zone lymphoma (with or without villous lymphocytes) (SMZL), and nodal marginal zone lymphoma. Despite a common cell of origin and similarities concerning a possible chronic antigenic stimulation, important differences in clinical presentation and evolution justify to consider each of these three entities separately, as it is made in WHO classification.

MALT Lymphomas. MALT lymphomas represent around 5% to 8% of NHL but up to half of primary gastric

lymphoma (23). Tumor cells appear to display a tissue-specific homing pattern. Proliferation seems to be dependent on the presence of activated, antigen-driven T lymphocytes, at least in initial stages. MALT lymphoma is characterized by a cellular heterogeneity including marginal zone centrocyte-like cells, monocytoid B cells, small lymphocytes, and plasma cells. Occasionally, large cells can be seen. Reactive follicles are usually present, with neoplastic cells occupying the marginal zone and/or the interfollicular region. In epithelial tissues, the marginal zone cells infiltrate the epithelium, forming lymphoepithelial lesions. Some degree of plasma differentiation is also often seen. Tumor cells express surface immunoglobulin (sIg), often cytoplasmic immunoglobulin (cIg), B-cell-associated antigens but not CD5, CD10, CD23, or CD43. Rearrangement of bcl-1 or bcl-2 is not seen.

If trisomy 3 (+3) occurs as the most frequent aberration (60%), this abnormality can be identified either as a complete +3 or as a partial trisomy 3 (trisomy 3q, tetrasomy 3q). Translocation (11;18)(q21;q21), involving API2 and MALT1 genes and t(1;14)(p22;q32), involving bcl-10 region are specific to MALT lymphoma. Translocation (11;18) is commonly associated with MALT lymphoma (13–35%) but t(1;14) is rare (1%). Other cytogenetic abnormalities are nonspecific being observed in other lymphomas. Translocation (14;18)(q32;q21), identical to the one seen in FL but involving the MALT1 gene and not the bcl-2 gene, is seen in 20% of MALT lymphoma.

Most patients with MALT lymphoma present with localized stage extranodal disease. Although the stomach is the most common site, many others have also been described such as lung, skin, thyroid, orbit, salivary glands, and other parts of the gastrointestinal tract. Many of them have histories of chronic antigenic stimulation or autoimmune disease (Sjögren's syndrome and Hashimoto's

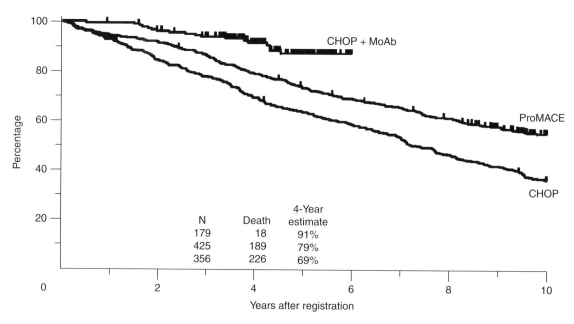

Figure 13.3 Follicular lymphoma and overall survival according to different treatment program. *Abbreviations*: CHOP, Cyclophosphamide, Hydroxydaunorubicin (Adriamycin), Oncovin (Vincristine), Prednisone/Prednisolone; ProMACE; MoAb, monoclonal antibody. *Source*: From Ref. 49.

thyroiditis). Infection with the following bacteria has been associated with a specific site of presentation: *H. pylori* and stomach, *Borrelia burgdorferi* and skin, *Chlamydia psittaci* and ocular adnexa, *Campylobacter jejuni* and small intestine. Dissemination of the tumor to other MALT sites, spleen or bone marrow, is seen at diagnosis in 30% of the cases but is more frequent in recurring disease (28). As in other indolent lymphomas, transformation into a large cell tumor can occur at time of relapse.

As MALT lymphomas are often localized, patients have usually been treated with surgery or local radiotherapy, depending on the disease site, but no prospective trial has validated these options. Relapses were observed in the same site or at other extranodal sites (28). Because of the diversity of locations, few, if any, studies looked at specific treatment except for gastric MALT lymphoma. Patients with gastric MALT lymphoma, without lymph node involvement on endoscopic ultrasonography, may be treated successfully with antibiotics (29,30). With two antibiotics (clarythromycin and amoxicillin or metronidazole) plus a proton pump inhibitor for 14 days, *H. pylori* is eliminated in 90% of the patients, and complete regression of the lymphoma is observed in nearly 80% of cases. However, some molecular abnormalities may persist, but do not require treatment. The influence of this treatment on survival has to be determined. Presence of t(11;18) is associated with lower response to antibiotics and more risk of relapse (31). The indolent nature of this lymphoma makes a conservative approach advisable, with antibiotic therapy as initial treatment being the choice. For patients with more advanced disease or in partial response or recurrence, chemotherapies such as chlorambucil, fludarabine, or rituximab yield good responses.

Nowadays, surgery is not recommended because gastrectomy may severely impair the patient's quality of life (29). Radiation therapy is a good choice for localized disease relapsing after first-line chemotherapy because of its efficacy and the near absence of long-term adverse effect (32).

Patients with nongastric MALT lymphoma associated with an infection can show response to antibiotics but success rate is unknown. Patients with localized nongastric MALT may be treated with surgery, local radiotherapy, or chemotherapy. Very few, if any, relevant prospective trials have been published. The choice of treatment depends on the site of the disease and consequences of treatment. Using chlorambucil (16 mg/m²/day, five days every month) for 6 to 12 months or rituximab 375 mg/m² IV every week for four weeks seems a good option. An overall response rate of 75% can be achieved. However, in patients with large tumor mass or an important large cell contingent, CHOP chemotherapy must be used. Rituximab has proven its efficacy in this lymphoma and may be added to chemotherapy. Patients with MALT lymphoma have a favorable outcome with five-year overall survival around 90%.

Splenic Marginal Zone Lymphoma. Patients with SMZL with or without villous lymphocytes are often elderly and present with massive splenomegaly, blood and bone marrow infiltration, but without lymph node or other visceral location (33). Immunologic cytopenia or M-component is frequent. An association with hepatitis C virus (HCV) infection has been shown. Tumor cells express surface immunoglobulin and sometimes cytoplasmic immunoglobulin (IgM, IgD), B-cell-associated antigens but not CD5,

• Avoid chemotherapy as long as possible

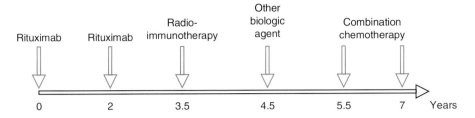

• Try to reach CR and have a long duration CR

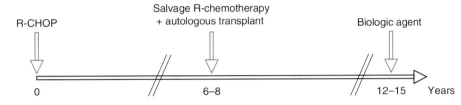

Figure 13.4 Philosophies in treatment of follicular lymphoma.

CD10, or CD23. They usually express CD11c, but they lack CD25 and CD103 (34). Splenectomy in case of large splenomegaly and delayed treatment when asymptomatic are the best solutions (35). When treatment is needed, HCV-positive patients can be treated with interferon ± ribavirin. When chemotherapy is considered, alkylating agents (chlorambucil or cyclophosphamide), fludarabine or rituximab, alone or in combination, can be used. Transformation to DLBCL can be seen in up to 10% of cases. The course of this disease is indolent with a median overall survival over 10 years.

Nodal Marginal Zone Lymphoma. Half of nodal MZL are seen in patients with MALT lymphoma and lymph node spread of the disease. However, tumors with the same features have been reported with primary localized or disseminated nodal involvement, and association with HCV has been noted. Patients with nodal MZL need to be treated, but no prospective study has yet described the best therapeutic modalities. We recommend radiation therapy for localized disease and CHOP plus rituximab for patients with disseminated disease. HDT with ASCT may be considered for patients with a high contingent of large cells or in relapse. A retrospective study from Lyon showed that these patients have a short TTF but may experience a long survival with five-year overall survival around 50% to 70% (30,36).

Lymphoplasmacytic Lymphoma/Waldenström Macroglobulinemia

Lymphoplasmacytic lymphoma (LPL)/Waldenström macroglobulinemia (WM) is a rare disease characterized as a malignant lymphoplasmo-proliferative disorder with monoclonal IgM production. There has been some debate whether WM should apply only to LPL with serum IgM concentration

superior to 30 g/L. However, irrespective of IgM concentration, LPL/WM is considered as a single clinicopathologic entity by most experts (37). Bone marrow infiltration is virtually present in all cases. It commonly involves lymph nodes and spleen. Extranodal infiltrates may occur but should be distinguished from MALT lymphoma. The immunophenotypic profile of lymphoplasmacytic cells in LPL/WM includes expression of pan-B cell antigen (CD19, CD20, CD22, CD79) with light-chain restricted surface IgM. CD10, CD23, and CD5 are usually negative, but 5% to 20% of patients appear to express CD5. Translocation t(9;14) involving PAX 5 gene has been reported in up to 50% of patients with LPL but apparently restricted to patients with nodal involvement without serum monoclonal protein.

Some patients present with hyperviscosity symptoms (headache, blurred vision, dizziness, and stroke) related to the monoclonal IgM, others with organomegaly (lymphadenopathy, splenomegaly, and hepatomegaly), anemia-related symptoms or constitutional symptoms. Chronic oozing of blood from nose is frequent. Peripheral neuropathy, cold agglutinin disease, and cryoglobulinemia can also occur.

Asymptomatic patients should be followed without treatment. Patients with symptoms related to the monoclonal protein may benefit plasma exchange. Systemic therapies include alkylating agents (chlorambucil), purine nucleoside analogues (fludarabine or cladribine), and rituximab. Abrupt increases in serum IgM level have been reported following initiation of rituximab. There are no data to recommend one treatment over the other and benefit of combination therapy is unknown. Other treatment options include thalidomide and interferon alpha. Lenalidomide, bortezomib, alemtuzumab, and many others are under study. Autologous and allogeneic hematopoietic stem cell transplantation can be considered in special circumstances, but experience is limited with these modalities.

Follicular Lymphoma

Follicular lymphoma is the second most common type of lymphoma and represents 20% to 25% of all lymphomas. They are composed of centrofollicular cells, a mixture of centrocytes (small cleaved centrofollicular cells) and centroblasts (large non-cleaved cells), interspersed with follicular dendritic cells. Centrocytes typically prevail and centroblasts are in the minority. The pattern of proliferation is usually follicular, but diffuse areas may be present and may sometimes predominate. The proportion of centroblasts and the size of centrocytes vary in different lymph nodes from the same patient. Histological subgroups with different outcomes have been described according to the percentage of each of the constituents, but these were considered irrelevant because the lymphoma growth is a continuous process, and it is difficult for this grading to be replicated by different groups of pathologists (23,38). However, cases with an important diffuse component (>50%) of large cells (grade 3b) have a worse outcome, similar to DLBCL and should be treated as DLBCL. Tumor cells are usually SIg$^+$, B-cell associated antigen$^+$ (CD19$^+$, CD20$^+$, or CD22$^+$), CD10$^+$, CD5$^-$, and CD23$^-$. Translocation t(14;18) involving the rearrangement of bcl-2 gene is present in 85% of the patients, resulting in abnormal expression of this anti-apoptosis gene. Histological transformation occurs in up to 70% of the patients at time of first progression or later. It is often associated with a succession of multiple genetic alterations, particularly mutations involving p53 and deletions of p16 (39).

Most patients have widespread disease at diagnosis and truly localized disease is rare. Few patients present with B symptoms or altered general status at diagnosis. Involved sites are predominantly lymph nodes, spleen, and bone marrow, and occasionally peripheral blood or extranodal sites. Bone marrow is involved in at least 60% of cases. Extranodal site involvement, other than bone marrow or blood, is often associated with more aggressive disease or histological progression. Nearly all patients have circulating bcl-2-rearranged cells.

Prognostic factors have been identified to predict survival of patients with follicular lymphoma. Follicular Lymphoma International Prognostic Index (FLIPI), a clinical prognostic index, divide patients into three different risk groups with overall 5- and 10-year survival ranging from 52% to 91% and 36% to 71%, respectively (40). FLIPI is composed of five prognostic factors: age more than 60 years, Ann Arbor stage III-IV, hemoglobin level inferior at 120 g/L, more that four nodal areas involved, and elevated serum LDH. Biological prognostic factors also exist, and recent advances identified the importance of follicular lymphoma microenvironment response in follicular lymphoma evolution (20,41).

Ten percent of all FL patients have a localized stage without large mass. With involved field radiotherapy, more than 95% of them achieve complete response but most of them relapse, sometimes years after the first manifestation. In one study, no treatment at all was associated with a similar outcome than radiation therapy (42). Chemotherapy must be used in these patients only after recurrence.

Patients with advanced FL are generally considered to have incurable disease. Treatment can have an impact on symptoms, progression-free survival, and perhaps overall survival. Because many patients are asymptomatic at diagnosis, observation without treatment is an option, as no curative treatment exists. A randomized trial from United Kingdom showed no difference in overall survival between a watch and wait policy and immediate systemic treatment in patients with low tumor burden asymptomatic advanced FL (43). A recommended approach for patient with low tumor burden disease is observation during the first six months after diagnosis, and in instance of rapid disease progression or symptomatic disease, initiation of treatment. Otherwise, a "watch and wait" strategy is currently the best one for these patients.

At least 50% of FL patients need to be treated at diagnosis. Treatment of choice is still a matter of discussion, especially with the introduction of new therapies. Monoclonal antibodies, as single agent or in combination with chemotherapy, have considerably changed FL treatment in the last decade. In front-line therapy, single-agent anti-CD20 rituximab achieve an overall response rate of 75%, with half of them being complete (44). It should be noted that maximal response can be delayed for up to six months. However, duration of response is usually only two years, not longer than watch and wait policy. Thus, longer treatment duration has been developed (see paragraph on maintenance), but no data show that this strategy is better than doing nothing until progression then chemotherapy associated with rituximab.

Another option is to use immunochemotherapy, a combination of a monoclonal antibody as rituximab, and chemotherapy. No single chemotherapy agent (e.g., chlorambucil) or combination regimens (e.g., cyclophosphamide, vincristine, prednisone ± doxorubicine, CVP, or CHOP) have shown survival advantage over the other. However, it can be argued that patients who achieve complete response at the end of first-line treatment have a longer survival, a longer time to treatment failure (TTF), and a lower probability of histological transformation at recurrence. As the achievement of complete response may happen more frequently with more aggressive regimen, CHOP is our preferred combination (Fig. 13.4). Fludarabine-based combinations allow a high response rate in relapsing and first-line patients, but TTF is not different from that obtained with other regimens, and this treatment is associated with more immunosuppression as well as difficulties in harvesting peripheral blood progenitor cells. Rituximab is associated with better results in untreated patient as well as in relapse setting. Four randomized trials have shown the benefit of adding rituximab to different chemotherapy combinations in untreated patient with FL (Table 13.3) (45–48). In these studies, rituximab was used with different regimens: CVP, CHOP, MCP (mitoxantrone, chlorambucil, and prednisolone), or CHVP-IFN (cyclophosphamide, doxorubicin, etoposide, prednisolone plus interferon-2a). All these studies demonstrated improvement in overall response rate, time to progression, and overall survival even with short follow-up considering FL. With these good results, rituximab with combination chemotherapy is now a standard in FL first-line treatment (Fig. 13.3). The regimen used in our institution is R-CHOP. However, as mentioned earlier, rituximab alone can be considered in certain circumstances.

For patients relapsing following first-line therapy without rituximab, a new chemotherapy regimen with the addition of rituximab is indicated (Fig. 13.5). If the front-line

Table 13.3 Randomized Studies Comparing Chemotherapy to Rituximab Plus Chemotherapy in Patients with Follicular Lymphoma

Reference	Setting	Treatment	Number of patients	Median follow-up (months)	Overall response rate/complete response rate (%)	Median progression-free survival (months)	Improvement in overall survival
Marcus et al. (46) and Hersey and Zhang (140)	First line	CVP vs. R-CVP	321	53	57/10 vs. 81/41	15 vs. 34[a]	Yes
Hiddemann et al. (47)	First line	CHOP vs. R-CHOP	428	18	90/17 vs. 96/20	31 vs. not reached[a]	Yes
Herold et al. (48)	First line	MCP vs. R-MCP	201	47	75/25 vs. 92/50	28.8 vs. not reached[a]	Yes
Salles et al. (45)	First line	CHVP+I vs. R-CHVP+I	358	60	85/59 vs. 94/75	35 vs. not reached[a]	Yes (in high risk patients)
Van Oers et al. (53)	Relapse/refractory	CHOP vs. R-CHOP[b]	465	39	75/16 vs. 85/30	20 vs. 33[a]	No
Forstpointner et al. (54)	Relapse/refractory mantle cell and follicular lymphoma	FCM vs. R-FCM[b]	147	18	58/13 vs. 79/33	10 vs. 16[a]	Yes

[a]Statistically significant.
[b]Second randomization for rituximab maintenance.

Table 13.4 Randomized Studies of Rituximab (R) Maintenance in Follicular Lymphoma

References	Setting	Treatment	Number of patients	Median follow-up (months)	Median progression-free survival (months)	Overall survival
Hainsworth et al. (51)	Relapse after chemotherapy induction with R single-agent	Observation vs. R maintenance	114	41	7.4 vs. 31[a]	No
Ghielmini et al. (52)	First line or relapse/refractory induction with R single-agent	Observation vs. R maintenance	202	35	12 vs. 23[a]	No
Hochster et al. (142)	Relapse/refractory induction with CVP or FC	Observation vs. R weekly × 4 every 6 months × 4	322	NA	2 year estimated PFS: 42% vs. 74%[a]	No
Van Oers et al. (53)	Relapse/refractory induction with CHOP or R-CHOP	Observation vs. R every 3 months for 2 years	334	33	23 vs. 52[a] (subgroup with R-CHOP induction)	Yes (for the entire cohort)
Forstpointner et al. (54)	Mantle cell and follicular lymphoma relapse/refractory with FCM or R-FCM induction	Observation vs. R weekly × 4 at 3 and 9 months post induction	176	26	26 vs. not reached[a] (subgroup of FL with R-FCM induction)	No

[a]Statistically significant.

therapy included rituximab, the benefit of rituximab in second line combination is unclear, but it is justify using it again if initial results were good. Single-agent therapy using rituximab is still an option even if already given before, with overall response rate up to 50%.

Rituximab maintenance after induction treatment in relapsed FL was studied by many, following single-agent rituximab, chemotherapy, or immunochemotherapy (Table 13.4). Following single-agent rituximab induction, maintenance improved progression-free survival but with no impact on time to next chemotherapy-based treatment and survival (51,52). Two groups studied rituximab maintenance following immunochemotherapy induction. Improvement in progression-free survival was seen in both studies

and even survival in one of them (53,54). With these results, two-year rituximab maintenance is recommended by many in relapse setting following immunochemotherapy. However, optimal duration of maintenance is unknown. Also, rituximab maintenance following immunochemotherapy in untreated patients is of unknown benefit, and a study in progress should answer the question.

High-dose therapy with ASCT has been used for several years in relapsing patients with either bone marrow or peripheral blood stem cells. It has enabled a significant prolongation of TTF over that obtained with standard treatments and even survival in one study (55,56). Currently, the use of rituximab in salvage regimen allows an in vivo purge and the reinjection of lymphoma-free stem cells.

Because of the activity of rituximab in first-line patients, this procedure will remain a good salvage possibility but not a standard first-line treatment. However, better results are achieved when high-dose therapy is done early in treatment plan, as following first relapse in eligible patients. The use of allogeneic stem cell transplantation is still a matter of debate, offering possibilities of long-term survival, but at the expense of high treatment related morbidities and mortalities. Interesting results with less early treatment mortalities are seen with nonmyeloablative conditioning regimen. However, graft-versus-host disease remains a concern.

Radiolabeled monoclonal antibodies are formed by conjugating a radioisotope to a monoclonal antibody and allowed delivery of radiation directly to the tumor. CD20 antigen remains the target of choice up to now. Two agents are approved for the treatment of NHL: [131]iodine-labeled tositumomab (Bexxar) and [90]yttrium ibritumomab (Zevalin). Good response rates were seen when used in relapsed or refractory FL even when patients were rituximab refractory (57,58). Introduction to initial therapy has been tried with interesting results (59). Their use in a consolidation strategy after first- and second-line therapy or part of high-dose therapy conditioning regimen is under study. Radioimmunoconjugates have shown efficacy in FL, but the best time to use them is still unknown.

Interferon-α (IFNα) recombinant has been used in association with either an initial chemotherapy regimen or as maintenance in responding patients. Some studies have shown disease-free and overall survival advantage, but with toxicities precluding its use in clinical practice, especially with the introduction of well-tolerated therapies as rituximab (60).

All patients eventually progress and die of their disease, 40% to 70% after histological transformation, with a median survival at least 15 years in recent series (61,62). Things may change again in the near future with the introduction of novel therapies.

Follicular lymphoma is characterized by the presence of bcl-2 gene rearrangement in more than 70% of the cases. It has been assumed that longer CR duration would result from the disappearance of this lymphoma marker, a status defined as a molecular response. However, molecular response studied in blood did not always correlate with clinical response and molecular response has been observed in patients with persisting enlarged lymph nodes. If patients in molecular response tend to have a longer TTF regardless of the clinical response, the presence of bcl-2-rearranged cells must be considered as a surrogate marker of tumor burden. In patients with disappearance of the bcl-2 gene rearrangement in blood and bone marrow, the number of lymphoma cells is below the detection power of PCR techniques. However, it is not synonymous with cure.

Mantle Cell Lymphoma

Mantle cell lymphoma (MCL) is a rare tumor comprising 5% to 8% of lymphomas. The tumor is composed exclusively of monomorphous small to medium-sized lymphoid cells with dispersed chromatin, scant pale cytoplasm, and inconspicuous nucleoli. The nuclei are irregular or cleaved but may be rounded. Usually mitoses are infrequent. The large blastoid cell variant has larger nuclei with more

dispersed chromatin and a high proliferation fraction. Proliferation is usually diffuse or vaguely nodular. Less commonly, a pure mantle zone pattern may be observed. Tumor cells are sIgM[+], usually IgD[+], B-cell-associated antigen[+], CD5[+], CD10[-], CD23[-], FMC7[+], and CD43[+]. The translocation t(11;14) involving the immunoglobulin heavy chain locus and the bcl-1 locus is present in 70% of cases by conventional cytogenetics (nearly all cases when studied by FISH) and results in over-expression of the PRAD1/CCND1 gene, a cell-cycle regulatory protein that encodes for cyclin D1. The diagnosis may be confirmed by the immunoexpression of cyclin D1.

This lymphoma occurs more frequently in older adults, with predominance in men. It is usually widely spread at diagnosis, with involvement of lymph nodes, spleen, bone marrow, peripheral blood, and extranodal sites, especially gastrointestinal tract (lymphomatous polyposis). Its clinical course is initially moderately aggressive but becomes progressively more so with time.

MCL patients do not respond very well to current therapeutic options (63). They often present partial regression of the lymphoma for 6–18 months and then progress, and die, for a median overall survival of three to four years. Recent data suggest however an improvement with a median overall of about five years (64). CHOP combined to rituximab in first-line patients was shown to be associated with a high response rate but not a longer survival than other regimens (65). Rituximab alone has been associated with good results in relapsing patients (66). Combination with high-dose aracytine might be more interesting than CHOP but is certainly more toxic (67). High-dose therapy with ASCT in patients responding to a combination regimen associated with rituximab is certainly a promising approach (68) (Fig. 13.2).

Outside randomized prospective trials, the following strategy is recommended: patients with localized disease may be treated with chemotherapy (R-CHOP) followed by involved field radiotherapy. Elderly patients with advanced disease should be treated with R-CHOP or, if there is any contraindication to anthracycline, with R-FC or rituximab, ifosfamide, plus etoposide (70) young patients may be treated with R-CHOP or a combination including aracytine and rituximab and, in instances of good response, high-dose therapy. Whatever the initial treatment, however, these patients will eventually progress and become resistant to chemotherapy.

Diffuse Large B-cell Lymphoma

Diffuse large B-cell lymphoma (DLBCL) comprises 40% of all lymphomas. It encompasses various histological subtypes, none of which optimally defined, and is often heterogeneous in morphology, genetics, and clinical presentation. These lymphomas are composed of large B cells with a round or variably cleaved nucleus, often with basophilic cytoplasm, and fairly marked mitotic activity. In most cases, the large cells are described as centroblasts (large cleaved cells). Other cell types are observed, such as large multilobated cells, large anaplastic B cells, or small noncleaved non-Burkitt cells (Burkitt-like lymphoma). Some variants may show abundant small reactive T cells and histiocytes or intravascular proliferation, which can cause diagnostic problems. Primary mediastinal large

B-cell lymphomas are composed of large cells with nuclei of variable appearance but clear cytoplasm surrounding by fibrosis. In most cases, it is still difficult if not impossible to subclassify these tumors. Distinction among morphologic variant of DLBCL has generally met poor intraobserver and interobserver reproducibility. Tumor cells are sIg$^\pm$, cIg$^\pm$, B-cell-associated antigens$^+$, CD45$^+$, CD5$^\pm$, and CD10$^\pm$. The bcl-2 gene is rearranged in 20% of the cases and c-myc in some cases. An anomaly of the long arm of chromosome 3 has been described and associated with bcl-6 rearrangement. Gene expression profiling (GEP), which allows to study thousand of genes expression at the same time, has been use in patients with DLBCL and showed two major patterns of gene expression. One group displays a germinal center like cell (GCC) signature and the other displays an activated B-cell (ABC) like signature. Their prognosis in terms of overall survival is markedly different with better results in GCC group (71).

Patients usually present with a rapidly enlarging nodal or extranodal mass. Up to 40% of cases are extranodal and all body sites may be involved. Disease is localized in 30% of the cases. Some locations are frequently associated with large mass, particularly mediastinum and abdomen.

About 70% of DLBCL patients who reach complete response may be cured, in contrast to almost none of those failing to do so. The ultimate aim then must be to reach complete response. Choice of therapy should be based on prognostic index such as IPI, alone or associated with new interesting parameters (10,16,18). Only some relapsing patients may be cured with salvage regimens, and therefore, cure must be provided with the first-line treatment advocating management in specialized centers.

Patients with early stage disease (stage I or II nonbulky, without adverse prognostic factors) have good prognosis: >80% to 90% complete response rate, <20% relapse rate, and 70% to 80% 10-year survival rate. These results are much better than those obtained with advanced stage disease. For a long time, CHOP has been the standard treatment, but in the past decade, new modalities have changed therapeutic options: increased dose/intensity CHOP-like regimens, combination with rituximab (Table 13.4) and high-dose therapy with autologous stem cell transplantation (ASCT).

Adding more drugs to standard CHOP regimen has failed to prove its interest (72), and increasing the dose intensity of CHOP has proven its value and remains a possible tool to increase response rate and decrease relapse rate (73). The regimen used in the GELA for 25 years, ACVBP, now has proven its superiority in terms of event-free and overall survivals compared with CHOP (74,75) (Figs. 13.6 and 13.7). The GELA studies used an approach, with four alterations of the CHOP regimen: a sequential consolidation after induction with the modified CHOP regimen, a shortening of the interval between courses to two weeks, an increase of doses, and a repeat of nonhematotoxic drugs on day 5 of each course (Fig. 13.5). The ACVBP regimen was used as standard arm in several randomized studies since 1987 and had shown its superiority over m-BACOD and CHOP for patients with poor risk lymphoma, and equivalence with HDT in patients with good risk lymphoma (76). It is actually unknown whether ACVBP will keep this advantage over CHOP with the introduction of rituximab in combination with chemotherapy (see paragraphs later). A study is in progress to answer this question. Others tried to improve results in keeping CHOP or CHOP-like chemotherapy but to shortened interval of administration from three weeks (CHOP 21) to two weeks (CHOP 14). This strategy improved results but it remains unknown whether CHOP 14 is better than CHOP 21 when rituximab is added to chemotherapy (77,78).

Addition of rituximab to chemotherapy increased remission among these patients (Table 13.5) (79–83) (Fig. 13.8). R-CHOP combines CHOP every three weeks for eight cycles with rituximab given on day 1 of each cycle. This regimen is associated with a dramatic increase in the survival of patients and has been shown to decrease the refractoriness to chemotherapy associated with bcl-2 protein expression (84). R-CHOP has become the reference regimen for patients with diffuse large B-cell lymphoma and for other B-cell lymphoma subtypes. Its use on a

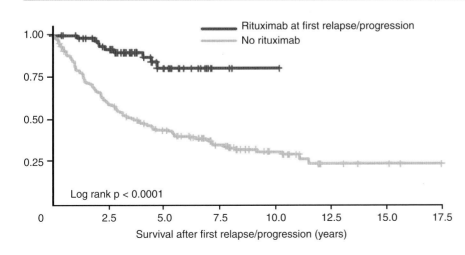

Figure 13.5 Overall survival in follicular lymphoma according to rituximab use at first relapse/progression. *Source*: From Ref. 50.

population-scaled basis decreases the mortality associated with DLBCL (85).

HDT with ASCT was tested in several settings in these patients after it has proven its interest in relapsing patients (see p. 254 Relapsing patients). Patients in partial response at the end of first-line chemotherapy may benefit from such a treatment too. For responding patients, several randomized studies allow to conclude that this treatment has no interest in patients with good risk lymphoma or slow response to chemotherapy. Some of these studies concluded that HDT with ASCT in first remission can improve survival for a subgroup of patients with high-risk lymphoma and who reached complete remission at the end of treatment (86,87). Currently, this treatment should be reserved for young patients with adverse prognostic factors.

From all data cited above, we may describe three large groups of patients. The first group has localized disease. These patients can be treated with standard treatments, either three courses of R-CHOP followed by involved field radiotherapy (88) or six to eight courses of R-CHOP or R-ACVBP regimen for those with more aggressive disease (89). However, no consensus exists about what should be considered standard treatment. For patients older than 60 years with stage I-II and age-adjusted IPI of 0, R-CHOP for four cycles without radiotherapy seems to be enough (90). More intensive treatments should be reserved for patients who do not achieve complete response or who relapse. As more than 80% of these patients are cured with these treatments, the only refinement may come for the description of some adverse prognostic parameters that will move poorer risk patients to other groups treated more intensively.

The second group comprises young patients with advanced disease. Best treatment for these patients is unknown. Treatment of reference is R-CHOP but other options such dose-intense R-CHOP-like regimens (R-CHOP 14, R-ACVBP) or HDT with ASCT exist. These treatments may have their place here, but there is no clear consensus on which treatment must be standard.

The third group comprises elderly patients, defined as patients not able to tolerate dose-intense regimens. In this setting, the recent GELA trial has settled the standard to eight cycles of R-CHOP (82). For patients older than 80 years and not able to tolerate intensive chemotherapy, dose-adjusted R-CHOP (mini R-CHOP) may be an option.

Other small groups of patients may be recognized, such as patients refractory to chemotherapy, defined as rapid progression after treatment discontinuation or progressive disease after initial courses. No parameters are able to identify these patients at diagnosis, except expression of bcl-2 protein. The addition of rituximab to chemotherapy may help to decrease the percentage of patients with refractoriness to chemotherapy (84).

Whether involved field radiotherapy in patients showing complete response may decrease the relapse rate in all patients or only in patients with large tumoral masses is debated. Some groups have presented better outcomes for patients treated with radiotherapy (91). However, the failure of radiation therapy to add to chemotherapy in localized disease, its long-term side effects, and the fact that persisting images may not reflect active disease do not favor this addition.

It is generally accepted that the definitive strategy for treating DLBCL patients has not yet been determined and that including patients in prospective, carefully designed, trials must be a rule of good clinical practice. Evaluation of response to treatment with early PET scan during chemotherapy may help to guide management and adapt therapy in the future. This strategy is actually evaluated in clinical studies.

Burkitt Lymphoma

Burkitt lymphoma (BL) is a highly aggressive NHL and is considered a B-cell mature neoplasm. Three clinical variants of BL have been described: endemic, sporadic, and immunodeficiency BL. Morphologically, BL consists of medium-sized monomorphic cells with a round nucleus, multiple nucleoli, and basophilic cytoplasm. Cytoplasmic lipid vacuoles are generally present. The tumor is highly proliferative with multiple mitoses, apoptotic cells, and macrophages. The cells are positive for surface immunoglobulin M ($sIgM^+$), express B antigens, and are $CD5^-$, $CD10^+$, $bcl-6^+$, and Tdt^+. All cases show translocation of the c-myc gene on chromosome 8 to the immunoglobulin heavy chain region on chromosome 14, t(8;14), or to the light chain region on chromosome 2, t(2;8), or chromosome 22, t(8;22), leading to the activation of c-myc. The plasmacytoid variant is more common in immunodeficient patients. Another variant called atypical Burkitt/Burkitt-like lymphoma shows high degree of apoptosis and high mitotic index as classical BL but also greater polymorphism in nuclear size and shape. Morphologic features can be intermediate between BL and DLBCL. Gene expression profiling can help to distinguish BL from DLBCL but is of limited access (92,93).

Sporadic BL is more common in children (40% of all child lymphomas) but accounts for 1% to 2% of lymphomas in adults. This clinical subtype is seen throughout the world. Most patients present with an abdominal tumor involving the cecum and mesentery, but some cases develop in ovary, breast, testis, or peripheral lymph node. Bone marrow or meningeal involvement is frequent affecting 50% to 70% and 20% to 40% of adults, respectively. Endemic BL occurs in specific areas (equatorial Africa or tropical areas with endemic malaria). The tumor is localized in the jaws or orbit in 50% of cases. Cases observed in endemic zones of Africa are associated with EBV infection in 100% of cases, which is different from the sporadic cases of Europe or the United States, where EBV infection is found only in 20% of the cases. Immunodeficiency associated BL is seen usually in association with HIV infection and associated with EBV in 25% to 40% of the cases.

Patients without bone marrow or CNS disease have a better outcome than those with these adverse locations, but all must be treated with regimens designed for children (94,95). These intensive regimens usually include high doses cyclophosphamide, cytarabine, methotrexate, and aggressive intrathecal CNS prophylaxis. Elderly patients with Burkitt lymphoma generally have a poor survival and may not tolerate intensive regimens proposed in young adults. The place of rituximab is this highly proliferative $CD20^+$ lymphoma has not yet be defined and in under study. Relapse usually occurs in the first year following treatment.

Mature T-cell Lymphomas (Table 13.2)
Mycosis Fungoides and Sézary Syndrome
Primary cutaneous lymphomas involve the skin without evidence of extracutaneous disease at the time of diagnosis. Around 75% of cutaneous lymphomas are of T-cell origin, and most of them are mycosis fungoides (MF) (96,97).

MF is characterized by infiltration of the epidermis by tumor cells, which are predominantly small to medium-sized cells with cerebriform nuclei. A minority of large cells can be seen. With disease progression, epidermotropism may be lost with more diffuse dermal infiltrate and tumor cells can increase in number and size. Most cases are CD4+, but rare CD8+ cases are reported. Other T-cell-associated antigens can be expressed as CD2, CD3, and CD5. CD7 expression is variable. If TCR genes are rearranged No specific genetic abnormality has been described yet.

MF is usually an indolent disease with evolution over years. Patients present with cutaneous patches that can progress to plaques and eventually nodules. Some present initially with generalized erythroderma, and others develop this state as disease progressed. Lymph node and visceral involvement are late occurrences, mostly in cases of histological transformation.

Sézary syndrome (SS) is defined by the historic triad of erythroderma, generalized lymphadenopathy, and blood involvement by the neoplastic T cells (Sézary cells). Blood involvement usually requires a number of at least 1000/mm³. Alternatively, demonstration of CD4:CD8 ratio greater than 10 or of a T-cell clone in blood can be sufficient to support the diagnosis of SS.

MF patients usually have a long survival although they rarely achieve complete response. Prognosis depends on the stage of the disease, with 10-year overall survival over 95% for patients with limited cutaneous disease, 42% for tumor stage disease, and 20% with proven lymph node involvement (96). SS follows an aggressive course with median survival between two and four years.

Patients with disease limited to the skin can be treated with topical measures as topical nitrogen mustard, electron beam therapy (local or total depending on the extent), or phototherapy with psoralen and ultraviolet A light (PUVA). As the disease progresses, other options are available as interferon, retinoid (bexarotene), combination therapy (PUVA+interferon, PUVA+bexarotene), and eventually systemic chemotherapy (HDAC inhibitors, cladribine, pentostatin, gemcitabine, liposomal doxorubicin, methotrexate). In any instance of disease progression toward large tumoral masses either cutaneous, in lymph nodes, or in visceral locations, chemotherapy should be preferred. Unfortunately, most patients will eventually fail to respond, develop large cutaneous tumors, or non-cutaneous tumoral sites, or have transformation into large cell lymphoma. New therapies such as denileukin diftitox (monoclonal antibody combined with toxin), alemtuzumab (monoclonal antibody anti-CD52), or vorinostat [histone deacetylase inhibitors (HDACi)] may have an interest in progressive disease. For patients presenting with SS, extracorporeal photophoresis and systemic therapies are recommended (98).

Peripheral T-cell Lymphoma
Peripheral T-cell lymphoma (PTCL) is not a single entity but includes several distinct clinical pathologic syndromes,

now well recognized in the WHO classification: angio-immunoblastic T-cell lymphoma, extranodal NK/T cell lymphoma-nasal type, enteropathy-type T-cell lymphoma, hepatosplenic γδ T-cell lymphoma, subcutaneous panniculitis-like T-cell lymphoma, anaplastic large cell lymphoma, CD30+ cutaneous proliferations, and HTLV-1 related lymphoma. Although many of these entities have been conclusively defined, some have been identified on a provisional basis only. These lymphomas account for 10% to 15% of all lymphomas in Europe and the United States but are more frequent elsewhere, e.g., Japan or East Asia. Their heterogeneity and the difficulties in differentiating between reactive and lymphomatous cells often make PTCL difficult to describe and classify. A feature common to all such lymphomas is the variability in presentation, with some cases being sufficiently atypical to suggest diseases other than lymphoma, resulting in diagnostic delay. Their clinical presentation is extremely heterogeneous, and very few trials have individualized these patients before treatment. They are usually treated like DLBCL patients but without rituximab and, unfortunately, a far worse outcome (100).

Angioimmunoblastic T-cell lymphoma (AITL) is a systemic disease with polymorphous infiltrate involving lymph nodes associated with a proliferation of follicular dendritic cells and a prominent arborization of high endothelial venules. Neoplastic cells are small to medium-sized and represent only a fraction of the infiltrate being mixed with small lymphocytes, eosinophils, plasma cells, histiocytes, and large lymphoid cells. Tumors cells express CD4+ and other T-cell antigens (CD2, CD3, CD5). CD10 and CXCL13 are also often expressed (101). Patients generally present at an advanced age with generalized lymph node hypertrophy, hepatosplenomegaly, fever, cutaneous reactions, and polyclonal hypergammaglobulinemia. Immunologic abnormalities are common. Optimal treatment is unknown. Prognosis is poor with long-term survival around 30% even with CHOP-like chemotherapy. The benefit of autologous stem cell transplantation on long-term survival is unknown (102).

Extranodal NK/T cell lymphoma (nasal type) is strongly associated with EBV and is seen predominantly in Asia. Most patients present with localized nasal mass with systemic disseminated disease being uncommon. This neoplasm shows a broad morphologic spectrum with a pleomorphic cellular infiltrate associated with angioinvasion and angiodestruction. CD56 is usually positive. This is an aggressive disease with a poor prognosis. A combination of chemotherapy (usually CHOP-like regimen) and radiotherapy is usually given. The sequence of treatment is unclear (103).

Enteropathy-type T-cell lymphoma often occurs in adults with a history of gluten enteropathy but can occur as a primary event. Jejunum and ileum are usually involved. Spread to distant sites is unusual at diagnosis. The infiltrate is again polymorph with the neoplastic cells showing the following immunophenotype: CD3+, CD7+, CD4-, CD8-, and CD103+. Small bowel obstruction and perforation are classic clinical presentations. Management includes resection when possible and chemotherapy. Results with CHOP are disappointing, but no regimen is known superior.

Hepatosplenic γδ T-cell lymphoma is a rare and aggressive disease. Median age at diagnosis is in the

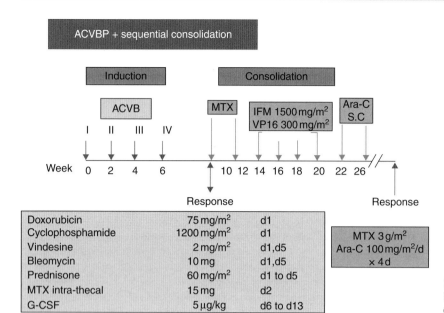

Doxorubicin	75 mg/m²	d1
Cyclophosphamide	1200 mg/m²	d1
Vindesine	2 mg/m²	d1,d5
Bleomycin	10 mg	d1,d5
Prednisone	60 mg/m²	d1 to d5
MTX intra-thecal	15 mg	d2
G-CSF	5 μg/kg	d6 to d13

Figure 13.6   Dose-intensive CHOP or ACVBP used in the LNH-84 protocol (76) followed by the sequential chemotherapy.

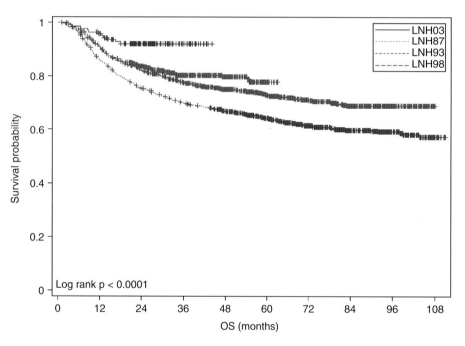

Figure 13.7   Overall survival in B-cell aggressive lymphoma treated with ACVBP in different GELA (Groupe d'étude des Lymphomes de l'Adulte) studies (LNH 1987-1993-1998-2003). *Abbreviations*: ACVBP, doxorubicin, cyclophosphamide, vindesine, bleomycin, and prednisone; OS, overall survival.

mid-thirties. Most of the time patients have advanced disease at presentation with liver, splenic, and bone marrow infiltration. Hemophagocytic syndrome can be observed. Prognosis is poor even with intensive chemotherapy.

Subcutaneous panniculitis-like T-cell lymphoma is also a rare disease and happens in the mid-thirties. Initial manifestation usually includes one or multiple subcutaneous nodules. Systemic symptoms such as fever and hemophagocytic syndrome are frequently reported. Evolution can be indolent, but sometimes aggressive. Five-year overall survival is around 60% (104). Combination chemotherapy and radiotherapy have been used, but the best therapeutic approach is unknown. However, good responses have been described.

Anaplastic Large Cell Lymphoma

Anaplastic large cell lymphoma (ALCL) accounts for 3% of adults NHL and 10% to 30% of pediatric lymphomas. ALCL has a large morphologic spectrum. Usually, the cells are large with a pleomorphic multilobed nucleus, multiple or large isolated nucleoli, and an abundant cytoplasm. Lymphohistiocytic and small cell variants have been described (105). Proliferation of these cells has a cohesive appearance and an affinity for lymph node sinuses. Tumor cells are CD30+, CD45±, EMA+, CD15−, and Alk1+; they are variably positive for T-cell antigens, as some cases show a null phenotype. A t(2;5) translocation (or a variant) is generally present leading to the expression of a NPM-ALK fusion protein; 10% show no evidence of gene rearrangement, and 90% show T-cell receptor gene rearrangement.

Two clinical presentations of ALCL are encountered: the first is systemic, with nodal and/or extranodal (sometimes cutaneous) involvement; the second is exclusively cutaneous, forming a continuum from lymphomatoid papulosis (not necessarily neoplastic despite being clonal) through lymphoma, usually Alk1−. The cutaneous variant may regress spontaneously over long periods before reemerging. In clinical presentation and course, the systemic ALCL is fairly similar to other large B- or T-cell lymphomas. In some cases, clinical manifestations may differ very little from those of mediastinal Hodgkin's disease with a large tumor, which renders the diagnosis fairly difficult.

Anaplastic T- or N/K-cell lymphomas are seen mostly in young adult patients. Patients with the systemic form often present with an aggressive picture, advanced stage and B symptoms, but they respond to dose-intense CHOP-like regimens, and 60% to 70% of them are disease-free at five years (14,106). Prognosis is different depending on Alk status: five-year overall survival of 75% for Alk+ and 50% for Alk− (107,108). Currently, the strategy used for DLBCL patients, except the use of anti-CD20 monoclonal antibody, is recommended. Patients with the cutaneous form have a better outcome, which will be described later.

Adult T-cell Lymphoma/Leukemia

Adult T-cell lymphoma/leukemia (ATL) is a T-cell neoplasm caused by HTLV-1. Tumor cells express T-cell-associated antigens (CD2, CD3, and CD5) but usually do not express CD7, and most are CD4+. TCR genes are rearranged and a clonally integrated HTLV-I genome is found in all cases.

Most cases occur in Japan, but an endemic focus is found in the Caribbean. The estimated risk to develop ATL following HTLV-1 infection is about 5%, with a latency period of several decades. Several clinical variants have been described: a leukemic form with high leucocyte count hepatosplenomegaly, hypercalcemia, and lytic bone lesions; a lymphoma form with lymphadenopathies without leukemia; a chronic form with isolated leucocyte count and skin rashes; and smoldering cases with mild lymphocytosis. Treatment generally includes combination chemotherapy regimens, but prognosis is usually poor.

Precursor B-cell and T-cell Neoplasms

Precursor B lymphoblastic leukemia (B-ALL)/lymphoblastic lymphoma (B-LL) and precursor T lymphoblastic leukemia (T-ALL)/lymphoblastic lymphoma (T-LL) are neoplasm of lymphoblasts committed to B- and T-cell lineage, respectively. Precursor B- and T-cell neoplasms are considered separately, but leukemia and lymphoma subtypes of each lineage are considered as a single disease

with different patterns of presentation. If the patient presents a mass lesion and 25% or fewer lymphoblasts in bone marrow, it is considered a lymphoma. Globally, B- and T-cell lymphoblastic lymphomas represent 2% of adult NHL.

Precursor B lymphoblastic lymphoma is an uncommon type of lymphoma representing 10% of lymphoblastic lymphoma, and most of them present in children or adolescents. Most frequent sites of involvement are the skin, bone, soft tissue, and lymph nodes. Unlike T-LL, mediastinal masses are unfrequent. B-ALL is a hundred times more frequent than B-LL. B-LL comprises lymphoblasts, which are cells slightly larger than small lymphocytes with a B phenotype (CD19+, CD79a+, and varying in their positivity for other B-cell antigens), TdT+, and HLA-DR+. Various cytogenetic abnormalities have been reported (109). Treatment should be the same as that for B-ALL.

Precursor T lymphoblastic lymphoma represents 90% of lymphoblastic lymphoma, and it is most frequent in adolescent and young adults. Mediastinal involvement is present in about two-third of cases. Other common sites involved include peripheral lymph node, pleural space, pericardium, bone marrow, and CNS. CNS is a frequent site of relapse without adequate prophylaxis (up to 30%). T-LL is composed of lymphoblasts undistinguishable from B-LL/B-ALL lymphoblasts on morphology alone. They have a T-cell phenotype (CD7+, CD3+, other T-cell antigens variable) and TdT+. Rearrangement of TCR genes is variable, and IgH gene rearrangement may be seen. Variable cytogenetic abnormalities have been reported but without prognostic significance. The recommended therapy for T-LL is the same as that for ALL with intensive chemotherapy and adequate CNS prophylaxis (110,111). With these modalities, five-year overall survival is around 50% in children. The value of mediastinal irradiation for patients with mediastinal involvement is unclear. Also, the benefit of high-dose therapy with autologous stem cell transplant in first complete response is unknown. In any case, the classical CHOP is not an effective therapy.

SPECIAL CLINICAL SITUATIONS

Elderly Patients

Elderly patients present some particularities compared with younger patients with respect to NHL histologies, comorbidities, tolerance to treatment, and prognosis. DLBCL and peripheral T-cell lymphoma, small lymphocytic lymphoma, lymphoplasmacytic lymphoma, and maybe splenic marginal zone lymphoma are seen more often in the elderly population. Other subtypes such as anaplastic large cell lymphoma are unusual in this group (112,113). Studies focusing on elderly population showed decrease in complete response rate and event-free survival. Survival of these patients is found to be consistently shorter than that of younger patients, and this difference persists after correction of survival data for cause of death that appeared unrelated to lymphoma (114). This shorter survival may be related to a tendency of physicians to administer reduced treatment and to poor tolerance of therapy, in itself related to poor performance status and the presence of associated disabilities (115).

As done in younger patients, the treatment of elderly patients with lymphoma has to be designed according to

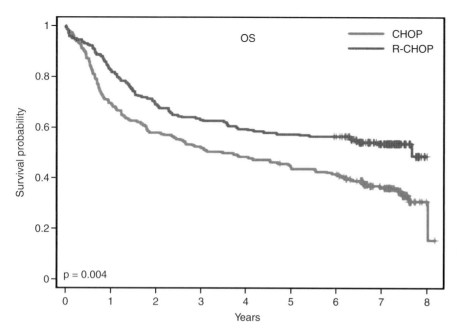

Figure 13.8 Overall survival with a median follow-up of seven years in LNH 98-5 study from GELA comparing CHOP with R-CHOP in elderly patients with diffuse large B-cell lymphoma. *Abbreviations*: CHOP, Cyclophosphamide, Hydroxydaunorubicin (Adriamycin), Oncovin (Vincristine), Prednisone/Prednisolone; OS, overall survival; R-CHOP, Rituximab, Cyclophosphamide, Hydroxydaunorubicin (Adriamycin), Oncovin (Vincristine), Prednisone/Prednisolone. *Source*: From Ref. 81.

lymphoma's histological subtype and the presence or absence of adverse prognostic factors. The special problems of treating elderly patients are specific to those with DLBCL, because these patients may not receive full high-dose chemotherapy regimens because of their age and concomitant diseases. However, the approach consisting to deliver an "age-specific" regimen has constantly failed to show any advantage (116). The gold-standard chemotherapy regimen for patients with DLBCL is now R-CHOP, and when doses were decreased because of advanced age, the CR rate decreased and the survival shortened (81,117). Treatment of elderly patients remains a constant challenge and appropriate evaluation is necessary to give treatment in function of biologic age rather than chronologic age. Multidisciplinary approach with geriatric evaluation can be very helpful.

Post-transplantation Lymphomas

The Epstein–Barr virus (EBV) has been implicated in the pathogenesis B-cell lymphoproliferative diseases (PTLDs) in immunosuppressed organ transplant recipients. The incidence is probably inferior to 1% in hematopoietic stem cell transplant with higher rates with HLA mismatched or T-cell depleted grafts. For solid organ transplant, incidence is usually under 2% but can be superior in cases needing more intense immunosuppression. Four groups of patients have been identified in PTLD (118): uncomplicated post-transplant infectious mononucleosis; benign polyclonal hyperplasia without evidence of malignant transformation; early malignant transformation into polyclonal polymorphic B-cell lymphoma with clonal cytogenetic abnormalities and immunoglobulin gene rearrangements; and monoclonal polymorphic B-cell lymphoma. The first two groups have infectious diseases that may be treated with antiviral drugs (acyclovir or gancyclovir) and/or reduction

of immunosuppression. Reduction of immunosuppression allows the regression of most PTLDs in the third group. Patients with monoclonal polymorphic lymphoma present frequently extranodal lesions and must be treated with a reduction of immunosuppression in combination with appropriate immunotherapy or chemotherapy. Rituximab is associated with good response without the toxic effects of chemotherapy, and it appears the actual standard. When chemotherapy is needed, R-CHOP is certainly the best current regimen (119). The place of EBV viral load screening by quantitative PCR analysis, and preemptive therapy is unclear. Late occurrences of lymphoma after transplantation are more likely to be unrelated to EBV infection and need to be treated as standard de novo DLBCL.

HIV-Infection-Related Lymphomas

Many different lymphoma types have been identified in AIDS patients, and high-grade B-cell pathologic type was the most frequent with 70% to 90% of cases. Diffuse large B-cell lymphoma including centroblastic, immunoblastic, and anaplastic variant, primary central nervous system lymphoma, Burkitt's lymphoma, primary effusion lymphoma, plasmablastic lymphoma, and PTLD associated with EBV are included in this category (120). Risk factors for the development of NHL include a low CD4 count. However, Burkitt's lymphoma happens in the context of CD4 count usually higher (>200 cells/μL). Lymphoma may occur in HIV-positive patients as the first manifestation of AIDS or in patients with a long history of AIDS-related infectious complications and poor performance status. In this last setting, lymphoma is usually extranodal, particularly with CNS involvement, but uncommon sites may be involved. The treatment of such patients is often palliative and they usually die of infectious complications associated with AIDS, sometimes potentiated by lymphoma treatment.

Lymphomas that occur as one of the first manifestation of AIDS are often seen in patients without severe infectious risk who may still have near normal CD4+ lymphocytes. Because of the prognosis of these patients has now improved with highly active antiretroviral therapy (HAART), their lymphoma must be treated with curative intent (121). Normally, the disease is disseminated, possibly with bone marrow or CNS involvement. Standard chemotherapy regimens as in non-HIV setting should be used. The addition of rituximab to chemotherapy is of uncertain value especially in patients with low CD4 counts, as increase in infectious complications happened in some studies.

TREATMENT STRATEGIES ACCORDING TO DISEASE SITE

It is widely believed that lymphomas may behave differently in certain sites, and this is certainly true with regard to initial manifestations of the disease and diagnostic procedures. However, no analysis has confirmed this peculiarity with respect to prognostic parameters, type of treatment required, or outcome. Whatever the initial site involved, treatment strategy is dictated by the histological subtype of the lymphoma and the presence of adverse prognostic parameters.

Gastrointestinal Tract Lymphomas

One half of gastrointestinal tract (GIT) lymphomas are small cell MALT lymphomas, which are commonly localized and have a very good outcome, and the other half are DBLCL or Burkitt's lymphoma and are associated with a poorer prognosis even if localized. However, a high proportion of gastric DLCL may occur as a transformation of a MALT lymphoma as witnessed by the persistence of a small cell component. Today, there is no agreement on the percentage of large cells required to support a diagnosis of transformation or on prognostic importance of the presence of these large cells. Patients with less than 20% of large cells may be treated with antibiotics as the patients with small cells.

Diagnosis is relatively easy in the stomach or colon with endoscopy, but laparotomy is often required for diagnosis of small bowel lymphomas. Small bowel lymphomas are characterized by their insidious course and an acute revelation by intestinal occlusion. In all cases, large surgical resection should be avoided, with surgical complications such as perforation or hemorrhage treated preventively by early adapted chemotherapy. These patients are treated like non-GIT patients with the same histological subtype. MALT, follicular, and mantle cell lymphomas are often disseminated, and surgery should be limited to the minimum. DLBCL patients may have a localized disease, and surgery is the only way to make the diagnosis. The most difficult disease to treat is the enteropathy-associated NK-cell lymphoma (122).

Primary CNS Lymphomas

Primary CNS lymphoma patients usually have localized disease and a DLBCL subtype. Surgical resection provides little therapeutic benefit. Radiotherapy allows a median survival of 12 months and is rarely curative. Complete response can be achieved with standard chemotherapy

regimens containing high-dose methotrexate (123,124). Radiotherapy can be associated to chemotherapy, but benefits are unclear and it increases neurotoxicity, especially for patients older than 60 years. The most effective regimen and the necessity of radiotherapy have yet to be defined. Inclusion of such patients in prospective trials is mandatory.

CNS relapse occurs in 5% of DLBCL and T-cell lymphoma patients, more frequently in LL and BL, and less so, and probably only after transformation, in indolent lymphomas. Thus, CNS prophylaxis is mandatory for LL and BL patients only. In DLBCL and T-cell lymphoma patients, an initial CSF examination is mandatory, particularly in patients with bone marrow infiltration or other adverse parameters. There is no curative treatment for CNS relapses, but high-dose methotrexate alone or combined with high-dose cytarabine yields some responses.

Skin Lymphomas

Aside from the MF/SS and secondary skin localizations of disseminated lymphomas, skin lymphomas are characterized by several entities (96). Primary cutaneous CD30+ lymphoproliferative disorders include primary cutaneous anaplastic large-cell lymphoma (C-ALCL) and lymphomatoid papulomatosis. These disorders have an excellent prognosis and may present spontaneous regression. Diffusion outside the skin occurs rarely, and these patients should not be treated as lymph node ALCL patients. Surgical excision or local radiotherapy is sufficient for localized C-ALCL and methotrexate for patients with multifocal skin disease. Cutaneous B-cell lymphomas include marginal zone lymphoma (MZL), follicle center lymphoma (FCL), and diffuse large B-cell lymphoma (DLBCL). Cutaneous MZL and FCL have an excellent prognosis and rare extracutaneous dissemination. An association between cutaneous MZL and *Borrelia burgdorferi* has been observed. Local therapy such as surgery or radiotherapy should be tried first if feasible, keeping chemotherapy for multiple sites or disseminated disease. At the other end, cutaneous DLBCL is an aggressive disease with frequent extracutaneous dissemination and inferior prognosis. Treatment should be the same as systemic DLBCL with polychemotherapy.

DLBCL Bone Lymphomas

DLBCL bone lymphomas may be localized to one site, disseminated in several bone sites or associated with non-bone localizations. These patients have to be treated with standard chemotherapy regimens adapted for DLBCL patients. The only special characteristic of these patients is the persistence of their bone alterations long after the disappearance of the lymphoma's cells, which makes it difficult to evaluate their response to treatment. PET scan may have a role here. The utility of local radiotherapy has not been demonstrated.

TREATMENT STRATEGIES ACCORDING TO RESPONSE TO INITIAL THERAPY

Standard chemotherapy regimens are unlikely to salvage many patients; more intensive modalities must be used.

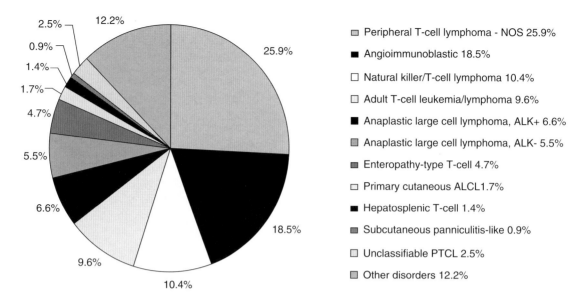

Peripheral T-cell lymphoma - NOS 25.9%

Angioimmunoblastic 18.5%

Natural killer/T-cell lymphoma 10.4%

Adult T-cell leukemia/lymphoma 9.6%

Anaplastic large cell lymphoma, ALK+ 6.6%

Anaplastic large cell lymphoma, ALK- 5.5%

Enteropathy-type T-cell 4.7%

Primary cutaneous ALCL 1.7%

Hepatosplenic T-cell 1.4%

Subcutaneous panniculitis-like 0.9%

Unclassifiable PTCL 2.5%

Other disorders 12.2%

Figure 13.9 Distribution of 1314 cases of peripheral T-cell and NK/T-cell lymphoma from 22 institutions around the world. *Source:* From Ref. 99. *Abbreviations:* ALCL, systemic anaplastic large cell lymphoma; PTCL, peripheral T-cell lymphomas.

High-dose therapy with autologous stem cell transplantation (ASCT) was first demonstrated for aggressive lymphomas but may be applied to indolent lymphomas as well.

Patients with Partial Response

Five to ten percent of patients will not respond to initial treatment, and 5% to 50% of them will achieve partial response, depending on the histology. However, outcome in non-responders and partial responders is fundamentally different. Patients who never responded to therapy have a rapidly fatal outcome and should be included in phase II trials testing new strategies. The prognosis of partial responders treated with conventional therapy is also poor, particularly for aggressive lymphomas, with only 0% to 25% of the patients becoming long-term survivors. Although secondary responses may be achieved in indolent lymphomas, they are usually only partial and not durable. The only difference between aggressive and indolent lymphoma patients is the respective percentages of patients who reach a PR and the duration of their responses after completion of a salvage regimen. Although encouraging results have been reported with the use of high-dose therapy with ASCT for patients in partial remission, the term PR corresponds to different status in the published series, and some of them with only the persistence of radiological abnormalities. PR must be defined as the persistence of lymphoma cells in bone marrow or lymph nodes in patients who had responded to initial therapy. PET scan may help to identify true PR from patients with CR but persisting masses. In elderly patients, local radiotherapy can be added if the persisting mass is localized, but we recommend to wait until progression and then to treat them palliatively.

Complete Response Patients with Persisting Masses

Patients with large tumors often present persisting mass on computed tomography (CT) scan after initial treatment, particularly in the mediastinum or abdomen. Their volume may be less than 25% of the initial tumor mass, or more considerable. Retrospective analyses in aggressive lymphoma patients have shown that most of these patients are already in complete remission but have persisting fibronecrotic tissue, and the problem facing physicians is how to recognize which patients have these non-tumoral lesions (125). This problem mostly exists in DLBCL patients, and residual mass is usually lymphomatous in other entities. Gallium scintigraphy may help if the tumor was positive before diagnosis, but PET scan has dramatically changed our conception of persisting images (5,126). Patients with a residual mass on CT scan and a fixation on PET scan have a partial response, but histological correlation should be done whenever possible, as false-positive results exist. If PR is confirmed, treatment plan include salvage chemotherapy plus HDT with ASCT if feasible. Patients with residual images on CT scan but without FDG fixation on PET scan have a true fibronecrotic mass and do not need further treatment.

Relapsing Patients

Around 40% of complete response lymphoma patients will subsequently relapse, and a higher percentage of patients in some subtypes such as FL, SLL, or LPL relapse. Relapses are observed more commonly during the first two years after completion of therapy. Duration of the first response and lymphoma response to the salvage chemotherapy regimen are major prognostic factors, although prognostic parameters that influenced outcome at diagnosis are also predictive of outcome after relapse. Numerous salvage

Table 13.5 Randomized Studies Comparing Chemotherapy to Rituximab Plus Chemotherapy in Untreated Patients with Diffuse Large B-cell Lymphoma

Reference	Setting	Treatment	Number of patients	Follow-up	Complete response rate	Event-free survival	Overall survival
Coiffier et al. (GELA) (82,141)	Elderly (60–80 years old)	CHOP vs. R-CHOP	399	5 years	63% vs. 76%	29% vs. 47%	45% vs. 58% (p < 0.0073)
Habermann et al. (Intergroup) (83)	Elderly (≥60 years old)	CHOP vs. R-CHOP (second randomization for responders with maintenance rituximab or not)	546	3.5 years	Not available	FFS 43% vs. 56% (p = 0.04)	No significant differences
Pfreundschuh et al. (MInT) (79)	18–60 years old, IPI 0-1	CHOP-like vs. R-CHOP like	824	3 years	68% vs. 86%	59% vs. 79%	84% vs. 93% (p = 0.0001)
Pfreundschuh et al. (RICOVER-60) (80)	61–80 years old	CHOP 14 vs. R-CHOP 14 (second randomization for 6 vs. 8 cycles)	1222	3 years	68–72% (6–8 cycles) vs. 78–76%	47–53% vs. 67–63%	68–66% vs. 78–73% (p = 0.0031 for 6 R-CHOP 14)

regimens that incorporate drugs not used in first-line therapy have been proposed (127). If 70% of the patients responded to salvage therapy, only 20% to 35% achieve second complete responses, and the median TTF is usually less than one year, with fewer than 10% of relapsed patients experiencing a long disease-free survival. Interpretation of clinical trials of salvage regimens is complicated because many patients with relapsed lymphoma died before receiving therapy or were not included in clinical trials.

Promising results of pilot series of high-dose therapy in relapsing DLBCL lymphoma patients have been confirmed by the results of the PARMA trial (128). High-dose therapy with ASCT is the only treatment that yields more than 5% long-term survival in relapsing patients, and it should be considered after first relapse in all patients younger than 65 years who respond to salvage chemotherapy (129).

Different modalities relevant to high dose therapy are not settled. Whether it is necessary to purge peripheral stem cells from persisting lymphoma cells and how to do it remains unknown. No trial has succeeded yet in showing a benefit for the ex vivo purge. However, in vivo purge before the harvest with rituximab seems to offer good-quality graft for B-cell NHL. Also, the best conditioning regimen and the role of total body irradiation have still to be defined.

High-dose therapy should be proposed to all patients in first progression after chemotherapy who respond to salvage therapy regardless of their lymphoma subtype because lymphoma cells may acquire resistance with progression, and subsequent complete responses are rare and of short duration. For relapsing patients who did not respond to salvage therapy, the utility of HDT is not demonstrated: it is estimated that 5% of them may benefit from such a treatment. Patients in second relapse may be treated with HDT if they continue to respond but they have a lower probability of remission than do the patients in first relapse. There is some evidence that late relapses are not associated with a better outcome than early

relapses and, thus, these patients should be offered the same treatment.

Histological Transformation
An initially indolent lymphoma who progress often undergoes histological transformation into a large cell or Burkitt-like lymphoma and a clinically aggressive disease with large tumor burden and high LDH level. These patients have a poor outcome and a median survival of about 12 months. They should be treated with R-CHOP or high-dose R-CHOP-like chemotherapy followed by high-dose therapy and ASCT (130).

Palliative Treatments
Even though complete remission is the ultimate aim at first, some patients need palliative treatments: for example, elderly patients with poor performance status or severe concomitant disease, truly refractory patients, relapsing patients for whom high dose therapy is not suitable, and patients progressing after high-dose therapy. In this setting, patients should be treated in the presence of clinical symptoms and an altered quality of life. The presence of lymphoma cells without disease symptoms is not a reason to treat these patients. If different chemotherapy regimens can be used, only those with low adverse event rates must be used. Oral treatments such as VP-16 or one-day combination chemotherapy should be preferred. In this setting, rituximab is an interesting drug for B-cell lymphoma patients because of its efficacy and its safety.

LONG-TERM TOXIC EFFECTS

As more and more patients are cured with current therapeutic strategies, the question of long-term adverse effects should be considered. As most of these patients have been cured by chemotherapy only, the frequency of such effects is lower than in Hodgkin's disease where most of the secondary late effects are due to radiation therapy. Patients

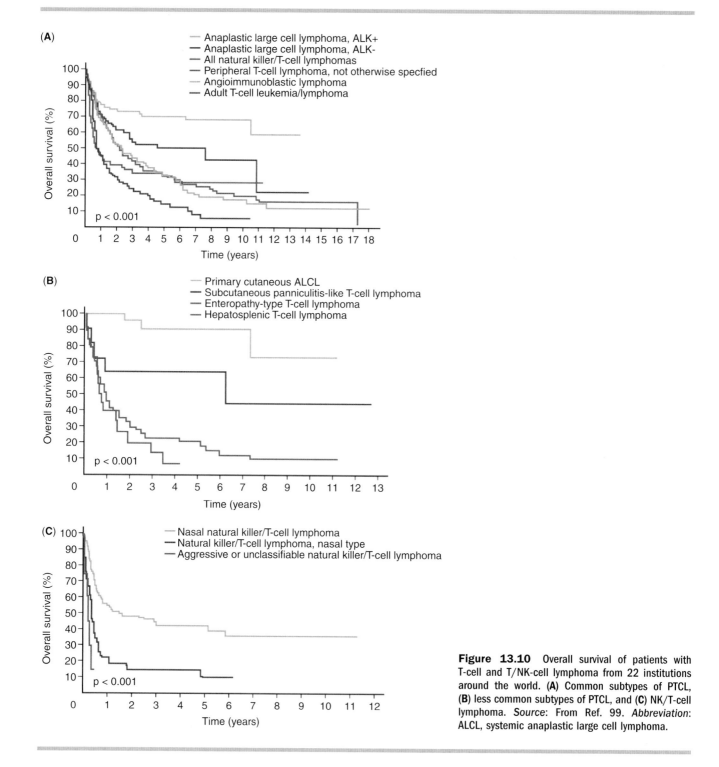

Figure 13.10 Overall survival of patients with T-cell and T/NK-cell lymphoma from 22 institutions around the world. **(A)** Common subtypes of PTCL, **(B)** less common subtypes of PTCL, and **(C)** NK/T-cell lymphoma. *Source*: From Ref. 99. *Abbreviation*: ALCL, systemic anaplastic large cell lymphoma.

with cured lymphoma should be followed regularly for years because late relapse may occur and unknown late adverse effects may appear.

Secondary Cancer

Secondary myelodysplastic syndrome or leukemia is observed in fewer than 2% of patients cured with first-line chemotherapy regimens including doxorubicin and cyclophosphamide (131). Other drugs such as etoposide may be more toxic but this remains to be demonstrated. Secondary leukemia is seen essentially in patients treated some agents like fludarabine or with high-dose therapy, particularly if they have received numerous regimens containing alkylating agents and/or total body irradiation (132,133). The exact incidence of this complication in patients receiving high-dose therapy is not known but probably inferior to 5%.

Secondary solid tumors appear to be rare. Their diversity and the time when they appear, whether before, after, or concomitant with the lymphoma, are compatible with coincidence. However, the number of solid tumors seems to increase with time in cured patients.

Fertility

One-third of lymphoma patients are younger than 35 years and would like to produce offspring if cured. In fact, patients treated with CHOP-like regimens do not suffer fertility problems, and most of them succeed in having children (134). Problems may occur only for older patients or those treated repeatedly for recurrences or with total body irradiation.

Ability to Resume a Normal Life

Young patients cured of a lymphoma usually resume a normal life without persisting adverse effects. They are able to work and must be encouraged to do so. Patients older than 50 years may have chronic fatigue and difficulty in performing strenuous labor or having sexual intercourse.

FUTURE DEVELOPMENTS

The treatment of lymphoma patients is not yet standardized, and many questions remain to be answered in prospective trials. As lymphoma biology is better understood, new drugs arrived in clinical trials and some of them could improve our therapeutic arsenal.

Immunotherapy

With the success encountered by adding anti-CD20 rituximab to chemotherapy, multiple monoclonal antibodies are in development (Table 13.6). Some are still targeting the CD20 antigen, but modification in antibody structure may allow better efficacy: ofatumumab (interesting results in FL and CLL) (135), veltuzumab, GA-101 are actually under study. Other monoclonal antibodies have different targets in order to improve efficacy: anti-CD22 (epratuzumab), anti-CD80 (galiximab), anti-CD40 (SGN-40 and HCD 122), and anti-CD4 (zanolimumab). Anti-CD22 linked with an antiobiotic (calicheamicin) or radioisotope (yttrium 90) are also under study.

Idiotype vaccination is another potential way to control lymphoma. Principles under vaccination are to isolate tumor-derived immunoglobulin idiotype and administer it to patients to induce immune response to lymphoma. This therapy is tested actually in FL following response to chemotherapy. Preliminary results from phase III studies are disappointing, and the future of such therapy is uncertain at least with our current knowledge.

IMiDs

This class of anticancer drugs called immunomodulating agents includes thalidomide and lenalidomide. Their mechanisms of action are unclear and are probably diverse including as example immunomodulation and angiogenesis inhibition. Lenalidomide has demonstrated impressive antitumor effect in several malignancies including multiple myeloma. Recent data of lenalinomide in treatment of lymphoproliferative disorders are promising (136).

Epigenetic Modification

Gene transcription regulation by histone and associated enzymes appear to play an important role in causing cancer. Histone deacetylase inhibitors (HDAC) have been introduced recently in treatment of lymphoma. Two molecules (romidepsin and vorinostat) are promising with good results in cutaneous T-cell lymphoma (137,138).

Intracellular Signaling

In recent years, many new drugs focusing on blockade of intracellular signaling by the inhibition of enzymes have showed impressive results in CML and renal cell carcinoma. Many targets and new molecules are under development in the field of lymphoma. Temsirolimus, a specific mTOR inhibitor, and enzastaurin, a protein kinase C beta inhibitor, represent some of these new molecules. Bortezomib, a proteasome inhibitor, is also under study.

Oncogene Modulation and Anti-oncogene as Lymphoma Treatment

Oncogene activation or tumor-suppressor gene inhibition is responsible for lymphoma development and progression

Table 13.6   Different Monoclonal Antibodies Currently Available for the Treatment of Patients with Lymphoma

Antibody	Antigen	Conjugate	Proven efficacy
Rituximab (MabThera, Rituxan)	CD20	None	Follicular lymphoma and DLCL in combination with chemotherapy
Ofatumumab	CD20	None	In testing
Veltuzumab	CD20	None	In testing
GA-101	CD20	None	In testing
Epratuzumab (Lymphocide)	CD22	None	In testing
SGN-40	CD40	None	In testing
Galiximab	CD80	None	In testing
Alemtuzumab (Campath)	CD52	None	Chronic lymphocytic leukemia
Zanolimumab	CD4	None	In testing
Ibritumomab tiuxetan (Zevalin)	CD20	Y-90	Progression after rituximab
Tositumomab (Bexxar)	CD20	I-131	Progression after rituximab

through numerous mechanisms, which are still only partially understood. Modulation of the activity of these genes could be a promising future challenge. Gene modulation may be attempted with cell surface receptor stimulation or inhibition, antisense therapy (e.g., bcl2 antisense) (139), genetic modulation. Few of these have demonstrated the efficacy and progressed to clinical application.

Drug Resistance

Several mechanisms of acquired resistance to anticancer drugs have been described, but multiple drug resistance (MDR) is the best known. Although fewer than 5% of lymphoma cells are MDR⁺ at diagnosis, the percentage increases in progressing patients. The precise role of drug resistance is unknown, but it may account for most of the observed failures; this needs to be analyzed in the future, as do inhibitors of the different mechanisms (140).

CONCLUSION

Lymphoma is a category of cancers comprising different entities, and several of them may be cured with adapted strategies based on disease risk, with complete cure being the ultimate aim. Complete remission is however not always possible, and it is usually achieved with first-line therapy, but high-dose therapy may be needed for relapsing or partial response patients. However, definitive strategies are still unknown, and involving patients in prospective trials is highly recommended. Better outcome may be observed in patients treated by physicians with extensive experience in this complicated disease. Physicians who treat fewer than 20 patients a year would be well advised to have regular contact with a referral center. Whatever the treatment and its results, lymphoma patients have to be followed for years for possible late adverse effects and late recurrences.

REFERENCES

1. Ries LAG, Melbert D, Krapcho M et al., eds. SEER Cancer Statistics Review, 1975–2004, National Cancer Institute. Bethesda, MD, 2007.
2. Pulte D, Gondos A, Brenner H. Ongoing improvement in outcomes for patients diagnosed as having non-Hodgkin lymphoma from the 1990s to the early 21st century. Arch Intern Med 2008; 168: 469–76.
3. Li YH, He YF, Jiang WQ et al. Lamivudine prophylaxis reduces the incidence and severity of hepatitis in hepatitis B virus carriers who receive chemotherapy for lymphoma. Cancer 2006; 106: 1320–5.
4. Besson C, Canioni D, Lepage E et al. Characteristics and outcome of diffuse large B-cell lymphoma in hepatitis C virus-positive patients in LNH 93 and LNH 98 Groupe d'Etude des Lymphomes de l'Adulte programs. J Clin Oncol 2006; 24: 953–60.
5. Mavromatis BH, Cheson BD. Pre- and post-treatment evaluation of non-Hodgkin's lymphoma. Best Pract Res Clin Haematol 2002; 15: 429–47.
6. Seam P, Juweid ME, Cheson BD. The role of FDG-PET scans in patients with lymphoma. Blood 2007; 110: 3507–16.
7. Juweid ME, Stroobants S, Hoekstra OS et al. Use of positron emission tomography for response assessment of lymphoma: consensus of the Imaging Subcommittee of International Harmonization Project in Lymphoma. J Clin Oncol 2007; 25: 571–8.
8. Federico M, Vitolo U, Zinzani PL et al. Prognosis of follicular lymphoma: a predictive model based on a retrospective analysis of 987 cases. Blood 2000; 95: 783–9.
9. Coiffier B, Salles G, Bastion Y. Prognostic factors in non-Hodgkin's lymphoma. In: Magrath IT, ed. The Non-Hodgkin's Lymphomas, 2nd edn. London: Adward Arnold Ltd, 1997: 739–68.
10. The international non-Hodgkin's lymphoma prognostic factors project. A predictive model for aggressive non-Hodgkin's lymphoma. N Engl J Med 1993; 329: 987–94.
11. Bastion Y, Berger F, Bryon PA et al. Follicular lymphomas: assessment of prognostic factors in 127 patients followed for 10 years. Ann Oncol 1991; 9: 123–9.
12. Coiffier B, Neidhardt-Berard EM, Tilly H et al. Fludarabine alone compared to CHVP plus interferon in elderly patients with follicular lymphoma and adverse prognostic parameters: a GELA study. Ann Oncol 1999; 10: 1191–7.
13. Coiffier B, Lepage E. Prognosis of aggressive lymphoma: a study of five prognostic models with patients included in the LNH-84 regimen. Blood 1989; 74: 558–64.
14. Armitage JO, Weisenburger DD. New approach to classifying non-Hodgkin's lymphomas: clinical features of the major histologic subtypes. J Clin Oncol 1998; 16: 2780–95.
15. Solal-Celigny P, Roy P. Follicular Lymphoma International Prognostic Index (FLIPI). In: 8th International Conference on Malignant Lymphoma, 12–15 June 2002, Lugano, Switzerland. Ann Oncol 2002: 18.
16. Lossos IS, Morgensztern D. Prognostic biomarkers in diffuse large B-cell lymphoma. J Clin Oncol 2006; 24: 995–1007.
17. Mounier N, Briere J, Gisselbrecht C et al. Estimating the impact of rituximab on bcl-2-associated resistance to CHOP in elderly patients with diffuse large B-cell lymphoma. Haematologica 2006; 91: 715–16.
18. Rosenwald A, Wright G, Chan WC et al. The use of molecular profiling to predict survival after chemotherapy for diffuse large-B-cell lymphoma. N Engl J Med 2002; 346: 1937–47.
19. Shipp MA, Ross KN, Tamayo P et al. Diffuse large B-cell lymphoma outcome prediction by gene-expression profiling and supervised machine learning. Nat Med 2002; 8: 68–74.
20. Dave SS, Wright G, Tan B et al. Prediction of survival in follicular lymphoma based on molecular features of tumor-infiltrating immune cells. N Engl J Med 2004; 351: 2159–69.
21. Gulmann C, Espina V, Petricoin E 3rd et al. Proteomic analysis of apoptotic pathways reveals prognostic factors in follicular lymphoma. Clin Cancer Res 2005; 11: 5847–55.
22. Jaffe ES, Harris NL, Stein H et al. World Health Organization Classification of Tumours: Pathology and Genetics of Tumours of Hematopoietic and Lymphoid Tissues. Lyon: IARC Press, 2001.
23. A clinical evaluation of the International Lymphoma Study Group classification of non-Hodgkin's lymphoma. The non-Hodgkin's lymphoma classification project. Blood 1997; 89: 3909–18.
24. Armitage JO, Weisenburger DD. New approach to classifying non-Hodgkin's lymphomas: clinical features of the major histologic subtypes. Non-Hodgkin's lymphoma classification project. J Clin Oncol 1998; 16: 2780–95.
25. Tsimberidou AM, Wen S, O'Brien S et al. Assessment of chronic lymphocytic leukemia and small lymphocytic lymphoma by absolute lymphocyte counts in 2,126 patients: 20 years of experience at the University of Texas M.D. Anderson Cancer Center. J Clin Oncol 2007; 25: 4648–56.
26. Zent CS, Ding W, Schwager SM et al. The prognostic significance of cytopenia in chronic lymphocytic leukaemia/

small lymphocytic lymphoma. Br J Haematol 2008; 141: 615–21.

27. Shanafelt TD, Geyer SM, Kay NE. Prognosis at diagnosis: integrating molecular biologic insights into clinical practice for patients with CLL. Blood 2004; 103: 1202–10.

28. Thieblemont C, Berger F, Dumontet C et al. Mucosa-associated lymphoid tissue lymphoma is a disseminated disease in one third of 158 patients analyzed. Blood 2000; 95: 802–6.

29. Zucca E, Bertoni F, Roggero E et al. The gastric marginal zone B-cell lymphoma of MALT type. Blood 2000; 96: 410–19.

30. Thieblemont C. Clinical presentation and management of marginal zone lymphomas. Hematology Am Soc Hematol Educ Program 2005: 307–13.

31. Liu H, Ruskon-Fourmestraux A, Lavergne-Slove A et al. Resistance of t(11;18) positive gastric mucosa-associated lymphoid tissue lymphoma to Helicobacter pylori eradication therapy. Lancet 2001; 357: 39–40.

32. Koch P, del Valle F, Berdel WE et al. Primary gastrointestinal non-Hodgkin's lymphoma: II. Combined surgical and conservative or conservative management only in localized gastric lymphoma—Results of the Prospective German Multicenter Study GIT NHL 01/92. J Clin Oncol 2001; 19: 3874–83.

33. Thieblemont C, Felman P, Callet-Bauchu E et al. Splenic marginal-zone lymphoma: a distinct clinical and pathological entity. Lancet Oncol 2003; 4: 95–103.

34. Matutes E, Oscier D, Montalban C et al. Splenic marginal zone lymphoma proposals for a revision of diagnostic, staging and therapeutic criteria. Leukemia 2008; 22: 487–95.

35. Thieblemont C, Felman P, Berger F et al. Treatment of splenic marginal zone B-cell lymphoma: an analysis of 81 patients. Clin Lymphoma 2002; 3: 41–7.

36. Berger F, Felman P, Thieblemont C et al. Non-MALT marginal zone B-cell lymphomas: a description of clinical presentation and outcome in 124 patients. Blood 2000; 95: 1950–6.

37. Owen RG, Treon SP, Al-Katib A et al. Clinicopathological definition of Waldenstrom's macroglobulinemia: consensus panel recommendations from the Second International Workshop on Waldenstrom's Macroglobulinemia. Semin Oncol 2003; 30: 110–15.

38. Hans CP, Weisenburger DD, Vose JM et al. A significant diffuse component predicts for inferior survival in grade 3 follicular lymphoma, but cytologic subtypes do not predict survival. Blood 2003; 101: 2363–7.

39. Elenitoba-Johnson KSJ, Gascoyne RD, Lim MS et al. Homozygous deletions at chromosome 9p21 involving P16 and P15 are associated with histologic progression in follicle center lymphoma. Blood 1998; 91: 4677–85.

40. Solal-Celigny P, Roy P, Colombat P et al. Follicular lymphoma international prognostic index. Blood 2004; 104: 1258–65.

41. Cerhan JR, Wang S, Maurer MJ et al. Prognostic significance of host immune gene polymorphisms in follicular lymphoma survival. Blood 2007; 109: 5439–46.

42. Advani R, Rosenberg SA, Horning SJ. Stage I and II follicular non-Hodgkin's lymphoma: long-term follow-up of no initial therapy. J Clin Oncol 2004; 22: 1454–9.

43. Ardeshna KM, Smith P, Norton A et al. Long-term effect of a watch and wait policy versus immediate systemic treatment for asymptomatic advanced-stage non-Hodgkin lymphoma: a randomised controlled trial. Lancet 2003; 362: 516–22.

44. Witzig TE, Vukov AM, Habermann TM et al. Rituximab therapy for patients with newly diagnosed, advanced-stage, follicular grade I non-Hodgkin's lymphoma: a phase II trial in the North Central Cancer Treatment Group. J Clin Oncol 2005; 23: 1103–8.

45. Salles G, Mounier N, De Guibert S et al. Rituximab combined with chemotherapy and interferon in follicular lymphoma patients: final analysis of the GELA-GOELAMS FL2000 Study with a 5-year follow-up. Blood 2007, abstract 792.

46. Marcus R, Imrie K, Belch A et al. CVP chemotherapy plus rituximab compared with CVP as first-line treatment for advanced follicular lymphoma. Blood 2005; 105: 1417–23.

47. Hiddemann W, Kneba M, Dreyling M et al. Front-line therapy with rituximab added to the combination of cyclophosphamide, doxorubicin, vincristine, and prednisone (CHOP) significantly improves the outcome for patients with advanced-stage follicular lymphoma compared with therapy with CHOP alone: results of a prospective randomized study of the German Low-Grade Lymphoma Study Group. Blood 2005; 106: 3725–32.

48. Herold M, Haas A, Srock S et al. Rituximab added to first-line mitoxantrone, chlorambucil, and prednisolone chemotherapy followed by interferon maintenance prolongs survival in patients with advanced follicular lymphoma: an East German Study Group Hematology and Oncology Study. J Clin Oncol 2007; 25: 1986–92.

49. Fisher RI, LeBlanc M, Press OW et al. New treatment options have changed the survival of patients with follicular lymphoma. J Clin Oncol 2005; 23: 8447-52.

50. Sebban C, Brice P, Delarue R et al. Impact of rituximab and/or high-dose therapy with autotransplant at time of relapse in patients with follicular lymphoma: a GELA study. J Clin Oncol 2008; 26: 3614-20.

51. Hainsworth JD, Litchy S, Shaffer DW et al. Maximizing therapeutic benefit of rituximab: maintenance therapy versus re-treatment at progression in patients with indolent non-Hodgkin's lymphoma—a randomized phase II trial of the Minnie Pearl Cancer Research Network. J Clin Oncol 2005; 23: 1088–95.

52. Ghielmini M, Schmitz SF, Cogliatti SB et al. Prolonged treatment with rituximab in patients with follicular lymphoma significantly increases event-free survival and response duration compared with the standard weekly × 4 schedule. Blood 2004; 103: 4416–23.

53. van Oers MH, Klasa R, Marcus RE et al. Rituximab maintenance improves clinical outcome of relapsed/resistant follicular non-Hodgkin lymphoma in patients both with and without rituximab during induction: results of a prospective randomized phase 3 intergroup trial. Blood 2006; 108: 3295–301.

54. Forstpointner R, Unterhalt M, Dreyling M et al. Maintenance therapy with rituximab leads to a significant prolongation of response duration after salvage therapy with a combination of rituximab, fludarabine, cyclophosphamide, and mitoxantrone (R-FCM) in patients with recurring and refractory follicular and mantle cell lymphomas: results of a prospective randomized study of the German Low Grade Lymphoma Study Group (GLSG). Blood 2006; 108: 4003–8.

55. Schouten HC, Qian W, Kvaloy S et al. High-dose therapy improves progression-free survival and survival in relapsed follicular non-Hodgkin's lymphoma: results from the randomized European CUP trial. J Clin Oncol 2003; 21: 3918–27.

56. Rohatiner AZ, Nadler L, Davies AJ et al. Myeloablative therapy with autologous bone marrow transplantation for follicular lymphoma at the time of second or subsequent remission: long-term follow-up. J Clin Oncol 2007; 25: 2554–9.

57. Fisher RI, Kaminski MS, Wahl RL et al. Tositumomab and iodine-131 tositumomab produces durable complete remissions in a subset of heavily pretreated patients with low-grade and transformed non-Hodgkin's lymphomas. J Clin Oncol 2005; 23: 7565–73.

58. Witzig TE, Gordon LI, Cabanillas F et al. Randomized controlled trial of yttrium-90-labeled ibritumomab tiuxetan

radioimmunotherapy versus rituximab immunotherapy for patients with relapsed or refractory low-grade, follicular, or transformed B-cell non-Hodgkin's lymphoma. J Clin Oncol 2002; 20: 2453–63.

59. Kaminski MS, Tuck M, Estes J et al. 131I-tositumomab therapy as initial treatment for follicular lymphoma. N Engl J Med 2005; 352: 441–9.

60. Rohatiner AZ, Gregory WM, Peterson B et al. Meta-analysis to evaluate the role of interferon in follicular lymphoma. J Clin Oncol 2005; 23: 2215–23.

61. Liu Q, Fayad L, Cabanillas F et al. Improvement of overall and failure-free survival in stage IV follicular lymphoma: 25 years of treatment experience at The University of Texas M.D. Anderson Cancer Center. J Clin Oncol 2006; 24: 1582–9.

62. Sacchi S, Pozzi S, Marcheselli L et al. Introduction of rituximab in front-line and salvage therapies has improved outcome of advanced-stage follicular lymphoma patients. Cancer 2007; 109: 2077–82.

63. Samaha H, Dumontet C, Ketterer N et al. Mantle cell lymphoma: a retrospective study of 121 cases. Leukemia 1998; 12: 1281–7.

64. Herrmann A, Hoster E, Dreyling M et al. Improvement of overall survival in mantle cell lymphoma during the last decades. In: American Society of Hematology Annual Meeting. Orlando, Florida, 2006.

65. Howard OM, Gribben JG, Neuberg DS et al. Rituximab and CHOP induction therapy for newly diagnosed mantle-cell lymphoma: molecular complete responses are not predictive of progression-free survival. J Clin Oncol 2002; 20: 1288–94.

66. Foran JM, Rohatiner AZS, Cunningham D et al. European phase II study of rituximab (chimeric anti-CD20 monoclonal antibody) for patients with newly diagnosed mantle-cell lymphoma and previously treated mantle-cell lymphoma, immunocytoma, and small B-cell lymphocytic lymphoma. J Clin Oncol 2000; 18: 317–24.

67. Khouri IF, Romaguera J, Kantarjian H et al. Hyper-CVAD and high-dose methotrexate/cytarabine followed by stem-cell transplantation: an active regimen for aggressive mantle-cell lymphoma. J Clin Oncol 1998; 16: 3803–9.

68. Dreyling M, Lenz G, Hoster E et al. Early consolidation by myeloablative radiochemotherapy followed by autologous stem cell transplantation in first remission significantly prolongs progression-free survival in mantle-cell lymphoma: results of a prospective randomized trial of the European MCL Network. Blood 2005; 105: 2677–84.

69. Thieblemont C, Antal D, Lacotte-Thierry L et al. Chemotherapy with rituximab followed by high-dose therapy and autologous stem cell transplantation in patients with mantle cell lymphoma. Cancer 2007; 104: 1434–41.

70. Tigaud JD, Demolombe S, Bastion Y et al. Ifosfamide continuous infusion plus etoposide in the treatment of elderly patients with aggressive lymphoma. A phase II study. Hematol Oncol 1991; 9: 225–33.

71. Rosenwald A, Wright G, Chan WC et al. The use of molecular profiling to predict survival after chemotherapy for diffuse large-B-cell lymphoma. N Engl J Med 2002; 346: 1937–47.

72. Fisher RI, Gaynor ER, Dahlberg S et al. Comparison of a standard regimen (CHOP) with three intensive chemotherapy regimens for advanced non-Hodgkin's lymphoma. N Engl J Med 1993; 328: 1002–6.

73. Coiffier B. Increasing chemotherapy intensity in aggressive lymphomas: a renewal? J Clin Oncol 2003; 21: 2457–9.

74. Tilly H, Lepage E, Coiffier B et al. Intensive conventional chemotherapy (ACVBP regimen) compared with standard CHOP for poor-prognosis aggressive non-Hodgkin lymphoma. Blood 2003; 102: 4284–9.

75. Coiffier B. Fourteen years of high-dose CHOP (ACVB regimen): preliminary conclusions about the treatment of aggressive-lymphoma patients. Ann Oncol 1995; 6: 211–17.

76. Tilly H, Mounier N, Lederlin P et al. Randomized comparison of ACVBP and m-BACOD in the treatment of patients with low-risk aggressive lymphoma: the LNH87-1 study. J Clin Oncol 2000; 18: 1309–15.

77. Pfreundschuh M, Trumper L, Kloess M et al. Two-weekly or 3-weekly CHOP chemotherapy with or without etoposide for the treatment of young patients with good-prognosis (normal LDH) aggressive lymphomas: results of the NHL-B1 trial of the DSHNHL. Blood 2004; 104: 626–33.

78. Pfreundschuh M, Trumper L, Kloess M et al. Two-weekly or 3-weekly CHOP chemotherapy with or without etoposide for the treatment of elderly patients with aggressive lymphomas: results of the NHL-B2 trial of the DSHNHL. Blood 2004; 104: 634–41.

79. Pfreundschuh M, Trumper L, Osterborg A et al. CHOP-like chemotherapy plus rituximab versus CHOP-like chemotherapy alone in young patients with good-prognosis diffuse large-B-cell lymphoma: a randomised controlled trial by the MabThera International Trial (MInT) Group. Lancet Oncol 2006; 7: 379–91.

80. Pfreundschuh M, Schubert J, Ziepert M et al. Six versus eight cycles of bi-weekly CHOP-14 with or without rituximab in elderly patients with aggressive CD20+ B-cell lymphomas: a randomised controlled trial (RICOVER-60). Lancet Oncol 2008; 9: 105–16.

81. Feugier P, Van Hoof A, Sebban C et al. Long-term results of the R-CHOP study in the treatment of elderly patients with diffuse large B-cell lymphoma: a study by the Groupe d'Etude des Lymphomes de l'Adulte. J Clin Oncol 2005; 23: 4117–26.

82. Coiffier B, Lepage E, Briere J et al. CHOP chemotherapy plus rituximab compared with CHOP alone in elderly patients with diffuse large-B-cell lymphoma. N Engl J Med 2002; 346: 235–42.

83. Habermann TM, Weller EA, Morrison VA et al. Rituximab-CHOP versus CHOP alone or with maintenance rituximab in older patients with diffuse large B-cell lymphoma. J Clin Oncol 2006; 24: 3121–7.

84. Mounier N, Briere J, Gisselbrecht C et al. Rituximab plus CHOP (R-CHOP) overcomes bcl-2-associated resistance to chemotherapy in elderly patients with diffuse large B-cell lymphoma (DLBCL). Blood 2003; 101: 4279–84.

85. Sehn LH, Donaldson J, Chhanabhai M et al. Introduction of combined CHOP plus rituximab therapy dramatically improved outcome of diffuse large B-cell lymphoma in British Columbia. J Clin Oncol 2005; 23: 5027–33.

86. Milpied N, Deconinck E, Gaillard F et al. Initial treatment of aggressive lymphoma with high-dose chemotherapy and autologous stem-cell support. N Engl J Med 2004; 350: 1287–95.

87. Haioun C, Lepage E, Gisselbrecht C et al. Survival benefit of high-dose therapy in poor-risk aggressive non-Hodgkin's lymphoma: final analysis of the prospective LNH87-2 protocol—A Groupe d'Etude des Lymphomes de l'Adulte Study. J Clin Oncol 2000; 18: 3025–30.

88. Miller TP, Dahlberg S, Cassady JR et al. Chemotherapy alone compared with chemotherapy plus radiotherapy for localized intermediate-and high-grade non-Hodgkin's lymphoma. N Engl J Med 1998; 339: 21–6.

89. Reyes F, Lepage E, Ganem G et al. ACVBP versus CHOP plus radiotherapy for localized aggressive lymphoma. N Engl J Med 2005; 352: 1197–205.

90. Bonnet C, Fillet G, Mounier N et al. CHOP alone compared with CHOP plus radiotherapy for localized aggressive lymphoma in elderly patients: a study by the Groupe d'Etude des Lymphomes de l'Adulte. J Clin Oncol 2007; 25: 787–92.

91. Aviles A, Delgado S, Nambo MJ et al. Adjuvant radiotherapy to sites of previous bulky disease in patients stage IV diffuse large cell lymphoma. Int J Radiat Oncol Biol Phys 1994; 30: 799–803.

92. Dave SS, Fu K, Wright GW et al. Molecular diagnosis of Burkitt's lymphoma. N Engl J Med 2006; 354: 2431–42.

93. Hummel M, Bentink S, Berger H et al. A biologic definition of Burkitt's lymphoma from transcriptional and genomic profiling. N Engl J Med 2006; 354: 2419–30.

94. Soussain C, Patte C, Ostronoff M et al. Small noncleaved cell lymphoma and leukemia in adults—a retrospective study of 65 adults treated with the lmb pediatric protocols. Blood 1995; 85: 664–74.

95. Mead GM, Sydes MR, Walewski J et al. An international evaluation of CODOX-M and CODOX-M alternating with IVAC in adult Burkitt's lymphoma: results of United Kingdom Lymphoma Group LY06 study. Ann Oncol 2002; 13: 1264–74.

96. Willemze R, Jaffe ES, Burg G et al. WHO-EORTC classification for cutaneous lymphomas. Blood 2005; 105: 3768–85.

97. Bouaziz JD, Bastuji-Garin S, Poszepczynska-Guigne E et al. Relative frequency and survival of patients with primary cutaneous lymphomas: data from a single-centre study of 203 patients. Br J Dermatol 2006; 154: 1206–7.

98. Trautinger F, Knobler R, Willemze R et al. EORTC consensus recommendations for the treatment of mycosis fungoides/Sezary syndrome. Eur J Cancer 2006; 42: 1014–30.

99. Armitage J, Vose J, Weisenburger D. International peripheral T-cell and natural killer/T-cell lymphoma study: pathology findings and clinical outcomes. J Clin Oncol 2008; 26: 4124-30.

100. Gisselbrecht C, Gaulard P, Lepage E et al. Prognostic significance of T-cell phenotype in aggressive non-Hodgkins lymphomas. Blood 1998; 92: 76–82.

101. Mourad N, Mounier N, Briere J et al. Clinical, biologic, and pathologic features in 157 patients with angioimmunoblastic T-cell lymphoma treated within the Groupe d'Etude des Lymphomes de l'Adulte (GELA) trials. Blood 2008; 111: 4463–70.

102. Kyriakou C, Canals C, Goldstone A et al. High-dose therapy and autologous stem-cell transplantation in angioimmunoblastic lymphoma: complete remission at transplantation is the major determinant of outcome-lymphoma working party of the European Group for Blood and Marrow Transplantation. J Clin Oncol 2008; 26: 218–24.

103. Li YX, Yao B, Jin J et al. Radiotherapy as primary treatment for stage IE and IIE nasal natural killer/T-cell lymphoma. J Clin Oncol 2006; 24: 181–9.

104. Project IT-CL. International peripheral T-cell and natural killer/T-cell lymphoma study: pathology findings and clinical outcomes. J Clin Oncol 2008; 26: 4124–30 (epublished ahead of print).

105. Falini B, Pileri S, Zinzani PL et al. ALK(+) lymphoma: clinico-pathological findings and outcome. Blood 1999; 93: 2697–706.

106. Tilly H, Gaulard P, Lepage E et al. Primary anaplastic large-cell lymphoma in adults: clinical presentation, immunophenotype, and outcome. Blood 1997; 90: 3727–34.

107. Gascoyne RD, Aoun P, Wu D et al. Prognostic significance of anaplastic lymphoma kinase (ALK) protein expression in adults with anaplastic large cell lymphoma. Blood 1999; 93: 3913–21.

108. Savage KJ, Harris NL, Vose JM et al. ALK-negative anaplastic large-cell lymphoma (ALCL) is clinically and immunophenotypically different from both ALK-positive ALCL and peripheral T-cell lymphoma, not otherwise specified: report from the International Peripheral T-Cell Lymphoma Project. Blood 2008; 111: 5496–504.

109. Maitra A, McKenna RW, Weinberg AG et al. Precursor B-cell lymphoblastic lymphoma. A study of nine cases lacking blood and bone marrow involvement and review of the literature. Am J Clin Pathol 2001; 115: 868–75.

110. Hoelzer D, Gokbuget N. Treatment of lymphoblastic lymphoma in adults. Best Pract Res Clin Hematol 2002; 15: 713–28.

111. Hoelzer D, Gokbuget N, Digel W et al. Outcome of adult patients with T-lymphoblastic lymphoma treated according to protocols for acute lymphoblastic leukemia. Blood 2002; 99: 4379–85.

112. The NHLClassification Project. Effect of age on the characteristics and clinical behavior of non-Hodgkins lymphoma patients. Ann Oncol 1997; 8: 973–8.

113. Thieblemont C, Grossoeuvre A, Houot R et al. Non-Hodgkin's lymphoma in very elderly patients over 80 years. A descriptive analysis of clinical presentation and outcome. Ann Oncol 2008; 19: 774–9.

114. Coiffier B. Treatment paradigms in aggressive non-Hodgkin's lymphoma in elderly patients. Clin Lymphoma 2002; 3: S12–18.

115. Peters FPJ, Lalisang RI, Fickers MMF et al. Treatment of elderly patients with intermediate- and high-grade non-Hodgkin's lymphoma: a retrospective population-based study. Ann Hematol 2001; 80: 155–9.

116. Tirelli U, Errante D, Vanglabbeke M et al. CHOP is the standard regimen in patients greater-than or equal-to 70 years of age with intermediate-grade and high-grade non-Hodgkin's Lymphoma. Results of a randomized study of the European Organization for Research and Treatment of Cancer Lymphoma Cooperative Study Group. J Clin Oncol 1998; 16: 27–34.

117. Picozzi VJ, Pohlman BL, Morrison VA et al. Patterns of chemotherapy administration in patients with intermediate-grade non-Hodgkin's lymphoma. Oncology 2001; 15: 1296–306.

118. Hanto DW. Classification of Epstein-Barr virus-associated posttransplant lymphoproliferative diseases. Implications for understanding their pathogenesis and developing rational treatment strategies. Annu Rev Med 1995; 46: 381–94.

119. Verschuuren EAM, Stevens SJC, Van Imhoff GW et al. Treatment of posttransplant lymphoproliatieve disease with rituximab: the remission, the relapse, and the complication. Transplantation 2002; 73: 100–4.

120. Mounier N, Spina M, Gisselbrecht C. Modern management of non-Hodgkin lymphoma in HIV-infected patients. Br J Haematol 2007; 136: 685–98.

121. Besson C, Goubar A, Gabarre J et al. Changes in AIDS-related lymphoma since the era of highly active antiretroviral therapy. Blood 2001; 98: 2339–44.

122. Gale J, Simmonds PD, Mead GM et al. Enteropathy-type intestinal T-cell lymphoma: clinical features and treatment of 31 patients in a single center. J Clin Oncol 2000; 18: 795–803.

123. DeAngelis LM, Seiferheld W, Schold SC et al. Combination chemotherapy and radiotherapy for primary central nervous system lymphoma: Radiation Therapy Oncology Group study 93-10. J Clin Oncol 2002; 20: 4643–8.

124. Ferreri AJM, Abrey LE, Blay JY et al. Summary statement on primary central nervous system lymphomas from the Eighth International Conference on Malignant Lymphoma, Lugano, Switzerland, June 12 to 15, 2002. J Clin Oncol 2003; 21: 2407–14.

125. Cheson BD, Horning SJ, Coiffier B et al. Report of an international workshop to standardize response criteria for non-Hodgkin's lymphomas. J Clin Oncol 1999; 17: 1244–53.

126. Cheson BD, Pfistner B, Juweid ME et al. Revised response criteria for malignant lymphoma. J Clin Oncol 2007; 25: 579–86.

127. Salles G, Shipp MA, Coiffier B. Chemotherapy of non-Hodgkin's aggressive lymphomas. Semin Hematol 1994; 31: 46–69.

128. Philip T, Guglielmi C, Hagenbeek A et al. Autologous bone marrow transplantation as compared with salvage chemotherapy in relapses of chemotherapy-sensitive non Hodgkin's lymphoma. N Engl J Med 1995; 333: 1540–5.

129. Shipp MA, Abeloff MD, Antman KH et al. International consensus conference on high-dose therapy with hematopoietic stem-cell transplantation in aggressive non-Hodgkin's lymphomas: report of jury. Ann Oncol 1999; 10: 13–19.

130. Williams CD, Harrison CN, Lister TA et al. High-dose therapy and autologous stem-cell support for chemosensitive transformed low-grade follicular non-Hodgkin's lymphoma: a case-matched study from the European bone marrow transplant registry. J Clin Oncol 2001; 19: 727–35.

131. Andre M, Mounier N, Leleu X et al. Second cancers and late toxicities after treatment of aggressive non-Hodgkin lymphoma with the ACVBP regimen: a GELA cohort study on 2837 patients. Blood 2004; 103: 1222–8.

132. Ruiz-Soto R, Sergent G, Gisselbrecht C et al. Estimating late adverse events using competing risks after autologous stem-cell transplantation in aggressive non-Hodgkin lymphoma patients. Cancer 2005; 104: 2735–42.

133. Metayer C, Curtis RE, Vose J et al. Myelodysplastic syndrome and acute myeloid leukemia after autotransplantation for lymphoma: a multicenter case-control study. Blood 2003; 101: 2015–23.

134. Elis A, Tevet A, Yerushalmi R et al. Fertility status among women treated for aggressive non-Hodgkin's lymphoma. Leuk Lymphoma 2006; 47: 623–7.

135. Coiffier B, Lepretre S, Pedersen LM et al. Safety and efficacy of ofatumumab, a fully human monoclonal anti-CD20 antibody, in patients with relapsed or refractory B-cell chronic lymphocytic leukemia: a phase 1-2 study. Blood 2008; 111: 1094–100.

136. Chanan-Khan AA, Cheson BD. Lenalidomide for the treatment of B-cell malignancies. J Clin Oncol 2008; 26: 1544–52.

137. Kim Y, Reddy S, Kim E et al. Romidepsin (depsipeptide) induces clinically significant responses in treatment-refractory CTCL: an international, multicenter study. Blood 2007 Abst 123 idem.

138. Olsen EA, Kim YH, Kuzel TM et al. Phase IIb multicenter trial of vorinostat in patients with persistent, progressive, or treatment refractory cutaneous T-cell lymphoma. J Clin Oncol 2007; 25: 3109–15.

139. O'Brien S, Moore JO, Boyd TE et al. Randomized phase III trial of fludarabine plus cyclophosphamide with or without oblimersen sodium (Bcl-2 antisense) in patients with relapsed or refractory chronic lymphocytic leukemia. J Clin Oncol 2007; 25: 1114–20.

140. Hersey P, Zhang XD. Overcoming resistance of cancer cells to apoptosis. J Cell Physiol 2003; 196: 9–18.

141. Coiffier B, Gisselbrecht C, Herbrecht R et al. LNH-84 regimen: a multicenter study of intensive chemotherapy in 737 patients with aggressive malignant lymphoma. J Clin Oncol 1989; 7: 1018–26.

142. Hochster H, Weller E, Gascoyne RD, et al. Maintenance rituximab after cyclophosphamide, vincristine, and prednisone prolongs progression-free survival in advanced indolent lymphoma: results of the randomized phase III ECOG1496 Study. J Clin Oncol 2009; 27: 1607–14.

14

Hodgkin Lymphoma

Sandra J. Horning

INTRODUCTION

Hodgkin lymphoma (HL) is an uncommon lymphoid malignancy with an incidence of about 3 per 100,000 in Western Europe and the United States. Occurring at all ages, the *incidence of HL* peaks in young adults, and a second, smaller peak is seen after age 60. The diagnosis is made based on an adequate tissue biopsy demonstrating multinucleate Reed-Sternberg cells and their mononuclear variants, which constitute only about 1% to 10% of the total cell population, in an appropriate cellular background (1). With modern diagnostic evaluation and therapy, HL is curable in every stage, leading to emphasis on minimizing adverse effects of treatment and optimizing survivorship. Although clinical factors are prognostic, they are not adequate to reliably identify individual patients at risk for treatment failure. Therefore, ongoing investigative efforts aim to adapt a therapy to early response, identify predictive tissue biomarkers at diagnosis, and develop novel therapeutics targeted to HL.

ETIOLOGY, BIOLOGY, AND PATHOLOGIC CLASSIFICATION

The cause of HL is unknown, but the B-cell tropic Epstein-Barr virus (EBV) has been implicated, as the clonal viral genome is detected in about 40% of HL cases, and EBV+ HL in young adults is associated with a history of infectious mononucleosis (2–4). However, EBV+ HL is more common in children and older adults, suggesting that the maturity of the immune system may be related. Genetic susceptibility also plays a role as indicated by the familial aggregation and the observation of a 100-fold increased risk in monozygotic twins when compared with dizygotic twins (5). HLA subtypes are also associated with reduced or increased risks of EBV+ HL (6). Together, these data support the hypothesis that HL may be related to a genetically associated immune response to an environmental pathogen.

The malignant Hodgkin/Reed-Sternberg cells do not resemble any normal hematopoietic cell by surface marker expression, and their relative scarcity in tissue samples complicated molecular analysis for years. Single-cell microdissection studies eventually elucidated the origin as a B-cell with nonproductively rearranged immunoglobulin heavy chains, down-regulated B-cell-specific transcription factors, and down-regulated signaling pathways (7). HL cells must rely on alternative survival and proliferative pathways, such as nuclear factor kappa B (NF-κB, via EBV or tumor necrosis receptor family members) and inhibition of the CD95 death pathway (through constituitive cellular Fas-associated death domain-like interleukin-1β-converting enzyme inhibitory protein, c-FLIP). HL manipulates its microenvironment (Fig. 14.1A) to suppress the immune response, attracting T helper and regulatory cells and reducing cytotoxic T and NK cells. Signals from the environment, acting through tumor necrosis factor receptors on HL cells, sustain HL through the activation of the NF-κB pathway. Despite the progress, understanding of the nature of the transforming events and the complex interaction of the genetic features, environmental factors, and the immune system of affected individuals remains incomplete and the subject of ongoing inquiry (8).

Classical HL is diagnosed by the morphologic appearance of multinucleate Reed-Sternberg cells (Fig. 14.1B) in an appropriate background of small lymphocytes, eosinophils, neutrophils, histiocytes, plasma cells, and fibroblasts. An adequate biopsy is required, and flow cytometry does not provide beneficial information. Classical HL includes four subtypes: nodular sclerosis, mixed cellularity, lymphocyte-rich, and lymphocyte-depleted (Table 14.1). Almost all cases express CD30, a marker of B-cell activation, and 87% express the myelomonocytic marker CD15, but the expression of the pan-B-cell marker CD20 is uncommon (5–25% cases). Faint PAX 5 expression is consistent with B lineage. Nodular sclerosis represents about two-thirds of cases in the developed world, whereas lymphocyte-depleted is rarely diagnosed. Lymphocyte-rich subtype is an uncommon, relatively recently defined entity (1). Nodular lymphocyte-predominant HL (NLPHL) is characterized by unique, malignant "popcorn" cells, which express the B-cell antigen CD20, but not CD15 or CD30. As described below, clinical features of HL vary with histologic subtype. The new World Health Organization classification of hematolymphoid malignancies includes a provisional diagnosis of a B-cell lymphoma, unclassifiable, with features intermediate between diffuse large B-cell lymphoma and classical HL (1). This diagnosis has features of HL (CD30[+], CD15[+] pleomorphic cells resembling Hodgkin cells) but also retains features of large cell lymphoma and is CD20[+]. Notably, the prominent inflammatory background of classical HL is sparse in this provisional entity.

CINICAL FEATURES, STAGING, AND DIAGNOSTIC EVALUATION

HL typically presents with painless supradiaphragmatic adenopathy, particularly in the low neck and supraclavicular

(A)

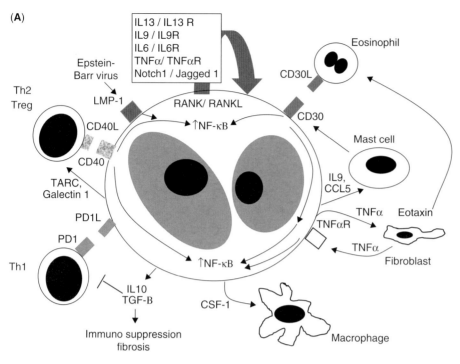

(B)

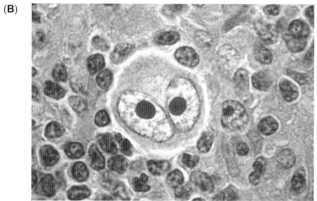

Figure 14.1 Hodgkin Reed-Sternberg cell and its microenvironment: **(A)** interactions that result in immunosuppression and favor survival; **(B)** photomicrography. *Abbreviations*: IL13, Interleukin-13; IL13R, Interleukin-13 receptor; IL9, Interleukin-9; IL9R, Interleukin-9 receptor; IL6, Interleukin-6; IL6R, Interleukin-6 receptor; NF-κB, Nuclear Factor kappa B; RANK, receptor activator for NFκB; LMP, latent membrane protein; TARC, thymus and activation regulated chemokine; PD1, programmed death-1; TGF-B, transforming growth factor beta; CSF, colony stimuating factor; TNF, tumor necrosis factor; CCL5 also known as RANTES (regulated on activation, normal T-cell expressed and secreted). *See Color Plate on Page xii.*

Table 14.1 Classification of Hodgkin Lymphoma

Name	Immunophenotype
Nodular lymphocyte-predominant	CD20+ CD30- CD15- Ig+
Classical	CD20-[a] CD30+ CD15+[b] Ig-
Nodular sclerosis	
Mixed cellularity	
Lymphocyte-rich	
Lymphocyte-depleted	
Grey zone/provisional	CD20+[b] CD30+[b] CD15+[b], Ig-
B-cell lymphoma, unclassifiable, with feature intermediate between diffuse large B-cell lymphoma and classical Hodgkin lymphoma	

[a]Infrequently positive.
[b]usually positive.

fossa. Mediastinal involvement is common. Most patients are asymptomatic, but a proportion has classic constitutional "B" symptoms of unexplained weight loss, fever, and drenching night sweats. Pruritus and alcohol-induced pain in involved lymph nodes are distinctive features in some patients. Nodular sclerosis subtype involves the mediastinum in 75% of cases and may present in limited or advanced stage. Older and immunodeficient patients are more likely to have constitutional symptoms, advanced disease, and mixed cellularity histology. NLPHL has a marked male predominance and presents with limited stage, peripheral adenopathy. Systemic symptoms and mediastinal involvement are uncommon in NLPHL. Lymphocyte-rich subtype shares many clinical features with NLPHL (9).

The four-stage Ann Arbor system was initially developed to facilitate curative radiation therapy and distinguish

Table 14.2 Diagnostic Procedures and Staging Criteria for Hodgkin Lymphoma

Recommended diagnostic procedures	Arbor staging system

Confirmation of diagnostic pathology
   Immunohistochemistry as indicated
History and physical examination
   Attention to constitutional symptoms
   Assessment of lymph nodes, spleen, liver
Chest radiograph with measurement of mediastinal
   mass ratio
CT scan of chest, abdomen and pelvis[a]
PET/CT scan whole body
Laboratory studies
   Complete blood count, differential
   Erythrocyte sedimentation rate
   Serum chemistry
Bone marrow biopsy (CS I-IIB, III, IV)
	I Involvement of a single lymph node region (I) or a single extralymphatic organ or site (I_E)
	II Involvement of two or more lymph node regions on the same side of the diaphragm
	     alone (II) or with involvement of limited, contiguous extralymphatic organ or tissue (II_E)
	III Involvement of lymph node regions on both sides of the diaphragm (III), which may
	     include the spleen (III_S) or limited, contiguous extralymphatic organ or site (III_E) or
	     both (III_{ES})
	IV Multiple or disseminated foci of involvement of one or more extralymphatic organs or
	     tissues, with or without associated lymph node involvement
	Modifying features
	A Asymptomatic
	B Drenching night sweats; fever >38°C; Loss of more than 10% body weight in
	     6 months
	X Bulky disease: >0.33 mediastinal mass ratio; >10 cm
	E Involvement of a single, contiguous, or proximal extranodal site

[a]May limit CT scan to areas positive by whole body PET/CT.

patients requiring systemic treatment (Table 14.2) (10). In 1989, bulky disease and extranodal (E) lesions were added to constitutional symptoms as modifying features (11). The dimensions of a mediastinal mass are expressed as the ratio of the maximum diameter of the mass over the thoracic diameter on a standing posterior–anterior chest radiograph. Practically, this measurement is now made by computed tomography scanning, and lesions greater than 10 cm are considered bulky. Each stage is given a designation of A (asymptomatic) or B, with symptoms of drenching night sweats, documented fever >38 degrees, and unexplained loss of 10% or more of body weight over the past six months.

Computed tomography of the chest, abdomen, and pelvis is the main radiographic procedure; the knowledge that HL typically involves an orderly progression from one nodal region to contiguous nodal sites should direct the radiologic review. A bone marrow biopsy is indicated in patients with B symptoms, subdiaphragmatic stage I-II presentation, advanced disease, age >60, and known immunodeficiency. Fluorodeoxyglucose positron emission tomography (FDG-PET) has assumed an increasing role in staging HL. FDG-PET alters the stage and treatment of HL in only a minority of patients (12). However, the ability of FDG-PET to distinguish metabolically active tissue from residual inactive (scar) tissue increases its predictive accuracy over

CT for response assessment (13). Nonetheless, false-positive results mandate that biopsy remain the standard for assessment of persistent disease and an essential procedure for evaluating unusual lesions or new sites of abnormal glucose uptake (13). Laboratory evaluation of new patients should include a complete blood count, metabolic panel, and erythrocyte sedimentation rate. As stated, a baseline chest X-ray is the standard by which mediastinal mass size is determined and can be useful in the long-term follow-up of patients.

PROGNOSTIC FACTORS

Prognostic factors for limited stage HL were initially based on the extent of staging and volume of radiation therapy (14). Table 14.3 shows the prognostic factors for limited disease as described by the German HL Study Group (GHSG), the European Organization for the Research and Treatment of Cancer (EORTC), and those commonly used in North America (15,16). Although historically based, these prognostic factors are important for the interpretation and translation of recent clinical trials in "favorable" and "unfavorable" limited stage HL that alter the dose and volume of radiation or the drugs and cumulative chemotherapy doses.

Table 14.3 Prognostic Factors for Hodgkin Lymphoma

Limited stage		Advanced stage
EORTC	GHSG	International collaborative study
Adverse prognostic factors		*Adverse prognostic factors*
MMR ≥0.35	MMR ≥0.35	Age ≥45 years
ESR >30 if symptomatic	ESR >30 if symptomatic	Stage IV
ESR >50 if asymptomatic	ESR >50 if asymptomatic	Male sex
>3 Ann Arbor sites	>2 Ann Arbor sites	White blood count ≥15,000/μl
Age ≥50	Extranodal disease	Lymphocyte count <600/μl or <8%
	Massive splenic disease	Albumin <4 g/dl
		Hemoglobin <10.5 g/dl
Presence of any factor is considered unfavorable		Factors summed to yield the international prognostic score
Two-thirds of limited stage patients have one or more adverse factors		75% of patients have a score of 1–3

Abbreviations: ESR, erythrocyte sedimentation rate; MMR, mediastinal mass ratio.

In advanced HL, (Table 14.3) seven prognostic factors, four based on laboratory assessment and three based on clinical features, are used to derive the International Prognostic Score of 0 to 7 (17). Most patients have a score of 2 to 3. The scoring system has proven to be very robust in the prediction of freedom from disease progression after initial treatment in multiple clinical trials. The international prognostic score aids in the interpretation of data from different studies and has been used for risk-adapted therapeutic strategies in advanced disease.

Interim FDG-PET scanning, after one to three cycles of combination chemotherapy, is emerging as an important indicator of treatment success in HL (18–20). In a consecutive series of 260 bulky and advanced HL patients scanned after two cycles of standard combination chemotherapy, FDG-PET-negative patients had a freedom from disease progression rate of >90% versus <20% in FDG-PET-positive patients (21). These results require broad confirmation for clinical practice but have led to a number of "risk-adapted" clinical trials based on interim PET results. Potentially, interim PET results can direct the use of intensive chemotherapy and radiotherapy more discriminately.

A variety of serum markers, host genetic factors, and tissue markers have been identified as prognostic factors of HL outcomes in correlative studies (22). Elevations in the serum levels of CD30 (from Hodgkin's cells), interleukin-10 (from Hodgkin's cells and host T-cells), tumor necrosis factor-alpha and its receptor (from Hodgkin's cells), and thymus and activating regulator chemokine (TARC, from Hodgkin's cells) have been associated with worse prognosis. Bcl-2 (in Hodgkin's cells), T regulatory, and cytotoxic T-cells (in the microenvironment) have emerged as the most robust tissue markers in a number of studies. Although host polymorphisms in interleukin-6 and interleukin-10 and polymorphisms that affect drug metabolism have been implicated, these studies have generally been less robust (22,23). Prospective assessment of the most promising markers through carefully designed trials is indicated.

TREATMENT
Limited Stage, Classical HL
Therapy for limited HL without risk factors (Tables 14.4 and 14.5) evolved over the past 10 to 15 years. Based on concern for serious radiation-related late effects (see below) and superior efficacy, combined modality treatment with brief chemotherapy and involved field radiotherapy (IFRT) supplanted the previous standard of extended field irradiation (EFRT: mantle plus para-aortic and splenic fields) in limited HL (64). A number of studies demonstrated the superiority of brief chemotherapy (two to three cycles) plus EFRT over the prior standard, EFRT alone (24–26). Subsequently, the Milan group reported that IFRT after four cycles of ABVD (doxorubicin, bleomycin, vinblastine, and dacarbazine) was as effective as EFRT, with 94% and 97% freedom from progressive disease (FFP) at 10 years, respectively (27). Similarly, the GHSG reported no advantage to EFRT over IFRT following three to four cycles of combination chemotherapy in prospective trials (28). Mature data from the EORTC/GELA H8U study also confirm that EFRT offers no benefit over IFRT after a limited course of chemotherapy (26).

To further address concerns for late effects of treatment in limited HL patients without risk factors, treatment programs have been designed to eliminate the risk of leukemia and sterility associated with chemotherapy using alkylating agents, to further reduce the cumulative exposure and duration of chemotherapy, and to decrease the dose of IFRT. Freedom from progression (FFP) more than 90% has been reported in favorable, limited HL by the Stanford and Manchester groups, with just eight and four weeks of chemotherapy, respectively, followed by IFRT (29,30). In interim analysis of the GHSG HD10 study, the FFP at two years was 96.6% and did not differ with two or four cycles of ABVD followed by IFRT (31). This study also randomly assigned patients to 20 or 30 Gy IFRT, and mature data are awaited to determine if the lower dose is equally effective. In a subsequent four-arm GHSG study, elimination of bleomycin and dacarbazine in the AV regimen or dacarbazine in the ABV regimen yielded inferior outcomes to the standard ABVD. On this basis, brief chemotherapy such as two cycles of ABVD with lower dose (~30 Gy) IFRT may be considered the standard therapy for limited classical HL with favorable characteristics. As discussed below, studies in progress seek to determine if interim PET scans can further refine the use of chemotherapy and radiotherapy.

The observation of second cancers and an increased risk of cardiac death associated with RT delivered in the 1970s and 1980s, together with the favorable long-term toxicity profile of ABVD relative to alkylating agent-based treatments, led to the study of chemotherapy alone in limited stage HL without risk factors. The National Cancer Institute of Canada (NCI-C) and the Eastern Cooperative Oncology Group (ECOG) tested ABVD alone in a complex study design, excluding very favorable or bulky disease patients. FFP at five years was 93% for RT-containing therapy compared with 87% for ABVD × 4–6 ($P = 0.006$) (32). No significant differences in event-free or overall survival were observed. It is difficult to compare these results with others because patients with favorable characteristics were randomized to EFRT (later known to be inferior to combined modality therapy) versus ABVD, with no difference in FFP observed in this subgroup. However, in patients with less favorable characteristics, combined modality with ABVD × 2 + IFRT was superior to ABVD ($P = 0.004$). Based upon the important primary endpoint of long-term survival and reduction in late adverse effects, proper interpretation of these results awaits long-term follow-up. In another study conducted by the EORTC/GELA (H9F), favorable limited stage patients were randomized to chemotherapy alone with epirubicin, bleomycin, vinblastine, and prednisone (EBVP) versus combined modality therapy. In this study, the EBVP alone arm was closed early due to inferior results ($P < 0.001$) (33). Thus, superior FFP results indicate that brief chemotherapy and IFRT should remain the standard for limited favorable HL, but mature analyses of late effects, second therapies, and overall survival with chemotherapy alone versus combined modality treatment will ultimately determine optimal management.

Patients with limited disease and adverse risk factors, such as bulky mediastinal disease and/or constitutional symptoms, require additional consideration (Table 14.5). It is important to note that patients with these unfavorable characteristics have been managed according to advanced

Table 14.4 Combination Chemotherapy for Hodgkin Lymphoma

Drug	Dose (mg/m^2)	Route	Schedule (days)	Cycle length (days)
COPP				28
Cyclophosphamide	650	IV	1,8	
Vincristine	1.4[a]	IV	1,8	
Procarbazine	100	PO	1–14	
Prednisone	40	PO	1–14	
ABVD				28
Doxorubicin	25	IV	1,15	
Bleomycin	10	IV	1,15	
Vinblastine	6	IV	1,15	
Dacarbazine	375	IV	1,15	
COPP/ABVD[b]				28
BEACOPP (Standard)				21
Bleomycin	10	IV	8	
Etoposide	100	IV	1–3	
Doxorubicin	25	IV	1	
Cyclophosphamide	650	IV	1	
Vincristine	1.4[a]	IV	8	
Procarbazine	100	PO	1–7	
Prednisone	40	PO	1–14	
BEACOPP (Escalated)				21
Bleomycin	10	IV	8	
Etoposide	200	IV	1–3	
Doxorubicin	35	IV	1	
Cyclophosphamide	1250	IV	1	
Vincristine	1.4[a]	IV	8	
Procarbazine	100	PO	1–7	
Prednisone	40	PO	1–14	
(G-CSF)	(+)	SQ	8+	
BEACOPP (14-day)[c]				14
STANFORD V				12 wk
Nitrogen mustard	6	IV	wk 1,5,9	
Doxorubicin	25	IV	wk 1,3,5,7,9,11	
Vinblastine	6	IV	wk 1,3,5,7,9,11	
Vincristine	1.4[a]	IV	wk 2,4,6,8,10,12	
Bleomycin	5	IV	wk 2,4,6,8,10,12	
Etoposide	60 × 2	IV	wk 3,7,11	
Prednisone	40 qod	PO	wk 1–10, taper	
G-CSF for dose reduction, delay				

[a]Capped at 2 mg.
[b]Alternate cycles of COPP with ABVD.
[c]Standard BEACOPP given every 14 days with growth factor support; Predoisone d1–7.

disease protocols in many studies. Two European groups established that EFRT provided no advantage to IFRT following a limited number of MOP/ABVD or COPP/ABVD cycles in unfavorable limited HL. The Milan group demonstrated the superiority of ABVD compared with MOPP, when either was given for six cycles sandwiched around EFRT, in CS IIA/B patients, a subset of whom had bulky mediastinal disease (34). As noted above, the subsequent trial from Milan, which included patients with bulky mediastinal disease, demonstrated the efficacy of ABVD × 4 + EFRT was the same as ABVD × 4 + IFRT (35). Likewise, the GHSG reported no advantage for EFRT over IFRT following two cycles of COPP/ABVD in stage I and II patients with risk factors (28). The Stanford group reported 96% FFP with the 12 week Stanford V chemotherapy regimen plus 36 Gy IFRT in bulky CS I-II A/B disease, although the patient numbers were small relative to the large multi-institutional trials (36). In interim analyses of

the EORTC/GELA H9U and the GHSG HD 11 studies, standard bleomycin, etoposide, doxorubicin, cyclophosphamide, vincristine, procarbazine, and prednisone (BEACOPP) was more toxic and no more effective than ABVD combined with ~30 to 36 Gy RT in this patient population (33,37). In addition, these results recommend combined modality treatment with a minimum of four cycles of ABVD chemotherapy and IFRT for limited classical HL with adverse risk factors (Table 14.5).

Advanced, Classical HL

Through a series of consecutive randomized trials conducted in the United States and Europe, ABVD chemotherapy was found to be superior to mustard, vincristine, procarbazine, and prednisone (MOPP) and less toxic than MOPP/ABVD or cyclophosphamide, vincristine, procarbazine, and prednisone (COPP)/ABVD regimens. Likewise, results from a

Table 14.5   Selected Randomized Clinical Trials in Hodgkin's Lymphoma

Study (N)	Treatment	FFS%	OS%	Follow-up (yr)
Limited stage, favorable, and unfavorable				
Milan (140)	4 ABVD + IFRT	94	96	12
	4 ABVD + STLI	93	94	
		P = NS	P = NS	
NCIC-ECOG (399)	4–6 ABVD	93	96	5
	RT-containing	87	94	
		P = 0.006	P = NS	
Limited stage, favorable				
EORTC/GELA H9F(783)	6 EBVP + 20-IFRT	88	98	4
	6 EBVP + 30-IFRT	85	100	
	6 EBVP	69	98	
		P = <0.001	P = 0.241	
GHSG HD10 (1370)	2 ABVD + 30-IFRT	No difference to date[a]	4	
	2 ABVD + 20-IFRT			
	4 ABVD + 30-IFRT			
	4 ABVD + 30-IFRT			
Limited stage, unfavorable				
EORTC/GELA H9U (808)	6 ABVD + 30-IFRT	91	95	4
	4 ABVD + 30-IFRT	87	94	
	4 BEACOPP + 30-IFRT	90	93	
		P = NS	P = NS	
GHSG HD11 (1422)	4 ABVD + 30-IFRT	No difference to date[a]	2.5	
	4 ABVD + 20-IFRT			
	4 BEACOPP + 30-IFRT			
	4 BEACOPP+ 20-IFRT			
Advanced stage				
GHSG HD9 (1201)	8 COPP/ABV + RT	69	83	5
	8 BEACOPP + RT	76	88	
	8 BEACOPP$_{esc}$ + RT	87	91	
		P < 0.002	P < 0.002	

[a]Interim analysis.
Abbreviations: ABVD, doxorubicin, bleomycin, vinblastine, dacarbazine; BEACOPP, bleomycin, etoposide, doxorubicin, cyclophosphamide, vincristine, procarbazine, prednisone; EBVP, epirubicin, bleomycin, vinblastine, prednisone.

United Kingdom trial studying more complex regimens indicated no advantage over ABVD (38). The GHSG compared standard and escalated BEACOPP (Tables 14.4 and 14.5) regimens, based on a mathematical model that predicted a clinical benefit with modest dose intensification, compared with their standard COPP/ABVD. The 5- and 10-year results from the HD9 study show superior freedom from treatment failure (P < 0.002) and overall survival (P < 0.002) of escalated BEACOPP compared to COPP/ABVD in IIB-IV HL (39,40). Escalated BEACOPP yielded superior freedom from treatment failure (FFTF) regardless of international prognostic score. The hematologic toxicity of BEACOPP was increased but manageable, requiring red cell and platelet transfusions and frequent hospitalization. Secondary leukemia was reported in four patients with standard BEACOPP, nine with escalated BEACOPP, and one with COPP/ABVD. Importantly, the HD9 study demonstrated a dose–response effect in advanced HL that can be achieved without stem cell support.

Subsequently, two relatively small studies tested BEACOPP (escalated and standard cycles) with ABVD in unfavorable and advanced HL, and these have been reported in abstracts (41). In both studies, BEACOPP achieved statistically superior FFP compared with ABVD,

but no difference in survival was observed at about four years of median follow-up. In the Italian Intergroup study, the design involved a planned cross over to high-dose chemotherapy for patients who had recurrent disease or failed to achieve a very good partial remission (41). Notably, these recent studies lacked the large sample size (n = 1201) of the GHSG HD9 study, which provided the statistical power to determine significant differences in survival despite small absolute differences. The EORTC is completing another important study of BEACOPP compared to ABVD in high IPS patients. It is important to note that patients >60 years do not tolerate BEACOPP, and in a small randomized experience from the GHSG, there was no benefit for BEACOPP compared to COPP/ABVD (42).

The role of radiotherapy in advanced HL has been debated over the years. Of note, two-thirds of patients in the GHSG HD9 study received radiotherapy for residual or bulky disease (39). A meta-analysis involving 1740 patients in 14 trials comparing combined modality treatment or chemotherapy alone found no benefit for radiotherapy in stage IV patients, and mortality was greater in patients treated with chemotherapy and radiotherapy (43). However, these conclusions were limited by the use of outmoded chemotherapy and radiotherapy, dominance by a few large trials and missing data. A GELA study reported similar outcomes for remission patients with advanced disease consolidated with two additional cycles of chemotherapy or radiotherapy, and an EORTC found no benefit for consolidative radiotherapy in advanced stage patients in complete remission following MOPP/ABV hybrid (44,45). Interim analyses of the GHSG HD12 study determined that radiotherapy did not improve FFTF after eight cycles of escalated or escalated/standard BEACOPP (46,47). Use of PET avidity at the conclusion of BEACOPP therapy to guide the use of RT in the GSHG HD15 study appears to be a reasonable strategy; just 12% of patients were irradiated using the study algorithm (47). Together, these data demonstrate that RT does not provide a clear benefit after a full course of doxorubicin-containing chemotherapy.

The Stanford group took another approach to bulky and advanced (II-IV) disease, limiting the duration of chemotherapy to 12 weeks, intensifying dose but reducing cumulative doses, and incorporating radiotherapy to sites of bulk (>5 cm) disease. Excellent institutional (Stanford, Memorial Sloan Kettering) and phase II cooperative group results with the Stanford V + RT regimen led to a large intergroup comparison of this approach with ABVD (48–50), the results of which are awaited. Meanwhile, in a small Italian study the use of Stanford V with variable radiotherapy was inferior to ABVD or another multidrug regimen, suggesting the important role of RT following brief chemotherapy (51). The recommended treatment for advanced HL should be based on achieving the least complicated cure as indicated by the FFP rate, anticipated acute and late complications, and overall survival. ABVD may be preferred for low or standard risk patients concerned about fertility and secondary cancers, as the incidence of refractory disease is low, the opportunity for salvage therapy exists, and the survival benefit remains unconfirmed. In interim analyses, potentially less toxic alterations of BEACOPP (4 standard + 4 escalated) and BEACOPP-14 appear to be equally effective although mature results are awaited (52). Several ongoing studies incorporate interim PET scans to drive therapeutic escalation or de-escalation in selected patients.

Nodular, Lymphocyte Predominant

In past, nodular lymphocyte-predominant HL (NLPHL) was often included with classical disease in prospective trials (53,54). The excellent prognosis for NLPHL has been demonstrated in multiple case series and the European Task Force report, where survivals for stage I and II disease were 99% and 94%, respectively, at eight years (55). Despite high survival rates, in this and prior analyses, late relapses were observed more frequently than in classical HL and, as such, adverse effects of multiple treatments have been of concern. Excision alone may be sufficient in some limited stage cases, but most are treated with IFRT. Advanced stage presentations are uncommon and significantly less favorable; these are usually managed as for classical disease. In a retrospective analysis, NLPHL patients participating in GHSG clinical trials had FFTF rates comparable to classical HL at five years; however, late relapses are more common in NLPHL than classical HL (53). Reliable expression of CD20 in NLPHL led groups at Stanford University and in Europe to study the therapeutic efficacy of rituximab (56,57). High response rates have been observed with just four rituximab injections, but a continuous pattern of relapse was observed thereafter. Longer courses of antibody treatment may result in more durable response (58). The misclassification of many NLPHL cases demonstrates the importance of expert hematopathology review (59). NLPHL can be difficult to differentiate from T-cell rich B-cell lymphoma, and reactive hyperplasia and progressive transformation of germinal centers can precede or follow a diagnosis of NLPHL (1). Transformation to diffuse large B-cell lymphoma has been reported in 3% to 5% of cases and a clonal association has been demonstrated (60). These attributes indicate the need for expert hematopathology review and a policy of re-biopsy for recurrent disease.

TREATMENT COMPLICATIONS AND SURVIVORSHIP

Appreciation of the late as well as early complications of treatment for HL has been an important force in shaping current treatment as well as investigational strategies. The major complications of RT include second cancers and cardiovascular disease. Reporting of these late effects is influenced by the latency period, which may require a minimum of 10 to 15 years of follow-up. The volume and dose of radiotherapy determine the risk of late effects, together with important cofactors (61). Second cancers principally involve the breast, lung, thyroid, soft tissue, bone, skin, and gastrointestinal tract. Age at treatment interacts with cofactors for selected sites such as tobacco use and alkylating agents for lung cancer and duration of menses for breast cancer (62–64). Thoracic RT confers an increased risk of cardiac disease, especially in doses more than 30 Gy, and recent data indicate that doxorubicin exposure is an important cofactor (65–68). Patients with HL have an increased risk of death from treatment complications that persists for more than 25 years, and younger patients are at risk for breast and colorectal cancer occurring at earlier ages (69). Appropriate monitoring and surveillance are important, particularly in patients treated with RT prior to 1990 (70).

The side effects of chemotherapy are related to specific drugs, their individual and cumulative doses, and potential drug interactions. Sterility and an increased risk of leukemia are associated with alkylating agents but are not generally observed with ABVD. In some series, an increased risk of solid cancers has been associated with alkylating agents as well as radiation therapy (71). Another form of secondary leukemia, which is notable for a shorter latency and a unique balanced translocation, has been reported with etoposide and has been associated with escalated BEACOPP (72). The relationship of this complication with individual and cumulative doses, schedule, and drug interactions is uncertain. Recent data from the GHSG show that BEACOPP results in male sterility and is associated with premature menopause (73,74). Although ABVD has little or no increased risk of secondary leukemia and has significantly less reproductive toxicity compared with the MOPP combination, recent data from a population-based study demonstrate a marked increase in relative risk of late cardiopulmonary toxicity, particularly in combination with mediastinal irradiation (67). Recent data also implicate doxorubicin in increasing late cardiotoxicity in combination with RT (75). It is hoped that interim PET scanning and the validation of biomarkers for efficacy and toxicity will afford limitation of cumulative drug exposures, more toxic chemotherapy regimens, and use and volume of RT to a subset of patients based on risk and benefit.

Other complications of treatment for HL include hypothyroidism secondary to neck RT, overwhelming sepsis after splenectomy or splenic RT, osteoporosis and osteonecrosis, and pulmonary toxicity. The latter has been related to cumulative bleomycin exposure and is more pronounced in older patients and in those exposed to granulocyte colony stimulating factors (76).

MANAGEMENT OF RECURRENT DISEASE

The success of second-line treatment is related to sensitivity to chemotherapy at relapse (determined by standard radiologic and PET criteria), initial remission duration, extent of disease and symptoms at relapse, presence of anemia at relapse, and number of prior treatments. Historically, recurrence after a full course of chemotherapy for advanced HL resulted in a <20% cure rate with second-line chemotherapy. Myeloablative chemotherapy and autologous transplantation is the preferred therapy, based on failure-free survival rates of 40% to 50% and two randomized trials that demonstrated the superiority of transplantation over second-line chemotherapy (77–80). The intensity of prior therapy may be prognostic; >65% of patients were estimated to be alive and disease-free at five years after Stanford V and radiotherapy, and the success of second-line therapy was greater after ABVD than after BEACOPP induction in a recent Italian study (36,41). Functional imaging with FDG-PET has also emerged as a highly significant prognostic factor for the success of myeloablative chemotherapy for recurrent HL (81). Historically, radiotherapy alone was effective second-line therapy only in selected cases, with most patients requiring a systemic approach (82,83).

Standard allogeneic transplantation for recurrent HL is associated with a lower risk of relapse than autologous transplantation, but this advantage is offset by higher transplant-related mortality. Reduced or nonmyeloablative conditioning prior to allogeneic transplantation results in lower transplant-related mortality, but at the expense of a higher relapse rate compared to myeloablative conditioning (84,85). Patients with longer remissions, chemosensitive disease, and more intense conditioning regimens have better reported outcomes. Evidence of activity of donor lymphocyte infusions in some patients and a favorable association of graft-versus-host disease with time to progression favor a graft-versus-host effect in HL. However, this procedure should continue to be evaluated in the context of prospective clinical trials (84).

The evolution from radiotherapy alone to combined modality therapy for limited disease has resulted in a lower rate of relapse but uncertainty as to the optimal management of relapse in this setting. An evaluation of patients relapsing after ABVD alone or RT-containing therapy in the NCIC-ECOG trial estimated that >90% patients were free of second progression or death at five years, whether managed at relapse with RT alone, combined modality, chemotherapy alone or high-dose therapy and autotransplantation (86). Less favorable results were reported by the GHSG, which found a 52% disease-free rate at 36 months

among patients who relapsed after brief chemotherapy and radiotherapy; the majority had systemic therapy and half were transplanted (87).

CONCLUSIONS AND FUTURE CONSIDERATIONS

As illustrated in Figure 14.2, outcomes have improved in HL over the past three decades. The continued challenge in HL is to define the most effective treatment with the fewest complications in risk-adapted strategies. The fact that HL can often be cured with second-line treatment results in a choice between more intensive primary therapy or a less intensive treatment with fewer complications but a higher rate of relapse. Counseling patients, who are increasingly involved in treatment selection, requires consideration of personal risk factors and preferences, prognostic factors, and response assessment during treatment. Although cure is a critical aim for all patients, overall survival, and quality of life are the ultimate endpoints.

Although overall cure rates and survivals have continuously improved, late effects of treatment continue to be of concern, and these unfavorably affect expected survival

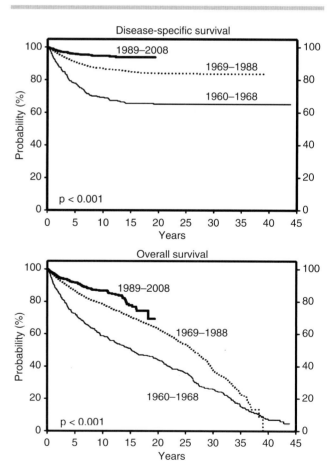

Figure 14.2 Disease-specific and overall survival according to era of treatment at Stanford University, significant gains in both Disease-specific survival (DSS) and overall survival (OS) were made with each era.

at 10 or more years. A major challenge is to monitor treated patients for decades, and engage them in ongoing care and research for optimal survivorship. The undesirable consequences of treatment in young HL patients have and continue to be a driving force in the development of prognostic biomarkers for efficacy and toxicity and novel targeted treatments. More effective therapies are required for older patients and those with recurrent and refractory disease. Understanding and prospectively defining the unique biologic attributes of these patients with suitable biomarkers is an ongoing challenge. Preliminary efficacy data have been reported with a variety of new agents including the histone deacetylase inhibitors, inhibitors of the mTOR pathway, and an anti-CD30 conjugated tubulin toxin. Studies of agents targeting angiogenesis, immune modulation, and other cell surface receptors or ligands are in progress. The constellation of progress in functional imaging, biomarkers, understanding of the basic biology of HL, and evolution of new targeted approaches hold great promise to take the prevention, diagnosis, and management of HL to the next level.

REFERENCES

1. Stein H. Hodgkin Lymphoma. In: Swerdlow S, Campo E, Harris NL et al., eds. WHO Classification of Tumours of Haematopoietic and Lymphoid Tissues, 4th edn. Lyon, France: International Agency for Research on Cancer, 2008.
2. Weiss LM, Strickler JG, Warnke RA et al. Epstein-Barr viral DNA in tissues of Hodgkin's disease. Am J Pathol 1987; 129: 86–91.
3. Hjalgrim H, Askling J, Rostgaard K et al. Characteristics of Hodgkin's lymphoma after infectious mononucleosis. N Engl J Med 2003; 349: 1324–32.
4. Alexander FE, Lawrence DJ, Freeland J et al. An epidemiologic study of index and family infectious mononucleosis and adult Hodgkin's disease (HD): evidence for a specific association with EBV+ve HD in young adults. Int J Cancer 2003; 107: 298–302.
5. Mack TM, Cozen W, Shibata DK et al. Concordance for Hodgkin's disease in identical twins suggesting genetic susceptibility to the young-adult form of the disease. N Engl J Med 1995; 332: 413–18.
6. Niens M, Jarrett RF, Hepkema B et al. HLA-A*02 is associated with a reduced risk and HLA-A*01 with an increased risk of developing EBV+ Hodgkin lymphoma. Blood 2007; 110: 3310–15.
7. Brauninger A, Schmitz R, Bechtel D et al. Molecular biology of Hodgkin's and Reed/Sternberg cells in Hodgkin's lymphoma. Int J Cancer 2006; 118: 1853–61.
8. Re D, Kuppers R, Diehl V. Molecular pathogenesis of Hodgkin's lymphoma. J Clin Oncol 2005; 23: 6379–86.
9. Anagnostopoulos I, Hansmann ML, Franssila K et al. European Task Force on Lymphoma project on lymphocyte predominance Hodgkin disease: histologic and immunohistologic analysis of submitted cases reveals 2 types of Hodgkin disease with a nodular growth pattern and abundant lymphocytes. Blood 2000; 96: 1889–99.
10. Carbone P, Kaplan H, Musshoff K. Report of the committee on the Hodgkin's disease staging. Cancer Res 1971; 31: 1860.
11. Lister TA, Crowther D, Sutcliffe SB et al. Report of a committee convened to discuss the evaluation and staging of patients with Hodgkin's disease: Cotswolds meeting [published erratum appears in J Clin Oncol 1990; 8: 1602.] [see comments]. J Clin Oncol 1989; 7: 1630–6.
12. Friedberg JW, Chengazi V. PET scans in the staging of lymphoma: current status. Oncologist 2003; 8: 438–47.
13. Juweid ME. Utility of positron emission tomography (PET) scanning in managing patients with Hodgkin lymphoma. Hematology Am Soc Hematol Educ Program 2006: 259–65, 510-1.
14. Hoppe RT, Coleman CN, Cox RS et al. The management of stage I—II Hodgkin's disease with irradiation alone or combined modality therapy: the Stanford experience. Blood 1982; 59: 455–65.
15. Löffler M, Mauch P, MacLennan K et al. The Second International Symposium on Hodgkin's Disease. Workshop I: Review on prognostic factors. Ann Oncol 1992; (3 Suppl 4): 63–6.
16. Tubiana M, Henry AM, Carde P et al. Toward comprehensive management tailored to prognostic factors of patients with clinical stages I and II in Hodgkin's disease. The EORTC Lymphoma Group controlled clinical trials: 1964–1987. Blood 1989; 73: 47–56.
17. Hasenclever D, Diehl V. A prognostic score for advanced Hodgkin's disease. International Prognostic Factors Project on Advanced Hodgkin's Disease. N Engl J Med 1998; 339: 1506–14.
18. Hutchings M, Loft A, Hansen M et al. FDG-PET after two cycles of chemotherapy predicts treatment failure and progression-free survival in Hodgkin lymphoma. Blood 2006; 107: 52–9.
19. Mikhaeel NG, Hutchings M, Fields PA et al. FDG-PET after two to three cycles of chemotherapy predicts progression-free and overall survival in high-grade non-Hodgkin lymphoma. Ann Oncol 2005; 16: 1514–23.
20. Gallamini A, Hutchings M, Avigdor A et al. Early interim PET scan in Hodgkin lymphoma: where do we stand? Leuk Lymphoma 2008; 49: 659–62.
21. Gallamini A, Hutchings M, Rigacci L et al. Early interim 2-[18F]fluoro-2-deoxy-D-glucose positron emission tomography is prognostically superior to international prognostic score in advanced-stage Hodgkin's lymphoma: a report from a joint Italian-Danish study. J Clin Oncol 2007; 25: 3746–52.
22. Hsi ED. Biologic features of Hodgkin lymphoma and the development of biologic prognostic factors in Hodgkin lymphoma: tumor and microenvironment. Leuk Lymphoma 2008; 49: 1668–80.
23. Ribrag V, Koscielny S, Casasnovas O et al. Pharmacogenetic study in Hodgkin's lymphomas reveals the impact of UGT1A1 polymorphisms on patient's prognosis. Blood 2009; 113: 3307–13.
24. Press OW, LeBlanc M, Lichter AS et al. Phase III randomized intergroup trial of subtotal lymphoid irradiation versus doxorubicin, vinblastine, and subtotal lymphoid irradiation for stage IA to IIA Hodgkin's disease. J Clin Oncol 2001; 19: 4238–44.
25. Engert A, Franklin J, Eich HT et al. Two cycles of doxorubicin, bleomycin, vinblastine, and dacarbazine plus extended-field radiotherapy is superior to radiotherapy alone in early favorable Hodgkin's lymphoma: final results of the GHSG HD7 trial. J Clin Oncol 2007; 25: 3495–502.
26. Ferme C, Eghbali H, Meerwaldt JH et al. Chemotherapy plus involved-field radiation in early-stage Hodgkin's disease. N Engl J Med 2007; 357: 1916–27.
27. Bonadonna G, Bonfante V, Viviani S et al. ABVD plus subtotal nodal versus involved-field radiotherapy in early-stage Hodgkin's disease: long-term results. J Clin Oncol 2004; 22: 2835–41.
28. Engert A, Schiller P, Josting A et al. Involved-field radiotherapy is equally effective and less toxic compared with extended-field radiotherapy after four cycles of chemotherapy in patients with early-stage unfavorable Hodgkin's lymphoma: results of the HD8 trial of the German Hodgkin's Lymphoma Study Group. J Clin Oncol 2003; 21: 3601–8.
29. Horning SJ, Hoppe RT, Breslin S et al. Very brief (8 week) chemotherapy (CT) and low dose (30 Gy) radiotherapy (RT)

for limited stage Hodgkin's disease (HD): preliminary results of the Stanford-Kaiser G4 study of Stanford V + RT. Blood 1999; 94(Suppl 1): 387a.

30. Radford JA, Williams MV, Hancock BW et al. Minimal initial chemotherapy plus involved field radiotherapy (RT) versus mantle field RT for clinical stage IA/IIA supra-diaphragmatic hodgkins disease (HD). Preliminary results of the UK Lymphoma Group LY07 trial. Proc Am Soc Clin Oncol 2003: 2304A.

31. Diehl V, Brillant C, Engert A et al. Reduction of combined modality treatment intensity in early stage Hodgkin's lymphoma: interim analysis of the HD 10 trial of the GHSG. ASH Annual Meeting Abstracts 2004; 104: 1307.

32. Meyer RM, Gospodarowicz MK, Connors JM et al. Randomized comparison of ABVD chemotherapy with a strategy that includes radiation therapy in patients with limited-stage Hodgkin's lymphoma: National Cancer Institute of Canada Clinical Trials Group and the Eastern Cooperative Oncology Group. J Clin Oncol 2005; 23: 4634–42.

33. Noordijk E, Thomas J, Ferme C et al. First results of the EORTC-GELA H9 randomized trials: the H9-F trial and H9U trial in patients with favorable or unfavorable early stage Hodgkin's lymphoma. Proc Am Soc Clin Oncol 2005: 6505A.

34. Santoro A, Bonadonna G, Valagussa P et al. Long-term results of combined chemotherapy-radiotherapy approach in Hodgkin's disease: superiority of ABVD plus radiotherapy versus MOPP plus radiotherapy. J Clin Oncol 1987; 5: 27–37.

35. Bonadonna G, Bonfante V, Viviani S, et al. ABVD plus subtotal nodal involved-field radiotherapy in early-stage Hodgkin's disease: long-term results. J Clin Oncol 2004; 22: 2835–41.

36. Horning SJ, Hoppe RT, Breslin S et al. Stanford V and radiotherapy for locally extensive and advanced Hodgkin's disease: mature results of a prospective clinical trial. J Clin Oncol 2002; 20: 630–7.

37. Klimm B, Engert A, Brillant C et al. Comparison of BEACOPP and ABVD chemotherapy in intermediate stage Hodgkin's lymphoma: results of the fourth interim analysis of the HD11 trial of the GHSG. Proc Am Soc Clin Oncol 2005: 6507A.

38. Johnson PW, Radford JA, Cullen MH et al. Comparison of ABVD and alternating or hybrid multidrug regimens for the treatment of advanced Hodgkin's lymphoma: results of the United Kingdom Lymphoma Group LY09 Trial (ISRCTN97144519). J Clin Oncol 2005; 23: 9208–18.

39. Diehl V, Franklin J, Pfreundschuh M et al. Standard and increased-dose BEACOPP chemotherapy compared with COPP-ABVD for advanced Hodgkin's disease. N Engl J Med 2003; 348: 2386–95.

40. Diehl V, Franklin J, Pfistner B et al. Ten year results of a German Hodgkin Study Group randomized trial of standard and increased dose of BEACOPP chemotherapy for advanced Hodgkin' lymphoma (HD9). Proc Am Soc Clin Oncol 2007: LBA8015.

41. Gianni AM, Rambaldi A, Zinzani PL et al. Comparable 3-year outcome following ABVD or BEACOPP first-line chemotherapy, plus pre-planned high-dose salvage, in advanced Hodgkin lymphoma: a randomized trial of the Michelangelo, GITIL and IIL cooperative groups. Proc Am Soc Clin Oncol 2008: abstract 8506.

42. Ballova V, Ruffer JU, Haverkamp H et al. A prospectively randomized trial carried out by the German Hodgkin Study Group (GHSG) for elderly patients with advanced Hodgkin's disease comparing BEACOPP baseline and COPP-ABVD (study HD9elderly). Ann Oncol 2005; 16: 124–31.

43. Loeffler M, Brosteanu O, Hasenclever D et al. Meta-analysis of chemotherapy versus combined modality treatment trials in Hodgkin's disease. International Database on Hodgkin's Disease Overview Study Group. J Clin Oncol 1998; 16: 818–29.

44. Ferme C, Sebban C, Hennequin C et al. Comparison of chemotherapy to radiotherapy as consolidation of complete or good partial response after six cycles of chemotherapy for patients with advanced Hodgkin's disease: results of the groupe d'etudes des lymphomes de l'Adulte H89 trial. Blood 2000; 95: 2246–52.

45. Aleman BM, Raemaekers JM, Tirelli U et al. Involved-field radiotherapy for advanced Hodgkin's lymphoma. N Engl J Med 2003; 348: 2396–406.

46. Diehl V, Schiller P, Engert A et al. Results of the third interim analysis of the HD12 trial of the GHSG: 8 courses of escalated BEACOPP versus 4 baseline courses of BEACOPP with or without additive radiotherapy for advanced stage Hodgkin's lymphoma [abstract]. Blood 2003; 102: 85.

47. Kobe C, Dietlein M, Franklin J et al. Positron emission tomography has a high negative predictive value for progression or early relapse for patients with residual disease after first line chemotherapy in advanced-stage Hodgkin lymphoma. Blood 2008; 112: 3989–94.

48. Hoppe RT, Advani RH, Ambinder RF et al. Hodgkin disease/lymphoma. J Natl Compr Canc Netw 2008; 6: 594–622.

49. Horning SJ, Williams J, Bartlett NL et al. Assessment of the Stanford V regimen and consolidative radiotherapy for bulky and advanced Hodgkin's disease: Eastern Cooperative Oncology Group pilot study E1492. J Clin Oncol 2000; 18: 972–80.

50. Horning SJ, Hoppe R, Advani R et al. Efficacy and late effects of Stanford V chemotherapy and radiotherapy in untreated Hodgkin's disease: mature data in early and advanced stage patients [abstract]. Blood 2005; 104: 92a.

51. Gobbi PG, Levis A, Chisesi T et al. ABVD versus modified Stanford V versus MOPPEBVCAD with optional and limited radiotherapy in intermediate- and advanced-stage Hodgkin's lymphoma: final results of a multicenter randomized trial by the Intergruppo Italiano Linfomi. J Clin Oncol 2005; 23: 9198–207.

52. Diehl V, Brillant C, Franklin J et al. BEACOPP chemotherapy for advanced Hodgkin's disease: results of further analyses of the HD9- and HD12- trials of the German Hodgkin Study Group (GHSG). ASH Annual Meeting Abstracts 2004; 104: 307.

53. Nogova L, Reineke T, Brillant C et al. Lymphocyte-predominant and classical Hodgkin's lymphoma: a comprehensive analysis from the German Hodgkin Study Group. J Clin Oncol 2008; 26: 434–9.

54. Nogova L, Reineke T, Eich HT et al. Extended field radiotherapy, combined modality treatment or involved field radiotherapy for patients with stage IA lymphocyte-predominant Hodgkin's lymphoma: a retrospective analysis from the German Hodgkin Study Group (GHSG). Ann Oncol 2005; 16: 1683–7.

55. Diehl V, Sextro M, Franklin J et al. Clinical presentation, course, and prognostic factors in lymphocyte-predominant Hodgkin's disease and lymphocyte-rich classical Hodgkin's disease: report from the European Task Force on Lymphoma Project on lymphocyte-predominant Hodgkin's disease. J Clin Oncol 1999; 17: 776–83.

56. Ekstrand BC, Lucas JB, Horwitz SM et al. Rituximab in lymphocyte-predominant Hodgkin disease: results of a phase 2 trial. Blood 2003; 101: 4285–9.

57. Schulz H, Rehwald U, Morschhauser F et al. Rituximab in relapsed lymphocyte-predominant Hodgkin Lymphoma: long-term results of a phase-II trial of the German Hodgkin Lymphoma Study Group (GHSG). Blood 2008; 111: 109–11.

58. Horning SJ, Bartlett NL, Breslin S et al. Results of a prospective phase II trial of limited and extended rituximab treatment in nodular lymphocyte predominant Hodgkin's disease (NLPHD). ASH Annual Meeting Abstracts 2007; 110: 644.

59. Rehwald U, Schulz H, Reiser M et al. Treatment of relapsed CD20+ Hodgkin lymphoma with the monoclonal antibody

rituximab is effective and well tolerated: results of a phase 2 trial of the German Hodgkin Lymphoma Study Group. Blood 2003; 101: 420–4.

60. Greiner TC, Gascoyne RD, Anderson ME et al. Nodular lymphocyte-predominant Hodgkin's disease associated with large-cell lymphoma: analysis of Ig gene rearrangements by V-J polymerase chain reaction. Blood 1996; 88: 657–66.

61. Hodgson DC, Koh ES, Tran TH et al. Individualized estimates of second cancer risks after contemporary radiation therapy for Hodgkin lymphoma. Cancer 2007; 110: 2576–86.

62. van Leeuwen FE, Klokman WJ, Stovall M et al. Roles of radiation dose, chemotherapy, and hormonal factors in breast cancer following Hodgkin's disease. J Natl Cancer Inst 2003; 95: 971–80.

63. Hill DA, Gilbert E, Dores GM et al. Breast cancer risk following radiotherapy for Hodgkin lymphoma: modification by other risk factors. Blood 2005; 106: 3358–65.

64. Travis LB. Evaluation of the risk of therapy-associated complications in survivors of Hodgkin lymphoma. Hematology Am Soc Hematol Educ Program 2007; 2007: 192–6.

65. Hancock SL, Tucker MA, Hoppe RT. Factors affecting late mortality from heart disease after treatment of Hodgkin's disease. JAMA 1993; 270: 1949–55.

66. Myrehaug S, Pintilie M, Tsang R et al. Cardiac morbidity following modern treatment for Hodgkin lymphoma: supraadditive cardiotoxicity of doxorubicin and radiation therapy. Leuk Lymphoma 2008; 49: 1486–93.

67. Swerdlow AJ, Higgins CD, Smith P et al. Myocardial infarction mortality risk after treatment for Hodgkin disease: a collaborative British cohort study. J Natl Cancer Inst 2007; 99: 206–14.

68. Travis LB, Gilbert E. Lung cancer after Hodgkin lymphoma: the roles of chemotherapy, radiotherapy and tobacco use. Radiat Res 2005; 163: 695–6.

69. Hodgson DC, Gilbert ES, Dores GM et al. Long-term solid cancer risk among 5-year survivors of Hodgkin's lymphoma. J Clin Oncol 2007; 25: 1489–97.

70. Hodgson DC. Hodgkin lymphoma: the follow-up of long-term survivors. Hematol Oncol Clin North Am 2008; 22: 233–44, vi.

71. Swerdlow AJ, Douglas AJ, Hudson GV et al. Risk of second primary cancers after Hodgkin's disease by type of treatment: analysis of 2846 patients in the British National Lymphoma Investigation. BMJ 1992; 304: 1137–43.

72. DeVore R, Whitlock J, Hainsworth JD et al. Therapy-related acute nonlymphocytic leukemia with monocytic features and rearrangement of chromosome 11q. Ann Intern Med 1989; 110: 740–2.

73. Sieniawski M, Reineke T, Nogova L et al. Fertility in male patients with advanced Hodgkin Lymphoma treated with BEACOPP: a report of the German Hodgkin Study Group (GHSG). Blood 2008; 111: 71–6.

74. Behringer K, Breuer K, Reineke T et al. Secondary amenorrhea after Hodgkin's lymphoma is influenced by age at treatment, stage of disease, chemotherapy regimen, and the use of oral contraceptives during therapy: a report from the German Hodgkin's Lymphoma Study Group. J Clin Oncol 2005; 23: 7555–64.

75. Aleman BM, van den Belt-Dusebout AW, De Bruin ML et al. Late cardiotoxicity after treatment for Hodgkin lymphoma. Blood 2007; 109: 1878–86.

76. Martin WG, Ristow KM, Habermann TM et al. Bleomycin pulmonary toxicity has a negative impact on the outcome of patients with Hodgkin's lymphoma. J Clin Oncol 2005; 23: 7614–20.

77. Horning SJ, Chao NJ, Negrin RS et al. High-dose therapy and autologous hematopoietic progenitor cell transplantation for recurrent or refractory Hodgkin's disease: analysis of the Stanford University results and prognostic indices. Blood 1997; 89: 801–13.

78. Reece DE, Connors JM, Spinelli JJ et al. Intensive therapy with cyclophosphamide, carmustine, etoposide +/− cisplatin, and autologous bone marrow transplantation for Hodgkin's disease in first relapse after combination chemotherapy [see comments]. Blood 1994; 83: 1193–9.

79. Linch DC, Winfield D, Goldstone AH et al. Dose intensification with autologous bone-marrow transplantation in relapsed and resistant Hodgkin's disease: results of a BNLI randomised trial. Lancet 1993; 341: 1051–4.

80. Schmitz N, Pfistner B, Sextro M et al. Aggressive conventional chemotherapy compared with high-dose chemotherapy with autologous haemopoietic stem-cell transplantation for relapsed chemosensitive Hodgkin's disease: a randomised trial. Lancet 2002; 359: 2065–71.

81. Elias Jabbour CH, Gregory Ayers, Rodolfo Nunez et al. Pretransplant positive positron emission tomography/gallium scans predict poor outcome in patients with recurrent/refractory Hodgkin lymphoma. Cancer 2007; 109: 2481–9.

82. Wirth A, Corry J, Laidlaw C et al. Salvage radiotherapy for Hodgkin's disease following chemotherapy failure [see comments]. Int J Radiat Oncol Biol Phys 1997; 39: 599–607.

83. Josting A, Nogova L, Franklin J et al. Salvage radiotherapy in patients with relapsed and refractory Hodgkin's lymphoma: a retrospective analysis from the German Hodgkin Lymphoma Study Group. J Clin Oncol 2005; 23: 1522–9.

84. Peggs KS, Anderlini P, Sureda A. Allogeneic transplantation for Hodgkin lymphoma. Br J Haematol 2008; 143:468–80.

85. Sureda A, Robinson S, Canals C et al. Reduced-intensity conditioning compared with conventional allogeneic stem-cell transplantation in relapsed or refractory Hodgkin's lymphoma: an analysis from the Lymphoma Working Party of the European Group for Blood and Marrow Transplantation. J Clin Oncol 2008; 26: 455–62.

86. Macdonald DA, Ding K, Gospodarowicz MK et al. Patterns of disease progression and outcomes in a randomized trial testing ABVD alone for patients with limited-stage Hodgkin lymphoma. Ann Oncol 2007; 18: 1680–4.

87. Sieniawski M, Franklin J, Nogova L et al. Outcome of patients experiencing progression or relapse after primary treatment with two cycles of chemotherapy and radiotherapy for early-stage favorable Hodgkin's lymphoma. J Clin Oncol 2007; 25: 2000–5.

15

Multiple Myeloma

Antonio Palumbo and Francesca Gay

EPIDEMIOLOGY AND ETIOLOGY

Multiple myeloma (MM) is an incurable malignant plasma cell disorder that constitutes 1% of all cancer and 10% of hematological neoplasms. Its worldwide incidence rates vary from 0.4 to 5 per 100,000, with a higher rate in males, in Western countries, and among African Americans. The incidence of MM increases considerably with age, with a median age at diagnosis of 66 years (age-adjusted incidence rates 2.1 vs. 30.1 in patients aged under and over 65 years, respectively) (1,2). The number of geriatric patients is expected to rise over time because of the increased life expectancy of the normal population.

Etiology is unknown, with no established lifestyle, occupational, or environmental risk factors. A genetic predisposition as well as exposure to radiation, chemicals, tobacco use, obesity, diet, and alcohol have been hypothesized as possible cause, but not yet demonstrated (2).

BIOLOGY AND PATHOGENESIS
Oncogenomics

Myeloma has complex heterogeneous cytogenetic abnormalities, most of which are of known prognostic significance (see "Prognosis"). Based on the pattern of chromosomal gain and losses, it can be subdivided into hyperdiploid (55–60%) and nonhyperdiploid karyotype (40–45%) (3).

Patients may present reciprocal chromosomal translocations, involving immunoglobulin H locus (14q32.3) and, less frequently, L locus (κ:2p12 or λ:22q11). In these translocations, various genes are juxtaposed to a strong immunoglobulin enhancer that disregulates their mRNA expression. The t(11;14)(q13;q32), present in 15% to 20% of patients, induces cyclin D1 over-expression, while t(6;14)(p21;q32) (5% of cases) increases cyclin D3 expression. The t(4;14) (p16.3;q32), present in about 15% patients, disregulates the Wolf-Hirschhorn syndrome candidate-1 and the fibroblast growth factor receptor-3 gene expression. Inhibition of fibroblast growth factor receptor-3 induces differentiation and apoptosis of plasma cells. The t(14;16)(q32;q23) disregulates the oncogene MAF, and t(14;20)(q32;q11) affects MAFB gene. Both translocations occur in 5% of patients. MAF increases MM cell proliferation and adhesion to bone marrow stromal cells.

Gain or loss of chromosomal regions occurs in all MM cases, which includes chromosome 13 deletion, loss of the short arm of chromosome 17 or of the short arm of chromosome 1, and gain or amplification of the long arm of chromosome 1 (4).

Many focal genetic lesions related to MM initiation and progression, involving tumor suppressor genes and oncogenes, have been identified from gene expression profiling studies (5,6).

Bone Marrow Microenvironment

The bone marrow microenvironment plays an essential role in MM pathogenesis. Recent studies have reinforced the relevance of extracellular matrix proteins (fibronectin, collagen, laminin, and osteopontin) and hematopoietic cells, stromal cells, endothelial cells, osteoclast, and osteoblast.

Adhesion to bone marrow stromal cells, mediated by various adhesion molecules (vascular cell adhesion molecule-4, intercellular adhesion molecule-1) directly stimulates, in both a paracrine and an autocrine manner, the production of cytokine and growth factors (interleukin-6, vascular endothelial growth factor, insulin growth factor-1) and activates an intracellular signaling cascade (involving extracellular signal-regulated kinase, janus kinase-2, activation of transcription-3-phosphatidilinositol-3-kinase and nuclear factor-κB). All these events promote tumor cell growth, survival, migration, and drug resistance. Secretion of angiogenetic factors, such us vascular endothelial growth factor, basic fibroblast growth factor, and hepatocyte growth factor, increased neo-angiogenesis. Receptor activator of nuclear factor-κB ligand produced by bone marrow stromal cells and macrophage inflammatory protein-1-alfa secreted by tumor cells stimulates osteoclastogenesis; osteoblastogenesis is inhibited by the secretion of interleukin-3 and Dickkopf-1 by MM cells and the secretion of hepatocyte growth factor by bone marrow stromal cells. Stimulation of osteoclastogenesis and inhibition of osteoblastogenesis promote osteolysis (7).

DIAGNOSIS

The diagnostic criteria have recently been updated for MM and the most common related-diseases (monoclonal gammopathy of undetermined significant (MGUS), smouldering MM (SMM) and plasmacytoma; Table 15.1 summarizes the diagnostic criteria of the other less-common disorders.

Diagnostic Work-up

Serum protein electrophoresis (SPEP) and urine protein electrophoresis (UPEP), on a 24-hours urine specimen, should be performed to screen the presence of monoclonal proteins. Immunofixation is necessary to determine the class of the

Table 15.1 Plasma Cell–Related Disorders (8)

Disorder	Disease definition
Plasma cell leukemia	Peripheral blood plasma cell count ≥2.0 ×10^9/L; ≥20% plasma cells in the peripheral blood differential white cell count. Primary: it presents in the leukemic phase; Secondary: it is leukemic transformation of a previously recognized MM.
Systemic AL amyloidosis	Presence in various tissues of amyloid derivated from the variable portion of monoclonal light chain, as a result of a clonal plasma cell proliferative disorder, plus evidence of an amyloid-related systemic syndrome (renal, liver, heart, gastrointestinal tract, or peripheral nerve involvement).
Waldenstrom macroglobulinemia	IgM monoclonal gammopathy with >10% bone marrow lymphoplasmacytic infiltration by small lymphocytes showing plasmacytoid or plasma cells differentiation and typical immunophenotype excluding other lymphoproliferative disorders.
POEMS Syndrome	Presence of a monoclonal plasma cell disorder, peripheral neuropathy, and at least one of the following seven features: osteosclerotic myeloma, Castleman disease, organomegaly, endocrinopathy (excluding diabetes mellitus or hypothyroidism), edema, typical skin changes, and papilledema.

Abbreviations: MM, multiple myeloma; POEMS, polyneuropathy, organomegaly, endocrinopathy, monoclonal-gammopathy, skin-changes.

monoclonal protein and to detect small amounts of proteins not relievable by electrophoresis. Quantification of the monoclonal protein by nefelometry completes the evaluation. Measurement of serum-free light-chain assay has been introduced into clinical practice to quantify κ and λ chains not bound to intact immunoglobulin. This assay is used to monitor patients with oligo/nonsecretory MM, light-chain MM, and primary amyloidosis. Diagnosis can be made by bone marrow aspirate and biopsy to demonstrate the infiltration of plasma cell in the bone marrow. Routine parameters including full blood count and blood chemistry (creatinine, calcium) and skeletal survey are used to determine the presence of organ damage. Magnetic resonance imaging (MRI) is more sensitive than skeletal survey to detect bone lesions: MRI is considered a second-level examination, suitable for patients with bone pain but with a negative skeletal survey and in case of suspected spinal cord compression. Computer tomography and MRI are indicated in case of suspected plasmacytoma. Diagnostic workup should be completed with prognostic markers: blood chemistry (β2-microglobulin, LDH, albumin), bone marrow cytogenetic, and fluorescent in situ hybridization.

Monoclonal Gammopathy of Undetermined Significance

MGUS is the most common plasma cell discrasia (3% of the population aged 50 years or older, with prevalence increasing according to age). It is an asymptomatic disorder characterized by

- monoclonal protein <3 g/dL;
- bone marrow plasma cells <10%;
- absence of end-organ damage attributable to plasma cell proliferation (8).

MGUS is associated with a lifelong risk of progression to MM or related disorders (1% per year), which does not diminish with time. Recognition is usually incidental, occurring when SPEP, UPEP, and immunofixation are performed in the workup of patients with a wide variety of medical conditions. The current standard of care is observation alone; patients may benefit from a risk-stratification [based on the size and type of monoclonal protein and serum-free light chain (9)] to guide follow-up; low-risk

patients can be rechecked in six months and then once every two years or only at the time of progression; all other patients need to be rechecked in six months, and then yearly thereafter.

Smouldering MM

SMM accounts for approximately 15% of all newly diagnosed MM. It is an asymptomatic condition whose recognition could be incidental. It is characterized by

- monoclonal protein (IgG or IgA) ≥3 g/dL;
- bone marrow plasma cells ≥10%;
- absence of end-organ damage attributable to plasma cell proliferation.

SMM is associated with a much higher lifelong risk of progression to MM or related disorders than MGUS (10% to 20% per year); patients must therefore be followed up closely (every three to four months), although they should not be treated until progression to symptomatic disease. Similar to MGUS, the type and size of monoclonal protein are an indicator of progression (8,10).

Symptomatic MM

Patients with symptomatic MM should be treated immediately. Symptomatic MM is defined by

- serum and/or urine monoclonal protein (in patients with no detectable monoclonal component, an abnormal serum-free light-chain ratio);
- bone marrow plasma cells ≥10%;
- evidence of end-organ damage attributable to plasma cell proliferation (*CRAB criteria*):
  - C: hypercalcemia (>11 mg/dL)
  - R: renal failure (creatinine >2 mg/dL)
  - A: anemia (hemoglobin <10.5 g/dL)
  - B: bone disease (lytic lesions or osteopenia) (11)

Anemia with fatigue is the more frequent feature at presentation, as well as bone pain secondary to bone disease. Hypercalcemia and renal failure require urgent treatment. Less frequently, patients present hepatomegaly and amyloidosis. Figure 15.1 shows frequencies of the main clinical

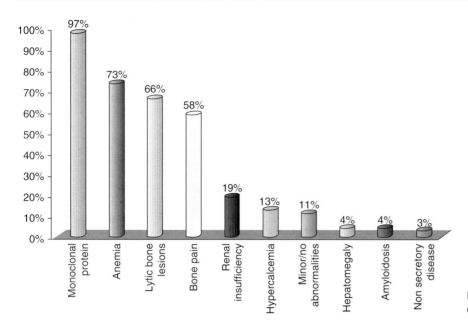

Figure 15.1 Main clinical presentation at diagnosis.

presentation at diagnosis. Recognition of organ damage and its correlation with MM is the first step to correctly suspect the evolution of MGUS or SMM to MM and to appropriately start therapy.

Plasmacytoma

Solitary plasmacytoma is rare; it is characterized by

- biopsy-proven solitary lesion of bone or soft tissue (most frequent upper respiratory tract, but it may virtually involve any organ) with evidence of clonal plasma cells;
- bone marrow not consistent with MM;
- normal skeletal survey and MRI of spine and pelvis;
- absence of end-organ damage attributable to plasma cell proliferation.

Treatment includes tumoricidal radiation. Patients are at the risk of progression to MM: the persistence of monoclonal protein after radiation is associated with an increased risk of progression. Progression generally occurs within three years (if it occurs), but patients must be followed up indefinitely (8).

PROGNOSTIC FACTORS

Albumin and β2-microglobulin have been identified has major prognostic factors and incorporated into a staging system. Cytogenetic analyses have shown prognostic activity, although they need to be validated in a large series of patients.

International Staging System

The current International Staging System (ISS) (Table 15.2) is a simple staging system using serum β2-microglobulin and albumin levels, because of the statistical power and the

wide availability of these two inexpensive laboratory tests. The ISS provides useful prognostic grouping regardless of age, therapy, and geographic area. Serum β2-microglobulin reflects tumor mass and renal function; in contrast, albumin levels reflect the effect of interleukine-6 produced by bone marrow microenvironment on the liver (12).

MM Biology

A prognostic correlation was found between cytogenetic abnormalities and survival. Patients with hyperdiploid MM tend to have a better prognosis than those with nonhyperdiploid disease (3). The t(14;16) and t(4;14) are associated with poor prognosis, whereas t(11;14) has a better prognosis. Deletion 13, deletion 17p, and gain or amplification of 1q have also been associated to poor prognosis (4).

A multivariate analysis including chromosomal aberrations [t(4;14) and deletion 17p] and β2-microglobulin values identified three patient subgroups with diverse outcomes: those lacking t(4;14) and deletion 17p, with a low β2-microglobulin have an excellent prognosis; patients presenting either t(4;14) or deletion 17p and high β2-microglobulin have a poor prognosis; all other patients have an intermediate prognosis (13).

Table 15.2 International Staging System (ISS) (12)

Stage	Criteria	Median survival (months)
I	β2 microglobulin <3.5 mg/L albumin ≥3.5 mg/L	62
II	not stage I or III[a]	44
III	β2 microglobulin ≥5.5 mg/L	29

[a]Two categories: β2 microglobulin <3.5 mg/L but albumin <3.5 mg/L; β2 microglobulin 3.5–5.5 mg/L irrespective of albumin.

Table 15.3 Response Criteria (11)

Response subcategory	Response criteria
CR	Negative immunofixation, disappearance of plasmacytomas, ≤5% bone marrow plasma cells
sCR	CR, normal free light-chain ratio, absence of clonal bone marrow plasma cells
VGPR	Monoclonal protein detectable by immunofixation but not on electrophoresis or ≥90% reduction in serum monoclonal protein plus urine monoclonal protein <100 mg/day
PR	≥50% reduction of serum monoclonal protein and reduction in urinary monoclonal protein by ≥90% or to <200 mg/24hr or ≥50% decrease in the difference between involved and uninvolved free light-chain levels or ≥50% reduction in plasma cells, ≥50% reduction in the size of plasmacytomas
SD	Not meeting criteria for CR, VGPR, PR, PD
PD	Increase of ≥25% in serum/urine monoclonal component, difference between involved and uninvolved free light-chain levels, bone marrow plasma cells percentage, development/increase in the size of new bone lesions or plasmacytomas, hypercalcemia

Abbreviations: CR, complete response; PD, progressive disease; PR, partial response; sCR, stringent CR; SD, stable disease; VGPR, very good partial response.

Gene expression profile improved molecular data-based patient stratification and prognostic staging (5,6).

Other factors related to a poor prognosis include plasma cell labeling index >3%, plasmablastic morphology, immunophenotype, high tumor burden, high LDH levels, and free light-chain ratio (14).

THERAPEUTIC CONSIDERATIONS
Selection of Therapy
Patients with symptomatic MM should be treated immediately. Treatment choice should be based on the patient's characteristics (age and presence of comorbidities) and on scientific evidence.

Patients younger than 65 years without relevant comorbidities that contraindicate high-dose therapy are candidates for autologous stem cell transplantation. Randomized trials have demonstrated superior response rate and survival in patients treated with high-dose therapy compared with those treated with conventional chemotherapy (15). All other patients should be treated with conventional chemotherapy plus new drugs. Standard treatment should always be supported by the evidence of improved progression-free survival (PFS), provided by a randomized trial. Smaller noncontrolled phase II studies should be considered as an important scientific evidence that need to be confirmed by randomized trials before deciding the standard of care. Table 15.3 summarizes the current response criteria. Tables 15.4 and 15.5 summarize the current acceptable regimens and the expected results for young and elderly patients.

Front-line Therapy in Young Patients
Induction Treatment
Vincristine+doxorubicin+dexamethasone (VAD) and dexamethasone alone were used for years as pretransplantation induction therapy. New drugs have recently been incorporated into pretransplantation regimens with promising preliminary results.

Thalidomide. A prospective randomized study compared thalidomide plus dexamethasone (TD) with VAD, showing a higher response rate after induction in patients treated with TD, although the benefit was not confirmed six months after autologous transplantation, since very good partial response (VGPR) rates were almost identical (16). Two randomized studies have demonstrated that TD is better than high-dose dexamethasone (HD): they reported higher response rates and prolonged time to progression (TTP) in patients receiving TD, not translated into overall survival (OS) improvement (17,18). The main toxicities related to thalidomide therapy are deep vein thrombosis (DVT) (12–26%) and peripheral neuropathy (2–7%). Based on these trials, the U.S. Food and Drug Administration (FDA) granted approval for TD for the treatment of newly diagnosed MM.

In two German-Dutch parallel phase III multicenter trials, the standard VAD regimen was compared with TD plus doxorubicin (TAD): higher VGPR rates after induction and after ASCT were reported, but results on survival are not yet available. Toxicities of the two regimens are comparable (19).

Bortezomib. A French randomized trial compared VAD with the association of bortezomib and HD (VD) as the induction regimen: preliminary results demonstrated that VD produced significantly higher pre- and post-transplantation VGPR rates (20). An ongoing Italian multicenter phase III trial compared VD plus thalidomide (VTD) with TD: data from the planned interim analysis showed that VGPR were significantly higher with VTD; this superiority was retained after the first transplantation (21). In both studies, additional follow-up is required to verify if this difference translate into a significant PFS advantage.

Doxorubicin combined with VD (PAD) are now being compared with VAD in another randomized trial; the results are not yet available, but different phase II studies (22,23) suggest a substantial activity of this regimen. Furthermore, it was investigated as part of induction regimen followed by reduced intensity autologous transplantation [Melphalan 100 mg/mq (Mel 100)] in elderly patients showing response rates similar to VD followed by melphalan 200 mg/mq (Mel 200) (20,24).

Lenalidomide. Lenalidomide plus HD (RD) was compared with HD alone in a double-blinded placebo-controlled trial: RD was demonstrated superior to HD in terms of responses and one-year PFS, while no differences in OS were reported (25). Another recent phase III study compared the combination of Lenalidomide plus low-dose

Table 15.4   Current Acceptable Induction and Consolidation/Maintenance Regimes and Expected Results for Young Myeloma Patients

	Regimen and doses	Response rate	Survival	References
Induction				
VAD	VCR: 0,4 mg days 1–4 Dox: 9 mg/m² days 1–4 Dex: 40 mg days 1–4, 9–12, 17–20 for three/four 4-wk cycles	CR: 2% ≥VGPR: 15–24% ≥PR: 54–71%	PFS: 90% at 12 months OS: 95% at 12 months	19,20
TD	Thal: 200 mg daily Dex: 40 mg days 1–4, 9–12, 17–20; or 40 mg/day for 4 days every other week for 2 months, then monthly for 2 months for three/four 3/4-wk cycles	CR: 4–5% ≥VGPR: 25% ≥PR: 49–79%	PFS/TTP: 50% at 17–22 months OS: 72% at 24 months	16,17,18,21
TAD	Thal: 200–400 mg days 1–28 Dox: 9 mg/m² days 1–4 Dex: 40 mg days 1–4, 9–12, 17–20 for three 4-wk cycles	CR: 4% ≥VGPR: 33% ≥PR: 72%	NA	19
VD	Bor: 1,3 mg/m² days 1,4,8,11 Dex: 40 mg days 1–4, 9–12 cycles 1–2; days 1–4 cycles 3–4 for four 4-wk cycles	≥VGPR: 50% ≥PR: 89%	PFS: 93% at 12 months OS: 97% at 12 months	20
VTD	Bor: 1,3 mg/m² days 1,4,8,11 Thal: 200 mg days 1–63 Dex: 40 mg days 1–2, 4–5, 8–9, 11–12 for three 3-wk cycles	≥VGPR: 60% ≥PR: 93%	NA	21
PAD/VDD	Bor: 1,3 mg/m² days 1,4,8,11 Dox: 9 mg/m² days 1–4 or PLD: 30 mg/m² day 4 Plus Dex: 40 mg days 1–4 (plus 8–11, 15–18 cycle 1 only) for four 3-wk cycles Or plus Dex: 20 mg days 1–2, 4–5, 8–9, 11–12, or 40 mg days 1–4 for six 3-wk cycles	CR: 12–24% ≥VGPR: 50–62% ≥PR: 89–97%	PFS: 50% at 29 months 91% at 12 months OS: 95% at 24 months	22,23,24
RD/Rd	Len: 25 mg days 1–28 Dex: 40 mg days 1–4, 9–12, 17–20 in a 5-wk cycles Len: 25 mg days 1–21 Dex: 40 mg days 1, 8, 15, 22 in a 4-wk cycles	CR: 22%	PFS: 77% at 12 months OS: 87–96% at 12 months	25,26
Consolidation				
Autologous transplant	Mel: 200 mg/m² + autologous stem cells	CR: 26–35% ≥VGPR: 55% ≥PR: 89–94%	EFS: 50% at 21–35 months OS: 66% at 45 months	27,28,30
	Mel: 100 mg/m² + autologous stem cells	≥PR: 77%	EFS: 50% at 28 months OS: 77% at 36 months	32
Reduced-intensity allogenic transplant	Nonmyeloablative total body irradiation + stem cells from HLA-identical sibling	CR: 55% ≥PR: 86%	EFS: 50% at 43 months OS: 78% at 48 months	30
	Nonmyeloablative chemotherapy + stem cells from HLA-identical sibling	≥VGPR: 62% ≥PR: 82%	EFS: 50% at 32 months OS: 50% at 35 months	31
Maintenance				
T-pamidronate	Thal: 50–400 mg daily Pamidronate: 90 mg at 4-wk intervals	≥VGPR: 67% ≥PR: 97%	EFS: 52% at 36 months OS: 87% at 48 months	33
TP	Thal: 200 mg daily (maximum 12 months) Prednisolone: 50 mg on alternate days	≥PR: 83–89%	PFS: 35% at 36 months OS: 86% at 36 months	34

Abbreviations: Bor, bortezomib; CR, complete response; Dox, doxorubicin; Dex, dexamethasone; EFS, event-free survival; Len, lenalidomide; Mel, melphalan; NA, not available; OS, overall survival; P, prednisolone; PAD, bortezomib-doxorubicin-dexamethasone; PFS, progression-free survival; PLD, pegilated lyposomal doxorubicin; PR, partial response; Rd, lenalidomide-low dose dexamethasone; RD, lenalidomide-high-dose dexamethasone; T, thalidomide; TAD, thalidomide-doxorubicin-dexamethasone; TD, thalidomide-dexamethasone; Thal, thalidomide; TP, thalidomide-prednisolone; TTP, time to progression; VAD, vincristine-doxorubicin-dexamethasone; VCR, vincristine; VD, bortezomib-dexamethasone; VDD, velcade-pegilated lyposomal doxorubicin-dexamethasone; VGPR, very good partial response; VTD, bortezomib-thalidomide-deamethasone; wk, week.

dexamethasone (Rd) with the RD: major grade 3 or higher toxic effects, including thrombosis (25% vs. 9%) and infections (16% vs. 6%), were significantly higher in the RD group, and one-year OS was significantly better with Rd. Increased mortality in the RD group was due to disease progression and side effects. Since the differences were confirmed in both younger and elderly patients, this study has major implications for the use of HD in newly diagnosed MM patients (26).

Consolidation and Maintenance

Results of a randomized trial comparing high-dose regimens suggest that Mel 200 should be the standard conditioning

Table 15.5 Current Acceptable Regimes and Expected Results for Elderly Patients or Young Patients Ineligible for High-Dose Therapy

Treatment	Regimen and doses	Response rate	Survival	References
MP	Mel: 0.25 mg/kg days 1–4; Pdn: 2 mg/kg days 1–4 for twelve 6-wk cycles Or Mel: 4 mg/m^2 days 1–7; Pdn: 40 mg/m^2 days 1–7 for six 4-wk cycles Or Mel: 9 mg/m^2 days 1–4; Pdn: 60 mg/m^2 days 1–4 for nine 6-wk cycles	CR: 1–5% ≥VGPR: 7–25% ≥PR: 31–50%	PFS/TTP: 50% at 14–21 months EFS: 27% at 24 months OS: 50% at 28–34 months 64% at 36 months	35,36,37,38, 39,40,41
MPT	Mel: 0.25 mg/kg days 1–4; Pdn: 2 mg/kg days 1–4; Thal: 100–400 mg/day for twelve 6-wk cycles +/– thal maintenance Or Mel: 4 mg/m^2 days 1–7; Pdn: 40 mg/m^2 days 1–7 for six 4-wk cycles; Thal: 100 mg daily until relapse or progressive disease	CR: 7–16% ≥VGPR: 22–43% ≥PR: 57–76%	PFS: 50% at 15–28 months EFS: 54% at 24 months OS: 50% at 28–52 months 80% at 36 months	37,38,39,40
VMP	Mel: 9 mg/m^2 days 1–4 Pdn: 60 mg/m^2 days 1–4 Bor: 1.3 mg/m^2 days 1,4,8,11,22,25,29,32 for the first four 6-wk cycles; days 1,8,15, 22 for the subsequent five 6-wk cycles	CR: 35% ≥VGPR: 45% ≥PR: 82%	TTP: 50% at 24 months	41
MPR	Mel: 0.18–0.25 mg/Kg days 1–4 Pdn: 2 mg/Kg days 1–4 for nine 4-wk cycles Len: 5–10 mg days 1–21 until relapse or progressive disease	CR: 24% ≥VGPR: 48% ≥PR: 81%	EFS: 95% at 12 months OS: 100% at 12 months	43

Abbreviations: Bor, bortezomib; CR, complete response; EFS, event-free survival; Len, lenalidomide; Mel, melphalan; MP, melphalan-prednisone; MPR, melphalan-prednisone-lenalidomide; MPT, melphalan-prednisone-thalidomide; OS, overall survival; Pdn, Prednisone; PFS, progression-free survival; PR, partial response; Thal, Thalidomide; TTP, time to progression; VGPR, very good partial response; VMP, bortezomib-melphalan-prednisone; wk, week.

regimen for eligible patients aged 65 years or younger (27). Tandem autologous transplantation offers better complete response (CR) rates compared with that of single transplantation: patients who achieved a CR after a single autologous transplantation experienced identical PFS to those who received a second transplant; by contrast, a second transplant is essential in patients achieving less than VGPR after the first one (28,29). Allogenic stem cell transplant offers substantial CR rate improvement and prolonged survival, although only a limited number of patients are eligible and it is associated with high treatment-related mortality. Tandem autologous transplantation plus reduced-intensity conditioning allograft was found to improve the outcome and reduce the treatment related mortality; an Italian study showed that patients with a HLA-matched sibling who received an autograft-allograft regimen had a significantly survival improvement in comparison with patients who underwent tandem autograft (30); a French study did not confirm these results (31).

Patients aged 65 to 70 years, with a good performance status and no relevant comorbidities, are eligible for a reduced-intensity autologous transplantation: a randomized trial comparing two courses of Mel 100 with standard MP showed longer three-year event-free survival (EFS) and OS in patients who underwent transplantation (32).

All randomized studies of transplantation were designed and implemented prior to the availability of new drugs, and therefore, the role of transplant may evolve in the future.

A variety of maintenance strategies have been investigated in patients whose diseases respond to autologous transplant, without univocal results. Two randomized studies (33,34) showed longer EFS and OS in patients treated with thalidomide (plus prednisolone or pamidronate) compared with patients who received no maintenance or pamidronate or prednisolone alone.

Front-line Therapy in Elderly Patients or Young Patients Ineligible for High-Dose Therapy

For elderly patients (older than 65 years) or young patients ineligible for high-dose therapy, the combination of oral melphalan and prednisone (MP) for years has been the conventional treatment. Despite better responses, no survival benefit has been reported with any other conventional chemotherapy. In a randomized trial, MP has been compared with melphalan plus dexamethasone (MD), HD, and HD plus interferon-α: improvement in PFS was reported in patients receiving melphalan as part of the induction treatment (both MP and MD) (35). Another randomized study compared MP with TD: despite a higher response rate with TD, patients treated with MP presented a significantly longer survival, particularly evident in patients older than 72 years. Patients on TD treatment had more extrahematological toxicity and early treatment discontinuation (36). Thus, melphalan or alkylating agents should always be included in the composition of treatment schema for newly diagnosed elderly patients. These results have provided the basis to combine the standard MP with novel agents.

Thalidomide. Four randomized (37–40) studies assessed the combination MP plus thalidomide (MPT), showing higher PR rates (57–76%) and longer PFS (median: 15–28 months) in patients treated with MPT compared with patients receiving MP; in two studies longer PFS translated into a significant improvement in OS. Thalidomide therapy was well tolerated; main toxicities were neuropathy, DVT, infections, and gastrointestinal toxicity, that, however, did not have a negative impact on survival, even in a very

Table 15.6 Current Acceptable Regimes and Expected Results for Relapsed Patients

Treatment	Regimen and doses	Response rate	Survival	References
VD	Bor: 1.3 mg/m² days 1,4,8,11 for eight 3-wk cycles; followed by days 1,8,15,22 for three 5-wk cycles Dex: 20 mg days 1–2, 4–5, 8–9, 11–12 in patients with progression after 2 cycles or PR after 4 cycles	CR: 6% ≥PR: 38% Improved response adding Dex in 18–33% of patients	TTP: 50% at 6 months OS: 80% at 12 months	44,45
V+PLD	Bor: 1.3 mg/m² days 1,4,8,11 PLD: 30 mg/m² day 4 for eight 3-wk cycles	CR: 4% ≥VGPR: 27% ≥PR: 44%	TTP: 50% at 9 months OS: 76% at 15 months	46
RD	Len: 25 mg days 1–21 Dex: 40 mg days 1–4, 9–12, 17–20 for the first four 4-wk cycles, then only days 1–4	CR: 14–16% PR: 60–61%	TTP: 50% at 11 months OS: 50% at 30 months	47,48
TD	Thal: 100–400 mg daily for a maximum of 12 months Dex: 40 mg for 4 days every other wk for 4 cycles and then monthly	PR: 65%	PFS: 47% at 12 months	49

Abbreviations: Bor, bortezomib; CR, complete response; Dex, dexamethasone; Len, lenalidomide; OS, overall survival; PFS, progression-free survival; PLD, pegylated lyposomal doxorubicin; PR, partial response; RD, lenalidomide-dexamethasone; TD, thalidomide-dexamethasone; Thal, thalidomide TTP, time to progression; VD, bortezomib-dexamethasone; VGPR, very good partial response; V+PLD, bortezomib-pegylated lyposomal doxorubicin; wk, week.

elderly population of patients aged >75 years (39). When compared with autologous transplantation (Mel 100) in patients aged 65 to 75 years old, MPT was associated with a significant improvement in survival and a significantly lower extrahematological toxicity (37).

Bortezomib. One randomized study compared MP with MP plus bortezomib (VMP). Preliminary results demonstrate that VMP was highly superior to MP for CR rate, TTP, and OS. The TTP benefit was seen consistently across patient subgroups, and its efficacy was not affected by renal function or high-risk disease (41), confirming the results of a phase II study evaluating the same regimen (42). This regime showed a significant increase in gastrointestinal toxicities, peripheral neuropathy, fatigue, and infections; DVT rate was low in both patient subgroups (41).

Lenalidomide. Lenalidomide plus MP (MPR) has been evaluated in a phase I/II study showing promising results (one-year PFS and OS of 95% and 100%, respectively); severe neutropenia was the most frequent adverse event; the incidence of nonhematologic adverse events was low (febrile neutropenia 9% and thromboembolism 5%) (43). A randomized double-blind trial comparing MP versus MPR is ongoing.

Treatment at Relapse

In relapsing patients, it is important to consider response and toxicities related to prior therapies: relapses occurring later than 18 months from previous therapy may be retreated with the same regimen, if well tolerated.

Bortezomib. Bortezomib is considered one of the standards of care for salvage therapy based on the results of a phase III trial comparing bortezomib and HD, reporting significant improvement in TTP and one-year OS in bortezomib-treated patients (44); addiction of dexamethasone was associated with improved responses (45). Recently, based on results of a phase III trial comparing bortezomib plus pegylated liposomal doxorubicin with bortezomib alone [showing that the use of the drug combination significantly extends both TTP and OS (46)], FDA has approved a regimen consisting of bortezomib plus pegylated liposomal doxorubicin for patients who have received at least one prior therapy (not including bortezomib).

Lenalidomide. RD has received FDA approval based on the results of two randomized studies comparing RD with HD in patients who have received at least one prior treatment, showing that the drug combination significantly improves TTP and OS (47,48).

Thalidomide. TD has been compared with HD in a phase III trial, and preliminary results demonstrated higher response rates and longer one-year PFS in patients treated with the two drugs (49).

Bortezomib, lenalidomide, and thalidomide can also be combined with doxorubicin, cyclophosphamide, or melphalan. A chemotherapy agent should be added in the presence of a suboptimal response to combination including new drugs and steroids; a sequential approach should be adopted, alternating different drugs in subsequent relapses. Combinations including chemotherapy regimes have shown higher response rates in comparison with dexamethasone alone, although randomized trials should confirm this preliminary evidence. Table 15.6 shows the current acceptable regimens and the expected results for relapsed patients.

ACKNOWLEDGEMENTS

We thank Antonella Bono and Tatiana Ouroussouff for technical assistance in preparing and editing the manuscript.

REFERENCES

1. Altieri A, Chen B, Bermejo JL et al. Familiar risk and temporal incidence trends of multiple myeloma. Eur J Cancer 2006; 42: 1161–70.
2. Alexander DD, Mink PJ, Adami HO et al. Multiple myeloma: a review of the epidemiologic literature. Int J Cancer 2007; 120: 40–61.
3. Smadja NV, Fruchart C, Isnard F et al. Chromosomal analysis in multiple myeloma: cytogenetic evidence of two different diseases. Leukemia 1998; 12: 960–9.
4. Hideshima T, Mitsiades C, Tonon G et al. Understanding multiple myeloma pathogenesis in the bone marrow to identify new therapeutic targets. Nat Rev Cancer 2007; 7: 585–98.

5. Carrasco DR, Tonon G, Huang Y et al. High-resolution genomic profiles define distinct clinico-pathogenetic subgroups of multiple myeloma patients. Cancer Cell 2006; 9: 313–25.

6. Shaughnessy JD Jr, Zhan F, Burington BE et al. A validated gene expression model of high-risk multiple myeloma is defined by deregulated expression of genes mapping to chromosome 1. Blood 2007; 109: 2276–84.

7. Podar K, Richardson PG, Hideshima T et al. The malignant clone and the bone-marrow environment. Best Pract Res Clin Haematol 2007; 20: 597–612.

8. Rajkumar SV, Dispenzieri A, Kyle RA. Monoclonal gammopathy of undetermined significance, Waldenström macroglobulinemia, AL amyloidosis, and related plasma cell disorders: diagnosis and treatment. Mayo Clin Proc 2006; 81: 693–703.

9. Rajkumar SV, Kyle RA, Therneau TM et al. Serum free light chain ratio is an independent risk factor for progression in monoclonal gammopathy of undetermined significance. Blood 2005; 106: 812–17.

10. Weber DM, Wang LM, Delasalle KB et al. Risk factors for early progression of asymptomatic multiple myeloma. Hematol J 2003; 4: S31, abstract P4.2.

11. Durie BG, Harousseau JL, Miguel JS et al. International uniform response criteria for multiple myeloma. Leukemia 2006; 20: 1467–73.

12. Greipp PR, San Miguel J, Durie BG et al. International staging system for multiple myeloma. J Clin Oncol 2005; 23: 3412–20.

13. Avet-Loiseau H, Attal M, Moreau P et al. Genetic abnormalities and survival in multiple myeloma: the experience of the Intergroupe Francophone du Myélome. Blood 2007; 109: 3489–95.

14. Fonseca R, San Miguel J. Prognostic factors and staging in multiple myeloma. Hematol Oncol Clin North Am 2007; 21: 1115–40.

15. Bensinger W. Stem-cell transplantation for multiple myeloma in the era of novel drugs. J Clin Oncol 2008; 26: 480–92.

16. Macro M, Divine M, Uzunhan Y et al. Dexamethasone + thalidomide (dex/thal) compared to VAD as a pre-transplant treatment in newly diagnosed multiple myeloma (MM): a randomised trial. Blood 2006; 108: abstract 57.

17. Rajkumar SV, Blood E, Vesole D et al. Phase III clinical trial of thalidomide plus dexamethasone compared with dexamethasone alone in newly diagnosed multiple myeloma: a clinical trial coordinated by the Eastern Cooperative Oncology Group. J Clin Oncol 2006; 24: 431–6.

18. Rajkumar SV, Hussein M, Catalano J et al. A multicenter, randomized, double-blind, placebo-controlled trial of thalidomide plus dexamethasone versus dexamethasone alone as initial therapy for newly diagnosed multiple myeloma. J Clin Oncol 2006; 24: 7517.

19. Lokhorst HM, Schmidt-Wolf I, Sonneveld P et al. Thalidomide in induction treatment increases the very good partial response rate before and after high-dose therapy in previously untreated multiple myeloma. Haematologica 2008; 93: 124–7.

20. Harousseau JL, Mathiot C, Attal M et al. VELCADE/dexamethasone (Vel/D) versus VAD as induction treatment prior to autologous stem cell transplantation (ASCT) in newly diagnosed multiple myeloma (MM): updated results of the IMF 2005/01 trial. Blood 2007; 110: abstract 139.

21. Cavo M, Patriarca F, Tacchetti P et al. Bortezomib (Velcade®)-thalidomide-dexamethasone (VTD) vs thalidomide-dexamethasone (TD) in preparation for autologous stem-cell (SC) transplantation (ASCT) in newly diagnosed multiple myeloma (MM). Blood 2007; 110: abstract 30.

22. Popat R, Oakervee HE, Hallam S et al. Bortezomib, doxorubicin and dexamethasone (PAD) front-line treatment of multiple myeloma: updated results after long-term follow-up. Br J Haematol 2008; 141: 512–16.

23. Jakubowiak AJ, Al-Zoubi A, Kendall T et al. Combination therapy with bortezomib (VELCADE), Doxil, and dexamethasone (VDD) in newly diagnosed myeloma: updated results of phase II clinical trial. Haematologica 2007; 92: 180–1.

24. Palumbo A, Avonto I, Patriarca F et al. Bortezomib, peylated-lyposomal-doxorubicin and dexamethasone followed by melphalan 100 mg/m^2 in elderly newly diagnosed patients: an interim analysis. Blood 2007; 110: abstract 138.

25. Zonder JA, Crowley J, Hussein MA et al. Superiority of Lenalidomide (Len) plus high-dose dexamethasone (HD) compared to HD alone as treatment of newly diagnosed multiple myeloma (NDMM): results of the randomized, double-blinded, placebo-controlled SWOG Trial S0232. Blood 2007; 110: 32a, abstract 77.

26. Rajkumar SV, Jacobus S, Callander N et al. A randomized trial of Lenalidomide plus high-dose dexamethasone (RD) versus Lenalidomide plus low-dose dexamethasone (Rd) in newly diagnosed multiple myeloma (E4A03): a trial coordinated by the Eastern Cooperative Group. Blood 2007; 110: abstract 74.

27. Moreau P, Facon T, Attal M et al. Comparison of 200 mg/m^2 melphalan and 8 Gy total body irradiation plus 140 mg/m^2 melphalan as conditioning regimens for peripheral blood stem cell transplantation in patients with newly diagnosed multiple myeloma: final analysis of the Intergroupe Francophone du Myélome 9502 randomized trial. Blood 2002; 99: 731–5.

28. Cavo M, Tosi P, Zamagni E et al. Prospective, randomized study of single compared with double autologous stem-cell transplantation for multiple myeloma: Bologna 96 clinical study. J Clin Oncol 2007; 25: 2434–41.

29. Attal M, Harousseau JL, Facon T et al. Single versus double autologous stem-cell transplantation for multiple myeloma. N Engl J Med 2003; 349: 2495–502.

30. Bruno B, Rotta M, Patriarca F et al. A comparison of allografting with autografting for newly diagnosed myeloma. N Engl J Med 2007; 356: 1110–20.

31. Garban F, Attal M, Michallet M et al. Prospective comparison of autologous stem cell transplantation followed by dose-reduced allograft (IFM99-03 trial) with tandem autologous stem cell transplantation (IFM99-04 trial) in high-risk de novo multiple myeloma. Blood 2006; 107: 3474–80.

32. Palumbo A, Bringhen S, Petrucci MT et al. Intermediate-dose melphalan improves survival of myeloma patients aged 50 to 70: results of a randomized controlled trial. Blood 2004; 104: 3052–7.

33. Attal M, Harousseau JL, Leyvraz S et al. Maintenance therapy with thalidomide improves survival in patients with multiple myeloma. Blood 2006; 108: 3289–94.

34. Spencer A, Prince HM, Roberts A et al. Thalidomide improve survivals when use after ASCT. Haematologica 2007; 92: abstract S7b.

35. Facon T, Mary JY, Pégourie B et al. Dexamethasone-based regimens versus melphalan-prednisone for elderly multiple myeloma patients ineligible for high-dose therapy. Blood 2006; 107: 1292–8.

36. Ludwig H, Tothova E, Hajek R et al. Thalidomide-dexamethasone versus melphalan prednisolone as first line treatment in elderly patients with multiple myeloma: second interim analysis. Haematologica 2007; 1: abstract 446.

37. Facon T, Mary JY, Hulin C et al. Melphalan and prednisone plus thalidomide versus melphalan and prednisone alone or reduced-intensity autologous stem cell transplantation in elderly patients with multiple myeloma (IFM 99-06): a randomised trial. Lancet 2007; 370: 1209–18.

38. Palumbo A, Bringhen S, Caravita T et al. Oral melphalan and prednisone chemotherapy plus thalidomide compared with melphalan and prednisone alone in elderly patients with multiple myeloma: randomised controlled trial. Lancet 2006; 367: 825–31.

39. Hulin C, Facon T, Rodon P et al. Melphalan-Prednisone-Thalidomide (MP-T) demonstrates a significant survival advantage in elderly patients >75 years with multiple myeloma compared with Melphalan and Prednisone (MP) in a randomized, double blind, placebo-controlled trial IFM 01-01. Blood 2007; 110: abstract 75.

40. Waage A, Gimsing P, Juliusson G et al. Melphalan-Prednisone-Thalidomide to newly diagnosed patients with multiple myeloma: a placebo controlled randomised trial phase 3 trial. Blood 2007; 110: abstract 78.

41. San Miguel JF, Schlag R, Khuageva N et al. MMY-3002: a phase 3 study comparing bortezomib-melphalan-prednisone (VMP) with melphalan-prednisone (MP) in newly diagnosed multiple myeloma. Blood 2007; 110: abstract 31.

42. Mateos M-V, Hernández J-M, Hernàndez M-T et al. Bortezomib plus melphalan and prednisone in elderly untreated patients with multiple myeloma: updated time-to-events results and prognostic factors for time to progression. Haematologica 2008; 93: 560–5.

43. Palumbo A, Falco P, Corradini P et al. Melphalan, prednisone, and lenalidomide treatment for newly diagnosed myeloma: a report from the GIMEMA--Italian Multiple Myeloma Network. J Clin Oncol 2007; 25: 4459–65.

44. Richardson PG, Sonneveld P, Schuster MW et al. Bortezomib or high-dose dexamethasone for relapsed multiple myeloma. N Engl J Med 2005; 352: 2487–98.

45. Jagannath S, Richardson PG, Barlogie B et al. Bortezomib in combination with dexamethasone for the treatment of patients with relapsed and/or refractory multiple myeloma with less than optimal response to bortezomib alone. Haematologica 2006; 91: 929–34.

46. Orlowski RZ, Nagler A, Sonneveld P et al. Randomized phase III study of pegylated liposomal doxorubicin plus bortezomib compared with bortezomib alone in relapsed or refractory multiple myeloma: combination therapy improves time to progression. J Clin Oncol 2007; 25: 3892–901.

47. Weber DM, Chen C, Niesvizky R et al. Lenalidomide plus dexamethasone for relapsed multiple myeloma in North America. N Engl J Med 2007; 357: 2133–42.

48. Dimopoulos M, Spencer A, Attal M et al. Lenalidomide plus dexamethasone for relapsed or refractory multiple myeloma. N Engl J Med 2007; 357: 2123–32.

49. Fermand JP, Jaccard A, Macro M et al. A randomized comparison of dexamethasone + thalidomide (Dex/Thal) vs Dex + Placebo (Dex/P) in patients (pts) with relapsing multiple myeloma (MM). Blood 2006; 108: abstract 3563.

16

Management of Gliomas, Medulloblastoma, CNS Germ Cell Tumors, and Carcinomas Metastatic to the CNS

Andreas F. Hottinger, Damien C. Weber, Marc Levivier, and Roger Stupp

INTRODUCTION

Primary tumors of the central nervous system need to be distinguished from metastatic lesions. Although primary brain tumors are relatively rare in adults, with a yearly incidence of approximately 10/100,000 representing only 2% of all malignancies, brain metastases (secondary brain tumors) are more common and present in almost one out of four patients with advanced stage cancer and in one-fourth of patients who die from cancer. The most common primary tumors are lung, breast carcinoma, and melanoma. An increasing incidence of both primary and secondary brain tumors since the 1970s has been suggested. This likely reflects greater access to imaging and improved neuroimaging techniques as well as better treatments and longer survival of cancer patients in general.

Neurological Signs and Symptoms

Symptoms related to intracranial tumors may be manifold and nonspecific (Table 16.1). Many patients with brain tumors have no or only minor symptoms for a long time, in whom the diagnosis may be fortuitous. Other patients may have abrupt onset of symptoms secondary to complications of the tumor such as seizure, increased intracranial pressure (e.g., obstructive hydrocephalus), intracranial bleeding, or ischemia. Except in the case of an acute event, the neurological examination is often normal, and a high index of suspicion is necessary. Headache is the most common symptom of a brain tumor. It is, however, nonspecific and may occur both in patients with increased or normal intracranial pressure. Some specific features should increase the suspicion of a tumor, such as new onset of headaches in middle-aged or older persons, daily headache on waking improving rapidly thereafter, change in pattern, character, or severity of a chronic headache, exacerbation of headache following coughing, sneezing, head movement, or exertion, acute headache followed by vomiting, or any headache with accompanying neurological deficit. Poorly described dizziness and tinnitus are also common complaints of patients with new brain tumors. Focal seizures, with or without secondary generalization, are the most common localized sign of a brain tumor and occur in about one-third of patients, in particular, if the tumor is localized close to the cortex. Conversely, about 20% of adults with inaugural seizures will have an underlying brain tumor. Possible focal findings include hemiparesis, aphasia, visual field loss, and sensory disturbances. Brain tumors may also be associated with cognitive or personality changes.

Patient Workup

The workup needs to answer a number of key questions: (a) Is it a single lesion, or are multiple lesions visible? (b) Does this patient have a known underlying disease (e.g., known active or previously treated cancer; immunosuppressive state (abscess, lymphoma), or (c) Is it surgically accessible for complete resection or debulking?

Multiple lesions are suggestive of a metastatic tumor, while a single mass may be either a primary or a metastatic brain tumor. The most frequent origin for a brain metastasis is primary lung and breast cancer, which can be detected by a standard chest-X-ray or a mammography and clinical breast examination. Brain metastases may also be due to occult renal cell cancer or previously unrecognized melanoma (e.g., resected "benign naevus" many years ago). In case of a single symptomatic CNS tumor, immediate resection will provide symptomatic relief and treatment as well as histological diagnosis. This is more efficient than extensive visceral workup aiming at identifying a putative primary tumor, whereas the ultimate treatment approach remains tumor resection in the brain. If a primary CNS lymphoma is suspected or an abscess cannot be ruled out, steroids should be withheld until surgical sampling.

Management of brain tumors requires a multidisciplinary team and coordinated diagnostic approach. For all decisions regarding the management of brain tumors, the performance status and neurological function plays an important role. Ideally, patients should be discussed upfront between neuroradiologists, pathologists, neurosurgeons, medical, neuro-, and radiation oncologists. This will allow the possibility of obtaining tumor tissue in an effective way to establish the correct diagnosis, maximum tumor debulking, and adequate postoperative therapy with radiation and/or chemotherapy.

In this chapter, the main features and treatments of primary and secondary (metastatic) brain tumors are summarized, and the management of primary CNS lymphoma is covered in chapter 16.

PRIMARY BRAIN TUMORS

Primary brain tumors are subdivided according to their localization: i.e., brain parenchyma, meninges, pituitary region,

Table 16.1   Common Signs and Symptoms of Brain Tumors

- No symptoms
- Headache
- Nausea/vomiting (especially on awakening)
- Changes of personality
- Memory loss
- Confusion
- Seizures
- Focal weakness
- Difficulty walking
- Visual disturbances
- Tinnitus

Table 16.2   WHO Histological Classification of Brain Tumors

Neuroepithelial tumors
- Astrocytic tumors
  - Pilocytic astrocytoma (grade 1)
  - Diffuse astrocytoma (grade 2)
  - Anaplastic astrocytoma (grade 3)
  - Glioblastoma (grade 4)
  - Pleomorphic xanthoastrocytoma
  - Subependymal giant cell astrocytoma
- Oligodendroglial tumors
  - Oligodendroglioma, low-grade (2) or anaplastic (grade 3)
- Ependymal tumors
  - Ependymoma, low-grade (2) or anaplastic (grade 3)
  - Myxopapillary ependymoma
  - Subependymoma
- Choroid plexus
  - Choroid plexus papilloma
  - Choroid plexus carcinoma
- Neuronal/mixed glial neuronal tumors
  - Gangliocytoma
  - Ganglioglioma
  - Dysembryoplastic neuroepithelial tumor
  - Central neurocytoma
- Pineal parenchymal tumors
  - Pineocytoma
  - Pineal parenchymal tumor of intermediate differentiation
  - Pineoblastoma
- Embryonal tumors
  - Medulloblastoma
  - Primitive neuroectodermal tumor (PNET)
  - Atypical teratoid/rhabdoid tumor

Tumors of cranial nerve
- Schwannoma
- Neurofibroma
- Malignant peripheral nerve sheath tumor

Meningeal tumors
- Meningioma
- Hemangiopericytoma
- Hemangioblastoma
- Melanocytoma

Germ cell tumors
- Germinoma
- Teratoma, mature or immature
- Mixed tumors
- Embryonal carcinoma
- Yolk sac tumor (endodermal sinus tumor)
- Choriocarcinoma

Primary CNS Lymphoma

Tumors of the sellar region
- Pituitary adenoma (not included in WHO CNS tumors)
- Craniopharyngioma
- Granular cell tumor

Cysts and tumor-like lesions
- Rathke cleft cysts
- Epidermoid cyst
- Dermoid cyst
- Colloid cyst of third ventricle

Metastatic tumors: not included in WHO CNS tumors

pineal region, or skull base. Definite diagnosis of primary brain tumors requires histopathological assessment and is based on the cell of origin of the tumor. The World Health Organization (WHO) classification is most commonly used, and regularly updated, most recently in 2006 (Table 16.2). The classification is based on histological features and architecture, with molecular markers being recognized and described, but not (yet) included as a standard diagnostic procedure. Within a tumor, differences in grade may be observed. The most malignant grade defines the diagnosis and will determine the prognosis. Because of the relative rarity of primary brain tumors, review by an experienced and specialized neuropathologist is recommended.

The incidence of primary brain tumors varies by race, age, sex, and geography. Brain tumors, with the exception of pituitary adenomas and meningiomas, are more common in Caucasians than in other ethnic groups. Men are at higher risk than women for developing most brain tumors, except for meningiomas (1).

Ionizing radiation and immune suppression are the two only unequivocal risk factors identified for the development of brain tumors. Many other risk factors (including electromagnetic fields, aspartame, exposure to petroleum derivatives or pesticides and tuberculosis, varicella zoster or simian virus 40 infections) have been reported in some smaller and nonconclusive studies. An increasing number of molecular genetic alterations have been identified in association with specific brain tumors (Fig. 16.1) (2). In summary, genetic changes involved in the pathogenesis of gliomas affect two major cell functions:

1. Overexpression of growth factors or their receptors [such as epithelial growth factor (EGF), or platelet-derived growth factor (PDGF)] that directly or indirectly activate signaling pathways such as RAS and AKT: Alternatively, inactivating mutations of tumor suppressors such as PTEN results in blocked inhibition of the same pathways.
2. Alteration of the cell cycle: Loss of inhibitors of the cell cycle such as INK4A, RB, p53, and others can also lead to tumor formation.

Further developments in genomics and proteomics will result in an exponential increase in the knowledge about brain tumors and should lead to the development of novel therapeutic strategies.

Gliomas account for over two-thirds of primary brain tumors, with glioblastoma being the most frequent primary brain tumor in adults. Gliomas arise from one of the basic types of glial cells: astrocytes, oligodendrocytes, and ependymal cells. The different types of gliomas have a number of common characteristics, notably their infiltrative growth pattern and absence of distinct margins, usually preventing complete resection. Genetic instability leads to

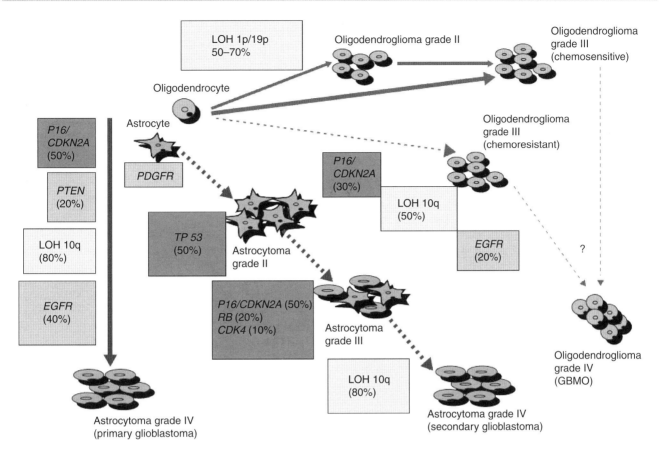

Figure 16.1 Molecular pathways of primary brain tumors. *Source*: From Ref. 2 with permission. *Abbreviations*: LOH, loss of heterozygosity; GBM, glioblastoma; GBMO, glioblastoma with oligodendroglial component. Dark grey squares correspond to genetic alterations of cell cycle control. TP53, mutation; RB, mutation; P16/CDKN2A, homozygous deletion; CDK4, amplification. Mid grey squares correspond to genetic alterations affecting signal transduction pathways. EGFR, amplification; PDGFR, overexpression; PTEN, mutation. Light grey squares correspond to loss of heterozygosity on chromosomes 1p/19q or 10q.

Surgery

Neurosurgery plays a central role in the management of most brain tumors. The goal of surgery in neuro-oncology is manifold:

- Diagnostic: To obtain adequate tissue for accurate histological diagnostic, to optimize prognosis and therapeutic choices.
- Symptomatic: To improve the neurological function, by relieving focal mass effect and intracranial hypertension.
- Therapeutic: Cytoreduction with complete or partial removal of the tumor. Some local therapies may also be delivered surgically (e.g., convection-enhanced delivery, carmustine-impregnated biodegradable wafers).

Several operative approaches and surgical techniques may be used to treat brain tumors. The choice will depend on the size and the location of the tumor, its radiological characteristics, the presumed histological diagnosis, as well as the age, general clinical status, and neurological symptoms of the patient. In the presence of a space-occupying lesion in the brain, general surgical principles prevail; however, they will be adapted on the basis of the specific type of tumor, i.e., whether benign or malignant, primary or secondary.

Advancement and new possibilities in modern medical imaging, as well as progress and developments in neurosurgical techniques and in neuro-anesthesia allow improved surgical performances, while reducing the operative risks and complications. Image-guided and computer-assisted neurosurgery plays an increasing role in the surgical management of brain tumors. Stereotaxic tumor localization allows performing accurate and safe biopsy in almost any area of the brain. Neuronavigation allows for improving the resection of brain tumors, thanks to accurate preoperative planning and more precise intraoperative guidance. Radiosurgery, which combines stereotaxis and radiation therapy, offers complementary or alternative therapeutic approaches, based on the same image-guidance principles. Modern software planning for stereotaxis, neuronavigation, and radiosurgery allows integrating multimodality images, including functional and metabolic data, such as PET scan.

Ideally, the goal of the neurosurgical procedure is to perform complete resection of the tumor and to cure the patient. Because the nervous system is a highly functional organ, this concept can only rarely be fulfilled, and the neurosurgical resection is limited by the functional areas surrounding the tumor and the risks of complications. Most benign extra-axial tumors, such as meningiomas or schwannomas, can be totally resected. In some instances, when the lesion is located in the skull-base and involves functional structures, such as cranial nerves or major vessels, the tumor cannot be resected in toto, and the residual disease may give rise to recurrence. Primary intracerebral tumors are infiltrating by nature, which often precludes complete resection. If the lesion is small and focal, located in a cerebral lobe, a lobectomy approach might allow the removal of the entire tumor, especially in low-grade glioma. In most cases, subtotal resection or debulking of the tumor is performed. Even in these cases, attempt to perform maximal resection is recommended, since it results in better survival. Secondary tumors, i.e., metastases of systemic cancers, are well-circumscribed lesions that may benefit of complete surgical removal. When the lesion is large and symptomatic due to mass effect, surgery will allow the most rapid clinical improvement. Surgery is often recommended for single brain metastasis.

Stereotactic biopsy, a relatively simple procedure allows for tissue diagnosis of deep seated unresectable tumors or when the patient's general condition does not allow surgical tumor resection. The risk of bleeding is estimated between 1% and 3%.

Radiation Therapy

Radiation therapy (RT) is an essential treatment modality for CNS tumors and is often combined with chemotherapy. RT induces (single and double strand) DNA breakage and ultimately induces apoptosis. The efficacy of RT depends on the delivery of adequate dose of RT to the target tissue, while sparing normal structures in the vicinity of the target volume.

RT is usually administered with photons delivered with a high-energy linear accelerator. Protons and charged heavy particles may also be used for the treatment of brain tumors. External beam radiotherapy is the most common RT-technique for brain tumors. It uses multiple spatially distributed intersecting beams to deliver RT to a defined 3D volume. Multiple equal doses of radiotherapy are administered, and patients must be immobilized in a fixation mask to ensure accuracy. Stereotactic RT regroups a number of techniques for the delivery of radiation beams to a very precise location. The two methods consist of (1) a multiheaded cobalt unit (gamma-knife) and (2) a linear accelerator capable of administering RT in multiple coplanar arcs or multiple coplanar beams in stereotactic conditions. Dose can be delivered in one fraction (i.e., radiosurgery) or with a conventional fractionation scheme (stereotactic fractionated RT). Particle beam radiotherapy uses heavy particles such as protons and neutrons. As these particles deposit their energy at the end of their trajectory through tissue (Bragg peak effect), this technique allows to precisely deliver the dose to the target volume. Proton therapy is restricted to the management of skull base tumors (chordoma and chondrosarcoma), pediatric brain tumors, and occasionally pituitary adenomas.

The side effects of RT are classified as acute, early delayed, and late complications. Acute reactions develop within hours to days of treatment and are typically caused by increased tumor associated edema, which may be treated with steroids. Early delayed complications, such as alopecia, skin erythema, and asthenia occur six weeks to six months following RT. Focal demyelination may induce transitory worsening neurological deficits. Furthermore, patients may present with fatigue and mild memory impairment. Radionecrosis and cognitive dysfunction are occasional late complications of RT, typically occurring years after completion of RT. The probability of developing radionecrosis and cognitive impairments increase with the total administered dose and dose per fraction, respectively. Provided that the brain-dose tolerance is considered, several prospective studies have shown that these complications are rare.

a tendency of malignant degeneration over time. Histologically, gliomas are graded from one to four. Grade 1 and 2 gliomas are often referred to as low-grade gliomas (or incorrectly benign gliomas), and grades 3 and 4 are described as high grade. Grade 1 gliomas are pilocytic astrocytomas almost exclusively seen in children; diffuse gliomas are either low-grade (grade 2) or anaplastic (grade 3), in its most aggressive form glioblastoma (grade 4). The prognosis and treatment is determined mainly by their histological grade, and to a lesser extent, also by the underlying cell type. Prognostic factors for a better outcome include younger age of the patient and tumor resectability. In elderly patients, tumors are often more aggressive and carry an inferior prognosis.

Glioblastoma

Glioblastoma (GBM)—in older terminology referred to as glioblastoma multiforme—is the most common and most aggressive of all primary brain tumors (3). It accounts for 12% to 15% of all intracranial neoplasms and 45% to 50% of all gliomas, with an incidence of 3–5:100,000 per year (3). It may affect patients of any age but is observed most commonly in individuals between age 45 and 65 years. There is a slight male preponderance (ratio 1.5:1). GBM usually develops in the subcortical white matter of the cerebral hemispheres, most commonly in the frontal and temporal lobes. It can however occur anywhere in the CNS, including the spinal cord. Most GBM arise de novo without recognizable precursor lesions (primary GBM).

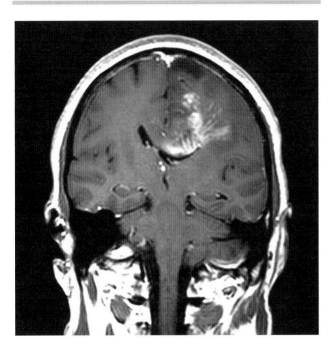

Figure 16.2 Radiological appearance of glioblastoma on MRI (gadolinium-enhanced T1-weighted MR image).

Anti-epileptic Drugs and Chemotherapy

A significant number of patients with high-grade gliomas and metastases develop seizures, especially if the tumor is localized close to the cortex and in the temporal, frontal, or parietal lobe. The seizures are typically simple partial, complex partial, or secondary generalized.

Antiepileptic drugs may induce overlapping toxicity with chemo- or radiation therapy [e.g., myelosuppression, dermatologic reactions, and radiosensitization. Many antiepileptic drugs (notably phenytoin, phenobarbital, carbamazeipin and its derivates) will induce the P450 hepatic enzymes thus increasing the metabolism of hepatically eliminated chemotherapeutic agents. This is less relevant for nitrosoureas, temozolomide, thiotepa, methotrexate, and corticosteroids (78)]. Conversely, many chemotherapeutic agents alter the metabolism of anticonvulsant agents. Thus, third-generation antiepileptic drugs should be the first choice in cancer patients.

Prophylactic administration of anticonvulsant medication in patients who never had a seizure has been abandoned; anticonvulsants prophylactically prescribed because of brain surgery should be tapered and discontinued in the first postoperative weeks (79).

Secondary GBM develop from lower-grade diffuse gliomas (WHO grade 2) or from anaplastic gliomas (WHO grade 3). Although the underlying genetic mechanisms involved in the pathogenesis is entirely different for primary and secondary GBM and can be determined on a molecular level, the two types cannot be distinguished histologically (Fig. 16.1). Similarly, prognosis and treatment are the same once a glioblastoma has been formally established. For practical purposes, we distinguish the more common de novo (primary) GBMs based on a short clinical history of symptoms lasting for less than three months, from patients with a longer evolution, symptoms dating back >6 months to years, or prior diagnosis of a lower-grade glioma. On magnetic resonance imaging (MRI), GBM appear as a heterogeneous enhancing mass with or without necrotic or cystic core. The margins are usually diffuse reflecting the invasiveness of the normal surrounding brain parenchyma of these tumors. Prominent peritumoral edema is common (Fig. 16.2). Histopathological confirmation of the diagnosis is mandatory and may allow further molecular tumor characterization. The latter is of increasing importance as novel, tailored, and targeted treatments emerge and, ideally, some tumor tissue should be conserved frozen at initial diagnostic procedure. GBM shows cellular and nuclear atypia, endothelial proliferation and, necrosis typically surrounded by radially oriented densely packed, small fusiform glioma cells in a pseudopalisading pattern.

Management of Newly Diagnosed GBM

Surgical resection to the extent that is safely feasible remains the first step in the management of glioblastoma. Strategies of primary (neoadjuvant) chemotherapy before surgery remain investigational and are unlikely to have an impact on resectability and outcome as long the commonly used agents provide objective response rates below 10%. Primary chemotherapy may be considered in patients with multifocal and inoperable disease requiring very large radiation fields or whole brain irradiation. Postoperative radiotherapy (or definitive radiotherapy in patients with unresectable disease) has been established more than 30 years ago, showing a modest but definite prolongation of median survival.

Chemotherapy in association with radiation has become the standard of care as first line therapy for GBM (Fig. 16.3). Temozolomide (TMZ) is administered orally at a continuous low dose (75 mg/m^2 daily, seven days per week) from the first to the last day of radiation therapy, up to a maximum of 49 days, together with concomitant radiotherapy (TMZ/RT). After a four-week break and a new MRI, adjuvant (better termed as "maintenance") TMZ treatment is given on a standard schedule (150–200 mg/m^2 daily x 5 days every 28 days) for up to six cycles (Fig. 16.3). In a landmark phase III trial conducted by the European Organization for Research and Treatment of Cancer (EORTC) and the National Cancer Institute of Canada Clinical Trials Group (NCIC), this regimen was compared to standard focal RT alone. Median survival was prolonged with the combined modality treatment from 12.1 months for patients receiving initially RT alone to 14.6 months for patients treated with TMZ/RT→TMZ (4). Although this increase in median survival is certainly modest, the increase of two-year survival rate from 10% to 27% for the TMZ/RT group is clinically relevant and the benefit persists with longer follow-up, although patients continue to recur and die of disease even after three to five years. At five years,

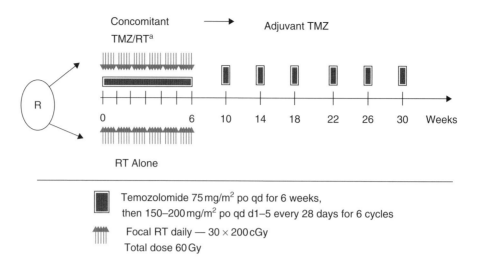

Concomitant TMZ/RT[a]   Adjuvant TMZ

R

0   6   10   14   18   22   26   30   Weeks

RT Alone

■ Temozolomide 75 mg/m² po qd for 6 weeks,
then 150–200 mg/m² po qd d1–5 every 28 days for 6 cycles

↟ Focal RT daily — 30 × 200 cGy
Total dose 60 Gy

Figure 16.3   Treatment regimen for GBM. [a]PCP prophylaxis was required for patients receiving TMZ during the concomitant phase.

10% of the patients treated initially with TMZ/RT were alive compared to only 2% with RT alone (5). Of importance, the improvement in survival from the early addition of chemotherapy can be seen in all clinical prognostic subgroups, although the absolute benefit is largest in the group of younger patients and those who have undergone prior tumor resection, which are known to be prognostically more favorable (6).

Retrospective molecular analysis of a representative subgroup of patients where adequate tumor tissue was available demonstrated that the benefit of the addition of TMZ chemotherapy is restricted mainly to patients whose tumors have a methylated methyl guanine methyl transferase (MGMT) gene promoter (7). MGMT is a ubiquitous DNA repair protein that can revert the damage induced by alkylating chemotherapy agents (e.g., TMZ) on the O6-position of the guanine. Methylation of the gene promoter (an epigenetic modification present in approximately 30–50% of GBM) will silence the gene and thus make the tumor cells more susceptible to alkylating agent chemotherapy. The predictive value of MGMT is currently being explored in a large randomized trial (RTOG0525/EORTC26052). If this is confirmed, different treatment strategies based on the molecular profile of their tumors may be proposed in the future to patients. One limitation to the implementation in the clinic is currently the lack of promising alternative strategies for patients whose tumors express the MGMT repair protein.

Most clinical trials for glioblastoma have restricted participation to patients younger than 65 to 70 years of age, as prognosis in older patients was considered particularly dismal. However, one-third of GBM patients are older than 65 years, and the management of these patients remains controversial. The benefit of radiotherapy in patients older than 65 years has recently been confirmed in a randomized trial comparing radiotherapy to best supportive care alone. Median survival was increased from 3.9 to 6.9 months and resulted in a better quality of life (8). A Canadian study showed equivalent survival rates in patients treated with hypofractionated RT more than 15 sessions compared to standard RT (9). These data suggest that elderly patients may, in the absence of significant comorbidity, benefit from a standard treatment approach or from accelerated RT. The role of chemotherapy in these patients is currently being evaluated in a number of ongoing trials.

Management of Recurrent Disease

At recurrence, therapeutic options remain limited. In all cases, the possibility of a new surgical resection must be reevaluated. For smaller tumors, radiosurgery or re-irradiation may be an option, although the benefits of these modalities have never been evaluated in prospective trials. A limitation of all localized treatments is the diffuse and infiltrative nature of recurrent glioma, likely to progress elsewhere rapidly even if controlled at the site of initial presentation. If available, inclusion into a clinical trial is certainly the most appropriate option.

As TMZ is used as a first line treatment in most patients, there are only few data available for the use of this agent in the recurrent setting. If there is a treatment interval of several months, successful re-treatment with TMZ has been reported (10), and treatment with a nitrosourea (lomustine, carmustine) may also be an option. Gliomas express high levels of vascular endothelial growth factor (VEGF), which is responsible, among others, for the vascular proliferation observed in GBM. Bevacizumab is a recombinant humanized antibody that binds to and inactivates the VEGF receptor. CPT-11 (Irinotecan®) is a topoisomerase I inhibitor that has by itself shown modest activity in the treatment of recurrent GBM with response rates of 0% to 18% (11). Recent reports from uncontrolled studies showed an unusually high response rate of 60%, a six-month progression-free survival rate of 40% to 50% and a median survival of nine months with the combination of bevacizumab and irinotecan (CPT-11) in patients with GBM and anaplastic astrocytomas (12).

Anaplastic Astrocytoma

Between 10% and 30% of all gliomas are anaplastic astrocytomas (AAs). The age group most affected is between 45 and 69 years. The male to female ratio is 1.2:1. The annual incidence is about 0.3 per 100,000. In population-based registries, AAs constitute 4% of all malignant nervous system tumors. Although most of the AAs are sporadic, certain inherited syndromes, such as neurofibromatosis types 1 and 2, tuberous sclerosis, and Li-Fraumeni syndrome predispose to developing astrocytomas. Anaplastic astrocytoma (WHO grade 3) is accompanied by genetic alterations, including loss of heterozygosity on chromosome 19 (13). Anaplastic astrocytomas frequently evolve from a less malignant precursor lesion and may further transform into glioblastomas.

Clinically, anaplastic astrocytomas are a heterogenous group of disease translating in very diverse outcomes. Although some anaplastic astrocytomas behave and evolve rapidly within a few months, others will have a more protracted course over two to four years. The median survival is approximately two years. Previously, clinical trials often included grade 3 tumors within a general treatment strategy of malignant gliomas that also included glioblastomas and the more favorable oligodendrogliomas. On MRI, anaplastic astrocytomas typically appear as solid masses with surrounding edema and mass effect. Contrast enhancement can be observed in 80% to 90% of cases. However, anaplastic astrocytomas without contrast uptake may be observed. The histopathological features of AAs are those of diffuse infiltrating astrocytomas with increased cellularity, distinct nuclear atypia, and increased mitotic activity. By definition, microvascular proliferation and necrosis are absent. Although there is usually a good concordance between pathologists in diagnosis for grade 4 tumors, disagreement in >30% of samples is common for anaplastic astrocytoma and other grade 3 tumors.

Treatment

Only few and insufficient data on outcome and optimal management are available from the literature. Initial studies suggested a benefit with the alkylating agent carmustine for patients with AAs exclusively (14), but this observation could not be confirmed in subsequent studies (15). Exclusive radiotherapy remains the standard of care, often in conjunction with adjuvant carmustine (BCNU) based on trials including all malignant glioma in the early 1980s. In daily practice, therapy is commonly prescribed in analogy to GBM despite the absence of definitive evidence. This approach is however debatable. One cannot assume that AA patients will benefit equally as those suffering from GBM. Moreover, the potential side effects of RT or of a prolonged treatment with an alkylating agent must be taken into account. For instance, transient (20%) and persisting (4%) myelosuppression was observed in patients with GBM (16). A number of studies have been designed in recent years to address this issue. A randomized RTOG trial (#9813) comparing RT and carmustine versus RT and TMZ has been closed because of insufficient accrual. An ongoing EORTC-Intergroup trial (CATNON) is comparing standard RT to TMZ/RT, RT→TMZ or TMZ/RT→TMZ, aiming also to answer the question whether concomitant chemoradiotherapy alone without prolonged maintenance therapy may account for improved outcome.

At recurrence, anaplastic astrocytomas have often transformed into a more aggressive variant and are commonly treated like recurrent GBM in function of the prior treatment exposure. In recurrent anaplastic astrocytoma, single TMZ has shown a high response rate of 35% in a large phase 2 trial (17).

Anaplastic Oligodendroglioma (WHO Grade 3) and Oligodendroglioma (WHO Grade 2)

Oligodendroglial tumors arise from oligodendrocytes or their precursors. They account for 2.7% of primary brain tumors and 9.5% of all gliomas. According to WHO criteria, oligodendrogliomas are classified into grade 2 oligodendroglioma and anaplastic oligodendroglioma (grade 3). The proliferation index is generally low (<5% MIB-1 positive cells) in grade 2 tumors and higher in grade 3 tumors (18). Mixed-type tumors with oligodendroglial and astrocytic features account for 5% to 10% of all gliomas (3). Given the differences in origin and prognosis, oligoastrocytomas and in particular oligodendrogliomas are considered as separate entities. The biological behavior and clinical prognosis of anaplastic mixed oligo-astrocytomas is similar to anaplastic astrocytomas. The therapeutic considerations are therefore identical for these tumors. Clear histological distinction of pure oligodendroglioma is not always possible. Pure oligodendroglioma with genetic loss on chromosomes 1p and 19q, recently identified as a translocation t(1p;19q), have a much more protracted natural history and are exquisitely sensitive to both radiation and chemotherapy treatment.

Grade 2 oligodendrogliomas are typically slow growing tumors, and 10-year survival rates of more than 50% may be observed. Favorable risk factors include absence of contrast enhancement on MRI, frontal localization, younger age at initial diagnosis, complete surgical resection, and high postoperative performance status. With current treatments, combining maximal surgery and RT, progression-free intervals of 2 to 2.5 years and median overall survival rates of four to five years are regularly achieved in grade 3 tumors, which may exceed seven years for patients with anaplastic oligodendroglial tumors with 1p/19q loss, compared with only three years for patients without the translocation (19).

Oligodendrogliomas show a T1 hypointense and T2 hyperintense well-demarcated lesion on MRI imaging with only little peritumoral edema. Contrast enhancement is rare and may be a sign of malignant transformation with a worse prognosis. Anaplastic oligodendrogliomas may show heterogeneous patterns due to variable presence of cystic degeneration, intratumoral hemorrhage, necrosis, and calcification.

Treatment

Based on the observation that recurrent oligodendroglial tumors are particularly responsive to combination chemotherapy with procarbazine, lomustine (CCNU), and vincristine (PCV), the RTOG in the United States and the EORTC in Europe launched two large randomized phase III trials investigating the value of (neo-)adjuvant PCV-chemotherapy before or after radiation for patients with newly diagnosed anaplastic oligoastrocytoma and oligodendroglioma (19,20). Both studies failed to demonstrate a significant improvement in overall survival, although a prolonged time to tumor progression was shown in the European study. Even in the subgroup of prognostically more favorable and presumably particularly chemosensitive pure oligodendroglioma with LOH 1p/19q, no advantage in favor of early chemotherapy could be shown. However, the much better overall prognosis and more protracted natural history could be confirmed for oligodendrogliomas with LOH 1p and 19q. These trials definitively establish oligodendroglioma with LOH1p/19q as a distinct pathologic entity. Chemotherapy appears to be of identical efficacy if given at the time of recurrence rather than upfront. The common practice of treating pure oligodendroglioma initially with chemotherapy, such as temozolomide, which has replaced the more toxic PCV regimen despite the absence of comparative clinical data, is not supported by available evidence (21,22). In particular for smaller tumors, a short course of six weeks of radiotherapy may be the easier and safer treatment than 6 to 12 months of potentially toxic chemotherapy. Alkylating agent chemotherapy may also be associated with clinically relevant long-term toxicity, e.g., myelodysplastic syndromes, secondary leukemias, and prolonged cellular immunosuppression with opportunistic infections. Patients with recurrent oligodendroglioma and oligoastrocytoma respond well to subsequent chemotherapy with PCV or TMZ.

Low-Grade Glioma (Diffuse Astrocytoma; WHO Grade 2)

Diffuse astrocytomas account for 10% to 15% of all gliomas and have an incidence rate of about 1.4/1 million population a year. Low-grade gliomas occur typically in adolescent children and young adults and are less common after the age of 40 years. The incidence rate decreases progressively from childhood into late adult life. Many patients present with seizures as single neurological manifestation. Often the disease is recognized fortuitously and may not require any specific treatment for many years. Similarly, the disease may have been present for a long time when it is first diagnosed. Mutations in p53 are found in two-thirds of patients affected by low-grade diffuse astrocytomas (WHO grade 2) (23).

The prognosis of low-grade gliomas is dependent on the tendency of these tumors to transform into more aggressive tumors in more than 60% of patients (18). The median survival for adults under treatment is in the range four to seven years, although some series report survival rates more than 10 years. Young age at diagnosis, MIB-1 index <5%, absence of neurological deficit and smaller size of lesion are associated with a more favorable clinical outcome (24). Gross total resection is also significantly correlated with longer survival. There are no validated prognostic factors that can predict malignant transformation.

The MR imaging typically shows a nonenhancing ill-defined hypointense lesion on T1-weighted images and a sharply demarcated hyperintense lesion with no or only minimal surrounding edema on T2-weighed images. The histopathology shows well-differentiated fibrillary or gemistocystic neoplastic astrocytes on the background of a loosely structured tumor matrix.

Treatment

Patients who present with seizures only and have typical radiographic features of a low-grade astrocytic glioma are often observed for a period of time with serial imaging before any surgical intervention is undertaken as long as the seizure disease can be controlled. Tissue is however required for a definitive diagnosis. This is preferably coupled with maximal surgical resection when feasible. For less accessible lesions, open or stereotactic biopsies are performed, aiming at the most aggressive part of the lesion, e.g., contrast enhancement if present. Patients with clinical progressive disease, such as uncontrolled seizure or patients with several risk factors for early tumor progression (incomplete resection, contrast enhancement or age >40, tumor ≥6 cm or tumors crossing the midline) (24) should be treated with RT up to 50 Gy. Higher doses have not shown any additional advantage, but an increase in toxicity in two randomized studies (25,26). Optimal timing of radiotherapy is commonly source for controversy. A randomized EORTC study (#22845) demonstrated equivalent survival outcome with an expectative and conservative approach compared with immediate irradiation. Thus, RT should preferably be given only at the time of clear clinical and radiological progression. This strategy allows to delay RT for an average of two to three years, and for more than seven years in one-third of the patients (27). The EORTC and NCIC are conducting a phase III trial to compare standard RT alone versus low-dose TMZ (75 mg/m^2/day for 21/28 days) as first-line treatment at tumor progression. The aim is to improve the overall outcome and to delay RT with potentially detrimental late neurocognitive toxicity in patients with a life expectancy of 5 to 15 and more years. In addition, tumor material is collected upfront and patients stratified for chromosomal loss on chromosome 1p/19q. This may allow to subsequently identifying patients with worse prognosis requiring more aggressive treatment and reassuring patient with true low-grade glioma that no active measure is needed.

Pilocytic Astrocytoma (WHO Grade 1)

Pilocytic astrocytomas (PA) account for less than 5% of all gliomas. These are typically pediatric brain tumors and more than 75% occur in patients younger than 20 years. These tumors are typically indolent and induce few neurological symptoms except for visual loss in case of optic gliomas. Pilocytic astrocytomas arise most commonly in the cerebellum, optic nerve or optic chiasm and more rarely in the basal ganglia and brainstem. Approximately 15% of optic nerve pilocytic astrocytomas are associated with neurofibromatosis. Supratentorial pilocytic astrocytomas have been associated with 80% to 100% 10-year survival rates following surgery. For cerebellar tumors, 95% disease-free survival at 25 years has been reported.

A complete resection is considered curative. Brainstem involvement is a negative prognostic factor. Leptomeningeal dissemination has been reported, with poor outcome. On MRI, these are well-circumscribed and contrast enhancing lesions, possibly with cystic formations. Only a minority are calcified. Gadolinium-uptake is common. Surprisingly, these tumors often show increased metabolic activity on PET scan, despite their low grade of proliferation. Histopathologic examination characteristically shows well-differentiated astrocytes, rosenthal fibers, bundles of neurofibrils, and microcysts. In these tumors, nuclear atypia and mitoses do not denote malignancy although rare pilocytic astrocytomas exhibit clinically malignant behavior.

Treatment

As pilocytic astrocytomas have well defined borders, surgical resection may be curative. Even after partial removal, symptoms improve in many patients and prolonged remissions may be observed. Therefore, if most of the tumor can be removed surgically, no further therapy should be instituted until there is clear evidence of progression. Management of pilocytic astrocytomas of the optic pathways remains controversial. Most resectable lesions should be excised, especially if vision is threatened. In case of recurrence, re-resection should be reconsidered. Unresectable or residual recurrent disease may be managed by radiation therapy with satisfactory control (28).

Brainstem Glioma

Gliomas arising in the brainstem comprise a heterogeneous set of neoplasms that may arise in the midbrain, pons, medulla, and upper cervical spine (29). Brainstem gliomas occur at any age, although 75% occur in children and adults younger than 20 years. In adults, brainstem gliomas are rare. Diffuse pontine astrocytomas represent about 80% of brainstem tumors. Histologically, these tumors are high-grade gliomas and have a uniformly poor prognosis (30). Focal brainstem gliomas typically arise in the midbrain or cervicomedullary junction. These tumors are most often low-grade tumors such as gangliogliomas, pilocytic, or fibrillary astrocytomas (30). Clinical symptoms usually start with cranial nerve palsies, especially diplopia that subsequently evolves to cause long tract signs. Hydrocephalus is uncommon. A number of factors have been found to be of prognostic importance for children with diffuse intrinsic brainstem gliomas. In general, patients with longer clinical history prior to time of diagnosis and those with more focal lesions, especially if localized in the midbrain and cervicomedullary junction tend to fare best. In practice, biopsy was performed for diffusely infiltrating brainstem gliomas that present with classic neuroimaging, given the high risk of significant disability should complications occur. Histology of brainstem gliomas spans the complete spectrum of differentiation from low-grade invasive astrocytoma to glioblastoma as seen in other parts of the brain. Neuroimaging, especially MRI and MR spectroscopy, often permits the differentiation of low-grade brainstem gliomas from high-grade lesions.

Treatment

The recognition of different subgroups of biologically distinct brainstem gliomas has allowed tailoring treatment. For instance, diffuse intrinsic gliomas that are highly infiltrative are not amenable to resection and should be treated with RT. On the other end of the spectrum, tectal gliomas show a prolonged natural history and may not require any specific therapy. Focal tumors of the cervicomedullary junction and dorsal exophytic gliomas may be resected safely (31). These exophytic tumors are more likely to be pilocytic astrocytomas or gangliogliomas with a better overall prognosis.

If surgically inaccessible, RT to a dose of 54 Gy in daily fractions of 1.8 Gy by external beam radiation to the lesion with a 0.5 to 1 cm margin is the treatment of choice in adults and children above 10 years (32). For children younger than 10 years with unresectable lesions, administration of chemotherapy may allow to delay RT. However, only few prospective clinical data are available for the use of chemotherapy in brainstem gliomas. The clinical practice has therefore been influenced by the management of supratentorial gliomas. In children with low-grade brainstem gliomas, weekly carboplatin/vincristine shows response rates of 40% (33) and two- and three-year survival rates of 75% and 68%, respectively. This regimen was compared with a TPCV regimen (6-thioguanine, procarbazine, lomustine, and vincristine) with similar results. Temozolomide is often used for the treatment of high-grade tumors in analogy to the positive results observed in supratentorial GBM.

Gliomatosis Cerebri (GC)

This diffuse glioma consists of exceptionally extensive infiltration of large areas of the CNS, with the involvement of at least three cerebral lobes. It usually displays an astrocytic phenotype, although oligodendroglioma and mixed oligoastrocytoma can also occur. The overall biologic behavior often corresponds to WHO grade 3, but a more indolent course may be observed in a sizable fraction of patients. All age groups and both genders may be affected with a peak incidence between 40 and 50 years. Presenting signs and symptoms vary considerably depending on the affected parts of the brain. The MRI typically shows diffuse enlargement of the involved cerebral structures without evidence of tissue destruction or focal tumor mass, which is best seen on T2 or FLAIR sequences. Classic histologic features include proliferation of small glial cells. The mitotic activity is typically low, however, with great variability. Necrosis and microvascular proliferation are generally absent in the classical variant. Like other gliomas, prognostic markers for better outcome include higher performance status, younger age, lower WHO grade, and histologic subtype.

Treatment

Radiation therapy usually involves large irradiation fields and may be associated with considerable toxicity and cognitive impairment. Therefore, chemotherapy (e.g., TMZ or PCV) is often considered as an alternative. Sanson reported a progression-free survival of 16 months in 63 patients and an overall survival of 29 months (34).

Ependymoma

Ependymomas account for less than 10% of CNS and 25% of spinal cord tumors occurring frequently in children and occasionally in adults. In children, the localization is mostly infratentorial, whereas in adults the majority of ependymomas arise in the subependymal space of the third ventricle. Diffuse cerebrospinal fluid (CSF) dissemination is common. Circulating tumor cells may obstruct CSF flow, leading to an increased intracranial pressure with headache, drowsiness, seizure, and focal neurological deficits or mimic brainstem lesions with deficits of multiple cranial nerves or of the cerebellum. On MRI, ependymomas often show a lesion that is hypointense on T1 and hyperintense on T2. Contrast enhancement is usually marked. Calcifications may be observed. All patients diagnosed with an ependymoma should have MRI imaging of the entire craniospinal neuraxis to exclude metastatic disease. CSF cytology performed two to three weeks after surgery is important in patients with posterior fossa lesions and those with high-grade anaplastic tumors as CSF dissemination affects both prognosis and treatment options. On histology, the ependymomas span a histologic appearance from low-grade differentiated lesions [myxopapillary ependymoma (WHO grade 1) or ependymoma (WHO grade 2)] to anaplastic (grade 3). Rarer subtypes include cellular, papillary tanacytic, epitheloid, and giant cell variants (18).

Treatment

The primary therapy is surgical resection, which can be curative if complete. Therefore, if postoperative imaging reveals residual disease, second-look surgery must be considered. For malignant (grade 3) tumors, or those with incomplete resection or recurrence, radiotherapy may be indicated. The role of chemotherapy in the management of ependymomas remains unclear. Minor activity was reported for a number of agents including cisplatin and etoposide, either alone or in combination (35,36). In children younger than three years, chemotherapy has been applied to try to delay RT. Adjuvant chemotherapy is not indicated outside clinical trials.

If the disease recurs, prognosis is grim and most patients will die within months of the relapse. A number of approaches may be offered including aggressive surgical re-resection, radiosurgery, re-irradiation, or palliative chemotherapy. High-dose chemotherapy with stem cell rescue has not demonstrated benefit in children with recurrent disease (37). The outcome is closely associated with the extent of surgical resection. Unlike most glial tumors, the prognosis of ependymomas is worse in children than in adults. This is probably related to the fact that posterior fossa ependymomas, which are more common in children, are less amenable to complete resection and are more often related to severe neurological disability. The overall prognosis of intracranial ependymomas, however, remains better than for other gliomas, with 5- and 10-year survival rates of about 80% and 50%, respectively (38).

Germ Cell Tumors

Germ cell tumors (GCTs) comprise a heterogeneous group of primary brain tumors occurring mainly in children and adolescents. They arise from pluripotent germinal cells and have an identical appearance and biological behavior to GCTs localized in the testes or ovaries. About half of the GCT are germinomas and can be commonly cured. The other half consists of nongerminomatous germ cell tumors (NGGCT: teratomas 20%, mixed tumors 20%, embryonal carcinoma, yolk salk tumors, and choriocarcinoma 10%) for which the prognosis is less favorable. GCTs are rare in Caucasians, representing about 0.5% to 3.4% of all primary intracranial neoplasms, but more common in Asians (2.1–9.4%). Males are two to four times more likely to develop

a germ cell tumor. Suprasellar tumors develop more frequently in females. All GCTs, with the exception of mature teratomas, are highly malignant but exquisitely responsive to chemo- and radiotherapy. Leptomeningeal spread occurs in 10% to 15% of cases. Many GCT secrete specific proteins that can be measured in the serum and CSF and may be useful for diagnosis and treatment surveillance. The different markers for each tumor type are summarized in Table 16.3.

Germinomas are composed of large round cells with vesicular nuclei, granular eosinophilic cytoplasm, and positive stain for placental alkaline phosphatase. NGGCTs commonly exhibit mixed histological features. Cytoplasmic and extracellular droplets that stain for alpha fetoprotein are diagnostic for yolk sac tumors. Choriocarcinomas are composed of bilaminar trophoblastic cells with high levels of beta-HCG and are prone to spontaneous hemorrhage. Mature teratomas are composed of fully differentiated tissues and are benign locally expansive neoplasms. Immature teratomas may have elements of sarcoma, carcinoma, or other nongerminatous germ cell tumors with a malignant behavior. Cytogenetic analysis often show the presence of an isochrome of the short arm of chromosome 12 [i(12p)]. This abnormality may be useful in the diagnosis of poorly differentiated neoplasms located in the midline.

Patients with pineal region tumors often present with features of obstructive hydrocephalus. Compression of the superior colliculus causes Parinaud's syndrome with light-near dissociation of pupillary response, limited upgaze, and convergence-retraction nystagmus. Compression of the superior cerebellar peduncle may result in ataxia or dysmetria. Because of the tumor location, endocrine dysfunction including growth failure, diabetes insipidus, and precocious puberty and visual abnormalities are frequent in sellar or suprasellar tumors.

On imaging, germinomas tend to be homogeneous and iso-intense to white matter on T1-weighted images and slightly hyperintense on T2 images. Teratomas and NGGCTs tend to infiltrate surrounding normal brain parenchyma. Areas of previous hemorrhages are typical of choriocarcinoma. In cases of a suspected germ cell tumor, imaging should include the brain and the complete spine. The CSF should be analyzed for cytology and tumor markers (alpha-fetoprotein, beta-HCG). This should be done ideally before surgical resection, or after an interval of at least two to four weeks after surgery due to potential contamination during the intervention. The gold standard for the diagnosis of GCT is histopathology, which mandates a surgical biopsy that must be sufficiently large to ensure adequate sampling, which is especially important in NGGCTs (39). Prognosis and treatment are determined by the most malignant histology within a tumor. In situations where elevated CSF markers clearly indicate the presence of a malignant GCT, a biopsy may not be indispensable (Table 16.3).

Treatment

The treatment modalities differ for pure germinomas, teratomas, and NGGCTs. Radical resection is warranted for mature teratoma, whereas surgery is not needed for pure germinomas.

Radiotherapy remains the treatment of choice for patients with pure germinoma and long-term survival

Table 16.3 Germ Cell Tumor Markers

	Alpha foetoprotein	Beta-human chorionic gonadotropin	Placental alkaline phospatase	Typical CSF findings
Germinomas	–	±	+	bHCG (slight elevation <50 mIU/ml)
NGGCT				
Teratoma				
• mature		–	–	
• immature	±	–	+	
Yolk sac tumors	+	–	±	aFP
Embryonal carcinoma	–	–	+	
Choriocarcinoma	–	+	±	bHCG

rates are more than 90% (40). The optimal dose and field of treatment remain controversial, total tumor doses of 45 to 50 Gy to the tumor are usual, with 20 Gy delivered to the lateral third and fourth ventricles, and an additional 30 Gy to the tumor bed in 1.8 Gy fractions. Depending on the clinical situation, the radiation field must include the ventricular system, the whole brain, or even the entire craniopsinal axis, given the tendency of these tumors to spread via the CSF. Given the high rate of neuroendocrine and cognitive sequelae as well as the risk of secondary malignancies of radiation therapy, systemic chemotherapy has been used in an attempt to reduce or delay the RT. Unfortunately, despite high response rates, chemotherapy alone is associated with high relapse rates. Greater success has been achieved using chemotherapy followed by RT (Table 16.4).

NGGCTs have a much worse prognosis than germinomas. They are primarily treated by chemotherapy, followed by focal RT for localized disease, and craniospinal RT for disseminated tumors. Short of prospective clinical trials for the rare CNS germ cell tumors, patients are commonly treated with the same regimens used for gonadal tumors. Platinum-based regimens are also the backbone for CNS tumors, but the observed cure rates of only 50% are inferior to testicular tumors (Table 16.4). In an international study, 71 mainly pediatric patients with intracranial GCT (26 with NGGCT) were treated with four 21-day cycles of carboplatin, etoposide, and bleomycin. Patients with a complete response were thereafter treated with two more cycles of the same therapy, whereas patients with incomplete responses received two additional cycles intensified with 65 mg/kg cyclophosphamide. Patients with NGGCT showed a response rate of 78%, with a two-year survival rate of 62%. Of the patients who progressed or recurred, half were successfully salvaged with RT or additional chemotherapy (41). Unfortunately, close to 10% of patients died of toxicity associated with the chemotherapy.

Patient with germinoma or NGGCT who recur or progress following primary treatment may be treated with chemotherapy and/or RT. Objective responses have been observed following a number of regimens including bleomycin/etoposide/cisplatin (BEP) or cisplatin/vinblastin/bleomycin (BVP) (42,43). Unfortunately, although responses may be observed even in patients previously treated with chemotherapy, they are usually short lived. Several groups have evaluated high dose chemotherapy with autologous stem cell rescue. Available data remain however scanty, and the value of high-dose consolidation remains unclear. RT may be most effective as part of a combined modality treatment (44).

Medulloblastoma

Medulloblastomas are the most common intracranial tumors of childhood, typically arising in the posterior fossa, and accounting for about 25% of childhood brain tumors. The incidence is about 0.5/100,000 children/year, peaking at age 7. In adults, medulloblastoma or the related primary neuro-ectodermal tumors (PNETs) are often found in the vermis or cerebellar hemisphere. Patients typically present with ataxia, dysmetria, or nystagmus and signs of increased intracranial pressure, including vomiting, headache, and possibly papilledema. If the tumor extends and compresses the brainstem, cranial nerve palsies, particularly of the VI and VII nerves may occur. Leptomeningeal dissemination may occur early in the disease course and cause widespread symptoms, including seizures, cranial nerve palsies, back pain as well as radicular sensory or motor deficits. Histological variants of medulloblastomas—including classic desmoplastic tumor, medullomyoblastoma, melanotic medulloblastoma, and cerebellar neuroblastoma—have currently no importance for the clinical management and outcome. The typical medulloblastoma shows densely packed cells with round or oval hyperchromatic nuclei and scant cytoplasm. MIB-1 is often higher than 20%. In children, a lesion localized in the vermis that is hyperdense on CT scan and hypointense on T1 and hyperintense on T2 with homogeneous and intense contrast uptake is highly suspicious of medulloblastoma. Hydrocephalus is a common finding. In adults, the tumor is usually localized in the cerebellar hemisphere. Hydrocephalus is uncommon, but a cyst may be evidenced. Enhancement is variable in adults. All patients with a medulloblastoma should be evaluated for metastatic disease with MRI of the entire craniospinal axis with contrast. The CSF should also be examined for the presence of malignant cells. Because of the risk of herniation, this procedure should however be reserved for two to three weeks after surgical removal of the tumor. Of note, CSF sampling through a shunt is inadequate, as the result may turn out negative despite the fact that lumbar CSF is clearly positive for malignant cells. Staging for medulloblastoma is summarized on Table 16.5 (45).

Table 16.4   Chemotherapy for Germ Cell Tumors

Treatment regimen	Number of patients	Responses	References
Germinomas			
Intracranial germinoma 2× Carboplatin (600 mg/m² i.v. day 1), etoposide (150 mg/m² i.v. days 1–3), ifosfamide (1.8 g/m² i.v. days 1–4) followed by RT 40 Gy	29	Event-free rate at 32 months: 93% Overall survival at 32 months: 100%	Baranzelli et al. (80)
Intracranial germinoma 4× alternating etoposide/carboplatin and etoposide/ifosfamide followed by 40Gy RT with CSI reserved for leptomeningeal dissemination	57	3-year event-free survival: 96% 3-year overall survival: 98%	Bouffet et al. (81)
Intracranial germinoma 2× Cisplatin (105 mg/m² i.v. day 1), Etoposide (150 mg/m² i.v. days 1–3), Cyclophosphamide (2 g/m² i.v. days 2–3), Bleomycin (15 mg/m² i.v. day 3) followed, if CR by 2× Carboplatin (AUC = 7, i.v. day 1–2), Etoposide (150 mg/m² i.v. days 1–3), Bleomycin (15 mg/m² i.v. day 3)	19	Event-free survival at 5 years: 47% Overall survival at 5 years: 68%	Kellie et al. (82)
CNS GCT Cisplatin (20 mg/m² i.v. days 1–5)/etoposide 100 mg/m² i.v. days 1–5) every 21 days followed by RT	17	No recurrences at 51 months	Buckner et al. (83)
Non germinomatous GCT			
4 cycles carboplatin/etoposide/bleomycin every 21 day, then if CR → 2 more cycles if less than CR → 2× cycles + cyclophosphamide (65 mg/kg) salvage with RT at time of POD	71 (26 with non germinomatous GCT)	Complete response rate: 78% 50% pts recurrence-free at 31 months	Balmaceda et al. (41)
6 cycles vinblastine/bleomycin/ carboplatin or etoposide/ carboplatin alternating with ifosfamide/etoposide	18	12 patients alive after 68 months, all but one with RT because of POD	Baranzelli et al. (44)
2 cycles cisplatin/etoposide/cyclophosphamide/ bleomycin (A), then 2× carboplatin, etoposide/bleomycin (B) then if CR: 1× A followed by 1× B if less than CR: second look surgery or RT	20	70% alive and free of disease at 6.3 years, (30% received RT because of POD)	Kellie et al. (84)

Treatment

Based on clinical staging criteria, the standard treatment for medulloblastoma has been surgery followed by craniospinal radiotherapy, resulting in five-year survival rates of 50% to 60%. The treatment is determined in part by the preoperative staging (see above and Table 16.5) and by the completeness of the surgical resection of the tumor: if there is a single tumor focus, complete resection should be aimed for. In case of widespread dissemination, a debulking operation to a residual volume of less than 1.5 cm is the preferred choice. Following surgery, patients are categorized either into average risk (age >3 and ≤21, absence of residual or residual tumor ≤1.5 cm, no evidence of metastatic disease in the neuraxis (negative MRI and CSF cytology done two to three weeks after surgery) or high-risk category (residual tumor >1.5 cm or staged as M1-M4) (Table 16.5).

All patients require whole neuroaxial radiation. RT at a dose of at least 55 Gy to the tumor has been shown to extend survival and may result in cures. In addition, it is recommended that high-risk patients receive 35 Gy to the entire brain and spinal cord, whereas 23.4 Gy may be sufficient for average risk patients. Despite this, almost 50% of patients die of early tumor recurrence. Moreover, many survivors develop significant neurocognitive impairment, growth delay, early puberty, and compromised spinal growth.

Medulloblastoma are also relatively chemosensitive. A variety of drugs have shown activity, in this type of tumor, including methotrexate, high-dose cyclophosphamide, and platinum derivates (46–48). A number of combination chemotherapies have been used with positive responses but little effect on survival. To date, none has been proven to be superior to a combination of weekly vincristine for eight weeks (starting during RT), followed by eight cycles of Lomustine and cisplatin every six weeks (beginning six weeks after RT) (49). To date, the adjunction of adjuvant chemotherapy for average risk patients has not improved survival. Many pediatric neurooncologists treat all patients with adjuvant therapy, given the 40% relapse rate at five years, the sensitivity of medulloblastoma to chemotherapeutic agents and the opportunity to reduce the dose of neuraxis RT. Although this regimen is well tolerated by children, this is not the case for adults. In adults, treatment is often based on an individual recurrence risk assessment. Standard risk patients (T1-3a, M0, and no residual disease after surgery, negative CSF cytology) are usually treated with 36 Gy craniospinal RT, supplemented by a boost of 18.8 Gy to the tumor bed. High-risk patients (T3b-4, any M+, or postoperative residual tumor) receive three to six cycles of a platinum-based chemotherapy regimen (e.g., cyclophosphamide, etoposide, and cisplatin) followed by craniospinal RT (50). Maintenance therapy is given if M+ disease is present. Long-term follow-up of the patients included in the study confirmed the better prognosis for patients with standard risk disease with five-year survival rates of 76% versus 61%, respectively. Since the inclusion of adjuvant chemotherapy in the management of high-risk disease, the prognosis has substantially improved (51). These results are similar to those observed in pediatric patients. Late recurrences even after 5 or 10 years have

Table 16.5 Staging of Medulloblastoma

Staging	
T1	Tumor <3 cm in diameter
T2	Tumor ≥3 cm in diameter
T3a	Tumor >3 cm in diameter with extension into aqueduct of sylvius and/or into foramen of luschka
T3b	Tumor >3 cm in diameter with unequivocal extension into the brainstem
T4	Tumor >3 cm in diameter with extension up past the aqueduct of sylvius and/or down past the foramen magnum
M0	No evidence of subarachnoid cells found in CSF
M1	Microscopic tumor cells found in CSF
M2	Gross nodular seeding in the cerebellar, cerebral subarachnoid space, or the third or lateral ventricles
M3	Gross nodular seeding in the spinal subarachnoid space
M4	Metastasis outside the cerebrospinal axis Residual tumor >1.5 cm postoperatively (considered high risk)

been observed, highlighting the importance of careful follow-up. The late toxicities of therapy must be taken into account and treatment involves a balance between maximizing cures and limiting long-term sequelae of treatment.

CNS METASTASES

Metastases to the central nervous system are often discussed as a separate disease entity. However, except for some particularities of the secondary localization in the brain, this is more a symptom and manifestation of the primary disease than a disease entity on its own. Unfortunately, most clinical trials aiming at optimizing treatment of brain metastases included many different tumor types, making the interpretation difficult and often not allowing definitive conclusions. In the following paragraphs, we will address some of the particularities of the management of central nervous metastases based on the limited evidence available. For specific information, the reader should refer to the respective chapters describing the underlying primary tumors in this textbook.

Brain Metastases

Brain metastases are detected in up to 40% of all cancer patients over the course of their disease (52). Brain metastases at initial diagnosis are more frequent in advanced stages of lung cancer and melanoma. In breast cancer, brain metastases are observed more frequently since survival has been prolonged with improved systemic treatments. For many agents and notably treatment with monoclonal antibodies (trastuzumab) the brain represents a sanctuary where these treatments do not adequately reach the target.

Symptoms depend on disease localization in the brain, exacerbated by the associated vasogenic edema. Seizures may occur in 10% to 20% of cases and up to 50% of patients with melanoma will develop seizures (53). Headache is an unspecific but common symptom. From a

practical point, any new neurological symptom or cognitive difficulties should warrant an active search for brain metastases in patients with known cancer.

Management and prognosis will be different in patients with a single or oligometastases compared with that in patients with diffusely disseminated disease, and thus adequate imaging is indispensable. MRI with contrast is the modality of choice as smaller asymptomatic metastases may go unrecognized on computer assisted tomography (CT). On imaging, metastases are usually round and homogeneously contrast-enhancing lesions. They may rarely be cystic or calcified. Intralesional hemorrhages are more common in melanoma, kidney cancer, and choriocarcinoma. Major, although unspecific arguments for the presence of brain metastases are the multiplicity of lesions, the localization at the gray-white matter junction, the sharp edge and the mismatch between a small lesion, and significant associated edema. These signs are however not specific and up to 10% of radiological diagnoses may be erroneous (52). If brain metastases are evidenced in a patient with a previously known cancer, there is usually no indication for further extensive workup or histological confirmation. To make adequate treatment decisions, the extent of the primary tumor has to be determined. In patients without known cancer, the workup should include a careful history and physical examination, e.g., removal of presumably benign naevi, in woman a breast examination, a chest X-ray and/or a CT scan of chest and upper abdomen. If the primary tumor cannot be easily detected, histological assessment of the CNS lesion may be most appropriate.

The aim of the treatment is to maintain the neurological functions of the patient to insure the best quality of life possible. Symptomatic treatments aim at the management of neurological dysfunctions and include steroids and antiepileptic medications. Antitumoral treatments include surgery, radiation therapy, stereotactic radiosurgery, and chemotherapy.

Surgery and Radiotherapy for Brain Metastases

Whole brain radiation therapy (WBRT) increases the overall survival two- to three-fold compared with best supportive care alone, but survival rarely exceeds six to nine months. Several prospective trials assessing the radiation dose or schedule have not shown an advantage of dose escalation or altered fractionation (54–56). Three prospective randomized trials have addressed whether the addition of surgery to WBRT will improve patient outcome. In two studies, median overall survival was improved when patients were treated with surgical resection of a single brain metastasis followed by whole brain radiotherapy (WBRT) compared with WBRT alone (median survival 9–10 months vs. 3–4 months) (57,58). The third study did not show a survival benefit for the surgical arm, which may be explained by a high proportion of patients with low performance status and active extra-cranial disease included in the study (59) and highlights the importance of adequate patient selection.

As an alternative to surgical resection, radiosurgery is frequently considered for smaller tumors. The addition of radiosurgery to WBRT has been addressed by the RTOG 9508 study. More than 330 patients (64% lung cancer) with

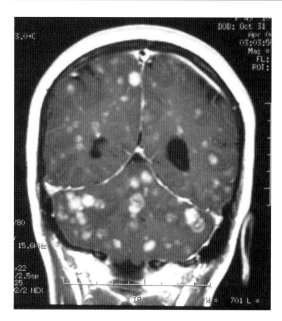

Figure 16.4 Radiological appearance of brain metastases on MRI (gadolinium-enhanced T1-weighted MR image).

one to three brain metastases were randomized to either WBRT alone or WBRT and radiosurgery (60). No difference in survival was observed for the entire cohort (median 6.5 vs. 5.7 months, p = 0.1356). However, a survival benefit was observed with the addition of radiosurgery for the subgroup of patients with a single metastasis (median survival 4.9 vs. 6.5 months; p = 0.04). Local control was significantly (p = 0.013) improved in the combined modality arm translating into a stable or improved performance status for a longer time. In a multivariate analysis, the recursive partioning analysis (RPA) class I tumors (patients with a controlled primary disease or brain only disease) was the only significant prognostic factor, independent of the number of brain metastases.

The role of surgery and/or radiosurgery in addition to WBRT has been investigated in a number of recent trials, and it is possible that WBRT is dispensable or can be postponed after surgery or radiosurgery, thereby avoiding potential acute and late toxicity. In one small multicenter trial, 95 patients were randomized to receive or not WBRT after complete resection of a single isolated brain metastasis. The recurrence rate in the brain was significantly reduced in the group receiving WBRT from 70% to 18% (p < 0.01). Although the overall survival was not significantly different, surgical patients were more likely to die because of neurological causes than patients treated with adjuvant WBRT (44% vs. 14%; p = 0.03) (61). In another underpowered trial, published in abstract form only, less than 100 patients were randomized to radiosurgery alone versus radiosurgery and WBRT versus WBRT alone. The observed OS was not significantly different in the three arms. In a recently published Japanese trial (62), 132 patients with one to four brain metastases were randomized to

radiosurgery ± WBRT. The primary endpoint was overall survival, which was not different between the two arms [one-year OS 38.5% and 28.4% in the combined modality and radiosurgery only arm (p = 0.42), respectively]. The one-year brain recurrence rate was however significantly increased in the radiosurgery only arm from 46.8% to 76.4% (p < 0.01). The rate of death due to neurological progression was identical (22.8% and 19.3% in the combined modality and radiosurgery only arm, respectively), while neurocognitive deterioration as measured with a mini-mental status exam, a questionable proxi in this situation, was delayed and attenuated with WBRT (63).

Two ongoing randomized trials address the outcome of patients treated with radiosurgery alone. More than 350 patients have been accrued in the EORTC 22952-26001 study comparing surgery or radiosurgery ± WBRT. Primary endpoint of this study is time to deterioration of the WHO performance status, with overall survival as a secondary endpoint. Preliminary results are presented at the ASCO annual meeting 2009. The North Central Cancer Treatment Study N0574 has already accrued over 100 of the 164 patients planned. The primary endpoint is the neuro-cognitive function tested by several neurocognitive tests.

Chemotherapy

Overall, the results of chemotherapy in the management of brain metastases remain disappointing, even though there have been reports of excellent responses in a number of chemosensitive cancers such as breast (cyclophosphamide, methotrexate, 5-FU based chemotherapies), small cell lung cancer (SCLC), or germ cell tumors (cisplatin based chemotherapies) (64–66). Although chemotherapy is not usually chosen as the initial treatment modality for brain metastases, there are some situations where starting treatment with chemotherapy may be appropriate. Studies of SCLC have shown that patients with synchronous presentation of systemic and CNS disease will have similar response rates in the brain and solid organs to initial chemotherapy regimens (66). It may be appropriate to initiate the best systemic therapy in a patient with symptomatic systemic disease and asymptomatic brain metastases.

Chemotherapy administered in conjunction with RT may have additive, synergistic, or radiosensitizing effects. The association of temozolomide with radiation has been shown to be well tolerated (67–69). Further studies are needed to confirm that this treatment may improve response rates and survival. Other radiosensitizers, such as modexafin gadolinium or efaproxiral, have failed to demonstrate an improved outcome in initial randomized trials of an unselected patient population with brain metastases (70).

Carcinomatous Meningitis

About 5% to 10% of patients with systemic cancer will eventually develop leptomeningeal carcinomatosis. It portends a dismal prognosis with median survival of about 4 to 16 weeks from time of diagnosis. Melanoma, breast and lung cancer, and hematologic and lymphoid malignancies are the most common origin of leptomeningeal

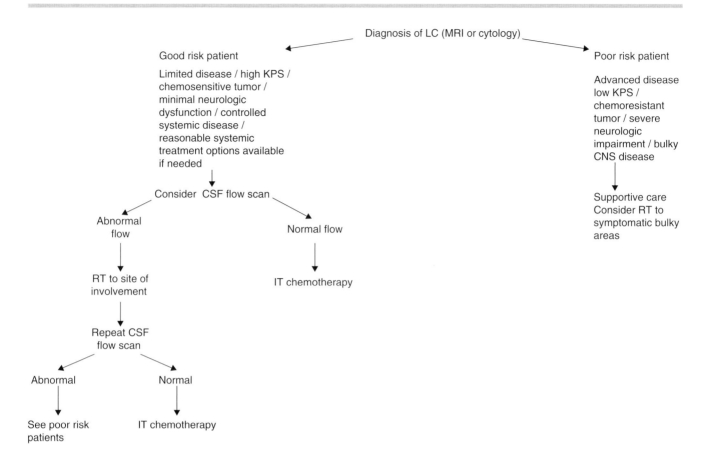

Figure 16.5 Suggested workflow for the management of leptomeningeal carcinomatosis. *Abbreviations*: CNS, central nervous system; CSF, cerebrospinal fluid; IT, intrathecal; KPS, Karnofsky performance scale; LC, leptomeningeal carcinomatosis; MRI, magnetic resonance imaging; RT, radiotherapy.

dissemination. Clinical signs of of meningeal irritation include headache, neck discomfort, nausea ± vomiting, and visual disturbances. Patients also commonly develop multiple cranial neuropathies and/or radicular neuropathies. The MRI of brain or spine can show leptomeningeal enhancement, typically in the form of linear cortical gyral enhancement following contrast administration. The cerebellar folia can also show similar patterns of enhancement. Neoplastic meningitis may also appear as bulky, nodular disease. In cases where the MRI is not diagnostic, lumbar puncture may provide cytologic evidence of the CSF dissemination of the cancer.

Untreated, carcinomatous meningitis of solid tumors will lead to death within a few weeks. Therapeutic options include RT, intrathecal or intraventricular chemotherapy, and high-dose systemic chemotherapy, provided the systemic disease is controlled and the patient has an adequate performance status. Randomized studies are not available to guide treatment. Figure 16.5 summarizes a practical approach. The type of primary malignancy, extent and control of systemic disease, performance status, neurological impairment, age of patient, history of prior CNS-directed therapy, and the presence or absence of abnormal CSF flow must be considered in the choice of therapy.

Intraventricular administration of methotrexate, cytarabine (Ara-c), and thiothepa have been reported (71–73). Response rates depend largely upon the type of primary tumor. Leptomeningeal carcinomatosis from breast cancer has shown the best results with response rates of up to 50% (71). In lung, digestive tract, or urogenital tract cancers, response rates of up to 30% have been reported. Unfortunately, recurrence is the rule, and in general survival remains poor. For instance in one study, 31 patients with carcinomatous meningitis showed median survival of 105 days with treatment of intrathecal slow release Ara-C, compared with 78 days for the 30 patients randomized to standard intrathecal methotrexate (p = 0.15) (72). In selected cases, oral temozolomide or high-dose IV methotrexate treatment may be considered, even though the evidence consists mostly of case reports (74–77). Radiotherapy is generally combined with intrathecal chemotherapy and is administered to symptomatic, bulky, or obstructive sites.

REFERENCES

1. Klaeboe L, Lonn S, Scheie D et al. Incidence of intracranial meningiomas in Denmark, Finland, Norway and Sweden, 1968–1997. Int J Cancer 2005; 117: 996–1001.

2. Behin A, Hoang-Xuan K, Carpentier AF et al. Primary brain tumours in adults. Lancet 2003; 361: 323–31.

3. DeAngelis LM. Brain tumors. N Engl J Med 2001; 344: 114–23.

4. Stupp R, Mason WP, van den Bent MJ et al. Radiotherapy plus concomitant and adjuvant temozolomide for glioblastoma. N Engl J Med 2005; 352: 987–96.

5. Stupp R, Hegi ME, Mason WP et al. Effects of radiotherapy with concomitant and adjuvant temozolomide versus radiotherapy alone on survival in glioblastoma in a randomized phase III study: 5 year analysis of the EORTC-NCIC trial. Lancet Oncol 2009 (epub ahead of print Mar 6).

6. Mirimanoff RO, Gorlia T, Mason W et al. Radiotherapy and temozolomide for newly diagnosed glioblastoma: recursive partitioning analysis of the EORTC 26981/22981-NCIC CE3 phase III randomized trial. J Clin Oncol 2006; 24: 2563–9.

7. Hegi ME, Diserens AC, Gorlia T et al. MGMT gene silencing and benefit from temozolomide in glioblastoma. N Engl J Med 2005; 352: 997–1003.

8. Keime-Guibert F, Chinot O, Taillandier L et al. Radiotherapy for glioblastoma in the elderly. N Engl J Med 2007; 356: 1527–35.

9. Roa W, Brasher PM, Bauman G et al. Abbreviated course of radiation therapy in older patients with glioblastoma multiforme: a prospective randomized clinical trial. J Clin Oncol 2004; 22: 1583–8.

10. Franceschi E, Omuro AM, Lassman AB et al. Salvage temozolomide for prior temozolomide responders. Cancer 2005; 104: 2473–6.

11. Prados MD, Lamborn K, Yung WK et al. A phase 2 trial of irinotecan (CPT-11) in patients with recurrent malignant glioma: a North American Brain Tumor Consortium study. Neuro Oncol 2006; 8: 189–93.

12. Vredenburgh JJ, Desjardins A, Herndon JE 2nd et al. Bevacizumab plus irinotecan in recurrent glioblastoma multiforme. J Clin Oncol 2007; 25: 4722–9.

13. Stupp R, Reni M, Gatta G et al. Anaplastic astrocytoma in adults. Crit Rev Oncol Hematol 2007; 63: 72–80.

14. Hildebrand J, De Witte O, Sahmoud T. Response of recurrent glioblastoma and anaplastic astrocytoma to dibromodulcitol, BCNU and procarbazine—a phase-II study. J Neurooncol 1998; 37: 155–60.

15. Hildebrand J, Gorlia T, Kros JM et al. Adjuvant dibromodulcitol and BCNU chemotherapy in anaplastic astrocytoma: results of a randomised European Organisation for Research and Treatment of Cancer phase III study (EORTC study 26882). Eur J Cancer 2008; 44: 1210–16.

16. Gerber DE, Grossman SA, Zeltzman M et al. The impact of thrombocytopenia from temozolomide and radiation in newly diagnosed adults with high-grade gliomas. Neuro Oncol 2007; 9: 47–52.

17. Yung WK, Prados MD, Yaya-Tur R et al. Multicenter phase II trial of temozolomide in patients with anaplastic astrocytoma or anaplastic oligoastrocytoma at first relapse. Temodal Brain Tumor Group. J Clin Oncol 1999; 17: 2762–71.

18. Louis DN, Ohgaki H, Wiestler OD et al. The 2007 WHO classification of tumours of the central nervous system. Acta Neuropathol 2007; 114: 97–109.

19. Cairncross G, Berkey B, Shaw E et al. Phase III trial of chemotherapy plus radiotherapy compared with radiotherapy alone for pure and mixed anaplastic oligodendroglioma: Intergroup Radiation Therapy Oncology Group Trial 9402. J Clin Oncol 2006; 24: 2707–14.

20. van den Bent MJ, Carpentier AF, Brandes AA et al. Adjuvant procarbazine, lomustine, and vincristine improves progression-free survival but not overall survival in newly diagnosed anaplastic oligodendrogliomas and oligoastrocytomas: a randomized European Organisation for Research and Treatment of Cancer phase III trial. J Clin Oncol 2006; 24: 2715–22.

21. van den Bent MJ, Taphoorn MJ, Brandes AA et al. Phase II study of first-line chemotherapy with temozolomide in recurrent oligodendroglial tumors: the European Organization for Research and Treatment of Cancer Brain Tumor Group Study 26971. J Clin Oncol 2003; 21: 2525–8.

22. Taliansky-Aronov A, Bokstein F, Lavon I et al. Temozolomide treatment for newly diagnosed anaplastic oligodendrogliomas: a clinical efficacy trial. J Neurooncol 2006; 79: 153–7.

23. Chawengchao B, Petmitr S, Ponglikitmongkol M et al. Detection of a novel point mutation in the p53 gene in grade II astrocytomas by PCR-SSCP analysis with additional Klenow treatment. Anticancer Res 2001; 21: 2739–43.

24. Pignatti F, van den Bent M, Curran D et al. Prognostic factors for survival in adult patients with cerebral low-grade glioma. J clin oncol 2002; 20: 2076–84.

25. Karim AB, Afra D, Cornu P et al. Randomized trial on the efficacy of radiotherapy for cerebral low-grade glioma in the adult: European Organization for Research and Treatment of Cancer Study 22845 with the Medical Research Council study BRO4: an interim analysis. Int J Radiat Oncol Biol Phys 2002; 52: 316–24.

26. Shaw E, Arusell R, Scheithauer B et al. Prospective randomized trial of low- versus high-dose radiation therapy in adults with supratentorial low-grade glioma: initial report of a North Central Cancer Treatment Group/Radiation Therapy Oncology Group/Eastern Cooperative Oncology Group study. J Clin Oncol 2002; 20: 2267–76.

27. van den Bent MJ, Afra D, de Witte O et al. Long-term efficacy of early versus delayed radiotherapy for low-grade astrocytoma and oligodendroglioma in adults: the EORTC 22845 randomised trial. Lancet 2005; 366: 985–90.

28. Debus J, Kocagoncu KO, Hoss A et al. Fractionated stereotactic radiotherapy (FSRT) for optic glioma. Int J Radiat Oncol Biol Phys 1999; 44: 243–8.

29. Recinos PF, Sciubba DM, Jallo GI. Brainstem tumors: where are we today? Pediatr Neurosurg 2007; 43: 192–201.

30. Fisher PG, Breiter SN, Carson BS et al. A clinicopathologic reappraisal of brain stem tumor classification. Identification of pilocystic astrocytoma and fibrillary astrocytoma as distinct entities. Cancer 2000; 89: 1569–76.

31. Epstein F, McCleary EL. Intrinsic brain-stem tumors of childhood: surgical indications. J Neurosurg 1986; 64: 11–15.

32. Schild SE, Stafford SL, Brown PD et al. The results of radiotherapy for brainstem tumors. J Neurooncol 1998; 40: 171–7.

33. Packer RJ, Ater J, Allen J et al. Carboplatin and vincristine chemotherapy for children with newly diagnosed progressive low-grade gliomas. J Neurosurg 1997; 86: 747–54.

34. Sanson M, Cartalat-Carel S, Taillibert S et al. Initial chemotherapy in gliomatosis cerebri. Neurology 2004; 63: 270–5.

35. Grundy RG, Wilne SA, Weston CL et al. Primary postoperative chemotherapy without radiotherapy for intracranial ependymoma in children: the UKCCSG/SIOP prospective study. Lancet Oncol 2007; 8: 696–705.

36. Geyer JR, Sposto R, Jennings M et al. Multiagent chemotherapy and deferred radiotherapy in infants with malignant brain tumors: a report from the Children's Cancer Group. J Clin Oncol 2005; 23: 7621–31.

37. Mason WP, Goldman S, Yates AJ et al. Survival following intensive chemotherapy with bone marrow reconstitution for children with recurrent intracranial ependymoma—a

report of the Children's Cancer Group. J Neurooncol 1998; 37: 135–43.

38. Schwartz TH, Kim S, Glick RS et al. Supratentorial ependymomas in adult patients. Neurosurgery 1999; 44: 721–31.

39. Regis J, Bouillot P, Rouby-Volot F et al. Pineal region tumors and the role of stereotactic biopsy: review of the mortality, morbidity, and diagnostic rates in 370 cases. Neurosurgery 1996; 39: 907–12.

40. Matsutani M, Sano K, Takakura K et al. Combined treatment with chemotherapy and radiation therapy for intracranial germ cell tumors. Childs Nerv Syst 1998; 14: 59–62.

41. Balmaceda C, Heller G, Rosenblum M et al. Chemotherapy without irradiation—a novel approach for newly diagnosed CNS germ cell tumors: results of an international cooperative trial. The First International Central Nervous System Germ Cell Tumor Study. J Clin Oncol 1996; 14: 2908–15.

42. Allen JC, Bosl G, Walker R. Chemotherapy trials in recurrent primary intracranial germ cell tumors. J Neurooncol 1985; 3: 147–52.

43. Siegal T, Pfeffer MR, Catane R et al. Successful chemotherapy of recurrent intracranial germinoma with spinal metastases. Neurology 1983; 33: 631–3.

44. Baranzelli MC, Patte C, Bouffet E et al. An attempt to treat pediatric intracranial alphaFP and betaHCG secreting germ cell tumors with chemotherapy alone. SFOP experience with 18 cases. Societe Francaise d'Oncologie Pediatrique. J Neurooncol 1998; 37: 229–39.

45. Packer RJ, Sutton LN, Elterman R et al. Outcome for children with medulloblastoma treated with radiation and cisplatin, CCNU, and vincristine chemotherapy. J Neurosurg 1994; 81: 690–8.

46. Prados MD, Warnick RE, Wara WM et al. Medulloblastoma in adults. Int J Radiat Oncol Biol Phys 1995; 32: 1145–52.

47. Greenberg HS, Chamberlain MC, Glantz MJ et al. Adult medulloblastoma: multiagent chemotherapy. Neuro Oncol 2001; 3: 29–34.

48. Abacioglu U, Uzel O, Sengoz M et al. Medulloblastoma in adults: treatment results and prognostic factors. Int J Radiat Oncol Biol Phys 2002; 54: 855–60.

49. Packer RJ, Gajjar A, Vezina G et al. Phase III study of craniospinal radiation therapy followed by adjuvant chemotherapy for newly diagnosed average-risk medulloblastoma. J Clin Oncol 2006; 24: 4202–8.

50. Packer RJ, Sutton LN, Goldwein JW et al. Improved survival with the use of adjuvant chemotherapy in the treatment of medulloblastoma. J Neurosurg 1991; 74: 433–40.

51. Brandes AA, Franceschi E, Tosoni A et al. Long-term results of a prospective study on the treatment of medulloblastoma in adults. Cancer 2007; 110: 2035–41.

52. Patchell RA. The management of brain metastases. Cancer Treat Rev 2003; 29: 533–40.

53. Byrne TN, Cascino TL, Posner JB. Brain metastasis from melanoma. J Neurooncol 1983; 1: 313–17.

54. Kurtz JM, Gelber R, Brady LW et al. The palliation of brain metastases in a favorable patient population: a randomized clinical trial by the Radiation Therapy Oncology Group. Int J Radiat Oncol Biol Phys 1981; 7: 891–5.

55. Borgelt B, Gelber R, Kramer S et al. The palliation of brain metastases: final results of the first two studies by the Radiation Therapy Oncology Group. Int J Radiat Oncol Biol Phys 1980; 6: 1–9.

56. Davey P, Hoegler D, Ennis M et al. A phase III study of accelerated versus conventional hypofractionated whole brain irradiation in patients of good performance status with brain metastases not suitable for surgical excision. Radiother Oncol 2008; 88: 173–6.

57. Patchell RA, Tibbs PA, Walsh JW et al. A randomized trial of surgery in the treatment of single metastases to the brain. N Engl J Med 1990; 322: 494–500.

58. Vecht CJ, Haaxma-Reiche H, Noordijk EM et al. Treatment of single brain metastasis: radiotherapy alone or combined with neurosurgery? Ann Neurol 1993; 33: 583–90.

59. Mintz AH, Kestle J, Rathbone MP et al. A randomized trial to assess the efficacy of surgery in addition to radiotherapy in patients with a single cerebral metastasis. Cancer 1996; 78: 1470–6.

60. Andrews DW, Scott CB, Sperduto PW et al. Whole brain radiation therapy with or without stereotactic radiosurgery boost for patients with one to three brain metastases: phase III results of the RTOG 9508 randomised trial. Lancet 2004; 363: 1665–72.

61. Patchell RA, Tibbs PA, Regine WF et al. Postoperative radiotherapy in the treatment of single metastases to the brain: a randomized trial. JAMA 1998; 280: 1485–9.

62. Aoyama H, Shirato H, Tago M et al. Stereotactic radiosurgery plus whole-brain radiation therapy vs stereotactic radiosurgery alone for treatment of brain metastases: a randomized controlled trial. JAMA 2006; 295: 2483–91.

63. Aoyama H, Tago M, Kato N et al. Neurocognitive function of patients with brain metastasis who received either whole brain radiotherapy plus stereotactic radiosurgery or radiosurgery alone. Int J Radiat Oncol Biol Phys 2007; 68: 1388–95.

64. Boogerd W, Dalesio O, Bais EM et al. Response of brain metastases from breast cancer to systemic chemotherapy. Cancer 1992; 69: 972–80.

65. Bokemeyer C, Nowak P, Haupt A et al. Treatment of brain metastases in patients with testicular cancer. J Clin Oncol 1997; 15: 1449–54.

66. Postmus PE, Smit EF. Chemotherapy for brain metastases of lung cancer: a review. Ann Oncol 1999; 10: 753–9.

67. Antonadou D, Paraskevaidis M, Sarris G et al. Phase II randomized trial of temozolomide and concurrent radiotherapy in patients with brain metastases. J Clin Oncol 2002; 20: 3644–50.

68. Addeo R, Caraglia M, Faiola V et al. Concomitant treatment of brain metastasis with whole brain radiotherapy [WBRT] and temozolomide [TMZ] is active and improves quality of life. BMC Cancer 2007; 7: 18.

69. Verger E, Gil M, Yaya R et al. Temozolomide and concomitant whole brain radiotherapy in patients with brain metastases: a phase II randomized trial. Int J Radiat Oncol Biol Phys 2005; 61: 185–91.

70. Mehta MP, Rodrigus P, Terhaard CH et al. Survival and neurologic outcomes in a randomized trial of motexafin gadolinium and whole-brain radiation therapy in brain metastases. J Clin Oncol 2003; 21: 2529–36.

71. Siegal T, Lossos A, Pfeffer MR. Leptomeningeal metastases: analysis of 31 patients with sustained off-therapy response following combined-modality therapy. Neurology 1994; 44: 1463–9.

72. Glantz MJ, Jaeckle KA, Chamberlain MC et al. A randomized controlled trial comparing intrathecal sustained-release cytarabine (DepoCyt) to intrathecal methotrexate in patients with neoplastic meningitis from solid tumors. Clin Cancer Res 1999; 5: 3394–402.

73. Jaeckle KA, Phuphanich S, Bent MJ et al. Intrathecal treatment of neoplastic meningitis due to breast cancer with a slow-release formulation of cytarabine. Br J Cancer 2001; 84: 157–63.

74. Raizer JJ, Hwu WJ, Panageas KS et al. Brain and leptomeningeal metastases from cutaneous melanoma: survival outcomes based on clinical features. Neuro Oncol 2008; 10: 199–207.

75. Ku GY, Krol G, Ilson DH. Successful treatment of leptomeningeal disease in colorectal cancer with a regimen of bevacizumab, temozolomide, and irinotecan. J Clin Oncol 2007; 25: e14–e16.

76. Carmona-Bayonas A. Concurrent radiotherapy and capecitabine, followed by high-dose methotrexate consolidation, provided effective palliation in a patient with leptomeningeal metastases from breast cancer. Ann Oncol 2007; 18: 199–200.

77. Lassman AB, Abrey LE, Shah GD et al. Systemic high-dose intravenous methotrexate for central nervous system metastases. J Neurooncol 2006; 78: 255–60.

78. Vecht CJ, Wagner GL, Wilms EB. Interactions between antiepileptic and chemotherapeutic drugs. Lancet Neurol 2003; 2: 404–9.

79. Glantz MJ, Cole BF, Forsyth PA et al. Practice parameter: anticonvulsant prophylaxis in patients with newly diagnosed brain tumors. Report of the Quality Standards Subcommittee of the American Academy of Neurology. Neurology 2000; 54: 1886–93.

80. Baranzelli MC, Patte C, Bouffet E et al. Nonmetastatic intracranial germinoma: the experience of the French Society of Pediatric Oncology. Cancer 1997; 80: 1792–7.

81. Bouffet E, Baranzelli MC, Patte C et al. Combined treatment modality for intracranial germinomas: results of a multicentre SFOP experience. Societe Francaise d'Oncologie Pediatrique. Br J Cancer 1999; 79: 1199–204.

82. Kellie SJ, Boyce H, Dunkel IJ et al. Intensive cisplatin and cyclophosphamide-based chemotherapy without radiotherapy for intracranial germinomas: failure of a primary chemotherapy approach. Pediatr Blood Cancer 2004; 43: 126–33.

83. Buckner JC, Peethambaram PP, Smithson WA et al. Phase II trial of primary chemotherapy followed by reduced-dose radiation for CNS germ cell tumors. J Clin Oncol 1999; 17: 933–40.

84. Kellie SJ, Boyce H, Dunkel IJ et al. Primary chemotherapy for intracranial nongerminomatous germ cell tumors: results of the second international CNS germ cell study group protocol. J Clin Oncol 2004; 22: 846–53.

17

Malignant Melanoma

Alexander M. M. Eggermont

TRENDS IN MELANOMA INCIDENCE

The incidence of malignant melanoma is increasing faster than any other solid tumor. In the United States, more than 62,000 new patients are diagnosed annually and about 8000 patients die each year (1). The recent publication of Cancer Incidence in Five Continents by the International Agency for Research on Cancer volume IX covers the period 1998–2002 and shows that the highest recorded incidence of cutaneous melanoma worldwide is in Queensland Australia ($56/10^5$ per year for men, and $41/10^5$ per year for women) and is also very high in New Zealand at 35 and $31/10^5$ per year, respectively, for men and women (2). In the United States, for non-Hispanic whites, these numbers are $19/10^5$ and $14/10^5$ per year for men and women, respectively. In Europe, incidence rates increase similarly and vary highly according to region (north-south gradient) and economic status (both north-south and west-east gradients). Incidence rates are highest in Switzerland, Austria, and the Scandinavian countries. Recent data show a steep rise in incidence in many east European countries, which reflects their rapid economic development over the last decades (3).

The main reason proposed for this increasing melanoma incidence over the last 40 years is greater exposure of pale Caucasian skin to natural ultraviolet radiation. A culture of sunbathing vacations from Scandinavia to Mediterranean or similar sunny destinations are believed to play a role. Short intermittent burning episodes of sun exposure have been identified by Elwood and others as a major melanoma risk factor (4). A problem in relating putative risk factors to the diagnosis of melanoma is the lack of knowledge on the latent period between initiating factors such as ultraviolet exposure and clinical appearance of a melanoma, which is measured in decades. Therefore, melanoma incidence will most likely continue to increase for at least the next 10 years (5). The observed increase in incidence particularly concerns elderly men, and for thin melanomas, young women of 20 to 40 years old (6). There is no clear evidence that sun avoidance campaigns have had a dramatic effect curbing this rise in incidence (7).

GENETIC AND ENVIRONMENTAL RISKS FOR MELANOMA

Melanoma risk factors are of a genetic or environmental nature with interaction between the two. Table 17.1 summarizes established and postulated risk factors for cutaneous melanoma. Around 5% of all invasive cutaneous melanomas occur in a familial setting with two or more close relatives affected, which indicates that in a small minority of melanoma patients, there are low prevalence–high penetrance genes involved. In addition, the typical phenotype of the melanoma patient, with pale Caucasian skin, red or blond hair, and blue eyes suggests that high prevalence–low penetrance genes such as MC1R may interact with environmental factors, particularly with sun exposure.

Melanoma Susceptibility Genes

About one-third of patients in melanoma families worldwide have an identifiable germline mutation in CDKN2A, a gene important in controlling entry into the cell cycle (8). A second melanoma susceptibility gene, CDK4, has been identified in five families to date worldwide (9), but in more than 50% of such families, no gene has been identified responsible for melanoma. The gene MC1R encodes for a protein involved in the production of eumelanin, which is responsible for dark coloring, and phaeomelanin, which is responsible for red hair and freckles. Studies suggest an interaction between mutated CDKN2A and MC1R (10,11). High prevalence–low penetrance genes such as MC1R are important in that they may be relevant to a much larger proportion of melanoma population compared with the small number of familial cases with CDKN2A mutations. Furthermore, common sequence variants on chromosome 20q11.22 seem to confer melanoma susceptibility (12). Also pigmentation gene variants ASIP and TYR have been reported to be associated with melanoma (13). The ASIP locus encodes the agouti signaling protein and TYR encodes for tyrosinase, so this report brings a molecular genetic explanation of the clinical observation of the association between melanoma, fair skin, and fair or red hair.

Skin Type and Naevi and Melanoma Risk

The likely melanoma patient is a pale-skinned Caucasian (phototype 1 and 2). High counts of banal melanocytic naevi are both associated with UV exposure and a major risk factor for sporadic melanoma. Also large atypical naevi, termed dysplastic naevi, is also an independent risk factor adding to melanoma risk.

Medical History and Melanoma Risk

There are conflicting studies that show either no increase or a significant increase in the risk for melanoma in renal

Table 17.1 Genetic, Medical, and Environmental Risk Factors for Cutaneous Melanoma

Genetic/medical history factors

Melanoma history
- Invasive cutaneous melanoma in one or more first-degree relatives
- Previous personal primary invasive melanoma

Presence of naevi
- Multiple banal melanocytic naevi (over 100)
- Three or more clinically atypical (dysplastic) naevi

Skin/hair phenotype
- Pale caucasian skin (skin types 1 or 2)
- Red, blond hair

Immunomodulation
- Increase after post-renal transplantation?
- Decrease after use of NSAIDs?

Environmental factors

Sun exposure history
- High solar exposure in early childhood (before age 10)
- History of sunburns
- Sunbathing holidays
- Sunbed use (especially before age 30)

Economic status/occupation
- Higher socioeconomic status?
- Airline crew?
- Exposure to pesticides?

transplant recipients receiving immunosuppressive drugs. A significant decrease in risk has been suggested in a recent case–control study of the use of oral nonsteroidal anti-inflammatory drugs use in melanoma patients and age-matched controls, suggesting that the regular use of this class of drugs is associated with reduced melanoma risk (14). Further studies are needed to confirm this finding.

Natural and Artificial UV Exposure and Melanoma Risk

On the one hand, short intense episodes of burning sun exposure appear to be a significant risk factor for melanoma, and on the other hand, cumulative ultraviolet exposure over the years may be involved especially in the lentigo maligna variety of melanoma. Whiteman and others postulated two distinct partly UV-induced pathways to melanoma that give rise to different clinical outcomes: the first involves intense intermittent exposure on the trunk of individuals who have large numbers of banal naevi and have melanoma diagnosed at a relatively young age, and the second is found in older individuals with chronic UV-exposure who may have a history of nonmelanoma skin cancer (15). This dual pathway concept is consistent with the observation of Thomas et al. that the *BRAF* gene mutations are more likely in melanoma of younger subjects with large numbers of naevi (type A) than in lesions on sun exposed skin of older patients (type B) (16).

On top of all this, the use of sunbeds has become very fashionable over the last decades. A recent meta-analysis of sunbed use and melanoma has concluded that overall sunbed exposure does add to melanoma risk (17).

Both sunbathing vacations and sunbed use are associated with the socioeconomic status, which has also emerged as a risk factor.

Occupation and Melanoma Risk

Chronic occupational sun exposure and working as a member of an airline crew have been reported to be associated with higher incidence rates of melanoma, as has the history of exposure to pesticides. These observations need to be confirmed by additional studies.

VISUAL DIAGNOSIS OF MELANOMA

Early diagnosis of melanoma should increase the cure rate. Melanomas develop in existing naevi in about 50% and as de novo lesions in the other 50%. Earlier public recognition of melanoma concentrates on simple guidelines, aimed mainly at superficial spreading lesions, which are the bulk of primary tumors. These guides include the U.S.-based ABCDEs of melanoma recognition and the Glasgow seven-point checklist (Table 17.2). Other useful simple aids to earlier diagnosis include the so-called ugly duckling sign, signifying a pigmented lesion, which is clearly distinct from other pigmented lesions on the same body site (18).

STAGING OF CUTANEOUS MELANOMA
The Current AJCC Staging System

The AJCC staging system is based on the evaluation of primary tumor (T), with Breslow thickness and ulceration as the major prognostic factor; the presence or absence of regional lymphatic metastases (N) and the number of involved lymph nodes as secondary factors of major prognostic significance; and distant metastases (M) with metastatic site and LDH levels as factors of major prognostic significance. The system divides patients into four groups (Tables 17.3 and 17.4) (19).

Stage I is limited to patients with low-risk primary melanomas, without any evidence of regional or distant metastases and is divided into stages IA and IB. Stage IA includes primary lesions ≤1 mm thick, without ulceration of the overlying epithelium or invasion of the reticular dermis or subcutaneous fat (Clark level IV or V). Stage IB includes primary lesions ≤1 mm thick with epithelial ulceration or invasion into Clark levels IV or V. It also includes primary lesions ≥1 mm and ≤2 mm thick without ulceration or invasion into Clark levels IV or V.

Stage II includes high-risk primary tumors, without the evidence of lymphatic disease or distant metastases and is divided into three subcategories. Stage IIA includes

Table 17.2 ABCD(Es) of Melanoma and Glasgow Seven-Point Checklist to Assist Accurate Preoperative Diagnosis of Cutaneous Malignant Melanoma

ABCDE	Glasgow seven-point checklist	
	Three major points	*Four minor points*
A—Asymmetry	Change in size	Diameter ≥6 mm
B—Border irregularity	Change in shape	Oozing or crusting
C—Color variation	Change in color	Inflammation
D—Diameter ≥6 mm		Itch
E—Elevation or enlargement or exudation		

Table 17.3 TNM Classification of Cutaneous Melanoma

Tumor (T) classification

TX	Primary tumor cannot be assessed (e.g., shave biopsy, regressed primary)
Tis	Melanoma in situ
T1	≤1.00 mm
	a: Without ulceration or level II/III
	b: With ulceration or level IV or V
T2	1.01–2.00 mm
	a: Without ulceration
	b: With ulceration
T3	2.01–4.00 mm
	a: Without ulceration
	b: With ulceration
T4	>4.00 mm
	a: Without ulceration
	b: With ulceration

Node (N) classification

N1	One lymph node
	a: Micrometastases[a] (clinically occult)
	b: Macrometastases[b] (clinically apparent)
N2	Two to three lymph nodes
	a: Micrometastases[a]
	b: Macrometastases[b]
	c: In-transit met(s)/satellite(s) without metastatic lymph nodes
N3	Four or more lymph nodes, metastatic or matted, or in-transit met(s)/satellite(s) with metastatic lymph node(s)

Metastasis (M) classification

M1	a: Distant skin, subcutaneous or lymph node metastases, normal LDH
	b: Lung metastases, normal LDH
	c: All other visceral metastases, normal LDH
	Any distant metastases, elevated LDH

[a]Micrometastases are diagnosed after elective or sentinel lymphadenectomy.
[b]Macrometastases are clinically detectable lymph node metastases confirmed by therapeutic lymphadenectomy, or lymph node metastases exhibiting gross extracapsular extension.
Source: Adapted from Ref. 19.

Table 17.4 AJCC 2002 Stage Groupings for Cutaneous Melanoma

Stage	Clinical stage grouping			Pathologic stage grouping		
0	Tis	N0	M0	pTis	N0	M0
IA	T1a	N0	M0	pT1a	N0	M0
IB	T1b	N0	M0	pT1b	N0	M0
	T2a	N0	M0	pT2a	N0	M0
IIA	T2b	N0	M0	pT2b	N0	M0
	T3a	N0	M0	pT3a	N0	M0
IIB	T3b	N0	M0	pT3b	N0	M0
	T4a	N0	M0	pT4a	N0	M0
IIC	T4b	N0	M0	pT4b	N0	M0
III△	Any T	N1-3	M0			
IIIA				pT1-4a	N1a	M0
				pT1-4a	N2a	M0
IIIB				pT1-4b	N1a	M0
				pT1-4b	N2a	M0
				pT1-4a	N1b	M0
				pT1-4a	N2b	M0
				pT1-4a/b	N2c	M0
				pT1-4b	N1b	M0
IIIC				pT1-4b	N2b	M0
				Any T	N3	M0
IV	Any T	Any N	M1	Any T	Any N	M1

Source: Adapted from Ref. 19.

lesions >1 mm and ≤2 mm thick with ulceration of the overlying epithelium and those >2 mm and ≤4 mm thick without epithelial ulceration. Stage IIB lesions are >2 mm and ≤4 mm thick with epithelial ulceration or >4 mm without ulceration. Stage IIC consists of primary lesions >4 mm with epithelial ulceration.

Stage III includes lesions with pathologically documented involvement of regional lymph nodes or the presence of in-transit or satellite metastases. Patients with one, two to three, and four or more affected lymph nodes are classified as having N1, N2, and N3 disease, respectively (Tables 17.1 and 17.2). Patients with in-transit or satellite metastases are classified as having N2 disease if lymph node involvement is not present, and as having N3 disease if lymph node involvement is present. In addition, microscopic versus macroscopic lymph node involvement is further subdivided as, for example, N1a versus N1b category, respectively. The presence of ulceration in the primary tumor remains an independent negative prognostic factor among patients with stage III disease, particularly those with microscopically involved nodes. Using these parameters, patients with stage III disease are divided into three subcategories: (a) Stage IIIA includes patients with one to three microscopically involved lymph nodes (N1a or N2a)

and with a nonulcerated primary tumor. (b) Stage IIIB includes patients with one to three microscopically involved lymph nodes (N1a or N2a) and with an ulcerated primary tumor; or patients with one to three macroscopically involved lymph nodes (N1b or N2b) and with a nonulcerated primary tumor; or patients with in-transit and/or satellite without metastatic lymph nodes (N2c). (c) Stage IIIC includes patients with four or more affected lymph nodes, matted lymph nodes, or the presence of in-transit metastases or satellite lesions in conjunction with lymph node involvement (N3); or patients with one to three macroscopically involved lymph nodes (N2b) and with an ulcerated primary tumor. Patients with clinical evidence of regional lymph node without a full regional lymph node dissection are classified as clinical stage III, and no further staging is applied.

Stage IV is defined by the presence of distant metastases, and patients are divided into three subcategories based on the metastasis location: M1a is limited to distant skin, subcutaneous tissues, or lymph nodes; M1b involves lung metastases; and M1c involves all other visceral sites. In addition, the presence of an elevated serum lactate dehydrogenase (LDH) in conjunction with any distant metastasis is classified as M1c disease.

Key Features of AJCC Staging System

The key features of the current 2002 AJCC staging system when compared with the prior 1997 system include (1) tumor thickness rather than level of invasion as a primary determinant for staging, (2) ulceration of primary tumor as a highly significant and independent negative prognostic factor, (3) grouping together satellite and in-transit metastases as a manifestation of lymphatic involvement rather than as an extension of primary tumor, and (4) the number of lymph node metastases as a more reliable and reproducible predictor of prognosis than size of involved lymph nodes (the number of lymph node metastases is used to divide patients with stage III disease, and lymph node involvement is further subdivided into micro- or macrometastatic), (5) separation of lung metastases from other visceral sites of involvement, based on an observed longer survival, and (6) elevated serum LDH as a negative prognostic factor for patients with metastatic disease.

SURGICAL MANAGEMENT
Extending Surgical Procedures for Primary Melanoma
Surgical management strategies in the treatment of primary melanomas have demonstrated that extended surgical procedures, e.g., wide margins (five randomized trials), elective lymph node dissection (four randomized trials), prophylactic isolated perfusion (one randomized trial), or sentinel node staging (one randomized trial), have no significant impact on survival (all trials reviewed in Ref. 20). The currently popular sentinel node biopsy (SNB) staging procedure needs a more detailed discussion.

Sentinel Node Biopsy
SN-status: Strongest Prognostic Factor in Melanoma
SN-status is the strongest prognostic factor in melanoma patients. Literature studies demonstrate five-year overall survival (OS) rates of 93% and 89% for SN-negative patients, and OS rates of between 67% and 64% for SN-positive patients (21,22).

SNB Staging Does Not Provide Survival Benefit
SNB is a staging procedure without impact on survival. The outcome of the MSLT-1 trial, comparing wide excision alone, where patients were followed up and underwent a delayed lymph node dissection (DLND) in case of subsequent clinical lymph node involvement versus WE + SNB, where patients with a positive SN underwent an immediate completion lymph node dissection (CLND), demonstrated clearly that at five years overall survival was virtually identical in both patient groups (86.6% for WE alone, and 87.1% for WE + SNB) (22). Comparison of the outcome in patients with a positive SN who underwent CLND with patients that underwent DLND in the WE-only group showed a survival benefit for the SN + CLND patients. These patient groups however are not directly comparable, and one may compare outcome in biologically different patient populations. It has become evident that not all SN-positive patients develop clinically node-positive disease, as patients with very small submicrometastases in the SN behave just like SN-negative patients (23) and may represent "clinically prognostically false-positive cases" (24).

SNB and Local Control
SN staging may improve long-term locoregional control in the lymph node basin compared with the patients who undergo DLND (22). Ultrasound of the regional lymph nodes may also be able to achieve this by detecting very small nonpalpable lymph node metastases, thus offering an alternative to a SN procedure (25). Some reports have

assumed an increased rate of in-transit metastasis after the SN procedure, but this has been refuted by the MSLT-1 trial and large data sets (22,26).

SN and Utility for Adjuvant Systemic Therapy Trials
SN staging is quite useful for stratifying patients in randomized systemic adjuvant therapy trials to create more homogeneous patient populations to determine whether adjuvant systemic therapies are of benefit. This will be further illustrated by the analyses of the EORTC 18952 and 18991 trials in the adjuvant therapy section below.

Conclusions Surgery of Primary
In conclusion, phase III randomized trials have shown that wide margins, elective lymph node dissections, SNB, and prophylactic isolated limb perfusions (ILPs) have not improved survival, and on the claim of providing a survival benefit cannot be considered standard of care in the routine management of primary melanoma.

SURGERY OF METASTATIC DISEASE
Therapeutic Lymph Node Dissection
The most frequently affected basins are the neck, axilla, and groin; the involvement of popliteal fossa or epitrochlear lymph nodes is rare. Lymphadenectomy may be curative or only prevent further relapse at that site. Both aims can only be achieved by meticulous removal of all involved and at-risk nodes. In general, this means dissection of all five levels of lymph nodes in the neck plus superficial parotidectomy if the primary site is thought to drain to parotid nodes, all three levels in the axilla, and the superficial, deep inguinofemoral and ilio-obturator nodes. Pelvic lymph nodes should be included if enlarged on preoperative imaging.

Therapeutic ILP for in-Transit metastasis
ILP is successful in treating highly morbid symptomatic in-transit metastasis. ILP, especially when melphalan is combined with TNF, is also highly effective in the symptomatic setting of multiple or bulky in-transit metastases, with CR rates of 70% and in the treatment of melphalan ILP failures with similarly high CR rates (27). The isolated limb infusion procedure is simpler and cheaper but confined to smaller limb volumina and has lower response rates (28).

Surgery for Distant Metastasis
The purpose of treatment of distant metastases is often palliation and its indication and utility is unfortunately underrated and underutilized. Surgery is the most effective means of providing this if it is technically feasible, if risk of morbidity and mortality is low, and if the patient is likely to live long enough to benefit. Good examples are single or localized metastases to the brain, bowel, lung, and sometimes liver. Completely resected single distant metastases may occasionally be associated with long survival (29). There is no prospective study comparing surgical with medical approaches to treatment of melanoma patients with a single or very few distant metastases.

Conclusions Surgery of Metastases

In conclusion, surgery remains the most effective treatment modality for metastatic disease. Radical lymphadenectomies for regional node basins have been standardized. ILPs for multiple in-transit metastases are effective, and resections of oligometastatic stage IV disease are to be considered in all patients with these clinical presentations.

SYSTEMIC ADJUVANT THERAPIES

Failure of Chemotherapy, Aspecific Immunostimulants, and Vaccines

Around 25 trials have been conducted evaluating chemotherapy or aspecific immunostimulants such as Bacillus Calmette-Guerin (BCG), *Corynebacterium parvum*, Levamisole, or combinations of these agents with dacarbazine in stage II-III melanoma. The trials were almost invariably underpowered yielding negative results with the exception of incidental nonrepeatable small-sized positive trials (reviewed in Ref. 20). None of five randomized trials with allogeneic melanoma cell-based vaccines demonstrated a significant impact on survival. The SWOG Melacine vaccine trial in stage II melanoma patients was negative overall but showed encouraging results in patients with particular HLA-types. A small trial with the ganglioside GM2 did show a benefit in a subset analysis of stage III patients who were seronegative for ganglioside antibodies prior to trial entry. This study led to the EORTC18961 trial in 1314 stage II patients, that was unblinded at the second interim analysis because of futility (DFS) and a significant trend for detrimental impact on survival (30). As a result of this, the outcome of the ECOG1694 trial, which compared the GMK-vaccine to high-dose IFN (HDI) treatment, is no longer interpretable (31). The significant difference between GMK-vaccine and HDI at the second interim analysis in that trial could be caused by a detrimental impact mediated by the vaccine. Unfortunately, these truly negative results have been observed also in other adjuvant trials. Both allogeneic cell lines–based Canvaxin trials in resected stage IV (496 patients) as well as in stage III (1166 patients) were unblinded early and stopped because of negative and even detrimental impact on survival (32).

Interferon Alpha

The failure of vaccine trials means that for years to come, interferon alpha is the only drug that will be used or considered to be used in the adjuvant setting. The evidence for its use is relatively complex and needs to be discussed in detail.

Individual High Dose-Intermediate Dose-Low Dose Trial Data

High-Dose IFN Trials. The comparative trials of HDI with observation in stage II and III (NCTCG, ECOG1684, ECOG1690, Sunbelt Trial) melanoma have demonstrated a consistent impact on disease-free survival (DFS) but not on overall survival (OS) (33–37) (Table 17.5). On the basis of the ECOG1684 trial (34), the use of HDI therapy was approved by both the FDA in the United States and EMEA in Europe for patients with high-risk melanoma (stage IIB-III). HDI is used in the United States but only in few European centers, because the impact of the therapy on overall survival is uncertain (35,36), and the toxicity and cost is relatively high. The recent Sunbelt trial (36) in the United States in SN-positive patients was negative. Also of importance is the outcome of the Hellenic trial demonstrating that four weeks of intravenous HDI was as good as the classical ECOG1684 one-year schedule of HDI, and much better tolerated (37).

Intermediate Dose IFN Trials. Intermediate doses of IFN (IDI) (Table 17.6) were tested in patients with stage IIB-III disease in the largest phase III trial to date (EORTC18952) (38). The results demonstrated a statistically insignificant 7.2% increase in distant metastasis-free interval (hazard ratio 0.83, 97.5% CI 0.66–1.03, p = 0.05) and a 5.4% increase in overall survival (OS, hazard ratio 0.85, 97.5% CI 0.68–1.07, p = 0.12) at 4.65 years of follow-up. However, the increase in OS was observed only in patients treated for 25 months with 5MU IFNα2b and not in those treated for 13 months with 10 MU IFNα2b (38). These results suggested that duration of therapy may be more important than dose. The Nordic trial in 800 patients reported a very similar impact of intermediate dose IFN, without the indication that two years was better than one year of treatment (39).

The question of treatment duration was addressed in the next EORTC trial (18991) in which 1256 patients were randomized to five years of pegylated interferon α2b (PEG-IFN) or observation alone (Tables 17.7 and 17.8) (30). In this trial, the dosing schedule is comparable to the HDI, but bioavailability of PEG-IFN may make it more

Table 17.5 High-Dose IFN Trials in Stage II/III Melanoma

Trial	Stage	Treatment	DFS	OS
NCTCG (33)	II-III	IFNα2a, 3 × 20 MIU/M2/wk, IM for 3 mo	5-yr; HR = 0.77; p = 0.19	5-yr; HR = 0.88; p = 0.40
ECOG 1684 (34)	IIB, III	IFNα2b, 20 MIU/qDays1–5/IV, for 4 wk, + 3 × 10 MIU/wk, SC, for 48 wk	6.9 yr; HR = 0.56 p = 0.0046	6.9 yr; HR = 0.68 p = 0.046
ECOG 1690 (35)	IIB, III	IFNα2b, 20 MIU/qDays1–5/IV, for 4 wk, + 3 × 10 MIU/wk, SC, for 48 wk	4.4 yr; HR = 0.90; p = 0.054	4.4 yr; HR = 1.07; p = 0.99
Sunbelt (36)	III SN+	IFNα2b, 20 MIU/qDays1–5/IV, for 4 wk, + 3 × 10 MIU/wk, SC, for 48 wk	5.3 yr; HR = 0.82; p = 0.46	5.3 yr; HR = 1.03; p = 0.90
Hellenic (37)	IIB, III	IFNα2b 15 MIU/qDays1–5/IV, for 4 wk vs. ECOG1684 schedule	3 yr; HR = 0.95; p = 0.70	3 yr; HR = 1.11; p = 0.52

Abbreviations: HR, hazard ratio; IM, intramuscular; IV, intravenous; MIU, million international units; SC, subcutaneous; yr, year.

Table 17.6   Intermediate Dose IFN Trials in Stage IIB/III

Trial	Stage	Treatment	DFS	OS
EORTC 18952 (38)	IIB-III	IFNα2b, 10 MIU/qDays1–5/SC, for 4 wk, + 3 × 10 MIU/wk, SC for 12 mo or 3 × 5 MIU/wk, SC for 24 mo	4.65-yr; HR = 0.81; p = 0.12	4.65-yr; HR = 0.88; p = 0.40
Nordic (39)	IIB, III	IFNα2b, 10 MIU/qDays1–5/SC, for 4 wk, + 3 × 10 MIU/wk, SC for 12 mo or 3 × 10 MIU/wk, SC for 24 mo	6 yr; HR = 0.83 p = 0.05	6 yr; HR = 0.88 p = 0.47

Table 17.7   Long Term Pegylated IFNα2b. *EORTC 18991*: Significant Impact of Pegylated Interferon α2b (PEG-IFN) on Disease-Free Survival (DFS) but Not on Distant Metastasis-Free Survival (DMFS) and Overall Survival (OS) in Patients with Stage III Melanoma

EORTC 18991 (40)	DFS	DMFS	OS
PEG-IFN[a]	45.6% (2.2)	48.2% (2.2)	56.8% (2.2)
Observation[a]	38.9% (2.2)	45.4% (2.3)	55.7% (2.1)
HR (95% CI)	0.82 (0.71–0.96)	0.88 (0.75–1.03)	0.98 (0.82–1.16)
p-Value	0.01	0.11	0.78

[a]4-year rate (SE).

Table 17.8   Long Term Pegylated IFNα2b. *EORTC 18991*: Significant Impact of Pegylated Interferon α2b (PEG-IFN) on Disease-Free Survival (DFS) and Distant Metastasis-Free Survival (DMFS) in Stage III Melanoma Patients with N1 Microscopic but Not N2 Macroscopic Nodal Involvement

EORTC 18991 (40)	DFS		DMFS	
	N1(micro)	N2(macro)	N1(micro)	N2(macro)
PEG-IFN[a]	57.7% (3.3)	36.3% (2.8)	60.5% (3.6)	38.7% (2.8)
Observation[a]	45.4% (3.5)	33.9% (2.6)	52.6% (3.5)	39.9% (2.7)
HR (99% CI)	0.73 (0.53–1.02)	0.86 (0.68–1.10)	0.75 (0.52–1.07)	0.94 (0.73–1.21)
p-Value	0.016	0.12	0.03	0.53

[a]4-year rate (SE).

comparable to high intermediate doses of IFN. PEG-IFN was administered for an induction period of eight weeks at 6 µg/kg body weight followed by long-term maintenance dosing of 3 µg/kg for the rest of five years. This was a registration study with relapse-free survival (RFS) as primary endpoint. RFS was significantly improved without a significant impact on distant metastasis-free survival (DMFS) or OS (Table 17.7). In patients with only microscopic involvement of regional lymph nodes (SNB-positive patients, N1), impact of the treatment was significant both for RFS and DMFS (Table 17.8), in contrast to a much smaller impact in those with palpable nodal involvement (N2). This significant impact was very similar to the observations in stage IIB and IIIN1 patients in the EORTC 18952 trial. This supports the importance and value of SN staging, which now identifies most of stage III patients.

Another clinical trial that addresses the duration of treatment only is currently analyzed. The trial of the Dermatologic Cooperative Oncology Group (DeCOG) compared administration of low-dose IFNα2a (3 × 3 MU/week) for 18 months—as approved in Europe—to administration for 60 months. No differences in terms of an improvement of disease-free or overall survival have been observed with the prolonged treatment duration (41).

Low-Dose IFN Trials. The impact of low-dose IFN (LDI) has been clearly established in stage II (42–44) but may be somewhat less substantial in stage III (45–47). In stage II, the LDI therapy has been particularly successful; a consistent and significant effect on DFS was observed in the French (42), Austrian (43), and Scottish (44) studies, with even a borderline significant effect on survival in the French trial (Table 17.9). LDI regimens of two and three years in stage IIB and III were tested in the Intergroup 1690 (35) and in the UKCCR Aim High trial (45) with quite modes results. Also, the WHO-16 trial, which evaluated three years of LDI in palpable nodes stage III patients, was negative both for DFS as well as for OS (46). Thus, it seems that earlier disease is more responsive to LDI than more advanced disease. In contrast, very recently, results of a DeCOG trial showed not only DFS but also OS benefit for LDI-treated patients compared to that in untreated controls in stage III patients, whereas the combination of LDI and dacarbazine did not demonstrate any benefit (47). Ultra low-dose IFN (1 MIU) was evaluated in the EORTC 18871 trial in stage II (>3 mm) and stage III patients and did not have any impact on DFS or OS (48). LDI (3 MIU) therapy was approved as an adjuvant therapy for stage II patients by the EMEA in Europe. The quite significant impact of

Table 17.9 Low-Dose IFN Trials in Stage II/III Melanoma

Trial	Stage	Treatment	DFS	OS
French (42)	II	IFNα2a, 3 × 3 MIU/wk for 18 mo	5-yr; HR = 0.75; p = 0.035	5-yr; HR = 0.72; p = 0.059
Austrian (43)	II	IFNα2a, 3 MIU/qday for 3 wk; 3 × 3 MIU/wk, for 12 mo	3.4 yr; HR = 0.62; p = 0.02	3.4 yr; HR = 0.83; p = NS
Scottish (44)	IIB, III	IFNα2b, 3 × 3 MIU/wk, for 6 mo	2-yr; HR = 0.72; p = 0.05	2-year; HR = 0.81; p > 0.2
ECOG 1690 (35)	IIB, III	IFNα2b, 3 × 3 MIU/wk, for 24 mo	5 yr; HR = 0.90; p = 0.17	5 yr; HR = 0.93; p = 0.81
UKCCR (45)	IIB, III	IFNα2a, 3 × 3 MIU/wk, for 24 mo	5 yr; HR = 0.94; p = 0.6	5 yr; HR = 0.91; p = 0.3
WHO-16 (46)	III	IFNα2a, 3 × 3 MIU/wk, for 36 mo	5 yr; HR = 0.95; p = 0.5	5 yr; HR = 0.96; p > 0.5
German (47)	III	IFNα2a, 3 × 3 MIU/wk, for 24 mo	4-yr; HR = 0.69; p = 0.018	4-yr; HR = 0.62; p = 0.0045
EORTC 18871 (48)	II-III	IFNα2b, 3 × 1 MIU/wk, for 12 mo	8 yr; HR = 0.96 p > 0.5	8 yr; HR = 0.96 p > 0.7

Table 17.10 Combination Trials with Low-Dose IFN

Trial	Combination	Stage	DFS	OS
Garbe et al. (47)	IFNα2a + dacarbazine[a]	III	4-yr; p = 0.97	4-yr; p = 0.75
Mitchell et al. (49)	IFNα2b + Melacine[b]	III	5-yr; p = 0.80	5-yr; p = 0.57
Hauschild et al. (50)	IFNα2b + interleukin-2[c]	II	6.6-yr; p = 0.93	6.6-yr; p = 0.93
Richtig et al. (51)	IFNα2a + isotretinoin[d]	II	5-yr; p = 0.25	5-yr; p = 0.80

Control arms: [a,d]low-dose IFN.
[b]high-dose IFN.
[c]observation.

IFN in stage II/III patient trials at the time when these patients were not SN-staged corresponds very well with the observations in the EORTC18952 and 18991 trials where the best benefit was observed in patients with positive sentinel nodes.

Combinational Trials with Low-Dose IFNα

Four prospective-randomized multicenter trials demonstrated that a combination of low-dose IFNα with other agents would not contribute to a better outcome for melanoma patients (Table 17.10). A DeCOG trial combined LDI with dacarbazine, both drugs given for two years in patients with stage III disease. Surprisingly, the combination of LDI plus dacarbazine diminished the treatment effects observed by LDI alone (47). Another randomized trial on 604 stage III melanoma patients combined Melacine with low-dose IFNα. This regimen was compared to high-dose IFNα2b alone. No differences, in terms of an improvement of RFS or OS, were observed (49). A DeCOG trial on LDI combined with low-dose interleukin 2 (IL-2) presented overlapping survival curves for DFS and OS compared to untreated controls (50). A randomized, double-blinded, placebo-controlled trial from Austria comparing LDI and isotretinoin to IFNα alone in stage II A/II B melanoma patients was stopped for futility (51). In conclusion, a combination of low-dose IFNα with various other agents, which might have an additional or synergistic effect, did not demonstrate any beneficial effect on either conventional LDI or observation alone.

Systematic Reviews and Meta-analyses

A systematic review of all trials (52), a meta-analysis of all trials (53), and a pooled data analysis of all HDI trials (54) demonstrated a consistent DFS improvement but no statistically significant impact on OS. A meta-analysis based on individual patient data, reported at the 43rd Annual Meeting of ASCO in 2007, confirmed the statistically significant benefit on DFS (7%) (55). It also demonstrated, for the first time, statistically significant impact on OS. However, this impact is extremely small and constitutes an absolute improvement of 3%. Moreover, this effect is partly due to the inclusion of trials ECOG1694, which had the ganglioside GM2 vaccine as a comparator arm (31). The validity of inclusion of this trial has been very recently questioned as the GMK vaccine in the EORTC18961 trial was associated with worse outcome (30). Another important finding from this meta-analysis is that the benefits of IFN were not clearly dose-related.

Lack of Useful Predictive Factors

Gogas and colleagues have reported that patients treated with adjuvant IFN who developed auto-antibodies against thyreoglobulin, antinuclear antibodies, or cardiolipin had a significantly better outcome than patients who did not develop these signs of autoimmunity (56). The development of markers that might predict who will mount a host immune response could be extremely important. The markers could be used to determine which patients to treat with IFN and for how long. An evaluation of the presence or emergence of autoantibodies in patients who participated in the EORTC 18952 and EORTC18991 trials did not confirm Gogas' observations (57,58).

Conclusions

The lack of beneficial drugs in stage IV melanoma is reflected by a lack of clearly effective adjuvant therapies for patients with stage II-III melanoma. After decades of research, cytotoxic drugs, immune stimulants, and vaccines have all failed to show any clinically meaningful impact in the adjuvant setting. IFNα is the only drug that is presently considered for adjuvant therapy and is used with various schedules in Europe, both in stage II and stage III patients. In the absence of a clear overall survival benefit, its role remains optional instead of standard of care. Adjuvant trials of bevacizumab and anti-CTLA4 (EORTC18071 in macroscopic stage III) were commenced in 2008, but results will not be known before 2011. Pegylated-IFN will be explored by EORTC (EORTC18081) in ulcerated, primary high-risk, stage II patients because of analyses of both EORTC 18952 and 18991 that suggest increased IFN-sensitivity in patients with primary ulcerated melanomas.

SYSTEMIC THERAPIES FOR STAGE IV DISEASE
Investigational Drugs in First Line for Metastatic Melanoma

It is sobering to see how little, if any, progress has been made over the last three decades in the systemic treatment of advanced metastatic melanoma. The response rate to the "standard" drug dacarbazine is probably inferior to 10%, and no treatment is good enough to be considered standard of care (59). Polychemotherapy, addition of tamoxifen, interferon, interleukin-2, or their combinations have all failed to improve survival in more than 27 phase III trials (60–88), which are summarized in Tables 17.11, 17.12, and 17.13. Also a recently conducted phase III trial (EORTC 180832) evaluating a dose-intensified administration of temozolomide (TMZ) versus a standard DTIC regimen failed to demonstrate a benefit for TMZ (89).

So new agents should be offered in first line to stage IV melanoma patients to identify active new agents. Moreover, vaccine therapy trials have yielded very low response rates and no indication of any impact on survival (90). In randomized trials, dendritic cells failed (91) as well as peptides in combination with IL-2 (92). The anti-CTLA4 antibody may be important alone, or in combination with cytokines and vaccines, as it fundamentally changes the balance between T-helper and T-supressor/T-regulatory cells and can change the immune response and immune status of melanoma patients and cause (lasting) tumor regressions (93). Unfortunately, the pivotal randomized trial of tremelimumab versus DTIC did not show a benefit over DTIC (94). The ipilimumab trials are ongoing and ipilimumab will also be evaluated in the adjuvant setting in stage III patients with macroscopically involved nodes (EORTC 18071).

The pro-apoptotic antisense drug oblimersen was evaluated in a very large phase III trial involving 777 patients.

Table 17.11   Randomized Trials Mono vs. Polychemotherapy ± Tamoxifen

Year (authors)	Regimen	#Pts	Median survival	Significance	Ref.
Chemotherapies					
1998 (Jungnelius et al.)	DV vs. DVC	326	5.9 vs. 7.2	NS	60
2002 (Jelić et al.)	D1CaV vs. D2CaV vs. VBIC vs. CaP	219	4 vs. 5 vs. 6 vs. 4	NS	61
2005 (Bafaloukos et al.)	TMZ vs. TMZ + C	132	11.5 vs. 12	NS	62
Chemotherapies involving Tamoxifen					
1992 (Cocconi et al.)	D vs. DT	117	6.5 vs. 11	p = 0.02	63
1996 (Rusthoven et al.)	BCB vs. DCBT	204	7 vs. 7	NS	64
1998 (Falkson et al.)	D ± T ± IFN	248	10 vs. 9 vs. 8 vs. 9.5	NS	65
1999 (Agarwala et al.)	D + Carbo ± T	56	7 vs. 4.6	NS	66
1999 (Creagan et al.)	DCaC ± T	184	6.8 vs. 6.9	NS	67
1999 (Chapman et al.)	D vs. DCBT	240	6.4 vs. 7.7	NS	68

Abbreviations: B, BCNU; BI, bleomycin; C, cisplatin; Ca, carmustine; carbo, carboplatin; D, dacarbazide; NS, not significant; P, procarbazine; T, tamoxifen; V, vinblastine.

Table 17.12   Randomized Trials Investigating Value of Addition of IFN to (Poly) Chemotherapy

Year (Author)	Regimen	#Pts	Median survival (months)	Significance	Ref.
1991 (Falkson et al.)	D ± IFN	64	9.6 vs. 17.6	p < 0.01	69
1993 (Thomson et al.)	D ± IFN	170	7.6 vs. 8.8	NS	70
1994 (Bajetta et al.)	D ± IFN[a]	242	11 vs. 11 vs. 13	NS	71
1998 (Falkson et al.)	D vs. D/IFN vs. D/T vs. D/IFN/T	258	10 vs. 9 vs. 8 vs. 9.5	NS	65
2000 (Middleton et al.)	D/IFN vs. DCBT	105	6.5 vs. 6.5	NS	72
2001 (Young et al.)	D ± IFN	61	7.2 vs. 4.8	NS	73
2005 (Kaufmann et al.)	TMZ ± IFN	282	8.4 vs. 9.7	NS	74
2005 (Vuoristo et al.)	D/nIFN vs. DCBT/IFN vs. D/rIFN vs. DCBT/rIFN	108	11 vs. 10 vs. 9 vs. 7.5	NS	75

[a]Dose 3 or 9 MIU.

Abbreviations: B, BCNU (carmustine); C, cisplatin; D, dacarbazine; IFN, interferon α; IL2, interleukin-2; n, natural; NS, not significant; r, recombinant; T, tamoxifen; TMZ, temozolomide; V, vinblastine.

Table 17.13   Randomized Trials with IL-2 or IL-2 + IFN Containing Regimens

Year (author)	Regimen	#Pts	Median survival (months)	Significance	Ref.
1993 (Sparano et al.)	IL2 ± IFN	85	10.2 vs. 9.7	NS	76
1997 (Keilholz et al.)	IL2/IFN ± C	133	9 vs. 9	NS	77
1998 (Johnston et al.)	CDBT ± IFN/IL2	65	5.5 vs. 5.0	NS	78
1999 (Dorval et al.)	C/IL2 ± IFN	117	10.4 vs. 10.9	NS	79
1999 (Rosenberg et al.)	CDT ± IFN/IL2	102	15.8 vs. 10.7	$p < 0.06$	80
2001 (Hauschild et al.)	D/IFN ± IL2	290	11 vs. 11	NS	81
2002 (Eton et al.)	CVD ± IFN/IL2	183	9.2 vs. 11.9	$p < 0.06$	82
2002 (Atzpodien et al.)	D/B/C/T ± IFN/IL2	124	13 vs. 12	NS	83
2002 (Agarwala et al.)	IL2 ± Histamine	305	9.1 vs. 8.2	NS	84
2002 (Ridolfi et al.)	CVD ± IFN/IL2	176	9.5 vs. 11.0	NS	85
2005 (Keilholz et al.)	CD/IFN ± IL2	363	9 vs. 9	NS	86
2006 (Bajetta et al.)	CVD ± IFN/IL2	139	12 vs. 11	NS	87
2008 (Atkins et al.)	CVD ± IFN/IL2	416	8.7 vs. 8.4	NS	88

Abbreviations: B, BCNU (Carmustine); C, cisplatin; D, dacarbazine; IFN, interferon α; IL2, interleukin-2; n, natural; NS, not significant; r, recombinant; T, tamoxifen; TMZ, temozolomide; V, vinblastine.

When given in combination with DTIC it improved response rates and progression-free survival rate significantly. Survival was not significantly improved. It appeared that all benefit occurred in the patient population with normal LDH levels, and the impact on survival was significant in this population (two-third of the total population) (95). A second pivotal trial is currently ongoing testing the same regimen in patients with LDH <0.8 UNL. Another apoptosis inducing agent [by way of increasing radical oxygen species (ROS)] is STA-4783 (Elesclomol). Synergy with taxol in animal models and a positive double-blind, randomized, placebo-controlled phase II trial comparing elesclomol + taxol with taxol alone has lead to the currently ongoing pivotal phase III trial with the same design (96). Another development regards sorafanib, a tyrosine kinase inhibitor, B-Raf inhibitor, with important anti-VEGFR2-mediated anti-angiogenic properties, which is currently evaluated in combination with caboplatin/taxol in a 800-patient phase III trial in first line (97). However, a rapid smaller phase III trial in second line failed to demonstrate a benefit for the same combination arm (98). In addition pivotal phase III trials are being developed for a nanoparticle albumen-bound paclitaxel (abraxane) formulation that has been approved for breast cancer (99) and for thymosin α1, a T-cell immune response–enhancing molecule.

More complex, but of fundamental importance, is the ongoing research how to utilize dendritic cells. Remarkable results have been reported by Rosenberg's group, with chemotherapy-lymphodepletion followed by adoptive transfer of autologous tumor-reactive lymphocytes in highly pretreated refractory melanoma patients. A response rate of 49% in 43 patients has been reported and should provide insight in what is crucial to obtain tumor regression in melanoma patients. When total body irradiation (TBI) of 2GY was added to the lymphodepletion conditioning protocol of the patients, a 52% response rate was observed in 25 patients and a 72% response rate in the next 25 patients when a TBI of 12GY was applied. Lymphodepletion conditioning of the patient seems to be the crucial element in this approach, which allows for the effective 100 to 1000-fold

in vivo expansion of short-term in vitro expanded T-cell cultures from tumor infiltrating lymphocytes (100).

CONCLUSIONS

There is no effective therapy for metastatic melanoma. Polychemotherapy or chemoimmunotherapy have not demonstrated survival benefits. Vaccines have shown thus far very little activity in stage IV disease. New drugs should be offered in first line to intensify the quest to identify effective agents. All efforts must be directed on science to improve our understanding of the biology of malignant melanoma. Too many wasteful phase III trials have been conducted with poor understanding of the mechanism of action of the involved drugs.

REFERENCES

1. http://seer.cancer.gov/statfacts/
2. Curado MP, Edwards B, Shin HR et al. eds. Cancer Incidence in Five Continents, vol. IX. IARC Scientific Publications No. 160. Lyon: IARC, 2007.
3. Karim-Kos HE, de Vries E, Soerjomataram I et al. Recent trends of cancer in Europe: a combined approach of incidence, survival and mortality for 17 cancer sites since the 1990s. Eur J Cancer 2008; 44: 1345–89.
4. Elwood JM, Gallagher RP. Body site distribution of cutaneous malignant melanoma in relationship to patterns of sun exposure. Int J Cancer 1998; 78: 276–80.
5. de Vries E, van de Poll-Franse LV, Louwman WJ et al. Predictions of skin cancer incidence in the Netherlands up to 2015. Br J Dermatol 2005; 152: 481–8.
6. Garbe C, Blum A. Epidemiology of cutaneous melanoma in Germany and Worldwide. Skin Pharmacol Physiol 2001; 14: 280–90.
7. http://www.health.qld.gov.au/hic/qcr2005/1982_03_text.pdf
8. Pho L, Grossman D, Leachman SA. Melanoma genetics: a review of genetic factors and clinical phenotypes in familial melanoma. Curr Opin Oncol 2006; 18: 173–9.

9. Soufir N, Ollivaud L, Bertrand G et al. A French CDK4-positive melanoma family with a co-inherited EDNRB mutation. J Dermatol Sci 2007; 46: 61–4.

10. Raimondi S, Sera F, Gandini S et al. MC1R variants, melanoma and red hair color phenotype: a meta-analysis. Int J Cancer 2008; 122: 2753–60.

11. Box NF, Duffy DL, Chen W et al. MC1R genotype modifies risk of melanoma in families segregating CDKN2A mutations. Am J Hum Genet 2001; 69: 765–73.

12. Brown KM, Macgregor S, Montgomery GW et al. Common sequence variants on 20q11.22 confer melanoma susceptibility. Nat Genet 2008; 40: 838–40.

13. Gudbjartsson DF, Sulem P, Stacey SN et al. ASIP and TYR pigmentation variants associate with cutaneous melanoma and basal cell carcinoma. Nat Genet 2008; 40: 886–91.

14. Curiel C, Gomex ML, Atkins T. Association between use of non steroidal anti-inflammatories and of melanoma: a case control study. J Clin Oncol Supplement 2007; 8500.

15. Whiteman DC, Watt P, Purdie DM et al. Melanocytic nevi, solar keratoses, and divergent pathways to cutaneous melanoma. J Natl Cancer Inst 2003; 95: 806–12.

16. Thomas NE, Edmiston SH, Alexander A. Number of naevi and early life ambient UV exposure are associated with B-RAF mutant melanoma. Cancer Epidemiol Biomarkers Prev 2007; 16: 991–7.

17. International Agency for Research on Cancer Working Group on artificial ultraviolet (UV) light and skin cancer. The association of use of sunbeds with cutaneous malignant melanoma and other skin cancers: a systematic review. Int J Cancer 2007; 120: 1116–22.

18. Grob JJ, Bonerandi JJ. The "ugly duckling" sign: identification of the common characteristics of nevi in an individual as a basis for melanoma screening. Arch Dermatol 1998; 134: 103–4.

19. Balch CM, Buzaid AC, Soong SJ et al. Final version of the American Joint Committee on Cancer staging system for cutaneous melanoma. J Natl Compr Canc Netw 2006; 4: 666–84.

20. Eggermont AMM, Gore M. Randomised adjuvant trials in melanoma: surgical and systemic. Semin Oncol 2007; 34: 509–15.

21. Gershenwald JE, Thompson W, Mansfield PF et al. Multi-institutional melanoma lymphatic mapping experience: the prognostic value of sentinel lymph node status in 612 stage I or II melanoma patients. J Clin Oncol 1999; 17: 976–83.

22. Morton DL, Thompson JF, Cochran AJ et al. Sentinel-node biopsy or nodal observation in melanoma. N Engl J Med 2006; 355: 1307–17.

23. van Akkooi AC, de Wilt JH, Verhoef C et al. Clinical relevance of melanoma micrometastases (<0.1mm) in sentinel nodes: are these nodes to be considered negative? Ann Oncol 2006; 17: 1578–85.

24. Thomas JM. Prognostic false-positivity of the sentinel node in melanoma [review]. Nat Clin Pract Oncol 2008; 5: 18–23.

25. Eggermont AMM. Reducing the need for sentinel node procedures by ultrasound examination of regional lymph nodes. Ann Surg Oncol 2005; 12: 3–5.

26. Pawlik TM, Ross MI, Thompson JF et al. The risk of in-transit metastasis depends on tumor biology and not the surgical approach to regional lymph nodes. J Clin Oncol 2005; 23: 4588–90.

27. Grünhagen DJ, Brunstein F, Graveland WJ et al. One hundred consecutive isolated limb perfusions with TNF-alpha and melphalan in melanoma patients with multiple in-transit metastases. Ann Surg 2004; 240: 939–47.

28. Thompson JF, Kam PC, Waugh RC et al. Isolated limb infusion with cytotoxic agents: simple alternative to isolated limb perfusion. Semin Surg Oncol 1998; 14: 238–47.

29. Testori A, Rutkowski P, Marsden J et al. Surgery and radiotherapy in the treatment of cutaneous melanoma. Ann Oncol 2008; in press.

30. Eggermont AM, Suciu S, Ruka W et al., EORTC melanoma group. EORTC 18961: post-operative adjuvant ganglioside GM2-KLH21 vaccination treatment vs observation in stage II (T3-T4N0M0) melanoma: 2nd interim analysis led to an early disclosure of the results. J Clin Oncol 2008; 26(Suppl): 9004.

31. Kirkwood JM, Ibrahim JG, Sosman JA et al. High-dose interferon alfa-2b significantly prolongs relapse-free and overall survival compared with the GM2-KLH/QS-21 vaccine in patients with resected stage IIB-III melanoma: results of intergroup trial E1694/S9512/C509801. J Clin Oncol 2001; 19: 2370–80.

32. Morton D, Mozzillo N, Thompson J et al. An international, randomised, phase III trial of BCG plus allogeneic melanoma vaccine (MCV) or placebo after complete resection of melanoma metastatic to regional nodes or distant sites. J Clin Oncol 2007; 25(Suppl): 8508.

33. Creagan ET, Dalton RJ, Ahmann DL et al. Randomized, surgical adjuvant clinical trial of recombinant interferon alfa-2a in selected patients with malignant melanoma. J Clin Oncol 1995; 13: 2776–83.

34. Kirkwood JM, Strawderman MH, Ernstoff MS et al. Interferon alfa-2b adjuvant therapy of high-risk resected cutaneous melanoma: the Eastern Cooperative Oncology Group Trial EST 1684. J Clin Oncol 1996; 14: 7–17.

35. Kirkwood JM, Ibrahim JG, Sondak VK et al. High- and low-dose interferon alfa-2b in high-risk melanoma: first analysis of intergroup trial E1690/S9111/C9190. J Clin Oncol 2000; 18: 2444–59.

36. McMasters KM, Ross MI, Reintgen DS et al. Final Results of the Sunbelt Trial. J Clin Oncol 2008; 26(May 20 Suppl): abstract 9003.

37. Gogas H, Dafni U, Bafaloukos D et al. A randomized phase III trial of 1 month versus 1 year adjuvant high-dose interferon alfa-2b in patients with resected high risk melanoma. J Clin Oncol 2007; 25: abstract 8505.

38. Eggermont AM, Suciu S, MacKie R et al. Post-surgery adjuvant therapy with intermediate doses of interferon alfa 2b versus observation in patients with stage IIb/III melanoma (EORTC 18952): randomised controlled trial. Lancet 2005; 366: 1189–96.

39. Hansson J, Aamdal S, Bastholt L et al. Results of the Nordic randomized adjuvant trial of intermediate-doe interferon alfa-2b in high-risk melanoma. Eur J Cancer Supplements 2007; 5: abstract 4.

40. Eggermont AM, Suciu S, Santinami M et al. Adjuvant therapy with pegylated interferon alfa-2b versus observation alone in resected stage III melanoma: final results of EORTC 18991, a randomised phase III trial. Lancet 2008; 372: 117–26.

41. Hauschild A, Volkenandt M, Tilgen W et al. Efficacy of interferon alpha 2a in 18 versus 60 months of treatment in patients with primary melanoma of >1.5mm tumor thickness: A randomized phase III DeCOG trial. J Clin Oncol 2008; 26(May 20 Suppl): abstract 9032.

42. Grob JJ, Dreno B, de la Salmonière P et al. Randomised trial of interferon alpha-2a as adjuvant therapy in resected primary melanoma thicker than 1.5mm without clinically detectable node metastases. Lancet 1998; 351: 1905–10.

43. Pehamberger H, Soyer HP, Steiner A et al. Adjuvant interferon alfa-2a treatment in resected primary stage II cutaneous melanoma. Austrian Malignant Melanoma Cooperative Group. J Clin Oncol 1998; 16: 1425–9.

44. Cameron DA, Cornbleet MC, Mackie RM et al. Adjuvant interferon alpha 2b in high risk melanoma—the Scottish study. Br J Cancer 2001; 84: 1146–9.

45. Hancock BW, Wheatley K, Harris S et al. Adjuvant interferon in high-risk melanoma: the AIM HIGH Study—United Kingdom Coordinating Committee on Cancer Research randomized study of adjuvant low-dose extended-duration interferon Alfa-2a in high-risk resected malignant melanoma. J Clin Oncol 2004; 22: 53–61.

46. Cascinelli N, Belli F, MacKie RM et al. Effect of long-term adjuvant therapy with interferon alpha-2a in patients with regional node metastases from cutaneous melanoma: a randomised trial. Lancet 2001; 358: 866–9.

47. Garbe C, Radny P, Linse R et al. Adjuvant low-dose interferon alpha-2a with or without dacarbazine compared with surgery alone: a prospective-randomized phase III DeCOG trial in melanoma patients with regional lymph node metastasis. Ann Oncol 2008; 19: 1195–201.

48. Kleeberg UR, Suciu S, Bröcker EB et al. EORTC Melanoma Group in cooperation with the German Cancer Society (DKG). Final results of the EORTC 18871/DKG 80-1 randomised phase III trial. rIFN-alpha2b versus rIFN-gamma versus ISCADOR M versus observation after surgery in melanoma patients with either high-risk primary (thickness >3mm) or regional lymph node metastasis. Eur J Cancer 2004; 40(3): 390–402.

49. Mitchell MS, Abrams J, Thompson JA et al. Randomized trial of an allogeneic melanoma lysate vaccine with low-dose interferon Alfa-2b compared with high-dose interferon Alfa-2b for resected stage III cutaneous melanoma. J Clin Oncol 2007; 25: 2078–85.

50. Hauschild A, Weichenthal M, Balda BR et al. Prospective randomized trial of interferon alfa-2b and interleukin-2 as adjuvant treatment for resected intermediate- and high-risk primary melanoma without clinically detectable node metastasis. J Clin Oncol 2003; 21: 2883–8.

51. Richtig E, Soyer HP, Posch M et al. Prospective, randomized, multicenter, double-blind placebo-controlled trial comparing adjuvant interferon alfa and isotretinoin with interferon alfa alone in stage IIA and IIB melanoma: European Cooperative Adjuvant Melanoma Treatment Study Group. J Clin Oncol 2005; 23: 8655–63.

52. Lens MB, Dawes M. Interferon alfa therapy for malignant melanoma: a systematic review of randomized controlled trials. J Clin Oncol 2002; 20: 1818–25.

53. Wheatley K, Ives N, Hancock B et al. Does adjuvant interferon-alpha for high-risk melanoma provide a worthwhile benefit? A meta-analysis of the randomised trials. Cancer Treat Rev 2003; 29: 241–52.

54. Kirkwood JM, Manola J, Ibrahim J et al. A pooled analysis of eastern cooperative oncology group and intergroup trials of adjuvant high-dose interferon for melanoma. Clin Cancer Res 2004; 10: 1670–7.

55. Wheatley K, Ives N, Eggermont AM et al. Interferon-α as adjuvant therapy for melanoma: An individual patient data meta-analysis of randomised trials. J Clin Oncol 2007; 25(Suppl): abstract 8526.

56. Gogas H, Ioannovich J, Dafni U et al. Prognostic significance of autoimmunity during treatment of melanoma with interferon. N Engl J Med 2006; 354: 709–18.

57. Bouwhuis M, Suciu S, Kruit W et al. Prognostic value of autoantibodies (auto-AB) in melanoma patients (pts) in the EORTC 18952 trial of adjuvant interferon (IFN) compared to observation (obs). J Clin Oncol 2007; 25(Suppl): abstract 8507.

58. Bouwhuis M, Suciu S, Testori A et al. Prognostic value of autoantibodies (auto-AB) in melanoma stage III patients in the EORTC 18991 phase III randomized trial comparing adjuvant pegylated interferon α2b (PEG-IFN) vs Observation. Eur J Cancer 2007; 5(Suppl): 11, abstract 13BA.

59. Eggermont AM, Kirkwood JM. Re-evaluating the role of dacarbazine in metastatic melanoma: what have we learned in 30 years? Eur J Cancer 2004; 40: 1825–36.

60. Jungnelius U, Ringborg U, Aamdal S et al. Dacarbazine–vindesine versus dacarbazine–vindesine–cisplatin in disseminated malignant melanoma. A randomised phase III trial. Eur J Cancer 1998; 34: 1368–74.

61. Jelić S, Babovic N, Kovcin V et al. Comparison of the efficacy of two different dosage dacarbazine regimens and two regimens without dacarbazine in metastatic melanoma: a single-centre randomized four-arm study. Melanoma Res 2002; 12: 91–8.

62. Bafaloukos D, Tsoutsos D, Kalofonos H et al. Temozolomide and cisplatin versus temozolomide in patients with advanced melanoma: a randomized phase II study of the Hellenic Cooperative Oncology Group. Ann Oncol 2005; 16: 950–7.

63. Cocconi G, Bella M, Calabresi F et al. Treatment of metastatic malignant melanoma with dacarbazine plus tamoxifen. N Engl J Med 1992; 327: 516–23.

64. Rusthoven JJ, Quirt IC, Iscoe NA et al. Randomized, double-blind, placebo-controlled trial comparing the response rates of carmustine, dacarbazine, and cisplatin with and without tamoxifen in patients with metastatic melanoma. National Cancer Institute of Canada Clinical Trials Group. J Clin Oncol 1996; 14: 2083–90.

65. Falkson CI, Ibrahim J, Kirkwood JM et al. Phase III trial of Dacarbazine versus Dacarbazide with Interferon Alpha2b versus Dacarbazide with Tamoxifen versus Dacarbazide with Interferon Alpha2b with Tamoxifen in patients with metastatic malignant melanoma: an Eastern Cooperative Oncology Study. J Clin Oncol 1998; 16: 1743–51.

66. Agarwala SS, Ferri W, Gooding W et al. A phase III randomized trial of dacarbazine and carboplatin with and without tamoxifen in the treatment of patients with metastatic melanoma. Cancer 1999; 85: 1979–84.

67. Creagan ET, Suman VJ, Dalton RJ et al. Phase III clinical trial of the combination of cisplatin, dacarbazine and carmustine with or without tamoxifen in patients with advanced malignant melanoma. J Clin Oncol 1999; 17: 1884–90.

68. Chapman PB, Einhorn LH, Meyers ML et al. Phase III multicenter randomized trial of the Dartmouth regimen versus dacarbazine in patients with metastatic melanoma. J Clin Oncol 1999; 17: 2745–51.

69. Falkson CI, Falkson G, Falkson HC. Improved results with the addition of interferon alfa-2b to dacarbazine in the treatment of patients with metastatic malignant melanoma. J Clin Oncol 1991; 9: 1403–8.

70. Thomson DB, Adena M, McLeod GRC et al. Interferon-alpha 2a does not improve response or survival when combined with dacarbazide in metastatic malignant melanoma: results of a multi-institutional Australian randomized trial. Melanoma Res 1993; 3: 133–8.

71. Bajetta E, Di Leo A, Zampino MG et al. Multicenter randomized trial of dacarbazine alone or in combination with two different doses and schedules of interferon alfa-2a in the treatment of advanced melanoma. J Clin Oncol 1994; 12: 806–11.

72. Middleton MR, Lorigan P, Owen J et al. A randomized phase III study comparing dacarbazine, BCNU, cisplatin and tamoxifen with dacarbazine and interferon in advanced melanoma. Br J Cancer 2000; 82: 1158–62.

73. Young AM, Marsden J, Goodman A et al. Prospective randomized comparison of dacarbazine (DTIC) versus DTIC plus interferon-alpha (IFN-alpha) in metastatic melanoma. Clin Oncol 2001; 13: 458–65.

74. Kaufmann R, Spieth K, Leiter U et al. Temozolomide in combination with interferon-alfa versus temozolomide alone in patients with advanced metastatic melanoma: a randomized, phase III, multicenter study from the Dermatologic Cooperative Oncology Group. J Clin Oncol 2005; 23: 9001–7.

75. Vuoristo MS, Hahka-Kemppinen M, Parvinen LM et al. Randomized trial of dacarbazine versus bleomycin, vincristine, lomustine and dacarbazine (BOLD) chemotherapy combined

with natural or recombinant interferon-alpha in patients with advanced melanoma. Melanoma Res 2005; 15: 291–6.

76. Sparano JA, Fisher RI, Sunderland M et al. Randomized phase III trial of treatment with high-dose interleukin-2 either alone or in combination with interferon alfa-2a in patients with advanced melanoma. J Clin Oncol 1993; 11: 1969–77.

77. Keilholz U, Goey SH, Punt CJ et al. Interferon alfa-2a and interleukin-2 with or without cisplatin in metastatic melanoma: a randomized trial of the European Organization for Research and Treatment of Cancer Melanoma Cooperative Group. J Clin Oncol 1997; 7: 2579–88.

78. Johnston SR, Constenla DO, Moore J et al. Randomized phase II trial of BCDT [carmustine (BCNU), cisplatin, dacarbazine (DTIC) and tamoxifen] with or without interferon alpha (IFN-alpha) and interleukin (IL-2) in patients with metastatic melanoma. Br J Cancer 1998; 77: 1280–6.

79. Dorval T, Negrier S, Chevreau C et al. Randomized trial of treatment with cisplatin and interleukin-2 either alone or in combination with interferon-alpha-2a in patients with metastatic melanoma: a Federation Nationale des Centres de Lutte Contre le Cancer Multicenter, parallel study. Cancer 1999; 85: 1060–6.

80. Rosenberg SA, Yang JC, Schwartzentruber DJ et al. Prospective randomized trial of the treatment of patients with metastatic melanoma using chemotherapy with cisplatin, dacarbazine, and tamoxifen alone or in combination with interleukin-2 and interferon alfa-2b. J Clin Oncol 1999; 17: 968–75.

81. Hauschild A, Garbe C, Stolz W et al. Dacarbazine and interferon alpha with or without interleukin 2 in metastatic melanoma: a randomized phase III multicentre trial of the Dermatologic Cooperative Oncology Group (DeCOG). Br J Cancer 2001; 84: 1036–42.

82. Eton O, Legha SS, Bedikian AY et al. Sequential biochemotherapy versus chemotherapy for metastatic melanoma: results from a phase III randomized trial. J Clin Oncol 2002; 20: 2045–52.

83. Atzpodien J, Neuber K, Kamanabroe D et al. Combination chemotherapy with or without s.c. IL-2 and IFN-alpha: results of a prospectively randomized trial of the Cooperative Advanced Malignant Melanoma Chemoimmunotherapy group (ACIMM). Br J Cancer 2002; 86: 179–84.

84. Agarwala SA, Glaspy J, O'Day SJ et al. Results from a randomized phase III study comparing combined treatment with histamine dihydrochloride plus interleukin-2 versus interleukin-2 alone in patients with metastatic melanoma. J ClinOncol 2002; 20: 125–33.

85. Ridolfi R, Chiarion-Sileni V, Guida M et al. Cisplatin, Dacarbazine with or without subcutaneous interleukin-2 and interferon alfa-2b in advanced melanoma outpatients: results from an Italian multicenter phase III randomized clinical trial. J Clin Oncol 2002; 20: 1600–7.

86. Keilholz U, Punt CJ, Gore M et al. Dacarbazine, cisplatin, and interferon-alfa-2b with or without interleukin-2 in metastatic melanoma: a randomized phase III trial (18951) of the European Organisation for Research and Treatment of Cancer Melanoma Group. J Clin Oncol 2005; 23: 6747–55.

87. Bajetta E, Del Vecchio M, Nova P et al. Multicenter phase III randomized trial of polychemotherapy (CVD regimen) versus the same chemotherapy (CT) plus subcutaneous interleukin-2 and interferon-alpha2b in metastatic melanoma. Ann Oncol 2006; 17: 571–7.

88. Atkins MB, Lee S, Flaherty LE et al. A prospective randomized phase III trial of concurrent biochemotherapy (BCT) with cisplatin, vinblastine, dacarbazine (CVD), IL-2 and interferon alpha-2b (IFN) versus CVD alone in patients with metastatic melanoma (E3695): An ECOG-coordinated intergroup trial. J Clin Oncol; in press.

89. Patel PM, Suciu S, Mortier L et al. Extended schedule, escalated dose Temozolomide versus Dacarbazine in stage IV malignant melanoma: final results of the randomized phase III study (EORTC 18032). Ann Oncol 2008; 19(Suppl 8): viii3 (Abstract LBA8).

90. Rosenberg SA, Yang JC, Restifo NP. Cancer-immunotherapy: moving beyond current vaccines. Nat Med 2004; 10: 909–15.

91. Schadendorf D, Ugurel S, Schuler-Thurner B et al. Dacarbazine (DTIC) versus vaccination with autologous peptide-pulsed dendritic cells (DC) in first-line treatment of patients with metastatic melanoma: a randomized phase III trial of the DC study group of the DeCOG. Ann Oncol 2006; 17: 563–70.

92. Sosman JA, Carrillo C, Urba WJ et al. Three phase II cytokine working group trials of gp100 (210M) peptide plus high-dose interleukin-2 in patients with HLA-A2-positive advanced melanoma. J Clin Oncol 2008; 26: 2292–8.

93. Weber J. Review: anti-CTLA-4 antibody ipilimumab: case studies of clinical response and immune-related adverse events [review]. Oncologist 2007; 12: 864–72.

94. Ribas A, Hauschild A, Kefford R et al. Phase III, open-label, randomized, comparative study of tremelimumab (CP-675,206) and chemotherapy [temozolomide (TMZ) or dacarbazine (DTIC)] in patients with advanced melanoma. J Clin Oncol 2008; 26(May 20 Suppl): abstract LBA9011.

95. Bedikian AY, Millward M, Pehamberger H et al. Oblimersen Melanoma Study Group. Bcl-2 antisense (oblimersen sodium) plus dacarbazine in patients with advanced melanoma: the Oblimersen Melanoma Study Group. J Clin Oncol 2006; 24: 4738–45.

96. Gonzalez R, Lawson DH, Weber RW et al. Phase II trial of elesclomol (formerly STA-4783) and paclitaxel in stage IV metastatic melanoma (MM): subgroup analysis by prior chemotherapy. J Clin Oncol 2008; 26: abstract 9036.

97. Flaherty KT. Chemotherapy and targeted therapy combinations in advanced melanoma. Clin Cancer Res 2006; 12: 2366s–70s.

98. Hauschild A, Agarwala SS, Trefzer U et al. Phase III randomized, placebo-controlled study of Sorafenib in combination with carboplatin and paclitaxel in second-line treatment in patients with unresectable stage III or stage IV melanoma. J Clin Oncol 2008; in press.

99. Gradishar WJ, Tjulandin S, Davidson N et al. Phase III trial of nanoparticle albumin-bound paclitaxelcompared with polyethylated castor oil-based paclitaxel in women with breast cancer. J Clin Oncol 2005; 23: 7794–803.

100. Dudley ME, Yang JC, Sherry R et al. Adoptive cell therapy for patients with metastatic melanoma: Evaluation of intensive myeloablative chemoradiation preparative regimens. J Clin Oncol 2008; 26: 5233–9.

18

Cancer of Unknown Primary Site

Gedske Daugaard, Anne Kirstine Møller, and Bodil Laub Petersen

In about 5% of all cancer patients, the primary origin of the tumor cannot be identified. Cancer of unknown primary site (CUP) ranks among the 10 most common malignancies and constitutes a heterogeneous clinical entity with regression of the primary tumor, development of early, uncommon, systemic metastases, and usually a poor prognosis. The biology of the disease is unknown, and it is not clear if CUP represents a distinct entity with specific genetic/phenotypic aberrations (1). The primary tumor is rarely identified in the period of subsequent follow-up, and less than 30% of patients have a primary site identified ante-mortem. Postmortem examination reveals a putative primary site in 60% to 80% of all patients.

Patients with CUP often undergo an extensive diagnostic workup using advanced immunohistochemical and imaging techniques for identifying the primary tumor site. In recent years, significant advances have occurred almost exclusively regarding the identification of subsets of patients who have clinical and pathologic features that require specific treatment strategies, which may translate into prolonged survival (2). Unfortunately, the majority of patients with CUP (approximately 85%) are not included in those favorable patient subsets, for whom diagnostic and therapeutic strategies are less obvious. Therefore, time-consuming and prolonged search often delays the initiation of treatment. Failure to identify the primary tumor might influence patient management, as tailored chemotherapeutic regimens and targeted agents for a number of solid tumors have increasingly been developed over the last decade.

Decisions confronting clinicians include which and how many investigations should be used to determine the primary site, and what the most cost-effective investigations are and which is the appropriate treatment.

The range of therapeutic options for patients with metastatic cancer continues to increase, and treatment decisions are based on tumor type, response rates, quality of life considerations, and survival data. Although the treatment outcomes of lymphoma and germ-cell tumors are clearly the most rewarding, effective treatment for several forms of carcinoma is now available and should be applied in appropriate settings.

Profiling of multiple gene expression in tumors is now possible because of the development of high-throughput DNA microarray platforms. Some molecular biology data suggest that each tumor maintains at least the basic genetic signature of the tissue of origin throughout clonal evolution and metastatic dissemination. Gene expression profiling may therefore enable an accurate identification of the site of origin of the tumor, and this could be an important tool in the treatment of CUP in the future.

CLINICAL INVESTIGATIONS

All patients should have a careful history taken and undergo a complete physical examination including head and neck, pelvic, and rectal examination, routine laboratory evaluation (blood counts and chemistry profile), urine analysis, and fecal occult blood test, although routine laboratory evaluation seldom shows any characteristic abnormalities in this group of patients (2,3). Specific investigations according to the site of lymph node metastases are described later in this chapter.

Radiological Studies

Using CT scans of the abdomen and pelvis, a primary tumor can be detected in 30% to 35% of patients. A CT scan of the thorax is also relevant in CUP patients, because lung cancer is one of the most common primary tumors identified in patients with CUP (1). In addition, CT scans can also be helpful in determining the extent of metastatic disease. CT scan of thorax, abdomen, and pelvis therefore constitutes the standard evaluation recommended in patients with CUP (3).

Endoscopic examinations should be performed only in patients with specific symptoms or signs. For example, patients with abdominal symptoms or occult blood in the stool should undergo endoscopic examination of the gastrointestinal tract (2,3).

Several studies have investigated position emission tomography (PET) using ^{18}F-fluorodeoxy-glucose (^{18}F-FDG PET) as a diagnostic tool in patients with CUP, particularly in patients with cervical lymph node metastases. Rusthoven et al. (4) and Seve et al. (5) have recently reviewed the literature of ^{18}F-FDG PET studies in CUP patients with cervical lymph node metastases and extracervical metastases, respectively. ^{18}F-FDG PET revealed a primary tumor, undetected by other modalities, in approximately 25% to 40% of patients and detected additional metastases in 27% to 37% (4,5). The majority of the studies were retrospective, and patients analyzed were few (9–47 patients with extracervical metastases). In addition, the patient selection, histology, and additional radiological diagnostic procedures varied highly between the reviewed studies (5). Despite these limitations, ^{18}F-FDG PET is recommended as an additional diagnostic tool to conventional workup in patients

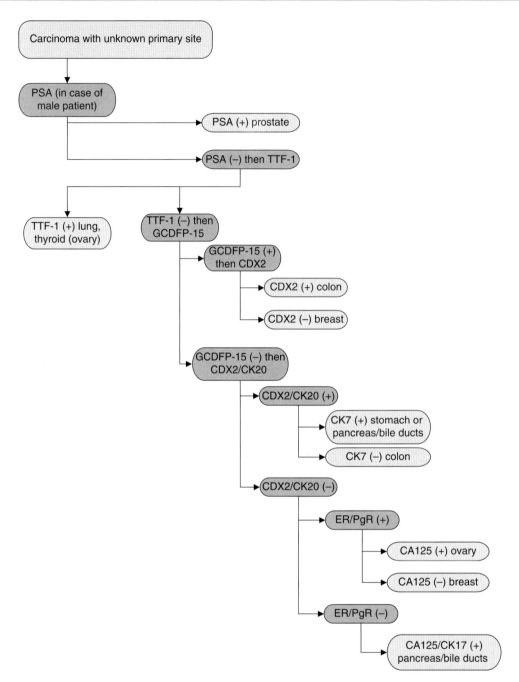

Figure 18.1 A diagnostic "decision tree" for carcinomas classified as CUP (identifiable germinal cell tumors, lymphomas, sarcomas, and primary hepatic carcinomas excluded). Applied markers are PSA (prostate specific antigen), TTF-1 (primarily lung), GCDFP-15 (breast), CDX2 (gastrointestinal tract), CK7, CK17 and CK20 (different expression in different epithelia), ER, PgR (hormone receptors), CA125 (certain types of adenocarcinoma). Based on data from Chu et al. (2005), Dennis et al. (2005), Park et al. (2007).

with CUP (6). In particular, it may be helpful in localizing head and neck tumors in CUP patients with cervical lymph node metastases. However, larger prospective studies are needed with more uniform inclusion criteria to evaluate the extent to which this investigation helps in the diagnosis of a primary tumor.

Recent papers have focused on the diagnostic value of combined ^{18}F-FDG PET/CT in patients with CUP. Most of the studies are retrospective and the sample size is small (range 21–68 patients). ^{18}F-FDG PET/CT has detected a primary tumor in 33% to 68% of the patients (7–11). ^{18}F-FDG PET/CT studies have been conducted in CUP patients only with cervical lymph node metastases (9,11), but in the majority of the studies, there was a high heterogeneity regarding patient selection, histology, and diagnostic workup (7,8,10). Larger prospective studies are needed to evaluate the value of ^{18}F-FDG PET/CT in patients with CUP, especially in patients belonging to the unfavorable subset (adenocarcinoma/carcinoma and multiple metastases), which constitutes the majority of CUP patients. ^{18}F-FDG PET/CT may help in guiding investigations early in the course; however, this also needs prospective evaluation.

Serological Tumor Markers

The use of serum tumor markers in the primary diagnostic work-up of cancer of unknown primary is limited, because of the lack of specificity and sensitivity. Some exceptions exist, though, and the measurement of PSA, AFP, and beta-HCG in male patients with CUP is recommended to exclude treatable extragonadal germ-cell tumors and metastatic prostate cancer (1,3). In female patients with pelvic tumors, the measurement of both CA125 and CEA can be very useful in helping to identify the primary site.

Other markers can be applied as an adjunct to monitoring response to therapy and detect recurrence. Biomarkers often used in this setting are PSA, AFP, beta-HCG, CA 125, CA 15-3, CA 19-9, and CEA. Few studies have examined serological tumor markers in patients with CUP. With the exception of AFP, the tumor markers (CEA, CA 19-9, CA 15-3, CA 125, and beta-HCG) were elevated in most of the patients. None of the markers were found to have a predictive value for response to chemotherapy or survival (12,13). These data suggest that patients with CUP have a non-specific overexpression of serum tumor markers. Once the measurement of tumor markers has been utilized in the initial diagnostic workup and exclusion of an established primary site, subsequent routine use of most tumor markers does not offer any significant diagnostic, prognostic, or predictive value in these patients.

Pathological Studies

Histology and Immunohistochemistry

Pathologic evaluation has been reported to be the most specific and cost-effective method to determine type and origin of CUP. The overall dominant morphological pattern of CUP is adenocarcinoma (50–70%), followed by poorly differentiated carcinoma (15–20%), squamous cell carcinoma, undifferentiated malignant tumor, and neuroendocrine carcinoma (each 5%). The major problem is to distinguish between different specific types of adenocarcinomas and undifferentiated carcinomas.

The primary site of metastatic adenocarcinoma is most frequently the breast, colon, lung, ovary, pancreas, prostate, and stomach, with a high representation of lung and pancreatic tumors (1).

Addition of immunohistochemistry to morphology using a limited panel of antibodies increases detection rate of primary site from 26% using morphology alone to 67% (14). The first step is to subdivide into differentiation subgroups (carcinoma, sarcoma, germ-cell tumor, lymphoma/leukemia, and melanoma). After primary subgrouping, a further identification can be attempted using other more specific markers (Fig. 18.1).

The primary antibody panel should combine the detection of site-specific antigens with the expression pattern of mucin antigens and intermediary filaments and in selected cases supplemented with markers of targeted therapy such as HER2.

Site-Specific Antigens, Intermediary Filaments, and Mucins

Prostate-specific antigen (PSA) is highly sensitive and specific for prostate cancer. PSA can be positive in the seminal vesicles, and weak positive reactions can be seen in pancreatic and salivary adenocarcinomas. Monoclonal PSA can be negative in high-grade tumors.

Thyroid transcription factor (TTF)-1 is found in pneumocytes and thyroid follicular epithelial cells. TTF-1 staining is not specific for lung but has been reported in neuroendocrine tumors, gastrointestinal, and ovarian cancer (15,16).

Gross cystic disease fluid protein (GCDFP)-15 is expressed in breast carcinomas, but also in carcinoma of salivary glands, colon, sweat glands, and prostate. This protein is considered a relatively specific marker for breast carcinoma although with a low sensitivity (17).

Estrogen and progesterone receptors (ER/PgR) are present in carcinomas of breast, ovary, and endometrium, but it is not specific for these sites, since especially ER can be demonstrated in carcinomas of lung, stomach, and thyroid (14).

Uroplakin III is a marker for urothelial cells with a high specificity and a moderate sensitivity for detection of primary and metastatic urothelial tumors (18).

CDX2 is an intestine-specific transcription factor and is expressed in the nuclei of normal colorectal tissue, colorectal adenocarcinoma, and mucinous types of adenocarcinomas of ovarian and lung origin in a homogeneous pattern (>75% tumor cell nuclei positive) (19).

Mucin antigens (MUCs). Mucins are high-molecular-weight glycoproteins synthesized by a broad range of epithelial tissues and designated MUCs. The expression pattern of MUC1, MUC2, and MUC5ac combined with the expression of CDX2 and CK17 is especially useful in distinguishing between pancreatic and gastrointestinal carcinomas (20).

Cytokeratins. CK7 and CK20, intermediary filaments present in epithelial cells, are the most widely examined antigens in the cytokeratin group comprising approximately 20 proteins. The differential expression pattern of these two cytokeratins can predict the site of primary tumor (21). For instance, CK7 positivity and CK20 negativity favors gynecological over gastrointestinal primary tumors, although exceptions exist. CK17 can be used to distinguish between pancreatic/biliary, esophageal, and GI carcinoma. The coexpression of CK7, CK17, MUC1, and MUC5ac is unique for pancreatobiliary tumors (22). CK5 is expressed in squamous cell carcinomas.

Markers of Targeted Therapy

The overexpression/amplification of HER2/neu is associated with a poor prognosis and shortened overall survival in patients with breast cancer (23). In CUP patients, HER2 overexpression has been reported in 4% to 35% of specimens examined. No correlation with clinicopathologic parameters and outcome between patients with overexpressing and nonoverexpressing HER2 tumors has been observed (23,24).

The epidermal growth factor receptor (EGFR or HER-1) is involved in the growth, differentiation, and proliferation of cancer cells. One-third to 80% of all solid tumors express EGFR (23). Three groups of investigators have evaluated the EGFR protein expression by immunohistochemistry in patients with CUP. EGFR was expressed in the majority of the tumors (66–75%), and EGFR overexpression was seen in 12% to 61% of the tumors (23–25). Massard et al. showed a correlation between EGFR expression and response to cisplatin-based chemotherapy (RRs were 50% and 22% in patients with EGFR-positive and EGFR-negative tumors, respectively) (24). Dova et al. studied EGFR gene mutations and amplification of exons 18, 19, and 21 in 50 CUP patients. They did not find any mutations or amplifications in these patients (25). A possible relationship between EGFR gene copy number, response to EGFR inhibitors, and survival has not yet been established in patients with CUP.

Tumor growth and metastasis is dependent on the recruitment of new blood vessels, i.e., angiogenesis. Angiogenesis is regulated by a diverse group of endogenous pro-angiogenic and anti-angiogenic factors. Of the identified angiogenic factors, VEGF is the most potent and specific and has been identified as a crucial regulator of both normal and pathologic angiogenesis. VEGF is overexpressed in many solid tumors and is frequently correlated with greater microvessel density (MVD), advanced disease stage, and poor survival (23).

The expression of VEGF in CUP patients was observed in 39% to 100%, and VEGF overexpression was seen in 26% to 83% of the tumors (23). Karavasilis et al. found a strong correlation between VEGF expression and MVD, and a high MVD score was seen more often in the unfavorable subset of CUP patients (26). Hillen et al. found that high MVD score was correlated to a shorter survival (27). In more recent studies, MVD and VEGF were not associated to any clinicopathological parameters (23).

Overexpression of c-Kit in CUP has been reported in 4% to 13% of the tumors examined but the expression was not correlated to any patient characteristics (23,24,28), and mutation in exon 11 of the KIT gene has not been observed (28).

In summary, the potential usefulness of these target proteins in CUP is at present not sufficiently documented (29).

Oncogenes and Tumor Suppressor Genes

Bcl2 and p53 are well-known proteins expressed in most cancer types. The bcl2 protein promotes tumor growth by inhibition of apoptosis. Briasoulis and colleagues (30) examined the expression of bcl2 in 47 samples of CUP and found bcl2 to be overexpressed in 40% of the tumors. However, this had no correlation to prognosis.

The tumor suppressor gene p53 is mutated in approximately 55% of all human cancers. Bar-Eli et al. (31) found by molecular methods that the frequency of p53 mutations in CUP was rather low (26%), suggesting that p53 mutations play a minor role in the development and progression of this tumor type. However, Briasoulis and colleagues employing immunohistochemistry found an overexpression of p53 in 53% of 47 samples of tumors of unknown primary (30).

It is very important that the results from immunohistochemistry are interpreted with caution. The differences in the expression of antigens in the different studies may in part be explained by the heterogeneity and small number of patients studied. The lack of standardized immunohistochemical methodology (antibody used, antigen retrieval, and scoring system) also contributes to the discrepant results (23).

Microarray Technology

Cancer is a genetic disease, propagated by acquisition of somatic mutations as well as inherited germline mutations. Gene-expression profiling through DNA microarray technology now allows the simultaneous measurement of the expression of thousands of genes in cancer cells (see chap. 1). This can be used to identify genetic changes relevant for (i) tumor growth and metastasis, (ii) anatomical origin, (iii) new therapeutic targets, and (iv) cancer subtype classification, which may help to predict response to treatment and prognosis (32).

Gene expression classifiers have been created to distinguish various solid tumors. Pentheroudakis and colleagues have reviewed the literature of published articles and conference abstracts regarding the classification of known primary tumors and their metastases as well as the identification of the primary site of CUP by DNA microarray technology (33). Thirteen reports have been published in the last five years. Different platforms and different complex mathematical modeling approaches have been used to identify a set of genes that could distinguish solid tumors of different origins—tissue specific genes (ranging from 10 to 16063 genes). The accuracy of predicting the anatomical site of origin in blinded experiments was 78% to 89% for known primary tumors (33) and for the corresponding metastases 73% to 87% (33,34). The latter data imply that metastatic lesions retain some of the molecular features of the primary tumor.

In patients with CUP, DNA microarray was able to suggest a primary site in 61% to 85% of the patients (33,35–37). The suggestions of primary sites were compared with clinicopathological characteristics of the patients. Pentheroudakis et al. also compared the relative incidence of primary tumors identified by autopsy and assigned by DNA microarray. Lung (27%) and pancreatic cancer (24%) constituted more than 50% of the primary tumors indicated at autopsy, with liver/bile duct (8%), kidney/adrenals (8%), tumors in the bowel (7%), and in the genital tract (7%). A primary tumor was identified in less than 1% of the cases in the bladder and breast. On the other hand, the most common cancers assigned by DNA microarray were breast (15%), pancreas (12.5%), bowel (12%), lung (11.5%), genital system (9%), and liver/bile duct (8%) (33). The explanations of the discrepancy of the relative incidence of known primary tumors found by these two modalities are many. First, the number of microarray studies conducted in patients with CUP is low and mostly originates from conference abstracts (four out of seven studies). Second, the patient number in these studies is small ranging from 11 to 76 patients (total 229 patients). Third, CUP is a heterogeneous group of cancer, and it is not known whether all studies have used the same definition of CUP. Fourth, the relative incidence of primary tumors assigned by microarray technology is derived primarily from one group, in which the exact patient number is unknown (33). However, even the diagnosis made at autopsy must also be considered a qualified guess.

MicroRNAs (miRNAs) are short, typically 22 nucleotides long noncoding RNAs capable of regulating gene expression at both transcription and at translation level. Each miRNA might regulate 200 genes. miRNAs have critical functions across various biological processes like cell differentiation, apoptosis, and in oncogenesis. It has been recently shown that miRNA expression profiles can classify human cancers with a high accuracy (89%) based on only 48 miRNAs (38). In a small group of poorly differentiated tumors, the miRNA classifiers were able to identify the primary origin (38).

Data on molecular identification of primary tumors in metastatic malignancies from known and unknown primary tumors by microarray technology are neither mature nor abundant, but are slowly accumulating. Further studies are needed to explore the biological characteristics of CUP and establish whether this group of tumors shares unique genetic and/or phenotypic anomalies. DNA microarray and miRNA profiles may become important diagnostic tools in CUP patients. In addition, these techniques may reveal new therapeutic targets and may be useful in prediction of response to therapy and prognosis.

PROGNOSTIC FACTORS

A few retrospective studies have evaluated prognostic factors in CUP patients, including sex, age, performance status, degree of weight loss, serum albumin level, liver metastases, and number of metastatic sites (39–41).

In a multivariate analysis, Seve et al. (41) found that liver metastases and serum albumin level were the most important prognostic factors. A group of good-risk patients (no liver metastasis and normal serum albumin levels) and a group of poor-risk patients (liver metastasis and/or low serum albumin levels) were identified with median survivals of 371 and 103 days, respectively (p < 0.0001). This classification has been validated further in an independent data set.

Culine and colleages (39) have developed another simple prognostic model using performance status and serum LDH levels. In patients with increased LDH and PS > 2, treatment outcome was poor. In a model by Ponce et al. (40), patients with liver metastases and a performance >2 had an overall survival of 1.9 months. Poor performance status is generally related to short survival in CUP patients.

TREATMENT ACCORDING TO LOCALIZATION/HISTOLOGY
Cervical Lymphadenopathy

Cervical lymph node metastases of squamous cell carcinoma from an unknown primary site constitute about 2% to 5% of all CUP patients. During treatment and follow-up the primary is identified in 10% to 30% of all cases (42,43). The most common occult primary sites include the oropharynx, oral cavity, and hypopharynx.

In patients with cervical adenopathy, a careful physical and fiber-optic endoscopy examination of the entire head and neck region is critical. Biopsies should be performed from all suspicious sites and include a tonsillectomy since up to 25% of primary tumors can be detected in this site (44).

The ability to find an occult primary site is improved with the use of CT, magnetic resonance imaging (MRI), or ^{18}F-FDG-PET (45) and Epstein-Barr virus (EBV) serology. In a prospective study, ^{18}F-FDG-PET indicated a primary tumor or metastatic sites in 30 of 60 patients. Primary tumor was confirmed in 18 of which 12 were located in the head and neck region (45). A therapeutic change of treatment was made in 25% as a consequence of ^{18}F-FDG-PET.

The treatment for squamous cell carcinoma of an unknown primary is still very controversial. The published studies are retrospective and include different treatment modalities like neck dissection, radiotherapy, chemoradiotherapy, or combination of these three modalities (42,46). In most cases, radiotherapy includes both sides of the neck and mucosal areas (46). Neck dissection alone has often been used in patients with N1 disease and combined treatment in more advanced disease.

The five-year disease-specific survival is between 50% to 80% (42,43,46). Macroscopic extracapsular spread is often a significant adverse prognostic factor together with the nodal stage (43).

Axillary Adenopathy

Occult primary breast cancer represents less than 1% of breast cancer. In women presenting with an axillary mass, clinical and radiological examinations should focus on the breast, and pathology evaluation should include measurement of estrogen and progesterone receptors and HER2 status. In patients with normal breast examination and mammography, MRI should be performed, since this technique can help identifying an occult primary breast cancer. Buchanan et al. (47) found a primary breast tumor in around half of the patients with axillary adenopathy, and no distant metastases by using MRI. All of these patients had negative results for mammography and ultrasound examination.

The management of patients with an occult breast cancer remains controversial. Only retrospective data are available (47,48). Most of these support an active treatment of the breast by either radiotherapy or mastectomy and that treatment should be identical to patients with breast cancer with similar nodal stage.

In the study by Buchanan (47), 72% of the patients were alive and without disease after four years.

Poorly Differentiated Carcinoma of Midline Structures

The terms "atypical teratoma" or "extragonadal germ-cell syndrome" have been used to describe carcinomas of unknown primary site, which have features reminiscent of gonadal germ-cell tumors. They predominantly occur in young males, frequently with pulmonary or lymph node metastases, and germ-cell markers such as alpha-fetoprotein and beta-HCG may be detected in serum or tissue sections. In this group of patients, complete response and long-term survival has been obtained by the use of regimens effective in the therapy of germ-cell tumors (49). In a series of 220 patients with undifferentiated carcinomas or poorly differentiated adenocarcinomas receiving cisplatin-based chemotherapy, 58 patients (26%) had complete response (49). Most of these patients did not have other clinical features of extragonadal germ-cell tumors. In the group of 42 patients with predominant tumor location in the retroperitoneum, results of treatment were considerably better (50% complete response rate), but only 14% long-term survivors (49) suggesting that some of the responsive patients in this group have histologically unrecognizable extragonadal germ-cell tumors.

If extragonadal germ-cell tumor remains a possible diagnosis, treatment with cisplatin-based chemotherapy is indicated.

Today, most patients with germ-cell tumors will be identified because of the progress in immunohistochemistry, and the majority of patients with increased tumor markers are probably not true germ-cell tumors, because carcinomas may also occasionally secrete germ-cell markers, and there could be alternative primary sites, e.g., the lung ("large cell carcinoma") and pancreas. This is supported by the study of Currow et al. (50) investigating 15 patients with increased markers. Not all were fit for treatment, and only one patient obtained complete remission.

In older patients (>60 years) with midline lymph node metastases, the response rate is 30% on platinum based chemotherapy, with a median overall survival of 10 months (51).

Neuroendocrine Tumors

In 10% to 15% of poorly differentiated carcinomas pathological examinations will identify neuro-endocrine features (49). The dominant site of tumor is often retroperitoneum, lymph nodes or mediastinum, but several other sites can also be seen. A broad spectrum of neuroendocrine neoplasia is now recognized. They can be divided into low-grade neuroendocrine tumors like carcinoid tumors, islet cell tumors, paragangliomas, and pheochromocytomas. A second group is the small cell carcinomas, and the third group includes the poorly differentiated neuroendocrine tumors. In the first group, treatment will depend on the clinical situation and consists of either local or systemic treatment or both. The second group of patients should be treated with combination regimens effective in the treatment of small cell lung cancer. In a study including 43 patients from the third group, a response rate of 77% were obtained with platinum-based chemotherapy and 18% remained continuously disease-free after two years (49). More recently, novel anti-angiogenic agents are showing promise in patients with neuroendocrine tumors, and further evaluation of this approach is appropriate.

Ascites in Female Patients with Metastatic Carcinoma of Unknown Primary

A presentation that merits particular attention is that of malignant ascites in middle-aged or elderly women in whom no primary site can be identified. Careful review of both cytology and cell block preparations of the ascites for any resemblance to an ovarian primary should be undertaken. The identification of the presence of a papillary pattern in histological specimens is most helpful. Based on

similarities in response to treatment, toxicity, and overall survival between patients with extraovarian peritoneal serous papillary carcinoma and those with papillary serous ovarian carcinoma, the treatment should be platinum based as offered to ovarian cancer (52). Long-term remission can be obtained in about 15% (49).

TREATMENT OF THE UNFAVORABLE CUP SUBSET

Chemotherapy has been a cornerstone of treatment for patients with CUP for many years, in the majority of the patients who belongs to the unfavorable subset.

Pavlidis has recently reviewed the major trials for the last 40 years (53). In the 1960s and 1970s, the regimens were mainly based on fluorouracil or doxorubicin. In the late 1980s, platinum-based regimens were introduced and the response rates and the median survival were improved. Since the late 1990s, regimens including new drugs such as gemcitabine, taxanes, and irinotecan have been tested in patients with CUP and shown promising results (53).

The results from prospective trials performed in patients with CUP after 2002 are summarized in Tables 1–3 (43,54–73). All trials were phase II studies using regimens with various combinations of two or three drugs. Few trials have included more than 100 patients (61,62,68) and most were nonrandomized. In the nonrandomized trials, the majority of the regimens contained platinum (13 out of 14 studies). The response rates ranged from 13% to 43% (mean 30%) and 0% to 13% (mean 5%) of the patients obtained complete remission. The median survival time ranged from 6.5 to 11.8 months, and the one-year and two-year survivals ranged from 26% to 43% (mean 34%) and 7% to 23% (mean 14%), respectively (Table 1).

Very few randomized studies have been conducted in patients with CUP in the recent years. These studies were small and unable to show any considerable differences in response rates or survivals (Table 2) (43,54,59,66,73).

Despite the lack of randomized trials comparing chemotherapy to best supportive care, the general opinion is that chemotherapy has improved survival in this heterogeneous group of cancers (5 months vs. 6–11 months) (74).

In the last five years, two second-line chemotherapy regimens have been published. The response rates were 10% and 29% and the median survival time was 4.5 and 8 months, respectively (Table 3) (63,70).

Targeted biological drugs have shown anti-tumor activity in various types of solid tumors, especially in combination with chemotherapy. Hainsworth et al. treated 51 patients with CUP with a combination of erlotinib and bevacizumab, and 73% of the included patients had previously received one or two chemotherapy regimens. The response rate was 10%. The median survival time was 7.4 months and 33% of the patients were alive at one year (75). Additional trials combining targeted biological agents and chemotherapy in first line treatment are thus warranted.

Although various studies have been made in recent years with existing and new drugs it is still not possible to make firm recommendations as to of the optimal treatment on the present data. However, when empirical chemotherapy is recommended, a regimen that contains platinum and taxanes or gemcitabine is a reasonable choice.

Table 18.1 First Line Chemotherapy Regimens in CUP Patients from 2002 to 2007

Regimen	Number of patients	Complete response (%)	Partial response (%)	Median survival (months)	The 1-year and 2-year survival (%)	Reference
MiPF	31	3	23	7.7	28 and 10	MacDonald et al. 2002 (64)
DC alternating with EP/GCSF	82	10	29	10	NR	Culine et al. 2002 (58)
GC_BP_L	120	4	21	9	42 and 23	Greco et al. 2002 (61)
PEG	30	13	23	7.2	26 (1-year)	Balaña et al. 2003 (55)
GD_X	36	3	37	10	43 and 7	Pouessel et al. 2004 (71)
C_BDE	102	6[a]	21[a]	9	35 and 18	Piga et al. 2004 (68)
P_LP	37	4	39	11	38 and 11	Park et al. 2004 (67)
P_LC_BE and GI_R	132	6	23	9.1	35 and 16	Greco et al. 2004 (62)
C_BP_L	22		23[a]	6.5	27 (1-year)	El-Rayes et al. 2005 (60)
GC_B	50		31	7.8	26 and 12	Pittman et al. 2006 (69)
D_XC_BG	63	13[a]	24[a]	11.8	NR	Mel et al. 2006 (abstract) (65)
C_BGC_A	33		39[a]	7.6	36 and 14	Schneider et al. 2007 (72)
I_RO_X	47	2[a]	11[a]	9.5	40 and 8	Briasoulis et al. 2008 (57)
$P_L(weekly)C_B$	42	5	13	8.5	33 and 17	Berry et al. 2007 (56)

[a]Response rate calculated by intention-to-treat analysis.
Abbreviations: C, cyclophosphamide; C_A, capecitabine; C_B, carboplatin; D, doxorubicin; D_X, docetaxel; E, etoposid; F, fluorouracil; G, gemcitabine; I_R, irinotecan; Mi, mitomycin C; NR, not reported; P, cisplatin; P_L, paclitaxel.

Table 18.2 Randomized Phase II Study in CUP Patients from 2002 to 2007

Regimens	Number of patients	Response rate (%)	Median survival (months)	The 1-year and 2-year survival (%)	Reference
PG vs. PI_R	80	55 vs. 38[a]	8 vs. 6	NR	Culine et al. 2003 (59)
F vs. F + Mi	88	12 vs. 20	6.6 vs. 4.7	28 vs. 21 (1 year)	Assersohn et al. 2003 (54)
P_LC_B vs. GV_L	92	22 vs. 21	10.7 vs. 6.9	31 vs. 22 (1 year)	Huebner et al. 2005 (abstract) (73)
PGP_L vs. PGV_L	66	48 vs. 42	9.6 vs. 13.6	NR	Palmeri et al. 2006 (66)

[a]Response rate calculated by intention-to-treat analysis.
Abbreviations: C_B, carboplantin; F, flururacil; G, gemcitabine; I_R, irinotecan; Mi, mitomycin; NR, not reported; P, cisplatin; P_L, paclitaxel; V_L, vinorelbine.

Table 18.3 Second Line Chemotherapy Regimens in CUP Patients from 2002 to 2007

Regimens	Number of patients	Response rate (%)	Median survival (months)	The 1-year and 2-year survival (%)	Reference
GD_X	15	29	8	NR	Pouessel et al. 2003 (70)
GI_R	40	10[a]	4.5	25 and 13	Hainsworth et al. 2005 (63)

[a]Response rate calculated by intention-to-treat analysis.
Abbreviations: D_X, docetaxel; G, gemcitabine; I_R, irinotecan; NR, not reported.

CONCLUSION

Patients presenting with CUP have a different pattern and frequency of metastases than would be expected in cases where the primary site is apparent at the time of presentation. The identification of the primary site in these cases differs according to whether data are obtained from postmortem examination or from molecular analysis of their genetic expression.

Time-consuming and costly radiological and imaging studies are often performed. No matter how extensive is the evaluation, the primary site is rarely identified. Accordingly, a selective search for treatable tumors is most appropriate and cost-effective. With adenocarcinomas, this will include prostate, breast, GI tract, lungs, thyroid, and ovary, and for undifferentiated tumors lymphomas, germ-cell and neuroendocrine tumors.

Close cooperation between an experienced pathologist and clinical oncologist is essential in the management of patients with unknown primary carcinoma. A comprehensive pathological examination is crucial, and, with undifferentiated tumors, this will include immunohistology, and sometimes electron microscopy, although the value of this is considered limited to a few cases such as sarcomas and neuroendocrine tumors. The usefulness of tumor markers in identifying the primary site of the tumor in patients with metastases of unknown origin is increasing with the number of available antibodies.

Provided that CUP indeed retain the characteristics of the primary tumor, the use of DNA microarray or miRNA profiles on metastatic tumor tissue potentially could play a significant diagnostic role in CUP patients and it may also reveal new therapeutic molecular targets. Implementation of mRNA and miRNA detection techniques in the routine clinical practice may direct treatment strategies for CUP patients allowing customized cancer therapies and may thereby avoid unnecessary and ineffective treatment.

The optimal treatment as of today cannot be determined. For patients without an identified treatable primary tumor the use of empirical chemotherapy using current drugs and schedules should be a matter of frank discussion between patient and physician. Evaluation of performance status is important and for those who will be eligible for chemotherapy a median survival of 6.5 to 11.8 months can be obtained, with 26% to 43% of the treated patients alive after one year from the time of diagnosis. Survival rates at two years are around 7% to 23% compared with a median survival of two to three months in an untreated population with unknown primary tumors.

Treatment of CUP patients continues to be a major challenge, especially the treatment of adenocarcinomas and undifferentiated carcinomas. Diagnostic strategies for this group of patients should be further defined, and the use of ^{18}F-FDG-PET/CT, DNA microarray, and miRNA as diagnostic tools in CUP should be clarified.

REFERENCES

1. Pavlidis N, Briasoulis E, Hainsworth J et al. Diagnostic and therapeutic management of cancer of an unknown primary. Eur J Cancer 2003; 39: 1990–2005.
2. Pavlidis N, Fizazi K. Cancer of unknown primary (CUP). Crit Rev Oncol Hematol 2005; 54: 243–50.
3. Briasoulis E, Pavlidis N. Cancers of unknown primary site: ESMO clinical recommendations for diagnosis, treatment and follow-up. Ann Oncol 2007; 18(Suppl 2): ii81–2.
4. Rusthoven KE, Koshy M, Paulino AC. The role of fluorodeoxyglucose positron emission tomography in cervical lymph node metastases from an unknown primary tumor. Cancer 2004; 101: 2641–9.
5. Seve P, Billotey C, Broussolle C et al. The role of 2-deoxy-2-[F-18]fluoro-D-glucose positron emission tomography in disseminated carcinoma of unknown primary site. Cancer 2007; 109: 292–9.
6. Fletcher JW, Djulbegovic B, Soares HP et al. Recommendations on the use of 18F-FDG PET in oncology. J Nucl Med 2008; 49: 480–508.
7. Ambrosini V, Nanni C, Rubello D et al. 18F-FDG PET/CT in the assessment of carcinoma of unknown primary origin. Radiol Med (Torino) 2006; 111: 1146–55.
8. Gutzeit A, Antoch G, Kuhl H et al. Unknown primary tumors: detection with dual-modality PET/CT-initial experience. Radiology 2005; 234: 227–34.
9. Nassenstein K, Veit-Haibach P, Stergar H et al. Cervical lymph node metastases of unknown origin: primary tumor

10. Pelosi E, Pennone M, Deandreis D et al. Role of whole body positron emission tomography/computed tomography scan with 18F-fluorodeoxyglucose in patients with biopsy proven tumor metastases from unknown primary site. Q J Nucl Med Mol Imaging 2006; 50: 15–22.
11. Wartski M, Le SE, Gontier E et al. In search of an unknown primary tumour presenting with cervical metastases: performance of hybrid FDG-PET-CT. Nucl Med Commun 2007; 28: 365–71.
12. Milovic M, Popov I, Jelic S. Tumor markers in metastatic disease from cancer of unknown primary origin. Med Sci Monit 2002; 8: MT25–30.
13. Yonemori K, Ando M, Shibata T et al. Tumor-marker analysis and verification of prognostic models in patients with cancer of unknown primary, receiving platinum-based combination chemotherapy. J Cancer Res Clin Oncol 2006; 132: 635–42.
14. Dabbs D, Silverman J. Immunohistochemical workup of metastatic carcinoma of unknown primary. Pathology Case Reviews 2001; 6: 146–53.
15. Nakamura N, Miyagi E, Murata S et al. Expression of thyroid transcription factor-1 in normal and neoplastic lung tissues. Mod Pathol 2002; 15: 1058–67.
16. Penman D, Downie I, Roberts F. Positive immunostaining for thyroid transcription factor-1 in primary and metastatic colonic adenocarcinoma: a note of caution. J Clin Pathol 2006; 59: 663–4.
17. Wick MR, Lillemoe TJ, Copland GT et al. Gross cystic disease fluid protein-15 as a marker for breast cancer: immunohistochemical analysis of 690 human neoplasms and comparison with alpha-lactalbumin. Hum Pathol 1989; 20: 281–7.
18. Kaufmann O, Volmerig J, Dietel M. Uroplakin III is a highly specific and moderately sensitive immunohistochemical marker for primary and metastatic urothelial carcinomas. Am J Clin Pathol 2000; 113: 683–7.
19. Werling RW, Yaziji H, Bacchi CE et al. CDX2, a highly sensitive and specific marker of adenocarcinomas of intestinal origin: an immunohistochemical survey of 476 primary and metastatic carcinomas. Am J Surg Pathol 2003; 27: 303–10.
20. Lau SK, Weiss LM, Chu PG. Differential expression of MUC1, MUC2, and MUC5AC in carcinomas of various sites: an immunohistochemical study. Am J Clin Pathol 2004; 122: 61–9.
21. Tot T. Adenocarcinomas metastatic to the liver: the value of cytokeratins 20 and 7 in the search for unknown primary tumors. Cancer 1999; 85: 171–7.
22. Chu PG, Schwarz RE, Lau SK et al. Immunohistochemical staining in the diagnosis of pancreatobiliary and ampulla of Vater adenocarcinoma: application of CDX2, CK17, MUC1, and MUC2. Am J Surg Pathol 2005; 29: 359–67.
23. Pentheroudakis G, Pavlidis N. Perspectives for targeted therapies in cancer of unknown primary site. Cancer Treat Rev 2006; 32: 637–44.
24. Massard C, Voigt JJ, Laplanche A et al. Carcinoma of an unknown primary: are EGF receptor, Her-2/neu, and c-Kit tyrosine kinases potential targets for therapy? Br J Cancer 2007; 97: 857–61.
25. Dova L, Pentheroudakis G, Georgiou I et al. Global profiling of EGFR gene mutation, amplification, regulation and tissue protein expression in unknown primary carcinomas: to target or not to target? Clin Exp Metastasis 2007; 24: 79–86.
26. Karavasilis V, Malamou-Mitsi V, Briasoulis E et al. Angiogenesis in cancer of unknown primary: clinicopathological study of CD34, VEGF and TSP-1. BMC Cancer 2005; 5: 25.
27. Hillen HF, Hak LE, Joosten-Achjanie SR et al. Microvessel density in unknown primary tumors. Int J Cancer 1997; 74: 81–5.

28. Dova L, Pentheroudakis G, Golfinopoulos V et al. Targeting c-KIT, PDGFR in cancer of unknown primary: a screening study for molecular markers of benefit. J Cancer Res Clin Oncol 2008; 134: 697–704.

29. Mano MS, Rosa DD, De AE et al. The 17q12-q21 amplicon: Her2 and topoisomerase-IIalpha and their importance to the biology of solid tumours. Cancer Treat Rev 2007; 33: 64–77.

30. Briasoulis E, Tsokos M, Fountzilas G et al. Bcl2 and p53 protein expression in metastatic carcinoma of unknown primary origin: biological and clinical implications. A Hellenic Co-operative Oncology Group study. Anticancer Res 1998; 18: 1907–14.

31. Bar-Eli M, Abbruzzese JL, Lee-Jackson D et al. p53 gene mutation spectrum in human unknown primary tumors. Anticancer Res 1993; 13: 1619–23.

32. Quackenbush J. Microarray analysis and tumor classification. N Engl J Med 2006; 354: 2463–72.

33. Pentheroudakis G, Golfinopoulos V, Pavlidis N. Switching benchmarks in cancer of unknown primary: from autopsy to microarray. Eur J Cancer 2007; 43: 2026–36.

34. Lenzi R, Rashid A, Ordonez N et al. Gene profiling validation for cancer using primary carcinoma samples. J Clin Oncol 2007; 25(18S): abstract 21130.

35. Bridgewater J, van LR, Floore A et al. Gene expression profiling may improve diagnosis in patients with carcinoma of unknown primary. Br J Cancer 2008; 98: 1425–30.

36. Qu K, Li H, Whetstone J et al. Molecular identification of carcinoma of unknown primary (CUP) with gene expression profiling. J Clin Oncol 2007; 25(18S): abstract 21024.

37. Varadhachary G, Talantov D, Jatkoe T et al. Prospective study of a 10-gene molecular assay to predict tissue of origin in patients with carcinoma of unknown primary (CUP). J Clin Oncol 2007; 25(18S): abstract 21096.

38. Rosenfeld N, Aharonov R, Meiri E et al. MicroRNAs accurately identify cancer tissue origin. Nat Biotechnol 2008; 26: 462–9.

39. Culine S, Kramar A, Saghatchian M et al. Development and validation of a prognostic model to predict the length of survival in patients with carcinomas of an unknown primary site. J Clin Oncol 2002; 20: 4679–83.

40. Ponce LJ, Segura HA, Diaz BR et al. Carcinoma of unknown primary site: development in a single institution of a prognostic model based on clinical and serum variables. Clin Transl Oncol 2007; 9: 452–8.

41. Seve P, Ray-Coquard I, Trillet-Lenoir V et al. Low serum albumin levels and liver metastasis are powerful prognostic markers for survival in patients with carcinomas of unknown primary site. Cancer 2006; 107: 2698–705.

42. Guntinas-Lichius O, Peter KJ, Dinh S et al. Diagnostic work-up and outcome of cervical metastases from an unknown primary. Acta Otolaryngol 2006; 126: 536–44.

43. Patel RS, Clark J, Wyten R et al. Squamous cell carcinoma from an unknown head and neck primary site: a "selective treatment" approach. Arch Otolaryngol Head Neck Surg 2007; 133: 1282–7.

44. Haas I, Hoffmann TK, Engers R et al. Diagnostic strategies in cervical carcinoma of an unknown primary (CUP). Eur Arch Otorhinolaryngol 2002; 259: 325–33.

45. Johansen J, Buus S, Loft A et al. Prospective study of 18FDG-PET in the detection and management of patients with lymph node metastases to the neck from an unknown primary tumor. Results from the DAHANCA-13 study. Head Neck 2008; 30: 471–8.

46. Beldi D, Jereczek-Fossa BA, D'Onofrio A et al. Role of radiotherapy in the treatment of cervical lymph node metastases from an unknown primary site: retrospective analysis of 113 patients. Int J Radiat Oncol Biol Phys 2007; 69: 1051–8.

47. Buchanan CL, Morris EA, Dorn PL et al. Utility of breast magnetic resonance imaging in patients with occult primary breast cancer. Ann Surg Oncol 2005; 12: 1045–53.

48. Khandelwal AK, Garguilo GA. Therapeutic options for occult breast cancer: a survey of the American Society of Breast Surgeons and review of the literature. Am J Surg 2005; 190: 609–13.

49. Fizazi K. Treatment of patients with specific subsets of carcinoma of an unknown primary site. Ann Oncol 2006; 17(Suppl 10): x177–80.

50. Currow DC, Findlay M, Cox K et al. Elevated germ cell markers in carcinoma of uncertain primary site do not predict response to platinum based chemotherapy. Eur J Cancer 1996; 32A: 2357–9.

51. Pentheroudakis G, Briasoulis E, Karavassilis V et al. Chemotherapy for patients with two favourable subsets of unknown primary carcinoma: active, but how effective? Acta Oncol 2005; 44: 155–60.

52. Bloss JD, Brady MF, Liao SY et al. Extraovarian peritoneal serous papillary carcinoma: a phase II trial of cisplatin and cyclophosphamide with comparison to a cohort with papillary serous ovarian carcinoma-a Gynecologic Oncology Group Study. Gynecol Oncol 2003; 89: 148–54.

53. Pavlidis N. Forty years experience of treating cancer of unknown primary. Acta Oncol 2007; 46: 592–601.

54. Assersohn L, Norman AR, Cunningham D et al. A randomised study of protracted venous infusion of 5-fluorouracil (5-FU) with or without bolus mitomycin C (MMC) in patients with carcinoma of unknown primary. Eur J Cancer 2003; 39: 1121–8.

55. Balaña C, Manzano JL, Moreno I et al. A phase II study of cisplatin, etoposide and gemcitabine in an unfavourable group of patients with carcinoma of unknown primary site. Ann Oncol 2003; 14: 1425–9.

56. Berry W, Elkordy M, O'Rourke M et al. Results of a phase II study of weekly paclitaxel plus carboplatin in advanced carcinoma of unknown primary origin: a reasonable regimen for the community-based clinic? Cancer Invest 2007; 25: 27–31.

57. Briasoulis E, Fountzilas G, Bamias A et al. Multicenter phase-II trial of irinotecan plus oxaliplatin [IROX regimen] in patients with poor-prognosis cancer of unknown primary: a hellenic cooperative oncology group study. Cancer Chemother Pharmacol 2008; 62: 277–84.

58. Culine S, Fabbro M, Ychou M et al. Alternative bimonthly cycles of doxorubicin, cyclophosphamide, and etoposide, cisplatin with hematopoietic growth factor support in patients with carcinoma of unknown primary site. Cancer 2002; 94: 840–6.

59. Culine S, Lortholary A, Voigt JJ et al. Cisplatin in combination with either gemcitabine or irinotecan in carcinomas of unknown primary site: results of a randomized phase II study—trial for the French Study Group on Carcinomas of Unknown Primary (GEFCAPI 01). J Clin Oncol 2003; 21: 3479–82.

60. El-Rayes BF, Shields AF, Zalupski M et al. A phase II study of carboplatin and paclitaxel in adenocarcinoma of unknown primary. Am J Clin Oncol 2005; 28: 152–6.

61. Greco FA, Burris HA III, Litchy S et al. Gemcitabine, carboplatin, and paclitaxel for patients with carcinoma of unknown primary site: a Minnie Pearl Cancer Research Network study. J Clin Oncol 2002; 20: 1651–6.

62. Greco FA, Rodriguez GI, Shaffer DW et al. Carcinoma of unknown primary site: sequential treatment with paclitaxel/carboplatin/etoposide and gemcitabine/irinotecan: a Minnie Pearl Cancer Research Network phase II trial. Oncologist 2004; 9: 644–52.

63. Hainsworth JD, Spigel DR, Raefsky EL et al. Combination chemotherapy with gemcitabine and irinotecan in patients

with previously treated carcinoma of an unknown primary site: a Minnie Pearl Cancer Research Network Phase II trial. Cancer 2005; 104: 1992–7.

64. Macdonald AG, Nicolson MC, Samuel LM et al. A phase II study of mitomycin C, cisplatin and continuous infusion 5-fluorouracil (MCF) in the treatment of patients with carcinoma of unknown primary site. Br J Cancer 2002; 86: 1238–42.

65. Mel JPM, Balaña C, López-Vega J et al. Phase II study of Docetaxel (D), Carboplatin (C) and Gemcitabine (G), in advanced tumors of unknown primary site. J Clin Oncol 2006; 24(18S): abstract 12028.

66. Palmeri S, Lorusso V, Palmeri L et al. Cisplatin and gemcitabine with either vinorelbine or paclitaxel in the treatment of carcinomas of unknown primary site: results of an Italian multicenter, randomized, phase II study. Cancer 2006; 107: 2898–905.

67. Park YH, Ryoo BY, Choi SJ et al. A phase II study of paclitaxel plus cisplatin chemotherapy in an unfavourable group of patients with cancer of unknown primary site. Jpn J Clin Oncol 2004; 34: 681–5.

68. Piga A, Nortilli R, Cetto GL et al. Carboplatin, doxorubicin and etoposide in the treatment of tumours of unknown primary site. Br J Cancer 2004; 90: 1898–904.

69. Pittman KB, Olver IN, Koczwara B et al. Gemcitabine and carboplatin in carcinoma of unknown primary site: a phase 2 Adelaide Cancer Trials and Education Collaborative study. Br J Cancer 2006; 95: 1309–13.

70. Pouessel D, Culine S, Becht C et al. Gemcitabine and docetaxel after failure of cisplatin-based chemotherapy in patients with carcinoma of unknown primary site. Anticancer Res 2003; 23: 2801–4.

71. Pouessel D, Culine S, Becht C et al. Gemcitabine and docetaxel as front-line chemotherapy in patients with carcinoma of an unknown primary site. Cancer 2004; 100: 1257–61.

72. Schneider BJ, El-Rayes B, Muler JH et al. Phase II trial of carboplatin, gemcitabine, and capecitabine in patients with carcinoma of unknown primary site. Cancer 2007; 110: 770–5.

73. Huebner G, Steinbach S, Kohne C et al. Paclitaxel (P)/carboplatin (C) versus gemcitabine (G)/vinorelbine (V) in patients with adeno- or undifferentiated carcinoma of unknown primary (CUP)—randomized prospective phase-II-trial. J Clin Oncol 2005; 23(16S): abstract 4089.

74. Greco FA, Hainsworth JD. Cancer of unknown primary site. In: DeVita V Jr, Hellman S, Rosenberg S, eds. Cancer Principles and Practice of Oncology. Philadelphia: Lippincott Williams and Wilkins, 2005: 2363–86.

75. Hainsworth JD, Spigel DR, Farley C et al. Phase II trial of bevacizumab and erlotinib in carcinomas of unknown primary site: the Minnie Pearl Cancer Research Network. J Clin Oncol 2007; 25: 1747–52.

76. Dennis JL, Hvidsten TR, Wit EC, et al. Markers of adenocarcinoma characteristic of the site of origin: development of a diagnostic algorithm. Clin Cancer Res 2005; 11: 3766–72.

77. Park SY, Kim BH, Kim JH, Lee S, Kang GH. Panels of immunohistochemical markers help determine primary sites of metastatic adenocarcinoma. Arch Pathol Lab Med 2007; 131: 1561-7.

19

Medical Emergencies

Luis Paz-Ares, Jesús Corral Jaime, Rocío García-Carbonero

INTRODUCTION

Cancer patients are at increased risk for life-threatening events because of a number of factors related both to the underlying malignancy and to the toxic effects of anticancer therapy. In addition, they may also experience other medical emergencies that may occur in individuals who do not have cancer. All three sources of medical complications should be considered in the diagnostic process before adequate management is instituted. This chapter will review the etiopathogenesis, clinical presentation, and management of the most common tumor-related emergencies. We will also briefly summarize one of the most common complications of antineoplastic therapy, febrile neutropenia. Other treatment-related complications are reviewed elsewhere in this book.

The management of an oncological complication follows the standard practice for a nononcological emergency: establishment of a diagnosis, evaluation of organ function, and prompt initiation of therapy. In addition, there are several other specific oncological factors that must be taken into consideration, as they may influence aggressiveness of management. These include the time scale of the event, cancer prognosis, prior clinical condition, patient's and family's opinion, and several legal and ethical issues. Overall, the aggressiveness of the therapeutic approach should be influenced by the reversibility of the event and by the probability of a reasonable survival with adequate quality of life for the patient.

METABOLIC EMERGENCIES
Hypercalcemia
Etiopathogenesis

Hypercalcemia is the most common life-threatening metabolic disorder associated with cancer, occurring in aproximately 10% of patients with malignant disease at some point during the disease course. Considering the general population, hyperparathyroidism is the most common cause of hypercalcemia in the outpatient setting, whereas neoplastic disease is the leading cause among hospitalized patients. The tumors most commonly associated with hypercalcemia include carcinomas of the breast, lung, kidney, head and neck, and esophagus, multiple myeloma, and other hematological malignancies (1).

Malignancy-associated hypercalcemia, even in patients with extensive osteolysis, is primarily mediated by humoral factors produced by tumor cells. The most common mediator is a peptide structurally related to parathyroid hormone (PTH): PTH-related peptide, which is present in aproximately 80% of hypercalcemic cancer patients. This peptide binds to PTH receptors in bone and kidneys, mimicking the biochemical abnormalities found in patients with hyperparathyroidism. Except for cases of parathyroid carcinoma, ectopic production of authentic PTH is exceptionally rare. Activation of receptor activator of nuclear factor-kappa-B ligand (RANKL), produced by either tumor cells, stromal cells, or cells of the immune system in response to PTHrp or interleukin, is another key process in malignancy-associated hypercalcemia. Prostaglandins, 1,25-dihydroxyvitamin D_3, and cytokines (tumor necrosis factor β, interleukin-1 and interleukin-6, transforming growth factors, colony-stimulating factors, etc.) may also play a role in the pathogenesis of cancer-related hypercalcemia (1–3).

Clinical Presentation and Diagnosis

Most hypercalcemic patients present with nonspecific symptoms, such as fatigue, nausea and vomiting, anorexia, and constipation. Polyuria, due to the impaired ability of renal tubules to concentrate urine induced by hypercalcemia, along with nausea and vomiting, leads to rapid dehydration and substantial worsening of the hypercalcemic state. The severity of symptoms is related not only to the magnitude of hypercalcemia, but also to the rate of calcium elevation; slow increases are better tolerated.

When severe hypercalcemia is present, neurological symptoms such as muscle weakness, hyporeflexia, lethargy, stupor, or coma may develop. Electrocardiographic changes (bradycardia, prolonged PR interval, shortened QT interval, widened T wave), and, in rare cases, sudden death from cardiac arrhythmias may also occur (1–2).

The diagnosis of hypercalcemia is confirmed by an elevated serum calcium level (>10.5 mg/dl). Because calcium is protein-bound, patients with hypoalbuminemia have spuriously low calcium levels. Conversely, patients with multiple myeloma may have pseudohypercalcemia, since elevated total serum proteins may increase the measured serum calcium erroneously. In such cases, quantification of ionized calcium is of great value, or, if this is not possible, different algorithms for albumin-corrected calcium values are available.

Treatment

The best treatment of cancer-related hypercalcemia is specific therapy directed at the underlying malignancy. However, most often, hypercalcemia develops in cases of widely metastatic tumors that are refractory to available therapy. Therefore, nonspecific measures should be instituted (Table 19.1).

Table 19.1 Treatment of Cancer-Related Hypercalcemia

Agent	Dose	Onset of action	Relative efficacy	Adverse effects	Comments
Pamidronate	60–90 mg 4 hr i.v. infusion	24–48 hr	60–75%	flu-like symptoms lymphopenia venous irritation	Decreases bone resorption Reduces skeletal events in myeloma/breast cancer
Zoledronate	4 mg 15 min i.v. infusion	<24 hr	80–90%	flu-like symptoms anemia nausea, constipation hypophosphatemia renal failure	Decreases bone resorption Reduces skeletal events in myeloma/breast/lung/ prostate cancer and other solid tumors
Gallium Nitrate	100–200 mg/m²/day 24 hr i.v. infusion up to 5 days	24–48 hr	5–80%	nephrotoxicity nausea/vomiting constipation	Decreases bone resorption
Calcitonin	2–8 UI/Kg s.c. or i.m. q 6–12 hr up to 2 days	1–4 hr	30%	nausea abdominal cramps hypersensitivity	Rapid onset of action Tachyphylaxis occurs quickly
Corticosteroids	40–100 mg/day of prednisone (or equivalent)	3–5 day	0–40% (depending on disease)	hyperglycemia gastritis osteopenia	Moderately active in myeloma, leukemia, and lymphoma
Isotonic saline	200–400 ml/hr	12–24 hr	20%	pulmonary edema	Corrects dehydration Promotes calciuresis

General Measures. Drugs that increase renal calcium reabsorption (thiazides) or decrease renal blood flow (non-steroidal antiinflammatory drugs, H_2-receptor antagonists), oral calcium supplementation, vitamin D, and retinoids should be discontinued. Immobilization tends to aggravate hypercalcemia and must be avoided if possible.

Intravenous Fluids and Diuretics. Intravenous isotonic saline infusion should be instituted to restore the extracellular fluid deficit. Volume expansion increases renal blood flow and calciuresis. Depending upon the severity of dehydration and patient cardiovascular and renal functions, saline solution may be infused at a rate of 200 to 500 ml/hr during the first hours until adequate urine output, and then reduced to 2 to 3 L daily in the following days. Careful monitoring is essential to prevent fluid overload. The use of furosemide, although it enhances calciuresis, should be restricted to balancing fluid intake and urine output in patients who have been fully rehydrated, because it increases the risk for developing hypovolemia, which could cause the hypercalcemic state to worsen. With these measures alone, only 20% to 30% of patients will become normocalcemic. Thus, treatment with antiresorptive drugs should be initiated early following rehydration (1,2).

Bisphosphonates. The bisphosphonates are pyrophosphate analogues that bind to hydroxyapatite crystals in the bone matrix and inhibit calcium release from bone by interfering with osteoclast activity. Unlike calcitonin and gallium nitrate, they do not have a direct activity on tubular calcium resorption in the kidney. Between 30% and 50% of the unmetabolized compound is recovered in the urine within 24 hours of intravenous administration. Most of the remaining drug is taken up by the bone, from which it is released very slowly. The oral bioavailability of bisphosphonates is very low (<2%), and their employment as oral therapy to maintain normocalcemia in cancer patients is discouraged (4).

Etidronate was the first bisphosphonate to be marketed, but it has largely been replaced by other bisphosphonates with demonstrated improved efficacy (1,4).

Clodronate is a second-generation bisphosphonate of intermediate potency available in Europe both as oral and as intravenous formulations. However, owing to the poor oral bioavailability, the use of repeated intravenous infusions every two to four weeks rather than oral therapy is preferred for the maintenance of normocalcemia after initial intravenous treatment. The recommended dose is 300 to 500 mg/day for three to five consecutive days, or a single dose of 900 to 1500 mg administered over four hours, achieving normocalcemia in more than 70% of patients. The effect occurs within two to three days, and the response may last 10 to 12 days. Rapid bolus injection may cause acute renal failure; slow intravenous infusion (one to two hours) is therefore recommended and is usually well tolerated (1,4). In the palliative setting clodronate may be given by subcutaneous infusion with mild local reaction as the main side effect.

Pamidronate is only available as an intravenous formulation in most European countries. The recommended dose is a single 60 to 90 mg two-hour infusion. Toxicity is generally mild. Transient febrile reactions, flu-like symptoms and lymphopenia occur frequently after the first infusion. Less common side effects include thrombophlebitis, asymptomatic hypocalcemia or hypophosphatemia, and ocular complications (uveitis and scleritis). Severe renal dysfunction reduces pamidronate clearance, but no dose adjustment is necessary because of the long elimination half-life from bone and the infrequent administration of the drug. Responses to pamidronate therapy are observed in 70% to 80% of patients with malignant hypercalcemia. The effect occurs within 24 to 48 hours, and the duration of response is commonly two weeks or longer (1,2,4).

In comparative studies, pamidronate produced higher rates of normocalcemia and responses of longer duration than etidronate, clodronate, and plicamycin (mithramycin). Moreover, in several randomized studies performed in patients with breast cancer or multiple myeloma, pamidronate administration, with or without systemic antineoplastic therapy, has significantly reduced and delayed the incidence of skeletal events, including pathological fracture, hypercalcemia, and the requirement for radiation therapy or bone surgery (1,2,4).

Zoledronate is a third-generation heterocyclic nitrogen-containing bisphosphonate that has shown to be up to 850-fold more potent than pamidronate in preclinical models. Randomized clinical trials have demonstrated that zoledronic acid provides a greater response rate (88% vs. 70%), faster onset of action (normalization of serum calcium by day 4 in 50% of patients vs. 33% of patients), and more prolonged response duration (median of 30 vs. 17 days) than pamidronate in the treatment of cancer patients with hypercalcemia (5). Furthermore, its mode of administration (a single 4 mg 15-minute intravenous infusion) improves patients' convenience while maintaining a similar safety profile. Consequently, zoledronic acid has superceded pamidronate disodium as the drug of choice for the treatment of hypercalcemia of malignancy (4,5). Adverse effects are infrequent too and consist of pyrexia, transient hypocalcemia, and renal function impairment. Close renal function monitoring is warranted and stepwise dose reductions recommended for creatinine clearance values of 50 to 60 ml/min (3.5 mg), 40 to 50 ml/min (3.3 mg), and 30 to 40 ml/min (3 mg), and the drug should not be used in patients with creatinine clearances below 30 ml/min. More recently, a new serious complication has been described associated with its use, the osteonecrosis of the jaw (1,2,4). Although initially reported in patients treated with zoledronic acid, it has also been observed after pamidronate therapy. The true incidence of osteonecrosis is unknown, although it is higher among myeloma patients (7–10%) and in those with recent teeth extractions or other invasive interventions of the jaw, particularly after prolonged drug exposure. Adequate dental health is therefore mandatory before bisphosphonate treatment, and caution is required beyond two years of therapy. Reinitiating bisphosphonate therapy in patients suffering from osteonecrosis is controversial and warrants further study.

Besides its effect on calcium homeostasis, zoledronate significantly contributes to reduce bone pain and decreases the incidence of skeletal events not only in breast cancer or myeloma patients, but also in patients with prostate cancer, lung cancer, and other solid tumors. In addition, preclinical studies suggest that zoledronic acid may also display anti-tumor and antiangiogenic properties. In line with these observations, recently communicated preliminary data of a randomized trial shows that zoledronic acid (4 mg i.v. q 6 months) improves disease-free survival in premenopausal women with hormone receptor positive breast cancer, decreasing not only the incidence of distant bone metastasis, but also locoregional recurrence and contralateral breast cancer. The role of bisphosphonate therapy will likely evolve as data from these and other ongoing studies mature.

Other bisphosphonates undergoing clinical testing include ibandronate, alendronate, tilundronate, and risendronate. Besides a decreased incidence of nephrotoxicity associated with ibandronate, they do not seem to provide any major advantages over other pyrophosphate analogues in clinical use (1,2,4).

Nonbisphosphonate Drugs. Gallium Nitrate binds to hydroxyapatite and causes a decrease in its solubility, rendering it more resistant to osteoclast-mediated bone resorption. Gallium nitrate also reduces renal tubular calcium resorption and stimulates bone formation in vitro. The recommended dose for the treatment of malignant hypercalcemia is 100 to 200 mg/m^2/day given as a 24-hour infusion for up to five days. Calcium serum levels begin to fall within 24 to 48 hours after drug administration, and normocalcemia is achieved within four to seven days in 70% to 90% of patients. Adverse effects include nephrotoxicity, nausea, vomiting, and constipation (1,2). Although randomized double-blind studies have demonstrated the superiority of gallium nitrate over etidronate, pamidronate, or calcitonin, its greater toxicity and more cumbersome mode of administration limits its use to the acute setting or to severe cases with bisphosphonate-refractory hypercalcemia (1,2).

Calcitonin is a natural peptide hormone, secreted by the thyroid gland, which decreases bone and renal tubular resorption of calcium. It is generally administered by the intramuscular or subcutaneous route, at a dose of 6 to 8 UI/kg every 6 hours. Its main advantage over other available drugs for the treatment of malignant hypercalcemia is its rapid onset of action (usually within two hours), but its hypocalcemic effect is weak (fewer than 30% of patients achieve normocalcemia), and response is not maintained for more than 48 hours despite continuous treatment. It is useful in the management of critically ill patients with acute severe hypercalcemia, in combination with gallium nitrate or zoledronate together with intravenous hydration (1,2).

Corticosteroids are moderately active hypocalcemic agents in patients whose underlying disease is responsive to steroids, such as myeloma, lymphoma, leukemia, and, to a lesser degree, breast carcinoma. Other treatments such as *mythramycin (plicamycin)* and *phosphates* have been largely replaced by bisphosphonates because of their lower efficacy and their unfavorable toxicity profile (1,2).

New Treatment Approaches. New pharmacological interventions involve the blockade of RANKL. RANKL is a key element in the differentiation, function, and survival of osteoclasts, which play an essential role in removing calcium from bone in response to PTH stimulation. RANKL is a transmembrane protein belonging to the TNF superfamily, widely expressed in bone and lymphoid tissues and on the surface of osteoblasts stimulated by osteotropic factors such as PTH, $1,25(OH)_2D_3$, or TNF-α (1,3). The extracellular domain binds to its specific receptor RANK, expressed on plasma membrane of monocyte-macrophage lineage osteoclast precursor cells, as well as in mature osteoclasts and dendritic cells, eventually promoting differentiation, activation, and survival of osteoclasts. The activity of RANKL is physiologically counterbalanced by circulating osteoprotegerin (OPG), which acts like a soluble decoy receptor of RANKL preventing its binding to RANK (1,3). Consistent with this, intravenous administration of OPG has shown potent hypocalcemic effects in murine models of humoral hypercalcemia, and are more effective in this setting than bisphosphonates. Preliminary data from small studies involving osteoporotic women suggest OPG safely reduces bone turnover. A fully humanized monoclonal antibody against RANKL, denosumab (AMG 162), has also demonstrated sustained decrease in bone resorption not only in women with osteoporosis but also in patients with multiple myeloma or breast cancer. Antibodies against PTHrp have been tested in preclinical models showing hypocalcemic effects. However, the role of these agents in the treatment of malignancy-associated hypercalcemia has not been evaluated in the clinical setting to date (1,3,6).

Summary

Malignant hypercalcemia is a frequent metabolic emergency in cancer patients that can be controlled in the majority of cases. Fluid replacement and treatment with bisphosphonates are the mainstay of therapy. Calcitonin and gallium nitrate, where available, may be added initially in critically ill patients with acute severe hypercalcemia. Zoledronate is the bisphosphonate of choice, administered by intravenous infusion every two to four weeks. Administration of zoledronic acid should also be considered for routine use together with systemic therapy in patients with solid tumors or multiple myeloma and osteolytic metastases, to reduce pain and delay skeletal complications. Anti-RANKL therapy is currently being evaluated in the clinical setting with encouraging preliminary results. The impact of these drugs on other cancer outcomes remains to be ellucidated.

Tumor Lysis Syndrome
Etiopathogenesis

The tumor lysis syndrome occurs as a result of rapid tumor cell lysis, with release of intracellular metabolites into the bloodstream at a rate that exceeds the excretory capacity of the kidneys. The major metabolic abnormalities seen in the tumor lysis syndrome are hyperkalemia, hyperuricemia, and hyperphosphatemia with hypocalcemia. It is more likely to occur in patients with preexisting renal dysfunction. The syndrome may be complicated by the propensity of uric acid and phosphates to precipitate in renal tubules and impair renal excretory function, which leads to further elevation of these metabolites, lactic acidosis and azotemia (1,7,8).

The tumor lysis is observed most frequently in patients with a large, high-proliferation-rate tumor that is highly sensitive to the cytotoxic effects of chemotherapy. This syndrome is most commonly associated with Burkitt's lymphoma, but it also occurs in other lymphoproliferative disorders such as high-grade non-Hodgkin's lymphoma, acute leukemia, and chronic myeloid leukemia in blast crisis. Anecdotal cases have also been reported in solid tumors such as small cell lung cancer, germ-cell tumors, breast cancer, medulloblastoma, and others (1,7,8).

Although the tumor lysis syndrome most often develops following the administration of chemotherapeutic agents, it may also occur following radiotherapy, hormonal therapy, or treatment with monoclonal antibodies or interferon, and occasionally it is seen spontaneously.

Clinical Presentation and Diagnosis

The signs and symptoms of tumor lysis syndrome are those caused by the electrolyte disturbances. Hyperkalemia may produce characteristic electrocardiographic changes, arrhythmias, and even cardiac arrest, which is the main cause of death in these patients. Hyperphosphatemia may cause the precipitation of calcium phosphate in renal tubules, which can impair renal function and further aggravate the syndrome. Hypocalcemia, which is thought to be

due to the precipitation of calcium phosphate in tissues because of hyperphosphatemia, is often asymptomatic; when severe, it may produce neuromuscular irritability, carpopedal spasms, altered mental status, and convulsions. Diagnosis is confirmed by laboratory tests demonstrating increased levels of serum uric acid, potassium and phosphate, and decreased serum calcium levels (1,7,8).

Treatment

The main treatment of tumor lysis syndrome is prevention. High-risk patients should be closely monitored, with electrolytes, creatinine, phosphate, and uric acid level determinations before treatment, and every 6 to 12 hours in the first days following therapy. Chemotherapy should be delayed until metabolic disturbances are corrected and the patient has been adequately hydrated with intravenous fluids (3000–4000 ml/day) for 24 to 48 hours. Ensuring an adequate urinary flow rate and maintaining a urine pH >7 with sodium bicarbonate are essential measures to increase the solubility of uric acid and minimize the chance of renal failure. Allopurinol reduces the incidence of nephropathy by inhibiting xanthine oxidase and thus decreasing the conversion of hypoxanthine and xanthine to uric acid. As it has no effect on preexisting uric acid, uric acid levels usually do not decrease until 48 to 72 hours after treatment. Allopurinol should be administered in patients at risk of tumor lysis syndrome in doses ranging from 300 to 900 mg/day, before chemotherapy, and during two to four days following treatment (doses should be reduced in cases of renal insufficiency). Parenteral administration (200–400 mg/m^2/day) may be required in patients with restricted oral intake. More recently, a new recombinant urate oxidase, rasburicase, has been developed for the prevention and treatment of hyperuricemia. Urate oxidase catalyzes the enzymatic oxidation of uric acid into allantoin, a readily excretable metabolite that is 5 to 10 times more soluble in urine than uric acid. At the recommended dose and schedule (0.15–0.2 mg/kg/day given as a 30-minute daily intravenous infusion for five days) it is well tolerated except for occasional instances of hemolytic anemia and methemoglobinemia observed in patients with glucose-6-phosphate dehydrogenase deficiency. Studies in both adults and children have shown that more tha 90% of patients achieve normalization of uric acid levels within four hours of rasburicase administration. There is no conclusive evidence, however, regarding its ability to reduce the need for dialysis. Its ability to lower preexisting elevated uric acid levels and the rapid onset of action, allowing patients to receive specific antineoplastic therapy with no delay, are distinct advantages that rasburicase possesses over allopurinol. Nevertheless, cost needs to be factored in the decision-making process due to its elevated price. Its use may be therefore restricted to patients presenting with hyperuricemia or to the prevention of tumor lysis syndrome in high-risk patients such as those with leukemias with white blood cell counts more than 50×10^3/mm^3 or lymphomas with lactate dehydrogenase levels greater than two to five times the upper limit of normal.

Hyperphosphatemia and its resultant hypocalcemia should be managed with oral phosphate binders such as aluminum hydroxide, 30 ml four times a day. If hyperkalemia develops, treatment with an oral sodium–potassium exchange resin or with combined insulin–glucose therapy should be initiated promptly. Calcium gluconate antagonizes the cardiac affects of hyperkalemia and can be especially helpful in patients with concomitant hypocalcemia. Persistent hypocalcemia is occasionally seen, even after hyperphosphatemia has been resolved, which may be due to low serum levels of 1,25-dihydroxyvitamin D_3. These cases should be treated with calcitriol. In severe cases (potassium ≥6 mmol/l, uric acid ≥10 mg/dl, phosphorus rapidly rising or ≥10 mg/dl, fluid overload, acutely worsening renal function, or highly symptomatic hypocalcemia), immediate hemodialysis is recommended (1,7,8).

Hypoglycemia
Etiopathogenesis
Tumor-induced hypoglycemia is commonly associated with insulin-secreting islet cell tumors, but it may rarely develop also in patients with large slowly growing mesenchymal tumors, hepatoma, and adrenocortical carcinoma. Several etiological mechanisms have been postulated: secretion of insulin or insulin-like substances, increased metabolism of glucose by the tumor, and failure of the regulatory mechanisms for glucose homeostasis. Insulin levels may be elevated in patients with hypoglycemia and islet cell cancers, but this is rarely observed in other neoplasms. Increased levels of substances with insulin-like activity have been measured in patients with hypoglycemia and nonislet cell malignancies. Increased glucose consumption by the tumor rarely leads to hypoglycemia if counter-regulatory mechanisms for glucose homeostasis are not impaired. However, in patients with large tumor burdens and extensive hepatic metastases, the combination of accelerated glucose utilization with impaired production may lead to hypoglycemia (1,7,9).

Clinical Presentation and Diagnosis
The clinical presentation of hypoglycemia is related to the degree and rate of glucose depression. Common symptoms include fatigue, diaphoresis, weakness, dizziness, and confusion, and tend to occur or worsen after fasting in the early morning or late afternoon. In severe acute cases (<40 mg/dl), patients may develop seizures, focal or diffuse neurological deficits, and coma.

Before assuming the diagnosis of tumor-induced hypoglycemia, one should exclude the more common causes of hypoglycemia: exogenous insulin use, oral diabetic agents, adrenal or pituitary insufficiency, ethanol abuse, or malnutrition. Despite a low serum glucose level, patients with insulinoma will have increased insulin and proinsulin levels. Patients with nonislet cell tumors will have normal to low insulin levels. Insulin-like plasma factors may be measured, where available, by bioassays or radioreceptor techniques. Artefactual hypoglycemia may occur in leukemia with high leukocyte counts, because of cellular glucose use in vitro (1,7,9).

Treatment
Specific antitumor therapy is the preferred treatment for hypoglycemia due to malignancy. Most insulin-secreting tumors are benign and can be removed by surgical intervention. Chemotherapy or diazoxide, a drug that inhibits insulin

secretion, have only modest efficacy in nonoperable patients. Nonislet cell tumors can sometimes be totally or partially resected, with resolution of hypoglycemia. When hypoglycemia is mild, increasing the frequency of meals may suffice. Intravenous infusion of glucose may be necessary in more severe cases while applying more specific measures. Corticosteroids may also provide temporary relief. In some instances, intermittent subcutaneous or intramuscular glucagon injections, or continuous infusions of glucagon with a portable pump, have been used successfully, particularly in patients with adequate glycogen stores (patients with insulinomas or with insulin-like products secreting tumors) (1,7,9). Glucose levels do not rise in response to glucagon when hypoglycemia is due to poor hepatic glycogen reserve/ liver failure.

Syndrome of Inappropriate Secretion of Antidiuretic Hormone (Siadh)
Etiopathogenesis
The syndrome of inappropriate secretion of antidiuretic hormone (SIADH) occurs in 1% to 2% of cancer patients. It is characterized by hyponatremia, low serum osmolality, and inappropriately high urine osmolality and sodium levels, caused by excessive production of antidiuretic hormone (ADH). Increased ADH levels produce excessive water reabsorption in the collecting ducts of the kidneys, and a mild increase in intravascular volume. Volume expansion increases renal perfusion, decreases proximal tubular sodium reabsorption, inhibits aldosterone secretion, and triggers the release of atrial natriuretic hormone. All these lead to hyponatremia, with inappropriately concentrated urine (1,7).

The most common causes of SIADH include pulmonary infections (pneumonia, tuberculosis, abscess), central nervous system diseases (mass lesion, stroke, infection, hemorrhage), drugs (cyclophosphamide, vincristine, opiates, thiazides, chlorpropramide, carbamazepine), and malignant diseases. Tumor-associated SIADH occurs mainly in patients with small cell carcinoma of the lung (10–15% of small cell lung cancer patients will develop clinically significant hyponatremia, which is associated with a poor prognosis), although it has also been reported in cancers of the prostate, adrenal cortex, gastrointestinal tract, and head and neck, and in carcinoid tumors, thymoma, lymphoma, and mesothelioma. Ectopic ADH secretion in patients with small cell lung cancer has been reported. All other conditions are associated with excessive ADH production in the posterior pituitary (1,7).

Clinical Presentation and Diagnosis
Many patients with SIADH are asymptomatic, and the disorder is discovered incidentally on routine blood electrolyte determinations. In mild cases, patients may report vague nonspecific symptoms such as fatigue, anorexia, nausea, myalgias, and headache. In more severe cases, when hyponatremia develops rapidly or the sodium falls below 115 mg/dl, altered mental status, confusion, seizures, and coma may develop. Psychotic behavior, pathological reflexes, papilledema, and even focal neurological signs have also been reported in cases of profound hyponatremia (1,7). Patients in whom hyponatremia develops rapidly are

more likely to present with severe clinical symptoms, although they can also tolerate a more rapid correction.

Before the diagnosis of SIADH can be established, other frequent causes of hyponatremia should be excluded, such as cardiac, hepatic or renal dysfunction, gastrointestinal fluid and electrolyte losses, adrenal insufficiency, hypothyroidism, or diuretics. Patients with plasma cell dyscrasias and elevated paraprotein levels may have artefactual hyponatremia. Once other causes of hyponatremia have been excluded, the diagnosis of SIADH is based on the demonstration of hyponatremia (<135 mmol/l), low serum osmolality (<280 mosmol/l), high urine sodium (>20 mmol/l), and osmolality (>200 mosmol/l) (1,7).

Treatment

The most effective therapy for SIADH is that directed at the underlying cause. Combination chemotherapy in patients with small cell lung cancer, radiotherapy and corticosteroids in patients with brain metastases, or discontinuation of the responsible agent in patients with drug-induced SIADH will revert the hyponatremia in most cases. If the etiology of excessive ADH secretion cannot be corrected, fluid intake restriction of 500 to 1000 ml/day generally produces normalization of serum sodium levels within 7 to 10 days. If fluid restriction is not effective or patients are unable to comply, treatment with demeclocycline may correct the hyponatremia by producing a dose-dependent nephrogenic diabetes insipidus. The main side effect is nephrotoxicity, generally mild and reversible. The recommended initial daily dose is 600 mg (lower in patients with liver or renal disease), divided into two or three doses per day. Doses may be increased up to 1200 mg if no response is observed. More recently, several vasopressin V2 receptor antagonists, such as lixivaptan, conivaptan, and tolvaptan, have been introduced into clinical practice and may emerge as additional therapeutic options for the management of this syndrome (10). In patients with coma or seizures, intravenous 3% hypertonic saline or isotonic saline infusion with furosemide should be instituted. The rate of rise in serum sodium should not be greater than 0.5 to 1 mmol/l/hr to minimize the risk of central pontine myelinolysis (1,7).

CARDIOVASCULAR EMERGENCIES
Superior Vena Cava Syndrome
Etiopathogenesis

Superior vena cava syndrome is the clinical expression of the obstruction of blood flow through the superior vena cava to the right atrium. The superior vena cava is the major drainage vessel for venous blood from the head, neck, upper extremities, and upper thorax, and its obstruction impairs blood return and increases venous pressure, causing facial and upper extremity edema, as well as pleural and pericardial effusions. In rare acute severe cases, tracheal, laryngeal, and brain edema may develop and cause death (11–13).

Superior vena cava syndrome may result from thrombosis, invasion, or compression of the superior vena cava by any pathological process that invades the lymphatics or other structures of the superior mediastinum. Nowadays, neoplasms account for 70% to 90% of cases of superior vena

cava syndrome. Bronchogenic carcinoma, predominantly small cell lung cancer, is the underlying malignancy in 50% to 70% of cases. The second most common tumor causing superior vena cava syndrome is lymphoma, especially diffuse large cell and lymphoblastic lymphoma, accounting for 8% to 20% of the cases. Other primary malignancies that may cause superior vena cava syndrome are mediastinal germ cell tumors and thymomas. Breast carcinoma is the most frequent metastatic neoplasm to cause superior vena cava syndrome. Up to 20% of the cases are due to nonmalignant conditions such as histoplasmosis, tuberculosis, sarcoidosis, goitre, idiopathic mediastinal fibrosis, or thrombosis of the superior vena cava in patients with central vein catheters or pacemakers. Superior vena cava syndrome is rare in children, and is usually iatrogenic, associated with indwelling catheters or surgery. When because of malignant diseases more than two-thirds of superior vena cava syndrome cases in children are caused by diffuse large cell or lymphoblastic lymphoma (11–13).

Clinical Presentation and Diagnosis

Superior vena cava syndrome is usually of insidious onset and is rarely a true oncological emergency. Patients generally complain of dyspnea, a sensation of fullness in the head, and swelling of the face, particularly around the eyes, trunk, and upper extremities, which tend to worsen when lying down or leaning forward. Other less frequent symptoms include headache, cough, chest pain, dysphagia, hoarseness, dizziness, visual disturbances, and fatigue. The most common findings on physical examination are neck vein distention, facial edema, plethora, cyanosis, arm and hand edema, tachypnea, and stridor. If the obstruction has developed slowly, collateral blood flow may be evident in the abdominal wall or in the upper chest and back. In cases with increased intracranial pressure, papilledema, confusion, seizures, or coma may develop (11–13).

Diagnosis of superior vena cava syndrome is usually clinically evident. The chest X-ray film shows a superior mediastinal widening or a right hilar mass in most cases. Only 16% of patients with superior vena cava syndrome have normal chest X-ray. Computed tomography (CT) is the most useful radiographic study, as it provides more detailed information such as the level of superior vena cava obstruction, the presence of superior vena cava thrombosis, collateral circulation, mediastinal adenopathies or masses, and other sites of unrecognized disease in the chest, and it may also help guide a fine-needle aspiration biopsy if histology has not yet been obtained. Contrast venography is usually reserved for patients in whom surgical bypass is considered. Radionuclide (technetium-99m) venography is an alternative minimally invasive method (13). At the time of presentation, fewer than 50% of patients have a known diagnosis of cancer. In the absence of severe airway obstruction, significantly elevated intracranial pressure, or cardiovascular collapse, etiological diagnosis should be established before definitive therapy. In patients with superior vena cava syndrome and small cell lung cancer, sputum cytology is diagnostic in up to two-thirds of patients and bronchoscopy in most of them. In the presence of pleural effusion, thoraconcentesis established the diagnosis of malignancy in 71% of cases. Bone marrow biopsy may provide the diagnosis in 25% of patients with small cell

mesothelioma. A computer-assisted tomography (CAT) scan of the chest is also useful, particularly in the setting of a newly diagnosed effusion, to define fluid loculations, mediastinal and/or hilar lymphadenopathy, pleural masses, and parenchymal disease. A bronchoscopy is indicated if an endobronchial lesion is suspected or if there is any radiographic sign of pulmonary atelectasis. Magnetic resonance imaging (MRI) may be helpful to define chest wall tumor invasion in the presence of malignant pleura effusion.

Thoracentesis is required to obtain pleural fluid for biochemical and cytological analysis, to relieve symptoms, and to determine the extent of lung expansion following pleural fluid drainage. MPEs are usually exudative (LDH > 200 U/ml, total protein > 3 g/dl, fluid:serum LDH ratio > 0.6 or fluid:serum protein ratio > 0.5) and contain red blood cells in one-third of cases. Low values of pleural fluid pH or glucose are associated with poorer prognosis. The first cytological examination is diagnostic in approximately 50% of patients. The diagnostic sensitivity of cytological examination is higher in patients with a previously known malignancy and may be improved with repeated thoracentesis. When multiple cytological examinations of pleural fluid are nondiagnostic, a pleural biopsy may be performed. Both thoracoscopic and image-guided biopsies have a far higher diagnostic yield than blind pleural biopsy (diagnostic in only 7–12% of cases). Thoracotomy is rarely necessary (16,18).

Treatment

Patients with malignant pleura effusion who have potentially responsive tumors should receive specific antineoplastic therapy as the primary therapeutic approach. It should be noted that pleural effusions of highly chemotherapy-sensitive tumors (i.e., lymphomas) may occasionally worsen with the first cycle of treatment and subsequently resolve. Therefore, in these tumor types, a rapid increase in the effusion following the initiation of therapy does not necessarily portend treatment failure. Thoracentesis is highly effective for acute relief of symptoms, but effusion recurrence occurs in 98% of patients within 30 days. Therefore, obliteration of the pleural space either by parietal pleurectomy or by the instillation of sclerosing agents is required for sustained relief. Response rates of 50% to 90%, defined as absence of fluid reaccumulation at one month, have been reported with tube thoracostomy followed by chemical pleurodesis. This requires complete pleural fluid drainage and reexpansion of the lung to allow apposition of the visceral and parietal pleura. The more recent use of small-bore catheters instead of the classical chest tubes seems to be equally effective, with less associated morbidity. Many different sclerosing agents have been employed, including talc, antibiotics (tetracycline, doxycycline, minocycline), antineoplastic drugs (bleomycin, doxorubicin, mitoxantrone, cisplatin, cytarabine), and biologic agents (interferon, interleukin-2, *Corynebacterium parvum*, streptococcal preparations) (16,19). The most extensively studied include tetracyclines, bleomycin, and talc. Several small randomized studies have shown talc to be more effective than tetracycline and bleomycin, and bleomycin to be superior to tetracycline. Although talc appears to be the most efficacious and inexpensive agent, most of the published experience involves its insufflation through a thoracoscope under general anesthesia, which increases costs and morbidity. For these reasons, some authors consider bleomycin the alternative of choice. More recently, talc has been used by aerosolization through a chest tube. A randomized CALGB study has demonstrated that it has similar efficacy than thoracoscopic talc insufflation while associated with improved safety profile and quality of life. The most common side effects of talc pleurodesis are fever (16%) and pain (7%). Empyema, pneumonitis, and respiratory failure may be observed rarely (20).

For malignant pleura effusion refractory to pleurodesis or associated with trapped lung, placement of an indwelling pleural catheter under local anesthesia may be considered, which allows intermittent drainage of effusions for prolonged periods of time on an outpatient basis. Randomized trials have shown this procedure has similar safety and efficacy than doxycycline sclerotherapy, requiring less hospitalization. Other alternative is a pleuroperitoneal shunt, which permits the patient to manually empty the pleural fluid into the peritoneal cavity and is associated with few complications and a success rate of 75% (16,19) (Fig. 19.1). However, the need for active pumping of the chamber a minimum of 400 times per day limits its usefulness to patients with excellent performance status. Finally, although effective in nearly 100% of cases, pleurectomy is rarely indicated because of its elevated morbidity (25%) and mortality (10%). It may be considered in patients with refractory effusions and trapped lung and significant expectation of survival or for those submitted to thoracotomy for other reasons (e.g., diagnosis).

Massive Hemoptysis
Etiopathogenesis

Massive hemoptysis is defined as expectoration of 600 ml or more of blood in 24 hours, or bleeding into the respiratory tree at a rate that presents a threat to life. Massive hemoptysis is uncommon, occurring in fewer than 5% of all patients with hemoptysis—but when it does occur, it is frequently fatal (35–70%) (21–23).

The most common causes of massive hemoptysis are tuberculosis, bronchiectasis, lung abscess, aspergilloma, and neoplasia. Bronchogenic carcinoma is the leading cause in patients older than 40 years. Although hemoptysis occurs with equal frequency among the different histological types of primary lung cancer, massive hemoptysis is most frequently associated with epidermoid carcinoma. These tumors tend to be large and angioinvasive, and to undergo spontaneous necrosis and cavitation. Bronchial adenomas may also produce massive hemoptysis because of their rich vascularity. Upper airway tumors, pulmonary metastases (from melanoma, breast, colon, or kidney cancer), and sarcomas rarely cause massive bleeding (21–23). Finally, hemoptysis in cancer patients may be also caused by nonmalignant conditions, such as fungal infections, thrombocytopenia, or other coagulation disorders. Some new antiangiogenic agents currently used in cancer care, such as bevacizumab, also increase the risk of bleeding, particularly in patients with central squamous lung cancer.

Clinical Presentation and Diagnosis

Massive expectoration of blood may produce symptoms secondary to hypovolemia and interference with alveolar gas exchange. Asphyxiation, rather than exanguination, is

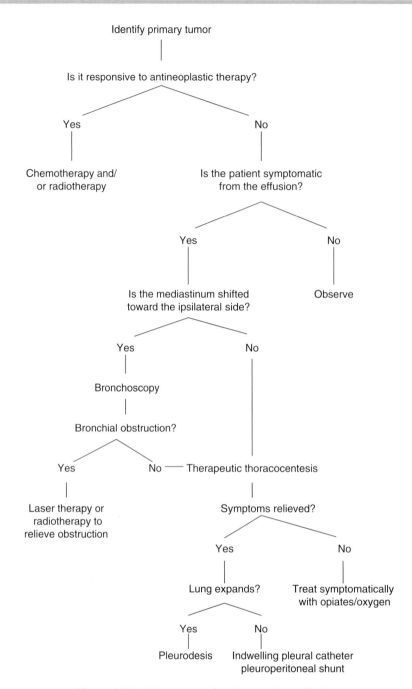

Figure 19.1 Management of malignant pleural effusions.

the principal threat. Assessment of respiratory and hemo-dynamic status and identification of the site of hemorrhage are the major objectives of diagnosis and management. Other sites of bleeding (oropharyngolaryngeal or gastroin-testinal tract) must be excluded. All patients with massive hemoptysis should undergo bronchoscopy, preferably during the active hemorrhage, to determine the site and cause.

Treatment

The most urgent measure in cases of massive hemoptysis is to maintain the patient's airway patency. Traditionally, the rigid bronchoscope has been the technique of choice

for the evaluation and management of massive hemoptysis, because of its larger diameter and better ability to suction, administer oxygen, and control the airway. The require-ment of general anesthesia and the inability to visualize the upper lobe bronchi are its major drawbacks. Flexible fiberoptic bronchoscopy, in contrast, allows the inspection of a much larger area of the bronchial tree and may be carried out under local anesthesia, although its ability to suction large amounts of blood and maintain oxygenation is more limited. Selective bronchial intubation of the unaf-fected lung and tamponade of the bleeding site with a balloon occlusion catheter (Fogarty) may be performed during bronchoscopy (22,23). General supportive measures should also be promptly instituted, such as rest, semi-upright positioning or positioning bleeding-side-down to prevent aspiration into the nonaffected lung, mild sedation, humidified oxygen, intravenous fluids, blood transfusion, and correction of coagulation disorders if they exist.

Surgical resection of the bleeding pulmonary segment remains the optimal definitive treatment of massive hemoptysis. Patients with controlled hemorrhage at the time of surgery have a mortality rate of 1% to 17%, whereas those with uncontrolled bleeding have a mortality rate of 20% to 40%. However, mortality rates of patients with massive hemoptysis managed with conservative nonsurgical measures have been reported to be 50% to 100% (21–23).

In patients who are not surgical candidates owing to poorly localized or nonlocalized bleeding, extensive neoplasm, prior pulmonary resection or inadequate pulmonary reserve, comorbid conditions, or overall prognosis, several nonoperative approaches may be effective in controlling active bleeding. Iced saline lavage through the rigid bronchoscope, prolonged tamponade with a Fogarty balloon catheter, or Nd:YAG laser therapy have been used successfully. Bronchial artery catheterization and embolization has been reported to control hemoptysis in up to 80% of patients. Currently, the most widely used particles for embolization are polyvinyl alcohol particles, which are non-biodegradable permanent embolic agents. The principal adverse effects of this procedure are spinal cord injury due to accidental embolization of the anterior spinal artery, and, less frequently, accidental visceral and extremity embolization. Hemoptysis may recur in up to 20% of patients. Recurrent bleeding during the first six months following embolization is usually due to undetected bronchial and systemic collaterals caused by diffuse pulmonary disease. Late recurrence is usually due to disease progression. Finally, palliative radiotherapy (e.g., 10Gy × 1) may be of value, benefiting 50% to 60% of patients with hemoptysis and lung cancer (21–23).

Airway Obstruction
Etiopathogenesis
Bronchial or lower airway obstruction is a frequent event in cancer patients, but is rarely life-threatening. Upper airway obstruction (hypopharynx, larynx, and trachea to the carina), in contrast, is less frequently encountered but represents a real oncological emergency.

Upper airway obstruction may result from multiple benign conditions that may be associated with malignancy, such as aspiration of a foreign body or food, tracheomalacia, tracheal stenosis, or edema, or, most commonly, may be caused directly by tumors involving the base of the tongue, tonsils, hypopharynx, larynx, thyroid, or the upper mediastinum. Primary tracheal neoplasms less often produce airway obstruction. In most instances, upper airway obstruction occurs in patients with a known diagnosis of cancer, although occasionally it may be the presenting sign of a small critically located lesion. The main cause of lower airway obstruction is primary carcinoma of the lung. Far less often, bronchial obstruction is caused by endobronchial metastasis from carcinomas of the breast, colon, or kidney or from melanoma (21,24).

Clinical Presentation and Diagnosis
The clinical manifestations of airway obstruction depend on the severity and location of the obstruction. Patients with upper airway obstruction usually present with dyspnea, apprehension, cough, drooling, stridor, diaphoresis, and tachycardia. In severe cases, the patient may become cyanotic and obtunded, bradycardia may develop, and stridor may disappear. Diagnosis and intervention are based solely on the clinical condition of the patient (25).

Lower airway obstruction frequently causes postobstructive pneumonitis. Dyspnea, hemoptysis, cough, fever, and wheezing are common findings. A chest X-ray or CT scan may reveal the presence of the tumor, pneumonic consolidations, atelectasis, or even lung collapse. In patients with unknown previous malignancy and a suspicious lesion on chest X-ray or a torpid response of a pneumonic consolidation to adequate antibiotic therapy, a bronchoscopy must be performed (25).

Treatment
In cases of acute life-threatening upper airway obstruction, urgent evaluation by an otolaryngologist and emergency low tracheostomy are indicated. Adjunct therapy with corticosteroids to reduce edema, supplemental oxygen and bronchodilators may also be useful. Once the airway patency has been addressed, a more thorough assessment of the underlying malignancy should be performed, to establish a specific treatment. Depending upon the histologic type, the site and extension of the neoplasm, and previous therapy, surgery, radiotherapy, and/or chemotherapy may be considered (21,24,25).

Lower airway obstruction does not usually require an emergency reestablishment of airway patency. Initial management should include supportive measures, such as supplemental oxygen, corticosteroids and bronchodilators, and antibiotics if there is any associated infection. Specific therapy for primary bronchial obstruction comprises surgery, radiotherapy, and/or chemotherapy, depending on tumor type and stage, and the patient's performance status. Placement of self-expandable metallic stents (SEMS), which can be done under local anesthesia using fiberoptic bronchoscopy, is a widely used alternative approach that provides prompt and durable palliation in unresectable patients with central airway obstruction. Uncovered stents, however, have the potential for granulation tissue formation and tumor in-growth along the length of the stent leading to re-occlusion of the lumen. The risk for these complications is lower with covered SEMS. Other disadvantage of metal stents is the difficulty moving them once deployed, making stent removal virtually impossible. Silicone stents are a cheaper alternative and have the advantage of being easily removed and exchanged when needed. This may be relevant in patients who respond to systemic antineoplastic therapy as their airway may be restored. The most common complication is stent migration (9.5%), followed by granulation tissue formation (8%) and mucous plugging (4%).

Recurrent endobronchial obstruction in patients who have received previous external-beam radiotherapy may be managed with several palliative approaches. Endoscopic laser therapy is a relatively easy technique and may quickly relieve symptoms in patients with incomplete obstruction of the trachea or mainstem bronchus. Obstruction recurrence, however, tends to occur rapidly, and repeated laser applications are associated with poorer efficacy and greater risk of complications. Potential adverse events include hemorrhage, perforation, and tracheo-esophageal or bronchopleural fistula (21,26). Endobronchial brachytherapy with radioactive isotopes (^{192}Ir or ^{60}Co) is another alternative for palliative treatment. An additional 20 to 40Gy may be safely administered in patients who have had prior external-beam irradiation. Palliation of symptoms may last longer than with laser therapy (21,27).

GASTROINTESTINAL EMERGENCIES
Bowel Obstruction
Etiopathogenesis
Bowel obstruction along with gastrointestinal bleeding is the most frequent reasons for emergency abdominal surgery in patients with malignancy. Neoplastic disease is the cause of bowel obstruction in 60% to 95% of cancer patients, in contrast to the 7% to 9% incidence of malignant obstruction in nonselected series. Colorectal, ovarian, and gastric malignancies are the most common primary tumors in patients who subsequently develop intestinal obstruction. About 10% to 30% of patients with colorectal cancer and 20% to 50% of ovarian cancer patients present or eventually develop bowel obstruction. Intestinal involvement due to metastatic cancer commonly presents as diffuse peritoneal carcinomatosis, being isolated gastrointestinal metastasis rarely observed. Breast cancer and melanoma are the most common nonabdominopelvic tumors causing bowel obstruction, which may occur many years since primary diagnosis of disease. Benign conditions may account for up 40% of cases of bowel obstruction in cancer patients, adhesions due to previous interventions being the most frequent cause. The site of obstruction is the small bowel in 60% of cases (28).

Clinical Presentation and Diagnosis
Patients with bowel obstruction usually present with constipation, abdominal distension, crampy pain, and intractable emesis, which may be feculent in cases of large bowel obstruction. Plain X-ray films of the abdomen (supine and upright or left lateral decubitus) and chest are important to confirm the diagnosis of bowel obstruction and to exclude perforation. Contrast X-ray studies are necessary only in selected cases (nondiagnostic plain abdominal films, atypical clinical findings or protracted course despite adequate management) and are contraindicated if perforation is suspected (28,29). Other radiological imaging, particularly CT, is also critical in determining the cause of obstruction, localization and extension, and possible therapeutic interventions.

Treatment
The management of patients with malignant bowel obstruction should be individually assessed, considering tumor localization, extension and biology, expected success of subsequent antineoplastic therapy, patient's functional status and overall prognosis, as well as his or her goals of care. Because it is rarely a true emergency, time

can and should be taken to come up with an appropriate treatment plan.

In the absence of fever, leukocytosis or peritonitis, a trial of conservative therapy should be considered for patients with bowel obstruction and incurable advanced disease. Conservative measures include intravenous hydration, correction of electrolyte imbalance, nasoenteric decompression and bowel rest, discontinuation or at least decrease of any medications that may interfere with bowel motility (especially narcotics), and treatment of distressing symptoms such as nausea or pain. Nonoperative management is successful in 12% to 29% of patients with cancer, although more than one-third of these develop recurrent obstruction and may eventually require surgical intervention. When conservative therapy fails, palliative nonsurgical interventions or surgical exploration are indicated.

The most commonly performed surgical procedures are bypass, stoma creation, and resection or lysis of adhesions. Surgical relief of symptoms is achieved in 55% to 96% of patients, and recurrence occurs in 9% to 33%. However, patients with malignant bowel obstruction are often poor surgical candidates due to advanced disease, malnutrition, hypoalbuminemia, and dehydration. In recent years, the armamentarium of endoscopic options has broadened considerably and now affords physicians a variety of nonsurgical means to palliate malignant obstruction of the gastrointestinal tract, including percutaneous gastrostomy (PEG), decompression tubes, endoscopic dilatation, enteral stents, and ablative methods such as diathermy, photodynamic therapy, laser therapy, and argon plasma coagulation (28–31). Colonic stenting is probably the most widely used option, either alone or as a bridge to elective surgery. It reduces morbidity and mortality rates as compared with emergency surgery and the need for colostomy formation; consequently, it is associated with shorter hospital stays and lower costs.

Perforation
Etiopathogenesis
Gastrointestinal perforation is a frequent surgical emergency in cancer patients. Perforation at a site involved by tumor is the cause in up to 60% of cases. Lymphoma is the most frequent malignant process associated with gastrointestinal perforation, accounting for about 50% of malignant causes. One-fifth of patients with primary gastrointestinal lymphoma develop perforation. Other less common causes are gastric and colon cancers. Occasionally, extraabdominal tumors such as melanoma and breast, lung, or ovarian cancers may metastasize to the intestinal wall and cause perforation. New antiangiogenic drugs recently developed for the treatment of cancer, such as bevacizumab, increase the risk for gastrointestinal perforation in patients with colorectal cancer, particularly when the primary tumor has not been surgically removed. Benign processes may also cause gastrointestinal perforation, such as peptic ulcer, postsurgical bowel anastomosis disruption, colonoscopy, colostomy irrigation, radiation enteritis, neutropenic colitis, diverticulitis, infection (cytomegalovirus, *Clostridium difficile*), and perforation proximal to an obstructing lesion (28).

Clinical Presentation and Diagnosis

Although contained perforations may present with moderate abdominal pain, most perforations freely communicate with the peritoneum and cause sudden severe abdominal pain, ileus and abdominal distension, fever, hypotension, tachycardia, and leukocytosis. Immunosuppression resulting from chemotherapy or steroid therapy may mask the usual signs and symptoms of gastrointestinal perforation and significantly delay diagnosis. Perforation of a hollow viscera is confirmed by demonstration of free air under the diaphragm on upright chest X-ray; however, 20% to 50% of patients with gastrointestinal perforation do not have free intraperitoneal air visualized. Gastrografin contrast X-ray studies and CT imaging may be useful in localizing the site of perforation and in planning surgery (28).

Treatment

Besides initial nasogastric decompression, fluid resuscitation, and broad-spectrum antibiotic therapy, prompt surgical intervention is mandatory in cases of gastrointestinal perforation. Gastroduodenal perforations are generally caused by acute ulceration, and are repaired with an omental patch. Chronic gastric ulcers should be biopsied and, if a frozen section shows malignancy, resected. Resection and primary anastomosis is the treatment of choice of most small bowel perforations. Perforations of the large bowel generally require resection, colostomy, and Hartman's procedure or mucous fistula. Intra-abdominal abscesses, which are frequently associated with chronic perforations, require aggressive surgical drainage (28,32).

Bleeding
Etiopathogenesis

The majority of gastrointestinal bleeding episodes in patients with malignancy are associated with benign processes. Gastritis and peptic ulcer disease (44–76%), followed by esophagitis and esophageal varices (11–17%), are the most common causes of gastrointestinal bleeding in cancer patients. Other conditions that less frequently produce gastrointestinal bleeding include Mallory–Weiss syndrome precipitated by chemotherapy-induced vomiting, viral enteritis, diverticulosis, angiodysplasia, and inflammatory bowel disease. Tumors are the source of bleeding in fewer than 25% of patients (32,33).

Clinical Presentation and Diagnosis

Upper gastrointestinal bleeding generally presents as hematemesis and melena, while hematochezia (recognizable blood mixed with stool) strongly suggests a bleeding source distal to the right colon. Orthostatic hypotension occurs when rapid blood loss exceeds 20% of blood volume. Tachycardia, hypotension, restlessness, and peripheral vasoconstriction are signs of shock, and indicate that supportive measures must be instituted immediately.

Whether bleeding is proximal or distal to the ligament of Treitz determines diagnostic and therapeutic modalities. If upper gastrointestinal bleeding is suspected, a nasogastric tube should be placed, and the stomach lavaged with room-temperature saline. Nasogastric tube aspiration is easy to perform and gives useful information: when positive, the bleeding source is proximal to the ligament of Treitz; when negative, a source proximal to the pylorus can be confidently excluded. Identification of a site of intraluminal bleeding should be attempted with esophagogastroduodenoscopy, proctosigmoidoscopy, or colonoscopy, depending on the site of bleeding. Upper gastrointestinal bleeding can be diagnosed accurately with oral endoscopy in up to 95% of patients. Capsule endoscopy may be indicated in patients with gastrointestinal bleeding of obscure origin after initial negative upper endoscopy and colonoscopy. The major advantage of endoscopy is that various therapeutic modalities may be used at the same time. If these techniques do not reveal the source of bleeding, other imaging studies are warranted. A technetium 99m-labelled red cell scan can localize the site of bleeding in 83% of patients if they are scanned sequentially at appropriately close intervals, since most hemorrhages are intermittent and the test material stays in the circulation for 24 to 48 hours. Angiography visualizes active bleeding at a rate >1 ml/min, and is diagnostic in only 50% to 65% of patients. It has the therapeutic advantage of allowing vasopressin infusion or embolization to control hemorrhage and is most useful when the suspected location is out of reach of conventional endoscopes (hemobilia or small bowel bleeding) (33,34).

Treatment

Since the majority of bleeding episodes from nonmalignant causes stop spontaneously, in most cases initial treatment consists of conservative medical management, which includes volume repletion and red cell transfusion, correction of coagulation and platelet abnormalities, and, in the case of upper gastrointestinal bleeding, gastric lavage with room-temperature saline to evacuate clotted blood and decompress the stomach, elimination of chemical offenders (nonsteroidal antiinflammatory agents, steroids, etc.), and initiation of surface-protective agents (antacids, H_2-receptor blockers, proton-pump inhibitors). If these conservative measures fail, endoscopic therapy with thermal contact devices or laser or injection treatments should be attempted. Intravenous infusions of vasopressin (especially for diffuse bleeding) or angiographic embolization are alternative options when endoscopic therapy is not effective or not feasible (small bowel bleeding). Surgery is indicated for failure of hemostasis after exhaustion of nonoperative treatment when a discrete source has been demonstrated or there is massive bleeding. Peptic ulcers that need surgical intervention are best treated with truncal vagotomy, pyloroplasty, and oversewing with plication of the ulcer bed. In cases of small bowel or colonic hemorrhage, resection of the involved bowel is generally simple and curative. Resection of a bleeding tumor is the preferred approach, when feasible, if a neoplastic lesion is the source of bleeding. When resection is not amenable, other operative alternatives should be considered, such as packing, direct suture ligation, ligation of arterial inflow, application of topical hemostatic agents, or fibrin glue delivered as an aerosolized spray. Angiographic embolization may be also used. Patients with widely metastatic disease are probably best managed with conservative measures (33,34).

UROLOGICAL EMERGENCIES

Hematuria

Etiopathogenesis

In most cancer patients, hematuria is associated with the presence of an indwelling device such as a Foley urethral catheter or a double-J ureteral stent. Local trauma from the catheter or bacterial urinary tract infection associated with a foreign body frequently causes minor hematuria. Simple urinary tract infection may also produce minor hematuria.

Gross hematuria, however, is often caused by urinary tract malignancies (kidney, urothelial tract, or prostate) or may be secondary to direct invasion of the urinary tract by colorectal and female genital cancers, or pelvic sarcomas (35,36). In addition, iatrogenic hemorrhagic cystitis is commonly observed as a side effect of chemotherapy or radiotherapy (37). Rarely, benign conditions such as a renal angiomyolipoma or an arteriovenous malformation are sources of massive hematuria. Finally, disorders of hemostasis (thrombocytopenia, coagulation abnormalities, etc.) can cause—or more often contribute to—significant hematuria.

Clinical Presentation and Diagnosis

The diagnosis of macroscopic hematuria is self-evident. Symptoms frequently encountered include voiding symptoms (frequency, urgency, and dysuria) and symptoms due to clot formation (pain or acute urinary retention). The evaluation should focus on risk factors (see Etiopathogenesis section) and on pelvic and rectal examination. Required laboratory tests include urinanalysis, urine culture, full blood count, prothrombin time, partial thromboplastin time, blood urea nitrogen, and creatinine. In some cases, pelvic and/or abdominal ultrasound, intravenous urography, and cystoscopy are indicated.

Treatment

Patients with severe hematuria require intravenous hydration, blood transfusion in the presence of severe anemia, discontinuation of anticoagulants, correction of coagulopathies, and insertion of a large-diameter urethral catheter (20–24°F) to allow bladder lavage and clot evacuation. If lavage is not effective, cystoscopy is indicated to disrupt the clots, inspect the urethra and bladder for a controllable source of bleeding, and fulgurate any bleeding vessels or tumor.

Further management depends on the primary diagnosis, extent of the tumor and prior treatment (36,37). Hematuria and urethral obstruction due to prostate cancer can generally be controlled by external-beam radiotherapy, or by transurethral resection and fulguration of the tumor. When massive hematuria is the result of a bladder carcinoma, transurethral resection, semi-emergency cystectomy, a Helmstein hydrostatic balloon or hypogastric artery embolization may be required. Treatment-related hematuria may require specific systemic therapy (e.g., mesna following hemorrhage caused by oxazophosphorines) or local measures (formalin instillations or 1% alum, hyperbaric oxygen).

Urinary Tract Obstruction

Oliguria and anuria are common problems in severely ill cancer patients with a wide range of diagnoses. Acute parenchymal injuries from a variety of toxic insults to the kidney, including anticancer drugs and other pharmacological agents, are frequent causes of oliguria and azotemia. Prerenal factors such as poor renal perfusion secondary to hypotension and low cardiac output may also be involved. However, many cases of renal failure in cancer patients are due to mechanical obstruction of the ureters or bladder neck by a variety of neoplastic processes.

Upper Tract Obstruction

Etiopathogenesis. Malignancy and stones are the two most common causes of upper urinary tract obstruction in cancer patients. Malignant ureteral obstruction may be caused by direct invasion of the ureteral wall by extrinsic compression by tumor or lymphatic metastases, or, rarely, by direct metastases to the ureter (35,36). Gynecological, prostate, urothelial, and colorectal cancers are commonly responsible (>80%). Other tumors such as breast or testicular carcinomas and lymphomas metastasize to the retroperitoneum or retroperitoneal lymph nodes and can produce the same picture. Benign causes of obstruction include radiation-induced retroperitoneal or periureteral fibrosis (1–3% at 20 years in patients with prostate or cervical cancer or Hodgkin's disease), surgical injury, and intrinsic ureteral obstruction following inadequately treated tumor lysis syndrome.

Clinical Presentation and Diagnosis. Clinical presentation depends upon the degree and rate of ureteral obstruction and on whether it affects one or both renoureteral systems. Acute obstruction of a ureter is generally manifested by severe flank pain produced by distension of the renal capsule and collecting system, or, less often, due to hyperperistalsis of the ureter. In contrast, chronic unilateral obstruction is usually asymptomatic and is detected incidentally during an X-ray evaluation. Bilateral ureteral obstruction (acute or chronic) is followed by oliguria and azotemia (weakness, fatigue, nausea, vomiting, mental status disturbances, etc.). Hematuria, nonspecific voiding symptoms (frequency, dysuria, incontinence), a palpable abdominal mass, and anuria are less commonly observed. For upper tract obstruction to result in renal dysfunction, the process must affect both kidneys, a solitary kidney or kidneys that are already partially compromised. Fever may be associated with urinary tract infection and sepsis, and ureteral fistula may lead to recurrent infection and abscesses.

In patients without symptomatic renal failure, renal disfunction is often discovered on routine blood chemistry analysis or ureteral obstruction is incidentally found on imaging procedures performed for other purposes. Less frequently, signs or symptoms of uremia may develop. During the initial evaluation, other causes of renal failure (prerenal or parenchymatous) need to be ruled out. Anuria secondary to urethral obstruction or a neurogenic bladder must be also excluded by bladder catheterization. Routine blood chemistry and urinanalysis will reveal the degree of renal dysfunction and electrolyte imbalances. Ultrasonography is a rapid, easy and readily available noninvasive method for diagnosing obstruction (hydronephrotic renal pelvis and intrarenal collecting system) (35,36). However, a negative examination does not rule out a ureteral obstruction, since marked dilatation of the proximal urinary tract may be delayed. Other tests that may be indicated include a CT scan, radionuclide scans, intravenous pyelogram, cystoscopy, and retrograde pyeloureterograms. This last exploration should be performed under sedation or light general anesthesia by a urologist, and is the most reliable method for diagnosing postrenal obstruction.

Treatment. Before instituting therapy for malignant ureteral obstruction, consideration must be given to the histology, treatment options and prognosis of the primary neoplasm, the presence of symptoms (e.g., pain or fever), the quality of life, and the socio-economic impact of prolonging the patient's life. The basis of treatment of malignant urinary obstruction includes general supportive therapy for renal failure (fluid balance, treatment of pH and electrolytic disturbances, hemodialysis if required, etc.), specific therapy of the primary neoplasm and measures of urinary diversion.

Urinary diversion may be accomplished by means of endoscopic, percutaneous, or surgical techniques (38,39). Endourological techniques allow the insertion of ureteral catheters or stents to bypass the obstructed ureter, dilatation of ureteral strictures, or removal of ureteral stones. Nowadays, internal indwelling flexible synthetic (silicone or polyurethane) stents with a double-J configuration (one end coiled in the bladder and the other end coiled in the renal pelvis) are most frequently used.

A percutaneous nephrostomy may also be performed under local or general anesthesia using ultrasonic guidance. A simple nephrostomy tube may be placed, or an indwelling ureteral stent may be passed anterogradely over a guidewire into the bladder, even if the retrograde approach has previously failed. Combination catheters with both distal (internal) and proximal (external) drainage capabilities are also available. Ideally, a percutaneous nephrostomy tube is replaced with an indwelling stent, which is more comfortable for the patient and is associated with fewer infections. The nephrostomy tube is clamped for 24 to 48 hours to ensure adequate internal drainage before removal, and the internal stents may subsequently be changed cystoscopically without repeating percutaneous procedures (38,39).

Open surgical procedures are associated with numerous complications. However, if endoscopic and percutaneous techniques fail, they may be considered in good prognosis patients. These include ureterolysis, cutaneous ureterostomy or nephrostomy, ureteral reimplantation into the bladder, creation of an intestinal conduit, and transureteroureterostomy (normal contralateral ureter). In rare instances, a nephrectomy may be required.

Once a urinary diversion has been performed, particular attention should be paid to postobstructive diuresis and natriuresis. Volume status and blood pressure should be monitored, as well as metabolic abnormalities.

The primary complications associated with either cystoscopic or percutaneous placement of ureteral stents are bleeding, infection, and obstruction. Bleeding is almost always minor and self-limiting. Although urinary tract infections should be treated with antibiotics, long-term use of antibiotics is not indicated, since sterilization is impossible and resistant organisms frequently develop. Stent incrustations and obstruction may occur; stent patency should be monitored by blood urea nitrogen and creatinine levels, and cystography, which normally demonstrates

reflux of contrast into the renal pelvis. Stent incrustations and obstruction may be minimized by hydration, treatment of infections, and frequent stent changes (every two to three months). Finally, long-term catheters may break, complicating their removal and replacement (38,39).

Lower Tract Obstruction

Etiopathogenesis. Bladder outlet obstruction leading to urinary retention is common in cancer patients and may be caused by mechanical factors involving the bladder neck or prostate, such as benign prostatic hyperplasia, urethral strictures, prostate, rectal or bladder cancer, or to a breakdown in the neurophysiologic function of the bladder. Urinary retention is observed in up to one-third of patients that undergo extensive pelvic surgery, such as abdominoperineal resection or radical hysterectomy, although nerve-sparing procedures have significantly reduced this risk. Iatrogenic causes of urinary retention such as anticolinergic drugs or Foley catheter obstruction should be excluded (35,36).

Clinical Presentation and Diagnosis. The main symptom of urinary retention is the inability to void. Occasionally, patients present incontinence due to overflow from the full bladder. Physical examination may reveal suprapubic tenderness and fullness. Ultrasound generally confirms the diagnosis.

Treatment. Urinary catheter placement rapidly relieves obstruction. Occasionally, cystoscopy is required to place the catheter. In difficult cases, suprapubic tube placement under ultrasound guidance may be performed. Patients are often effectively treated with a variety of pharmacologic agents, such as alpha-adrenergic receptor blockers. Chronic intermittent catheterization is preferred when feasible to permanent catheterization in these often debilitated patients (35,36).

NEUROLOGICAL EMERGENCIES
Increased Intracranial Pressure
Etiopathogenesis
The skull is a closed space containing three relatively noncompressible substances: blood, brain, and cerebrospinal fluid. Consequently, small volume increases of any of these substances easily lead to increased intracranial pressure. When the intracranial pressure reaches levels that compromise cerebral perfusion or cause a shift in intracranial contents that distorts brainstem centers, patients may rapidly deteriorate and die.

Brain metastases are the most frequent cause of increased intracranial pressure in cancer patients. In adults, the most common metastatic tumors in the brain are lung (40%) and breast cancer (15%) (40). Other neoplasms frequently encountered include melanoma, renal, testicular, and gastrointestinal carcinomas. Cerebral volume may increase also as a consequence of hemorrhage, ischemia, infection, or autoimmune inflammatory processes. Intratumoral bleeding occurs more commonly in melanomas, choriocarcinomas, renal cell carcinomas, and papillary thyroid cancer. Coagulopathies predispose to subdural bleeding. Patients with leukemias and blast counts more than $4 \times 10^5/\mu l$ can develop diffuse cerebral edema and increased intracranial pressure due to leukostasis. Subependimal or leptomeningeal masses located at "bottle-neck" of spinal fluid pathways such as the foramen of Monro or the aqueduct of Sylvius also raise pressure by obstructing spinal fluid flow. Leptomeningeal carcinomatosis leads to communicating hydrocephalus due to decreased reabsorption of spinal fluid. Dural sinus stenosis from dural metastases, as well as dural sinus thrombosis or extracranial venous outflow obstruction (internal jugular vein or superior vena cava compression) may also cause increased intracranial pressure.

Clinical Presentation and Diagnosis

General symptoms of high intracranial pressure include headache (typically a constant ache that worsens on waking), nausea, vomiting, drowsiness, and blurred vision from papilledema. However, if pressure elevation is diffuse, the patient may be asymptomatic. In general, slowly expanding neoplasms produce fewer symptoms than those that are rapidly enlarging. Focal neurological deficits and seizures may occur, depending upon the location of tumor deposits. Patients with chronically elevated intracranial pressure may develop cognitive decline, precipitate micturition, and gait apraxia.

Pressure gradients between different cranial compartments may develop and produce brain herniation syndromes. Transtentorial temporal lobe (uncal) herniation usually compresses the ipsilateral brainstem, causing a depressed level of consciousness, ipsilateral dilated pupil, and contralateral hemiplegia. Tonsillar herniation is rare, but may compress the brainstem, causing a stiff neck, a depressed level of consciousness, and eventually death. Shift of the anterior cingulate gyrus under the falx cerebri (subfalcian herniation) is often asymptomatic. If posterior fossa lesions block cerebrospinal fluid pathways, hydrocephalus with expansion of the ventricles and compression of the brain occurs, causing headache and a depressed level of consciousness.

The diagnosis of increased intracranial pressure is suggested by the symptoms and signs listed above, and imaging studies generally confirm the diagnosis and provide relevant etiologic information. The most readily available study is a brain CT scan, which is useful to define the number, size, and location of lesions, and also reveals whether there is associated edema, hemorrhage, shift of the midline structures, or ventricular dilatation. MRI provides more precise neuroanatomic information and may better determine the cause of increased intracranial pressure. Spine MRI should be considered in patients with unexplained communicating hydrocephalus. If minute structural lesions within or surrounding the cerebral aqueduct are suspected, cerebrospinal fluid flow studies (Cine-MRI) may be performed if available. Magnetic resonance is also an adequate method to visualize obstruction or infiltration of dural

venous sinuses. Angiography is currently reserved for exceptional indications. Cerebral perfusion may be monitored by transcranial Doppler sonography in patients with increased intracranial pressure in intensive care units. Lumbar puncture should not be performed in any patient with suspected or documented intracranial mass lesion accompanied by a mass effect. However, once the intracranial pressure has been normalized, cerebrospinal fluid analysis may be undertaken if indicated (i.e., cryptococcal meningitis).

Treatment

Acutely deteriorating patients with increased intracranial pressure and in whom herniation is a threat and requires immediate treatment (Table 19.3). Elevation of the head to 30 degrees provides optimal venous return and decreased arterial pressure. Ensuring airway patency is of vital importance. Most comatose patients will require intubation. Once the patient has been intubated, hyperventilation [arterial P_{CO_2}, (Pa_{CO_2}), lowered to 25–30 mmHg] is the most effective method of lowering intracranial pressure by inducing cerebral vasoconstriction and decreasing the brain blood volume. The peak effect of hyperventilation occurs within 2 to 30 minutes and persists for 48 to 72 hours, when renal compensation of the respiratory alkalosis occurs. Other maneuvers to reduce the intracranial pressure include the elevation of serum osmolality with mannitol (25–100 g intravenously; 20% solution) until serum osmolality reaches 320 mosmol/l. Above this level, significant toxicity may occur. Steroids (e.g., dexamethasone 100 mg intravenous bolus followed by 25 mg/6 hr) are administered acutely, but take hours to achieve their full effect. They are effective agents when increased intracranial pressure is caused by vasogenic edema. Once treatment is under way, an emergency CT scan should be performed. Emergency surgery may be life-saving for patients with brain metastases, intracranial hemorrhage, or other mass lesions. Obstructive hydrocephalus constitutes a neurosurgical emergency. Rapid neurological deterioration with cerebral herniation require immediate placement of an external ventriculostomy. If the cause of fluid obstruction cannot be definitively treated, a permanent drainage of cerebrospinal fluid through a ventriculoperitoneal shunt or endoscopic placement of a third ventriculostomy can be considered. Shunting should be avoided in patients with leptomeningeal carcinomatosis to avoid peritoneal tumor seeding. However, most acutely decompensated patients are stabilized by medical therapy, permitting definitive and disease-specific treatment to be undertaken electively.

Most cases, notwithstanding, are less severe and do not require such intensive therapy. Generally, the association of general measures (fluid restriction, avoidance of hypotonic solutions, etc.) and steroid therapy (dexamethasone 10–20 mg initially, followed by 4 mg/4–6 hr) dramatically

---

Table 19.3 Management of Severely Increased Intracranial Pressure

1. Mantain airway patency: intubate stuporous and comatose patients and lower Pa_{CO_2} to 25 mmHg
2. Mannitol: administer 25–100 g intravenously as soon as possible (20% solution)
3. Dexamethasone: administer 100 mg intravenously as soon as possible followed by 25 mg q6h
4. Emergency CT scan
5. Consider surgical decompression (if indicated and feasible)

improve symptoms of increased intracranial pressure. The indication of anticonvulsants to all patients with central nervous system malignant disease to prevent seizures is controversial.

Tumor-specific treatment options include surgery, radiotherapy and, less frequently, chemotherapy. The selection of the most appropriate intervention for the individual patient is dependent upon a careful evaluation of the extent of intracranial disease, as well as an understanding of patient and tumor characteristics that are important determinants of prognosis. Patients with a solitary metastases in an operable location, good performance status, control of the primary tumor, and absence of extracranial metastases should undergo surgery (41). Surgical resection plays also an important role in establishing the diagnosis and reversing life-threatening complications from brain metastases (intracranial hypertension, seizures, and focal neurological deficits). Radiosurgery may provide an acceptable noninvasive alternative to surgical exeresis for patients with fewer than three metastases and lesions smaller than 3 cm without a cystic component or obstructive hydrocephalus (42). This therapeutic approach also offers the potential of treating patients with surgically inaccessible tumors. Whole-brain radiotherapy (WBRT) after surgery or radiosurgery improves local control of brain metastases although it does not have an impact on patient's survival and its potential long-term neurocognitive morbidity is not negligible (40–43). WBRT alone is the treatment of choice in patients with multiple brain metastases or an active systemic disease and in patients with single brain metastasis not amenable to surgery or radiosurgery (40,43). Cranial irradiation provides improvement or reversal of neurological symptoms in about 70% of patients that often lasts for the rest of their lives. Finally, the role of chemotherapy in the treatment of brain metastases is restricted to certain tumor types that are particularly sensitive to cytotoxic drugs, such as germ cell tumors, lymphoma, breast cancer, and small cell lung carcinoma.

Spinal Cord Compression
Etiopathogenesis
Compression of the spinal cord or cauda equina by tumor is, after brain metastasis, the most common neurological complication of advanced cancer. It affects about 5% to 10% of all cancer patients, and in up to 20% of cases, it is the first manifestation of malignancy (mostly non-Hodgkin lymphoma, myeloma, and lung cancer). This complication is particularly relevant in clinical practice, since it may lead to irreversible functional loss (paraplegia, incontinence) with important consequences for patients' quality of life and survival.

Spinal cord compression may be caused by epidural, leptomeningeal, or intramedullar metastases. The majority of cases result from vertebral body hematogenous metastasis with secondary extension into the epidural space. Lung, breast, and prostate cancers usually produce spinal cord compression through this mechanism. Sometimes, a tumor metastasizes to the epidural space without bone involvement. About 10% to 15% of cases of epidural spinal cord compression are due to direct extension of paraspinal tumors (lymphoma, myeloma, soft tissue sarcoma, head and neck and colon cancers) through intervertebral foramina to the lateral epidural space. Less often, spinal cord compression may develop from direct invasion of the spinal cord by primary spinal cord tumors (neurilemmomas, meningiomas, gliomas, etc.), by leptomeningeal infiltration (lung and breast cancers, lymphoma, and leukemia) or by intramedullary cord metastasis (lung and breast cancers, melanoma, and lymphoma).

The distribution of spinal cord compression locations correlates with the proportion of vertebral body mass in each spinal segment (10% cervical, 70% thoracic, and 20% lumbosacral). Two or more contiguous vertebral bodies are involved by metastatic disease in about 25% of patients with spinal cord compression. Synchronous unexpected sites of epidural disease have been found in up to one-third of patients in whom the whole axial skeleton is investigated.

Clinical Presentation and Diagnosis
Back pain is the first symptom of spinal cord compression in more than 90% of patients (44). The pain is constant and progressive, and may be local (at the involved area of the spine), radicular (radiating into arm, trunk, or leg), or both. The aching may be present several months before neurological signs develop and is exacerbated by coughing, sneezing, the Valsalve maneuver, or flexion of the neck, and is relieved by sitting. During physical examination, an attempt should be made to reproduce the patient's pain by spine percussion, gentle neck flexion, and straight-leg raising (Lasegue maneuver).

Motor dysfunction is the second most common initial feature of epidural spinal cord compression, but it usually follows the onset of pain by weeks to months. Weakness is most obvious in proximal muscles of the lower extremities, so the patient may complain of difficulty in rising from low chairs or a toilet seat. At this stage of spinal cord compression, tone in the lower extremities is usually increased. Deep tendon reflexes are hyperactive and the plantar responses are extensor. Proximal weakness might suggest myopathy, but in that disorder proximal upper extremities are usually also weak, tendon reflexes and muscle tone are normal and sensory changes are absent. When the conus medullaris is the site of compression, bladder dysfunction may be the first and only sign. Both the patient and the physician may fail to recognize that frequent small voidings may be a sign of urinary retention. However, the cauda equina syndrome is typically characterized by asymmetric painful lumbosacral polyradiculopathy, a patchy sensory deficit corresponding to multiple lumbar and sacral nerve roots, and bladder and bowel incontinence. This syndrome should be distinguished from infiltration of the lumbosacral plexus or the corresponding peripheral nerves originating from it (femoral or sciatic nerve).

Sensory symptoms include numbness and paresthesias. A sensory level to pinprick should be determined. Varicella zoster eruption may occur at the dermatological level of epidural metastasis. More seldom, compression of spinocerebellar pathways can lead to gait or truncal ataxia mimicking cerebellar disease.

All cancer patients with back pain should be assumed to have spinal cord compression until proven otherwise. An urgent evaluation is indicated when physical examination suggests myelopathy, when X-ray films indicate more than 50% vertebral body collapse or pedicle erosion (three-quarters of patients have epidural disease), or when local and radicular pain are present (one-half of patients have epidural disease). Differential diagnosis should be made from other disorders that may mimic spinal cord compression in patients with cancer, such as epidural or subdural hemorrhage, epidural lipomatosis, bilateral plexopathy, muscle strain, disc herniation, spinal stenosis, and osteoporotic compression fracture.

Plain X-ray films, CT and bone scans are not sufficiently sensitive for the diagnosis of spinal cord compression. Nowadays, MRI has become the imaging test of choice. It allows imaging of the entire spine and visualization of the parenchyma of the spinal cord, and gives information regarding paraspinal disease. The technique is noninvasive and very sensitive, and is able to demonstrate small metastases to the vertebral column. Gadolinium contrast administration may cause vertebral body metastases to become isointense with adjacent normal bone, obscuring the lesion, so the scan should be performed before contrast is administered, and regions of interest revisualized afterwards. When MRI is nondiagnostic or equivocal, further imaging techniques may be required. Myelography is the diagnostic procedure of choice when MRI is not available or contraindicated. It may also be more effective in detecting small epidural deposits, particularly when they are located laterally in the spinal canal. Bone scan is most useful as a screening procedure for bone metastases. However, its lack of resolution and specificity is inadequate to appropriately diagnose and localize spinal cord compression. When spinal cord compression is the first manifestation of cancer, a whole body CAT scan (with positron emission tomography if available) may be considered to determine the extent of disease and help localize the primary tumor to guide further diagnostic workup and therapy. Biopsy of spinal bone metastases is mandatory prior to initiation of therapy in patients with no other known tumor deposits accessible to pathologic examination.

Treatment

The goals of treatment of spinal cord compression are palliation of pain, neurological improvement, and bone stabilization (45). Therapy is most effective if begun prior to the onset of symptoms, and in the absence of neurological deterioration. The degree of neurological recovery is inversely proportional to the extent and duration of the neurological deficit. Treatment should be instituted rapidly and includes corticosteroids in nearly all patients. Radiation therapy, surgery, and/or chemotherapy should be selectively used based on type, location, and stage of the tumor, neurological status, prior treatment history, and bone stability. Palliative symptomatic therapy may be the only care provided in patients with widespread disease and poor performance status.

Corticosteroids. Corticosteroids may alleviate pain and stabilize or improve neurological deficits through a transient, dose-dependent reduction in vasogenic spinal cord edema. Less frequently, their oncolytic effect (particularly in lymphoma) may relieve cord compression by shrinking tumors. Pain is often relieved within hours, but neurological dysfunction usually responds less strikingly than when corticosteroids are used to treat brain metastases. There is

no consensus regarding the best loading dose and maintenance regimen for steroids in the management of spinal cord compression. After an initial intravenous bolus, doses of up to 10 mg every six hours are most commonly used. It is uncertain whether protocols using higher doses (initial 100 mg i.v. bolus followed by 96 mg divided into four doses for three days with subsequent rapid taper) are more effective in achieving pain control or improving neurologic symptoms, and they are associated with a higher incidence of complications (gastroduodenal ulcer, insomnia, euphoria, hallucinations, etc.). Higher doses may be used in patients with severe neurological impairment at diagnosis or with rapidly progressive motor symptoms.

Surgery. Surgical treatment has been traditionally reserved for radioresistant tumors, symptomatic progression despite optimal radiotherapy, cord compression resulting from pathologic fracture, spinal instability, lack of a prior histological diagnosis of cancer, posteriorly located tumors or tumors located within previously irradiated fields.

In the past, posterior exposure with simple laminectomy (removal of the posterior elements of the spinal column) at the level of cord compression has been a common approach. However, most of the spinal metastases that cause spinal cord compression are located in the vertebral body, which is anterior to the spinal cord. Therefore, a laminectomy does not remove the tumor and often does not result in immediate decompression. In addition, laminectomy can cause secondary destabilization of the spine. Thus, an anterior approach for surgical decompression is favored in selected patients. This allows tumor resection and spinal stabilization if necessary. Results of several uncontrolled surgical series and one meta-analysis suggest that direct decompressive surgery is superior to radiotherapy alone (45). More recently, a randomized trial has proven that in appropriately selected cases, the percentage of patients who were able to walk after treatment was significantly higher in the group that were treated with surgery and radiotherapy compared with the group that only received radiotherapy (84% vs. 57%; p = 0.001), and their functional status was maintained for a longer period of time (46). In addition, overall survival was also significantly prolonged in the surgery group (median survival 126 vs. 100 days; p = 0.003). Therefore, the combination of a surgical approach and radiotherapy may be indicated in selected patients with symptomatic spinal cord compression and only one area of spinal cord compression.

Radiotherapy. Radiotherapy has been the most frequently utilized treatment for patients with spinal cord compression, either alone (many patients are poor surgical candidates due to comorbid conditions, advanced cancer or multiple vertebral body metastases) or in combination with surgery (45).

Once the site of spinal cord compression has been identified, emergency radiotherapy is to be started to a volume that includes two vertebral bodies above and below that site. Alternatively, radiation treatment may be initiated during the following two weeks of decompressive surgery. Various schedules have been applied with comparable results. Most frequently used protocols generally consist of 5 to 10 applications of 3 to 4 Gy. In the palliative setting, single fractions of 8 Gy may be preferable. More recently, stereotactic radiosurgery of spinal metastases has shown to be feasible and is currently under clinical evaluation. Patients who recompress in-field after radiotherapy may be considered for re-irradiation, especially if more than six weeks have elapsed since the completion of their last course.

Chemotherapy. With or without radiotherapy, cytotoxic therapy can be useful in some patients with chemosensitive tumors, most often lymphomas and occasionally other solid tumors. All patients with spinal cord compression caused by a tumor for which effective antineoplastic agents are available should be treated with these agents. If pain is the only symptom, chemotherapy alone can be tried first. If myelopathy is present, corticosteroids and radiotherapy with or without surgery should be the primary therapeutic approach unless the tumor is known to be exquisitively chemosensitive.

HEMATOLOGICAL EMERGENCIES

Febrile Neutropenia

Etiopathogenesis

Cancer patients are at increased risk for infection as a consequence of immune function impairment and loss of barrier integrity related to both their underlying malignancy and the toxic effects of anticancer therapy. The association of neutropenia and infection continues to be the most common life-threatening complication of chemotherapy and a major cause of morbidity and mortality in this patient population (47,48).

Febrile neutropenia is defined as a neutrophil count of <500 cells/mm³ or a count of <1000 cells/mm³ with a predicted decrease to <500 cells/mm³ in association with a single oral temperature of ≥38.3°C (101°F) or a temperature of ≥38.0°C (100.4°F) for ≥1 hour. The degree and duration of neutropenia closely correlate with the risk of serious infectious complications. Between 48% and 60% of neutropenic patients who become febrile have an established or occult infection, and up to 20% of febrile patients with neutrophil counts below 500/mm³ present bacteremia.

The major pathogens causing infection in neutropenic patients are predominantly bacteria and fungi that normally colonize the body surfaces. Viral and parasitic infections are much less common and usually develop in patients with a greater degree of myelosuppression. There has been, however, a significant change over the past three decades in the pattern of pathogens involved in the infectious complications of neutropenic patients. During the 1960s through the mid 1970s, the majority of microbiologically documented infections in neutropenic patients were caused by gram-negative bacilli, particularly *Escherichia coli*, *Klebsiella* spp., and *Pseudomonas aeruginosa*. Since then, however, gram-positive microorganisms have emerged as the predominant pathogens, being now responsible for up to two-thirds of bacteremias documented in neutropenic patients. The two major gram-positive bacteria accounting for this change have been *coagulase negative staphylococci*, mainly associated to the widespread use of indwelling intravascular catheters, and *viridans streptococci*, particularly in patients receiving prophylaxis with quinolones or with substantial mucosal

damage from chemotherapy. In addition, some new pathogens have emerged (*Leuconostoc* spp., *Corynebacterium jeikeium*, *Rhodococcus* spp., etc.) and are now responsible for an increasing proportion of infections in neutropenic cancer patients.

Of greater concern is the emergence of antibiotic-resistant bacteria due to the widespread prophylactic and therapeutic use of broad-spectrum antibiotics (48). In fact, a very recent trend towards a growing incidence of gram-negative infections has been observed in some centers. It is unclear, however, whether this could be due to a decreasing use of quinolone prophylaxis or rather with a greater incidence of quinolone resistance. Furthermore, an increasing number of extended-spectrum β-lactamases are being reported in *Klebsiella* spp., *Enterobacter* spp., and *E. coli*, which render these organisms resistant to most β-lactams, although most of them are still sensitive to fourth generation cephalosporins (cefepime) and to carbapenems. More recently, β-lactamases that confer resistance to carbapenems have been identified in some gram-negative rods such as *P. aeruginosa* and *Acinetobacter* spp. Quinolone-resistant *P. aeruginosa* has also been described. Finally, there are some strains of these nonfermenter gram-negative bacilli and other pathogens such as *Stenotrophomona maltophilia* that have been found to be resistant to all broad-spectrum antibiotics empirically used for treatment of neutropenic fever except polymyxins. Among gram-positive cocci, oxacillin-resistant *staphylococci* and penicillin- and macrolide-resistant *Streptococcus pneumonie* and *viridans group streptococci* are commonly encountered in many institutions. More worrisome, however, is the emergence of enterococci (particularly *Enterococcus faecium*) with high-level resistance to aminoglycosides (precluding the synergistic interaction with penicillins), high-level resistance to ampicillin, and resistance to vancomycin (VRE). VRE may account for up to one-third of all enterococcal infections at some institutions, and are associated with high morbidity and mortality rates. As the eradication of gastrointestinal colonization by VRE is difficult to achieve, efforts to prevent transmission are of utmost importance among hospital personnel.

The prevalence of many of these infections is greatly determined by antibiotic policies within institutions. On the other hand, knowledge of the particular hospital epidemiological data regarding the relative incidence of different pathogens and their antimicrobiological susceptibility patterns is essential to select an adequate initial empirical antibiotic regimen both for prophylaxis and treatment. Appropriate surveillance monitoring to detect changes in a timely manner and infection-control measures to reduce intrahospital spread are also essential measures for infection control.

Clinical Presentation and Diagnosis

Both the presentation and management of infection in the neutropenic patient differ from infection in other settings. Predominant sites of infection largely depend upon the location and size of the tumor, and the site and nature of medical devices and surgical procedures. However, signs and symptoms of infection may be subtle because of the diminished inflammatory response associated with myelosuppression, and fever is often the only presenting sign.

Even a meticulous initial evaluation is able to identify the source of infection in only one-third of the patients.

Baseline evaluation should include a detailed history and physical examination, with careful documentation of prior infectious complications, epidemiologic exposures, concomitant medication associated with increased likelihood of opportunistic pathogens (i.e., corticosteroids, cyclosporin), and type of chemotherapy regimen received and time elapsed since its administration, as this can provide some estimate regarding the expected degree and duration of neutropenia. Initial workup should also include blood counts with differential leukocyte counts, blood and urine chemistries, a chest radiograph, at least two sets of blood cultures, and microbiological investigation of any clinically suspicious site. If a central venous catheter is in place, some investigators recommend to obtain blood samples for culture from each lumen and from a peripheral vein, although a peripheral blood culture is believed to be enough by others. Little information is usually gained from routine cultures of the anterior nares, oropharynx, urine, and rectum in the absence of symptoms. However, they may provide useful information for epidemiologic infection control purposes (i.e., anterior nasal cultures may reveal colonization with methicillin-resistant *Staphylococcus Aureus*, penicillin-resistant *pneumococcus* or *Aspergillus* species; rectal cultures may yield *Pseudomonas aeruginosa*, multidrug-resistant gram-negative bacilli or vancomycin-resistant *enterococci*). It is critical to reevaluate the patient regularly during the febrile neutropenia episode to monitor response to therapy and to identify evolving signs of infection that may not have been present at baseline evaluation.

Treatment

Conventional Management. Because of the high likelihood of occult infection, and the potential for rapid progression to severe sepsis, empiric broad-spectrum antibiotic therapy should be rapidly initiated in neutropenic patients at the onset of fever. Indeed, prompt hospitalization and administration of empirical broad-spectrum antibiotics has effectively improved the outcome of these patients (47,48). Several broad spectrum antibiotics can be safely used in monotherapy for the treatment of fever and neutropenia, including third- or fourth- generation cephalosporins (ceftazidime, cefepime), carbapenems (imipenem, meropenem), and combinations of broad-spectrum penicillins with β-lactamase inhibitors (piperacillin-tazobactam). A meta-analysis of 33 randomized trials comparing different antipseudomonal beta-lactams as empirical single-agent therapy for febrile neutropenia concluded that cefepime was associated with slightly higher overall mortality, and carbapenems with fewer treatment modifications but a higher rate of adverse events, particularly pseudomembranous colitis (49). Combination antibiotic therapy including an antipseudomonal agent and an aminoglycoside does not improve outcome as empirical therapy and results in increased toxicity; its use should be therefore reserved for patients with hemodynamic instability or at high risk for antibiotic-resistant gram-negative bacterial infections, based on local susceptibility patterns or individual patient's history. Ciprofloxacin is an acceptable alternative to aminoglycosides in patients with renal failure. The combination of vancomycin plus aztreonam may be considered in patients allergic to β-lactams.

If fever resolves, antibiotics should be continued until resolution of neutropenia. If neutropenia persists, treatment should be continued for a minimum of seven days (14 days for some authors). A switch to oral regimens (ciprofloxacin with amoxicillin/clavulanate) may be considered in clinically stable patients. Persistent fever per se is not an indication to modify initial empirical antibacterial regimen. Antibiotics should be modified based on clinical evolution and/or microbiological findings. This is generally required in 30% to 50% of episodes.

Despite the increased incidence of infections caused by gram-positive cocci experienced over the past few decades, randomized studies do not demonstrate a clear benefit to the routine empirical use of vancomycin or teicoplanin in the absence of documented gram-positive infections. The Infectious Disease Society of America (IDSA) recommend the use of glycopeptides as part of the initial empiric therapeutic regimen only in the following settings: at institutions where fulminant gram-positive bacterial infections are common; in clinical situations associated with increased risk of *viridans streptococci* infections (patients receiving prophylaxis with quinolones or with substantial mucosal damage from chemotherapy); and in patients with clear clinical signs of catheter-related infections, known colonization with penicillin-resistant *pneumococci* or meticillin-resistant *staphylococci*, or patients with hypotension or cardiovascular impairment (48). Empiric vancomycin should be discontinued after three to four days if no gram-positive infection is microbiologically documented. Although a glycopeptide is often empirically added to patients with persistent fever of unknown origin, there is little evidence in the literature to support this practice. Carbapenems or piperacillin/tazobactam are acceptable alternative agents with adequate coverage against oral flora in patients at high risk for viridans streptococci infections. More recently, linezolid has shown to have broad-spectrum activity against gram-positive pathogens including vancomycin resistant *enterococci*. In patients with neutropenic fever and a proven or suspected infection due to a gram-positive organism, linezolid has proven to be equally effective as vancomycin with somewhat lower renal toxicity. However, the FDA issued a Safety Alert in March 2007 because linezolid was associated with an increased number of deaths in a randomized study conducted in seriously ill patients with catheter-associated bacteremia compared with vancomycin, oxacillin, or dicloxacillin. In this study, mortality rates did not differ among treatment arms in patients with gram-positive infections; however, it was higher in patients treated with linezolid among those with infections due to gram-negative organisms alone, due to mixed gram-positive and negative bacteria, or with no documented infection at study entry. For these reasons, empiric linezolid use should be restricted for patients who are known to be VRE carriers with severe sepsis, or in clinical situations where a resistant Gram-positive pathogen is present or highly suspected.

Patients with persistent fever and neutropenia despite broad-spectrum antibiotic therapy are at significant risk of invasive fungal infections that are highly lethal. Randomized studies suggested that the addition of empirical amphotericin B in neutropenic patients with persistent fever reduced the incidence of fungal infections and fungal-related deaths. The lipid formulations of amphotericin B (amphotericin B in lipid complex, amphotericin B colloidal dispersion, and liposomal amphotericin B) have comparable efficacy and are less nephrotoxic than conventional amphotericin B. In addition, the azoles fluconazol, itraconazol, and voriconazol have also shown to be equally effective and less toxic than amphotericin B for the empirical treatment of patients with neutropenia and persistent fever. However, no definitive data are available regarding their relative efficacy in the treatment of documented fungal infections in neutropenic patients. Because of the limited activity of fluconazole against Aspergillus species and some non-albicans Candida species, this agent should not be used in patients with such documented infections or at high risk for developing them. More recently, caspofungin has demonstrated efficacy in the treatment of patients with invasive fungal infections, including cases resistant to amphotericin B. In randomized trials conducted in patients with persistent fever and neutropenia, it has shown to be as effective and better tolerated than liposomal amphotericin B, with lower rates of renal toxicity or infusion-related events. Moreover, among patients with baseline fungal infections, caspofungin was associated with a higher proportion of successful outcome including survival for seven days after the completion of therapy.

Risk-Based Therapy. An increased understanding of risk factors influencing outcome of febrile neutropenia has allowed the identification of subgroups of patients within this heterogenous clinical entity at a low risk of medical complications and death who may benefit from alternative simplified treatment strategies.

In the pivotal retrospective study by Talcott et al., a risk assessment model for episode outcome was developed using clinical variables that could be assessed within 24 hours of presentation of fever and neutropenia. This model was later prospectively validated in 444 episodes from two different U.S. institutions (50). Patients were stratified in four groups: Group 1 comprised neutropenic patients already hospitalized at the onset of fever; Group 2 included outpatients with concurrent comorbidities; Group 3 consisted of outpatients with progressive or uncontrolled cancer; and Group 4 were all nonhospitalized febrile neutropenic patients without any significant comorbidities or progressive disease (Table 19.4). Serious medical complications and death occurred in 34% and 10% of patients with risk factors (groups 1–3), while there were observed in only 5% and 0% of patients in the low-risk group (group 4), respectively. More recently, the Multinational Association of Supportive Care in Cancer (MASCC) has developed an internationally validated numeric risk-index scoring system to identify low-risk febrile neutropenic cancer patients based on a prospective study that included 1351 patients from 20 institutions in 15 countries (Table 19.4) (51). A MASCC risk-index score >21 identified low-risk patients with a positive predictive value of 91%, a specificity of 68%, and a sensitivity of 71%. Sensitivity is greater in this model than in Talcott's model (71% vs. 30%) at the price of a loss in specificity (68% vs. 90%), although the overall misclassification rate is lower (30% vs. 59%). Of note, the rate of identification of patients as being at low risk is substantially increased compared with the Talcott's model (63% vs. 26%).

Alternative treatment strategies with improved cost-effectiveness and toxicity profile are being evaluated in this low-risk population (52). Two adequately sized multicenter randomized studies, one from Europe and one from the United States, have demonstrated that hospital-based oral antimicrobial therapy consisting of a combination of ciprofloxacin and amoxicillin-clavulanate is as safe and effective as standard intravenous regimens in patients with low-risk febrile neutropenia (53). Amoxicillin-clavulanate may be substituted with clindamycin in patients allergic to β-lactams.

The availability of broad-spectrum oral quinolones has also enabled clinicians to change from parenteral to oral regimens allowing earlier patient discharge or outpatient care (52). As fluoroquinolone use in children is controversial due to the potential increased risk of arthropathy, management with oral cefixime has been assayed in pediatric populations. This antibiotic, however, is no longer available in the United States and other western countries. Although some limited experiences including a number of

Table 19.4 Risk Models for Stratification of Risk in Febrile Neutropenic Patients

	Talcott's model (50)	MASCC model (51)		
		Characteristic	Weight	
High risk	Group 1: Inpatients	Burden of illness		A MASCC risk-index score <21 identifies high-risk patients
	Group 2: Serious comorbidity	• No or mild symptoms	5	
	Group 3: Uncontrolled cancer	• Moderate symptoms	3	
		No hypotension	4	
		No chronic obstructive pulmonary disease	4	
		Solid tumor or no previous fungal infection	4	
		No dehydration	3	
		Outpatient status	3	
		Age ≤60 years	2	
Low risk	Group 4: Outpatients with none of the above mentioned risk features			A MASCC risk-index score >21 identifies low-risk patients

Abbreviation: MASCC, multinational association for supportive care in cancer.

uncontrolled studies and some small randomized trials suggest that these strategies may be feasible and safe in selected settings, large multicenter randomized trials are needed to demonstrate its safety and efficacy in the general medical community. These alternative therapeutic approaches lessen the need for intravenous-access devices, decrease the incidence of nosocomial infections with aggressive and resistant pathogens, reduce drug related toxicity, improve patients quality of life and convenience for their family or caregivers, lower costs of treatment, and allow a more efficient utilization of health care resources. However, the potential risks of developing serious complications that cannot be adequately managed at home, the risk of noncompliance and inadequate monitoring, and the potential intolerance to oral treatment (emesis, diarrhea) need to be carefully assessed to ensure the success of risk-based therapy. A key component of outpatient management includes therefore readily accessible trained staff and adequate infrastructure 24 hours per day. A proposed risk-based therapeutic algorithm is summarized in Figure 19.2.

A risk-based approach should also be applied to the use of colony-stimulating factors (CSFs) in this setting. As the degree and the duration of neutropenia are key factors closely related with the risk and outcome of infection, the role of CSFs has been widely evaluated in this patient population. Several randomized studies have demonstrated that the use of CSFs reduces the duration of neutropenia, but this benefit has not been always associated with advantages in other more meaningful clinical endpoints (hospital stay, episode complications, cost, or mortality) (54,55). A recent meta-analysis of randomized trials evaluating the role of CSFs in conjunction with antibiotic therapy for the management of patients with established febrile neutropenia concluded, however, that CSFs significantly shortened neutrophil recovery and hospital stay, with a trend towards a reduction in infection-related mortality. Last American Society for Clinical Oncology (ASCO) guidelines recommend that the therapeutic use of CSFs for established neutropenic fever should be considered in patients at high risk for infection-related complications or who have prognostic factors predictive of a poor clinical outcome (54). These high risk features include an expected profound or prolonged neutropenia, age greater than 65 years, uncontrolled primary disease, pneumonia, sepsis syndrome, invasive fungal infection, or being hospitalized at the time of fever onset. Nevertheless, infectious complications in cancer patients may be better prevented by the prophylactic use of cerebrospinal fluid in conjunction with chemotherapeutic regimens associated with a high risk of inducing neutropenic fever (greater than 20%). The rationale and indications for cerebrospinal fluid prophylaxis is however beyond the scope of this chapter.

Disseminated Intravascular Coagulation (Dic)
Etiopathogenesis
Disseminated intravascular coagulation (DIC) is characterized by the generalized activation of the coagulation system leading to widespread intravascular formation of fibrin and thrombotic occlusion of small and midsize vessels. This may ultimately cause multiorgan failure as generalized intravascular coagulation can compromise organ blood

supply and induce severe hemodynamic and metabolic disturbances. In addition, the subsequent consumption of clotting factors and platelets may result in hemorrhagic complications.

This hemostatic disorder occurs in up to 15% of patients with cancer and results from increased generation of thrombin, suppression of physiologic anticoagulation, and impaired fibrinolysis mediated by several proinflammatory cytokines. A distinct form of DIC is frequently encountered in patients with acute promyelocytic leukemia, which associates a hyperfibrinolytic state to the mentioned widespread activation of coagulation. Except for this particular malignant disease, acute DIC in cancer patients is rare and frequently the result of other predisposing conditions (i.e., septicemia), whereas chronic forms of DIC are more commonly encountered (56).

The generalized formation of thrombin in DIC is mediated by the extrinsic pathway involving tissue factor and activated factor VIIa. Tissue factor is expressed on the surface of tumor cells and may be expressed on mononuclear cells in response to proinflammatory cytokines, although the exact source of this factor is not always clear. Interleukin-6 seems to be the main cytokine involved in the activation of coagulation, whereas tumor necrosis factor is the principal mediator of the anticoagulation pathway and fibrinolysis derangements. Solid tumor cells can also express other procoagulant molecules, such as cancer procoagulant, a cysteine protease with factor X-activating properties. In addition, different physiologic inhibitors of coagulation such as antithrombin III, protein C, and tissue factor pathway inhibitor (TFPI) are markedly reduced in DIC as a result of cytokine-mediated impaired activity, decreased synthesis or increased degradation leading to suppression of anticoagulation. Finally, an increase in the plasma levels of plasminogen-activator inhibitor type 1 (PAI-1) inhibits the fibrinolytic system, which cannot be counteracted by the fibrinolytic activity induced by the widespread formation of fibrin (56).

Clinical Presentation and Diagnosis
DIC is an acquired disorder that occurs in a wide variety of clinical conditions, including sepsis, trauma, vascular disorders (giant hemangioma, aortic aneurysm), obstetrical complications (amniotic-fluid embolism, abruptio placentae), reactions to toxins, immunologic disorders (transplant rejection, transfusion reaction, or severe allergic reaction), and malignant diseases (myeloproliferative diseases, solid tumors). The clinical presentation of acute DIC consists of hemorrhagic and/or thrombotic events. The specific clinical features will depend on the site, nature, and severity of these events. The range of hemorrhagic complications may extend from minor bleeding from mucosal or cutaneous surfaces to extensive life-threatening hemorrhage involving visceral sites or central nervous system. Hypercoagulable manifestations may include deep vein thrombosis, Trousseau's syndrome, pulmonary embolism, purpura fulminans, nonbacterial thrombotic endocarditis, or acral ischemia.

Laboratory evaluation demonstrates prolongation of clotting times, such as prothrombin time (PT), partial thromboplastin time (PTT), thrombin time, and reptilase time, thrombocytopenia, with platelet counts generally

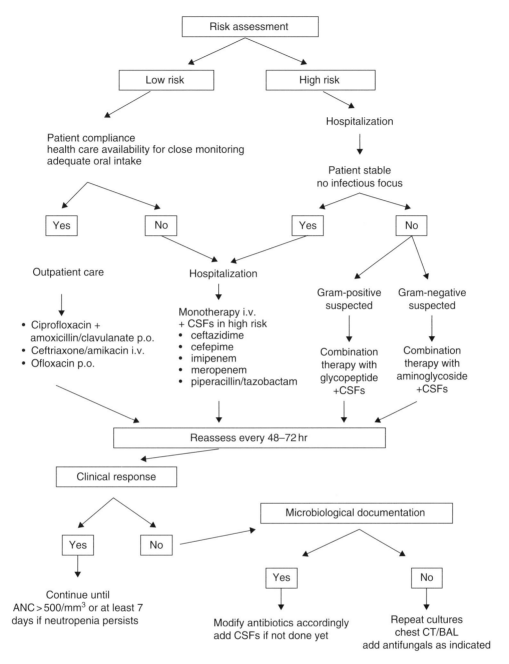

Figure 19.2 Risk-based therapeutic algorithm for febrile neutropenia.

below 100,000/mm³ or rapidly declining, and elevated levels of fibrin degradation products (FDPs) (56). Hypofibrinogenemia may be observed in severe cases although plasma fibrinogen levels often remain within the normal range because this protein is an acute-phase reactant. However, as no single laboratory test available today is sufficiently accurate to allow a definite diagnosis of DIC, a scoring system has been developed by the subcommittee on DIC of the International Society of Thrombosis and Haemostasis (Table 19.5) (57). This scoring system has been prospectively validated with sensitivity and specificity values around 95%. Serial coagulation tests may also help in establishing the diagnosis of DIC. Measurement of low

plasma levels of inhibitors of coagulation such as antithrombin III or protein C may provide useful prognostic information. More specialized assays include the measurement of soluble fibrin or different tests for measuring the generation of thrombin (determination of prothrombin activation fragment F_{1+2} or thrombin-antithrombin complexes) (56). These tests may be useful in the diagnosis of DIC in certain clinical situations, although they are generally not essential and not widely available.

Finally, several now available monitoring devices assessing the viscoelastic properties of whole blood, i.e., thrombelastography, rotation thrombelastometry, and Sonoclot analysis, may overcome some limitations of routine

Table 19.5   Algorithm for the Diagnosis of Disseminated Intravascular Coagulation (DIC)

Score global coagulation test results
 1. Platelet count (>100 × 10^9/l = 0, <100 × 10^9/l = 1, <50 × 10^9/l = 2)
 2. Elevated fibrin-related marker (e.g., fibrin degradation products or D-dimer) (no increase, 0; moderate increase, 2; strong increase, 3)[a]
 3. Prolonged prothrombin time (<3 secs = 0, >3 but <6 secs = 1, >6 secs = 2)
 4. Fibrinogen level (>1.0 g/l = 0, <1.0 g/l = 1)
Calculate score
   If >5: compatible with overt DIC
   If <5: no overt DIC; repeat next 1–2 days

[a]In most prospective validation studies, D-dimer assays were used and a value above the upper limit of normal (0.4 μg/l) was considered moderately elevated, whereas a value >10 times the upper limit of normal (4.0 μg/l) was considered as a strong increase.

coagulation tests. These devices are particularly useful to rapidly identify hypo- and hypercoagulable states in the perioperative setting and can also help guide pro- and anticoagulant therapies.

Treatment

Effective specific treatment of the underlying disorder is essential for successful outcome of DIC. However, supportive treatment specifically aimed at the coagulation abnormalities is also often required. In the setting of asymptomatic DIC, it is reasonable to observe the patient closely while identifying and treating precipitating factors and the underlying condition. Supportive measures will differ depending upon the clinical presentation of DIC. Treatment with heparin is probably useful in patients who present with thrombotic complications, particularly those with clinically overt thromboembolism, purpura fulminans, or acral ischemia, whereas its use in the presence of hemorrhage is contraindicated. Unfractionated heparin is usually administered at doses of 300 to 500 U/hr as a continuous intravenous infusion, although low-molecular-weight heparin may also be used. More recently, prophylactic low doses of heparin have been evaluated in patients with severe sepsis with a trend towards lower mortality rates for heparin-treated patients as compared with placebo. Concentrates of coagulation inhibitors, such as antithrombin III, have shown in controlled clinical trials to improve disseminated intravascular coagulation and organ function, although an improved survival has been less consistently demonstrated (56). Its use, nevertheless, is generally reserved for patients with severe DIC due to its elevated cost. Randomized studies have also established the clinical efficacy of activated protein C in normalizing coagulation activation during severe sepsis, significantly reducing mortality rates particularly in patients with DIC. Novel antithrombin III-independent inhibitors of thrombin are also being tested with promising results, although the increased risk of bleeding observed with these new drugs may limit their clinical use. Other recently developed drugs such as recombinant tissue factor pathway inhibitor, despite early promising results, have failed to show a survival impact in controlled clinical trials.

On the contrary, replacement therapy with platelets, fresh-frozen plasma, and/or cryoprecipitate may be necessary in patients presenting with bleeding symptoms or who require an invasive procedure that may increase their risk of bleeding (56). Platelet transfusions are indicated in

patients who bleed when platelet counts fall below $50 × 10^9$/L. In nonbleeding patients, a much lower threshold for platelet transfusion is generally used ($10–20 × 10^9$/L). Large volumes of plasma may be required to correct the coagulation defect. Coagulation factor concentrates, such as prothrombin complex concentrate, can obviate this problem, although these compounds lack essential factors, such as factor V. Specific deficiencies in coagulation factors, such as fibrinogen, can be corrected by the administration of purified coagulation factor concentrates. The use of antifibrinolytic agents is discouraged with the exception of patients with acute promyelocytic leukemia or other patients with DIC associated with primary or secondary hyperfibrinolysis. In addition, all-trans retinoic acid, a vitamin A derivative that promotes terminal differentiation of leukemic promyeloblasts, induces bone marrow and cytogenetic complete response in 64% to 96% of patients with acute promyelocytic leukemia with rapid correction of the coagulopathy in these patients.

Microangiopathic Hemolytic Anemia
Etiopathogenesis

Microangiopathic hemolytic anemia is characterized by microvascular thrombotic lesions that result in hemolytic anemia, thrombocytopenia, and blood vessel occlusion that gives rise to tissue ischemia and end-organ damage. Depending on whether renal or brain lesions prevail, two pathologically indistinguishable but clinically different entities have been described: the hemolitic uremic syndrome (HUS) and the thrombotic thrombocytopenic purpura (TTP). What triggers the formation of platelet aggregates in the microvasculature has not been entirely elucidated. Several causes have been proposed, including defects of platelets or plasma components and endothelial cell damage. The HUS usually occurs as a single episode in children often preceded by gastroenteritis caused by cytotoxin-producing gram-negative bacteria, most commonly *E. coli* O157:H7 (58). These bacteria can contaminate meat, milk, cheese, and other types of insufficiently cooked or pasteurized food. They produce Shiga exotoxin that binds with high affinity to ceramide receptors in the membranes of glomerular, colonic, and cerebral epithelial or endothelial cells, renal mesangial and tubular cells, and monocytes and platelets. This stimulates epithelial cells and monocytes to secrete cytokines and chemokines, induces endothelial cells to secrete unusually large multimers of von Willebrand factor (VWF), activates platelets and may also increase tissue factor on endothelial and epithelial-cell surfaces. Once the A subunit of Shiga toxin is internalized to cells, it is converted to a glycosidase whose actions ultimately result in cell death. Familial forms of HUS, however, are generally recurrent and are associated with defective production of the complement control protein factor H. This results in overactivation of C3, which may potentiate autoantibody-mediated or immune-complex-mediated glomerular injury. On the other hand, recent evidence suggests that the abnormal processing of VWF multimers may play a central role in the etiopathogenesis of TTP (59). Indeed, the absence of normal VWF-cleaving protease activity gives rise to unusually large VWF multimers that would trigger platelet aggregation. The VWF-cleaving protease has now been identified as a new member of the ADAMTS family of metalloproteases, designated ADMATS13. The acquired form of TTP is associated with inhibitory autoantibodies against ADMATS13, and the congenital chronic relapsing form is caused by mutations in the ADAMTS13 gene, resulting in a constitutional deficiency (59). These findings not only provide a rationale for the previously empirical plasma exchange therapy (removal of the inhibitory antibodies and large VWF multimers, and replacement of the deficient protease with the plasma infused), but may also help in developing more rational and targeted treatment strategies.

Microangiopathic hemolytic anemia occurs in up to 6% of patients with metastatic carcinomas (most frequently from gastric, breast, or lung primaries), and it may develop in patients with minimal disease (especially gastric cancer) treated with mitomycin C (5–15% incidence) or, less commonly, other cytotoxic agents, antibodies, or immunotoxins. It has also been reported after total-body irradiation and after allogeneic bone marrow, kidney, liver, heart, or lung transplantation. The etiopathogenesis of these microangiopathies is unknown, although direct glomerular endothelial damage and immune complex formation have been postulated as potential mechanisms involved (58).

Clinical Presentation and Diagnosis

Microangiopathic hemolytic anemia has often an insidious onset and typically presents with Coombs-negative hemolytic anemia and severe thrombocytopenia. The clinical features are diverse and reflect the anatomic site involved. Renal failure is the main predominant feature of HUS, although it may also occur in TTP. Neurological symptoms observed in TTP often fluctuate and range from headaches, personality changes, and sensorimotor deficits, to impaired consciousness and coma. Gastrointestinal ischemia is also commonly encountered and may manifest as abdominal pain and nausea or vomiting. Chest pain, congestive cardiac failure, cardiac arrhythmias, and myocardial infarction may as well be observed. Rash, fever, hypertension, and noncardiogenic pulmonary edema can occur in association with chemotherapy-induced microangiopathic hemolytic anemia. Symptoms may be precipitated or worsened by blood transfusions (58,59).

Laboratory findings include thrombocytopenia, hemolytic anemia with negative direct antiglobulin test, red cell fragmentation, reticulocytosis (reflecting the increased red blood cell turnover), elevated lactate dehydrogenase, and possibly biochemical evidence of renal or liver impairment representing ischemic organs (58,59). The predominant source of lactate dehydrogenase elevation is ischemic injured tissues rather than red cells undergoing intravascular hemolysis. Prolongation of clotting times is not generally a feature of microangiopathic hemolytic anemia, but it may occur in severe cases if a secondary DIC develops as a consequence of extensive intravascular hemolysis or tissue necrosis.

Treatment

The mainstay of therapy is plasma exchange, which should be initiated within 24 hours of presentation as treatment delays significantly increase therapeutic failures and mortality rates (58,59). An exchange volume of 1 to 1.5 times the calculated plasma volume (45–80 ml/kg) is generally recommended, although the optimal volume or duration of therapy remain to be elucidated. The advent of this therapy has dramatically reduced mortality rates from 70–90% to 20–30%. Paraneoplastic microangiopathic hemolytic anemia may respond to effective antineoplastic therapy and the causal cytotoxic agent should be discontinued in chemotherapy-induced cases. Blood product administration should be avoided (58,59). Staphylococcal protein A immunoperfusion to remove the circulating immune complexes may be successful in some instances. Corticosteroids, platelet inhibitors, heparin, or immunosuppressive agents have not clearly shown to be effective (58,59). Greater therapeutic success may be expected when microangiopathic hemolytic anemia occurs as a manifestation of the underlying cancer rather than as a complication of therapy, and among them, in patients with lower tumor burdens than in those with widely disseminated disease.

ORTHOPEDIC EMERGENCIES

Bone Metastases

Etiopathogenesis

Skeletal metastases are the major oncological orthopedic complication, present in 70% of patients who die of cancer. The most common primary tumors are breast (>50%), lung, kidney, prostate, and thyroid carcinomas. Skeletal metastases are commonly associated with disabling pain and pathological fracture. The risk of the latter is correlated with the type of bone destruction (osteolytic lesions are at higher risk than osteoblastic ones), the extent of the lesion, and the anatomical location (40% of all pathological fractures occur in the proximal femur) (60).

Bone metastasis follows complex molecular interactions that enable tumor cells to detach from the primary site, invade the extracellular matrix, intra-vasate, extra-vasate, and proliferate within bone. Normal bone remodeling maintains an appropriate balance between the action of osteoclasts (bone-resorbing cells) and osteoblasts (bone-forming cells). Skeletal malignancies, including bone metastases, disrupt the OPG-RANKL-RANK signal transduction pathway and promote enhanced osteoclast formation, thereby accelerating bone resorption and inducing bone loss. This osteolysis in turn leads to the release of bone-derived growth factors, contributing to a "vicious cycle" in which interactions between tumor cells and osteoclasts not only lead to increased osteoclastogenesis and osteolytic activity, but also to aggressive growth and behavior of the tumor cells (60).

Clinical Presentation and Diagnosis

The morbidity associated with metastatic bone disease includes pain that may require opiates, hypercalcemia, pathologic fracture, spinal cord compression, and the need for radiotherapy and/or surgery, which are often referred to as skeletal-related events. Pain is the most frequent symptom from bone metastases and is typically well localized, worsening at night or with weight-bearing activity. Functional pain due to mechanical weakness may be a marker for bone at risk of fracture. Pathologic fractures are also common events, as they may occur in more than one-third of patients with metastatic breast carcinoma or hormone-refractory prostate cancer. Hypercalcemia and spinal cord compression have already been discussed elsewhere in this chapter.

About 50% of bone must be destroyed before a metastatic lesion can be detected radiographically. In the spine, plain films typically show the absence of a pedicle with the "winking owl sign." Technetium bone scanning is the most sensitive and cost-effective diagnostic test for bone metastasis, although traumatic or inflammatory changes may give false-positive results (10% rate), and lesions with barely any osteoblastic activity, such as those seen in multiple myeloma, may give false-negative tests. A CT scan is the best imaging modality to characterize the size of a bone lesion and extent of cortical involvement. It therefore provides relevant information to evaluate bone stability and the risk of fracture, and to plan surgical therapy. MRI is the preferred procedure to assess the extent of vertebral and epidural involvement in patients with metastatic deposits in the spine and pelvis, particularly when associated with neurological compromise.

Treatment

Bone metastases that do not cause pain or do not confer a significant risk of impending bone fracture or spinal cord compression may be managed with the specific systemic therapy, generally in association with bisphosphonates, for the underlying disease. Bisphosphonates prevent skeletal related events in patients with bone metastasis secondary to multiple myeloma, breast carcinoma, prostate cancer, and other solid tumors. New pharmacological interventions involve the blockade of RANKL. RANKL is a key element in the differentiation, function, and survival of osteoclasts. A fully humanized monoclonal antibody against RANKL, denosumab (AMG 162), has demonstrated sustained decrease in bone resorption in patients with osteoporosis, multiple myeloma, or breast cancer, and is currently undergoing broad clinical evaluation.

The treatment of choice for localized metastatic bone pain is radiotherapy. Radiotherapy is effective in relieving bone pain, preventing impending fractures, and promoting healing in pathological fractures. Hematological and gastrointestinal side effects are usually mild and transient. The therapeutic schedules most commonly used include an 8-Gy single fraction administration, 20 Gy given in five daily treatments (4 Gy/day), and 30 Gy given in 10 daily fractions (3 Gy/day). These regimens are considered equivalent in terms of pain control and narcotic relief, although the need for re-treatment and pathologic fracture rates seem somewhat lower with protracted dose-fractionation schedules (61). However, greater convenience and lower costs favor the shorter administration schemes. Radiotherapy provides pain relief in the majority of patients, and more than 50% eventually achieve complete pain control. Re-irradiation of previously irradiated sites may benefit selected patients, particularly after an initial period of response. Widefield or half-body external beam radiation has been used in patients with multiple painful bone metastases with acceptable toxicity. Administration of systemic radionuclides may be also considered to alleviate pain in patients with diffuse bone disease, or in previously irradiated patients. Strontium-89 and Samarium-153, given as a single intravenous administration on an outpatient basis, are the agents most commonly used in clinical practice (62). Overall pain reduction is achieved in 60% to 80% of patients. Reversible myelosuppression, particularly thrombocytopenia, is the most common toxic effect, with nadir counts four to six weeks after injection. Repeat doses with intervals of 6 to 12 weeks are feasible and effective providing further pain relief in many patients.

However, severely painful lesions require special intervention to relieve pain, ease nursing care, allow early mobilization, and restore function. Surgical intervention should be considered in patients with a reasonable life expectancy and failure of conservative therapy (including radiotherapy), or a pathological or impending fracture. Lesions with a high risk of fracture include lytic lesions involving more than 2.5 cm of the cortex in long bones, or painful intramedullary lesions greater than 50% of the cross section of the bone. In small lesions, blind intramedullary nailing with local irradiation may provide appropriate fixation and pain relief. In larger lytic lesions, intramedullary nailing supplemented by methyl methacrylate resin to fill the defect is recommended. In the presence of extensive bone destruction, segmental resection and replacement by an endoprosthesis may be required (63).

Finally, some limited experiences have shown that radiofrequency ablation or cryoablation of bone metastases may induce longlasting palliation in patients with refractory bone metastases or in those who are ineligible to conventional treatments.

REFERENCES

1. Fojo AT. Metabolic emergencies. In: DeVita VT, Lawrence TS, Rosenberg SA, eds. Cancer: Principles and Practice of Oncology, 8th edn. Philadelphia: Lippincott-Raven, 2008: 2446–54.
2. Lumachi F, Brunello A, Roma A et al. Medical treatment of malignancy-associated hypercalcemia. Curr Med Chem 2008; 15: 415–21.
3. Hofbauer LC, Neubauer A, Heufelder AE. Receptor activator of nuclear factor-kappaB ligand and osteoprotegerin: potential implications for the pathogenesis and treatment of malignant bone diseases. Cancer 2001; 92: 460–70.
4. Lambrinoudaki I, Christodoulakos G, Botsis D. Bisphosphonates. Ann N Y Acad Sci 2006; 1092: 397–402.
5. Saad F. New research findings on zoledronic acid: survival, pain and antitumour effects. Cancer Treat Rev 2008; 34: 183–92.
6. Roodman GD, Dougall WC. RANK ligand as a therapeutic target for bone metastases and multiple myeloma. Cancer Treat Rev 2008; 34: 92–101.
7. Spinazzé S, Schrijvers D. Metabolic emergencies. Crit Rev Oncol Hematol 2006; 58: 79–89.

8. Coiffier B, Altman A, Pui CH et al. Guidelines for the management of pediatric and adult tumor lysis syndrome: an evidence-based review. J Clin Oncol 2008; 26: 2767–78.

9. De Groot JW, Rikhof B, van Doorn J et al. Non-islet tumour-induced hipoglycaemia: a review of the literature including two new cases. Endocr Relat Cancer 2007; 14: 979–93.

10. Palm C, Pistrosch F, Herbrig K et al. Vasopressin antagonists as aquaretic agents for the treatment of hyponatremia. Am J Med 2006; 119(7 Suppl 1): S87–S92.

11. Keefe DL. Cardiovascular emergencies in the cancer patient. Semin Oncol 2000; 27: 244–55.

12. Yahalom J. Superior vena cava syndrome. In: DeVita VT, Lawrence TS, Rosenberg SA, eds. Cancer: Principles and Practice of Oncology, 8th edn. Philadelphia: Lippincott-Raven, 2008: 2427–34.

13. Wilson LD, Detterbeck FC, Yahalom J. Clinical practice. Superior vena cava syndrome with malignant causes. N Engl J Med 2007; 356: 1862–9.

14. Watkinson AF, Yeow TN, Fraser C. Endovascular stenting to treat obstruction of the superior vena cava. BMJ 2008; 336: 1434–7.

15. Gray BH, Olin JW, Graor RA et al. Safety and efficacy of thrombolytic therapy for superior vena cava syndrome. Chest 1991; 99: 54–9.

16. Nguyen DM. Malignant effusions of the pleura and the pericardium. In: DeVita VT, Lawrence TS, Rosenberg SA, eds. Cancer: Principles and Practice of Oncology, 8th edn. Philadelphia: Lippincott-Raven, 2008: 2523–33.

17. Retter AS. Pericardial disease in the oncology patient. Heart Dis 2002; 4: 387–91.

18. Neragi-Miandoab S. Malignant pleural effusion, current and evolving approaches for its diagnosis and management. Lung Cancer 2007; 55: 253–4.

19. Walker-Renard PB, Vaughan LM, Sahn SA. Chemical pleurodesis for malignant pleural effusions. Ann Intern Med 1994; 120: 56–64.

20. Dresler CM, Olak J, Herndon JE 2nd et al. Cooperative Groups Cancer and Leukemia Group B; Eastern Cooperative Oncology Group; North Central Cooperative Oncology Group; Radiation Therapy Oncology Group. Phase III intergroup study of talc poudrage vs talc slurry sclerosis for malignant pleural effusion. Chest 2005; 127: 909–15.

21. Aurora R, Milite F, Vander Els NJ. Respiratory emergencies. Semin Oncol 2000; 27: 256–69.

22. Corder R. Hemoptysis. Emerg Med Clin North Am 2003; 21: 421–35.

23. Thompson AB, Teschler H, Rennard SI. Pathogenesis, evaluation and therapy for massive hemoptysis. Clin Chest Med 1992; 13: 69–82.

24. Wood DE. Management of malignant tracheobronchial obstruction. Surg Clin North Am 2002; 82: 621–42.

25. Chen K, Varon J, Wenker OC. Malignant airway obstruction: recognition and management. J Emerg Med 1998; 16: 83–92.

26. Unger M. Endobronchial therapy of neoplasms. Chest Surg Clin N Am 2003; 13: 129–47.

27. Kohek PH, Pakisch B, Glanzer H. Intraluminal irradiation in the treatment of malignant airway obstruction. Eur J Surg Oncol 1994; 20: 674–80.

28. Schnoll-Sussman F, Kurtz RC. Gastrointestinal emergencies in the critically ill cancer patient. Semin Oncol 2000; 27: 270–83.

29. Ripamonti C, Twycross R, Baines M et al. Clinical-practice recommendations for the management of bowel obstruction in patients with end-stage cancer. Support Care Cancer 2001; 9: 223–33.

30. Ripamonti CI, Easson AM, Gerdes H. Management of malignant bowel obstruction. Eur J Cancer 2008; 44: 1105–15.

31. Khot UP, Lang AW, Murali K et al. Systematic review of the efficacy and safety of colorectal stents. Br J Surg 2002; 89: 1096–102.

32. Runkel NS, Schlag P, Schwartz V et al. Outcome after emergency surgery for cancer of the large intestine. Br J Surg 1991; 78: 183–8.

33. Savides TJ, Jensen DM, Cohen J et al. Severe upper gastrointestinal tumor bleeding: endoscopic findings, treatment and outcome. Endoscopy 1996; 28: 244–8.

34. Kovacs TO, Jensen DM. Recent advances in the endoscopic diagnosis and therapy of upper gastrointestinal, small intestinal, and colonic bleeding. Med Clin North Am 2002; 86: 1319–56.

35. Strope SA, Hafez KS. Urologic emergencies. In: DeVita VT, Lawrence TS, Rosenberg SA, eds. Cancer: Principles and Practice of Oncology, 8th edn. Philadelphia: Lippincott-Raven, 2008: 2455–60.

36. Russo P. Urologic emergencies in the cancer patient. Semin Oncol 2000; 27: 284–98.

37. West NJ. Prevention and treatment of hemorrhagic cystitis. Pharmacotherapy 1997; 17: 696–706.

38. Kouba E, Wallen EM, Pruthi RS. Management of ureteral obstruction due to advanced malignancy: optimizing therapeutic and palliative outcomes. J Urol 2008; 180: 444–50.

39. Yachia D. Recent advances in ureteral stents. Curr Opin Urol 2008; 18: 241–6.

40. Patchell RA. The management of brain metastases. Cancer Treat Rev 2003; 29: 533–40.

41. Patchell RA, Tibbs PA, Walsh JW et al. A randomized trial of surgery in the treatment of single metastases to the brain. N Engl J Med 1990; 322: 494–500.

42. Sperdutto PW, Scott C, Andrews D et al. A phase III trial comparing whole brain irradiation alone versus whole brain irradiation plus stereotactic surgery for patients with one to three brain metastases. Int J Radiat Oncol Biol Phys 2002; 51: 3.

43. Berk L. An overview of radiotherapy trials for the treatment of brain metastases. Oncology 1995; 9: 1205–12.

44. Baehring JM. Spinal cord compression. In: DeVita VT, Lawrence TS, Rosenberg SA, eds. Cancer: Principles and Practice of Oncology, 8th edn. Philadelphia: Lippincott-Raven, 2008: 2441–6.

45. Loblaw DA, Perry J, Chambers A et al. Systematic review of the diagnosis and management of malignant extradural spinal cord compression: the Cancer Care Ontario Practise Guidelines Initiatives Neuro-Oncology Disease Site Group. J Clin Oncol 2005; 23: 2028–37.

46. Patchell R, Tibbs PA, Regine WF et al. Direct decompressive surgical resection in the treatment of spinal cord compression caused by metastatic cancer: a randomised trial. Lancet 2005; 366: 643.

47. Bodey GP, Rolston KVI. Management of fever in neutropenic patients. J Infect Chemother 2001; 7: 1–9.

48. Garcia-Carbonero R, Paz-Ares L. Antibiotics and growth factors in the management of fever and neutropenia in cancer patients. Curr Opin Hematol 2002; 9: 215–21.

49. Paul M, Yahav D, Fraser A et al. Empirical antibiotic monotherapy for febrile neutropenia: systematic review and meta-analysis of randomized controlled trials. J Antimicrob Chemother 2006; 57: 176–89.

50. Talcott JA, Siegel RD, Finberg R et al. Risk assessment in cancer patients with fever and neutropenia: a prospective, two-center validation of a prediction rule. J Clin Oncol 1992; 10: 316–22.

51. Klastersky J, Paesmans M, Rubenstein EB et al. The Multinational Association for Supportive Care in Cancer risk index: a multinational scoring system for identifying low-risk febrile neutropenic cancer patients. J Clin Oncol 2000; 18: 3038–51.

52. Kern WV. Risk assessment and treatment of low-risk patients with febrile neutropenia. Clin Infect Dis 2006; 42: 533–40.

53. Kern WV, Cometta A, De Bock R et al. Oral versus intravenous empirical antimicrobial therapy for fever in patients with granulocytopenia who are receiving cancer chemotherapy. International Antimicrobial Therapy Cooperative Group of the European Organization for Research and Treatment of Cancer. N Engl J Med 1999; 341: 312–18.

54. Smith TJ, Khatcheressian J, Lyman GH et al. 2006 update of recommendations for the use of white blood cell growth factors: an evidence-based clinical practice guideline. J Clin Oncol 2006; 24: 3187–205.

55. Garcia-Carbonero R, Mayordomo JI, Tornamira MV et al. Granulocyte colony-stimulating factor in the treatment of high-risk febrile neutropenia: a multicenter randomized trial. J Natl Cancer Inst 2001; 93: 31–8.

56. Levi M, Ten Cate H. Disseminated intravascular coagulation. N Engl J Med 1999; 341: 586–92.

57. Toh CH, Hoots WK. SSC on disseminated intravascular coagulation of the ISTH. The scoring system of the Scientific and Standardisation Committee on Disseminated Intravascular Coagulation of the International Society on Thrombosis and Haemostasis: a 5-year overview. J Thromb Haemost 2007; 5: 604–6.

58. Moake JL. Thrombotic microangiopathies. New Engl J Med 2002; 347: 589–600.

59. Allford SL, Hunt BJ, Rose P et al. Guidelines on the diagnosis and management of the thrombotic microangiopathic haemolytic anaemias. Br J Haematol 2003; 120: 556–73.

60. Coleman RE. Metastatic bone disease: clinical features, pathophysiology and treatment strategies. Cancer Treat Rev 2001; 27: 165–76.

61. Sze WM, Shelley M, Held I et al. Palliation of metastatic bone pain: single fraction versus multifraction radiotherapy—a systematic review of the randomised trials. Cochrane Database Syst Rev 2004; CD004721.

62. Finlay IG, Mason MD, Shelley M. Radioisotopes for the palliation of metastatatic bone cancer: a systematic review. Lancet Oncol 2005; 6: 392–400.

63. Harrington KD. Orthopedic surgical management of skeletal complications of malignancy. Cancer 1997; 80: 1614–27.

20

Symptom Control and Palliative Care

Shirley H. Bush and Eduardo Bruera

INTRODUCTION

The main objective of palliative care is to improve the quality of life for both patients with life-threatening illness and their families (1). Patients with advanced cancer may experience physical, psychosocial, and spiritual difficulties throughout their illness, which will have an impact on their overall quality of life. Palliative care is also applicable in conjunction with other therapies, such as chemotherapy or radiation therapy, early in the course of an illness and continues beyond the death of a patient, with bereavement support provided to families.

When this same approach to symptom control and psychosocial support is integrated into the care of patients receiving potentially curative or life-prolonging treatment, the term supportive care is sometimes used.

The first step in the symptom control of advanced cancer patients is continuous, multidimensional assessment. This is the cornerstone of effective palliative care and is accomplished through an interdisciplinary approach. Physicians must work together with many other health care professionals, such as psychologists, pastoral care workers, social workers, nurses, occupational therapists, physiotherapists, and dieticians, to provide holistic care and support not only to the patient but also to family members.

This chapter begins with a general overview of patient assessment and examples of tools used. Sections detailing some of the major symptoms observed in palliative care patients follow, including descriptions of their assessment and management. Finally, the chapter concludes with recommendations for improving symptom control.

ASSESSMENT

Simple validated symptom assessment tools are the most appropriate for advanced cancer patients. Patients are often fatigued and experiencing significant symptoms that make it too difficult to complete a time-consuming and complex assessment tool. The tool should be an instrument that assesses for the presence of multiple symptoms. In addition to the identification and evaluation of the intensity of symptoms, assessment tools may also monitor the effectiveness of therapy and screen for adverse effects of medication. Systematic assessment using a tool will detect a significantly higher number of symptoms as compared with open-ended questions (2). Assessment tools should be utilized regularly, especially when patients develop new symptoms,

experience an increase in intensity of preexisting symptoms, or when there has been a change in therapy.

Multidimensional Assessment

There are three steps involved in the experience of symptoms by a patient: production, perception, and expression. Production is caused predominantly by the cancer itself and cannot be measured directly. Examples of this are the nociceptive input from bone metastases or the stimulation of J receptors in the lung in patients with dyspnea. Perception takes place at the level of the central nervous system, and, like symptom production, it cannot be measured directly. Perception is influenced by the action of endorphins and inhibitory pathways.

Symptom expression is the target for all our assessment and therapy. However, symptom expression between patients with similar disease pathology and the same initial level of production can be very different. Symptom expression is also influenced by other factors such as mood disorders, delirium, cultural background, personal beliefs, social support, chemical coping, and somatization.

It is important to identify the extent to which different factors are influencing the expression of a symptom of an individual patient at a particular point in time. This will enable the delivery of effective targeted therapy by the interdisciplinary team. For example, two patients may both give a subjective rating of 8 out of 10 for fatigue. The major contributors to the fatigue of patient 1 are cachexia, anemia, and deconditioning. Correction of these factors will have minimal impact on the fatigue experienced by patient 2, whose major contributor is depression. Patients often present with multiple coexisting and interrelated symptoms requiring simultaneous assessment and management. For a thorough multidimensional evaluation of the patient, several different assessment tools may be needed. Some examples are listed below.

Edmonton Symptom Assessment System

The Edmonton Symptom Assessment System (ESAS) is used to quantitatively evaluate the patient's subjective perception of a number of symptoms. The ESAS has been validated and routinely records multiple symptoms: pain, fatigue, nausea, depression, anxiety, drowsiness, appetite, shortness of breath, and feeling of well-being (3). The patient rates each of these symptoms on a scale of 0 to 10, where 0 means that the symptom is absent and 10 rates it as the worst possible severity. Ideally, patients fill out their own ESAS, but if needed, it can be completed with the assistance of their caregiver (family or health care professional). As patients with advanced cancer usually have multiple symptoms, the determination of the intensity of each symptom using the ESAS allows the team to initially focus on the management of highly rated symptoms and to monitor the responsiveness to interventions.

The Memorial Delirium Assessment Scale

The Memorial Delirium Assessment Scale (MDAS) is a validated 10-item, four-point clinician-rated scale (possible range, 0–30) designed to quantify delirium severity in patients with cancer and other medically ill patients (4). Scale items assess disturbances in arousal and level of consciousness, as well as several areas of cognitive functioning (e.g., memory, attention, orientation, disturbances in thinking) and psychomotor activity. The resulting scale integrates behavioral observations and objective cognitive testing and takes approximately 10 minutes to administer.

CAGE

Alcoholism occurs in 5% to 15% of the general population and approximately 20% of hospitalized patients but remains undiagnosed in more than two-thirds of patients (5). The CAGE questionnaire is a brief tool designed to screen for alcoholism (6). CAGE is a mnemonic for

- Have you ever felt that you should Cut down on your drinking?
- Have you ever been Annoyed by people criticizing your drinking?
- Have you ever felt bad or Guilty about your drinking?
- Have you ever had a drink first thing in the morning or a drink to get rid of a hangover (Eye opener)?

The validity of this test decreases if it is done after having asked the patient about the quantity of alcohol or drug ingested, so it is strongly recommended to perform the CAGE questionnaire first. Occasionally, if patients are not currently using alcohol, they respond in the negative, interpreting the questions as only referring to the present or recent past. This is minimized by stressing that the questions refer to the patients' lifetime.

CAGE positivity, with two or more questions answered in the affirmative, indicates the possibility of chemical coping. In the palliative care setting, the identification of chemical coping is important because opioid analgesics share a similar reward brain pathway with alcohol (with partial mediation of both by endorphins). Patients with a history of chemical coping have a higher risk of using opioid analgesics as a means of coping with stress.

Functional Assessment

Functional assessment is an independent predictor of survival prognosis (7). It is also essential information for planning the venue of care, which can be in the home, inpatient palliative care unit or inpatient hospice, or acute hospital setting. Two complementary tools, the Edmonton Functional Assessment Tool (EFAT) (8) and the Functional Independence Measure (FIM) (9), can be used to evaluate the functional status of patients with advanced cancer. The EFAT is more focused on the identification

and quantifying the intensity of the factors contributing to functional impairment, whereas the FIM evaluates the different functions of the patients' daily activity in more detail.

Psychosocial Assessment

Psychosocial distress, especially caused by mood disorders such as depression and anxiety, frequently goes undiagnosed, causes significant distress to patients and their families, and affects the symptom control in patients. The factors responsible for psychosocial distress need to be identified to provide appropriate therapy. This includes asking questions about family and social support, financial difficulties and "unfinished business," cultural issues influencing the illness experience and care needs, loss of autonomy and control, emotional or existential/spiritual distress, and fears regarding death and the dying process. The most effective way to assess and alleviate psychosocial distress is through using an interdisciplinary approach. The role of social workers, case managers, pastoral care workers, and psychologists, among others, is of vital importance.

PAIN

Pain occurs in 70% to 90% of cancer patients with advanced disease (10). Although in approximately 90% of patients, pain can be adequately controlled using common pain management measures, at least 20% of cancer patients have significant pain at the end of life (11). Reasons for this include inadequate assessment and inadequate knowledge about pain pathophysiology and its appropriate treatment. In addition, ongoing misconceptions held by physicians and patients regarding opioids lead to underprescription of these drugs. Pain control is often inadequate, as only "as needed" doses or too low doses of the regular baseline opioid are prescribed, and at times, the frequency of dosing is insufficient. Common concerns are fear of addiction (psychological dependence), causing excessive drowsiness or respiratory depression, and hastening death. It should be emphasized that when prescribed in appropriate doses to control cancer pain, opioids do not hasten death. Pain appears to be antagonistic of opioid-induced sedation and respiratory depression.

Pain Assessment

For the appropriate management of cancer pain, a detailed pain assessment is essential, identifying the cause, pathophysiology, and intensity for each pain reported by the patient. For patients experiencing persistent pain despite appropriate therapy, multidimensional assessment and psychosocial evaluation is mandatory (see section "Multidimensional Assessment").

Causes of Pain

The most common cause of pain in advanced cancer patients is the primary cancer itself or metastases. Pain may be due to the anticancer therapy such as postsurgical injury to peripheral nerves and postradiotherapy- (e.g., radiation fibrosis, myelopathy, osteoradionecrosis, mucositis) and chemotherapy-related pain syndromes (e.g., polyneuropathy, mucositis). A minority of patients have pain due to debility or concurrent disorder (e.g., postherpetic neuralgia, constipation, osteoarthritis, musculoskeletal pain).

Types of Pain

Cancer pain is categorized according to different anatomical and pathophysiological pain mechanisms (12). The mechanistic categories are nociceptive, comprising superficial somatic, deep somatic, and visceral pain, and neuropathic pain. Pain can be described as mixed when there is more than one pathophysiology.

The nociceptive pain mechanism occurs through stimulation of superficial or deep tissue receptors (nociceptors) with the afferent impulse propagated along the ascending spinothalamic nociceptive pathways. Superficial somatic pain arises from skin and mucosa (e.g., malignant ulcers, stomatitis), and deep somatic pain from bones, joints, muscles, organ capsules, pleura, and peritoneum (e.g., bone metastases, liver capsule distension or inflammation). Somatic pain is usually well localized with local tenderness. Visceral pain involves solid or hollow organs and deep abdominal or mediastinal tumor masses, but it is poorly localized and may be referred.

Neuropathic pain arises from a disturbance of neural pathways (e.g., compression, invasion, destruction, or dysfunction) in the peripheral or central nervous system. Neuropathic pain has many different characteristics and is often difficult for patients to describe. Dysesthetic pain (e.g., deafferentation) is constant but can also fluctuate and has a burning sensation. It is usually localized but sometimes radiates (e.g., post herpetic neuralgia). Lancinating pain is paroxysmal with a sharp, shooting quality (e.g., trigeminal neuralgia). (See sections "Adjuvant Therapy" and "Nonpharmacological Therapy").

"Episodic pain" is a term to describe the transitory exacerbation of pain that changes with time, which can be classified into three subtypes: activity and movement-related (also referred to as incidental or incident pain), spontaneous, and "end-of-dose failure" (13). The term "breakthrough pain" has also been used to describe this phenomenon of a transitory increase in pain (14). The prevalence of episodic pain is in the range of 40% to 70%. The mean time to peak is three minutes with a mean duration of 15 to 30 minutes, but can be as long as two or even four hours. The parenteral and transmucosal routes, for drugs with appropriate pharmacodynamic properties, have a faster onset of action for "rescue" analgesia than the oral route for management of episodic pain (13).

Both neuropathic and episodic pain present challenges to usual pain management.

Identification of Poor Cancer Pain Prognostic Factors

The presence of poor prognostic factors should be an indication to physicians that they may encounter difficulties in controlling the patient's pain. Assessment tools have been developed to evaluate cancer pain prognosis such as the Cancer Pain Prognostic Scale (CPPS) and the revised Edmonton Staging System (rESS) (15,16).

Poor prognostic factors for cancer pain are as follows:

- History of alcoholism and drug abuse
- History of somatization as primary coping strategy or as a result of affective disorders such as anxiety or depression
- Tolerance, defined as a significant increase in opioid dose over time (e.g., an increase in 5% or greater of the daily baseline dose on consecutive days)
- Neuropathic pain
- Incidental pain/episodic pain

A lack of awareness of these factors can result in an unnecessary and inappropriate rapid dose escalation of medications, especially opioids, and drug toxicities.

Pharmacotherapy
Mild Pain

For patients with mild pain, physicians can start therapy with a nonopioid drug such as paracetamol (acetaminophen in the United States) or a weak opioid such as codeine. Paracetamol acts centrally, acting as a cyclo-oxygenase (COX) inhibitor in the brain (17). It does not affect platelet function and has no gastrointestinal toxicity. This makes it an ideal option for advanced cancer patients, and it can be used with an additive effect for patients taking opioids for moderate to severe pain (18). Typical doses are 500 to 1000 mg orally every four to six hours. The maximum recommended daily dose is 4 g. It should be used with caution in patients with severe hepatic impairment.

The dose of codeine is 30 to 60 mg orally every four hours and as needed for episodic pain. Codeine is usually ineffective in patients (5–10% of Caucasians and 1–2% of Asians) lacking the enzyme CYP2D6 needed for the metabolism of codeine.

Nonsteroidal anti-inflammatory drugs (NSAIDs) may be used alone or in addition to opioid therapy. They act by the inhibition of the COX enzyme peripherally, and evidence suggests that they may have a central effect (19). NSAIDs also exhibit a ceiling effect. The coxibs are preferentially selective for COX-2 and have a low gastroduodenal toxicity. All coxibs probably have a prothrombotic tendency, so they should be prescribed with caution, especially for patients at risk of heart disease or with peripheral vascular disease. (In 2004, rofecoxib was withdrawn worldwide due to concerns over an increase in serious thrombotic events). Caution should also be shown when prescribing any NSAID for a long period.

Combination preparations of paracetamol/opioid and NSAID/opioid are available in some countries. However, their rigid dose formulation not only limits opioid dose escalation but also increases the risk of toxicity of the associated drug at higher doses. Ongoing pain despite maximal titration is an indication for the use of a stronger opioid in a different formulation.

Moderate and Severe Pain

Patients experiencing moderate or severe pain will require treatment with a strong opioid. This decision should be based on pain severity and not on prognosis. Morphine, a potent mu-agonist, is generally the strong opioid of choice for cancer pain management. Morphine is not recommended in renal failure due to the accumulation of potentially toxic metabolites (20). Other commonly used strong opioids include hydromorphone, oxycodone, fentanyl, and methadone (Table 20.1).

Concerns about opioid addiction are usually unfounded as advanced cancer patients who have appropriate treatment with opioids and have no history of chemical coping are at minimal risk of becoming addicted. Patients on chronic opioid therapy may show signs of opioid withdrawal if the dose is abruptly reduced or discontinued (physical dependence). To avoid opioid withdrawal symptoms (agitation, tremulousness, fever, diaphoresis, mydriasis, tachycardia, and muscle and abdominal cramping) the opioid dose should be tapered at a rate of 20% per day.

Initiation of Opioid Therapy

Therapy should be initiated with an immediate-release (IR) opioid. The preferred route is oral, but the parenteral route may be necessary for rapid titration in cases of severe acute pain or in situations where the oral route is not possible (e.g., dysphagia, bowel obstruction, depressed conscious state) (Fig. 20.1). The recommended oral starting dose should be rapidly titrated over two to four days until the pain is controlled before changing to a maintenance opioid regimen (Fig. 20.2). Patients with severe pain may need higher starting doses. Physicians should always prescribe an IR opioid (usually 10% of the daily dose) as a "rescue" dose for episodic pain that is not controlled by the regular scheduled baseline analgesic. In some countries, a "rescue" dose of 16% (one-sixth) of the 24-hour dose has been recommended, which is equivalent to the four-hourly dose of morphine. More recent studies suggest that an individual's "rescue" dose should be found by titration (13).

The increase of the daily opioid dose depends on the number of "rescue" doses needed to "top-up" baseline analgesia. If a patient needs more than three extra doses of IR opioid, the dose for the following day should be the sum of the regular scheduled doses plus the "rescue" doses. It is not necessary to increase the regular daily opioid dose if patients are requiring less than three extra "rescue" doses.

Opioid therapy should not routinely be initiated with slow-release (SR) preparations or long half-life opioids. These opioids are difficult to titrate and take time to reach their full effect when patients will usually need more rapid pain relief. The most common adverse effects on commencing morphine are nausea and vomiting, drowsiness, constipation, and confusion. The first two usually resolve after

Table 20.1   Strong Opioids Used in Palliative Care

Morphine
Diamorphine (United Kingdom only)
Oxycodone
Hydromorphone
Methadone
Fentanyl (including oral transmucosal fentanyl citrate)
Sufentanil
Alfentanil
Buprenorphine [Transdermal (TD)—not United States]

Example
1. Assess the patient.
2. Schedule an immediate-release (IR) opioid on a regular basis and extra doses for breakthrough pain.
   The recommended starting doses are as follows:
   • Morphine 10mg orally (5mg i.v./s.c.) every 4hours and 5mg orally (2.5mg i.v./s.c.) as needed for breakthrough pain.
   • Hydromorphone 2mg orally (1mg i.v./s.c.) every 4hours and 1mg orally (0.5mg i.v./s.c.) as needed for breakthrough pain.
   • Oxycodone 5mg orally every 4hours and 2.5–5mg orally as needed for breakthrough pain (i.v./s.c. formulations are not available in all countries).
Note: Use lower initial dose of opioid if patient is frail and elderly or opioid naive.
   e.g., Morphine 5mg orally every 4hours.
3. Prescribe an antiemetic and laxative to prevent and to treat nausea and constipation.
   • Metoclopramide: 10mg every 4–6hours and 10mg every 2hours for breakthrough nausea
     or
   • Haloperidol: 1.5mg orally at night.
   • Laxative: Sennoside 8.6mg, 1–2 tablets b.d. (b.i.d.).
4. Frequently assess for efficacy and side effects.

Figure 20.1   Initiation of opioid therapy.

Example
1. In order to determine the new daily dose, it is necessary to calculate the total 24-hour opioid dose of the previous day (regular scheduled dose plus as needed "rescue" doses for breakthrough pain).
   e.g., if the patient was receiving 10 mg of morphine every 4 hours and needed 5 doses of 6 mg for breakthrough pain (approx. 10% of the daily dose), then the total dose is 90 mg [calculated by: 60 mg of the scheduled dose (10 mg × 6) plus 30 mg of morphine for the breakthrough pain (6 mg × 5)].
2. The new daily dose is divided by 6 to make 4-hourly doses. The new as needed "rescue" dose is 10% of the new daily dose.
   e.g., The new daily dose of morphine is 90 mg, administered as 15 mg every 4 hours. The new "rescue" dose is 9 mg (10% of the daily dose).
3. Continue with laxatives.
4. Continue with antiemetics if necessary. (It may be possible to cease them after the first week).
5. Continue frequent assessment.
Note: It is not necessary to increase the daily dose of opioid if the patient needs less than three "rescue" doses for breakthrough pain per day.

Figure 20.2   Titration of opioid dose.

---

three to five days, but constipation is usually ongoing. Therefore, it is common practice to prescribe as needed or regular antiemetics, such as metoclopramide or haloperidol (particularly for the first three to five days) and laxatives (for the duration of use of all opioids), to prevent and treat nausea and vomiting and constipation, respectively.

Some opioids have no role in the palliative care setting. Meperidine (pethidine) is not suitable for chronic pain relief, as it has a relatively short duration of action (two to three hours). It also has a neurotoxic metabolite, normeperidine (norpethidine), which can accumulate with repetitive dosing and cause myoclonus and even seizures, particularly in patients with renal failure. Mixed agonist-antagonist analgesics, such as pentazocine, nalbuphine, and butorphanol, also should not be used. They have a dose-related ceiling effect, whereby increasing the dose beyond that point will only increase their side effects and not increase analgesia. In addition, pentazocine often causes psychotomimetic effects.

Maintenance Therapy

Once pain is controlled, immediate-release IR opioids can be changed to a slow-release SR preparation (Fig. 20.3). This has the advantage of less frequent administration and fewer tablets. It is highly recommended to continue with the same opioid on conversion (e.g., IR morphine to morphine-SR).

The transdermal fentanyl patch requires special consideration, and it should only be initiated if pain is stable as it typically takes 12 hours to reach systemic analgesic concentrations, with steady state usually reached by the second patch application. Therefore, it is crucial to continue the previous regular opioid for 12 to 18 hours after commencing treatment with a fentanyl patch. Likewise, fentanyl concentrations decrease slowly after patch removal, so once treatment with a fentanyl patch has been discontinued, it is necessary to wait about 8 to 12 hours before commencing a new opioid.

At times, disease progression or the development of tolerance necessitates upward titration of the maintenance opioid dose. If pain improves because of response to other treatment modalities, e.g., after radiotherapy, or if the patient develops opioid toxicity with satisfactory pain control, then downward titration is indicated. A patient experiencing refractory adverse effects with a particular opioid may require a change in the maintenance opioid (see section "Opioid Rotation/Substitution").

Opioid Toxicity

The most common adverse effects of treatment with opioids are sedation, nausea, constipation, and dry mouth. Severe sedation that persists for several days after initiation of opioid therapy can be treated with psychostimulants, such as methylphenidate (21). The usual methylphenidate dose is 5 to 10 mg in the morning with 5 mg at noon, but some patients find it beneficial to also take afternoon or evening doses (22). Other less-common opioid side effects include pruritus and urinary retention.

Opioids may also induce neurotoxicity. Adverse effects on CNS include hallucinations, delirium, hyperalgesia (an increased response to a stimulus which is normally painful), generalized myoclonus (transient involuntary contractions of muscle/s), and tonic-clonic seizures (23). Neurotoxicity is usually seen in patients receiving high doses of opioids, prolonged opioid administration, previous borderline cognition, and in patients with renal failure. The treatment of opioid neurotoxicity includes hydration (in an attempt to increase renal elimination of the parent drug and metabolites), opioid rotation or switching (see section "Opioid Rotation/Substitution"), and in some cases, opioid reduction. Patients should also be assessed for other causes of neurotoxicity and reversible causes treated if appropriate. For patients with renal failure, there is a high possibility of metabolite accumulation, especially with morphine and diamorphine, and alternative opioids such as fentanyl and methadone are recommended (20).

Opioid Rotation/Substitution

A switch in opioid is indicated if pain control has not been achieved despite high opioid doses, if the patient has developed tolerance to the opioid, or if refractory adverse effects or toxicity to the currently administered opioid develop (24). Examples of refractory adverse effects with morphine are persistent nausea and vomiting, confusion, drowsiness, myoclonus, and refractory constipation. The development of significant renal impairment in a patient on morphine usually necessitates a change in the opioid.

Opioid rotation aims to improve pain relief by reversing opioid tolerance (25). Opioid rotation (or substitution) is a strategy also used for toxicity reduction (24). In carrying out opioid rotation, it is important to consider the interindividual variations in oral bioavailability, pharmacokinetics of opioids, and incomplete cross-tolerance between opioids. Opioid conversion tables are widely available to assist with the switch from one opioid to another (26–29). They have been developed using mainly data from single- and repeated-dose studies in patients with acute pain and some chronic studies. Therefore, the equianalgesic dose of the new opioid should be reduced

---

Example

Once the 24-hour dose of opioid has been established, the patient can be changed over to a slow-release opioid preparation. The main reason for doing this is the convenience of less frequent drug administration.

The slow-release (SR) opioids are:
- Morphine-SR, Oxycodone-SR, Hydromorphone-SR every 12 hours.
- Morphine-SR every 24 hours (for once daily preparations).
- Transdermal Fentanyl every 72 hours.

1. If the opioid is not changed (morphine IR to morphine SR), the 24-hourly dose remains unchanged.
   e.g., The equivalent of 90 mg of immediate release (IR) morphine per day is 90 mg of slow release (SR) morphine every 24 hours or 45 mg administered every 12 hours, depending on the SR preparation used.
2. For "rescue" analgesia for breakthrough pain, physicians should use only IR opioids at 10% of the daily opioid-SR dose.
   e.g., For a patient on morphine-SR 45 mg every 12 hours, give morphine-IR 9 mg as needed.
3. Continue with laxatives.
4. Continue with antiemetics if necessary.
5. Continue frequent assessment.

Figure 20.3 Changing to slow-release (SR) opioids.

by approximately 30% as a precaution, and the patient should be closely monitored.

Methadone, an opioid with unique characteristics, is increasingly being used as a second-line opioid for cancer pain (30). Methadone is a synthetic mu-delta opioid agonist and a relatively potent antagonist at N-methyl-D-aspartate (NMDA) receptors in the spinal dorsal horn, which have an important role in opioid tolerance, central sensitization, and neuropathic pain. It is a lipophilic drug with excellent oral bioavailability of approximately 80%. It is metabolized in the liver, where it may interact with inducers and inhibitors of the cytochrome P450 system, to inactive metabolites. Caution is therefore needed for co-administration of methadone with other drugs that affect the cytochrome P450 system, especially the CYP 3A4, and possibly the 2D6 and other isoenzymes. Methadone can be used in patients with renal failure without the need for dose adjustment. There is considerable interindividual variation in the pharmacokinetics of methadone leading to wide ranging differences in plasma half-life, from 8 hours up to 150 hours. With chronic dosing, methadone has a duration of action of 6 to 12 hours.

The onset of action of oral methadone is rapid (under 30 minutes) (31). However, it is not recommended to increase the dose more frequently than every three to four days due to the delay in reaching full effect. Conversion to methadone from other opioids is complex and the ratio varies according to the total 24-hour opioid dose used previously (32). The conversion ratio of oral morphine to oral methadone varies from 3:1 to 20:1 depending on the prior morphine dose. The higher the previous dose of morphine, the higher the methadone potency (Table 20.2). Specialist palliative care input is strongly advised.

Methadone is available in a variety of formulations: tablet, liquid, suppository, and injection enabling oral, rectal, intravenous, and subcutaneous administration. Oral methadone is very cost effective as it is 10 to 20 times cheaper than other opioids. The potential for subcutaneous site reactions from infusions of methadone may be attenuated by the use of dexamethasone or hyaluronidase (see section "Subcutaneous Route"). Another strategy is to administer subcutaneous methadone intermittently (33).

Adjuvant Therapy

Some patients will continue to have opioid refractory cancer-associated pain despite optimal opioid titration for baseline pain. This often occurs in cases of neuropathic or movement-related pain. The addition of adjuvant drugs

should be considered when good analgesia has not been achieved and when opioids have been titrated to the level of dose-limiting toxicity. New analgesic interventions should preferably be added one at a time and at an initial low dose for those medications that have sedative adverse effects. An adequate trial should be given and the medication ceased if not effective after optimal titration. Table 20.3 lists commonly used adjuvant drugs.

Patients with either multiple bone metastases and severe movement-related episodic pain, mucositis, or neuropathic pain have responded to ketamine, an NMDA receptor antagonist, given as a "burst" subcutaneous infusion for three to five days (34).

Nonpharmacological Therapy

Anesthetic or neurosurgical interventional techniques may be considered in patients who have refractory pain despite comprehensive multidisciplinary management or have intolerable toxicity associated with usual pharmacological treatments. Techniques used include celiac plexus/splanchnic block for abdominal visceral pain, e.g., pancreatic cancer pain, spinal (intrathecal or epidural) analgesia with opioids and local anesthetic, e.g., for neuropathic or plexopathy pain, and percutaneous or open cordotomy for lower extremity pain (35).

Nonpharmacological approaches can be helpful and include physical therapies for musculoskeletal pain (e.g., massage, ultrasound, hydrotherapy, electro acupuncture, and trigger point injection) and psychological techniques (e.g., guided imagery, relaxation, hypnosis, biofeedback, and other cognitive or behavioral methods).

DELIRIUM

Delirium is a neuropsychiatric syndrome characterized by a disturbance of consciousness with a reduced ability to focus, sustain, or shift attention, changes in cognition or perceptual disturbances that occur over a short period of time and fluctuate over the course of the day (36). It occurs in the presence of an underlying organic derangement.

Table 20.2   Conversion Table: Morphine to Methadone

Oral morphine dose (mg)	Conversion ratio of oral morphine to oral methadone (mg morphine: mg methadone)
<100	3:1
101–300	5:1
301–600	10:1
601–800	12:1
801–1000	15:1
>1001	20:1

Table 20.3   Commonly Used Adjuvant Drugs

- Amitriptyline/nortriptyline 10–25 mg at bed time, titrated up to 150 mg, if needed, for neuropathic pain.
- Gabapentin 100 mg t.d.s (t.i.d.), titrated up to 300 mg t.d.s. for neuropathic pain [up to 900 mg q.d.s (q.i.d.) in severe cases].
- Dexamethasone 4–10 mg p.o./i.v./s.c. b.d.–t.d.s. and then tapered for neuropathic, bone, and visceral pain.
- Pregabalin 75 mg b.d. (b.i.d.) titrated up to 300 mg b.d. (start with 25–50 mg b.d. in debilitated patients and titrate slowly) for neuropathic pain.
- NSAIDs for bone pain and inflammatory pain.
- Pamidronate 90 mg i.v. every 4 weeks or zoledronic acid 4–8 mg i.v. every 4 weeks for bone pain and hypercalcemia.
- Baclofen 10 mg t.d.s. for painful muscle spasms.
- Methylphenidate 5–10 mg in the morning and 5 mg at noon for opioid sedation.
- Antibiotics (parenteral route if possible) for painful infections, especially in patients with head and neck cancers or perineal disease.

The etiology of delirium is often multifactorial (Fig. 20.4). Three subtypes of delirium have been described according to the level of psychomotor activity: hyperactive, hypoactive, and mixed. Delirium is present in 26% to 44% of advanced cancer patients at the time of admission to an acute care hospital or palliative care unit, and more than 80% of patients will develop delirium in the last hours and days before death (37). The presence of delirium is an independent factor in predicting short-term survival of patients with advanced cancer (37).

Delirium and its recall are an important source of distress to patients, family caregivers, and health care professionals (38). Delirium challenges patient assessment and impairs patient communication with family and professional caregivers. Nursing staff may misinterpret the signs of patients with agitated delirium as increased pain intensity and administer extra unnecessary doses of opioids, potentially increasing the delirium severity (39).

Diagnosis of Delirium and Assessment

Delirium is frequently misdiagnosed and under recognized, especially hypoactive delirium (40). Hypoactive delirium may be inaccurately diagnosed as depression. Subsequent treatment with an antidepressant could exacerbate the delirium. It may also be difficult in the elderly to distinguish delirium from dementia, which is a known risk factor for the development of delirium. Routine and frequent cognitive assessment of patients is necessary for the early diagnosis and monitoring of delirium. See section "The Memorial Delirium Assessment Scale."

Diagnosis and Therapy of Reversible Causes

Although delirium may herald the terminal phase, it has been shown to be reversible in about 50% of episodes (41).

Therefore, reversible causes should be identified, and patients should be given appropriate treatment with simple interventions (Fig. 20.4). Physicians should conduct a careful clinical examination looking for signs of sepsis, dehydration, and side effects of medication, especially opioids, and other potential causes of delirium. If appropriate, blood tests (e.g., full blood count, electrolytes, calcium, renal, and liver function) and chest X-ray may be performed.

Medication side effects should be managed with discontinuation of the implicated drug if possible. For delirium secondary to opioids, the opioid should be rotated (substituted) (see section "Opioid Rotation/Substitution"). If a patient has good pain control, then a decrease in the opioid dose should be considered as the patient may be receiving an excessive dose for their pain management needs. Dehydration should be treated with the administration of parenteral fluids (intravenous or subcutaneous) (see section "Subcutaneous Route"). Treatment options should be discussed with the patient and their family to ascertain their wishes before proceeding with further therapies. Suitable antibiotics may be commenced for infection/sepsis. Hypoxic patients should receive oxygen and the underlying cause treated if appropriate. Hypercalcemia may be treated with hydration with saline and bisphosphonates. For brain tumor or metastases, then high-dose corticosteroids and radiotherapy can be considered.

Nonpharmacological Therapy of Delirium

Simple environmental measures may help in the management of patients with delirium (42). These include ensuring a physically safe environment, minimizing noise and excessive light, the presence of familiar objects, and enlisting the family to assist with re-orientation. Family caregivers observe patient behaviors and experience distress more frequently than do health care professionals and will

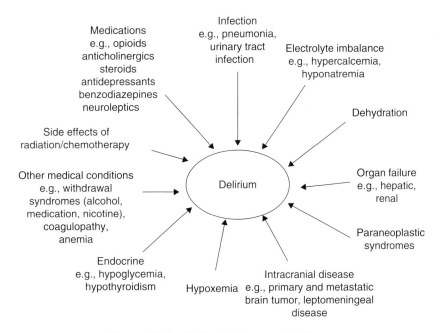

Figure 20.4   Multifactorial causes of delirium.

require ongoing education and support (43). Patients will also require reassurance to help reduce their distress.

Pharmacological Therapy of Delirium

The symptomatic therapy of delirium in advanced cancer patients should be considered a short-term measure, while reversible causes are investigated and treated. Haloperidol is the usual first line neuroleptic agent, although there is limited evidence from randomized clinical trials (44). It is a potent dopamine blocking neuroleptic and has limited anticholinergic effects. Haloperidol is a very effective medication for the treatment of hyperactive and mixed delirium and has also been used for hypoactive delirium (45). It is versatile to use with many routes of administration: oral (p.o.), subcutaneous (s.c.), intravenous (i.v.), and intramuscular (i.m.). To treat agitation, initial doses of haloperidol 1 to 2 mg p.o./s.c./i.v. every six hours and 1 to 2 mg every two hours as needed are usually effective. The haloperidol dose should be titrated to effect and can be used as a continuous infusion. Sometimes more frequent dosing is necessary to control severe agitation. The majority of patients will show improvement in their hyperactive symptoms within three to five days. If there is no significant response, a more sedating neuroleptic such as chlorpromazine or methotrimeprazine (levomepromazine) should be tried.

Newer neuroleptics, the atypical antipsychotics such as risperidone, olanzapine, and quetiapine, are another treatment option for delirium (46). They have the advantage of fewer extrapyramidal adverse effects, few drug interactions, and they can be administered once or twice daily. Olanzapine may cause rapid weight gain, hyperglycemia, and raise cholesterol and triglyceride levels (47). With risperidone treatment in elderly dementia patients, there is a significantly increased risk of cerebrovascular events (48). There is a parenteral formulation of olanzapine for intramuscular injection, which has also been administered by the subcutaneous route in some units (49).

Occasionally, patients with ongoing severe agitation that has been refractory to the above treatments will require deeper sedation. Medications used to achieve this are midazolam as a continuous subcutaneous or intravenous infusion and phenobarbital (phenobarbitone) (50,51).

DYSPNEA

Dyspnea or shortness of breath is a common symptom in patients with advanced cancer and is frequently present at the end of life. Dyspnea is a subjective sensation. Therefore, it is not uncommon for patients with advanced cancer to feel short of breath in the absence of either a respiratory condition (e.g., pneumonia, pulmonary embolism, pleural effusion, and others) or visible/audible respiratory distress (e.g., use of accessory muscles, raised respiratory rate, and respiratory noises/stridor). The reverse may also occur. Patients may exhibit respiratory distress or a thoracic condition, but not experience dyspnea. Consequently, it is essential to specifically ask patients if they feel short of breath. Therapy should focus on the alleviation of the subjective sensation, rather than the improvement of patients' respiratory effort or the correction of abnormalities in blood gases or pulmonary function.

Causes of Dyspnea

Dyspnea is frequently multicausal. It may be the result of the tumor itself, e.g., bronchial obstruction, atelectasis, pleural effusion, carcinomatous lymphangitis, superior vena cava obstruction, and cardiac tamponade secondary to a malignant pericardial effusion. It may also be due to effects of oncological treatment e.g., pneumonitis or fibrosis post radiotherapy or chemotherapy. In addition, non-malignant causes are frequent complications in patients with advanced cancer, such as pneumonia, pulmonary embolism, anemia, and pneumothorax (Fig. 20.5).

Muscle weakness has been proposed as the cause for dyspnea in patients without an evident underlying cause (52). Cachexia-anorexia syndrome, frequently present in patients with advanced cancer, can result in muscle weakness and consequently dyspnea (see section "Cachexia/Anorexia Syndrome in Cancer Patients"). Psychological issues such as anxiety may induce or exacerbate the sensation of dyspnea.

Assessment of Dyspnea

The subjective symptom of dyspnea must be differentiated from objective signs such as tachypnea or use of accessory muscles. Dyspnea can be evaluated using simple tools such as visual analog, numerical, and verbal rating scales.

As with other symptoms, the expression of dyspnea can be enhanced by many other factors, including anxiety and delirium (see section "Multidimensional Assessment"). These factors should be taken into account to avoid the administration of excessive medication, which will increase the likelihood of side effects without improved therapeutic benefit.

Therapy

Whenever possible, identified reversible causes of dyspnea should be treated. However, in palliative care, it is important to consider the burden/benefit of treatment and patient comfort before performing any invasive procedure. Superior vena cava obstruction syndrome can be treated with high-dose steroids, chemotherapy, radiotherapy, or stent placement. Carcinomatous lymphangitis is treated with corticosteroids and occasionally with aggressive chemotherapy. Significant pleural effusions can be drained. In patients with good performance status, pleurodesis should be considered, as there is almost a 100% recurrence rate at one month after pleural aspiration alone (53). Chemical sclerosants, such as talc, are needed for successful pleurodesis (53). Pericardial fluid can be drained by closed needle pericardiocentesis or via surgical incision. Antibiotics can be instigated for the treatment of pneumonia. Exacerbations of chronic obstructive airways disease may respond to management with bronchodilators, corticosteroids, and antibiotics. For patients with symptomatic anemia, blood transfusion may be indicated. For pulmonary embolism, anticoagulation is the appropriate therapy.

There is some evidence that oxygen therapy can provide symptomatic relief in cancer patients who are hypoxemic, but not in those who are nonhypoxemic (54). Oxygen therapy via nasal prongs may be better tolerated

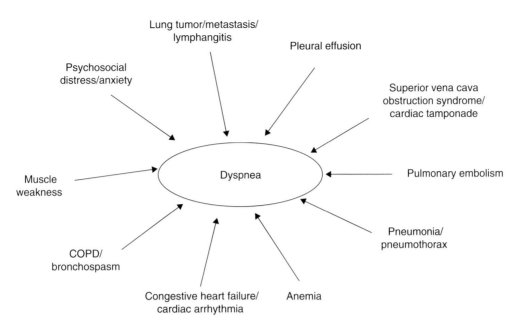

Figure 20.5 Multifactorial causes of dyspnea.

than by mask. Administration of air via nasal prongs to patients with advanced cancer may also provide similar symptomatic relief to oxygen, including hypoxemic patients (55).

Oral and parenteral opioids relieve dyspnea (56). Morphine is the most studied opioid. The management of dyspnea with opioids is similar to that of pain (see section "Initiation of Opioid Therapy"). The starting dose of morphine for opioid naïve patients is 5 to 10 mg p.o. (or 2.5–5 mg s.c.) every four hours and 2.5 to 5 mg p.o. (or 2.5 mg s.c.) hourly as needed for "breakthrough" or incident dyspnea on exertion (Lower doses of opioid should be used in frail and elderly patients). If patients are experiencing ongoing dyspnea, their maintenance dose of opioid should be increased. Opioids administered by nebulization have been reported by some authors to be effective in the management of dyspnea. However, they have not demonstrated significant efficacy in several studies (56). Simple saline nebulizers often provide symptomatic relief.

Health care professionals are often concerned about using opioids for symptomatic management of dyspnea. Appropriate doses of opioids can be used safely in patients with advanced cancer or other terminal diseases, including opioid-naïve patients, without causing opioid-induced respiratory depression (57). Opioid therapy can provide excellent subjective improvement in dyspnea with no obvious change in objective signs. Frequently, patients will report feeling comfortable although their respiratory rate remains high. This information is very useful to help reduce distress in families.

Benzodiazepines may play a role where anxiety is a significant factor. However, there is no good evidence to support their routine use in the management of dyspnea (56).

Nonpharmacological interventions are also helpful for symptomatic relief of dyspnea (58). Use of a fan helps by creating air movement and facial cooling. Breathlessness clinics have been shown to significantly improve patients' breathlessness, activity levels, and distress levels (59). Fear and anxiety in patients should be addressed. It is also important to provide education and support to families to reduce their anxiety, including discussion of expected changes in breathing pattern as the patient enters the terminal phase.

CACHEXIA/ANOREXIA SYNDROME IN CANCER PATIENTS

Cachexia/anorexia is a complex metabolic syndrome characterized by weight loss, lipolysis, muscle wasting, and fatigue. The body image changes that result from this syndrome can cause substantial psychological distress to the patient and family. The social activity of eating is lost with the act of eating and feeding also having a large cultural significance.

Cachexia may occur in up to 80% of patients with advanced cancer. Patients with this syndrome are more susceptible to medication side effects and have an increase in morbidity and mortality (60).

Mechanism of Cachexia

For many years, there was a misconception that cachexia was due to increased energy requirements of the cancer. However, recent research has shown that cachexia is due to a catabolic state related to the interaction between tumor byproducts and the release of cytokines by the host. In addition, in some patients this condition is aggravated by a decreased food intake (Fig. 20.6). The cancer releases proteolytic and lipolytic factors (61). The host, in response to the cancer, produces several pro-inflammatory cytokines including tumor necrosis factor (TNF-α), interleukin (IL)-1, IL-6, and interferon. These cytokines are secreted by macrophages and lead to weight loss, anorexia, and protein and fat breakdown (61).

Decreased food intake contributes to cachexia, especially in patients with problematical nutrition such as patients with cancer of the head and neck, esophagus, gastrointestinal tract, or unresolved symptoms such as severe nausea and vomiting and bowel obstruction. For other patients, decreased food intake plays only a minor role.

Assessment of Cachexia

Cachexia is the involuntary weight loss of more than 10% of a patient's premorbid weight. Nutritional status can be assessed by measuring skin fold thickness, mid upper arm circumference, and bioelectrical impedance. Practical laboratory tests, such as albumin and C-reactive protein (CRP) may also correlate with prognosis (62). Anorexia can be assessed using visual analog or numerical rating scales, measuring the patient's subjective loss of appetite. Anorexia is a multidimensional symptom with many causes (Fig. 20.7). Patients should be assessed for all reversible contributors to anorexia. Common related symptoms are fatigue and dyspnea.

Management of Cachexia

Nutritional support is of limited benefit in most cases of cancer-related cachexia (63). However, it can prolong survival in patients whose cachexia results primarily from decreased oral food intake, e.g., patients with head and neck cancer. In this subgroup of patients, medically assisted nutrition is usually administered by the enteral, rather than parenteral, route. The gastrostomy route (PEG) should be considered for advanced cancer patients requiring prolonged enteral nutrition.

Parenteral nutrition has no advantages over enteral nutrition in patients with functional bowel and should not be used routinely (64). It is expensive, complicated to administer and has a higher morbidity than enteral nutrition, e.g., sepsis, electrolyte and glucose imbalance.

Families often feel an obligation to increase their loved ones oral intake to "build them up" with the assumption that this will prevent further weight loss. Force-feeding of the patient by the well-intentioned family often exacerbates nausea in the patient and causes psychological distress and conflict. Explanation of the metabolic changes occurring with anorexia should be given to the patient and family with clarification that simply increasing oral food intake is unlikely to prolong life in a patient with advanced cancer. Patients should be encouraged to eat small amounts of their desired foods for comfort and enjoyment.

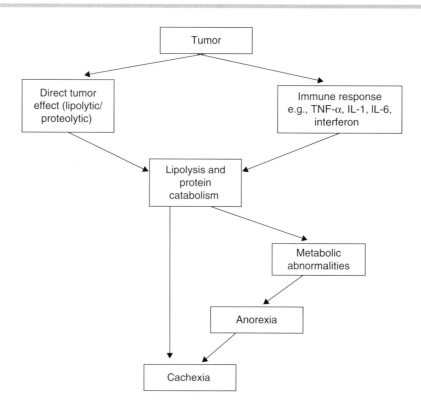

Figure 20.6 Mechanism of cachexia.

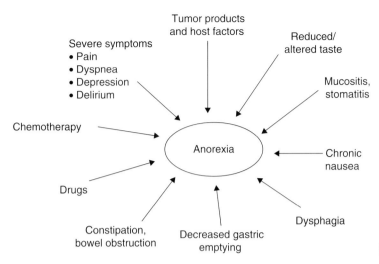

Figure 20.7 Multifactorial causes of anorexia.

Pharmacological Interventions

In cachexic patients with chronic nausea, regular metoclopramide can improve appetite and food intake (65) (see section "Nausea and Vomiting"). For the management of cachexia/anorexia syndrome, the two most commonly used agents are corticosteroids and progestagens.

Corticosteroids, such as dexamethasone, increase patient's appetite, food intake, sensation of well-being and performance status. These beneficial effects are short-term only, lasting approximately four weeks, and do not increase patients' weight (66). In addition, steroids have many side effects including glucose intolerance, proximal myopathy, insomnia, agitation, euphoria, depression, steroid psychosis, development of cushingoid features, and increased infection risk. Therefore, prolonged use of steroids is not recommended. The usual dose of dexamethasone for appetite stimulation is 4 to 8mg orally daily (in the morning or as divided doses). The smallest effective dose should be used, and if no benefit is obtained within a week, it should be ceased.

Progestagens used in the pharmacological management of cachexia/anorexia include megestrol acetate and medroxyprogesterone. Megestrol acetate improves appetite in up to 80% of patients. It also increases weight in approximately 20% of treated patients (mostly due to increased fat tissue) and sensation of well-being (67). Symptomatic improvement in appetite occurs within the first week of therapy, but weight gain may take several weeks. Dose-related symptom improvement starts at 160mg/day. A dose of approximately 480 to 800mg/day of megestrol acetate is thought to be optimal for weight gain. However, in a recent Cochrane review, there was insufficient information to ascertain an optimal dose (68). Megestrol acetate is also an expensive drug (up to 20 times more expensive than dexamethasone).

For planned long-term use, megestrol acetate is probably preferable to corticosteroids. In a randomized comparison study, megestrol acetate (800mg/day) had less toxicity than dexamethasone (0.75mg four times daily) and also a trend toward better improved appetite and better weight gain (69). However, there was a higher rate of deep vein thrombosis in the megestrol acetate treated group. Megestrol acetate should not be used in patients with a history of thromboembolic disease. Other side effects of megestrol acetate include peripheral edema, hyperglycemia, and adrenal suppression. Symptomatic adrenal insufficiency with hypogonadism in male patients with cancer has also been described (70).

Medroxyprogesterone acetate may also improve appetite and weight at doses of 1000mg/day (equivalent to megestrol 160mg/day) (71).

Other pharmacological agents are currently being investigated as treatments for cachexia/anorexia syndrome (Table 20.4). As cachexia has multiple contributors, future research is warranted on the effects of combined therapies, including diet, physical activity, anti-inflammatory drugs, appetite stimulants, and anabolic (androgenic) steroids.

Table 20.4 New Emerging Therapies for Cachexia/Anorexia Syndrome

- Thalidomide
- Melatonin
- Testosterone (and derivatives e.g., oxandrolone)
- Cannabinoids
- Growth hormone
- NSAIDs
- TNF inhibitors
- Ghrelin
- L-carnitine
- Polyunsaturated fatty acids (eicosapentaenoic acid—EPA)

FATIGUE

Fatigue has been defined as a subjective feeling of tiredness, weakness or lack of energy with both a physical and cognitive dimension (72). It is one of the most common symptoms in patients with advanced cancer and is associated with a decline in performance status. It is important to identify fatigue as it adversely impacts on quality of life and is also associated with the severity of both physical symptoms (pain, dyspnea, insomnia, anorexia, drowsiness) and psychological symptoms (anxiety and depression) (73).

Causes of Fatigue

Cancer-related fatigue is a multidimensional syndrome that has multiple causes and contributing factors (Fig. 20.8). Cancer induces pro-inflammatory cytokines such as interleukin (IL)-1, IL-6, and tumor necrosis factor (TNF-α) and interferon, which are involved in the mechanism of fatigue and other symptoms such as cachexia and anorexia, fever, anemia, and depression (74).

Cachexia/anorexia syndrome, present in approximately 80% of patients with advanced cancer, causes progressive loss of fat and especially skeletal muscle (see section "Cachexia/Anorexia Syndrome in Cancer Patients"). Muscle wasting also contributes to fatigue (61). Immobility, including prolonged bed rest, leads to deconditioning with loss of muscle mass which reduces tolerance to both exercise and daily activities. Anemia, common in patients with advanced cancer, may be secondary to bleeding, myelosuppression related to cancer therapy, bone marrow infiltration, malnutrition and cytokines produced by the tumor. Profound fatigue can result from severe anemia (hemoglobin <8 g/dL). Psychological factors, such as depression and anxiety, may cause or exacerbate fatigue. Pre-existing medical comorbidities, such as congestive heart failure, end-stage respiratory disease, renal, and hepatic failure, will also increase fatigue. Male patients with advanced cancer or on long term opioid therapy may develop symptomatic hypogonadism (75,76).

Assessment of Fatigue

In a nonspecialized setting, such as oncology departments, screening for fatigue can be performed with single-item questions such as "Do you feel unusually tired or weak?" (72). The patient's subjective assessment of the severity of their fatigue can be quantified using visual analog or numerical rating scales. In addition, as fatigue is a multidimensional model, multiple symptoms should be assessed simultaneously using multidimensional questionnaires, e.g., ESAS (see section "Assessment"). Other longer and more detailed instruments are used in the research setting. These include the 13-item fatigue subscale (which can be used as a stand alone questionnaire) of the Functional Assessment of Chronic Illness Therapy (FACIT) measurement system, and brief fatigue inventory (BFI) (77,78). The EORTC QLQ-C30 has a three-item fatigue subscale (79), which measures the physical dimension of fatigue; so, it may not be suitable for a palliative care patient population (80).

Management of Fatigue

After identifying potential contributors to fatigue, specific reversible causes should be treated. These include pain, anemia, dehydration, infection, cachexia, depression, and endocrine abnormalities, such as hypothyroidism, and hypogonadism. Androgen replacement therapy is currently being trialed in hypogonadic male patients for the management of fatigue.

Among nonpharmacological interventions, aerobic exercise has been shown to be effective in reducing fatigue in patients receiving cancer treatment and cancer survivors (72). Most trials have been done in patients with good

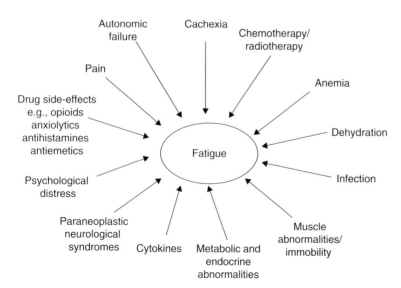

Figure 20.8   Multifactorial causes of fatigue.

performance status, so it is suggested that exercise training is adapted in patients with reduced performance status and gradually increased as tolerated. Input from physical and occupational therapists is warranted.

Pharmacological Management

As with cachexia/anorexia, symptomatic pharmacological management of fatigue includes corticosteroids and progestational agents (see section "Cachexia/Anorexia Syndrome in Cancer Patients"). Psychostimulants have also been used.

Corticosteroids decrease fatigue by an unknown mechanism. They have a beneficial effect for only a short period (two to four weeks). After this period, corticosteroids are not only ineffective, but potential side effects of myopathy and infections will worsen fatigue (see section "Cachexia/Anorexia Syndrome in Cancer Patients"). The usual doses are 20 to 40 mg/day of prednisone or its equivalent dose of dexamethasone.

Megestrol acetate may improve fatigue and activity levels in patients with advanced cancer (67) (see section "Cachexia/Anorexia Syndrome in Cancer Patients").

The psychostimulant medication, methylphenidate has been used to treat a variety of symptoms in advanced cancer patients. These include treatment of opioid-induced sedation, depression, and hypoactive delirium as well as improving cognition and potentiating the analgesic effect of opioids (81). Studies have shown methylphenidate to be more effective than placebo in the management of cancer related fatigue (82). Tolerance to methylphenidate may develop (21).

NAUSEA AND VOMITING

Nausea and vomiting is common in patients with advanced cancer, with a frequency of 40% to 70%, and reported by patients as having a profound negative impact on their quality of life. These symptoms can occur independently of each other, or as part of a continuum with stages of nausea, retching, and vomiting. Nausea is associated with hypersalivation, increased respiratory and heart rates, hypotension, and sweating. Retching occurs when the gut contents are sucked into the lower esophagus, and the diaphragm contracts against a closed glottis. Newer antiemetic regimens can prevent chemotherapy induced vomiting in 70% to 80% of patients, but are less effective in controlling nausea (83).

Mechanism of Nausea and Vomiting

The mechanism of nausea and vomiting is complex with vomiting occurring as part of a protective reflex pathway.

Centrally, the chemoreceptor trigger zone (CTZ) is located in the area postrema, in the floor of the fourth ventricle in the medulla, where there is effectively no blood brain barrier (84). The capillaries of the area postrema have a leaky fenestrated endothelium, and permit direct chemical communication between blood and subarachnoid cerebrospinal fluid. The CTZ is connected to the vomiting center (VC) by neural pathways, with sensory information processed in the tractus solitarius and its nucleus. The CTZ may also send outputs directly to VC efferent components.

The VC, a neuroanatomical region, is situated in adjacent coordinated sites in the lateral reticular formation of the medulla and also receives afferents from the gastrointestinal tract, thorax, vestibular system, thalamus, higher brain stem, and cerebral cortex. Integration of emetogenic stimuli with parasympathetic activity and stimulation of the motor efferent pathways from the VC causes vomiting to occur.

Although there are at least 17 different receptors, some of them tend to be more predominant in certain zones. The principal receptor in the CTZ is dopamine D_2, whereas the principal VC receptors are histamine H_1 and muscarinic cholinergic Ach_m, and other receptors such as serotonin type 2 ($5HT_2$). Both these zones have serotonin type 3 receptors, $5HT_3$. Neurokinin-1 (NK-1) receptors, predominantly located in areas of the brain stem involved in emesis, are normally activated by substance P and contribute to the emetic response secondary to chemotherapy.

Chemotherapeutic agents cause nausea and vomiting by: activation of the CTZ (e.g., release of neurotransmitter such as dopamine, serotonin, substance P), gastrointestinal mucosa damage or stimulation of gastrointestinal neurotransmitter receptors (e.g., serotonin, $5HT_3$), through cortical and vestibular mechanisms and by alteration of taste and smell (85). Chemotherapy-induced nausea is categorized as acute, delayed, or anticipatory. In acute emesis, vomiting occurs 0 to 24 hours after therapy. Emesis is delayed if it starts 24 or more hours after chemotherapy. Anticipatory or conditioned emesis begins before chemotherapy treatment. Patients often have a history of poor control of vomiting with prior chemotherapy, and patients with a history of motion sickness are also predisposed (86).

Assessment of Nausea and Vomiting

The intensity of nausea should be determined by using assessment tools such as numerical or visual analog scales. The frequency and timing of vomits should also be recorded. Nausea and vomiting usually have multiple underlying causes (Fig. 20.9).

A review of the patient's history, associated symptoms, and drug history will often identify the likely cause(s). Frequently under diagnosed, severe constipation is a common cause of nausea. The medication regimen should be inspected for opioids and chemotherapeutic agents. A physical examination should be conducted to rule out other possible causes such as oral and esophageal infection, bowel obstruction, and brain tumor. Laboratory and clinical investigations, e.g., electrolytes, serum calcium, renal and liver function, and abdominal X-ray, should be done according to the suspected underlying cause and appropriate to the patient's illness trajectory.

Therapy

Reversible causes should be corrected wherever possible. For example, opioid substitution should be considered if there is persistent nausea and vomiting as a side effect of opioid treatment. Hypercalcemia, hyponatremia, and hypokalemia should be corrected and oral/esophageal infections treated. Proton pump inhibitors can provide symptomatic relief for gastroesophageal reflux disease, dyspepsia, and peptic ulcer disease. Severe constipation should be treated, and decompression may be required for

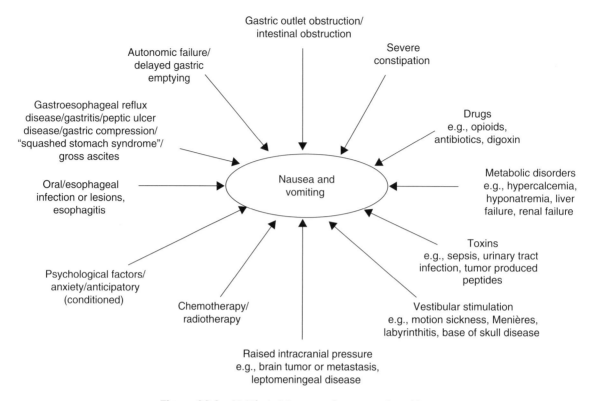

Figure 20.9   Multifactorial causes of nausea and vomiting.

mechanical bowel obstructions. Raised intracranial pressure due to brain tumor or metastasis can be treated with corticosteroids and cranial irradiation.

General measures for management include avoiding the smell of cooking food, trying easily digested foods, and small attractive meals. Patients may need assistance to sit upright in bed, or out of bed, for meals. Acupuncture point stimulation reduces acute chemotherapy-induced vomiting, and acupressure may reduce acute nausea (87). Behavioral therapy with systematic desensitization is recommended for anticipatory (conditioned) emesis with chemotherapy, where there is also a role for lorazepam or alprazolam (86).

Pharmacological management is often guided by considering the potential cause(s) of nausea and vomiting in each case and utilizing known receptor site antagonism by antiemetic drugs (88). Common clinical pictures have also been used to guide treatment in a specialist inpatient palliative care unit (89). However, there is currently little research evidence to support this (90). A nonoral route, e.g., continuous subcutaneous infusion (CSCI), should be used for the management of vomiting or persistent nausea and the patient reevaluated at regular intervals for efficacy. For refractory nausea and vomiting, combinations of parenteral antiemetics targeting different receptor sites are often used in clinical practice. Parenteral rehydration may be required.

Metoclopramide and domperidone have both central (block D_2 receptors in CTZ) and peripheral effects. They are

prokinetics and stimulate gastric and intestinal motility, which appears to be mediated by local release of acetylcholine and may cause colic if used in complete mechanical bowel obstruction. Antimuscarinics will block this peripheral prokinetic effect, making it counterproductive to give them concurrently (91). There is minimal risk of extrapyramidal effects with domperidone, as it does not normally cross the blood–brain barrier. Metoclopramide is the most commonly used antiemetic medication in palliative care. It is also a $5HT_4$ receptor agonist and acts as a $5HT_3$ receptor antagonist at higher doses. As opioids produce emesis by acting centrally (via CTZ) and peripherally (reduce motility throughout gastrointestinal tract), metoclopramide is often the first choice antiemetic for preventing and treating opioid-induced nausea and vomiting. (However, in some countries, haloperidol is used for this indication due to its more potent central inhibitory effects). The usual dose of metoclopramide is 10 mg p.o./s.c./i.v. every four hours, or by continuous infusion, up to 120 mg/24 hours.

Haloperidol is a potent specific D_2 receptor antagonist at CTZ. It has a long half-life, so is often given as a 1 to 3 mg nocte maintenance dose. Extrapyramidal adverse effects are unusual at low doses, <5 mg/24 hours.

Cyclizine and diphenhydramine are antihistaminic antimuscarinic antiemetics acting on the H_1 receptor in the VC and vestibular system. They are a useful option if the patient's nausea and vomiting has a vestibular component and also in cases of intestinal obstruction or raised intracranial pressure. In practice, antihistaminic antimuscarinic anti-emetics are often used in conjunction with haloperidol, providing broader receptor blockade. Cyclizine has the advantage of subcutaneous administration, but some patients do experience skin irritation. Common doses of cyclizine used in clinical practice are 25 to 50 mg p.o. every eight hours and 100 to 300 mg/24 hours by CSCI.

In contrast to cyclizine, promethazine hydrochloride is not only a long-acting antihistamine but also a phenothiazine. In view of this, in addition to antihistaminic and antimuscarinic cholinergic properties, promethazine also has antidopaminergic activity. However, its CTZ antagonism is much weaker than that of haloperidol.

Prochlorperazine is a "broad spectrum" antiemetic with coverage at D_2, H_1, Ach_m (weak) and α_1 adrenoreceptors. It may cause extrapyramidal adverse effects. Unfortunately, its use is limited as it is too irritant to be administered by the subcutaneous route. Rectal suppositories are available and can be particularly useful in the community setting. Levomepromazine (methotrimeprazine) is a more sedating phenothiazine than prochlorperazine. In addition to the same broad receptor coverage of prochlorperazine, as listed above, it also is a potent $5HT_2$ receptor antagonist. The usual antiemetic dose is 6.25 to 25 mg/24 hours. (Higher doses can be used in the management of agitation.)

Corticosteroids, such as dexamethasone, are known for their intrinsic antiemetic effect and also because they increase the antiemetic properties of other medications (92). The mechanism is not well defined. Corticosteroids are usually added to current antiemetic medication in refractory cases, as second line therapy. Dexamethasone is administered in a dose ranging from 8 mg each morning to 10 mg p.o./s.c./i.v. twice a day. To avoid the common adverse effect of insomnia, the latest scheduled dose should be no later than 14:00 hours. Once control is achieved, rapid dose tapering is indicated.

Octreotide, a synthetic somatostatin analog, can play a useful role in the management of inoperable intestinal obstruction and is more effective than hyoscine butylbromide (93). It reduces both gastrointestinal motility and secretions, with consequent reduction in gut distension, nausea stimulus, and number of daily vomits. Reported effective daily doses are 0.1 to 0.6 mg, given by CSCI or intermittent subcutaneous boluses (94). Hyoscine butylbromide remains a useful alternative in reducing vomiting in malignant intestinal obstruction as it also reduces intestinal secretions, in addition to associated colic pain. It is a widely available (but not in the United States) peripherally acting antimuscarinic and is much cheaper than octreotide.

Hyoscine hydrobromide is an antimuscarinic with both central and peripheral actions. It is used as a prophylactic treatment for motion sickness and also in the management of inoperable intestinal obstruction. However, unlike hyoscine butylbromide, the hydrobromide salt may cause sedation and delirium, as it crosses the blood–brain barrier. A transdermal patch formulation is still available in some countries.

$5HT_3$-Receptor antagonists are indicated for nausea and vomiting during treatment with chemotherapy and radiotherapy and to prevent postoperative emesis. They have also been used in the management of ongoing vomiting, especially from chemical, cerebral, and gut causes, when first line antiemetics have failed (95). Headache is a very common adverse effect in up to 20% of patients and constipation is also common (96).

More recently, an antiemetic regimen with aprepitant, a neurokinin-1(NK-1)-receptor antagonist, has been shown to be more effective than a regimen with ondansetron and dexamethasone for the prevention of chemotherapy-induced nausea and vomiting (CINV) (97). Aprepitant inhibits CYP3A4 and induces CYP2D6 leading to potential drug interactions. European and American guidelines now recommend the use of aprepitant in CINV (86,98). Before chemotherapy of high emetic risk, the three-drug combination of a $5HT_3$ serotonin receptor antagonist, dexamethasone, and aprepitant is recommended.

Cannabinoids have antiemetic effects. Their use in routine clinical practice is limited because of their undesirable effects such as drowsiness and hallucinations.

CONSTIPATION

Constipation is defined as the passage of small hard stools infrequently and with difficulty and is a prevalent symptom in patients with advanced cancer. It occurs in 40% to 70% of patients referred to a palliative care service and nearly 90% of patients on oral strong opioids (99). Constipation is frequently under diagnosed and potential complications are usually underestimated by physicians. Frequency of bowel action is a poor guide to colonic function, so simply asking patients when their bowels last opened does not provide enough information to aid management. Stool form and consistency, as assessed by the Bristol stool form scale, have been shown to be well correlated with intestinal transit time and fecal output (100).

Clinical Manifestation

Constipation causes abdominal bloating and colic pain and often leads to increased flatulence. It may cause nausea and anorexia, and rarely vomiting. Untreated constipation may result in fecal impaction, and associated "overflow diarrhea." This diarrhea is due to the production of mucus by the rectum in addition to bacterial liquefaction of fecal material proximal to the obstruction. As a result, patients have frequent passage of small amounts of watery feces or the continuous seepage of moist stool and mucus. This situation can deteriorate if the patient is treated with antidiarrheal medications, as this will lead to further constipation. Constipation is a recognized precipitant for delirium in the elderly (40). Patients with constipation may also experience rectal pain from associated rectal fissure and hemorrhoids, and tenesmus.

Colonic perforation is a rare life-threatening complication. Fecal impaction can cause increased pressure on the bowel wall, resulting in ischemic necrosis of the mucosa leading to pain and bleeding. When severe, perforation may occur. The use of corticosteroids may increase the risk of this fatal complication.

Assessment of Constipation

Physicians need to assess patients' bowel habits regularly. In the evaluation, they should include questions about the consistency and quantity of the stool, difficulty in defecation, and symptoms related to constipation, such as abdominal bloating and pain, or nausea. Factors contributing to constipation should also be reviewed (Fig. 20.10).

Examination is important and includes a rectal examination, especially if low fecal impaction suspected. A plain abdominal X-ray can be helpful if the diagnosis is difficult.

Therapy

Physicians should proactively manage constipation and prevention is crucial. In the non-pharmacological management of constipation, patients should be encouraged to toilet regularly at the same time each day and make use of the gastrocolic reflex that occurs shortly after eating. Patients should endeavor to maintain adequate hydration and not accept constipation as a consequence of anorexia. A private environment for toileting should be available and patients should be assisted to sit upright with feet on the ground where possible.

Prophylactic oral laxatives should be prescribed, or an existing laxative regimen adjusted, for all patients commencing strong opioids. Docusate 50 mg and sennosides 8.6 mg, one to two tablets p.o. b.d., is a commonly used combined preparation with both fecal softening and stimulant actions. The dose of laxative should be titrated according to the patient's response, and may need increasing up to two to four tablets every six hours to produce a regular bowel action without straining every one to three days. However, the role of docusate is controversial. A recent nonrandomized study in two cohorts of hospitalized cancer patients receiving docusate plus sennosides or sennosides alone showed that the docusate plus sennosides bowel protocol was less effective and more expensive (101). An increase in

opioid dose often necessitates an increase in laxative dose (99). (Methadone and fentanyl are less constipating than morphine) (26,102). If docusate-senna or sennosides alone are not effective when used in increasing doses, then another laxative such as lactulose or polyethylene glycol should be added. (These two laxatives may also be preferable in patients unable to tolerate senna because of colic). Lactulose is an osmotic laxative so patients will need to have a reasonable fluid intake. It can cause abdominal bloating and flatulence. The usual lactulose dose of 10 to 30 ml p.o. b.d. may need increasing to 30 ml six hourly. Low dose polyethylene glycol (macrogol) and electrolytes is an oral "iso-osmotic" laxative that can also be used in the management of fecal impaction (103). If intestinal obstruction is suspected, stimulant laxatives should be ceased and only laxatives with a softening action used.

At times, rectal measures are needed in addition if oral laxatives are ineffective. Glycerin/glycerol suppositories soften the stool and bisacodyl suppositories stimulate propulsive activity. Mini-enemas are useful in patients with advanced cancer because of their small volume, and hence better tolerated than the administration of large volume high enemas, which is often exhausting for frail patients. Manual disimpaction may sometimes be necessary.

There has been recent interest in the use of peripherally acting mu-opioid antagonists. Methylnaltrexone and alvimopan have been shown to be more effective than placebo in reversing constipation and opioid-induced increased gastrointestinal transit time, but their long-term efficacy and safety is currently unknown (104). In view of concerns of an increase in cardiovascular events in patients treated with alvimopan compared with placebo, the U.S. Food and Drug Administration (FDA) has recently approved it for use in

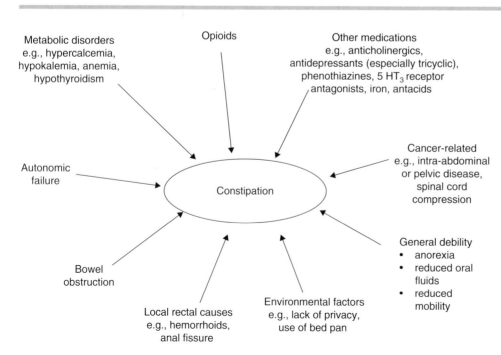

Figure 20.10 Multifactorial causes of constipation.

the United States with a Risk Evaluation and Mitigation Strategy (REMS) for hospitalized bowel surgery patients only (www.fda.gov). A recent double-blind, randomized study in patients with advanced illness and opioid-induced constipation has shown that subcutaneous methylnaltrexone in a dose of 5 mg or greater was significantly more effective than a dose of 1 mg (105). Approximately 50% of patients had a laxation response within four hours after the first dose (≥5 mg). Methylnaltrexone did not reduce analgesia or cause opioid withdrawal symptoms but there were mild gastrointestinal adverse events, such as abdominal pain, diarrhea, flatulence, and nausea. Methylnaltrexone recently received FDA approval in the United States for opioid-induced constipation in patients with advanced illness.

SUBCUTANEOUS ROUTE

When a patient with advanced cancer is unable to take oral medications or fluids, or when a rapid effect of a medication is needed, the subcutaneous route is an effective option for most medications. It is particularly useful in the community setting where there is limited administration of intravenous medications and fluids but where medications are often given by continuous subcutaneous infusion (CSCI). It is also less invasive and less restrictive for the patient and can be maintained over prolonged periods of time. Responsible family caregivers can be trained to administer intermittent subcutaneous injections of medications (106).

Common sites for placing butterfly needles (25 or 23 gauge) are the anterior chest wall and anterior abdominal wall. (Edematous areas should be avoided). The needle should be inserted at 30° to 45° into the subcutaneous tissue. With nonirritant drugs, subcutaneous sites may last up to seven days (107). If frequent resiting is needed (i.e., <48 hours), a plastic cannula could be trialed instead of a metal butterfly needle. With known irritant drugs, the solution should be diluted as much as is practicable or changed to a less irritant alternative medication. A low dose of dexamethasone (e.g., 0.5–1 mg) can be added last to the syringe (if compatible with the already diluted drug solution) (108).

The subcutaneous route may also be used for medically assisted hydration. One liter of fluid a day usually provides adequate hydration, due to altered fluid homeostasis in advanced cancer patients. Suitable fluids are normal saline or two-thirds dextrose (5%) and one-third normal saline solution. Fluids can be infused over 24 hours, overnight or as boluses of 250 ml over an hour, three or four times a day. The last method is less restrictive for the patient and family.

ETHICAL ISSUES IN PALLIATIVE CARE AT THE END OF LIFE
Palliative Sedation

Palliative sedation therapy is the use of proportionate sedation to reduce patient consciousness to achieve symptom control at the end of life for intractable symptoms that have remained refractory to all possible treatments and cause intolerable suffering (109). Appropriately titrated palliative sedation to relieve intractable distress in the dying is an ethically and legally accepted intervention and is distinct from euthanasia as the aim is to relieve suffering and not to shorten life. Consultation with palliative care experts is advisable before initiating palliative sedation therapy (109). Drugs used for palliative sedation include midazolam, levomepromazine (methotrimeprazine), lorazepam, phenobarbital (phenobarbitone), and propofol (109).

"Respite" sedation is a planned temporary sedation that is reversed and may be used to break a cycle of patient distress associated with a temporarily uncontrolled symptom (110).

Patient Desire for Hastened Death

Patients may express a desire for hastened death, but are often not intending a literal request for euthanasia/assisted suicide. The factors associated with this desire are often complex and more often related to psychosocial and existential distress rather than pain or other physical symptoms (111). Following on from a recent systematic review, multidisciplinary recommendations on approaches to responding to patients making a "desire to die" statement have been published (112). Therapeutic communication is a key principle.

Euthanasia and Assisted Suicide

Currently, there is much ongoing discussion around the world in both medicine and society regarding this issue, with euthanasia and assisted suicide legalized in some countries.

Euthanasia is killing on request and has been defined as "a doctor intentionally killing a person by the administration of drugs, at that person's voluntary and competent request," whereas physician-assisted suicide has been defined as "a doctor intentionally helping a person to commit suicide by providing drugs for self-administration, at that person's voluntary and competent request" (113).

In this overview chapter of palliative care, it is not possible to discuss this controversial area in great depth, but the interested reader is referred to some seminal articles to help inform this topical debate (113–115).

SUMMARY

The symptoms reviewed here are some of the primary symptoms experienced by palliative care patients. This review is by no means exhaustive. The continued goal of palliative care is to address all symptoms adversely affecting quality of life and to recognize when medical treatment has become increasingly burdensome and is disproportionately interfering with patients' quality of life as they approach the end of life. Future directions should continue to focus on interdisciplinary collaboration and to further research to improve therapies for the symptom control of palliative care patients.

ACKNOWLEDGEMENTS

Eduardo Bruera is supported in part by National Institutes of Health grant numbers RO1NR010162-01-A1, RO1CA122292-01, RO1CA124481-01.

REFERENCES

1. WHO 2002: WHO definition of palliative care. Available at: http://www.who.int/cancer/palliative/definition/en/ [Accessed 13 June 2008].
2. Homsi J, Walsh D, Rivera N et al. Symptom evaluation in palliative medicine: patient report vs. systematic assessment. Support Care Cancer 2006; 14: 444–53.
3. Bruera E, Kuehn N, Miller MJ et al. The Edmonton Symptom Assessment System (ESAS): a simple method for the assessment of palliative care patients. J Palliat Care 1991; 7: 6–9.
4. Breitbart W, Rosenfeld B, Roth A et al. The Memorial Delirium Assessment Scale. J Pain Symptom Manage 1997; 13: 128–37.
5. Bruera E, Moyano J, Seifert L et al. The frequency of alcoholism among patients with pain due to terminal cancer. J Pain Symptom Manage 1995; 10: 599–603.
6. Mayfield D, McLeod G, Hall P. The CAGE questionnaire: validation of a new alcoholism screening instrument. Am J Psychiatry 1974; 131: 1121–3.
7. Viganò A, Dorgan M, Buckingham J et al. Survival prediction in terminal cancer patients: a systematic review of the medical literature. Palliat Med 2000; 14: 363–74.
8. Kaasa T, Loomis J, Gillis K et al. The Edmonton Functional Assessment Tool: preliminary development and evaluation for use in palliative care. J Pain Symptom Manage 1997; 13: 10–19.
9. Keith RA, Granger CV, Hamilton BB et al. The functional independence measure: a new tool for rehabilitation. Adv Clin Rehabil 1987; 1: 6–18.
10. Portenoy RK, Lesage P. Management of cancer pain. Lancet 1999; 353: 1695–700.
11. Zech DF, Grond S, Lynch J et al. Validation of World Health Organization Guidelines for Cancer Pain Relief: a 10-year prospective study. Pain 1995; 63: 65–76.
12. Ashby MA, Fleming BG, Brooksbank M et al. Description of a mechanistic approach to pain management in advanced cancer. Preliminary report. Pain 1992; 51: 153–61.
13. Bush SH. Episodic pain. In: Bruera E, Higginson IJ, Ripamonti C et al., eds. Textbook of Palliative Medicine. London: Hodder Arnold, 2006: 505–11.
14. Portenoy RK, Hagen NA. Breakthrough pain: definition, prevalence and characteristics. Pain 1990; 41: 273–81.
15. Hwang SS, Chang VT, Fairclough DL et al. Development of a cancer pain prognostic scale. J Pain Symptom Manage 2002; 24: 366–78.
16. Fainsinger RL, Nekolaichuk CL, Lawlor PG et al. A multicenter study of the revised Edmonton Staging System for classifying cancer pain in advanced cancer patients. J Pain Symptom Manage 2005; 29: 224–37.
17. McQuay HJ, Moore A. Non-opioid analgesics. In: Doyle D, Hanks G, Cherny NI et al., eds. Oxford Textbook of Palliative Medicine, 3rd edn. New York: Oxford University Press, 2004: 342–9.
18. Stockler M, Vardy J, Pillai A et al. Acetaminophen (paracetamol) improves pain and well-being in people with advanced cancer already receiving a strong opioid regimen: a randomized, double-blind, placebo-controlled cross-over trial. J Clin Oncol 2004; 22: 3389–94.
19. Mercadante S. The use of anti-inflammatory drugs in cancer pain. Cancer Treat Rev 2001; 27: 51–61.
20. Murtagh FE, Chai MO, Donohoe P et al. The use of opioid analgesia in end-stage renal disease patients managed without dialysis: recommendations for practice. J Pain Palliat Care Pharmacother 2007; 21: 5–16.
21. Bruera E, Brenneis C, Paterson AH et al. Use of methylphenidate as an adjuvant to narcotic analgesics in patients with advanced cancer. J Pain Symptom Manage 1989; 4: 3–6.
22. Bruera E, Driver L, Barnes EA et al. Patient-controlled methylphenidate for the management of fatigue in patients with advanced cancer: a preliminary report. J Clin Oncol 2003; 21: 4439–43.
23. Ripamonti C, Bruera E. CNS adverse effects of opioids in cancer patients. CNS Drugs 1997; 8: 21–37.
24. Mercadante S, Bruera E. Opioid switching: a systematic and critical review. Cancer Treat Rev 2006; 32: 304–15.
25. Foley KM. Controversies in cancer pain. Medical perspectives. Cancer 1989; 63: 2257–65.
26. Hanks G, Cherny NI, Fallon M. Opioid analgesic therapy. In: Doyle D, Hanks G, Cherny NI et al., eds. Oxford Textbook of Palliative Medicine, 3rd edn. New York: Oxford University Press, 2004: 316–41.
27. Indelicato RA, Portenoy RK. Opioid rotation in the management of refractory cancer pain. J Clin Oncol 2002; 20: 348–52.
28. Ripamonti C, Groff L, Brunelli C et al. Switching from morphine to oral methadone in treating cancer pain: what is the equianalgesic dose ratio? J Clin Oncol 1998; 16: 3216–21.
29. Ayonrinde OT, Bridge DT. The rediscovery of methadone for cancer pain management. Med J Aust 2000; 173: 536–40.
30. Bruera E, Sweeney C. Methadone use in cancer patients with pain: a review. J Palliat Med 2002; 5: 127–38.
31. Fisher K, Stiles C, Hagen NA. Characterization of the early pharmacodynamic profile of oral methadone for cancer-related breakthrough pain: a pilot study. J Pain Symptom Manage 2004; 28: 619–25.
32. Ripamonti C, De Conno F, Groff L et al. Equianalgesic dose/ratio between methadone and other opioid agonists in cancer pain: comparison of two clinical experiences. Ann Oncol 1998; 9: 79–83.
33. Centeno C, Vara F. Intermittent subcutaneous methadone administration in the management of cancer pain. J Pain Palliat Care Pharmacother 2005; 19: 7–12.
34. Jackson K, Ashby M, Martin P et al. "Burst" ketamine for refractory cancer pain: an open-label audit of 39 patients. J Pain Symptom Manage 2001; 22: 834–42.
35. Cramond T. Invasive techniques for neuropathic pain in cancer. In: Bruera E, Portenoy RK, eds. Topics in Palliative Care, Volume 2. New York: Oxford University Press, 1998: 63–86.
36. American Psychiatric Association (APA). Diagnostic and Statistical Manual of Mental Disorders, 4th edn. Washington DC: American Psychiatric Association, 2000.
37. Centeno C, Sanz A, Bruera E. Delirium in advanced cancer patients. Palliat Med 2004; 18: 184–94.
38. Breitbart W, Gibson C, Tremblay A. The delirium experience: delirium recall and delirium-related distress in hospitalized patients with cancer, their spouse/caregivers, and their nurses. Psychosomatics 2002; 43: 183–94.
39. Bruera E, Fainsinger RL, Miller MJ et al. The assessment of pain intensity in patients with cognitive failure: a preliminary report. J Pain Symptom Manage 1992; 7: 267–70.
40. Young J, Innouye SK. Delirium in older people. BMJ 2007; 334: 842–6.
41. Lawlor PG, Gagnon B, Mancini IL et al. Occurrence, causes, and outcome of delirium in patients with advanced cancer. A prospective study. Arch Intern Med 2000; 160: 786–94.
42. Zimberg M, Berenson S. Delirium in patients with cancer: nursing assessment and intervention. Oncol Nurs Forum 1990; 17: 529–38.
43. Bruera E, Bush SH, Willey J et al. Impact of delirium and recall on the level of distress in patients with advanced cancer and their family caregivers. Cancer 2009 Feb 24. [Epub ahead of print].
44. Seitz DP, Gill SS, van Zyl LT. Antipsychotics in the treatment of treatment of delirium: a systematic review. J Clin Psychiatry 2007; 68: 11–21.

45. Platt MM, Breitbart W, Smith M et al. Efficacy of neuroleptics for hypoactive delirium. J Neuropsychiatry Clin Neurosci 1994; 6: 66–7.

46. Boettger S, Breitbart W. Atypical antipsychotics in the management of delirium: a review of the empirical literature. Palliat Support Care 2005; 3: 227–37.

47. Jayaram MB, Hosalli P, Stroup S. Risperidone versus olanzapine for schizophrenia. Cochrane Database Syst Rev 2006; CD005237. DOI: 10.1002/14651858.CD005237. pub2

48. Schneider LS, Dagerman K, Insel PS. Efficacy and adverse effects of atypical antipsychotics for dementia: meta-analysis of randomized, placebo-controlled trials. Am J Geriatr Psychiatry 2006; 14: 191–210.

49. Delgado-Guay M, Curry E, Bruera E et al. Subcutaneous olanzapine for hyperactive or mixed delirium in a comprehensive cancer center. Palliat Med 2008; 22: 457, poster abstract 191.

50. Burke AL, Diamond PL, Hulbert J et al. Terminal restlessness— its management and the role of midazolam. Med J Aust 1991; 155: 485–7.

51. Stirling LC, Kurowska A, Tookman A. The use of phenobarbitone in the management of agitation and seizures at the end of life. J Pain Symptom Manage 1999; 17: 363–8.

52. Kongragunta VR, Druz WS, Sharp JT. Dyspnea and diaphragmatic fatigue in patients with chronic obstructive pulmonary disease. Responses to theophylline. Am Rev Respir Dis 1988; 137: 662–7.

53. Antunes G, Neville, Duffy J et al. BTS guidelines for the management of malignant pleural effusions. Thorax 2003; 58: 29–38.

54. Bruera E, de Stoutz N, Velasco-Leiva A et al. Effects of oxygen on dyspnoea in hypoxaemic terminal-cancer patients. Lancet 1993; 342: 13–14.

55. Philip J, Gold M, Milner A et al. A randomized, double-blind, crossover trial of the effect of oxygen on dyspnea in patients with advanced cancer. J Pain Symptom Manage 2006; 32: 541–50.

56. Viola R, Kiteley C, Lloyd NS et al. The management of dyspnea in cancer patients: a systematic review. Support Care Cancer 2008; 16: 329–37.

57. Clemens KE, Quednau I, Klaschik E. Is there a higher risk of respiratory depression in opioid-naive palliative care patients during symptomatic therapy of dyspnea with strong opioids? J Palliat Med 2008; 11: 204–16.

58. Booth S, Moosaci SH, Higginson IJ. The etiology and management of intractable breathlessness in patients with advanced cancer: a systematic review of pharmacological therapy. Nat Clin Pract Oncol 2008; 5: 90–100.

59. Hately J, Laurence V, Scott A et al. Breathlessness clinics within specialist palliative care settings can improve the quality of life and functional capacity of patients with lung cancer. Palliat Med 2003; 17: 410–17.

60. Ma G, Alexander HR. Prevalence and pathophysiology of cancer cachexia. In: Bruera E, Portenoy RK, eds. Topics in Palliative Care, Volume 2. New York: Oxford University Press, 1998: 91–129.

61. Strasser F. Pathophysiology of the anorexia/cachexia syndrome. In: Doyle D, Hanks G, Cherny NI et al., eds. Oxford Textbook of Palliative Medicine, 3rd edn. New York: Oxford University Press, 2004: 520–33.

62. Elahi MM, McMillan DC, McArdle CS et al. Score based on hypoalbuminemia and elevated C-reactive protein predicts survival in patients with advanced gastrointestinal cancer. Nutr Cancer 2004; 48: 171–3.

63. Klein S, Koretz RL. Nutrition support in patients with cancer: what do the data really show? Nutr Clin Pract 1994; 9: 91–100.

64. Mercadante S. Parenteral versus enteral nutrition in cancer patients: indications and practice. Support Care Cancer 1998; 6: 85–93.

65. Pereira J, Bruera E. Chronic nausea. In: Bruera E, Higginson I, eds. Cachexia-Anorexia in Cancer Patients. Oxford: Oxford University Press, 1996: 23–37.

66. Gagnon B, Bruera E. A review of the drug treatment of cachexia associated with cancer. Drugs 1998; 55: 675–88.

67. Bruera E, Ernst S, Hagen N et al. Effectiveness of megestrol acetate in patients with advanced cancer: a randomized, double-blind, crossover study. Cancer Prev Control 1998; 2: 74–8.

68. Berenstein EG, Ortiz Z. Megestrol acetate for treatment of anorexia-cachexia syndrome. Cochrane Database Syst Rev 2005; CD004310. DOI: 10.1002/14651858.CD004310. pub2.

69. Loprinzi CL, Kugler JW, Sloan JA et al. Randomized comparison of megestrol acetate versus dexamethasone versus fluoxymesterone for the treatment of cancer anorexia/cachexia. J Clin Oncol 1999; 17: 3299–306.

70. Dev R, Del Fabbro E, Bruera E. Association between megestrol acetate treatment and symptomatic adrenal insufficiency with hypogonadism in male patients with cancer. Cancer 2007; 110: 1173–7.

71. Simons JP, Aaronson NK, Vansteenkiste JF et al. Effects of medroxyprogesterone acetate on appetite, weight, and quality of life in advanced-stage non-hormone-sensitive cancer: a placebo-controlled multicenter study. J Clin Oncol 1996; 14: 1077–84.

72. Radbruch L, Strasser F, Elsner F et al. Fatigue in palliative care patients—an EAPC approach. Palliat Med 2008; 22: 13–32.

73. Yennurajalingam S, Palmer JL, Zhang T et al. Association between fatigue and other cancer-related symptoms in patients with advanced cancer. Support Care Cancer 2008; (epub ahead of print). DOI 10.1007/s00520-008-0466-5.

74. Kurzrock R. The role of cytokines in cancer-related fatigue. Cancer 2001; 92(6 Suppl): 1684–8.

75. Strasser F, Palmer JL, Schover LR et al. The impact of hypogonadism and autonomic dysfunction on fatigue, emotional function, and sexual desire in male patients with advanced cancer: a pilot study. Cancer 2006; 107: 2949–57.

76. Rajagopal A, Vassilopoulou-Sellin R, Palmer JL et al. Symptomatic hypogonadism in male survivors of cancer with chronic exposure to opioids. Cancer 2004; 100: 851–8.

77. Yellen SB, Cella DF, Webster K et al. Measuring fatigue and other anemia-related symptoms with the Functional Assessment of Cancer Therapy (FACT) measurement system. J Pain Symptom Manage 1997; 13: 63–74.

78. Mendoza TR, Wang XS, Cleeland CS et al. The rapid assessment of fatigue severity in cancer patients: use of the Brief Fatigue Inventory. Cancer 1999; 85: 1186–96.

79. Aaronson NK, Ahmedzai S, Bergman B et al. The European Organization for Research and Treatment of Cancer QLQ-C30: a quality-of-life instrument for use in international clinical trials in oncology. J Natl Cancer Inst 1993; 85: 365–76.

80. Knobel H, Loge JH, Brenne E et al. The validity of EORTC QLQ-C30 fatigue scale in advanced cancer patients and cancer survivors. Palliat Med 2003; 17: 664–72.

81. Sood A, Barton DL, Loprinzi CL. Use of methylphenidate in patients with cancer. Am J Hosp Palliat Care 2006; 23: 35–40.

82. Minton O, Stone P, Richardson A et al. Drug therapy for the management of cancer related fatigue. Cochrane Database Syst Rev 2008; CD006704. DOI: 10.1002/14651858.CD006704. pub2

83. Jordan K, Schmoll HJ, Aapro MS. Comparative activity of antiemetic drugs. Crit Rev Oncol Hematol 2007; 61: 162–75.

84. Mannix KA. Palliation of nausea and vomiting. In: Doyle D, Hanks G, Cherny NI et al., eds. Oxford Textbook of Palliative Medicine, 3rd edn. New York: Oxford University Press, 2004: 459–68.

85. Berger AM, Clark-Snow RA. Chemotherapy-related nausea and vomiting. In: Berger AM, Shuster JL, Von Roenn JH, eds. Principles and Practice of Palliative Care and Supportive Oncology, 3rd edn. Philadelphia, PA: Lippincott Williams and Wilkins, 2007: 139–49.

86. American Society of Clinical Oncology Guideline for Antiemetics in Oncology: update 2006. Available at: http://www.asco.org/guidelines/antiemetics [accessed 24 April 2008].

87. Ezzo JM, Richardson MA, Vickers A et al. Acupuncture-point stimulation for chemotherapy-induced nausea or vomiting. Cochrane Database Syst Rev 2006; CD002285. DOI: 10.1002/14651858.CD002285.pub2

88. Stephenson J, Davies A. An assessment of aetiology-based guidelines for the management of nausea and vomiting in patients with advanced cancer. Support Care Cancer 2006; 14: 348–53.

89. Bentley A, Boyd K. Use of clinical pictures in the management of nausea and vomiting: a prospective audit. Palliat Med 2001; 15: 247–53.

90. Glare P, Pereira G, Kristjanson LJ et al. Systematic review of the efficacy of antiemetics in the treatment of nausea in patients with far-advanced cancer. Support Care Cancer 2004; 12: 432–40.

91. Twycross R, Back I. Nausea and vomiting in advanced cancer. European Journal of Palliative Care 1998; 5: 39–45.

92. Grunberg SM. Antiemetic activity of corticosteroids in patients receiving cancer chemotherapy: dosing, efficacy, and tolerability analysis. Ann Oncol 2007; 2: 233–40.

93. Mercadante S, Ripamonti C, Casuccio A et al. Comparison of octreotide and hyoscine butylbromide in controlling gastrointestinal symptoms due to malignant inoperable bowel obstruction. Support Care Cancer 2000; 8: 188–91.

94. Ripamonti CI, Easson AM, Gerdes H. Management of malignant bowel obstruction. Eur J Cancer 2008; 44: 1105–15.

95. Currow DC, Coughlan M, Fardell B et al. Use of ondansetron in palliative medicine. J Pain Symptom Manage 1997; 13: 302–7.

96. Perez EA, Hesketh P, Sandbach J et al. Comparison of single-dose oral granisetron versus intravenous ondansetron in the prevention of nausea and vomiting induced by moderately emetogenic chemotherapy: a multicenter, double-blind, randomized parallel study. J Clin Oncol 1998; 16: 754–60.

97. Warr DG, Hesketh PJ, Gralla RJ et al. Efficacy and tolerability of aprepitant for the prevention of chemotherapy-induced nausea and vomiting in patients with breast cancer after moderately emetogenic chemotherapy. J Clin Oncol 2005; 23: 2822–30.

98. Roila F, Hesketh PJ, Herrstedt J. Prevention of chemotherapy- and radiotherapy-induced emesis: results of the 2004 Perugia International Antiemetic Consensus Conference. Ann Oncol 2006; 17: 20–8.

99. Sykes NP. The relationship between opioid use and laxative use in terminally ill cancer patients. Palliat Med 1998; 12: 375–82.

100. Lewis SJ, Heaton KW. Stool form scale as a useful guide to intestinal transit time. Scand J Gastroenterol 1997; 32: 920–4.

101. Hawley PH, Byeon JJ. A comparison of sennosides-based bowel protocols with and without docusate in hospitalized patients with cancer. J Palliat Med 2008; 11: 575–81.

102. Mancini IL, Hanson J, Neumann CM et al. Opioid type and other clinical predictors of laxative dose in advanced cancer patients: a retrospective study. J Palliat Med 2000; 3: 49–56.

103. Wirz S, Klaschik E. Management of constipation in palliative care patients undergoing opioid therapy: is polyethylene glycol an option? Am J Hosp Palliat Care 2005; 22: 375–81.

104. McNicol ED, Boyce D, Schumann R et al. Mu-opioid antagonists for opioid-induced bowel dysfunction. Cochrane Database Syst Rev 2008; CD006332. DOI: 10.1002/14651858.CD006332.pub2

105. Portenoy RK, Thomas J, Moehl Boatwright ML et al. Subcutaneous methylnaltrexone for the treatment of opioid-induced constipation in patients with advanced illness: a double-blind, randomized, parallel group, dose-ranging study. J Pain Symptom Manage 2008; 35: 458–68.

106. Lee L, Headland C. Administration of as required subcutaneous medications by lay carers: developing a procedure and leaflet. Int J Palliat Nurs 2003; 9: 142–9.

107. Brenneis C, Michaud M, Bruera E et al. Local toxicity during the subcutaneous infusion of narcotics (SCIN). A prospective study. Cancer Nurs 1987; 10: 172–6.

108. Reymond L, Charles MA, Bowman J et al. The effect of dexamethasone on the longevity of syringe driver subcutaneous sites in palliative care patients. Med J Aust 2003; 178: 486–9.

109. de Graeff A, Dean M. Palliative sedation therapy in the last weeks of life: a literature review and recommendations for standards. J Palliat Med 2007; 10: 67–85.

110. Rousseau P. Palliative sedation in the management of refractory symptoms. J Support Oncol 2004; 2: 181–6.

111. Hudson PL, Kristjanson LJ, Ashby M et al. Desire for hastened death in patients with advanced disease and the evidence base of clinical guidelines: a systematic review. Palliat Med 2006; 20: 693–701.

112. Hudson PL, Schofield P, Kelly B et al. Responding to desire to die statements from patients with advanced disease: recommendations for health professionals. Palliat Med 2006; 20: 703–10.

113. Materstvedt LJ, Clark D, Ellershaw J et al. Euthanasia and physician-assisted suicide: a view from an EAPC Ethics Task Force. Palliat Med 2003; 17: 97–101, discussion 102–79.

114. Hurst SA, Mauron A. The ethics of palliative care and euthanasia: exploring common values. Palliat Med 2006; 20: 107–12.

115. Emanuel EJ, Fairclough DL, Emanuel LL. Attitudes and desires related to euthanasia and physician-assisted suicide among terminally ill patients and their caregivers. JAMA 2000; 284: 2460–8.

21

Psycho-oncology and Communication

Darius Razavi and Alain Ronson

INTRODUCTION

It is now widely accepted that cancer and its treatments constitute a stress factor imposed to cancer patients and their relatives to a significant extent, leading to adjustment efforts (or coping) and possibly psychopathological disturbances. There is a remarkable heterogeneity in patients' responses to these stress factors. A prevalence of psychopathological disturbances in cancer patients has been reported in many studies. In 1983, the Psychosocial Collaborative Oncology Group observed a prevalence rate of 47% of psychiatric disorders in a cohort of cancer patients (inpatient and outpatient populations of three cancer centers) (1). Most importantly, this rate was approximately twice that reported for psychiatrics disorders in medical patients, and three times the modal estimate for the general population reported in the literature. As a diagnostic category, adjustment disorders accounted for 68% of all diagnoses. Other diagnoses were major affective disorders (13%), organic mental disorders (8%), personality disorders (7%), and anxiety disorders (4%). Most patients with psychopathological disturbances have depression or anxiety as the principal symptom. Most of these conditions are treatable disorders. It should be recalled at this level that cancer patients have an increased risk of suicide compared with the risk found in the general population, particularly during the first year after diagnosis. Therefore, the assumption that emotional distress, one of the most frequent expressions of a difficulty to cope or a psychopathological disturbance, is just a foreseeable and ordinary "reaction" to cancer has to be reconsidered. Finally, cancer affects not only the patients, but also their relatives to a significant extent. The important prevalence of psychological problems and psychopathological disturbances that have been reported in oncology underlines the need for psychological and psychopharmacological interventions designed specifically for cancer patients and their significant others. Preserving the quality of life of the patients and their families as much as possible has become a major goal in cancer care. These issues will be addressed in the "Psycho-oncology" section of this chapter.

It is now widely recognized that the way doctors communicate with their patients affects not only the adequacy of the clinical interview and the detection of psychological disturbance, but also patients' compliance and satisfaction with care. The failure to identify many of the patients' problems seems mostly related to insufficient psycho-oncological knowledge and deficient communication skills among health professionals who care for these patients and their families. Moreover, it is often recognized that caring for cancer patients is highly stressful, and the

stressors include critical decisions, errors yielding important consequences, breaking bad news, numerous therapeutic failures, administration of treatments with serious side effects, contacts with mutilated/disfigured patients, emotionally loaded relationships, and death of the patients. Many of these stressors imply communication with patients, relatives, and colleagues. They may lead to the development of burnout, which may influence quality of care, occupational life, and/or institutional functioning. Interventions and strategies have been proposed to help physicians to deal with cancer care: support groups and training opportunities. Communication skills training programs are probably the best cost-effective ways of reducing stress in cancer care and of improving patient satisfaction with care. These issues will be addressed in the "Communication" section of this chapter.

It should be recalled that advances in the psycho-oncology and communication fields remain dependent on progress in psychology, psychiatry, and oncology. In addition, there are numerous areas and method of research in these fields and that a large volume of published work is available. This chapter will address only some of the core psychological, psychopathological, and communication issues directly related to the oncological practice. This chapter will include some psychobiological considerations, which may be in close interdependence with some of the issues discussed.

PSYCHO-ONCOLOGY
Acute Stress Reactions

Cancer patients are often facing sustained stressful situations. Patients may experience also periods of extreme stress. Cancer and its treatment may thus be considered as chronic stressors. Hospitalization, illness, surgical, and nonsurgical procedures are stressful to all patients. Pain, disability, or death anticipation challenges human adjustment. Some stressors, such as marital, job difficulties, or financial problems, are not related to medical problems. Many significant stressors related or not related to cancer may generate acute stress reactions. Acute responses to the stressors comprise fear responses along with adjustment effort to novelties and losses. Acute stress reactions usually subside within hours or days. Symptoms of acute stress reactions usually appear within minutes of the impact of the stressful events (cancer diagnosis for example) and disappear within two or three days: inattention, daze, numbness, and inability to understand what is happening are frequent during the first hours, followed by either withdrawal, agitation, fear, or anxiety. These responses facilitate support recruitment, sharing emotions, and appraisal of cancer-related events and their consequences.

Biological stress responses are unconditioned protective responses. The stress response includes an arousal of the autonomic system and an activation of the hypothalamic–pituitary–adrenal (HPA) axis. The main mediators of the stress responses are catecholamines and glucocorticoids, respectively. This neuroendocrine response is essential for the maintenance of stability under stress. Homeostasis is defined by narrow variations of vital biological parameters during an acute stress, and allostasis refers to maintaining stability throughout a chronic stress. Allostatic load is defined as the cost inflicted to the organism (brain and body) during chronic stress (2). Allostatic load has been linked with structural and functional brain changes: in particular, neuronal growth and survival as well as dendritic branching may be altered in the hippocampus. These changes may explain numerous cognitive and emotional manifestations of cancer patients. Glucocorticoids may be chronically in excess because of reduced feedback signals from an altered hippocampus. The damage of the hippocampus—which results from chronic exposure to stress hormones—maintain a state of HPA axis hyperactivity. The production of glucocorticoids may also be decreased, resulting in a failure to restrain inflammatory responses (HPA axis and immune system are linked by numerous functional relationship) (3). The concept of allostatic load may be useful to study the potential consequences of cancer and treatment-related stress on psychological outcomes. The concept of allostatic load may also be useful to study the potential consequences of psychological stress on cancer disease outcomes; overproduction of pro-inflammatory cytokines may have, for example, an impact on tumor biology and cancer course and prognosis (4). A recent review of published results indicates that stress-related psychosocial factors are associated with poorer survival and higher mortality (5). Allostatic load may also be linked with several other outcomes that can significantly worsen the burden of cancer and its treatment, for example, cardiovascular and metabolic damages, bone demineralization, etc.

Adjustment Disorders

Cancer and its treatments are stressful life events, causing a significant change in the lifestyle leading to continued unpleasant circumstances, which may result in an adjustment disorder. Adjustment disorders are thought to arise as a direct consequence of stressors, trauma, and losses associated with the diagnosis and the treatment. Adjustment disorders should be differentiated from acute stress reactions, which are transient disorders of significant severity. Adjustment refers to efforts and processes aimed at managing demands of stressors. It involves the use of internal or external resources and the use of coping and problem-solving strategies. It involves also changes in established patterns of functioning, world views, and coping methods. Adjustment disorders are states of subjective distress and emotional disturbance interfering with social functioning and performance. They appear usually within one month of the occurrence of a stressful event and their duration does not usually exceed six months. Manifestations include depression, anxiety, and feelings of inability to cope, loss of control, and low self-esteem. A diagnosis of adjustment disorder should be considered in patients who have symptoms of anxiety or depression, who are experiencing a major psychosocial stressor and who do not meet the criteria for an anxiety disorder, a depressive disorder or a post-traumatic stress disorder.

Vulnerability factors are unfortunately not available. Even if it has not been clearly demonstrated, patients with a previous history of such a disorder or a complicated prolonged psychological reaction to stressors, trauma, and losses may be at increased risk for developing these disorders. Inherited and acquired alterations of the HPA axis can determine how the individual responds to stressors during adult life: in particular, stressors occurring early in life have a profound effect on the HPA axis. Patients suffering from preexisting HPA axis hyperactivity might be more vulnerable to the development of emotional disturbances in the context of cancer (6), a finding that, if confirmed, would give strong support—through the identification of predictive factors—for the preventive use of psychological or pharmacological interventions in patients at increased risk for psychological morbidity.

Depressive Disorders

The clinical presentation of depressive disorders includes psychological and somatic symptoms: dysphoric and diurnal mood changes, feelings of hopelessness and helplessness, suicidal ideation, guilt, poor concentration, and rarely, delusional thoughts. Somatic symptoms like constipation, insomnia, pain, fatigue, anorexia, and psychomotor retardation or agitation are not reliable signs in cancer patients, since they can be caused by cancer or its treatment. Depression may cause amplification of physical symptoms, increased functional impairment and poor treatment adherence. Patients with a family or a personal history of depression are certainly at greater risk of developing a depression during the course of cancer. As in the general population, alcohol abuse is also a risk factor for depression, a fact that is also illustrated by the higher incidence of depression in patients with head and neck cancer. Patients with pancreatic cancer also have a higher depression (7); the cause for this phenomenon is still unknown, but a paraneoplastic syndrome is suspected. Other common causes for the development of depressive symptoms in cancer patients include chronic unrelieved pain, medication (corticosteroids, vincristine, interferon, cimetidine, and others), metabolic alterations (like hypercalcemia), or damage to the central nervous system by cancer lesions.

The differential diagnosis of depression includes sadness, adjustment disorders with depressed mood, grief, and delirious states with depressed affect. If the psychological symptoms described above are present for at least two weeks and the cognitive state of the patient is not altered, then the diagnosis of depression is likely and a treatment should be considered. It may sometimes be very difficult to diagnose depression in cachectic cancer patients with advanced disease, and confirmation of the diagnosis by a psychiatrist may become necessary. The diagnostic criteria for depression overlap frequently with anxiety disorders and there is moreover a frequent anxiety and depression comorbidity. Certain criteria have been suggested to be of use for diagnosing major depressive syndromes in medical patients (8). Somatic items of usual criteria, such as problems with appetite and sleep, fatigue, and complaints about lessened concentration, could be replaced by psychological items such as fearfulness or depressed appearance, social withdrawal or decreased talkativeness, self pity, pessimism, etc.

Depressive syndromes are heterogeneous and their etiologies diverse. Genetic predispositions are thought to interact with environmental risk factors such as stressful life events. The pathogenesis of depression includes beside abnormal cognitive styles, abnormal activity of the HPA axis, alterations in neurotrophic signaling, abnormal hippocampal neurogenesis. There are moreover numerous potential bidirectional relationships between cancer and depression. Stress response dysregulation (in particular glucocorticoids), frequently found in the context of depression, may, in theory, negatively influence the course and prognosis of cancer through several mechanisms: shunting of glucose availability in favor of cancer cells, promotion of oncogene expression, impaired immunological surveillance (9). Although such influences may be considered in theory, it should be recalled that the effect size of these potential influences should be carefully studied.

Anxiety Disorders

Anxiety may have several different meanings and may apply to different thought, feelings, and behaviors. Anxiety alerts to changes and involves the anticipation of future danger. Anxiety is thus usually useful to avoid potential danger and to prepare for further coping and action. A reasonable degree of anxiety can be adaptive. Often, psychological response systems may become dysregulated (over- or underactive), leading to an incapacity to habituate to repeated stressors or to a defective extinction of stress responses after end of threat (a suggested mechanism of post-traumatic stress disorder). Anxiety may therefore grow progressively, become extreme, and interfere with coping, and then becomes a disorder. Anxiety can manifest in different forms: prolonged worries, intrusive thoughts, irrational fears, panic, phobia, obsession, compulsion, etc. The onset of anxiety disorders may precede the cancer diagnosis or may be reactivated by the stressors associated with cancer. Anxiety disorders are frequently met in oncology, and are associated with numerous and intense cancer worries and with functioning impairment.

Postchemotherapy physical discomfort (nausea and vomiting) is often associated with anxiety. During the course of chemotherapy, an important percentage of patients become therefore sensitized to treatment, reporting anxiety, depression, nausea, and fatigue in anticipation of chemotherapy. Symptoms can be conditioned: patients may develop conditioned symptoms responses to clinic cues as a result of the repeated pairing of the clinic environment (conditioned stimulus) with infusions of chemotherapy (unconditioned response) (10). It should be recalled that anxiety can also be a symptom of an underlying medical conditions or a substance induced symptom (corticoids for example).

In the recent years, a growing body of literature has supported the notion that a diagnosis of cancer or cancer recurrence represents a traumatic event, potentially leading to the development of post-traumatic stress disorders. Cancer-related events are often of sudden onset and frequently unexpected. They are also associated with physical discomfort and a sense of helplessness. Post-traumatic stress disorder occurs as a delayed or protracted response to an extremely stressful event or situation. Typical symptoms include episodes of repeated reliving of the trauma in intrusive memories, nightmares, and avoidance of activities and situations reminiscent of the trauma or its causes. There is thus commonly fear and avoidance of what reminds the original trauma. Moreover, the patient may also avoid situations to which he or she attributes the stressful event. There may be acute outbursts of fear, panic, or aggression. Anxiety and depression are also common. Finally, emotional numbing and autonomic hyperactivity are core components of the clinical picture of post-traumatic stress disorder (PTSD). Studies have confirmed the existence of a full-blown PTSD in up to 20% of cancer patients (11).

Genetic variations may predispose an individual to anxiety disorders (for example, serotonin transporter gene variations may lead to low serotonin levels). Neural circuits and stress hormones are implicated in the modulation of fear memory strength and in the development of anxiety disorders. Neural circuits that modulate fear and anxiety have been identified, and their dysfunctions are thought to underline anxiety disorders. Patients with anxiety disorders are showing greater activity than matched controls in the amygdala and insula: these structures are associated with exaggerated fear responses. Patients with PTSD are showing hypoactivation in the dorsal and the rostral anterior cingulate cortex and the ventromedial prefrontal cortex (12): these structures are considered to play a role in the regulation of emotions.

Sickness Behavior

Cancers, infections, and inflammatory processes can induce many symptoms called "sickness behavior." There are many bidirectional relations among brain, immune, and endocrine functions that may explain the development of a "sickness behavior": anhedonia, anxiety, irritability, anergia, anorexia, fatigue, cognitive disturbances, and distress like symptoms. The physiological processes underlying the development of these symptoms include different neuro-immune-endocrine mechanisms. It has been suggested that the activation of the pro-inflammatory cytokine system in cancer patients is associated with this syndrome (13). The effect of pro-inflammatory cytokines on the central nervous system is one of the mechanism underlying the development of sickness symptoms in patients with infection and cancer or in patients treated with radio-, chemo-, and immunotherapy. Thus, patients have to cope with these symptoms (14).

Patients with subclinical symptoms, such as sadness, pessimistic thoughts, and sleep disturbances, prior to initiating cytokine treatment are more likely to become clinically depressed during the course of the cytokine therapy (15). The "sickness behavior" involves several clinical clusters probably reflecting separate underlying pathways, as suggested by differential responses of psychological and cognitive disturbances, pain, fatigue, and anorexia to an antidepressant drug (paroxetine) (16). These data suggest that psychological pretreatment characteristics—for example, depressive symptoms—may predict the side effect profile associated with some cancer treatments.

Psychological Interventions

The feasibility and effectiveness of using psychological and psychopharmacological interventions for preventing psychological problems and psychopathological disturbances in cancer patients should be considered at each phase of the course of the illness. There is some evidence that psychological and psychopharmacological interventions may prevent and allow a better management of adverse symptoms associated with cancer and its treatment (17). For example, chemotherapy may be considered as a severe stressor, and it could be useful to assess psychological and pharmacological interventions designed to reduce, retard, or prevent these consequences.

Specific assessment methods for the screening of psychological problems and psychological disturbances in oncology are available. Screening may identify patients who could be helped with psychological or psychopharmacological interventions. In addition, early recognition of these conditions among family members and caregivers improve the quality of care. The fact that effective methods of treatment are available for several psychological problems and psychopathological disturbances associated with cancer is another argument that justifies the implementation of a screening procedure. Are specific and sensitive screening methods available at a reasonable cost? The performance of screening methods has been widely studied. Most of the methods tested have been self-administered questionnaires because standardized interviews require time and training: the Hospital Anxiety and Depression Scale (18) and the Distress Thermometer (19) are the most frequently used screening methods. These screening instruments generally take less than 15 minutes to complete and have proven to be quite acceptable to most patients. At this point, most of the screening efforts have been focused on anxiety, depression, and psychological distress, which are the most frequent symptoms of adjustment disorders and anxiety, and depressive disorders associated with the diagnosis of cancer and its treatment and evolution. Studies that assess the performance of the screening methods report a sensitivity and specificity of around 75%.

It is important to recall that a precise and comprehensive assessment of the psychological problems and psychopathological disturbances and a good understanding of the social situation are of utmost importance before any psychological or psychopharmacological intervention. An in-depth interview allows to establish a diagnosis of psychological disturbance and to clarify past and present problems. A careful assessment of the symptoms of psychopathological disturbances described above is needed. The fact that psychopathological disturbances in cancer patients remain underdiagnosed is often related to the physician's fear to ask direct questions about the feelings of their patients: patients do not feel such questions to be stressful as long as they are posed in an emphatic way and most patients feel relief when talking about their feelings.

All psychological interventions are dealing with the following question: what can be done to help the cancer patient cope? Despite the multiplicity of approaches and the objectives they openly declare (i.e., to reduce psychological morbidity, enhance quality of life, improve communication, provide information, and teach skills), their purpose can be summarized as an optimization of the patient's adaptation to the consequences of the disease. Psychological interventions have different aims: prevention, restoration, and support. First, preventive interventions are designed to avoid the development of predictable psychological problems or psychopathological disturbances. Second, restorative interventions refer to actions used to control or eliminate residual psychological problems or psychopathological disturbances. Third, supportive interventions are planned to lessen the number and the amplitude of problems and disturbances. Psychological interventions are often multidisciplinary, with a variety of content. The type of psychological intervention ranges from information and education to more sophisticated support programs including directive (behavioral or cognitive) therapies or nondirective (dynamic) therapies. These interventions may be combined with the prescription of psychopharmacological interventions. Psychological interventions may thus range from the information and support provided by physicians or nurses to the use of techniques performed by well-trained psychologists and psychiatrists. Psychological interventions can be divided schematically according not only to their degree of directivity (non-directive vs. directive) but also to their form (individual, family, or group). There is much evidence that most of these interventions are effective but that their effects are frequently limited (effect of small or medium size) (20).

Directive techniques include mainly behavioral and cognitive therapies. Behavioral therapies are based on conditioning theories. They involve precise observation of behavior and use directive methods to achieve determined goals. Their results can be observed directly by the disappearance or persistence of the symptom. The positive effects of the behavioral techniques in treating adverse reactions are rather well documented by controlled studies. These techniques are especially effective for anticipatory nausea and vomiting related to cancer chemotherapy. They have been proposed for treating anxiety and depression and for treating or controlling psychological reactions secondary to painful procedures and cancer pain and adverse reactions to treatments (21). Cognitive therapy deals with present problems and tries to identify maladaptive thoughts, irrational beliefs, and inner factors that are responsible for psychological problems or psychopathological disturbances. Once identified, these thoughts are confronted with reason and reality. Self-monitoring automatic thoughts, restructuring, and teaching coping strategies are commonly used with cancer patients.

Nondirective techniques include information, counseling, and supportive or dynamic psychotherapy. Providing information is the first step in helping patients cope with cancer. Information on diagnosis, prognosis, treatments, and long-term sequels is given by physicians in the first line, but can be further delivered by other medical staff members and completed by members of self-help associations. Information can be provided to the patient alone or to the patient in the presence of family members, or even to family members apart from the patient. A tailored and step-by-step information is often needed as the perception of information by the patient or his family may be distorted by psychological factors, especially in the case of negative information. Counseling is a special form of help performed by trained persons whose purpose is to listen to the patients, help them express and understand their feelings about cancer, and encourage them to cope with their current situation. This technique is an attempt to provide cancer patients with first-line support and continuity when no other more-specialized help is available. Two models of psychotherapy are used with the cancer patient: supportive and dynamic. These two types of interventions need the development of a trusting relationship that allows free communication. Supportive psychotherapy is aimed at restoring or maintaining at least the status quo in crisis: patients' sense of safety, self-esteem, adaptative defenses, and hope are therefore supported. Supportive psychotherapy helps the patient to tolerate and to regulate a wider range of affects and to limit impulsivity and destructiveness (self or other). It supports reality testing and challenges unrealistic ideas. Dynamic psychotherapy, based on psychoanalytic or psychodynamic models, is useful when patients wish to explore further their reactions and feelings and to promote personality development.

Psychopharmacological Interventions

Clinical experience supports the usefulness of psychotropic medications in oncology. The efficacy of some psychotropic medications have been tested: mianserine (22), fluoxetine, and methylphenidate (23) have been tested for treating depression, and alprazolam (24) and lorazepam (25) have been tested for treating phobic nausea and vomiting related to chemotherapy. A double-blind, placebo-controlled study has shown that patients receiving fluoxetine reported significantly less psychological distress at the end of the study than patients receiving the placebo (26). In another double-blind, placebo-controlled trial (27), advanced cancer patients were randomly assigned to receive fluoxetine or placebo for 12 weeks. The antidepressant induced significant improvement of quality of life and reduction of depressive symptoms.

Psychotropic medications are generally well tolerated. Drug interactions and altered pharmacokinetics due to the intake of other medications are possible. Clinicians should be careful to possible pharmacokinetic and pharmacodynamic interactions. In a sample of breast cancer patients of known cytochrome P450 2D6 genotype, for example, the antidepressant paroxetine was shown to decrease plasma concentrations of an active tamoxifen metabolite. Among commonly prescribed antidepressants, paroxetine, fluvoxamine, and fluoxetine are potent inhibitors of various cytochrome P450 isoenzymes, while the inhibitory potential of sertraline and citalopram is said to be minimal and not relevant, respectively (28). Venlafaxine and mirtazapine are also weak inhibitors and may, therefore, be used safely with regard to drug interactions (29).

Moreover, one should continue to pay close attention to the unresolved question of lowered or increased cancer risk potentially associated with the use of antidepressants. It can be concluded from the available body of preclinical drug trial and epidemiologic studies that an association between antidepressant use and risk of cancer promotion could neither be excluded nor be established. Further studies specifically addressing this question are strongly needed given the widespread use of antidepressant. The prescription of antidepressants for the treatment of mood and anxiety disorders should be recommended in the meanwhile, since their benefits in reducing level of distress, risk of suicide, and improving quality of life probably exceed the risk of cancer promotion. However, ongoing uncertainties should encourage restraint in the systematic preventive use of psychotropic drugs.

COMMUNICATION
Communication Problems

Physicians are facing everyday communication problems with patients and their relatives: breaking bad news (diagnosis, prognosis, and imminent death), uncontrolled chronic pain, compliance problems, distress, informed consent, euthanasia request, and suicidal ideation. The way to cope with these problems are influenced by physicians' attitudes and self-efficacy about communication, such as fear of death, fear of the unknown, fear of being unable to respond to patients questions, and fear of reactivating patients' distress. Frequently, physicians find hard to communicate appropriately with patients, or to do so without taking too much time. They frequently express a need for communication strategy guidelines to be more patient-centered. Although different definitions are available (30), patient-centeredness can be defined as physicians' behaviors that enable the patient to express his or her perspective on illness and treatment and health-related behavior, his or her symptoms, concerns, ideas, and expectations.

Good communication with a cancer patient is essential in facilitating his or her best possible adjustment. For instance, it enables the patient to anticipate problems, assists rehabilitation, and avoids unnecessary distress (31). For some patients, good communication provides an opportunity to prepare for death, which is sometimes more bearable than a future that is uncertain. Some skills form the basis for a good communication: it implies that physicians use facilitating behaviors (i.e., behaviors that aim to elucidate the patient's perspective on illness and treatment) and avoid inhibiting or blocking behaviors (i.e., behaviors that restrain the patient from expressing his or her view) such as leading or multiple questions, premature information, or reassurance (32). There are three main types of communication skills: evaluative (open and open directive questions, assessing, checking, summarizing), informative (step-by-step information giving), and supportive skills (listening, acknowledging, reassurance giving, empathy, educated guesses). Effective communication is achieved by using appropriately evaluative, informative, and supportive skills. An appropriate combination and sequence of these three different types of skills are useful for obtaining a patient history, breaking bad news, conveying information about treatment, eliciting needs and concerns, reassuring patients, and monitoring the adaptation of patients and their relatives (33).

For assessing the patients' problems, physicians may use open questions, clarification, and checking. Effective communication is facilitated by using open questions, questions with a psychological focus, clarification of psychological aspects, screening questions, and educated guesses (34). Conversely, communication is inhibited by closed questions, leading questions, and by focusing solely on physical aspects. The avoidance of clarifying patients' problems, concerns, and needs may lead to give information, advice, and reassurance prematurely, before the patients' problems concerns and needs have been fully explored. Listening to patients is the only way to evaluate their problems, concerns, needs, and personal resources. Listening is a very difficult task. Listening is facilitated by using techniques that encourage the patient to express him/herself (calm attitude, silence, etc.). Listening requires an empathic attitude, which makes possible to build confidence between the patient and his/her physician, and to obtain information on the emotions and perceptions of the patient. Assessment skills should be integrated into the process of evaluating, for example, the patient's need for information. This process must include an assessment of what the patient already knows and what she or he wishes to know. A step-by-step information should be provided with a step-by-step assessment of what has been understood. After the transmission of an information, these assessments offer an opportunity to check whether the information has been understood.

One of the core component of support is the attention given to patients' present and potential future problems, concerns, and needs. Support is often offered without any previous assessment of these problems, concerns, and needs. Physicians are therefore experiencing difficulties to identify their exact nature and extent and to feel and to recognize their patients emotional reactions. Precise identification and assessment of the patient's problems, concerns, and needs are essential and constitute the first phase of an active support. It enables physicians to understand patients' feelings, and if possible, to anticipate their future reactions: this cognitive understanding underlines the concept of empathy, which is conceptually different from sympathy, which is underlined by physicians' emotional feeling of patients emotions. This understanding may avoid the development of patients' consecutive distress, which is a frequent consequence of a loss of control over poorly assessed outside events: the physician-assisted reevaluation of implications associated with reality often enables the patient to regain control. Reassurance is another core component of support. Reassurances are interventions that focus on, internal resources (for example on the patient's capacity to meet the challenges) or on external resources (for example the possibility of responding to an experimental treatment). Other core components of support include verbal and nonverbal strategies such as setting up the interview and the relationship and the use of silence and empathy.

Learning Communication Skills

Training programs are being developed to improve physicians' communication skills. Cognitive (e.g., theoretical information), experiential (e.g., case-history discussions), behavioral (e.g., role-playing exercises) training techniques are used to teach the essential skills of good communication. Training can range from one-day courses to longer curricula, which require mild to intensive involvement of participants. Most are residential workshops that take place during the weekend and are increasingly organized away from the working environment. There may

be other potential positive effects of these trainings for physicians (attitudes, quality of care, coping with stress, professional growth) and for patients (satisfaction with care, detection of their needs, compliance with treatment, quality of life).

Experiential techniques include case-history discussions, staff observations, and supervisions. During a training session, case-history discussions give the physicians the opportunity to present and analyze practical situations in all their complexity. The benefits of this technique are outlining the personal strategies in communication; heightening the self-awareness of physicians, clarifying the areas to be explored to determine the nature and the extent of the patients' problems; and finally, it also offers opportunities for exchanging information with colleagues about psychological aspects, which is often lacking in clinical practice. To be effective, this technique has to be used in small group sessions to stimulate discussion.

Behavioral techniques include role-playing exercises, patient interviews under observation, and walking rounds. Role-play has been widely used for teaching communication skills. It consists of asking participants during a training session to play different roles (patient, family, nurse, physician, etc.) and then to discuss the simulate interview. Identification with roles enables participants to observe and analyze feelings, attitudes, perceptions, and behaviors induced by clinical practice. It also helps in experimenting with communication strategies, like setting up the interview, getting the patient talk, controlling an interview, using assessment questions before informing, and reassuring. Role-playing is perhaps one of the most formative techniques, but trainers must use the tool carefully, with clear instructions in the secure context of small groups. When scripts are proposed, they should be as close as possible to clinical practice and realistic situations. The use of audio-visual techniques such as videotaped role-playing and video- or audio-taped patient interviews are useful.

In the last two decades, several communication skills training programs have been tested for their efficacy (35–38). In these studies, the main aim of the training programs was to promote the knowledge and the use of communication skills that are able to promote better patient care. Results of these studies have allowed to draw some conclusions as regards training techniques and their effects. Results of these studies confirm the usefulness of communication skills training programs. As it could have been expected, a dose-effect of training on some communication skills learned was found. To be effective, training should include learner-centered, skills-focused, and practice-oriented techniques, be organized in small group (no more than six), and be long enough (at least 20 hours) (39). Training programs should include consolidation sessions to ensure transfer of learned skills to clinical practice (40): a key challenge is to help physicians apply what they have learned in their clinical practice. Consolidation workshops are therefore useful. Distance-learning approach may be also used for individual feedback of audiotape material. Finally, two-way radios are being developed that will enable health care professionals to be supervised during their live interviews with patients or relatives.

CONCLUSIONS

Because of the recognition of the high prevalence of psychological problems and psychopathological disturbances associated with cancer and its treatments, numerous programs are available to prevent and alleviate these disturbances. The respective indications of psychological interventions, psychotropic medications, or both, are based on clinical experience and controlled prospective studies. Research is still needed to improve interventions efficacy. The first step should be to recognize the respective usefulness of single psychological or pharmacological intervention in specific situations along with the best supportive care of the patients. The second step should be to compare different interventions for their efficacy, cost, and feasibility in a cancer setting. The third step should be to test for the possible superior effectiveness of combinations (e.g., nondirective technique with directive technique, individual psychological support with family support, psychological support with psychotropic medication).

To improve the psychological care of cancer patients, physicians must be trained in basic interviewing, assessment, and counseling skills. All physicians should be able to detect and clarify key verbal and nonverbal cues that patients and relatives express (e.g., concerns, problems, and needs), to control the interview and maintain its focus, to acquire precision in assessment strategies (e.g., dates, names, symptom intensity), and to explore emotionally loaded concerns (e.g., wish to die, prognosis, death) in a manner that is helpful and not too distressing or painful. Communication skills training programs designed for physicians dealing regularly with cancer patients and their significant others should be available in all health care settings devoted to cancer care. Consolidation training programs should be available to stimulate the implementation of learned skills. A special effort should also be devoted to help physicians to acquire complementary skills to respond more adequately to the complex problems encountered in oncology. These trainings should prepare physicians to cope with the complexities of difficult clinical situations such as breaking bad news and discussing ethical dilemmas (e.g., informed consent, euthanasia, "do-not resuscitate" orders, deciding curative and palliative treatments).

REFERENCES

1. Derogatis LR, Morrow GR, Fetting J, et al. The prevalence of psychiatric disorders among cancer patients. JAMA 1983; 249: 751–4.
2. McEwen BS. The neurobiology of stress: from serendipity to clinical relevance. Brain Res 2000; 886: 172–89.
3. Miller AH, Ancoli-Israel S, Bower JE, et al. Neuroendocrine-immune mechanisms of behavioral comorbidities in patients with cancer. J Clin Oncol 2008; 26: 971–82.
4. Gidron Y, Ronson A. Psychosocial factors, biological mediators, and cancer prognosis: a new look at an old story. Curr Opin Oncol 2008; 20: 386–92.
5. Chida Y, Hamer M, Wardle J, et al. Do stress-related psychosocial factors contribute to cancer incidence and survival? Nat Clin Pract Oncol 2008; 5: 466–75.
6. Capuron L, Raison CL, Musselman DL, et al. Association of exaggerated HPA axis response to the initial injection of interferon-alpha with development of depression during interferon-alpha therapy. Am J Psychiatry 2003; 160: 1342–5.
7. Passik SD, Roth AJ. Anxiety symptoms and panic attacks preceding pancreatic cancer diagnosis. Psychooncology 1999; 8: 268–72.
8. Endicott J. Measurement of depression in patients with cancer. Cancer 1984; 53(10 Suppl): 2243–9.
9. Spiegel D, Giese-Davis J. Depression and cancer: mechanisms and disease progression. Biol Psychiatry 2003; 54: 269–82.
10. Bovbjerg DH, Montgomery GH, Raptis G. Evidence for classically conditioned fatigue responses in patients receiving chemotherapy treatment for breast cancer. J Behav Med 2005; 28: 231–7.
11. Gurevich M, Devins GM, Rodin GM, et al. Stress response syndromes and cancer: conceptual and assessment issues. Psychosomatics 2002; 43: 259–81.
12. Etkin A, Wager TD. Functional neuroimaging of anxiety: a meta-analysis of emotional processing in PTSD, social anxiety disorder, and specific phobia. Am J Psychiatry 2007; 164: 1476–88.
13. Raison CL, Miller AH. Depression in cancer: new developments regarding diagnosis and treatment. Biol Psychiatry 2003; 54: 283–94.
14. de Ridder D, Geenen R, Kuijer R, et al. Psychological adjustment to chronic disease. Lancet 2008; 372: 246–55.
15. Capuron L, Ravaud A, Miller AH, et al. Baseline mood and psychosocial characteristics of patients developing depressive symptoms during interleukin-2 and/or interferon-alpha cancer therapy. Brain Behav Immun 2004; 18: 205–13.
16. Capuron L, Gumnick JF, Musselman DL, et al. Neurobehavioral effects of interferon-alpha in cancer patients: phenomenology and paroxetine responsiveness of symptom dimensions. Neuropsychopharmacology 2002; 26: 643–52.
17. Razavi D, Delvaux N, Farvacques C, et al. Prevention of adjustment disorders and anticipatory nausea secondary to adjuvant chemotherapy: a double-blind, placebo-controlled study assessing the usefulness of alprazolam. J Clin Oncol 1993; 11: 1384–90.
18. Razavi D, Delvaux N, Farvacques C, et al. Screening for adjustment disorders and major depressive disorders in cancer in-patients. Br J Psychiatry 1990; 156: 79–83.
19. Mitchell AJ. Pooled results from 38 analyses of the accuracy of distress thermometer and other ultra-short methods of detecting cancer-related mood disorders. J Clin Oncol 2007; 25: 4670–81.
20. Jacobsen PB, Jim HS. Psychosocial interventions for anxiety and depression in adult cancer patients: Achievements and challenges. CA Cancer J Clin 2008; 58: 214–30.
21. Redd WH, Montgomery GH, et al. . Behavioral intervention for cancer treatment side effects. J Natl Cancer Inst 2001; 93: 810–23.
22. van Heeringen K, Zivkov M. Pharmacological treatment of depression in cancer patients. A placebo-controlled study of mianserin. Br J Psychiatry 1996; 169: 440–3.
23. Macleod AD. Methylphenidate in terminal depression. J Pain Symptom Manage 1998; 16: 193–8.
24. Greenberg DB, Surman OS, Clarke J, et al. Alprazolam for phobic nausea and vomiting related to cancer chemotherapy. Cancer Treat Rep 1987; 71: 549–50.
25. Malik IA, Khan WA, Qazilbash M, et al. Clinical efficacy of lorazepam in prophylaxis of anticipatory, acute, and delayed nausea and vomiting induced by high doses of cisplatin. A prospective randomized trial. Am J Clin Oncol 1995; 18: 170–5.
26. Razavi D, Allilaire JF, Smith M, et al. The effect of fluoxetine on anxiety and depression symptoms in cancer patients. Acta Psychiatr Scand 1996; 94: 205–10.
27. Fisch MJ, Loehrer PJ, Kristeller J, et al. Fluoxetine versus placebo in advanced cancer outpatients: a double-blinded trial of the Hoosier Oncology Group. J Clin Oncol 2003; 21: 1937–43.

28. Jin Y, Desta Z, Stearns V, et al. CYP2D6 genotype, antidepressant use, and tamoxifen metabolism during adjuvant breast cancer treatment. J Natl Cancer Inst 2005; 97: 30–9.

29. Spina E, Scordo MG, D'Arrigo C. Metabolic drug interactions with new psychotropic agents. Fundam Clin Pharmacol 2003; 17: 517–38.

30. Mead N, Bower P. Patient-centredness: a conceptual framework and review of the empirical literature. Soc Sci Med 2000; 51: 1087–110.

31. Lienard A, Merckaert I, Libert Y, et al. Factors that influence cancer patients' anxiety following a medical consultation: impact of a communication skills training programme for physicians. Ann Oncol 2006; 17: 1450–8.

32. Zandbelt LC, Smets EM, Oort FJ, et al. Patient participation in the medical specialist encounter: does physicians' patient-centred communication matter? Patient Educ Couns 2007; 65: 396–406.

33. Merckaert I, Libert Y, Delvaux N, et al. Factors that influence physicians' detection of distress in patients with cancer: can a communication skills training program improve physicians' detection? Cancer 2005; 104: 411–21.

34. Maguire P, Faulkner A, Booth K, et al. Helping cancer patients disclose their concerns. Eur J Cancer 1996; 32A: 78–81.

35. Razavi D, Delvaux N, Marchal S, et al. The effects of a 24-h psychological training program on attitudes, communication skills and occupational stress in oncology: a randomised study. Eur J Cancer 1993; 29A: 1858–63.

36. Maguire P, Booth K, Elliott C, et al. Helping health professionals involved in cancer care acquire key interviewing skills--the impact of workshops. Eur J Cancer 1996; 32A: 1486–9.

37. Fallowfield L, Jenkins V, Farewell V, et al. Efficacy of a cancer research UK communication skills training model for oncologists: a randomised controlled trial. Lancet 2002; 359: 650–6.

38. Delvaux N, Razavi D, Marchal S, et al. Effects of a 105 hours psychological training program on attitudes, communication skills and occupational stress in oncology: a randomised study. Br J Cancer 2004; 90: 106–14.

39. Merckaert I, Libert Y, Razavi D, et al. Communication skills training in cancer care: where are we and where are we going? Curr Opin Oncol 2005; 17: 319–30.

40. Razavi D, Merckaert I, Marchal S, et al. How to optimize physicians' communication skills in cancer care: results of a randomized study assessing the usefulness of post training consolidation workshops. J Clin Oncol 2003; 21: 3141–9.

22

Inherited Predisposition to Cancer: Genetic Counseling and Clinical Management

Diana M. Eccles

INTRODUCTION

Genetic predisposition to cancer has been recognized for over a century. In the last few decades, the underlying genetic basis for many of these striking familial cancer clusters has been discovered. The revolution in molecular genetic technology during this time has been instrumental in understanding how and which genetic factors influence cancer risks. Some 20% to 30% of patients presenting with common malignancies like breast or colon cancer will have a blood relative who has been diagnosed with the same disease. High-penetrance, dominantly inherited cancer predisposition syndromes are important to recognize because of the substantial risks of cancer especially at young ages. However, as the genes that lead to cancer predisposition are discovered, it is now apparent that less than 5% of all breast or colon cancers arise predominantly because of the inheritance of a single high-penetrance gene mutation (Fig. 22.1). More recently, it has become clear that much of the familial clustering of common cancers, and even many cancers where there is no family history, arise because of a combination of several genetic variants that are frequent in the population and that each increases the risk by a fractional amount above the population's average risk (common, low penetrance alleles) (1–4). The information emerging about these common genetic variants is relevant to a much larger proportion of cancers although the individual absolute associated risks are quite small (5). However, ultimately as more is learned about interactions between this type of gene and the environment and tumor biology, there may be future opportunities to target individuals who might benefit from preventive strategies including chemoprevention (6). These polymorphic genetic variants clearly modify the risk of cancer for a carrier of a high-penetrance gene mutation (7), and variants that influence long-term prognosis are now being identified (8).

The challenge for the immediate future is to understand how all these genetic variants interact and to develop risk assessment models that take genes, environment, interactions, and outcomes into account. This will ultimately enable individuals to receive targeted, rather than general, advice to guide choices about surveillance, prevention, and treatment of cancer. Cancer genetics clinical services focus largely on risk assessment and management for individuals likely to have highly penetrant genetic predisposition syndromes; the family history here is a useful guide to potential modifying factors within a family. Genetic testing is aimed at clarifying future cancer risks for an individual and their relatives. Genetic testing for low-penetrance alleles is not currently clinically useful but may become so when all significant risk alleles have been identified and prospective studies have confirmed their clinical validity. Finally, increasing knowledge of the influence of inherited traits on cancer biology and treatment outcomes will allow oncologists to tailor cancer treatments taking into account the heritable factors.

This chapter explains the broad general concepts and principles that are useful to help in assessing any cancer patient who might have a genetic predisposition to cancer. Some more common genetic cancer predisposition syndromes are then described in a little more detail. These have been selected, as they are sufficiently frequent that the oncologists may come across them from time to time during their regular clinical practice.

INHERITED PREDISPOSITION TO CANCER

The presence of one or more common genetic variant might increase the risk of an individual developing cancer by a similar magnitude to many of the known epidemiological risk factors (1.1–1.5 times the population average risk). The cancer risk however does increase with each additional risk allele, confirming the concept that familial cancer clusters are often due to polygenic influences. In contrast, cancers seen as a result of the highly penetrant but much less-common cancer predisposition syndromes due to single gene mutations are often diagnosed at unusually young ages, are associated with multiple primary cancers in the same individual, and may have treatment implications (see p.386–388). Recognition of a genetic contribution to cancer in the oncology clinic and specifically recognition of the likelihood of an underlying high-risk genetic syndrome will have substantial implication for the wider family of that patient.

RARE MUTATIONS, HIGH PENETRANCE

Less than 5% of all cancers arise because of an inherited mutation in a single gene that confers a high lifetime chance that cancer will develop. This type of highly penetrant gene mutation often gives rise to a striking clustering of cancers amongst blood relatives including young onset, multiple primaries, and many affected relatives. Highly penetrant cancer predisposition genes have considerable clinical implications for the individual, and their diagnosis and management will be the focus of this chapter. Figure 22.2

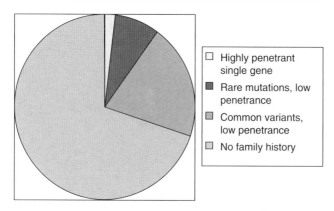

Figure 22.1 Breast cancer cases and estimated proportion of cases due to genetic susceptibility alleles.

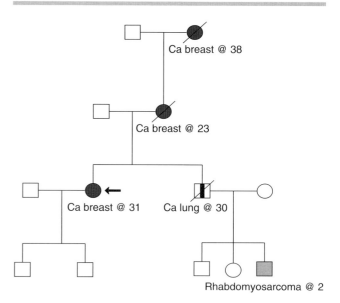

Figure 22.2 A family history due to classic Li Fraumeni Syndrome.

shows a family history due to a mutation in the TP53 gene. This was one of the earliest dominant cancer predisposition genes in which the underlying gene defect was identified (9). TP53 is fundamental to the recognition of DNA damage, cell cycle arrest, and apoptosis (10). This gene is commonly mutated somatically in cancer cells, but inherited mutations are rare. Inherited mutations in the TP53 gene give risk to a condition known as the Li Fraumeni Syndrome first recognized as an association between childhood soft tissue sarcomas and very young onset breast cancer in mothers of these children (11). The spectrum of cancers in this condition is wide, the penetrance is very high, and there is a 10% to 20% risk of childhood malignancy (12). Fortunately LFS is rare (although the incidence is not well defined it certainly affects fewer than 1 in 2000 people. From an oncology perspective though it is more prevalent amongst young breast cancer patients and may underlie up to 7% of breast cancer cases diagnosed before 30 years of age (13).

RARE MUTATIONS WITH LOW PENETRANCE

By understanding and exploring pathways of relevance to cancer development in general, several genes have recently been discovered that when mutated confer a relatively small (around two fold) increase in risk compared with the general population risk. These mutations are rare and in many cases were already known to cause much more severe recessively inherited diseases in individuals who inherit two faulty copies (homozygotes or compound heterozygotes for a mutation). There are several examples of such genes including Ataxia Telangiectasia known initially due to the childhood onset recessive disease but now clearly demonstrated to increase the breast cancer risk in carriers of a single ATM gene mutation a increased childhood malignancy risk and developmental anomalies (14–16). There may be many such genes in which rare mutations lead to a measurable but modest increase in cancer risk, but finding these before cancer develops would currently require full sequencing of potentially many hundreds of genes (many of which are not yet known to be associated with an increased risk). Furthermore,

the management of an individual with a low or even moderate level of increase in cancer risk is still largely based on encouraging a healthy lifestyle and early introduction of cancer surveillance tests. Guidelines advocating surveillance for genetic risks, especially in the moderate increase category, are often based on expert opinion, local resources, and interest, rather than irrefutable evidence of a benefit from the tests advocated. Since many of these mutations affect genes important for DNA repair, it is important to consider whether the risk/benefit ratio of repeated exposure to ionizing radiation, sometimes from quite young ages, is in favor of an overall benefit.

COMMON VARIANTS WITH LOW PENETRANCE

Advances in molecular genetic technologies have lead to the recent completion of many genome wide association studies in a variety of diseases including common cancers. These studies use large numbers of cases with controls (many thousands often) to compare the frequency of genetic variants (usually single nucleotide polymorphisms or SNPs) across the entire genome. Those that occur more commonly in cases than controls, after appropriate statistical corrections, are associated with an increased risk of developing the disease (although are not necessarily causative). Typically these common genetic variants individually confer very small increases in risk (of the order of 1.3–1.5 fold), but appear to act in a multiplicative way so that several risk alleles can potentially increase the cancer associated risk to as much as twice the average population risk (6). Over the next decade, it is likely that many more risk alleles will be identified, and the challenge will be to determine how these interact with each other and with environmental factors in order for them to be applicable in risk determination in the clinic. For the time being, the family history is likely to be as good a guide as genetic testing to risks caused by this type of low-penetrance allele.

None of these genes acts in isolation; high- and low-penetrance genes are likely to interact with each other in a variety of ways as well as being influenced by environmental factors, thereby modifying gene expression and disease penetrance. Even for high-penetrance genetic predisposition then, genetic testing can provide an indication of risk level on the basis of the presence or absence of a single potent genetic risk factor but cannot accurately predict for an individual absolutely if, when and where cancer will develop. Increasingly, it will be possible to study the influence of genetic variants on long-term outlook following cancer diagnosis. Such variants may act by driving phenotypic tumor features that are known to be associated with prognosis, may influence treatment response, or may act independently of these mechanisms. It will be important for these studies to secure DNA samples from individuals entering clinical trials where comprehensive clinical data can be correlated with genetic data.

WHOM TO REFER FOR GENETIC INVESTIGATION

The family pedigree remains the mainstay of genetic risk assessment at all stages from the general practitioner through to the specialist genetic service. As a general rule, the average age at the onset is usually more than a decade younger for cancer in hereditary predisposition syndromes than for the disease in the general population. The following broad principles should alert the oncologist to the possibility of an underlying genetic predisposition to cancer in a patient presenting with malignancy:

- Unusually young age at cancer diagnosis
- More than one primary cancer (bilateral in paired organs or two or more separate primary sites)
- A family history involving multiple affected relative with the same or a related cancer on the same side of the family

However, a striking family history is not always apparent, and a family history of cancer can be obscured for many reasons:

- Small family size
- Genetic or environmental modifiers that have substantially reduced cancer risks for gene carriers in the family
- Paternity not being as stated
- Individual with cancer was adopted or is not in contact with their family
- Paternal transmission of a cancer predisposition predominantly affecting females
- Maternal transmission of a cancer predisposition predominantly affecting males

FAMILIAL CLUSTERING OF CANCERS

Cancer is a common disease affecting one in three individuals in their lifetime. It follows that many individuals are likely to have one or more relative affected by cancer in an extended family. Older/typical age at onset, a variety of primary cancer sites, and evidence of substantial

environmental risk (e.g., smoking and lung cancer) are less likely to be due to high penetrance single genes and more likely to be due to clustering of low-penetrance risk alleles in the family. Patients who have later onset disease and one or two affected relatives at typical ages are less likely to carry a high-risk single gene mutation. However, the increase in risk to other relatives, even if likely to be due to lower penetrance genes, may warrant some additional surveillance strategy above what is offered in the general population.

GENETIC ASSESSMENT

Where the possibility of a single dominant genetic cancer predisposition syndrome is suspected, then referral for further investigation to the clinical genetics service is indicated. The genetic assessment of the cancer family history involves confirmation of key diagnoses where possible to make an accurate assessment of the risk that the cancer predisposition may be hereditary. This helps in making decisions about whether to initiate genetic testing and to advise the individual and their family of the probability of developing the disease and the options available to manage increased cancer risks.

The initiation of genetic testing requires careful consideration of which gene(s) to test and the chance of finding a pathogenic mutation. If genetic testing is undertaken, the clinical interpretation and communication of the results requires careful consideration of the family history and context. Using genetic test information, individuals can be advised of cancer risks and ways in which the genetic condition can be prevented, avoided, or ameliorated.

GENETIC TESTING
Searching for a Pathogenic (Disease Causing) Mutation in Each Family

It is important to recognize that when genetic testing to find a faulty gene is initiated, there are very few situations in which this testing can *exclude* the possibility of a strong genetic predisposition. For a genetic test to be used to exclude a diagnosis of genetic predisposition to cancer, all mutations in all the genes that could possibly predispose to the diagnosis must be detectable (this is almost never true for cancer predisposition genes). The most appropriate starting point for genetic testing is the individual in the family who is most likely to carry the predisposition (this means someone in the family who has been diagnosed with a relevant cancer). For example, a family with a strong history of colon cancer could be due to a mutation in one of a dozen or more genes. Mutations are scattered throughout the coding sequence of these gene: some may be present in the intronic (noncoding) parts of the gene or may affect regulatory sequences, and these intronic and regulatory sequences are not routinely examined in diagnostic testing. Not finding a mutation when a genetic syndrome is suspected may be due to many factors:

- The causative mutation was missed with the technique(s) used.
- The wrong gene was tested.

- The individual tested was a phenocopy (their cancer arose by chance but the rest of the cancers in the family were due to a shared gene mutation not present in the tested individual).

Solutions to these problems might be the following:

- New molecular detection techniques e.g., the development of a robust functional assay that tests the integrity of the molecular pathway in which several gene mutations may lead to the same phenotypic effect
- Identification of all genes that can cause the same phenotypic endpoint
- Testing of a second individual in the family who is likely to be a gene carrier

Predictive Genetic Testing

In this situation, an unaffected family member who is at risk of having inherited a mutation that has been identified in an affected relative is offered a genetic test to clarify their risks (Table 22.1). The probability that the individual has inherited the gene mutation depends on the closeness of relationship to the nearest gene carrier (50% *a priori* risk for first degree relative, 25% for second-degree relatives, and so on). This probability is modified by the ages of the individual to be tested and any intervening unaffected relatives. Once predictive testing has been completed, the tested individual will know their genetic status. For a gene carrier, we can predict a high lifetime chance of developing the relevant cancer(s) (assuming the test is for a rare highly penetrant pathogenic mutation). For an individual who does not carry the gene mutation, the risks are similar to general population risks.

SPECIFIC GENETIC SYNDROMES
Hereditary Breast and Ovarian Cancer

For a patient presenting with young onset breast cancer, genetic predisposition should be considered, as it has implications for future cancer risks for that individual and for their close relatives. Families with four or more affected close relatives with young-onset breast and/or ovarian cancer are likely to be due to a mutation in either the *BRCA1* or *BRCA2* genes. On the other hand, polygenic susceptibility accounts for more than half of families with three or fewer breast cancers particularly where age at onset is similar to that in the general population. Figure 22.3 shows a typical pedigree caused by an inherited mutation in the *BRCA1* gene. The occurrence of ovarian cancer and young-onset breast cancer in four close relatives is highly likely due to a shared mutation in the *BRCA1* gene (or possibly the *BRCA2* gene). The pedigree illustrated in Figure 22.4 is more likely due to polygenic influences (older average age of onset, unaffected intervening female relatives).

Genetic Testing

There are several methods for assessing the likelihood that a pedigree has occurred because of an underlying inherited mutation in *BRCA1* or *BRCA2*. Available methods have variable sensitivity and provide a guide to clinical management but none are specific in relation to an individual (17).

Table 22.1 Predictive Testing for Cancer Predisposition

What will the test result mean for the individual?	A predictive test for a known high risk predisposition gene can tell a person they have a high lifetime risk for the related cancer(s) or that their risk is similar to the population risk. Genetic tests can refine risk assessment but cannot predict with certainty when and where a cancer will occur. They may provide information that helps inform not only choices about risk management but also discussion with the oncologist about cancer treatment.
Is there any means to avoid or ameliorate the consequences if the high risk mutation has been inherited?	The individual must be fully informed about the risk of cancer and the options for surveillance and prevention including the level of evidence that any proposed intervention will be effective. Sometimes a consultation with a surgeon may be appropriate as part of the information gathering process—this may be offered before testing but is more typically part of the detailed exploration of risk reducing surgery options for someone testing positive for a high risk gene.
What is the risk of transmission to other family members?	Some individuals will choose to have genetic testing so that they can inform their children or other relatives whether they need be concerned about genetic cancer risks. If this is the main motivation for seeking testing then their relatives should be involved in the decision about testing. Some may not wish to know and in a situation where there is no known effective intervention available to ameliorate the risk, the genetic information may cause unresolvable anxiety for some individuals—others will find that just knowing gives them a sense of control.
How will the information affect important family relationships?	Where a cancer predisposition syndrome leads to childhood onset of disease and where early surveillance or surgery is clinically important (e.g., the FAP) then testing is usually offered at the age when the intervention will start for gene carriers. Complex responses can arise to genetic testing outcomes reflecting often longstanding background family dynamics, health beliefs, and experience of the genetic disease. Testing of children for adult onset disorders is usually not appropriate and may pose particularly difficult ethical dilemmas. Discuss how the information will be transmitted to the wider family (a general letter giving a brief summary of the genetic condition in the family and advising relatives to seek genetic advice can be useful)
Is the individual seeking testing particularly at risk for an adverse reaction to the test outcome?	A supportive relative, partner, or close friend present through the genetic counseling process is very valuable. Individuals or families with no support or who are psychologically vulnerable may benefit from additional input from an experienced clinical psychologist.

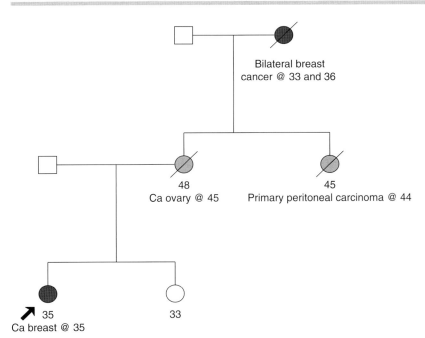

Figure 22.3 A typical family history due to an inherited BRCA1 mutation.

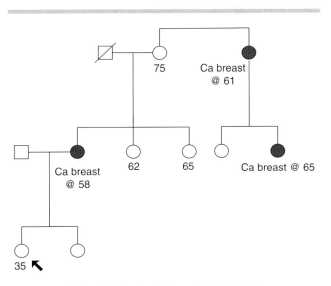

Figure 22.4 Familial non-BRCA1/BRCA2.

Table 22.2 Main Sites of Increased Cancer Risk and Estimated Cumulative Penetrance[a]

Cancer site	BRCA1 (risks are % risk to age 70) (52,53)	BRCA2 (52,53)
Breast	44–78%	31–56%
Ovary	18–54%	2.4–19%
Prostate	May be small increase but conflicting evidence	7.5% (by age 70 years)

[a]Figures are the percentage of gene carriers likely to develop the cancer by age 70 (52,53).

Objective likelihood estimates however perhaps provide a more equitable approach to the fair distribution of the cost of mutation testing if this is conducted as part of a publicly funded healthcare service (18). Furthermore objective assessments of likelihood, where a threshold of likelihood is applied before molecular genetic investigations are initiated, will inevitably find mutations in families with additional factors that increase risk. Additional risk factors in the family are likely to mean the family members can expect a similar higher gene penetrance and in this stimulation more radical interventions such as surgical prevention may be favoured.

As genetic testing becomes cheaper, it may be tempting to request more and more genetic investigations to identify mutations in these genes. However, as the likelihood of finding a pathogenic mutation decreases, the possibility that a variation in the usual wild type sequence of the gene will be found coincidentally becomes relatively greater. These variations in sequence arise as a result of occasional miscopying of DNA during reproduction and are often entirely coincidental to the disease phenotype. However, if the particular mutation in the gene has not been observed to be common in the population from which the patient was drawn, the interpretation of the significance of the variant becomes difficult and can lead to inappropriate consequences. Careful reporting and interpretation by scientists and clinicians with specific expertise in this area is essential to avoid misinterpretation of genetic test results (19).

Hereditary breast and ovarian cancers due to a pathogenic mutation in the *BRCA1* and *BRCA2* genes leads to a high lifetime cancer risks summarized in Table 22.2.

Risk Management

Guidelines vary depending on the country of origin. At present, there is no clear evidence that screening reduces mortality in hereditary breast and ovarian cancer. Breast screening using a combination of mammography, and MRI does detect early breast cancers although a mortality benefit has not yet been demonstrated (20,21). Current approaches to ovarian screening have not so far been shown to lead to earlier detection of the typical serous papillary cystadenocarcinoma of the ovary that develops in *BRCA1* and *BRCA2* gene carriers and new approaches to ovarian screening are needed (22,23). High-risk gene carriers should be encouraged to consider risk reducing salpingo-oophorectomy once childbearing is complete. There is a substantial risk of finding early ovarian or fallopian tube malignancy in gene carriers who undergo risk reducing salpingo-oophoerectomy, so very careful surgical operative procedures are required to minimize the risk of spreading occult malignancy at surgery and a thorough histopathological examination of the removed ovaries and fallopian tubes is essential (24). If occult malignancy is identified, this will require formal staging and may require consideration of adjuvant chemotherapy.

Benefits of Bilateral Salpingo-Oophorectomy

Bilateral oophorectomy may be a therapeutic option to reduce endogenous estrogen for patients presenting with ER positive breast cancer, but the same caveats about careful operative procedures, inclusion of fallopian tubes in the resection, and careful postoperative tissue examination apply. Bilateral oophorectomy has been shown to reduce the future risk of new primary breast cancer for both *BRCA1* and *BRCA2* gene carriers if carried out before the natural menopause (25,26).

Disadvantages of Bilateral Oophorectomy

The risk of menopausal symptoms, which for some women may severely compromise the quality of life, may be a disincentive to early oophorectomy. With no prior history of breast cancer or perhaps where a clearly ER and PR negative breast cancer was diagnosed in the past, low-dose estrogen replacement therapy until the menopause (with endometrial protection as appropriate) should be an option for women who find severe menopausal symptoms are having a significant impact on their quality of life (26). Some women at high risk of developing breast cancer will elect to have bilateral risk-reducing mastectomies, usually with immediate reconstruction although the rate of risk reducing mastectomies varies widely between countries (27).

Hereditary Nonpolyposis Colorectal Cancer (HNPCC or Lynch Syndrome)

Figure 22.5 shows a typical pedigree due to an inherited mutation in the mismatch repair gene hMSH2. There are more than three individuals affected by colon cancer in more than one generation and the average age at first diagnosis is less than 50 years. Endometrial cancer is also highly suggestive of Lynch syndrome (28). Other tumors are also seen more frequently than one would expect by chance including urothelial transitional cell carcinomas,

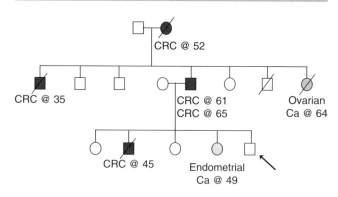

Figure 22.5 Lynch syndrome.

ovarian cancer (often mucinous or endometrioid types), hepatobiliary cancers, small intestinal, and gastric adenocarcinomas (29). Breast and CNS tumors are an infrequently reported association. Keratoacanthomas and both benign and malignant tumors of sebaceous glands are reported in some families and were noted to be a part of the Muir Torre syndrome now known to be part of the HNPCC spectrum.

HNPCC is caused by mutations in one of a family of mismatch repair genes. There are several mismatch repair genes, but the three most commonly implicated in the genetic diagnosis are *hMLH1*, *hMSH2*, and a somewhat smaller proportion of families being due to *hMSH6*. The latter tends to have lower and later penetrance for colon cancer and a more striking endometrial cancer occurrence (28). Biallelic mutations in another mismatch repair gene, *PMS2*, leads to a high risk of primitive neuroectodermal tumors of the CNS in infancy, and can be recognized due to the skin manifestations of multiple café au lait patches and neurofibromas that are more typically seen in Neurofibromatosis Type 1 (16). There may be no family history of colorectal cancer; the penetrance of these mutations in the heterozygous state is not known but is probably not high (both parents of an affected child will carry one faulty copy of the gene and will therefore be heterozygous for the condition).

Polyposis Syndromes

Familial adenomatous polyposis (FAP) is the most frequent hereditary Polyposis syndrome at an estimated incidence of about 1 in 10,000. The underlying gene fault is an inactivating mutation in the APC tumor suppressor gene. The condition is transmitted as a dominant trait with very high penetrance (30). In classic FAP, hundreds to thousands of premalignant adenomatous colonic polyps develop throughout the colon due to somatic mutation in the remaining wild type copy of the gene. Management comprises isolating the mutation for a newly diagnosed individual and offering predictive testing to all relatives. Lower GI colonoscopy is offered from around the time of puberty or before if symptoms arise. Total colectomy is currently the best option to prevent colorectal cancer, and there are a number of surgical options including laparoscopic colectomy (31). Extracolonic manifestations include skin epidermoid cysts, desmoids tumors, gastric fundus polyps, adenomas and carcinoma of the duodenum especially around the Ampulla of Vater, osteomas especially in the skull bones and supernumerary teeth. There is some correlation between the position of the mutation in the gene and disease manifestations, and this can lead to variable clinical presentation (32,33).

A recently discovered genetic condition that clinically can mimic FAP is due to biallelic mutation in the base excision nucleotide repair gene, *MutYH* (34). This is a recessive condition (both copies of the gene need to be mutated before the phenotype appears). This diagnosis should be considered in individuals or sibling presenting with multiple colonic adenomatous neoplasms where neither parent is affected.

There are other rare dominantly inherited conditions that can lead to clustering of GI cancers in families including the following:

- Juvenile polyposis caused by mutations in *BMPR1A*, *SMAD4*, and other genes (polyps are often characteristic of juvenile polyposis but can be very variable) (35,36)
- Peutz Jegher syndrome caused by mutations in STK11 (this diagnosis is usually accompanied by characteristic freckling of skin and mucosal membranes) (37)
- Hereditary mixed polyposis (polyps are usually a mixture of adenomas and hyperplastic polyps, some cases may be caused by mismatch repair gene mutations) (30).

Diagnosis

A careful review of the clinical and pathological features of the index case and possibly expert review of the colorectal pathology is often key to making the correct diagnosis and guiding appropriate genetic testing (30).

Genetic Testing for Colon Cancer Genes

As for most other genes that give rise to cancer predisposition the initial step is to select an individual from the family who clearly has a relevant phenotype and is willing to give a blood sample for testing. For a common disease like colon cancer, it is important to recognize that colon cancer will also occur by chance and selection of the best option for testing is the person in the family most likely to be a gene carrier (for example the case with the youngest age at diagnosis or multiple primary cancers). In some situations, detailed pathology review and additional tumor testing may help select cases for genetic testing. For example, in Lynch syndrome, the presence of microsatellite instability and loss of expression of one of the mismatch repair proteins in tumor tissue helps to guide genetic analysis of the family and can be useful particularly where the family history is not particularly striking (38). Next, the diagnostic lab oratory scientific staff should be properly instructed about the likely clinical diagnosis and the likely gene to be affected; this will depend on family structure, type and pattern of disease, and additional clinical features. Mutation analysis can then be targeted toward the appropriate gene(s). A mutation that differs from the wild type and is predicted to lead to a truncated or absent protein product confirms the diagnosis and provides a predictive test for at risk relatives. Not finding a mutation

does not refute a clinical diagnosis and may occur for the same reasons as outlined on p. 381.

Management

Guidelines for surveillance, prevention, and treatment are developed to take into account the cancer risks and the typical ages of presentation observed in a genetic condition. Many conditions that lead to a high genetic risk of developing cancer are rare, so in any one center, there is often limited experience. Guidelines may develop out of a group with a particular research interest, and may also be agreed by large international consortia. There are inevitably country and center variations, which are sometimes shaped by experience rather than constructed by a systematic review of evidence of benefit but for the more common genetic conditions surveillance protocols are largely evidence- and consensus-based.

For HNPCC, most guidelines advocate colonoscopy surveillance every one to two years starting at 25 years for those who carry the gene mutation (39).

For FAP, screening starts at 10 to 12 years of age annually and when polyps become numerous a subtotal or total colectomy is the treatment of choice. A subtotal colectomy requires continuing surveillance of the remaining rectum (31).

For other polyposis syndromes in general, surveillance also starts in the teens with colonoscopy and continues annually until polyp load or dysplasia result in the need for prophylactic removal of the colon.

For familial colorectal cancer predisposition, examination of the colonic pathology (see tumour pathology section) and the clinical picture can help to weigh against a diagnosis of HNPCC or one of the polyposis syndromes. In such families polygenic etiology is the most likely explanation; like breast cancer, this will be the explanation for the majority of families with two or three: cancers where onset is after 50 and affected relatives are interspersed with older unaffected relatives. Colonic tumors are usually microsatellite stable (MSS), and a less intensive surveillance regimen is indicated in these families (40).

Hereditary Renal Carcinoma

For a patient presenting with renal carcinoma at an unusually young age or where there was more than one renal tumor in the same individual or there are other family members affected with renal cancer, there may be an underlying genetic explanation. Review of the renal tumor cell type(s) can be valuable. Table 22.3 summarizes some of the genetic conditions that can present with renal carcinoma, the type of pathology typically seen, and the associated features.

TUMOR PATHOLOGY

Knowledge about histopathological tumor type may help guide genetic investigations to an underlying genetic diagnosis.

Breast Cancer

BRCA1 and BRCA2 tumors are typically of higher histological grade than average (BRCA1 tumors are often

Table 22.3 Possible Genetic Diagnoses for Patients with Multiple or Very Young Onset Renal Tumors

Syndrome	Gene (location)	Pathology of renal tumors	Associated features
Von Hippel Lindau disease	VHL (3p25)	Clear cell carcinoma, adenomas, and cysts	Retinal, cerebellar and spinal angiomas, pancreatic cysts, pheochromocytomas
Birt-Hogg-Dubé syndrome	Folliculin (17p11.2)	Oncocytomas and all other types	Fibrofolliculomas of skin, spontaneous pneumothorax due to congenital bullae
Familial papillary renal cell carcinoma	c-MET (7q31)	Multiple bilateral papillary renal cell carcinomas	
Tuberous sclerosis	TSC1, Hamartin (9q34) TSC2, Tuberin (16p13)	Angiomyolipomas	CNS hamartomas and gliomas, cardiac rhabdomyomas angiofibromas (face), ungual fibromas
Chromosomal translocation, chromosome 3	3p (not the VHL locus)	Multiple bilateral clear cell renal carcinomas	

grade 3, ER, PR, and HER2 negative tumors), more detailed immunophenotyping shows that they are typically but not exclusively similar to the basal subgroup of breast tumors (41). BRCA2 tumors are less distinctive but tend to be of higher nuclear grade and are more often ER and PR positive and are usually HER2 negative (42). Familial non-BRCA1/BRCA2—mostly due to polygenic and environmental factors—is typically lower grade (43). None of the pathological features is diagnostic of an underlying BRCA1 or BRCA2 mutation but can help to weight the probability of finding a mutation in a high-risk predisposition gene.

Colorectal Neoplasia

Review of the type of colorectal polyps found in family members can be helpful for example hyperplastic polyps are rare in FAP but more likely in HNPCC. Multiple juvenile polyps are suggestive of JPS, but these are can be reported as inflammatory or hyperplastic or many other types of polyp (36).

For HNPCC, the pathology can be critical. The tumors arise due to loss of the ability to repair copying errors arising as a result of in misaligned DNA commonly seen in areas of repetitive DNA sequence. Accumulation of replication errors is the underlying molecular pathology in cancer generally and colonic neoplasia in Lynch syndrome progresses rapidly to carcinoma once initiated. The underlying deficiency in DNA repair can be demonstrated by examining the colon cancer for signs of mismatch repair deficiency.

Antibodies to the proteins produced by each of the mismatch repair genes can be used to examine protein expression with immunohistochemistry. Loss of expression of an MMR protein (Fig. 22.6A) implies loss of normal function which may be due entirely to somatic loss of function or may be due to an underlying inherited mutation in one copy followed by loss of the second copy due to somatic mutation or epigenetic silencing (38).

Mismatch repair deficiency due to loss of function in both copies of a mismatch repair gene in the tumor, manifests as multiple additional alleles in tumor DNA compared with normal tissue. DNA repair is effective in tissues where there is still one normal copy of the MMR gene (Fig. 22.6B).

No evidence of microsatellite instability in a colorectal tumor (a microsatellite stable or MSS tumor) may be due to any of the following possible explanations:

- There is no underlying mismatch repair gene deficiency.
- The tumor tested arose by chance (i.e., is a phenocopy) other members of the family or other tumors from the individual may show MMR deficiency.
- There is too much normal tissue mixed with tumor cells to be able to observe the MSI phenotype.

Immunohistochemistry can be used to stain tumor tissue for mismatch repair gene protein products. Loss of expression of one or more of the mismatch repair genes is indicative of loss of function in one of the mismatch repair genes. This tumor-based testing can be useful in assessing whether a colon cancer is likely to have arisen due to an underlying error in one of the mismatch repair genes. This might have arisen somatically or it might be an inherited predisposition. Somatic loss of function due to hypermethylation of the hMLH1 mismatch repair gene accounts for some 10% to 15% of all colorectal cancers. In the context of a young-onset tumor or a family history of the disease, MSI and aberrant expression of one of the MMR proteins warrants referral of the individual to the clinical genetic services for further investigation including genetic testing after appropriate counseling (38).

Where the likelihood is low that the colorectal cancer has arisen due to a mismatch repair gene defect or one of the polyposis syndromes, colonic surveillance guidelines suggest a later start and less frequent colonoscopy surveillance and this is often guided by the pattern of cancers and age at onset for the family seeking advice.

Gynecological Malignancies

Ovarian cancer can arise as part of a genetic predisposition syndrome—most commonly hereditary breast and ovarian cancer (HBOC—due to BRCA1 or BRCA2) or HNPCC. In *BRCA1* and *BRCA2* gene carriers the most common histological type of ovarian cancer is serous papillary cystadenocarcinomas which typically present at advanced stages and do not appear to be amenable to early detection using current approaches (23). Ovarian tumors of borderline

(A)

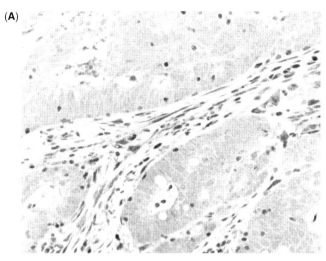

(B)

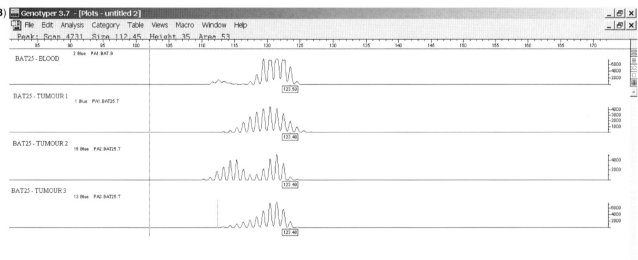

Figure 22.6 **(A)** Immunohistochemistry, colon tumor block stained with antibodies to hMSH2 showing loss of nuclear staining in tumor tissue and normal (brown) staining in stromal cells; *See Color Plate on Page xii.* **(B)** DNA extracted from blood shows a range of alleles due to some slippage during DNA amplification by PCR. The three DNA samples extracted from tumors from the same patient show clear evidence of microsatellite instability with multiple additional alleles (peaks) compared to blood, this is particularly obvious in tumor 2.

malignant potential are underrepresented and this patho-logical subtype of ovarian cancer contributes very little to the estimate of likelihood of finding an underlying *BRCA1* or *BRCA2* mutation (44).

In HNPCC the ovarian tumors are more frequently mucinous or endometrioid (unpublished data) and more likely to present at earlier stages than in *BRCA1* and *BRCA2* (44). Endometrial cancer risk is higher than ovarian cancer risk for women with Lynch syndrome, and of course, the two may occur coincidentally.

SYSTEMIC TREATMENTS

Cytotoxic treatments in general exert their therapeutic effect by damaging DNA to destroy the ability of rapidly dividing cells to proliferate. Many of the genes that predispose to cancer are genes involved in DNA repair mechanisms. The genetic predisposition syndromes are relatively uncommon and probably underdiagnosed and any single oncologist will have limited experience of patients with genetic predisposition to cancer.

When a cancer is diagnosed the treatment options discussed are aimed at around reducing the risk of meta-static disease developing. There is a trade off between tox-icity of treatment (both short and long term), either surgical or cytotoxic and the benefit of treatment in terms of reduc-ing the risk of recurrence. With hereditary cancer there is the additional concern about an increased risk of further primary tumors that may encourage more extensive sur-gery. The likelihood of developing metastatic disease from the presenting cancer and the treatment options for that must be clearly discussed and ideally separated from dis-cussion about the likelihood of developing a new primary cancer at some time in the future and options for reducing that risk. The patient must understand this difference and which management option applies to which risk in order to make a rational choice about treatment options.

Currently, there is no evidence that acute toxicity from cytotoxic treatments is increased in the more frequently encountered cancer predisposition syndromes, specifically BRCA1 and BRCA2 and the Lynch syndrome. However, there is evidence that the cytotoxic agents employed in managing the cancers may be more or less effective than average because of the particular subtype of cancer that these patients are more likely to develop. For example, *BRCA1* gene carriers tend to develop breast cancers that fit into the basal subgroup and may be relatively resistant to mitotic spindle poisons such as taxanes and have increased sensitivity to platinum salts (46,47). Prognosis for patients with MSI tumors is improved overall and there appears to be little survival benefit for giving adjuvant 5FU to a patient with a colon cancer due to a mismatch repair gene defect although further data are needed in this area both for sporadic and HNPCC associated MSI colon cancers (48).

The tumor types seen in association with hereditary predisposition also have their sporadic counterpart, prob-ably due in the main to somatic silencing of the relevant gene as part of the multistep process of carcinogenesis (49,50). Development of novel therapies that target an under-lying genetic defect that is predictably present in cancers arising in those with a strong genetic predisposition provides great promise for the near future. Furthermore, the geneti-cally predisposed population provides an excellent group in which to test approaches to cancer prevention (51). Novel therapies may be most useful in numerical terms to pre-venting or treating sporadic cancers of the same type. For example, the PARP inhibitor class of drugs was developed and entered clinical trials very quickly compared to many more conventional cytotoxic drugs (52). The enzyme PARP is involved in repairing single strand DNA breaks; when breaks in a single strand of DNA are not efficiently repaired by the cell a double strand break ensues. Double strand break repair requires a range of proteins including BRCA1 and BRCA2 to be present. When cells have no normal functioning BRCA1 or BRCA2 and experience excessive single strand DNA breaks due to inhibition of the PARP enzyme, mitotic chaos follows. One normally functioning copy of the gene seems to be sufficient for double strand break repair so the only effect of the drug is in BRCA null (cancer) cells.

SUMMARY

The oncologist is in a good position to identify individuals with a genetic predisposition to cancer and initiate referral to genetic services for further investigation. The family history is the key tool for evaluating genetic risks however there are certain features in an individual cancer patient that might suggest the possibility of a high risk genetic predisposition. Recognition of genetic predisposition to cancer is important to manage risks for other family mem-bers and increasingly will become relevant for the targeted treatment of the cancer patient her/himself.

ACKNOWLEDGMENTS

I thank Dr. Adrian Bateman HNPCC immunohistochem-istry (Fig. 6A) and Dr. Ester Cross for the MSI illustration (Fig. 6B).

REFERENCES

1. Easton DF, Pooley KA, Dunning AM et al. Genome-wide association study identifies novel breast cancer susceptibility loci. Nature 2007; 447: 1087–93.
2. Hunter DJ, Kraft P, Jacobs KB et al. A genome-wide associa-tion study identifies alleles in FGFR2 associated with risk of sporadic postmenopausal breast cancer. Nat Genet 2007; 39: 870–4.
3. Tomlinson IP, Webb E, Carvajal-Carmona L et al. A genome-wide association study identifies colorectal cancer susceptibil-ity loci on chromosomes 10p14 and 8q23.3. Nat Genet 2008; 40: 623–30.
4. Eeles RA, Kote-Jarai Z, Giles GG et al. Multiple newly iden-tified loci associated with prostate cancer susceptibility. Nat Genet 2008; 40: 316–21.
5. Bodmer W, Bonilla C. Common and rare variants in multi-factorial susceptibility to common diseases. Nat Genet 2008; 40: 695–701.
6. Pharoah PD, Antoniou AC, Easton DF et al. Polygenes, risk prediction, and targeted prevention of breast cancer. N Engl J Med 2008; 358: 2796–803.
7. Antoniou AC, Spurdle AB, Sinilnikova OM et al. Common breast cancer-predisposition alleles are associated with breast

cancer risk in BRCA1 and BRCA2 mutation carriers. Am J Hum Genet 2008; 82: 937–48.

8. Fagerholm R, Hofstetter B, Tommiska J et al. NAD(P)H: quinone oxidoreductase 1 NQO1(*)2 genotype (P187S) is a strong prognostic and predictive factor in breast cancer. Nat Genet 2008; 40: 844–53.

9. Malkin D, Li FP, Strong LC et al. Germ line p53 mutations in a familial syndrome of breast cancer, sarcomas, and other neoplasms. Science 1990; 250: 1233–8.

10. Lane DP. Cancer. p53, guardian of the genome. Nature 1992; 358: 15–16.

11. Li FP, Fraumeni JF Jr, Mulvihill JJ et al. A cancer family syndrome in twenty-four kindreds. Cancer Res 1988; 48: 5358–62.

12. Olivier M, Goldgar DE, Sodha N et al. Li-fraumeni and related syndromes: correlation between tumor type, family structure, and TP53 genotype. Cancer Res 2003; 63: 6643–50.

13. Gonzalez KD, Noltner KA, Buzin CH et al. Beyond Li Fraumeni Syndrome: Clinical Characteristics of Families With p53 Germline Mutations. J Clin Oncol 2009; 27: published online Feb 9th.

14. Seal S, Thompson D, Renwick A et al. Truncating mutations in the Fanconi anemia J gene BRIP1 are low-penetrance breast cancer susceptibility alleles. Nat Genet 2006; 38: 1239–41.

15. Renwick A, Thompson D, Seal S et al. ATM mutations that cause ataxia-telangiectasia are breast cancer susceptibility alleles. Nat Genet 2006; 38: 873–5.

16. De Vos VM, Hayward BE, Charlton R et al. PMS2 mutations in childhood cancer. J Natl Cancer Inst 2006; 98: 358–61.

17. Antoniou A, Hardy R, Walker L et al. Predicting the likelihood of carrying a BRCA1 or BRCA2 mutation: validation of BOADICEA, BRCAPRO, IBIS, Myriad and the Manchester scoring system using data from UK genetics clinics. J Med Genet 2008; 45: 425–31.

18. Hopper JL, Dowty JG, Apicella C et al. Towards more effective and equitable genetic testing for BRCA1 and BRCA2 mutation carriers. J Med Genet 2008; 45: 409–10.

19. Plon S, Eccles DM, Easton D et al. IARC unclassified genetic variants working group. Sequence variant classification and reporting: recommendations for improving the clinical utility of cancer susceptibility genetic test results. Hum Mutat 2008; 29: 1282–91.

20. Leach MO, Boggis CR, Dixon AK et al. Screening with magnetic resonance imaging and mammography of a UK population at high familial risk of breast cancer: a prospective multicentre cohort study (MARIBS). Lancet 2005; 365: 1769–78.

21. Kuhl CK. High-risk screening: multi-modality surveillance of women at high risk for breast cancer (proven or suspected carriers of a breast cancer susceptibility gene). J Exp Clin Cancer Res 2002; 21(3 Suppl): 103–6.

22. Stirling D, Evans DG, Pichert G et al. Screening for familial ovarian cancer: Failure of current protocols to detect ovarian cancer at an early stage according to the International Federation of Gynecology and Obstetrics System. J Clin Oncol 2005; 23: 5588–96.

23. Hogg R, Friedlander M. Biology of epithelial ovarian cancer: implications for screening Women at high genetic risk. J Clin Oncol 2004; 22: 1315–27.

24. Callahan MJ, Crum CP, Medeiros F et al. Primary fallopian tube malignancies in BRCA-positive women undergoing surgery for ovarian cancer risk reduction. J Clin Oncol 2007; 25: 3985–90.

25. Kauff ND, Domchek SM, Friebel TM et al. Risk-reducing salpingo-oophorectomy for the prevention of BRCA1- and BRCA2-associated breast and gynecologic cancer: A multicenter, prospective study. J Clin Oncol 2008; 26: 1331–7.

26. Rebbeck TR, Friebel T, Wagner T et al. Effect of short-term hormone replacement therapy on breast cancer risk reduction after bilateral prophylactic oophorectomy in BRCA1 and BRCA2 mutation carriers: the PROSE Study Group. J Clin Oncol 2005; 23: 7804–10.

27. Metcalfe KA, Lubinski J, Ghadirian P et al. Predictors of contralateral prophylactic mastectomy in women with a BRCA1 or BRCA2 mutation: The Hereditary Breast Cancer Clinical Study Group. J Clin Oncol 2008; 26: 1093–7.

28. Lynch HT, Boland CR, Rodriguez-Bigas MA et al. Who should be sent for genetic testing in hereditary colorectal cancer syndromes? J Clin Oncol 2007; 25: 3534–42.

29. Watson P, Vasen HF, Mecklin JP et al. The risk of extra-colonic, extra-endometrial cancer in the Lynch syndrome. Int J Cancer 2008; 123: 444–9.

30. Jass JR. Colorectal polyposes: from phenotype to diagnosis. Pathol Res Pract 2008; 204: 431–47.

31. Vasen HF, Moslein G, Alonso A et al. Guidelines for the clinical management of familial adenomatous polyposis (FAP). Gut 2008; 57: 704–13.

32. Eccles DM, van der LR, Breukel C et al. Hereditary desmoid disease due to a frameshift mutation at codon 1924 of the APC gene. Am J Hum Genet 1996; 59: 1193–201.

33. Spirio LN, Samowitz W, Robertson J et al. Alleles of APC modulate the frequency and classes of mutations that lead to colon polyps. Nat Genet 1998; 20: 385–8.

34. Al-Tassan N, Chmiel NH, Maynard J et al. Inherited variants of MYH associated with somatic G:C-->T:A mutations in colorectal tumors. Nat Genet 2002; 30: 227–32.

35. Chow E, Macrae F. A review of juvenile polyposis syndrome. J Gastroenterol Hepatol 2005; 20: 1634–40.

36. Aretz S, Stienen D, Uhlhaas S et al. High proportion of large genomic deletions and a genotype phenotype update in 80 unrelated families with juvenile polyposis syndrome. J Med Genet 2007; 44: 702–9.

37. McGarrity TJ, Amos C. Peutz-Jeghers syndrome: clinicopathology and molecular alterations. Cell Mol Life Sci 2006; 63: 2135–44.

38. Hampel H, Frankel WL, Martin E et al. Screening for the Lynch syndrome (hereditary nonpolyposis colorectal cancer). N Engl J Med 2005; 352: 1851–60.

39. Vasen HFA, Moslein G, Alonso A et al. Guidelines for the clinical management of Lynch syndrome (hereditary nonpolyposis cancer). J Med Genet 2007; 44: 353–62.

40. Dove-Edwin I, de Jong AE, Adams J et al. Prospective results of surveillance colonoscopy in dominant familial colorectal cancer with and without Lynch syndrome. Gastroenterology 2006; 130: 1995–2000.

41. Lakhani SR, Reis-Filho JS, Fulford L et al. Prediction of BRCA1 status in patients with breast cancer using estrogen receptor and basal phenotype. Clin Cancer Res 2005; 11: 5175–80.

42. Phillips KA. Immunophenotypic and pathologic differences between BRCA1 and BRCA2 hereditary breast cancers. J Clin Oncol 2000; 18(21 Suppl): 107S–12S.

43. Lakhani SR, Gusterson BA, Jacquemier J et al. The pathology of familial breast cancer: histological features of cancers in families not attributable to mutations in BRCA1 or BRCA2. Clin Cancer Res 2000; 6: 782–9.

44. Evans DG, Young K, Bulman M et al. Probability of BRCA1/2 mutation varies with ovarian histology: results from screening 442 ovarian cancer families. Clin Genet 2008; 73: 338–45.

45. Prat J, Ribe A, Gallardo A. Hereditary ovarian cancer. Hum Pathol 2005; 36: 861–70.

46. Quinn JE, Kennedy RD, Mullan PB et al. BRCA1 functions as a differential modulator of chemotherapy-induced apoptosis. Cancer Res 2003; 63: 6221–8.

47. Bhattacharyya A, Ear US, Koller BH et al. The breast cancer susceptibility gene BRCA1 is required for subnuclear assembly

of Rad51 and survival following treatment with the DNA cross-linking agent cisplatin. J Biol Chem 2000; 275: 23899–903.

48. Ribic CM, Sargent DJ, Moore MJ et al. Tumor microsatellite-instability status as a predictor of benefit from fluorouracil-based adjuvant chemotherapy for colon cancer. N Engl J Med 2003; 349: 247–57.

49. Turner NC, Reis-Filho JS, Russell AM et al. BRCA1 dysfunction in sporadic basal-like breast cancer. Oncogene 2007; 26: 2126–32.

50. Domingo E, Laiho P, Ollikainen M et al. BRAF screening as a low-cost effective strategy for simplifying HNPCC genetic testing. J Med Genet 2004; 41: 664–8.

51. Burn J, Bishop DT, Mecklin J-P et al. A randomised controlled trial of aspirin and resistant starch to prevent colorectal neoplasia in Lynch Syndrome (HNPCC): The CAPP2 Study. N Engl J Med 2008; in press.

52. McCabe N, Turner NC, Lord CJ et al. Deficiency in the repair of DNA damage by homologous recombination and sensitivity to poly(ADP-ribose) polymerase inhibition. Cancer Res 2006; 66: 8109–15.

53. Antoniou A, Pharoah PD, Narod S et al. Average risks of breast and ovarian cancer associated with BRCA1 or BRCA2 mutations detected in case series unselected for family history: a combined analysis of 22 studies. Am J Hum Genet 2003; 72: 1117–30.

54. Levy-Lahad E, Friedman E. Cancer risks among BRCA1 and BRCA2 mutation carriers. Br J Cancer 2007; 96: 11–15.

Appendix

Gianluca Del Conte and Cristiana Sessa

Glossary of Terminology Used in Clinical Pharmacokinetics

Absolute bioavailability is the fraction of drug absorbed upon extravascular administration in comparison to the dose administered.

Area under the curve (AUC∞) is a measure of quantity of unchanged drug absorbed and in the body, calculated as the integral of drug plasma or blood levels over time from zero to infinity.

Bioavailability (F) is the fraction of drug systemically available, defined as both the fraction of the administered dose absorbed and the fraction of absorbed dose reaching systemic circulation in the presence of first-pass effect.

Central compartment is the sum of all body regions (organs and tissue) in which the drug concentration is in instantaneous equilibrium with that in blood or plasma. Blood or plasma is always part of the central compartment.

Compartment is a mathematical entity that can be described by a definite volume and a concentration of drug contained in it. In pharmacokinetics, experimental data are explained by fitting them to compartmental models.

Cumulative urinary excretion curves are plots of the actual cumulative amounts of drug and/or its metabolites excreted into urine versus time after administration.

Disposition is the loss of drug from the central compartment due to distribution into other compartments and/or elimination and metabolism.

Dose or concentration dependence refers to a change of one or more of the pharmacokinetic processes of absorption, distribution, metabolism, and excretion with increasing dose or concentration.

Elimination half-life (T$_{1/2}$) of a drug is the time required for the drug levels (in blood, plasma or serum) to decline by 50% after equilibrium (between plasma and tissue) is reached. Loss of drug from the body, as described by the biologic half-life, means the elimination of the administered parent drug molecule (not its metabolites) by urinary excretion (renal clearance), metabolism (metabolic clearance), or other pathways of elimination (lung, skin, etc.). It includes T$_{1/2}$α (distribution) and T$_{1/2}$β (terminal). T$_{1/2}$ may be influenced by dose, variation in urinary excretion (pH), intersubject variation, age, protein binding, concomitant drugs, and liver and renal functions.

Enzyme induction is the increase in enzyme content or rate of enzymatic processes resulting in faster metabolism of a compound. It may increase clearance and decrease biologic half-life.

Enzyme inhibition is the decrease in rate of metabolism of a compound, usually by competition for an enzyme system. It may increase biologic half-life and decrease clearance of a drug.

First-pass effect is the phenomenon in which some drugs are already *metabolized* (not chemically degraded) between site of absorption and reaching systemic circulation. It may occur in the gut wall, mesenteric blood, and/or in the liver, upon oral and deep rectal administration.

Hepatic clearance (CL$_H$) is the hypothetical volume of distribution in liters of the unmetabolized drug that is cleared in one minute via the liver. It depends on intrinsic hepatic clearance and liver blood flow.

Loading dose, priming dose or initial dose is the dose used in initiating therapy to rapidly achieve therapeutic concentrations. The need for a loading dose depends on biological half-life, dosing interval, and therapeutic concentration to be achieved.

Mean residence time (MRT) is the average time that the drug stays in the body or plasma.

Nonlinear kinetics or saturation kinetics refer to a change of one or more of the pharmacokinetic parameters during absorption, distribution, metabolism, or excretion caused by saturation or overloading because of increasing doses.

Peak concentrations (C$_{max}$) is the maximal concentration of a drug achieved in plasma or in blood after drug administration.

Peripheral compartment is the sum of all body regions (i.e., organs, tissues, or parts of them) to which a drug is eventually distributed, but is not in instantaneous equilibrium with the central compartment.

Plasma clearance (CL) can be defined as the volume of plasma that is completely cleared of drug per unit time.

Protein binding is the phenomenon that occurs when a drug combines with plasma protein to form a reversible complex. Some drugs can be displaced from protein binding by other compounds of higher affinity for the protein-binding sites. Protein binding is of clinical significance (i.e., with regard to displacement, volume of distribution, metabolism) when it exceeds 80% to 90%. It is the unbound drug that is in equilibrium with the biophase (FF).

Renal clearance (CL$_R$) is the hypothetical plasma volume in liters (volume of distribution) of the unmetabolized drug that is cleared per unit time via the kidney. Renal clearance is affected by renal blood flow, urinary pH, and the net effects of tubular reabsorption and secretion.

Steady-state (C$_{ss}$) is the concentration of drug in blood and tissue on multiple dosing when input and output are at equilibrium or during a constant-rate intravenous infusion.

Time to peak concentration (T$_{max}$) is the time until C$_{max}$ is reached from drug administration.

Total body clearance (CL$_b$) is an overall measure of the body's drug removal rate. CL$_b$ is the result of all drug removal processes, including renal clearance of the unchanged drug and metabolic clearance. CL$_b$ is the hypothetical volume of distribution in liters of the unmetabolized drug which is cleared per unit of time (L/min or L/hr) by any pathway of drug removal (renal, hepatic, and other pathways of elimination); it is a proportionality constant relating absorbed dose and steady-state blood, plasma, and serum concentration.

Volume of distribution at steady state (V$_{dss}$) is the hypothetical volume of body fluid that would be required to dissolve the total amount of drug at the same concentration as that found in blood or plasma. It is a proportionality constant that relates the amount of drug in body to the serum or plasma concentration.

List of abbreviations

Drugs	Other
2-Cda: cladribine	
2-CdATP: 2-chlorodeoxyadenosine triphosphate	
2-F-ara-AMP: fludarabine phosphate	
	4E-BP1: factor 4E binding protein 1
5-CHO-FH$_4$: 5-formyltetrahydrofolate (leucovorin)	**5′DFCR**: 5′-deoxy-5-fluorocytidine
5-FU: 5-fluorouracil	**5′DFUR**: 5′-deoxy-5-fluorouridine
6-MP: 6-mercaptopurine	
6-TG: 6-thioguanine	
6-TGN: 6-thioguanine nucleotides	
A: androgen	**AAGP**: α-I-acid glycoprotein
AG: aminoglutethimide	**ADA**: adenosine deaminase
AI: aromatase inhibitors	**ADCC**: antibody-dependent cell-mediated cytotoxicity
AMSA: amsacrine	**AG**: antigen
Ara-C: cytarabine	**AICAR**: aminoimidazole carboxamide ribonucleotide transformylase
	ALL: acute lymphoblastic leukemia
	ALT: alanine transaminase
	AML: Acute myeloid leukemia
	ANC: absolute neutrophil count
	AP: alkaline phosphatase
	APC: 7-ethyl-10-[4-*N*-(5-aminopentanoic acid-1-piperidino]carbonyloxycamptothecin
	APL: acute promyelocytic leukemia
	AR: androgen receptor
	Ara-U: uracil arabinoside
	Ara-CTP: cytosine arabinoside triphosphate
	ARDS: acute respiratory distress syndrome
	AST: aspartate aminotransferase
	ATP: adenosine triphosphate
BLM: bleomycin	**basic FGF**: basic fibroblast growth factor
	BBB: blood-brain barrier
	b.i.d: bis in die
	BM: bone marrow
	BMT: bone marrow transplantation
	BP: blood pressure
	BUN: Blood Urea Nitrogen
CTX: cyclophosphamide	**CBC**: complete blood count
	CDC: complement-dependent cytotoxicity
	CdR kinase: deoxycytidine kinase
	CGCL: Cockcroft-Gaultt creatinine clearance
	CH$_2$-FH$_4$: reduced-folate cofactor
	CHF: cardiac heart failure
	CI: continuous infusion
	CLL: Chronic lymphocytic leukemia
	CNS: central nervous system

Drugs	Other
CTX: cyclophosphamide (*Continued*)	**COMT**: catechol-*O*-methyltransferase
	COPD: chronic obstructive pulmonary disease
	CPK: creatine phosphokinase
	CR: complete remission
	Cr: serum creatinine
	CRC: colorectal cancer
	CrCL: creatinine clearance
	CSF: cerebrospinal fluid
	CTCL: cutaneous T-cell lymphoma
	Cyd deaminase: cytidine deaminase
	CYP450: cytochrome P450
	CVC: central venous catheter
DACT: dactinomycin	**dATP**: deoxyadenosine triphosphate
dCF: pentostatin (2-deoxycoformycin)	**dCTP**: deoxycytidine-5′-triphosphate
DDP: cisplatin	**DES**: diethylstilbestrol
dFdC: difluorodeoxycytidine	**dFdCTP**: difluorodeoxycytidine triphosphate
dFdU: difluorodeoxyuridine	**DHFR**: dihydrofolate reductase
DHAD: mitoxantrone	**DIC**: disseminated intravascular coagulation
DNR: daunorubicin	**DL**: dose-limiting
DTIC: dacarbazine	**dNTP**: deoxynucleotide triphosphate
DOX: doxorubicin	**DPD**: dihydropyrimidine dehydrogenase
	DSB: double strand breaks
	dTTP: deoxythymidine triphosphate
	DVT: deep venous thrombosis
	DXM: dexamethasone
E: estrogen	**EGF**: epidermal growth factor
EDTA: ethylenediaminetetraacetic acid	**EGFR**: epidermal growth factor receptor
EPI: epirubicin	**EIA**: enzyme-inducing anticonvulsant
	ER: estrogen receptors
FT: tegafur	**F-DHU**: 5-fluorodihydrouracil
FUDR: floxuridine	**FdUMP**: 5-fluoro-2′deoxyuridine-5′monophosphate
	FH$_4$: reduced folates
	FISH: fluorescence in situ hybridization
	FN: febrile neutropenia
	FPGS: folylpolyglutamate synthethase
	FUMP: 5-fluorouridine-5′monophosphate
	FUTP: 5-fluorouridine-5′-triphosphate
GEM: gemcitabine	**G-CSF**: granulocyte colony-stimulating factor
	GARFT: glycinamide ribonucleotide transformylase
	GFR: glomerular filtration rate
	GI: gastrointestinal
	GIST: gastrointestinal stromal tumors
	Gn: gonadotrophin
	GnRH: gonadotrophin-releasing hormone
HMM: hexamethylmelamine	**H$_2$O$_2$**: hydrogen peroxide
HN$_2$: mechlorethamine	**HACA**: human anti-chimeric antibodies
HU: hydroxyurea	**HAI**: intrahepatic arterial infusion
	Hb: hemoglobin
	HD: high-dose
	HER: human epidermal growth factor receptor
	HGPRTase: hypoxanthine-guanine phosphoribosyl transferase
	HIF: hypoxia-inducible factor
	HSC: hematopoietic stem cells
	HSR: hypersensitivity reaction
	HUS: hemolytic uremic syndrome

Drugs	Other
IDA: idarubicin **IFO**: ifosfamide	**ICH**: immunohistochemistry **IGF-1**: insulin-like growth factor 1 **ILD**: interstitial lung disease **INR**: international normalized ratio **Interpt.**: interpatient **Intrapt**: intrapatient **IP**: intraperitoneal **IT**: intrathecal
LV: leucovorin **L-PAM**: melphalan	**LDH**: lactice acid dehydrogenase **LFTs**: liver function tests **LHRH**: luteinizing hormone-releasing hormone **LVEF**: left ventricular ejection fraction
MGA: megestrol acetate **MMC**: mitomycin C **MPA**: medroxyprogesterone acetate **MTIC**: methyltriazeno-imidazole-4-carboxamide **MTX**: methotrexate	**MAB**: monoclonal antibody **MAOI**: monoamine-oxidase inhibitors **MAP**: mitogen-activated protein **MDR**: multidrug resistance **MDS**: myelodisplastic syndrome **mFBP**: membrane folate-binding protein **MM**: multiple myeloma **MMR**: mismatch repair enzyme complex **MOA**: Monoamine oxidase **MTD**: maximum tolerated dose **mTOR**: mammalian target of rapamycin
NVB: navelbine	**N**: nausea **NAD**: nicotinamide adenine dinucleotide **NCI-CTC**: National Cancer Institute's-Common Toxicity Criteria **NF-κB**: nuclear factor κB **NHL**: non-Hodgkin's lymphoma **NPC**: 7-ethyl-10-(4-amino-1-piperidino)carbonyloxycamptothecin **NSCLC**: non-small cell lung cancer **N&V**: nausea and vomiting **NV**: normal value **O_2^-**: superoxide **O^6-AT**: DNA-O^6-alkylguanine-DNA alkyltransferase **OH$^-$**: hydroxyl radical
PDN: prednisone	**PB**: premature beats **PBSC**: peripheral blood stem cell support **PCP**: pneumocystis carinii pneumonia **PD**: pharmacodynamic **PDGF**: platelet-derived growth factor **PE**: pulmonary embolism **PEG**: polyethylene glycol **P-gp**: P-glycoprotein **P13-K**: phosphatidylinositol 3-kinase **PK**: pharmacokinetics **PKC**: protein kinase C **PML**: promyelocytic leukemia **PMN**: polymorphonucleated cells **PNS**: peripheral nervous system **PO**: per os **PPAR**: peroxysome proliferation activator inhibitor receptor **PRCA**: pure red cell aplasia **PRPP**: phosphoribosylpyrophosphate **PT**: prothrombin time **Pt**: platelets **Pts**: patients

Drugs	Other
PDN: prednisone (*Continued*)	**RAR**: retinoic acid receptor
	RA-APL: retinoic-acid-Antiphospholipid syndrome
	RBC: red blood cells
	RCC: Renal Cell Carcinoma
	RD: recommended dose
	RES: reticuloendothelial system
	RIA: radioimmunoassay
	RNR: ribonucleotide reductase
	RT: radiotherapy
	RXR: retinoid X receptor
	SC: subcutaneously
	SCF: stem cell factor
	SCT: stem cell transplant
	SERMs: selective estrogen receptor modulator
	SIADH: secretion of inappropriate antidiuretic hormone
	SIRS: systemic inflammatory response syndrome
	SPECT: single photon emission tomography
	SPN: sensory peripheral neuropathy
	STAT: signal transducers and activators of transcription
TAM: tamoxifen	**TE**: thromboembolic disorders
THU: tetrahydrouridine	**TGF-β**: transforming growth factor β
TOR: toremifene	**t.i.d**: ter in die
	TK: tyrosine kinase
	Thd Pase: thymidine phosphorylase
	TLS: tumor lysis syndrome
	TNFα: tumor necrosis factor-α
	TPMT: thiopurine methyltransferase
	TS: thymidylate synthase
	TSH: thyroid-stimulating hormone
VCR: vincristine	**V**: vomiting
VLB: vinblastine	**VEGF**: Vascular endothelial growth factor
VM26: teniposide	**VOD**: veno-occlusive disease
VP16: etoposide	
	WBC: white blood count
	XO: xanthine oxidase

1 ALKYLATING AGENTS
1.1 Nitrogen Mustard

Name, chemistry, relevant features	Mechanism of action	Pharmacology and dose modifications
Meclorethamine (HN₂) Mustargen®	Prototype of bifunctional alkylating agent: covalent bond of the alkyl group to N_7 of guanine with formation of DNA-interstrand cross-links between two guanines located in the opposite strands.	Chemical transformation into highly reactive compounds, rapidly bound to tissues; degradation by spontaneous hydrolysis; PK not studied.
Cyclophosphamide (CTX) Endoxana® cyclic phosphamide ester of HN₂.	Hepatic CYP-450 activation to highly reactive metabolites (acrolein: bladder irritant; phosphoramide mustard: alkylating moiety) causing DNA-interstrand cross-links.	PO well absorbed; biphasic plasma disappearance with $T_{1/2}\beta$ of 4–6.5 hr after 6–80 mg/kg; renal excretion of metabolites; high degree of interpt. variation in metabolism; only CTX measured in CSF. Special populations *Renal impairment* Cr CL <20 ml/min: ↓ dose 50–75%.
Ifosfamide (IFO) Mitoxana® analogue of CTX; oxazophosphorine HN₂	In comparison with CTX, slower hepatic activation to acrolein and active ifosforamide mustard (which causes DNA-interstrand cross-links) and higher proportion of inactive dechloroethylated metabolites.	High degree of interpt./intrapt. Variability of PK and metabolism. $T_{1/2}$ 15 hr, 60% of dose as unchanged drug in urine after single dose of 5 g/m². Induction of IFO metabolism after 3 days of IV bolus or CI treatment with increase of CL due to production of dechloroethylated species; decreased urinary fraction (12–18% of dose) of unchanged IFO after repeated doses. Comparable serum AUCs and urinary fractions of IFO and metabolites after IV bolus and CI administration; no effect of DXM on IFO metabolism. Special populations *Renal impairment* Cr CL <20 ml/min: ↓ dose 50–75%.
Mesna Sodium mercaptoethane sulfonate Uromitexan® IV formulation.	Selective urinary tract protectant for oxazophosphorine-type alkylating agents by binding of the SH moiety to acrolein.	Dimerization in blood to the inactive disulfide dimesna, reduced back to mesna in renal tubules and excreted in urine; 10% protein bound. 40% and 30% urinary excretion of free-thiol mesna after IV and PO administration; lower but more prolonged (between 12 and 24 hr) urinary excretion of free-thiol mesna after PO administration than IV.
Mesna Uromitexan® PO formulation.	Same as that of the IV formulation.	Urinary C_{max} 1–2 hr. Special populations Age: ↑ Risk of urinary toxicity of IFO/CTX in elderly.
Melphalan (L-PAM) Alkeran® Synthetic product from phenylalanine and HN₂.	Bifunctional alkylating activity with formation of DNA-interstrand cross-links. Preference of alkylation for guanine adjacent to other guanines.	60–90% protein bound mainly to albumin; variable PO absorption (mean 60%), lower after food ingestion, peaking within 2 hr. $T_{1/2}\alpha$ of 6–8 min and $T_{1/2}\beta$ of 40–60 min; no dose dependent variable PK. Inactivation by nonenzymatic hydrolysis; 50% of dose in 24 hr urine. Special populations *Renal impairment* No guideline available but expect ↑ myelotoxicity.
Chlorambucil Leukeran® Aromatic derivative of HN₂.	Bifunctional alkylating activity; major metabolite phenylacetic acid mustard with alkylating activity.	Rapid ~100% absorption, lower after food ingestion, peaks within 2–4 hr, >90% protein bound; $T_{1/2}$ 1.5 hr. Metabolized in liver; 1% urinary excretion.

Drug interactions	Route, schedule, and recommendations	Toxicity
	<u>Local vesicant on extravasation.</u> In case of leakage: infiltration of the area with sterile isotonic Na-thiosulfate (1/6 molar) and application of ice compresses for 6–12 hr. <u>IV:</u> 0.4 mg/kg (10–12 mg/m^2) every 4–6 wk; 6 mg/m^2 days 1 and 8 every 4 wk (MOPP).	Neutropenia and thrombocytopenia (after about 8 days, for 10–20 days); acute severe prolonged N&V; phlebitis; rare severe allergic reactions; maculopapular rash.
<u>With CYP-450 inducers:</u> potential but of unknown clinical relevance (barbiturates) or blockers (glucocorticoids); detoxification with Mesna.	<u>PO:</u> 50–100 mg/m^2 daily. <u>IV:</u> 1000–1500 mg/m^2 every 3 wk. <u>IV HD:</u> 7000 mg/m^2 (MTD) (IV hydration + Mesna).	DL neutropenia after 8–14 days, recovering within 10 days; N&V (delayed with IV therapy); alopecia; hemorrhagic cystitis (prevented by adequate pre- and post hydration). Thrombocytopenia; SIADH (more common at >50 mg/kg); cardiotoxicity (↑ incidence in case of prior anthracyclines, large single infusions, glutathione depleting agents).
See CTX. <u>With nephrotoxic drugs:</u> (DDP) ↑ renal damage. <u>With CNS active agents</u> (including narcotics, some antiemetics): ↑ CNS toxicities, methylene blue to reverse and prevent CNS toxicities.	<u>Adequate hydration</u> before, up to 72 hr after to avoid hemorrhagic cystitis. <u>IV:</u> short (1–3 hr inf.) or CI: 1.2–1.5 g/m^2 days 1–3 or days 1–5 every 3–4 wk; 24 hr CI: 5 g/m^2. <u>IV HD (CI):</u> 3–4 g/m^2 on days 1–4 (MTD).	DL hemorrhagic cystitis prevented with hydration and Mesna; 50% myelosuppression with cumulative anemia; >50% N&V; >80% alopecia; 12% CNS toxicity with confusion, lethargy, seizures, hallucinations, possibly due to inactive metabolites, ↑ CNS toxicity in elderly/pts with renal impairment; 60% nephrotoxicity (tubular), ↑ risk in children. Similar toxicities, but of ↑ incidence and degree.
Incompatible in solution with DDP; does not affect the antitumor activity of other cytotoxic agents. **Caution** ↑ Risk of urinary toxicity in pts with prior pelvic RT, urinary infection, and prior hemorrhagic cystitis.	<u>IFO IV short infusion:</u> 60% daily total dose divided into three doses (each 20%), 15 min before (always IV), 4 and 8 hr later (40% single dose if given PO). <u>IFO CI:</u> same equal dose (directly mixed), continue up to 12 hr after the end of IFO. <u>CTX-HD</u> (>10 mg/kg) 2–3 hr infusion: 100% daily total dose in repeated doses, each 20% total dose, 1st dose always IV 15 min before CTX, then every 6 hr from start up to 24 hr from end.	PO: N&V if given undiluted; in case of V within 1 hr, redose IV. False ↑ of urinary chetones. HSR with skin reaction, itching, edema, rare anaphylaxis.
	<u>PO:</u> 400 mg capsules. Dose: double IV dose at each dosing; in case of CI give 40% dose at the end, then at 4, 8, and 12 hr from end. First dose 2 hr before starting IFO/CTX.	
<u>With cyclosporine:</u> ↑ risk of nephrotoxicity.	<u>PO</u> (daily dose at one time and fasting): 1 mg/kg total dose over 5 days every 4–5 wk. <u>IV:</u> 8 mg/m^2 every 4–5 wk. <u>IV HD:</u> 40–200 mg/m^2 (MTD: 180 mg/m^2).	Delayed (after 2–3 wk) neutro-thrombocytopenia (recovery up to 6 wk); probably more leukemogenic than other alkylators. Rare: N&V, diarrhea. Earlier neutropenia (days 6–16); mucositis; diarrhea; alopecia; N&V. 2% HSR after repeated courses.
	<u>PO:</u> 0.1–0.2 mg/kg (4–10 mg total) daily for 3–6 wk.	Neutropenia; high incidence of secondary leukemia after prolonged treatment.

Name, chemistry, relevant features	Mechanism of action	Pharmacology and dose modifications
Prednimustine Ester conjugate of chlorambucil and prednisolone	Alkylation of DNA, as for chlorambucil; ↑ lipid solubility and cellular uptake than chlorambucil.	50% F with rapid and extensive presystemic degradation to component drug moieties.

1.2 Alkyl Sulfonate

Busulfan Myleran® Alkyl sulfonate; chemically unrelated to HN_2.	Polyfunctional alkylating agent, producing cross-links between two DNA strands and DNA protein cross-links. Lack of sequence specificity of alkylation.	Good PO absorption; no dose dependent $T_{1/2}$ of 2.5 hr. Extensive liver metabolism with production of several species; methanesulfonic acid as main excretion species in urine; CSF concentrations after high dose comparable to those in plasma.

1.3 Ethylenimines

Thiotepa N,N',N''-triethylenethiophosphoramide; can be administered by any parenteral route.	Polyfunctional alkylating agent with three aziridine groups. Intracellular release of aziridine and generation of ethylenimonium ions acting as monofunctional alkylating agents; the different functional groups induce DNA-interstrand cross-links.	40% protein bound; rapid activation by CYP450 to main metabolite TEPA, less cytotoxic and with longer terminal $T_{1/2}$ (5 hr); 24% of dose excreted in 24 hr urine. Possible metabolic saturation at highest doses studied (6–7 mg/kg). Advantages of IT over IV administration still to be verified. After IV, CSF levels equivalent to those in plasma. **Special populations** *Liver impairment* No guideline available but use with caution.
Hexamethylmelamine Altretamine Hexalen® Triazene ring with dimethylamino groups at each of the three carbons.	Still unknown, possibly DNA alkylation; structurally similar to triethylenemelamine.	>90% protein bound; variable PO absorption with T½ of 0.5–3 hr. Rapid demethylation by microsomal CYP450; $T_{1/2}\beta$ 3–10 hr; 60–70% of dose in 24 hr urine as metabolites.

1.4 Nitrosoureas

BCNU Carmustine® Chloroethylnitrosourea.	DNA chloroethylation with formation of inter-/intrastrand cross-links between guanine and cytosine on the opposite strands; carbamoylation of proteins through isocyanate molecules.	Rapid biotransformation with $T_{1/2}\alpha$ and $T_{1/2}\beta$ of 6 and 70 min; partial metabolization in liver to inactive species with prolonged plasma levels; PK not dose-dependent; 30% of dose in 24 hr urine. BBB rapidly crossed; >50% plasma levels in CSF.
CCNU Lomustine® Chloroethyl-cyclohexylnitrosourea.	Same as that of BCNU.	Rapid absorption, decomposition, and metabolism in liver with parent drug never detectable; C_{max} of metabolites within 3 hr. 50% of dose in 12 hr urine as degradation products; >30% plasma levels in CSF.
Methyl-CCNU Semustine® 4-Methyl derivative of CCNU.	Same as that of BCNU.	Rapid absorption, decomposition and metabolism in liver with parent drug never detectable; C_{max} of metabolites within 1–6 hr. 60% of dose eliminated in 48 hr urine as metabolites; >30% plasma levels in CSF.

Drug interactions	Route, schedule, and recommendations	Toxicity
	<u>PO:</u> 40 mg daily divided into 3–4 portions.	Dose-dependent prolonged myelosuppression; mild steroidal side-effects.
Prophylaxis of seizures after high dose with EIAs (phenytoin and phenobarbital).	<u>PO:</u> 4–8 mg daily for weeks (higher dose for higher WBC count; weekly counts; stop for WBC between 10,000–20,000; restart when WBC count rises again).	Selective neutropenia, after 11–30 days, recovering in 3–7 wk; hyperpigmentation of skin; interstitial pneumonitis; rare: aplastic anemia, cataracts after prolonged treatment.
	<u>HD:</u> 4 mg/kg on days 1–4 (MTD: 640 mg/m^2).	DL hepatotoxicity with VOD and ↑ LFTs, severe myelosuppression, moderate (92%) to severe (7%) N&V; generalized seizures.
Inhibition of pseudocholinesterase activity with ↑ effect of succinylcholine.	<u>IV bolus:</u> 0.3–0.4 mg/kg every 1–4 wk.	Dose-related and cumulative myelosuppression with short WBC and longer Pt nadir; DL mucositis, hyperpigmentation of skin, hepa-totoxicity; confusion, somnolence.
	<u>IV HD:</u> 500–1125 mg/m^2 (MTD: 1000 mg/m^2).	
↑ Absorption from body cavities in presence of infiltration/ inflammation of mucosa (RT).	<u>Intrapleural, intrapericardial:</u> 60 mg at ≥1 wk interval.	Rare myelosuppression.
	<u>Intravesical:</u> 30–60 mg/wk × 4.	Lower abdominal discomfort, bladder irritability.
	<u>IT:</u> 15 mg at ≥1 wk interval.	
<u>With CYP450 inducers:</u> (Phenobarbitone) with ↓ antitumor effect. <u>With concomitant IMAO:</u> severe orthostatic hypotension.	<u>PO:</u> single agent, 260 mg/m^2 on days 1–14 every 4 wk; combination, 150–200 mg/m^2 on days 1–14 every 4 wk. (four divided daily doses).	DL N&V, ↓ if taken after meals; cumulative CNS somnolence, mood disorders, hallucinations, dizziness; PNS, mainly sensory toxicity; reversible mild leukopenia.
<u>With cimetidine:</u> ↑ myelosuppression.	<u>IV</u> (1–2 hr inf.): 200 mg/m^2 every 6 wk.	Delayed (after 3–6 wk) potentially cumulative myelosuppression; acute severe N&V; burning pain in the vein; flushing; mild reversible hepatic toxicity; pulmonary fibrosis with long-term therapy, ↑ risk for cumulative doses >1400 mg/m^2. Possible delayed onset (>10 yr after) in cured children having received cranial RT.
	<u>IV HD:</u> 1200 mg/m^2 (MTD 1050 mg/m^2) (single agent) split into two fractions at 12 hr intervals; 300–600 mg/m^2 (combination).	DL pulmonary (interstitial pneumonitis and fibrosis) and hepatic (VOD) toxicities.
Same as those of BCNU.	<u>PO:</u> 100–130 mg/m^2 (single agent) every 6–8 wk on <u>empty stomach.</u>	Delayed (after 3–6 wk) potentially cumulative myelosuppression; acute N&V; mild reversible hepatic toxicity; ↑ risk of second malignancy after long-term therapy. Rare, cumulative (after 1100 mg/m^2) pulmonary fibrosis, possible delayed onset (>10 yr after) in cured children having received cranial RT.
	<u>PO:</u> 125–200 mg/m^2 every 6 wk on <u>empty stomach.</u>	Same as those of CCNU.

Name, chemistry, relevant features	Mechanism of action	Pharmacology and dose modifications
Streptozocin Zanosar® Glucosamine-1-methyl nitrosourea; water soluble.	DNA methylation; carbamoylation of proteins through isocyanate molecules; inhibition of O^6-AT; inhibition of key enzymes in gluconeogenesis.	Rapid and extensive metabolism; no intact drug after 3 hr; prolonged $T_{\frac{1}{2}}$ of metabolites. 20% of dose in 24 hr urine as metabolites; BBB rapidly crossed. Special populations *Renal impairment* Cr CL <25 ml/min: ↓ dose by 50–75%.

1.5 Triazenes

Dacarbazine (DTIC) Dacarbazine NP DTIC-Dome® Dimethyl-triazeno-imidazole-carboxamide	Methylation of DNA by MTIC formed by N-demethylation of DTIC. Photodecomposition products also responsible for cytotoxicity in vitro of questionable importance in vivo.	20% protein bound; rapid hepatic microsomal activation ($T_{\frac{1}{2}}$ of intact drug: 40 min); light sensitive with photodecomposition. 40% of drug eliminated in 24 hr urine; BBB poorly crossed. Special populations *Renal and Liver impairment* No guideline available, but prepare to ↓ dose.

1.6 Imidazotetrazines

Temozolomide Temodal® Imidazotetrazine-derivative; analogue of DTIC; methyl derivative of mitozolamide.	Prodrug; converted to cytotoxic MTIC through chemical process (instead of metabolic activation as for DTIC). ↑ Induction of O^6-alkylguanine adducts with depletion of O^6-AT; schedule-dependent antitumor activity.	100% F reduced by food, rapidly absorbed within 1 hr; $T_{\frac{1}{2}}\beta$ 1.8 hr, linear PK. Wide tissue distribution; crosses BBB (30% ratio CSF/plasma AUC). No accumulation with daily dosing; clearance not affected by anticonvulsants (with exception of valproic acid), H2 blockers, barbiturates, DXM but 5% lower in women with greater myelosuppression. Special populations *Renal impairment* No guideline available but caution in pts with severe impairment.

2 PLATINUM COMPOUNDS

Cisplatin (DDP) Cis-diamminedichloroplatinum (II) Inorganic planar coordination complex.	DNA binding of aquated species with formation of DNA inter-/intrastrand cross-links; binding to SH groups of critical enzymes. Mechanisms of resistance include ↓ cellular drug accumulation, cytosolic inactivation by thiol-containing compounds, enhancement of DNA repair, overexpression of some proto-oncogenes and loss of DNA MMR enzymes.	90% protein bound; active species produced within the cell by aquation hydrolysis. Triphasic disappearance of total platinum with $T_{\frac{1}{2}}\gamma$ of 5.4 days and high tissue distribution. 90% renal excretion mainly by glomerular filtration; 40% of dose excreted in 24 hr urine; poor CSF penetration. Special population *Age* ↑ Risk of neurotoxicity in >65 yr due to ↓ renal function. *Renal impairment.* Cr CL 50–70 ml/min: use mannitol and increase hydration to ↑ diuresis. Cr CL < 50 ml/min: use with caution.
Carboplatin (CBDCA) 1,1-Cyclobutanedicarboxylato(2-)-0,0′-platinum (II) Carboplatin NP Paraplatin® Second generation platinum compound; 10-fold more water soluble than DDP.	Same as that of DDP; slower reactivity with DNA and lower potency than DDP; mechanisms of resistance possibly similar to those of DDP.	Lower relative rate of activation than DDP; $T_{\frac{1}{2}}$ of ultrafilterable platinum of 170 min; triphasic disappearance of total platinum with $T_{\frac{1}{2}}\beta$ and $T_{\frac{1}{2}}\gamma$ of 1.5 hr and 5.8 days; 30% plasma levels in CSF after IV treatment; 70% of dose as parent in 24 hr urine; plasma clearance of ultrafilterable species correlated to GFR. Special population *Renal impairment* Doses are based on Cr CL as estimate of GFR (Calvert formula).

Drug interactions	Route, schedule, and recommendations	Toxicity
↑Risk of nephrotoxicity with potentially nephrotoxic drugs; ↑ risk of glucose intolerance with corticosteroids; ↑ effect of DNA-reactive anticancer agents through inactivation of O^6-AT; prolongation of the T$_{\frac{1}{2}}$ of DOX requiring its dose reduction.	Local vesicant on extravasation. IV (30–60 min inf.) single agent: 1 g/m^2 every week × 4–6 wk with 4-wk rest; combination: 500 mg/m^2 on days 1–5 every 6 wk. **Warning** Adequate hydration before and after each course and monitoring of renal function (serial urinalysis for proteinuria).	DL cumulative nephrotoxicity due to tubular damage with proteinuria, glycosuria, and hypophosphatemia; acute, severe, cumulative N&V; occasional diarrhea and hepatotoxicity with ↑ LFTs and hypoalbuminemia; acute hypoglycemia; burning pain in the vein; mild myelosuppression and hepatotoxicity.
↑ Activation with CYP-450 activity inducers (barbiturates).	IV (15–30 min inf.): single agent, 250 mg/m^2 on days 1–5 every 3–4 wk. **Warning** Avoid direct sun exposure for 24 hr after DTIC; ↓ vein irritation and pain if DTIC given protected from light.	Acute, severe N&V; flu-like syndrome after 1 wk; sunlight-reaction with facial flushing, pain on the head and hands; mild myelosuppression and hepatotoxicity.
Possible synergism with antitumor agents with similar mechanism of action to deplete O^6-AT; possible synergism with ionizing radiations.	PO: 150–200 mg/m^2 on days 1–5 every 4 wk (fasting, single-dose). Heavily pretreated pts: 150 mg/m^2 on days 1–5 every 4 wk; non heavily pretreated adult and pediatric pts: 200 mg/m^2 on days 1–5 every 4 wk; Dose reductions by 50 mg/m^2 daily according to ANC/Pt nadirs, do not reduce below 100 mg/m^2.	DL myelotoxicity (mainly neutropenia and thrombocytopenia) with delayed nadir >20 days and recovery in 7–14 days; 50 % N&V (severe 10%); 30 % fatigue and malaise.
Could delay excretion of drugs eliminated through kidneys (MTX, BLM, IFO). With concomitant nephrotoxic drugs (aminoglycosides, amphotericin B): ↑ renal toxicity. With concomitant SH-containing agents (sodium thiosulfate, amifostine, glutathione): ↓ renal toxicity. With taxanes: ↑ incidence of peripheral neuropathy.	IV: (30–60 min inf.): standard dose 50–100 mg/m^2 every 3 wk; 20 mg/m^2 on days 1–5 every 3 wk, with pre-/post hydration to ↑ diuresis and prevent renal toxicity. HD: 120 mg/m^2 single day every 3 wk 40 mg/m^2 on days 1–5 every 3 wk (with hypertonic saline; nephroprotective agents). IP: 90–270 mg/m^2 (with pre-/post hydration).	Dose-dependent, early (after 1–24 hr), severe, and delayed (after 24–120 hr) N&V; acute tubular damage with hypomagnesemia; cumulative subclinical tubular damage with ↓ Cr CL; cumulative peripheral sensory neuropathy (paresthesias, sensory loss) slowly reversible; 30% irreversible. Same toxicities but ↑ incidence and degree; dose-dependent high-frequency hearing loss and myelotoxicity (anemia); rare, focal encephalopathy and retinal toxicity.
Dose modifications Calvert formula Adults: total dose (mg) = target AUC × (GFR + 25); pretreated pts AUC: 4–6 mg/ml/min; untreated pts AUC: 6–8 mg/ml/min. Children: total dose (mg) = target AUC × [GFR^a + 0.36 × BW (kg)]. (^{a}GFR as estimated by ^{51}Cr-EDTA or 24 hr urine collection or Cockcroft-Gault equation).	IV (30–60 min inf.): Standard dose Adult untreated pts/Calvert formula; single agent, AUC 6–8 mg/ml/min every 3–4 wk; combination, AUC 4–5 mg/ml/min every 3–4 wk (without hydration). HD: Single agent, 2000 mg/m^2 (MTD) (with hydration); combination, AUC 11–20 mg/ml/min.	DL cumulative thrombocytopenia after 2–3 wk, recovering within 2 wk; moderate N&V after 6–12 hr; myelotoxicity, cumulative peripheral neuropathy; allergic reactions after very high cumulative doses, no cross reactivity with DDP; transient ↑ in hepatic enzymes. DL hepatotoxicity, nephrotoxicity with loss of serum electrolytes, reversible vision loss.

Name, chemistry, relevant features	Mechanism of action	Pharmacology and dose modifications
Oxaliplatin Eloxatin® Trans-l-diaminocyclohexane oxalatoplatinum.	Same as that of DDP with bulkier DNA adducts; activity in cancer cell lines and murine models resistant to DDP because of deficiency of MMR activity and enhanced replicative bypass.	95% protein bound; at the end of inf. 50% accumulated (nonexchangeable) in RBC and 50% in plasma (33% ultrafilterable); triphasic disappearance of ultrafilterable platinum with $T_{\frac{1}{2}}\beta$ and $T_{\frac{1}{2}}\gamma$ of 16.3 hr and 273 hr; 54% of dose in 48 hr urine. High CL by tissue binding and renal CL_R (34%) correlated with GFR. Extensive nonenzymatic biotransformation to cytotoxic/noncytotoxic species. ↑ AUC of ultrafilterable platinum if Cr CL < 60 ml/min. No need of ↓ dose if Cr CL > 20 ml/min. No cumulation of total plasma platinum with repeated administrations.

3 ANTITUMOUR ANTIBIOTICS

Bleomycin sulfate (BLM) Mixture of sulfur containing glycopeptides; formed by a DNA-binding fragment and an iron-binding portion. Activation through O_2 binding.	DNA binding with production of single and double-strand breaks; DNA damage affected by specific repair enzymes, gluta-thione, ionizing radiation. BLM inactivated by BLM hydrolase; pulmonary toxicity due to low enzyme concentration and high O_2 tension. When used intrapleurally acts as sclerosing agent.	10% protein bound; $T_{\frac{1}{2}}$ of 2–3 hr; rapid tissue inactivation, lower in skin and lung with 50% of dose in 24 hr urine, mainly as inactive species. C_{max} with IM administration after 30–60 min, 1/3 of that after IV; 45% systemic absorption after intrapleural administration. Special population *Renal impairment* Cr CL ≤ 30 ml/min: ↓ dose by 50%.
Mitomycin C (MMC) Mitomycin C Kyowa® A purple antibiotic isolated from *Streptomyces caespitosus*.	Activation to bifunctional alkylating agent with formation of DNA interstrand cross-links and oxygen free radicals. Activation by chemical reducing agents, enzymatic reduction, exposure to acidic pH: Possible preferential activation in hypoxic environment.	Rapid plasma disappearance due to tissue distribution and liver metabolism; $T_{\frac{1}{2}}\beta$: 25–90 min; <10% of dose in 24 hr urine, 23% hepatic extraction with HAI administration. Special population PK unchanged if liver/renal impairment.
Dactinomycin (DACT) Cosmegen Lyovac® Phenoxazine pentapeptide antibiotic.	DNA intercalation of the planar multi-ring phenoxazone between guanine–cytosine base pairs with inhibition of RNA synthesis. Radiosensitizer.	5% protein bound; by RIA, biphasic disappearance with $T_{\frac{1}{2}}$ of 35 hr, longer in case of liver impairment; minimally metabolized, does not cross BBB; 30% of dose in urine and feces as intact drug within 1 wk.

4 ANTIMICROTUBULE AGENTS

4.1 Vinca Alkaloids

Vinblastine sulfate (VLB) Vinblastine NP Velbe® Sulfate salt of a dimeric alkaloid from *Vinca rosea*; formed by two multi-ringed units (catharanthine and vindoline) with methyl side chain on vindoline.	Binding to a specific site on tubulin with prevention of polymerization, inhibition of microtubule assembly and mitotic spindle formation. Involved in MDR phenomenon through P-gp overexpression.	80% protein bound; rapidly distributed into tissues with triphasic disappearance ($T_{\frac{1}{2}}\gamma$ 19–25 hr); partially metabolized in liver to deacetyl VLB; 80% of dose excreted unchanged in bile. Special population *Liver impairment* ↓ Dose if obstructive liver disease.
Vincristine sulfate (VCR) Vincristine NP Oncovin® Sulfate salt of a dimeric alkaloid from *Catharanthus rosea* As VLB with formyl side chain on vindoline.	Same as that of VLB.	48% protein bound; rapidly distributed into tissues with triphasic disappearance; liver metabolism with 70% of dose in 72 hr feces. Special population *Liver impairment* Bilirubin up to 3 mg/ml: ↓ 50% dose.

Drug interactions	Route, schedule, and recommendations	Toxicity
Additive or synergistic effects in vitro and in vivo with 5-FU, TS inhibitors, CPT-11. Incompatible with normal saline, alkaline solution (5-FU).	<u>IV</u> (2 hr inf.): <u>Single agent</u>, 130 mg/m^2 every 3 wk; <u>combinations</u>, 85 mg/m^2 every 2 wk.	DL peripheral neuropathy (mainly hands/feet and perioral) of two types: Type 1—acute early onset, reversible within 14 days, sensory, enhanced by cold contact; Type 2—persistent >14 days paresthesia, dysesthesia, and deficit in proprioception with functional impairment, cumulative, reversible at discontinuation (complete recovery only in 41% within 8 mo). Incidence overall neuropathy single agent: 82%, 19% persistent, with functional impairment 12%; 10% and 50% of risk of developing it after 6 and 9 cycles; 65% N&V (gr 3-4 11%), 30% diarrhea (gr 3-4 4%), 10% neutropenia. Rare: HSR.
↑ Risk of pulmonary toxicity with hyperoxia, concomitant RT, nephrotoxic drugs with ↓ excretion of BLM.	<u>IV bolus</u>: 10–20 mg/m^{2a} per week. <u>IM, SC</u>: Same dose as IV, with antipyre-tics/steroids to prevent fever. <u>IV CI</u>: 5–10 mg/m^2 on days 1–4 every 3 wk. <u>Intrapleural</u>: 60–120 U (50% of dose in the systemic circulation). Avoid NSAID against chest pain. ^{a}mg = unit.	IV: Acute DL stomatitis; 50% fever and chills; 50% cumulative skin hyperpigmentation. Mild to moderate alopecia. Rare, HSR (1% of lymphoma pts) and Raynaud's phenomenon. Low-dose hypersensitivity pneumonitis responsive to steroids. 10% late chronic pneumonitis up to irreversible interstitial fibrosis (dry cough, dyspnea, rales, basilar infiltrates), ↑ incidence for cumulative dose >250 U, age >70 yr, COPD, thoracic RT, hyperoxia during surgical anesthesia; role of steroids uncertain.
<u>With concomitant DOX</u>: ↑ Risk of cardiotoxicity.	Local vesicant on extravasation. <u>IV bolus</u>: Single agent, 20 mg/m^2 every 6–8 wk; combination, 10 mg/m^2 every 6–8 wk. <u>Intravesical</u>: 20 mg × 3 per week.	Delayed (after 3–8 wk) cumulative leuko- and throm-bocytopenia, cumulative anemia; partial alopecia. Rare: HUS with thrombocytopenia, renal and cardiac failure: ↑ Risk for cumulative dose >50 mg, exacerbated by RBC transfusions, rarely reversible, steroids ineffective (52% lethal). Rare, severe interstitial pneumonitis with lung infiltrates.
Unexpected hepatic toxicity after hepatotoxic agents (halothane, enflurane).	Local vesicant on extravasation. <u>IV (bolus)</u>: Single agent, 500 μg (maximum 15 μg/kg) on days 1–5 every 4 wk; combination, 500 μg on days 1–2.	DL myelotoxicity with leuko-thrombocytopenia in 1 wk and nadirs up to 3 wk. Severe, prolonged (up to 24 hr) N&V; 30% stomatitis and diarrhea; alopecia; late radiation recall toxicity (mainly skin, but also GI, liver, lung). Immunosuppression.
	Local vesicant on extravasation. <u>IV (bolus)</u>: 4 mg/m^2 to begin with, increased to 6 mg/m^2 per week. Prophylaxis of constipation: use lactulose.	DL leukopenia after 5–10 days, recovering within 7–14 days. Neurotoxicity with constipation and abdominal pain; less frequent, peripheral neuropathy, jaw pain, urinary retention, ↑ incidence if underlying neurological problems; stomatitis and mild alopecia.
↑ Accumulation of MTX in tumor cells.	Local vesicant on extravasation. <u>IV (bolus)</u>: 0.4–1.4 mg/m^2 (maximum 2 mg total dose) per week. <u>IV (CI)</u>: Single agent, 0.5 mg/m^2 on days 1–5; combination, 0.4 mg/m^2 days 1–4 (VAD regimen) every 3 wk.	DL cumulative neurotoxicity, with SPN (paresthesias, loss of deep tendon reflexes); less frequent, autonomic effects with abdominal pain and constipation; ↑ inci-dence if underlying neurological problems); 20% alopecia. Rare SIADH.

Name, chemistry, relevant features	Mechanism of action	Pharmacology and dose modifications
Vinorelbine (NVB) Navelbine® Semisynthetic derivative of VLB with structural modifications on the catharanthine ring.	Same as VLB; ↓ activity on axonal microtubules with possibly ↓ neurotoxicity.	80–90% protein bound; rapid tissue distribution with triphasic disappearance ($T_{1/2}\gamma$ 27–40 hr); high liver uptake; hepatic metabolism by CYP3A in two metabolites, one active (desacetyl metabolite); main hepatic excretion. PK unchanged by age; F, mean 27% $\pm$ 14; C_{max} after 1.5 hr and large first-pass effect. No food effect on oral absorption. Special population *Liver impairment* Bilirubin > 2 × NV: ↓ dose by 50%.

4.2 Taxanes

Name, chemistry, relevant features	Mechanism of action	Pharmacology and dose modifications
Paclitaxel Taxol® Diterpene from bark and leaves of *Taxus brevifolia*; poor water solubility, need of vehicle with 50% polyoxyethylated castor oil (Cremophor EL) and 50% ethanol.	Promotes microtubule assembly of tubulin dimers and stabilizes microtubule dynamics with inhibition of cell proliferation, blockade of mitosis and induction of apoptosis. Resistance related to P-gp overexpression and mutations of tubulin, slower rate of microtubule assembly, overexpression of Bcl-2. ↑ In vitro cytotoxicity after longer exposure time. In vitro sensitizing effect to ionizing radiation. Effective in vitro concentrations (≥0.1 µmol/l) achieved in man at the end of infusion.	>90% protein bound; rapid tissue uptake with triphasic plasma disappearance and extensive liver metabolism at the taxane ring through CYP2C8 and CYP3A4; main metabolite inactive 6-OH paclitaxel. High biliary secretion and low intestinal absorption of paclitaxel and metabolites. Non-linear PK in humans, mainly caused by Cremophor EL; C_{max} and AUC not proportional to dose, because of saturable distribution, metabolism, and elimination. Neutropenia related to the time plasma concentrations of ≥0.05–0.1 µmol/l are maintained. Does not cross BBB. After IP treatment: low V_d, slow peritoneal CL, prolonged significant IP and plasma concentrations. Special populations *Liver impairment* Liver enzymes >2 <10 × NV or bilirubin 2–5 × NV: ↓ dose to 90 mg/m² (3 hr inf.). *Renal impairment* No need of dose ↓.
Docetaxel Taxotere® Semisynthetic paclitaxel derivative from needles of *Taxus baccata*; more water soluble than paclitaxel; Tween 80 in the solution.	Same mechanisms of action and resistance as paclitaxel. Schedule independent antitumor activity; in vitro sensitizing effect to ionizing radiation.	>90% protein bound; linear PK up to 115 mg/m² with triphasic plasma disappearance ($T_{1/2}\beta$ and $T_{1/2}\gamma$ of 38 min and 12 hr); extensive liver metabolism with oxidations of the C13 side chain and production of inactive metabolites; high interpt. variability of metabolism and PK. 74% of dose excreted in feces as metabolites, 5% in urine; CL ↓ 27% in pts with ↑ transaminases; CL is independent predictor of severe and febrile neutropenia in population of PK study. Special population *Liver impairment* AP >2.5 × NV and transaminases >1.5 × NV: ↓ dose by 25%. Bilirubin, AP ↑ >6 × NV or transaminases >3.5 × NV: discontinue.
Paclitaxel protein-bound particles for injectable suspension ABRAXANE® Albumin-bound form of paclitaxel.	Same mechanism of action as paclitaxel.	89–98% protein bound. 20% excreted into feces. 4% of the dose excreted into urine. Hepatic metabolism as paclitaxel. Biphasic PK. $T_{1/2}$: ~27 hr. Linear AUC between 80 and 375 mg/m². CL_b: 15 l/hr/m². V_d: 632 l/m². CL and V_d are larger than paclitaxel (43% and 53% higher respectively). Special populations Liver impairment Data not available.

Drug interactions	Route, schedule, and recommendations	Toxicity
Potential interactions with inducers/ inhibitors of CYP3A.	Local vesicant on extravasation. IV (5–10 min inf.): Single agent, 30 mg/m^2 weekly with ↓ dose according to myelotoxicity; combination, 25 mg/m^2 weekly with cisplatin every 4 wk. PO (soft-gel capsules): 60 mg/m^2 per week per 3 wk, then ↑ to 80 mg/m^2 per week if no severe neutropenia.	DL non-cumulative neutropenia (90%; 36% G 4) after 7–10 days, recovering within 7–14 days; 25% SPN with decreased deep tendon reflexes; 35% constipation; 40% N&V (2% severe); 12% alopecia; 10% chemical phlebitis; 27% fatigue. PO: 50% N&V (15% severe); >50% diarrhea; 6% G 2–4 neutropenia.
In vitro effects on metabolism of concomitant CYP450 isoenzyme substrates (cyclosporin, steroids, macrolide antibiotics, benzodiazepines, barbiturates, anticonvulsant drugs, fluconazole). With doxorubicin: ↑ Incidence of CHF with paclitaxel (3 hr inf.) and DOX (bolus > 380 mg/m^2 cumulative dose). With cisplatin: ↑ Peripheral neuropathy. With concomitant EIAs: ↓ C$_{ss}$ and ↓ systemic toxicity in pts receiving 96 hr infusion paclitaxel.	Premedication: Steroids, histamine H1- and H2-receptors antagonists (day −1, day 1). IV (3 hr inf.): 175 mg/m^2 every 3 wk. IV (24 hr inf.): 135 mg/m^2 every 3 wk. HD (+G-CSF): Good risk pts 200–250 mg/m^2 every 3 wk. IV weekly (1–3 hr inf.): 90–100 mg/m^2 per week. IV CI (96 hr): 140 mg/m^2 (without premedication). IP: 82.5–125 mg/m^2 every 3 wk.	DL non-cumulative neutropenia (50% G 4) after 7–10 days, recovering in 1 wk; total alopecia (within 2–4 wk); 60% dose-dependent myalgia (8% severe) after 2–3 days for 3–4 days; 60% dose-dependent cumulative SPN (3% severe), slowly reversible; 41% HSR (<2% severe); 12% hypotension; 23% ECG abnormalities (sinus bradytachycardia, PB) usually asymptomatic, not requiring interventions; radiation recall skin reaction. Schedule-dependent neutropenia and mucositis, ↑ with 24 hr infusion. DL cumulative SPN, onycholysis. DL mucositis, onycholysis. DL abdominal pain.
Specific substrates of CYP4503A isoenzymes (erythromycin, ketoconazole, nifedipine) could modify CL.	Premedication: DXM 8 mg b.i.d. for 3 days (from day 1). IV (1 hr inf.): Single agent, 60–100 mg/m^2 every 3 wk; combination, 75–100 mg/m^2 every 3 wk. Weekly: 36 mg/m^2 per week × 3 every 4 wk.	DL: Non-cumulative neutropenia (80% G 3-4, 11% febrile neutropenia) after 8 days, recovering within 1 wk; 76% total alopecia (within 2–4 wk), 62% asthenia (5% severe), 50% SPN (4% severe), 47% skin reactions (5% severe), 39% diarrhea (5% severe), 15% acute HSR (2% severe); 64% fluid retention (6% severe) due to capillary protein leak syndrome, after a median cumulative dose of ≥400 mg/m^2. Steroids useful to ↓ severity of skin reactions and of fluid retention (after a median dose of 800 mg/m^2), and to avoid severe HSR. Rare: Radiation recall phenomena, ischemic colitis. DL fatigue and asthenia; rare peripheral edema and neuropathy; uncommon mild neutropenia and onycholysis.
Potential interaction with CYP2C8 and CYP3A4 substrates.	IV 30 min inf.: 260 mg/m^2 every 3 wk. No premedication to prevent HSR because of the lack of cromophor.	80% neutropenia (9% severe), 2% febrile neutropenia, 2% thrombocytopenia, 33% anemia. 90% alopecia, 71% SPN, 47% asthenia (8% severe), 44% myalgia (8% severe), 26% diarrhea (10% severe), 18% V, 10% fluid retention, 4% HSR.

Name, chemistry, relevant features	Mechanism of action	Pharmacology and dose modifications

4.3 Epothilones

Ixabepilone
IXEMPRA®

Semisynthetic analogue of epothilone B, with a chemically modified lactam substitution.

Binding β-tubulin subunits with suppression of dynamic instability of αβ-II and αβ-III microtubules, low in vitro susceptibility to multiple drug resistance mechanisms such as MRP-1 and P-gp.

In vitro binding to human proteins from 67% to 77%. Extensively metabolized in the liver, main route of metabolism via CYP3A4, 30 metabolites excreted into human urine and feces. ~86% of the dose is eliminated within 7 days in feces (65% of the dose) and urine (21% of the dose). Linear PK for doses from 15 to 57 mg/m², $T_{1/2}$: ~52 hr, no accumulation in plasma, V_{dss} >1000 L.

Special population
In case of liver impairment the combination with capecitabine is controindicated in pts with AST or ALT >2.5 × ULN or bilirubin >1 × ULN due to increased risk of toxicity and neutropenia-related death. If moderate hepatic impairment, start at 20 mg/m², dosage possibly escalated in subsequent cycles up to, but no more than 30 mg/m² if tolerated. In patients with AST or ALT >10 × ULN or bilirubin >3 use not recommended; limited data available for patients with baseline AST or ALT >5 × ULN.

5 ENZYME INHIBITORS: TOPOISOMERASE II INHIBITORS

5.1 Anthracyclines, Anthracenediones

Doxorubicin (DOX)
Doxorubicin Rapid Dissolution

Hydroxyl daunorubicin; anthracycline antibiotic constituted by water-soluble aminosugar (daunosamine) linked to planar anthraquinone nucleus (adriamycinone) site of electron transfer reactions.
Same structure as DNR with hydroxyacetyl group C_8.

Cytotoxicity due to: (1) DNA intercalation of aglycone between base pairs with inhibition of nucleic acid synthesis; (2) Topo II inhibition; (3) Generation of hydroxyl radicals (relevant mainly for cardiac toxicity) through (a) redox cycling of quinone with production of O_2^-, H_2O_2, and OH^-, which bind to DNA and cell membrane lipids; (b) formation of drug-metal (Fe^{2+}, Cu^{2+}) complexes, which catalyze and bind to DNA and cell membranes. Cardiomyopathy possibly related to (3) because of destruction of detoxifying glutathione peroxidase by DOX and relative deficiency of scavenging enzymes in heart. Involved in MDR phenomenon through P-gp overexpression and Topo II alterations.

75% protein bound with rapid tissue distribution; triphasic plasma disappearance ($T_{1/2}\gamma$ of DOX and metabolites: 25–28 hr). Main metabolite DOXOL produced by ubiquitous (mainly liver) aldoketo reductase, less active than DOX; 7-deoxyaglycones, inactivation species produced mainly in liver, conjugated and excreted into bile and urine. 40% of dose excreted in bile and 5% in 7-day urine.

Special populations
Liver impairment
Bilirubin >1.25–2.0 × NV: ↓ dose by 50%.
Bilirubin >2.0–4.0 × NV: ↓ dose by 25%.
No verified guidelines for abnormal transaminases: caution suggested.

Daunorubicin (DNR)

Anthracycline antibiotic constituted by daunosamine linked to planar daunomycinone.

Same as DOX.

Rapid and extensive tissue binding with triphasic plasma disappearance ($T_{1/2}\gamma$: 18 hr). Metabolic pathways similar to DOX; main plasma metabolite DNR-OL with higher AUC and longer $T_{1/2}\gamma$ than DNR. 40% of dose as DNR and metabolites in bile and <25% in urine.

Special populations
Renal impairment
Cr >1.5 × NV: ↓ dose by 50%.
Liver impairment
↓ Dose if severe liver impairment; guidelines not validated.

Drug interactions	Route, schedule, and recommendations	Toxicity
With CYP3A4 Inhibitors: ↓ Dose 20 mg/mq or washout period after discontinuation. **With CYP3A4 Inducers:** ↓ I concentrations to subtherapeutic levels. **With Capecitabine:** Not clinically significant PK interactions.	IV (3 hr inf.): every 3 wk. Single agent 40 mg/m². Maximum calculated dose on BSA 2.2 m². Premedication: 1 hr before treatment with H1 antagonist and a H2 antagonist. If HSR: Corticosteroids (IV 30 min before inf. or PO 60 min before inf.).	Most common adverse reactions (≥20%): 63% SPN (14% G3–4) fatigue/asthenia, myalgia/arthralgia, alopecia, N&V, stomatitis/mucositis, diarrhea, and musculoskeletal pain.
Compatible with IV BLM, VLB, VCR, CTX; incompatible with DXM, 5-FU, heparin. With CYP450 inducers: ↑ CL. With MDR modulators: ↓ CL through P-gp inhibition. With MMC, CTX, paclitaxel, Ca antagonists: ↑ Risk of cardiotoxicity. With dexrazoxane: ↓ risk of cardiotoxicity.	**Local vesicant on extravasation.** IV (bolus) intermittent: Single agent, 60–75 mg/m² every 3 wk; combination, 50–60 mg/m² every 3 wk. IV (bolus) weekly: 20 mg/m² per week. IV CI (72–96 hr) (central IV line): 60 mg/m² every 3 wk. **Warning** Recommended maximum cumulative dose (dose associated <10% risk of CHF). Cardiac risk factors (combination CT, prior mediastinal RT, age >70 yr, pre-existing heart disease). IV bolus intermittent: Cumulative dose: ≤450 mg/m²; 300–400 mg/m² if cardiac risk factors. IV bolus weekly & IV CI: Cumulative dose: ≤700 mg/m²; 550 mg/m² if cardiac risk factors.	DL neutropenia after 10–14 days, recovering in 1 wk; acute, dose-dependent N&V; total alopecia within 3 wk; hyperpigmentation of skin and nails; radiation recall; venous flare reactions. Rare, stomatitis. Cardiotoxicity: Dose independent: reversible, acute (after hours or days): arrhythmias (with non-specific ST segment and T-wave changes, AV blocks, A tachyarrhythmia; more rarely, acute pericarditis/myocarditis. Dose-related: Irreversible cumulative, delayed, chronic cardiomyopathy with CHF responsive to diuretics, digitalis, ACE inhibitors. Serial determinations of LVEF by MUGA/ECHO to minimize the risk of cardiotoxicity (base-line, 300, 450 mg/m², then after each dose). Discontinue treatment if ≥10% ↓ of baseline to a level below normal. Endomyocardial biopsy findings predictive of subsequent CHF. More frequent stomatitis.
Compatible with IV Ara-C, hydrocortisone; incompatible with DXM and heparin. With MDR modulators: ↓ CL through P-gp inhibition.	**Local vesicant on extravasation.** IV (bolus): Single agent, 60 mg/m² on days 1–3 every 4 wk; combination, 30–45 mg/m² on days 1–3 every 4 wk. Children: 25 mg/m² per week. **Warning** Recommended maximum cumulative dose (dose associated <10% risk of CHF). Cardiac risk factors (combination CT, prior mediastinal RT, age >70 yr, pre-existing heart disease) Single agent, combination: ≤550 mg/m²; ≤300 mg/m² if risks factors.	DL myelotoxicity after 10–14 days, recovering in 3 wk; early, moderate N&V; total alopecia within 3 wk; hyperpigmentation of skin, radiation recall and venous flare reaction as for DOX. Cardiotoxicity: Acute and cumulative delayed as for DOX; children and infants are more susceptible.

Name, chemistry, relevant features	Mechanism of action	Pharmacology and dose modifications
Idarubicin (IDA) Zavedos® Demethoxy-DNR; DNR analogue lacking -OCH_3 at 4th position on the aglycone; ↑ lipophilicity with ↑ cellular uptake; 6–8-fold more potent than DNR in animal models.	(1) and (2) same as those of DOX; (3) less prominent.	97% protein bound (parent and metabolites); high tissue uptake, triphasic plasma disappearance ($T_{1/2}\gamma$ 18 hr), primary biliary excretion, extensive metabolism to 13-OH derivative IDOL with comparable activity and $T_{1/2}\gamma$ of 72 hr; F 30–50%; C_{max} of IDA after 1–4 hr and IDOL after 3–8 hr; first-pass effect with higher AUC ratio IDOL/IDA than after IV; accumulation of IDOL after daily doses. Special populations *Liver impairment* LFTs >1.25–2 × NV: ↓ dose by 50%. LFTs >2–5 × NV: ↓ dose 75%; guidelines not validated. *Renal impairment* Cr >1.5 × NV; ↓ dose by 50%.
Epirubicin (EPI) Pharmorubicin® Epimer of DOX with 4′-OH on daunosamine in equatorial rather than axial position; ↑ lipophilicity, ↑ β-glucuronidation to inactive compounds with ↓ cardiotoxicity, ↑ CL, and ↓ potency.	(1) and (2) same as those of DOX; (3) less prominent due to ↑ glucuronides production escaping redox cycling and free radical formation. Involved in MDR phenomenon.	77% protein bound; extensive liver metabolism with EPI and 13-OH derivative (epirubicinol) with formation of inactive glucuronides rapidly excreted. Triphasic plasmatic disappearance with $T_{1/2}\gamma$ of 40 hr; 50% of dose excreted in the bile in 4 days and <20% into urine. Special populations *Liver impairment* Bilirubin 1.2–3 mg/dl or AST 2–4 × NV: ↓ dose by 50%. Bilirubin >3 mg/dl or AST >4 × NV: ↓ dose by 75%.
Doxorubicin HCl liposome Caelyx® DOX encapsulated in pegylated (STEALTH®) liposomes.	Longer circulation times; higher concentrations in tumor tissues in animal models than DOX, possibly due to enhanced permeability and retention.	Linear PK up to 20 mg/m^2; $T_{1/2}$: 74 hr. In comparison to DOX: higher CL (0.030 L/hr/m^2), lower V_d (1.93 L/m^2 equal to plasma volume), greater AUC, similar metabolism. Special populations: *Age* No differences. *Liver impairment* At cycle 1: Bilirubin 1.2–3 mg/dl: ↓ dose by 25%; bilirubin > 3 mg/dl: ↓ dose by 50%. At 2nd cycle if 1st cycle well tolerated: ↑ dose by 25%. *Renal impairment* Cr CL 30–156 ml/min: no modifications.
Mitoxantrone (DHAD) Novantron® Synthetic dihydroxyanthracenedione constituted by a tricyclic planar hydroxyquinone analogue and two identical aminoalkyl side chains.	See DOX: (1) and (2) same; (3) less prominent because of lack of redox cycling and ↓ potential of cardiotoxicity. Involved in MDR phenomenon.	78% protein bound; rapid tissue distribution with linear triphasic plasma disappearance (median $T_{1/2}\gamma$ 75 hr); primary hepatobiliary elimination with 25% of dose in feces and 11% of dose in urine of 5 days. Special populations *Liver impairment* ↓ Dose if severe liver impairment; guidelines not validated.

Drug interactions	Route, schedule, and recommendations	Toxicity
	Local vesicant on extravasation. IV (10–15 min inf.): 12 mg/m² on days 1–3 every 4 wk. **Warning** Recommended maximum cumulative dose (dose associated <10% risk of CHF). Cardiac risk factors (combination CT, prior mediastinal RT, age >70 yr, pre-existing heart disease). Single agent or combination: ≤ 150 mg/m²; ↓ dose if risk factors. PO: leukemia; single agent, 25 mg/m² on days 1–3 every 4 wk; combination or solid tumors, 15 mg/m² on days 1–3 every 4 wk.	10 mg/m² myelotoxic as 60 mg/m² of DOX. DL neutropenia after 10 days, recovering in 2 wk; 82% mild to moderate N&V; 50% mucositis; 75% alopecia, usually partial; 20–30% ↑ transient LFTs; venous flare reactions. Cardiotoxicity: Dose-related cumulative delayed as that of DOX and DNR but with better therapeutic index. PO: 60% G 1–2 N&V; 15% diarrhea; 40% alopecia; ↑ toxicity after single dose than repeated daily doses.
Do not mix heparin or fluorouracil; do not mix with other drugs in the same syringe; avoid prolonged contact with alkaline pH solution because of hydrolysis. With cimetidin: ↑ AUC by 50% and ↓ decrease plasma clearance by 30%; avoid concomitant use.	**Local vesicant on extravasation.** IV (10–15 min inf.): standard dose, single agent: 90 mg/m² every 3 wk; combination, 60–75 mg/m² every 3 wk. **Warning** Recommended maximum cumulative dose (dose associated <10% risk of CHF). Cardiac risk factors (combination CT, prior mediastinal RT, age >70 yr, pre-existing heart disease). Single agent, combination: ≤900 mg/m²; ≤540 mg/m² if risks factors. HD (30–60 min inf.) days 1–2: total dose, single agent, 120–150 mg/m²; combination, 120 mg/m² + CSF or 200 mg/m² + PBSC.	Acute side effects comparable to those of DOX with dose ratio of DOX:EPI of 1:1.2 for hematological, 1:1.5 for non-hematological toxicities, 1:1.8 for cardiotoxicity. Dose-related cumulative delayed cardiotoxicity as for DOX; serial LVEFs by MUGA/ECHO (baseline, 300–400 mg/m², 600–700 mg/m², then after each dose) to minimize the risk of cardiotoxicity (4% at ≤950 mg/m², 15% at 1000 mg/m²). Secondary AML: cumulative risk 0.2% and 0.8% at 3 and 5 yr when used with other DNA-damaging cytotoxics. DL mucositis; 90% G 4 neutropenia; severe N&V; total alopecia.
No drug interaction studies. Do not mix with other drugs.	**Local vesicant on extravasation.** IV: Infuse initially at 1 mg/min to minimize risk of reactions. AIDS-KS: 30 min inf.—20 mg/m² every 3 wk; solid tumors: 60 min inf.—50 mg/m² every 4 wk. **Warning** Cumulative cardiotoxic dose not defined: in metastatic front line pts monitor cardiac functions after >600 mg/m² in naive and 450 mg/m² in DOX-pre-treated pts.	Dose-dependent cumulative skin toxicity with palmar-plantar erythrodysesthesia, possibly due to preferential accumulation in flexure, pressure areas, palms (40% at 50 mg/m², 17% G 3), usually appearing after 2–3 cycles, recovering in 2–4 wk, steroids possibly useful:↓ incidence at ≥4 wk intervals and by avoiding pressure, high temperature for 1 wk after treatment, pyridoxine possibly useful. 34% asthenia; 30% stomatitis (9% G 3–4); 20% alopecia; 10% infusion reactions (occasional HSR); 5% G 3–4 N&V; 10% G 3 neutropenia (solid tumors); <10% cardiac-related AE, lower risk of cardiotoxicity compared to DOX at cumulative equiactive doses; evaluation of long-term cardiac effects ongoing.
	Local vesicant on extravasation. IV (10–15 min inf.): Single dose, 12–14 mg/m² every 3 wk; combination, 10 mg/m² every 3 wk; leukemia: 12 mg/m² days 1–3. **Warning** Recommended maximum cumulative dose (dose associated <10% risk of CHF) Cardiac risk factors (combination CT, prior mediastinal RT, age >70 yr, pre-existing heart disease) Cumulative dose (risk of <10% CHF): ≤140 mg/m²; ≤120 mg/m² if risk factors. HD: 60–80 mg/m².	DL neutropenia after 12 days, with recovery in 1 wk; 37% malaise; 30% G 1–2 N&V; 20% alopecia; 8% mucositis. Cumulative delayed cardiotoxicity as for DOX after higher cumulative equitoxic doses. Similar treatment and monitoring. Secondary AML: Cumulative risk 1.1% and 1.6% at 5 and 10 yr when used with other DNA-damaging cytotoxics and RT.

Name, chemistry, relevant features	Mechanism of action	Pharmacology and dose modifications

5.2 Epipodophyllotoxins and Aminoacridines

Etoposide (VP16) Vepesid® Semisynthetic derivative of podophyllotoxin with epipodophyllotoxin linked to a glucopyranoside with methyl group; made more water-miscible by organic solvents (Tween 80, polyethylene glycol).	Topo II inhibition with stabilization of the DNA-TOPO II complex and production of DNA double-strand breaks. Cytotoxicity, phase and schedule dependent; lower repeated doses more effective than higher single dose. Involved in MDR phenomenon through P-gp overexpression and Topo II alterations (↓ activity, point mutations).	95% protein bound; biphasic disappearance with $T_{1/2}$ of 6–8 hr; linear PK also at high doses. 44% of dose in feces and 56% (mainly parent compound) in urine of 5 days; hepatic metabolism with production of less active hydroxy acid metabolites, glucuronide and/or sulfate conjugates in urine. Dose-dependent, variable F (50–75%) up to 200 mg total dose; lower at >200 mg. Measurable CSF levels of parent compound and metabolites after high-doses. Special populations ↓ Cr CL, ↓ albumin, age > 65 yr: ↓ dose.
Etoposide phosphate Etopophos® Water-soluble prodrug of etoposide, completely converted to etoposide in vivo.	Same as that of etoposide.	Same as that of etoposide.
Teniposide (VM26) (Vumon®) Same as etoposide with a thienylidene group on the glucopyranoside.	Same as that of etoposide.	>99% protein bound; triphasic disappearance with $T_{1/2}\gamma$ of 20 hr; 86% eliminated by hepatic metabolism (metabolites mostly unknown), 20% of dose in 24 hr urine; ↓ CL_R than etoposide. Special populations *Liver impairment* Bilirubin 1–2.5 mg/dl: ↓ dose by 50%. Bilirubin >2.5 mg/dl: ↓ dose by 75%.
Amsacrine (m-AMSA) Amsidine® Synthetic aminoacridine derivative.	DNA intercalation of the three coplanar rings. Topo II inhibition with production of DNA double-strand breaks occurring at base sequences different from those of etoposide and anthracyclines.	98% protein bound; biphasic CL with $T_{1/2}\alpha$ of 30 min. and $T_{1/2}\beta$ of 7 hr; extensive liver metabolism with production of alkylthiol derivative excreted in urine (35% of dose) and bile (50% of dose); metabolites still cytotoxic. Longer $T_{1/2}$ (17 hr) if liver impairment with ↑ stomatitis and myelotoxicity. Special populations *Liver impairment* Bilirubin 1–2.5 × NV or AST 2–5 × NV: ↓ dose by 50%. Bilirubin >2.5 × NV or AST >5 × NV: ↓ dose further or discontinue. *Renal impairment* Need of ↓ dose uncertain.

6 ENZYME INHIBITORS: TOPOISOMERASE I INHIBITORS
6.1 Camptothecins

Irinotecan (CPT-11) (Campto®) Hydrochloride trihydrate; semisynthetic derivative of camptothecin. Water soluble precursor of the lipophilic metabolite SN38.	Topo I inhibition with production of single-strand DNA breaks. Antitumor activity not schedule dependent. Converted primarily in liver to active and inactive metabolites by at least two known pathways. (1) By carboxylesterase to SN38, 1000-fold more potent, subsequently inactivated by glucuronidation to SN 38G. Both CPT-11 and SN38 undergo pH dependent reversible hydrolysis from active form lactone (closed ring) to carboxylate (inactive open ring). (2) By CYP3A to oxidative metabolites: APC (500-fold less potent than SN 38) and NPC, excreted in bile.	High interpt. variability due to individual variations of metabolic pathways activity (See Mechanism) and polymorphism of UGT enzyme (responsible for SN38 glucuronidation). Protein binding: 50% CPT-11, 95% SN38. For both, linear PK up to 350 mg/m², unchanged after repeated cycles. SN38 AUC values <10% of CPT-11; excretion 28% total urinary with CPT-11 and SN38 as main products; 24% fecal excretion. Relationship between AUC (CPT-11 and SN38) and % of ↓ of ANC. Special populations Guidelines for 3-wk schedule only. *Liver impairment* Bilirubin >1 mg/dl: keep dose <145 mg/m². Bilirubin NV but AST >3 × NV: start dose at 225 mg/m², then ↑ if no toxicity. *Gilbert's syndrome with mutation of UGT1A1* ↓ Dose to 200 mg/m² every 3 wk. *Renal impairment* Cr >1.6–3.5 mg/dl: start at 225 mg/m², then ↑ if no toxicity.

Drug interactions	Route, schedule, and recommendations	Toxicity

Drug interactions	Route, schedule, and recommendations	Toxicity
<u>With DDP, HD-CBDCA, cyclosporin A:</u> ↓ CL. <u>With concomitant EIAs:</u> ↑ CL.	<u>IV</u> (30–60 min inf.): 100–120 mg/m^2 on days 1–3 or on days 1–5 every 3–4 wk. <u>IV HD</u> (500 mg/hr inf.): single agent, 60 mg/kg (preparatory for BMT), 3000 mg/m^2 (MTD); combination, 400–800 mg/m^2 on days 1–3. <u>IV</u> (72 hr CI): 150 mg/m^2 daily. <u>PO</u> 100 mg (50 mg × 2) daily, in untreated pts, days 1–14; pretreated pts, days 1–10 every 4 wk.	DL non-cumulative neutropenia after 10–12 days, recovering within 7–10 days; N&V; less frequent, exacerbation of pre-existing VCR neuro-pathy, diarrhea. Rare hypotension, flushing. High-dose: DL myelotoxicity, mucositis, severe N&V. DL neutropenia after 3 wk, recovering in 1 wk; mild to moderate N&V; total alopecia after repeated cycles. <u>All schedules:</u> ↑ Risk of secondary monoblastic leukemia with balanced 11q 23 translocations, short latency period, no preleukemic phase for cumulative doses of ≥2 g/m^2. High-dose DDP, alkylating agents, RT as additional risk factors.
Same as that of etoposide.	<u>IV</u> (5 min inf.) (solution of higher concentration than for etoposide): 50–100 mg/m^2 on days 1, 3, and 5. <u>IV HD:</u> (2 hr inf.) highest safe dose, 1000 mg/m^2 on days 1 and 2.	Comparable to those expected from etoposide. 3% HSR (chills, rigors, bronchospasm, and dyspnea); 2% flushing; 3% skin rashes.
	<u>IV</u> (30–60 min inf.): *single agent*, 60 mg/m^2 on days 1–5 every 3–4 wk; *combination* (children ALL), 165 mg/m^2 × 2 per wk × 4 (with Ara C).	DL neutropenia after 7–10 days, recovering within 1 wk; moderate N&V; alopecia; mucositis; chemical phlebitis. Rare type I HSR. Secondary leukemias as after etoposide.
Incompatible with chloride ion (Cl).	**Local vesicant on extravasation.** <u>IV</u> (2 hr inf.): *Single agent*, 100–125 mg/m^2 on days 1–5 every 3–4 wk; *combination*, 70–90 mg/m^2 on days 1–5 every 3–4 wk.	DL neutropenia after 11–13 days, recovering in 7–10 days; 30% N&V; 10% stomatitis; 10% diarrhea; 10% abdominal pain; alopecia; phlebitis. Less frequent: ↑ of LFTs, dizziness, headache. 1% cardiotoxicity (acute arrhythmias, longer QT); possible risk factors: hypokalemia, prior anthracyclines.
No PK interactions with DDP, 5-FU, Etoposide and OXA. In vitro ↓ CYP3A metabolism with CYP3A4 substrates (loperamide, ketoconazole, ondansetron) of unknown clinical relevance. <u>With EIAs:</u> ↑ CL (phenytoin, carbamazepine, phenobarbital, pyrimidone, felbamate). <u>With valproate:</u> ↓ SN38 glucuronidation. **Warning** Concomitant anticonvulsant therapy: allowed gabapentin, lamotrigine; *not* allowed: phenytoin, carbamazepine, phenobarbital, pyrimidone, felbamate.	All schedules: <u>IV</u> 90 min inf. <u>Single agent</u> Every 3 wk: 300–350 mg/m^2. weekly: 125 mg/m^2 × 4, every 6 wk. <u>Combination</u> Every 2 wk: 180 mg/m^2. <u>LOD treatment:</u> Treat at 1st episode of loose stools with loperamide (4 mg immediately, then 2 mg every 2 hr until diarrhea-free for 12 hr), and hydrate. Weekly schedule: 125 mg/m^2	Diarrhea principally of two types. Type 1: Early-onset diarrhea-cholinergic syndrome (EOD-CS) (during or within 24 hr from inf.), associated with rhinitis, salivation, miosis, diaphoresis, preventable by atropine (IV or SC 0.25–1 mg). Type 2: Late onset diarrhoea (LOD) (>24 hr) lasting for 5–7 days. Single agent G3–4 toxicity by schedule: *Intermittent:* 22% LOD, 22% neutropenia, 15% asthenia, 14% N&V, 12% EOD-CS, 12% CNS symptoms, 5% anorexia. *Weekly:* 7%EOD-CS, 31% LOD, 31% neutropenia, 16% N, 14% asthenia, 12% V, 7% anorexia, 2% CNS symptoms.

Name, chemistry, relevant features	Mechanism of action	Pharmacology and dose modifications
Topotecan (Hycamtin®) 9-dimethylaminomethyl-10-hydroxycamptothecin; water-soluble semi synthetic derivative of camptothecin.	Topo I inhibition with production of single-strand DNA breaks; pH dependent hydrolysis with predominance of lactone (active species) at pH <7.0; less active open-ring. Active N-desmethyl metabolite in plasma produced by CYP. Higher antitumor activity in experimental models after CI/repeated than single bolus administrations.	50% of drug as carboxylate (80% after 18 hr) at the end of short infusion; wide tissue distribution; biphasic disappearance of lactone ($T_{\frac{1}{2}}\beta$: 3 hr) with linear PK highly variable. Main renal excretion (60–70% total drug in 24 hr urine); 30–40% penetration into CSF in children; positive correlation between total AUC and % $\downarrow$ of ANC. Special population *Renal impairment* Cr CL 20–39 ml/min: $\downarrow$ dose by 50%; no data in case of Cr CL <20 ml/min. *Liver impairment* No need of $\downarrow$ dose.

7 ENZYMES

L-Asparaginase Kidrolase® Enzyme isolated from *Escherichia coli* (commercial). Crisantaspase Enzyme isolated from *Erwinia chrysanthemi*, available for patients with HSR to *E. coli* enzyme.	Hydrolyzes L-asparagine with inhibition of protein synthesis, delayed DNA and RNA synthesis in tumor cells dependent on exogenous asparagine. Resistance due to high intrinsic asparagine synthetase activity.	Minimal tissue distribution due to large size/highly ionized state, production of binding antibodies; plasma levels proportional to dose; slow variable CL with $T_{\frac{1}{2}}\beta$ of 8–30 hr. Minimal urinary/biliary excretion; cumulation with daily dosing. Plasma levels after IM 50% of those after IV with longer $T_{\frac{1}{2}}\beta$ ~40 hr.
PEG Asparaginase Oncaspar® PEG conjugate of L-asparaginase to prevent uptake by RES with $\downarrow$ probability of developing antibodies while prolonging $T_{\frac{1}{2}}$.	Same as that of asparaginase; 50% enzymatic activity of the parent compound.	Longer $T_{\frac{1}{2}}$ than parent compound (5.7 days).

8 ANTIMETABOLITES
8.1 Antifolates

Leucovorin (LV) 5-CHO-FH$_4$; reduced form of folic acid (racemic mixture); active L-LV.	Provides cells with FH$_4$ depleted because of DHFR inhibition by MTX.	90% absorption after PO up to <50 mg total dose, then 75%; T_{max} 0.5 hr. Crosses BBB, rescue delayed for $\geq$24 hr after IT treatment.
Raltitrexed Tomudex® Quinazoline folate analogue.	Potent and selective inhibitor of TS, forms polyglutamates, 100-fold more potent than parent compound and retained within cells.	93% protein bound; triphasic disappearance with $T_{\frac{1}{2}}\beta$ and $T_{\frac{1}{2}}\gamma$ of 1.7 hr and of 198 hr; long $T_{\frac{1}{2}}\gamma$ due to intracellular deglutamation and release from tissues. Not metabolized. Excreted unchanged in urine (40–50%) and 15% in feces, about 50% retained in tissues. Special populations *Renal impairment* $\uparrow$ re-treatment interval to 4 wk and reduce dose according to Cr CL: Cr CL 55–65 ml/min: $\downarrow$ dose by 25%. Cr CL 25–54 ml/min: $\downarrow$ dose equivalent to ml/min (e.g., if 30 ml/min, give 30% full dose). Cr CL < 25 ml/min: discontinue.

Drug interactions	Route, schedule, and recommendations	Toxicity
Same as those of CPT 11. With DDP: ↑ Neutropenia if Topotecan given after DDP. With EIAs: ↑ CL (concomitantly phenytoin).	IV (30 min inf.): Single agent, 1.5 mg/m² on days 1–5 every 3 wk; combination, 0.75 mg/m² on days 1–5 every 3 wk. If G-CSF is used, start at least 24 hr from last dose.	DL neutropenia (78% G 4) after 10–12 days, recovering in 1 wk; 37% severe anemia after 15 days; 27% severe thrombocytopenia after 15 days; 32% diarrhea; 54% cumulative fatigue; 60% mild to moderate N&V; 49% dose-related cumulative alopecia.
With MTX: ↓ MTX toxicity through inhibition of protein synthesis, causing prevention of cells entry into S phase and ↓ polyglutamation. With concomitant steroids: ↑ hyperglycemia. With VCR and PDN: ↑ toxicity of IV schedule.	Corticosteroids, epinephrine, and O₂ available during/after infusion. IV (30 min inf.) induction: 5000 IU/m² on days 1–14; 6000 IU/m² × 3 per wk. IM maximum volume 2 ml.	35% HSR (skin rash, arthralgia, fever, chills, anaphylaxis); ↑ incidence with repeated doses, doses > 6000 IU/m², IV route. Erwinia in case of HSR, with still possibility of HSR t. GI toxicity (mild N&V, anorexia, cramps) and early hepatic toxicity with ↑ enzymes and ↓ protein synthesis rapidly reversible (albumin, fibrinogen, prothrombin, antithrombin III with thrombosis, ↓ Factors V and VIII); pancreatitis with normal lipase and amylase; hyperglycemia; hypercalcemia; renal damage with ↑ BUN; CNS symptoms (lethargy, disorientation, fatigue, confusion).
	IM (preferred due to lower incidence of toxicity) every 2 wk in combination: adult and children with BSA ≥0.6 m²: 2500 IU/m²; children with BSA <0.6 m²: 82.5 IU/kg. **Warning** IM maximum volume 2 ml.	↓ Incidence of HSR (with IM): 18% overall, 32% in previously hypersensitive pts (5% G 3–4), 10% in naive patients (2% G 3–4).
	With MTX See high-dose MTX. With 5-FU (short inf.) 20–200 mg/m² on days 1–5.	
	IV (15 min inf.): 3 mg/m² every 3 wk. **Warning** Avoid concomitant use of folates, tubular secreted drugs (e.g., NSAIDs), and highly protein bound drugs (e.g., warfarin). Serial checks of liver and renal function tests.	DL prolonged diarrhea (38%, 10% G 3–4) and neutropenia (13%); 49% asthenia (5% G 3–4); 58% N&V (9% G 3–4); 16% ↑ LFTs, 12% mucositis (2% G 3–4); 6% alopecia.

Name, chemistry, relevant features	Mechanism of action	Pharmacology and dose modifications
Methotrexate (MTX) Folic acid analogue; 4-amino, 10-methyl analogue of aminopterin.	Tight-binding inhibitor of DHFR with depletion of intracellular FH_4, necessary for synthesis of purines (through GAR and AICAR transformylases) and thymidylate (through TS) with inhibition of DNA and RNA synthesis. MTX and FH_2 polyglutamated by FPGS, higher in some tumors than in normal cells. DHFR, GAR, AICAR, and TS directly inhibited by polyglutamates. MTX enters cells through reduced folate carrier and mFBP, with higher affinity for FH_4 than for MTX. Mechanisms of resistance to MTX include impaired membrane transport, defective polyglutamation, and alteration of DHFR due to $\uparrow$ expression or $\downarrow$ binding affinity. High-dose therapy based on different distribution of transport carrier systems between tumor and normal cells, with passive diffusion of MTX into tumor cells and selective rescue of normal cells by LV. LV intracellularly converted to 10-CHO-FH_4, which competes with polyglutamated species for DHFR; the dose of LV to rescue normal cells depends on MTX concentration; MTX cytotoxicity depends on drug concentration and duration of exposure. Therapeutic concentrations: 1×10^{-6} mol/L.	60% protein bound; thriphasic plasma disappearance with $T_{1/2}\gamma$ of 8–10 hr, longer if $\downarrow$ Cr CL and third space fluid collections. 60–100% urinary excretion after high-dose MTX through glomerular and tubular processes with drug CL_R comparable to Cr CL; 40% of drug in 24 hr urine as 7-hydroxy-MTX, poorly soluble in acidic pH. Biliary excretion <10% drug clearance. Well absorbed after PO doses of $\leq 25\,mg/m^2$, erratic F at higher doses and in children. With HD ($8\,g/m^2$) therapeutic concentrations achieved in CSF and maintained much longer than with IT. After IT administration, $T_{1/2}$ of 12–18 hr with delayed CL and $\uparrow$ myelo-neurotoxicity if active meningeal disease. HD or IT treatment for meningeal prophylaxis; through Ommaya reservoir (therapeutic). Special populations *Age* $\uparrow$ Sensitivity in elderly due to $\downarrow$ renal function. *Renal impairment* Cr CL $\leq 80\,ml/min$: $\downarrow$ dose; Cr CL <50 ml/min: discontinue. *Liver impairment* No need of $\downarrow$ dose.
Pemetrexed (Alimta®) L-Glutamic acid, *N*-[4-[2-(2-amino-4,7-dihydro-4-oxo-1*H*-pyrrolo[2,3-*d*]pyrimidin-5-yl)ethyl] benzoyl] disodium salt.	Simultaneous inhibition of TS (primary target), DHFR and GARFT (secondary targets) reverted by thymidine and hypoxanthine in combination; enters cells through mainly reduced folate carrier and mFBP; polyglutamated by FPGS, with >100 fold greater affinity for TS than monoglutamate. In mice, dietary folic acid protects from toxicity without $\downarrow$ efficacy.	Linear PK; $\downarrow$ Cr CL results in $\downarrow$ CL_p and $\uparrow$ AUC. Not metabolized to an appreciable extent, 70–90% excreted unchanged in 24 hr urine. $T_{1/2}\beta$ 3.5 hr, small V_d, CL not affected by PO folic acid, IM vitamin B12 or concomitant DDP. Inverse relationship between severity of neutropenia and AUC; $\downarrow$ ANC nadir also occurring in presence of baseline $\uparrow$cystathionine and $\uparrow$ homocysteine levels (markers of vitamin B12 and folate deficiency); vitamin supplementation effective in $\downarrow$ toxicity. Special population *Renal impairment* CrCL $\geq 45\,ml/min$: no dose adjustment; CrCL <45 ml/min: no data available but caution.

Drug interactions	Route, schedule, and recommendations	Toxicity
↑ Toxicity with salicylates, sulfonamides, phenytoin due to protein binding displacement; with probenecid, penicillins, cephalosporins, aspirin, NSAIDs due to inhibition of tubular secretion. With antitumor agents: ↓ toxicity of asparaginase if MTX given first ↑ therapeutic activity of 5-FU, VCR, or AraC if MTX given first; ↑ levels of 6-MP if MTX given first. With RT: ↑ Risk of soft tissue necrosis and osteonecrosis.	Standard dose IV (bolus): 30–50 mg/m² per week. HD **Warning** Implement: (1) IV fluids and urinary alkalinization: keep urinary pH >7 ml/min; ↑ diuresis at least 12 hr before and up to ≥48 hr after, monitor Cr CL (must be ≥60 ml/min). (2) MTX plasma levels monitoring to guide duration and amount of (3). (3) LV rescue: Start 2–24 hr after MTX until MTX levels are <5 × 10⁻⁸ M. Jaffe regimen *Dose:* 50–250 mg/kg 6 hr inf. *Rescue:* Start 2 hr from the end of MTX with LV 15 mg/m² IM every 6 hr × 7, then according to MTX level at 48 hr for 8 doses. MTX level at 48 hr LV mg/m² ≥5 × 10⁻⁷ M 15 ≥1 × 10⁻⁶ M 100 ≥2 × 10⁻⁶ M 200 Repeat after 48 hr and continue up to <5 × 10⁻⁸ M. PO: 15–20 mg/m² × 2 per week. IT: >3 yr old: 12 mg total dose every 2–7 days. **Warning** Do not use preservative containing solutions.	Leuko-thrombocytopenia after 4–14 days; stomatitis; diarrhea; ↑ toxicity in dehydrated, malnourished pts. HD: Acute: reversible nephrotoxicity; N&V; maculopapular rash (up to 5 days after); oral stomatitis (after 3–7 days) preceding myelotoxicity, both reversible within 2 wk; ↑ LFTs, reversible within 2 wk; fever. Transient encephalopathy with paresis, aphasia, and seizures within 6 days, recovering in 72 hr. PO: chronic toxicities, hepatic fibrosis, interstitial infiltrates. IT: Acute chemical arachnoiditis; 10% *subacute* neurotoxicity (motor paralysis, cranial nerve palsies); *chronic* demyelinating encephalopathy (dementia, limb spasticity; ↑ with concomitant cerebral RT).
No interaction with aspirin, or DDP. With NSAID: ↓ CL (20%) and ↑AUC (20%) with ibuprofen. **Caution** Concomitant NSAID use in renal impairment (Cr CL 45–79 ml/min); avoid NSAIDs with short T½ for 2 days before, the day of, and 2 days following pemetrexed administration. No information for long-acting NSAIDs; avoid NSAIDs with long T½ for 5 days before, the day of, and 2 days following pemetrexed administration.	IV (10 min inf.) every 3 wk: 500 mg/m² with vitamin supplementation (vitamin B12 IM 1000 µg, 1–3 wk before and every 9 wk during study; folic acid PO 350–1000 µg starting 1–3 wk before and continuing until 30 days after discontinuation). Skin rash prophylaxis: PO DXM 4 mg b.i.d. days 1–2.	G 3–4 toxicities in withNSCLC pts receiving vitamin supplementation: 5% neutropenia, 4% anemia, 2% thrombocytopenia, 2% ALT elevation, 5% fatigue, 3% N, 2% febrile neutropenia, 1% stomatitis, 1% rash, 0.5% diarrhea.

Name, chemistry, relevant features	Mechanism of action	Pharmacology and dose modifications

8.2 Pyrimidine Analogues

5-Fluorouracil (5-FU)

Uracil analogue with fluorine atom substituted for H at C_5 of the pyrimidine ring.

Intracellular activation to: (1) FdUMP with inhibition of TS (ternary complex with CH_2-FH_4) and inhibition of DNA synthesis and repair; (2) FUMP, metabolized to FUTP, with incorporation into RNA, altering RNA functions; (3) FdUMP phosphorylated to FdUTP with incorporation into DNA.
(1) Is probably the principal mechanism with long $T_{1/2}$ (6 hr) of ternary complex.
Resistance due to deletion of activating enzymes, relative deficiency of CH_2-FH_4, alterations in TS, ↑ activity of catabolic enzymes. Pattern of 5-FU metabolism different in different normal tissues and tumor types; mechanism of cytotoxicity also related to drug concentration and time of exposure.

Erratic F, also because of first-pass effect. After IV bolus $T_{1/2}\beta$ 6–20 min with <1 μM (cytotoxic) within few hours; non-linear PK at higher doses, with ↓ non-renal CL due to saturation of catabolism. Crosses BBB; T_{max} 30 min. Rapid catabolism (50% of dose) in liver and in tissues to F-DHU by DPD; main biliary excretion of 5-FU and catabolites; extensive catabolism also extrahepatic. 50% of dose cleared through liver first-pass after HAI or IV portal infusion. After IP treatment 300:1 gradient between IP: IV concentrations due to slow peritoneal absorption and rapid liver metabolism with low systemic toxicity.
Improvement of therapeutic index by adapting 5-FU dose to AUC in H & N pts receiving 5-FU (96 hr inf.) and DDP in a multicentric randomized study.

Special populations
Liver impairment
Omit if bilirubin >4 × NV.
Pharmacogenomic
↑ risk of life-threatening toxicities at standard doses in DPD-deficient persons; present in some degrees in 3% of patients.

UFT
Uftoral®

Tegafur (FT) and uracil in a molar ratio of 1:4. FT is 5-FU linked to furan ring (dehydroxylated ribose sugar), to be administered with LV.

FT activated to 5-FU in liver, inactivated to F-DHU by DPD; uracil supposed to inhibit subsequent catabolism in liver with possibly higher concentrations in tumor than in blood or normal tissues.

FT: 52% protein bound. Rapid variable absorption; T_{max} 0.3–3 hr; after 5 days AUC and C_{ss} of 5-FU after UFT equivalent to those achieved with CI of 5-FU; no accumulation after repeated doses; <20% FT excreted in urine.
Undergoes microsomal oxidation by CYP2A6.

Special population
PK in liver/renal impairment not studied.

Floxuridine (FUDR)

2-Deoxy-5-fluorodeoxyuridine; deoxy-ribonucleoside of 5-FU.

Prodrug of 5-FU; transformed to 5-FU or to FdUMP. Similar mechanism of action as that of 5-FU.

Given by HAI, higher first-pass extraction (90%) than 5-FU (40%) with ↓ systemic toxicity; PK data not available.

Special population
↓ dose in pts with liver impairment, prior pelvic RT, prior alkylators.
Guidelines not available.

Drug interactions	Route, schedule, and recommendations	Toxicity
Incompatible in solution with any acidic agent; incompatible with diazepam, Ara-C, DOX, MTX. <u>With LV:</u> stabilization of the FdUMP-TS-folate ternary complex; *with* <u>dipyridamole</u> (inhibitor of thymidine uptake): ↓ dTTP and ↑ FdUMP; <u>with MTX</u> (if given before 5-FU): ↑ FUMP and FUTP; <u>with IFN</u> and <u>with cisplatin:</u> mechanism of synergism still uncertain; <u>with allopurinol</u> (300 mg t.i.d.): (selective inhibition of 5-FU anabolism in normal tissues), to prevent toxicity; <u>with delayed high-dose uridine</u> to prevent myelo-suppression.	*Protect from light* <u>IV (bolus) single agent:</u> 400–500 mg/m² (12 mg/kg) on days 1–5 every 3–4 wk; 500 mg/m² per week (15 mg/kg). Maximum recommended daily dose = 800 mg. <u>Combination with LV</u> <u>Low dose</u> IV (bolus): 425 mg/m² on days 1–5 immediately after LV (bolus) 20 mg/m² on days 1–5 every 4–5 wk. <u>HD</u> IV (bolus): 375 mg/m² on days 1–5 1 hr after LV (30 min inf.) 500 mg/m² on days 1–5 every 3 wk. IV (CI): 1000 mg/m² on days 1–5 every 3–4 wk. Prolonged CI: 200 mg/m² per day until toxicity (× 4–5 wk). HAI or IV portal infusion IP 500 mg/L. PO not recommended.	Toxicity and clinical efficacy partly related to schedule of administration. DL neutropenia (31% G 3–4) after 9–14 days; 7% stomatitis; 6% diarrhea (IV fluids and ↓ dose at subsequent cycles if >3 discharge/day), excessive lacrimation. Less frequent, skin hyperpigmentation, radiation recall with erythema, moderate alopecia; transient blurring of vision, eye ocular toxicity with lacrimation, nasal discharge. Rare, neurologic disturbances with somnolence and cerebellar ataxia (more frequent after high-dose and LV combination); cardiac toxicity with chest pain, ECG changes consistent with myocardial ischemia, ↑ serum enzymes, (↑ risk in pts with pre-existing heart disease). <u>IV + LV:</u> ↑ frequency of myelosuppression, stomatitis and neurological disturbances. <u>CI:</u> DL stomatitis and diarrhea; slowly reversible hand-foot syndrome (34% G 3–4) incidence related to duration of infusion, pyridoxine (50–150 mg/day) possibly useful; 20% epigastric pain and gastric ulcerations; ↑ frequency of cardiac toxicity. <u>HAI or IV portal:</u> mild mucositis and GI symptoms; biliary sclerosis with cholestatic jaundice; catheter related complications (thrombosis of the gastroduodenal artery with necrosis of intestinal epithelium, hemorrhage, perforation).
<u>With halogenated antiviral agents</u> Severe myelosuppression and CNS toxicity.	PO: 300 mg/m² daily on days 1–28 plus LV 90 mg daily on days 1–28 every 5 wk (daily doses of both drugs divided into 3 doses given every 8 hr), 1 hr before or 1 hr after meals. **Warning** Give the highest dose of UFT in the morning and lower doses in the afternoon or evening, if the total number of UFT capsules cannot be evenly divided. **Caution** *In pts with history of heart disease.* *In pts receiving drugs affecting CYP2A6 activity.*	DL GI toxicity (2% diarrhea, 3% N&V, 5% anorexia, mucositis); 3.5% asthenia; fatigue; leukopenia.
<u>Narrow margin of safety CI.</u>	<u>CI HAI:</u> 0.2 mg/kg on days 1–14 every 4 wk. **Warning** <u>Contraindications</u> Poor nutritional state, ↓ BM function, potentially serious infections. **Caution** Possibility of severe toxic reaction: deliver first course as inpatient.	Catheter-related complications and drug-related hepatic toxicity as those of HAI and IV portal 5-FU: N&V, diarrhea, stomatitis, localized erythema, ↑ LFTs, gastritis, cramps, abdominal pain, intra-/extra hepatic sclerosis, BM depression, GI ulceration. Discontinue therapy promptly in case of first signs of cardiac ischemia, stomatitis, initial leukopenia, intractable vomiting, and diarrhea.

Name, chemistry, relevant features	Mechanism of action	Pharmacology and dose modifications
Capecitabine Xeloda® 5-deoxy-5-fluoro-N-[(pentyloxy) carbonyl]-cytidine; rationally designed oral fluoropyrimidine carbamate.	Same as that of 5-FU; tumor-selective agent with ↓ risk of toxicity than with systemic 5-FU. 5′-DFUR in tumor converted by Thd Pase to 5-FU, further catabolized by DPD; efficacy in xenografts correlated with ratio of Thd Pase to DPD; tissue distribution of activating enzymes in monkeys, but not in rodents, comparable to humans. In xenografts, 5-FU concentrations in tumor > than in plasma and healthy tissues and > than after equitoxic doses of 5-FU. Antitumor activity correlated with total dose given.	<60% protein binding; rapid (T_{max} 1–2 hr); rapid and almost complete absorption of unchanged drug in fasting conditions, 70% with food. Selectively metabolized in liver to 5′-DFCR by carboxylesterase, then converted to 5′-DFUR by cytidine deaminase in liver and tumor. 5′-DFUR is then activated to 5-FU mainly in liver and at tenor site (See Mechanism). 84% of dose in urine 24 hr, 96% over 7 days. In xenografts, ↑ antitumor activity of combinations of capecitabine than of combinations of 5-FU. Special populations *Age* No impact on PK, but monitor >80 yr for ↑ risk of diarrhea. *Renal impairment* Cr CL 30–50 ml/min: ↓ dose by 25%. Cr CL < 30 ml/min: discontinue. *Liver impairment* Unknown. *Pharmacogenomic* As with 5-FU ↑ risk of G 4 toxicities at standard doses in persons with DPD deficiency (3% incidence).
Cytarabine **(cytosine arabinoside; Ara-C)** Cytosar® Deoxycytidine antagonist with arabinose instead of deoxyribose.	Activated to Ara-CTP in tumor cells by sequential kinase activity; degraded to inactive Ara-U by widely distributed deaminases. Ara-CTP acts by inhibiting DNA polymerase and DNA repair and by incorporation into DNA; possible differentiating effects on leukemic cells at lower doses. Cytotoxicity dependent on duration of exposure and rate of DNA synthesis. Enters cells by facilitated nucleoside transport system at standard doses, by passive diffusion at ↑ doses. Resistance due to deficiency of CdR kinase, ↑ of dCTP pools, ↑ cytidine deaminase activity, ↓ nucleoside transport sites, ↓ intracellular retention of Ara-CTP. In AML or ALL pts, Ara-C uptake, Ara-CTP formation, and retention in blasts are determinants of response.	13% protein bound; after IV bolus C_{max} 10 μM after 100 mg/m², proportionally higher up to 3 g/m² (2 hr inf.) (>100 μM). Rapid plasma elimination with $T_{\frac{1}{2}}\alpha$ of 10–15 min and $T_{\frac{1}{2}}\beta$ of 30–150 min; 70–80% of dose in urine as Ara-U; Ara-U predominates in plasma with $T_{\frac{1}{2}}\beta$ of 3–6 hr. After CI of 0.1–2 g/m² daily proportional increase of C_{ss} up to 5 μM; rapid increase of plasma levels with toxicity at higher doses due to saturation of deamination. After SC or CI, >2-fold higher AUC than after IV bolus. Crosses BBB with C_{ss} CSF 20–40% of those in plasma within 24 hr of CI. After 50 mg/m² IT, C_{max} of 1 mm with >0.1 μM for 24 hr, $T_{\frac{1}{2}}\beta$ of 3 hr. Drug concentration and duration of exposure primary determinants of toxicity. Special populations *Renal impairment* At high dose, ↓ dose if ↑ Cr because of ↑ risk of neurotoxicity.
Cytarabine liposome DepoCyt® Cytarabine encapsulated into spherical multivescicular lipid-based particles (Depo Foam) for IT administration only. Depo Foam particles release drug by erosion and are biodegradable and metabolized.	As cytarabine; sustained-release formulation, direct administration into CSF.	After 50 mg IT, CSF peak levels of free cytarabine within 5 hr; $T_{\frac{1}{2}}\alpha$ ~10 hr, $T_{\frac{1}{2}}\beta$ ~141 hr; free cytarabine concentration >0.02 μg/ml for >14 days; negligible systemic exposure due to rapid Ara-U conversion in plasma.

Drug interactions	Route, schedule, and recommendations	Toxicity
	<u>PO</u> intermittent schedule, <u>single agent</u> and <u>combination</u> same dose: 2500 mg/m² daily in two divided doses for 2 wk, followed by 1-wk rest, every 3 wk. Each dose taken with water 12 hr apart within 30 min from end of meal. **Warning** Do not use in pts with known hypersensitivity to 5-FU.	DL 50% diarrhea (15% severe), 54% hand-foot syndrome (17% severe), 48% hyperbilirubinemia (23% severe), 43% N (4% severe), 41% fatigue (8% severe), 35% abdominal pain (10% severe), 27%V (4% severe), 25% stomatitis (3% severe), 13% neutropenia (3% severe), neurological (<10%).
Synergism with antitumor agents producing DNA breaks because of inhibition of DNA repair (alkylating agents, DDP, VP16, AMSA); synergism with RNR inhibitors (thymidine, HU, fludarabine) because of ↓ dCTP pools. Incompatible with heparin, insulin, MTX, 5-FU, penicillin, and methylprednisolone.	*Standard dose* <u>IV</u> (12 hr inf.): 100 mg/m² b.i.d. on days 1–5 or 7 or on days 1–7. *High-dose* <u>IV</u> (3 hr inf. >200 mg/m²): 2–3 g/m² b.i.d. on days 1–6. *Low dose* <u>SC or IV</u> (bolus or CI): 5–20 mg/m² daily × 2–3 wk. <u>IT</u>: 30 mg/m² × 2 per week until CR, then one additional dose.	<u>SD:</u> DL myelosuppression with biphasic leukopenia; initial nadir after 7–9 days, second nadir after 12–15 days, recovering within 2–3 wk. Frequent acute GI toxicity (N&V, abdominal pain, diarrhea); stomatitis and intrahepatic cholestasis. Flu-like syndrome with rashes, myalgia, fever, appearing 6–12 hr post-treatment. <u>HD:</u> 20% neurotoxicity with reversible cerebellar (10%) and cerebral dysfunction (somnolence, confusion); ↑ risk if >36 g/m² total dose, >50 yr old, ↑ creatinine; repeat neurological examination daily; ↓ incidence with longer infusion. Severe myelotoxicity; mucositis; total alopecia; diarrhea; typhlitis and necrotizing colitis. Conjunctivitis (prophylactic steroids drops up to 48 hr after last dose), sometimes hemorrhagic, with slowly reversible visual acuity problems. Rare, pulmonary toxicity with non-cardiogenic edema. DL myelosuppression. IT: fever, headache, chemical arachnoiditis with vomiting, seizures with transient paraplegia. Rare: myelopathic syndrome.
	<u>IT</u> (1–5 min bolus): 50 mg. <u>Induction and consolidation:</u> every 2 wk. <u>Maintenance:</u> every 4 wk. <u>Prophylaxis:</u> DXM b.i.d. 4 mg days 1–5, 2 mg day 6, 1 mg day 7.	Acute neurotoxicity within 5 days from treatment: 25% headache; 18% chemical arachnoiditis (neck rigidity or pain, meningism), ↓ with steroids prophylaxis,↑ with concomitant RT/CT; 19% N, 17% V, fever, back pain; transient ↑ of CSF proteins and WBC after administration.

Name, chemistry, relevant features	Mechanism of action	Pharmacology and dose modifications
Gemcitabine (d FdC) Gemzar® 2′2′-Difluorodeoxy-cytidine; fluorine-substituted Ara-C analogue.	Intracellularly activated to dFdCTP by CdR kinase with accumulation and prolonged retention. Inhibition of DNA synthesis through incorporation into DNA (masked chain termination) and inhibition of RNR with depletion of dNTP, which compete with dFdCTP for incorporation into DNA (self-potentiating mechanism). Depletion of dNTP lead also to: (1) $\uparrow$ rate of dFdC phosphorylation; (2) $\downarrow$ activity of cytidine deaminase, self-potentiating mechanisms.	Low protein binding; linear PK; for 30 min inf., biphasic disappearance with $T_{\frac{1}{2}}$ of 8 min due to tissue inactivation by cytidine deaminase (mainly liver and kidney) to dFdU; 77% of dose as dFdU in urine. Saturable accumulation process of dFdCTP; $\uparrow$ intracellular concentrations possibly achieved by longer drug exposure; longer infusion associated with $\uparrow V_d$ and longer $T_{\frac{1}{2}}$. **Special populations** *Renal impairment* $\uparrow$ risk of HUS, monitor closely.

8.3 Purine Analogues

6-Mercaptopurine (6-MP) Puri-Nethol® Analogue of hypoxanthine with thiol substituted for 6-OH group.	Intracellularly activated to: (1) 6-MP ribose phosphate by HGPRTase with inhibition of de novo purine synthesis and then → (2) 6-TGN nucleotides with incorporation into RNA and DNA and production of DNA strand breaks. Catabolism through oxidation to 6-thiouric acid by XO, and by methylation to 6-CH$_3$ MP by TPMT.	30% protein bound; 20% highly variable F because of extensive first-pass metabolism. After PO, C_{max} (1 μM) at 1–2 hr, $T_{\frac{1}{2}}$ 1–1.5 hr, >5-fold variable AUC. Primary CL_H, $\downarrow$ dose if abnormal liver function. Intracellular concentrations of metabolites highly variable; genetic polymorphism of TPMT activity with correlation with therapeutic and toxic effects; higher activity of TPMT with low 6-TGN concentrations and $\uparrow$ relapse rate; TPMT-deficient pts with $\uparrow$ 6-TGN in hematopoietic tissues and possibly fatal myelosuppression. Availability of PCR-based methods to identify pts who need $\downarrow$ dose. After IV, $\uparrow$ bioavailability, $\downarrow$ variability of plasma levels, cytotoxic levels in CSF.
6-Thioguanine (6-TG) Lanvis® Analogue of guanine with thiol substituted for 6-OH group.	Same as 6-MP. Intracellularly activated to (1) and (2). Catabolism with desulphuration and deamination followed by oxidation to thiouric acid; unlike 6-MP, 6-TG is not inhibited by the XO inhibitor allopurinol.	Erratic F ($\downarrow$ after food ingestion) with T_{max} of 2–4 hr, 10-fold variation in plasma levels and $T_{\frac{1}{2}}\beta$ of 90 min. Main CL_H. **Special populations** *Liver impairment* Guidelines not available but $\downarrow$ dose suggested. Inherited deficiencies of TMPT and HGRPT (Lesh Nyhan syndrome): $\downarrow$ dose suggested.
Pentostatin (dCF) Nipent® 2-Deoxycoformycin.	Irreversible inhibition of ADA, with accumulation of dATP in lymphoid cells, subsequent inhibition of RNR and DNA synthesis. Very high levels of ADA, which deaminates adenosine and 2-deoxyadenosine to inosine and 2-deoxyinosine, in lymphatic tissues and circulating T cells.	4% protein bound; biphasic plasma disappearance with $T_{\frac{1}{2}}\alpha$ of 8–7 min and $T_{\frac{1}{2}}\beta$ of 5 hr. 80–90% ADA inhibition in peripheral lymphocytes after single dose of 4 mg/m². 80–100% of dose excreted unchanged in urine. **Special populations** *Costitutional* $\downarrow$ PS risk factor for toxicity. *Renal impairment* Cr CL 48–60 ml/min: $\downarrow$ dose 50%. Cr CL < 48–60 ml/min: $\downarrow$ dose 50%, discontinue.

Drug interactions	Route, schedule, and recommendations	Toxicity
Cytotoxicity reversed by exogenous deoxycytidine; synergistic effect in vitro/in vivo of concomitant DDP and RT. With radiosensitizer: no available guidelines but ↓ dose if concomitant RT and avoid concomitant use in NSCLC. With warfarin: ↑ anticoagulant effect of warfarin.	IV (30 min inf.): single agent: 1000 mg/m^2 per week × 7 followed by 1 wk rest, then weekly × 3 every 4 wk; 1000 mg/m^2 per week × 3 every 4 wk. Combination with DDP: 1250 mg/m^2 days 1,8 every 3 wk or 1000 mg/m^2 days 1, 8, 15 every 4 wk.	DL non-cumulative myelotoxicity (25% G 3–4 neutropenia, 5% thrombocytopenia); 75% ↑ LFTs, 10% G 3–4; 65% mild to moderate N&V; 40% mild "flu-like syndrome," 1.5% severe; 30% maculopapular rash; 30% peripheral edema. 15% alopecia; 8% diarrhea; 7% stomatitis; ↑ non-hematological side effects after more frequent administrations. *Rare*: severe <u>pulmonary effects</u> including edema, interstitial pneumonitis (1%), or ARDS: discontinue drug, steroids might be effective; <u>HUS</u> in presence of anemia with evidence of microangiopathic hemolysis, elevation of bilirubin or LDH, severe thrombocytopenia and/or ↑ Cr.
Synergism with inhibitors of de novo purine synthesis (MTX) given before because of ↑ PRPP, cofactor for HGPRT. With allopurinol: Allopurinol is a XO inhibitor. ↑ toxicity with concomitant use, ↓ dose by 50–75%. With hepatotoxic drugs: ↑ hepatic toxicity with concomitant use. With warfarin: inhibition of anticoagulant effect of warfarin. With aminosalicylate derivatives: in vitro evidence of TPMT inhibition, potential ↑ leukopenia. With trimethoprim and sulfamethoxazole: Increased risk of hematological toxicity with trimethoprim and with co-trimoxazole.	PO Children: 2.5 mg/kg daily (70 mg/m^2); adults: 80–100 mg/m^2 daily. **Warning** Discontinue if rapid WBC or Pt fall.	PO: DL myelosuppression after several weeks of treatment; 25% GI toxicity; rare, drug fever, rash, hepatic toxicity with intrahepatic cholestasis and parenchymal necrosis. Regular monitoring of LFTs with drug discontinuation at early signs.
With allopurinol: no interaction. With concomitant hepatotoxic drugs: ↑ hepatic toxicity. With TMPT inhibitors: (sulfalazine, olsalazine) ↑ toxicity, avoid concomitant use.	PO: daily, single dose on an empty stomach. Refer to protocol by which pt is being treated for dose and duration.	DL myelosuppression; less GI and hepatic toxicity than after 6-MP.
With concomitant nephrotoxic agents: ↑ renal toxicity. With vidarabine: biochemical interaction, possible ↑ of toxicities due to inhibition of degradation. With fludarabine and HD-CTX: fatal toxicities after treatment in combination.	IV (20–30 min inf.): 4 mg/m^2 every 2 wk. Pre- and post hydration: 500 ml of IV pre-/post hydration to ↑ diuresis. **Warning** Serial monitoring of renal function.	60% leukopenia (neutro, lympho), 32% thrombocytopenia; 38% prolonged immunosuppression with infections; 53% N&V from 12 up to 48 hr post treatment; 30–40% neurological (lethargy and fatigue) and renal (↑ Cr) toxicities, both dose-dependent; 43% cutaneous rash; 21% pruritus; 19% myalgia; 17% diarrhea; 10% chills. *Rare*: keratitis, hepatic disorders (2%).

Name, chemistry, relevant features	Mechanism of action	Pharmacology and dose modifications
Cladribine (2CdA) Leustatin® 2-Chloro-deoxyadenosine; ADA-resistant deoxyadenosine analogue.	Prodrug intracellularly activated to 2-CdATP by CdR kinase, with accumulation in lymphocytes because of ↑ kinase. In dividing cells, CdATP inhibits RNR with inhibition of DNA synthesis. In resting cells, CdATP causes DNA strand breaks with NAD and ATP depletion, which can trigger apoptosis. ↑ Cytotoxicity after prolonged exposure.	20% protein bound; 97% and 37% F after SC and PO; triphasic plasma disappearance with T$_½$ 7.5–32 hr; 10–30% excretion in 24 hr urine. After SC similar variable AUC than after PO and IV (2 hr inf.). No accumulation after repeated doses. Prolonged intracellular retention in CLL after IV. Crosses BBB: CSF levels 25% of plasma.
Fludarabine phosphate (2-F-ara-AMP) Fludara® 2-Fluoro-arabinosyl-adenosine monophosphate; fluorinated nucleotide analogue of the antiviral vidarabine; ADA resistant; water soluble.	Rapidly converted in plasma to active form 2-F-araA, which enters cells by facilitated nucleoside transport intracellularly activated to F-ara-ATP by CdR kinase. F-ara-ATP inhibits enzymes (DNA polymerase α, RNR and DNA primase) for DNA synthesis and repair by incorporation into DNA and can trigger apoptosis. Resistance due to low CdR kinase activity, ↓ capacity for nucleoside transport, changes in target enzymes.	19–29% protein bound; triphasic plasma disappearance of 2-F-araA with T$_½$$\gamma$ of 20 hr with accumulation after repeated administrations; 23% of dose in urine; CL correlated to Cr CL. In human blasts F-ara-ATP peaks 4 hr after the infusion, with median T$_½$ value of 15 hr, higher than those needed for enzyme inhibition. Cellular PK unchanged after repeated doses. Special populations *Age* ↑ risk of CNS toxicity in >60 yr age or with pre-existent neurological disorders. *Renal impairment* Cr CL 30–70 ml/min: ↓ dose by 50%. Cr CL < 30 ml/min: discontinue.
Clofarabine Clolar® 2-Chloro-9-(2-deoxy-2-fluoro-β-D-arabinofuranosyl)-9H-purin-6-amine.	Inhibits DNA synthesis by: (1) decreasing cellular dNTP pools through inhibition of RNR, (2) by terminating DNA chain elongation, (3) inhibiting repair through inhibition of DNA polymerases.	47% protein bound. 49–60% dose excreted unchanged into urine. Very limited metabolism (0.2%), metabolized intracellular to active triphosphated metabolite by deoxycytidine kinases. Non-compartmental analysis, CL: 28.8 l/hr/m^2, T$_½$ 5.2 hr. Special populations *Renal and liver impairment* Data not available.

9 MISCELLANEOUS AGENTS

Anagrelide HCl Agrylin® 6,7-dichloro-1,5-dihydroimidazo[2,1-b]quinazolin-2(3H)-onemonohydrochloride monohydrate.	Dose-dependent ↓ in Pt production possibly due to specific interference in the megakaryocyte post-mitotic phase; inhibition of Pt aggregation at higher doses; no significant effects on RBC or WBC.	T$_{max}$ 1 hr, T$_½$ 3 days, does not accumulate in plasma after repeated administrations; ↑ F with fasting; extensive metabolism with 70% of dose excreted in urine with <1% parent compound. Special populations *Renal impairment* Cr ≥ 2 mg/dl: serial monitoring of Cr.
Arsenic trioxide Trisenox® As$_2$O$_3$	Mechanism of action not fully elucidated. *In vitro*: apoptosis in human PML cells, damage or degradation of the fusion protein PML-RAR alpha. Used in pts with t(15,17) translocation or (PML-RAR)-α gene expression.	PK of the active trivalent arsenic species not characterized. Complex metabolism, including reduction by arsenate reductase to trivalent arsenic, methylation by methyltransferases not of the P450 family, mostly in liver, to mono- and dimethyl metabolite. Arsenic is stored mainly in liver, kidney, heart, lung, hair, and nails. Special population *Renal impairment* No data available, but caution because arsenic is eliminated through the kidney.

Drug interactions	Route, schedule, and recommendations	Toxicity
	<u>Hairy cell leukemia</u> <u>IV</u> (CI): 0.01 mg/kg daily on days 1–7 (single dose). <u>SC</u> bolus (0.1 mg/kg daily on days 1–5) could replace IV administration; double dose if given PO.	Dose-related severe neutropenia (70%) and anemia (37%) after 1–2 wk with recovery within 4 wk; prolonged depression (up to 6–8 mo) of CD4+ cells and prolonged BM hypocellularity; 69% fever with 32% febrile neutropenia; 28% documented infections (50% viral and fungal); 45% fatigue; 27% cutaneous rash; 28% N; 22% headache; 19% injection site reactions.
<u>With concomitant dCF</u> High risk of pulmonary toxicity. <u>With Fludarabine</u> ↑ cellular Ara-CTP levels pretreated in pts.	<u>IV</u> (30 min inf.): 25 mg/m² on days 1–5 every 4 wk. **Cautions** Monitor for hemolysis while on treatment (See Toxicity). High-dose schedule discontinued because of 36% irreversible delayed severe CNS toxicity (blindness, coma, and death).	DL cumulative myelosuppression recovering within 4 wk in 60% of pts, but occasionally prolonged; trilineage BM hypoplasia or aplasia reported; 33% immunosuppression with infections; 60% fever; 36% N&V; 21% CNS toxicity with weakness and somnolence; less common, visual disturbance, agitation, paresthesia 15% skin rash; 15% diarrhea; 10% malaise; rare, ↑ liver enzymes (1%), ↑ Cr (1%). Autoimmune hemolytic anemia can occur after ≥1 course, do not rechallenge, steroids might not be effective.
No known interactions.	Pediatric Dose <u>IV</u> (2 hr inf.): 52 mg/m² days 1–5 every 2–6 wk. Adults <u>IV</u> (2 hr inf.): 40 mg/m² days 1–5 every 4 wk. **Warning** Give concomitant IV fluids throughout the 5 days. Discontinue if SIRS (due to cytokine release, e.g., tachypnea, tachycardia, hypotension, pulmonary edema).	52 mg/m²: 10% neutropenia (10% severe). 27% transient ↓ LVEF. 40% G 3–4 ↑ AST-ALT, 15% G 3–4 ↑ bilirubin, 6% G 3–4 ↑ creatinine. 83% V, 75% N, 57% febrile neutropenia, 53% diarrhea, 47% pruritus, 46% headache, 41% dermatitis, 41% fever, 38% rigors, 36% abdominal pain, 34% tachycardia, 31% fatigue, 31% anorexia, 29% limb pain, 29% hypotension, 20% edema, 18% stomatitis, 15% sepsis. Uncommon: Capillary leak syndrome and SIRS.
<u>With sucralfate:</u> Potential interference with absorption.	<u>PO:</u> 0.5 mg o.i.d. or 1 mg b.i.d. for at least 1 wk, subsequently modified to maintain a Pt count < 600,000 × mm³; dosage to be ↑ by 0.5 mg daily per week up to a maximum of 10 mg daily or 2.5 mg single dose, usual dose 1.5–3 mg. Response start within 7–14 days of proper dosage. ↑ of Pt count usually 4 days from treatment stop. Monitor Pt every other day week 1, then weekly.	Dose related: 44% headache; 26% diarrhea; 23% asthenia; 20% edema; 17% abdominal pain. **Warning** Vasodilating and positive inotropic properties: 27% palpitation; 8% tachycardia; possible CHF, migraine, syncope, thrombosis. **Caution** In pts with known/suspected heart disease. Pretreament cardiovascular assessment.
None known. **Caution** In pts receiving other drugs known to prolong QT intervals (e.g., certain antiarrhythmics or thioridazine).	<u>Adult and children >5 yr</u> <u>IV</u> infusion (1–2 hr): 0.15 mg/kg daily *Induction* Until BM remission or for 60 days maximum. *Maintenance* Maximum 25 doses in 5 wk, starting 3–6 wk from completion of induction. <u>Acute vasomotor reaction</u> ↑ infusion length to 4 hr. <u>APL syndrome</u> DXM IV 10 mg b.i.d. for at least 3 days. **Warning** Before treatment check ECG and electrolytes: QTc < 500 ms, P > 4 mEq/l, Mg > 1.8 mg/dl.	*Most severe:* <u>APL differentiation syndrome:</u> fever, dyspnea, ↑ weight, pulmonary infiltrates, pleural or pericardial effusions, leukocytosis; <u>ECG abnormalities:</u> 38% QT prolongation within 1–5 wk with normalization by 8th week, 13% G 3–4 ↓ P and Mg; rare, complete AV block, torsade de pointes potentially fatal; 5% <u>HSR</u>, 3% severe. *Most common:* Generally mild, reaction at injection site (pain, erythema, edema); 55% tachycardia, 58–75% N&V, 43% diarrhea, 58% abdomimal pain (10% G 3–4), 60% headache (3% G 3–4), 63% fatigue (5% G 3–4), 63% fever (5% G 3–4), 43% dermatitis, 33% pruritus, 40% edema, 38% rigors, 25% chest pain (5% severe); 25–30% arthralgia/myalgia (5–8% G 3–4); hematologic: 50% leukocytosis, 12% G 3–4 thrombocytopenia, 13% G 3–4 hyperglycemia.

Name, chemistry, relevant features	Mechanism of action	Pharmacology and dose modifications
Hydroxyurea (HU) Hydroxycarbamide/Hydroxyurea NP Hydrea® $CH_4N_2O_2$.	Enters cells by passive diffusion; inhibits RNR with depletion of ribonucleotides and inhibition of DNA synthesis and repair. Radiation sensitizer.	Well absorbed; T_{max} 1 hr, 50% of dose transformed in liver and excreted in urine and as respiratory CO. $T_{\frac{1}{2}}$ 3.5–4 hr. Degraded by urease of intestinal bacteria; metabolism unknown; 55% excreted by renal route. Crosses BBB and third space fluids with peaks in 3 hr. Special populations *Renal impairment* According to GFR: GFR > 50 ml/min: 100% of dose; GFR 10–50 ml/min: ↓ dose by 50%; GFR < 10 ml/min: discontinue.
Procarbazine *N*-methylhydrazine; structure similar to MAO inhibitors.	Prodrug; generates several reactive free radicals, with direct damage to DNA through auto-oxidation, chemical decomposition and CYP450 mediated metabolism; generates also methyldiazonium with monofunctional alkylating activity. Also DNA methylation mainly at N^7-O^6 of guanine with extent of O^6 methylation correlated to O^6-AT activity.	Completely absorbed with peak concentrations in plasma and in CSF in 1 hr. Rapidly concentrated and metabolized ($T_{\frac{1}{2}}\beta$ 10 min) in liver and kidney with 75% of dose excreted as metabolites in 24 hr urine. Special populations *Renal and liver impairment* No guidelines available but ↓ dose.
Trabectedin Yondelis® Marine compound from *Ecteinascidia turbinata*.	Binds to the minor groove of DNA, bending the helix toward major groove. Affects functions of transcription factors, DNA binding proteins, and DNA repair pathways.	Multiple-compartment disposition model with extensive tissue distribution. 94–98% protein bound. V_d 5000 l; metabolized by CYP3A4; renal elimination < 1%, 58% excreted in feces. $T_{\frac{1}{2}}$ 180 hr. CL ~35 l/hr. 51% interpts. variability. Special populations No effect of renal impairment. *Hepatic impairment* Potential higher systemic exposure → close monitoring. Dose modifications ↓ dose in case of ↑ AST/ALT and AP between cycles.

Drug interactions	Route, schedule, and recommendations	Toxicity
With RT: radiation recall reactions independent from timing of RT (may be before, concomitant, or even after HU administration). With didanosine: ↑ incidence of pancreatitis and neurotoxicity. With Ara-C: modulation of Ara-C activity, with ↑ production of Ara-CTP and incorporation into DNA. With 5-FU: antagonist effect, with ↓ FdUMP due to inhibition of RNR. Additive effect with 5-FU and LV because of ↓ dUMP pool competing with FdUMP for binding to TS.	*CML* PO: 20–30 mg/kg daily; discontinue if WBC < 2.5 × 10^9/l or Pt < 100 × 10^9/l. Radiosensitizer: 80 mg/kg as a single dose, every 3 days from at least 7 days before radiation.	DL leukopenia, after a median of 10 days, recovering at discontinuation; maculopapular rash and facial erythema; LFT abnormalities; drowsiness; transient renal function abnormalities.
Weak MAOI: avoid concomitant use of sympathomimetic drugs (isoproterenol, ephedrine, tricyclic antidepressants, gingseng, tyramine rich foods (dark beer, cheese, red wine, bananas), MOA and COMT inhibitors (↑ effect with headache, hypertensive crisis, tremor, palpitations). With alcohol: disulfiram-like reaction (severe GI toxicity, headache). With antitumour agents: possible interaction through inhibition of CYP450 system and depletion of O^6-AT.	PO: 100 mg/m² daily on days 1–14 every 4 wk (MOPP regimen). **Warning** Start at low dose and then escalate daily to minimize GI toxicity.	DL delayed myelosuppression (mainly thrombocytopenia after up to 4 wk); acute GI toxicity (N&V, diarrhea), with tolerance after continued administration; flu-like syndrome at the beginning of treatment; allergic reactions with skin rash and pulmonary infiltrates (controlled with low-dose cortisone); CNS disturbances (paresthesia, headache, insomnia). Late toxicities: azoospermia, anovulation, ↑ incidence of second tumors after MOPP + RT.
CYP3A4 inhibitors: ↑ T concentrations. Avoid concomitant treatment with strong CYP3A4 inhibitors.	IV (24 hr inf.): 1.5 mg/m² every 3 wk. Premedication: IV 20 mg DXM 30 min prior to prevent toxicity before the therapy. **Warning** Central venous line is strongly recommended. Alcohol intake should be avoided. Higher risk of rhabdomyolysis in case of CPK > 2.5. Do not use in pts with ↑ bilirubin.	*Most common:* 77% early reversibile neutropenia (50% severe), 2% febrile neutropenia, 13% severe thrombocytopenia, <1% bleeding events, 13% severe anemia; 45% hepatic toxicity (severe ↑ ALT/AST increases; peak values on day 5 and recovery by day 15), 23% hyperbilirubinemia (1% severe). <1% severe hepatic injury. 26% CPK elevations (4% severe). <1% CPK ↑ in association with rhabdomyolysis with severe liver impairment and/or renal impairment. In case of rhabdomyolysis: start immediately parenteral hydration, urine alkalinization, and dialysis. 63% N (6% severe), 38.5% V (6.5% severe). 10% severe fatigue/asthenia. 3% alopecia.

Name, chemistry, relevant features	Mechanism of action	Pharmacology and dose modifications

10 TARGETED THERAPY
10.1 Growth Factors
10.1.1 HER

Name, chemistry, relevant features	Mechanism of action	Pharmacology and dose modifications
Herceptin Trastuzumab® Recombinant, humanized, IgG$_1$ MAB against the extracellular domain of the erb-B2 receptor (HER2).	Binds to HER2 with inhibition of proliferation and mediation of ADCC. HER2 protein overexpression tested by ICH assays (e.g., HercepTest); HER2 gene amplification tested by FISH assays (e.g., PathVysion).	Minimum serum concentration associated with optimal tumor growth inhibition: 20 µg/ml. **IV weekly at RD** T$_{½}$ 28.5 days, CL 0.225 l/day, V$_d$ 2.95 l; high interpt. variability for CL (43%); C$_{ss}$ reached at about weeks 16–32 (mean through concentration 79 µg/ml)concomitant chemotherapy (anthracyclines plus cyclophosphamide, paclitaxel or cisplatin) did not influence CL. **IV every 3 weeks at RD** T$_{½}$ 18–27 days, CL 0.203 l/days, C$_{ss}$ reached at about 24 wk (mean through concentration 66 µg/ml).
Pertuzumab Fully humanized mAb based on the human IgG1 framework sequences.	Blocks the association of HER2 with other HER family members, including EGFR, HER3, and HER4.	Bicompartmental model. CL ~0.24 l/day. T$_{½}$ ~17 days. V$_d$ 2.7–3.11 l.
Lapatinib Tykerb® Member of the 4-anilinoquinazoline class of KI. Monohydrate of the ditosylate salt, chemical name N-(3-chloro-4-{[(3-fluorophenyl) methyl]oxy}phenyl)-6-[5-({[2-(methylsulfonyl)ethyl]amino} methyl)-2-furanyl]-4-quinazolinamine bis(4-methylbenzenesulfonate) monohydrate.	Inhibitor of the intracellular TK domains of both ErbB1 and ErbB2. No cross-resistance with trastuzumab in vitro.	>99% protein bound (to albumin and AAGP). Extensively metabolized by CYP3A4 and CYP3A5. Excreted predominantly in feces (27%), renal excretion is negligible. Incomplete and variable oral absorption, ↑ with food. T$_{max}$ 4 hr. C$_{ss}$ by day 6–7, T$_{½}$ 24 hr.

10.1.2 EGF

Name, chemistry, relevant features	Mechanism of action	Pharmacology and dose modifications
Cetuximab Erbitux® Recombinant chimeric human IgG1 MAB.	High affinity binding to the extracellular domain of EGFR with internalization of the receptor and downregulation. Exhibits also ADCC. In vitro additive effects with cytotoxics, biological agents, RT. Synergistic activity in combination with CPT-11 in CRC xenografts refractory to single agent CPT-11. Relapse not correlated to EGFR expression. EGFR overexpression tested by ICH assays. Response inversely correlated with activating KRAS/RAF mutation.	Non-linear PK at doses >200 mg/m^2. Vss 2–3 l/m^2, T$_{½}$ 112 hr at the RD 400/250 mg/m^2; C$_{ss}$ achieved after 3 wk of treatment. **Special populations** *Age* No age effect. *Others* Not studied in children, in patients with renal or moderate to severe liver impairment (AST and/or ALT >2.5 NV, or bilirubin >1.5 × NV).

Drug interactions	Route, schedule, and recommendations	Toxicity
In vitro, in vivo synergistic effects with DDP, VP16, and docetaxel; additive with paclitaxel, anthracyclines, NVB.	IV weekly: loading dose (90 min inf.): 4 mg/kg; maintenance (30 min inf.) 2 mg/kg. IV every 3 weeks: loading dose (90 min inf.): 8 mg/kg; maintenance (90 min inf.): 6 mg/kg. **Warning** Pre-existing cardiac conditions or with prior cardiotoxic therapies: baseline cardiac assessment (EKG + Echo or Muga). Pre-existing pulmonary compromise. Do not administer as an IV push or bolus. Do not mix or dilute with other drugs; do not mix with dextrose solutions.	*Most common:* mild, less frequently moderate: 42% asthenia, 36% fever, 32% chills, 26% ↑ cough, 26% headache, 25% diarrhea, 23% dyspnea, 20% infections, 18% rash, 14% insomnia. *Most serious:* cardiomyopathy 5% severe CHF (responsive to cardiac medications) with dyspnea, peripheral edema and ↓ LVEF; discontinue treatment in pts with symptomatic CHF; 19% in combination with anthracyclines, HSR including anaphylaxis and pulmonary symptoms mainly during initial infusion, rechallenge with steroids and antihistamines; infusion reaction during 1st infusions with chills, fever, nausea, vomiting, hypotension (40% mild to moderate); pulmonary events most frequent in elderly.
No interactions with capecitabine and docetaxel.	IV (60 min inf.): loading dose 840 mg. IV (30 min inf.): maintenance 420 mg every 3 wk.	Most common: 58% diarrhea, 32% fatigue, 31% N, 24% abdominal pain, V, 19% anorexia, 17% rash, 14% asymptomatic ↓ LVEF, 13% constipation, 12% dyspnea, 12% edema, 12% asthenia, 11% cough, 11% headache, 11% anemia, 11% arthralgia, 10% back pain. Uncommon: severe HRS.
With strong CYP3A4 inhibitors: decrease dose to 500 mg/day. With strong CYP3A4 inducers: increase dose from 1250 mg/day up to 4500 mg/day based on tolerability. Avoid fenitoin, fenobarbital, carbamazepine (inducers), etoconazole, and antivirals (inhibitors).	PO: 1250 mg o.i.d. continuously, taken at least 1 hr before or 1 hr after a meal. **Warning** QTc to be regularly assessed.	With capecitabine *Most common (>20%)* 65% diarrhea (19% G 3), 44% N (2% G 3), 26% V (2% G 3), 53% hand-foot syndrome (12% G 3), 28% rash (2% G 3), 14% stomatitis. Rare <10% ↓ LVEF.
No PK interaction with CPT-11, DDP, Gemcitabine, Paclitaxel, Docetaxel.	IV (2 hr inf.): 400 mg/m² day 1, then 1 hr inf. 250 mg/m² weekly. Premedication with antihistamine 30–60 min prior the 1st dose. Skin reactions: if occurrence prolong retreatment interval, ↓ dose, and use symptomatic topical steroids. **Warning** Resuscitation equipment available during administration. Monitor HR, BP during the infusion, up to 1 hr after.	*Most common:* 89% acne-like rash (12% severe), correlated with response to treatment, mostly during the first week, lasting for >90 days in 50% of pts, resolving in 50% of pts within 30 days after discontinuation. 40% pruritus (2% severe), 21% nail changes. *Other common G 3–4:* 16% dyspnea, 14% abdominal pain, 11% asthenia, 33% fatigue. 55% hypomagnesemia (17% severe), 13% infections with neutropenia. 4 % HSR, occurring at 1st infusion in 80% of cases, mainly moderate, with fever, chills, rash, dyspnea, cough, back pain; controlled by ↓ infusion rate; if severe, discontinue treatment permanently. Immunogenicity: 4% HACA, not clinically relevant.

Name, chemistry, relevant features	Mechanism of action	Pharmacology and dose modifications
Panitumumab Vectibix® Recombinant, human Mab anti-EGFR.	Inhibits binding of ligands for EGFR. Response not correlated to EGFR expression; response inversely correlated with activating K-RAS/RAF mutation.	Linear PK for doses > 2 mg/kg. C_{ss} reached by the third infusion. $T_{1/2}$ 7.5 days (range: 3.6–10.9 days). Special populations Liver impairment No data available.
Gefitinib Iressa® Synthetic anilinoquinazoline. N-(3-chloro-4-fluorophenyl)-7-methoxy-6-(3-morpholinopropoxy) quinazolin-4-amine).	Selective EGFR-TK inhibitor; EGFR inhibition maintained for 24 hr with need of chronic treatment; no correlation between EGFR expression and xenograft sensitivity; correlation with response and EGFR mutations in exons 18, 19, and 21.	90% protein bound. F 60% not altered by food; slow absorption with C_{max} at 3–7 hr, plasma Css achieved within 10 days, with 56% and 30% interpt./intrapt.: variability. $T_{1/2}$: 48 hr. Extensively distributed: V_{dss} 1400 l after IV Extensively metabolized by CYP3A4; 86% excretion in feces, very limited renal elimination of parent and metabolites (<4%). Special populations No relationship with body weight, age, gender, ethnicity, renal function. *Liver impairment* Not relevant if mild to severe. No data available for non-cancer related impairment.
Erlotinib Tarceva® N-(3-ethynylphenyl)-6,7-bis(2-methoxyethoxy)-4-quinazolinamine, monohydrochloride.	Direct and reversible inhibition of HER1/EGFR TK, and EGFR-dependent proliferation at nanomolar concentrations. In animals, 0.5 µg/ml plasma concentrations associated with EGFR inhibition and antiproliferative activity; after oral administration, maximum inhibition 1 hr, >70% for >12 hr; response correlated with EGFR expression.	>90% protein bound to albumin and AAG; rapid absorption after oral administration with T_{max} 3–4 hr; 60% F ↑ up to 100% with food, $T_{1/2}$ 36 hr, C_{ss} 1.20 mg/ml reached within 7–8 days; no drug accumulation after 150 mg daily dosing. Metabolism: predominantly hepatic through CYP3A4 and CYP3A5; principal active metabolite OSI-420; by other P450 systems also in tumor tissues. Excretion: 83% in feces, 8% in urine.

10.1.3 VEGF

Bevacizumab Avastatin® Recombinant humanized IgG1 MAB anti-VEGF.	Binds to VEGF inhibiting interaction to receptor (Flt1 and KDR).	$T_{1/2}$ 20 days (range 11–50 days); time to Css 100 days. Special population *Age, gender* No adjustment required for age, gender. *Others* No information available in case of renal or liver impairment.

Drug interactions	Route, schedule, and recommendations	Toxicity
	IV(1 hr inf.): 6 mg/kg every 14 days. IV (90 min inf.): doses >1000 mg. **Warning** Do not administer as an IV push or bolus. Limit sun exposure for risk of skin reactions.	*Most common*: 90% skin-related toxicities (16% G 3–4). 65% erythema, 57% acne, 57% pruritus, 29% nail tox, 25% skin exfoliation, 9% hair tox. 4% infusion reaction: (1% G 3–4). 25% fatigue (4% G 3–4), 25% abdominal pain (7% G 3–4), 23% N, 21% diarrhea, 12% edema. 39% hypomagnesemia (2% G 3–4). *Most severe*: <1% pulmonary fibrosis (as potential risk factors: pulmonary fibrosis and interstitial pneumonitis).
With CYP3A4 inhibitors or inducers: itraconazole (inhibitor) ↑ 85% AUC; with rifampicin (inducer) ↓ 88% AUC, ↑ dose to 500 mg to be considered. With drugs ↑ gastric pH: potential reduction of plasma concentrations. With warfarin: INR elevations and/or bleeding events.	PO: 250 mg fixed daily dose. Interrupt treatment temporarily: (maximum 14 days) for G 3–4: diarrhea, ↑ LFTs, skin rashes; any grade eye symptoms. Discontinue treatment for acute onset or worsening of pulmonary symptoms (dyspnea, cough, fever).	*Very common*: 48% G 1–2 diarrhea, 13% N, 12% G 1–2 V, 56% G 1–2 pustular skin rash, rarely itchy. *Common*: 30% G 1–2 ↑ AST/ALT, 7% anorexia, 6% G 1 asthenia, 2% conjunctivitis. *Uncommon* (0.1 to <1%): corneal erosion; 2% ILD, 33% fatal, as interstitial pneumonitis and alveolitis with cough and fever, acute onset, higher mortality in case of concurrent idiopathic pulmonary fibrosis. ILD has occurred in pts with prior RT (31% of cases), prior CT (57%), no previous therapy (12%). In case of aberrant eye-lashes they should be removed.
With CYP3A4 inducers: ↓ AUC by 2/3. With CYP3A4 strong inhibitors: ↑ AUC by 2/3. With warfarin: INR elevations.	PO: 150 mg daily continuously. 1 hr before or 2 hr after food. Treatment for skin rash: steroid creams, topical antibiotics or systemic antihistamines. Interrupt treatment temporarily if diarrhea (administer loperamide), severe skin reactions. Discontinue treatment permanently if ILD.	*Most common*: 75% cutaneous rash (8% ≥G 3), 54% diarrhea (9% ≥G 3), 52% fatigue (18% ≥G 3), 42% dyspnea (28% G 3–4), 33% N (3% G 3), 32% cough (4% G 3–4), 24% infection, 17% stomatitis, 13% pruritus, 13% dry skin, 12% conjunctivitis. *Uncommon*: 1% ILD (as for gefitinib).
With CPT-11 (potential): 33% ↑ concentration of SN-38 in pts receiving bevacizumab in combination with irinotecan/LV/5-FU (IFL) and ↑ of G 3–4 diarrhea: extent and reasons of interaction uncertain.	In combination with: CPT-11/LV/5-FU. IV (90 min inf.): 5 mg/kg once every 2 wk until disease progression. Start treatment at least 28 days after surgery. If surgery: wait at least 20 days from last administration. **Warning** Do not administer as an IV push or bolus. Higher risk of TEE in >65 yr old pts; GI perforation in pts with intestinal subocclusion; hemorrhage in pts with squamous NSCLC, recent history of hemoptosis, ongoing hemorrhage. Discontinue permanently: in case of GI perforation, wound dehiscence, serious bleeding, nephritic syndrome, hypertensive crisis, HSR (no data on rechallenge). Temporary suspension: in case of severe proteinuria.	*Most common*: (it refers to the combination with IFL) : 61% abdominal pain (8% severe), 60% hypertension (7% severe), 52% V, 43% anorexia, 34% severe diarrhea, 32% stomatitis, 26% dizziness, 24% hemorrhage, 15% weight loss, 10% asthenia, 9% DVT (9% severe). 37% leukopenia, 21% severe neutropenia, 36% proteinuria. *Most serious*: 2–4% GI perforation (potentially fatal), 1% wound healing complications (15% if surgery after bevacizumab; hemorrhage: 4.7% severe usually massive hemoptysis (in NSCLC pts), rare GI, subarachnoid, and stroke; *TE*: possibly ↑; hypertension crisis, nephrotic syndrome; 2% CHF: ↑ risk (14%) with concomitant DOX; <3% HSR; <0.1% RPLS (reversible posterior leukoencephalopathy syndrome) with neurological disorders, lethargy, confusion, visual disturbances.

Name, chemistry, relevant features	Mechanism of action	Pharmacology and dose modifications
Sorafenib Nexavar® Tosylate salt of sorafenib. 4-(4-{3-[4-Chloro-3-(trifluoromethyl) phenyl]ureido}phenoxy)*N*2-methylpyridine-2-carboxamide 4-methylbenzenesulfonate.	Inhibitor of multiple intracellular (w-BRAF and m-BRAF, CRAF) and cell surface kinases (KIT, FLT-3, RET, VEGFR-1, and PDGFR-β).	99.5% protein bound. Metabolized primarily in the liver by CYP3A4, and glucuronidated by UGT1A9. Eight metabolites identified (five in plasma). The main metabolite is the pyridine *N*-oxide with potency similar to sorafenib (9–16% of circulating species at C_{ss}). Excretion: 77% in feces, 19% in urine as glucuronidated metabolite, 51% of dose unchanged in feces. F 38–49%, with a high-fat meal F ↓ by 29%. $T_{1/2}$ 25–48 hr. C_{ss} achieved by day 7. T_{max} 3 hr. Linear PK up to 400 mg b.i.d. Dose modifications: If necessary dose may be reduced to 400 mg o.i.d. If additional dose reduction is required it may be reduced to a 400 o.i.d. every other day. Special populations Liver impairment In pts with HCC with mild or moderate impairment AUC are 23–65% lower than in pts with other tumor types.
Sunitinib malate Sutent® Malate salt of sunitinib, Butanedioic acid, hydroxy-, (2S)-, compound with *N*-[2-(diethylamino) ethyl]-5-[(Z)-(5-fluoro-1,2-dihydro-2-oxo-3*H*-indol-3-ylidine)methyl]-2,4-dimethyl-1*H*-pyrrole-3-carboxamide.	Multiple inhibitor of TKI receptors: PDGFRα and PDGFRβ, vascular endothelial growth factors (VEGFR1, VEGFR2, and VEGFR3), stem cell factor receptor (KIT), Fms-like tyrosine kinase-3 (FLT3), colony stimulating factor receptor Type 1 (CSF-1R), and the glial cell-line derived neurotrophic factor receptor (RET).	Protein binding of Sunitinib and Sunitinib malate in vitro: 95% and 90%. Metabolism: primarily by CYP450 to primary active metabolite (23–37% of total exposure), further metabolized by CYP3A4. Elimination: 61% in feces, 16% in urine. CL/F: 34–62 l/hr with a 40% interpts. variability. Linear PK beetween 25 and 100 mg, AUC and C_{max} increase proportionally with dose. T_{max}: 6–12 hr. No food effect on F. V_d/F: 2230 l.
Vandetanib *N*-(4-bromo-2-fluorophenyl)-6-methoxy-7-[(1-methylpiperidin-4-yl)methoxy]quinazolin-4-amine.	Inhibition of VEGFR, EGFR, and RET TK with mainly angiogenic effect.	Metabolism by CYP3A4 to *N*-demethyl and *N*-oxide metabolites, HEPATIC (44%) and renal (25%). Linear PK. T_{max} 4–10 hr. CL 11 l/hr. V_d 3000 l $T_{1/2}$ 10 days. C_{ss} by day 28. Special populations *Renal impairment* ↑ by 1.5 and by 2 fold in case of mild/moderate and severe renal impairment respectively.

10.1.4 CD20

Rituximab Mabthera® Chimeric anti-CD20 IgG k MAB with murine variable and human constant regions.	High affinity binding to CD20 (human B-lymphocyte-restricted differentiation Ag, Bp35), on pre-B, mature B, and in >90% NHL B cells. CD20 is not internalized upon binding, neither shed nor found in blood. Mechanism of action not fully understood, via ADCC and CDC. Within few days ↓ of peripheral CD20+ cells with recovery beginning after 6 mo.	Linear PK; ↓ CL with drug accumulation after multiple infusions, $T_{1/2}$ 29 days after 2nd dose, detectable serum levels up to 3–6 mo after treament completion. Metabolism not understood. Special population *Age* No age effect. *Others* ↑ risk of cytokine release and TLS if WBC > 50×10^9/mm³ or high tumor burden (>25×10^9/mm³ circulating tumor cells).

Drug interactions	Route, schedule, and recommendations	Toxicity
With compound glucuronidated by UGT1A1 and UGT1A9: the concomitant administration of Sorafenib results in their ↑ AUC. With Docetaxel: 36–80% ↑ in docetaxel AUC and a 16–32% increase in docetaxel C_{max}. With Doxorubicin: 21% increase in the AUC of doxorubicin. With Fluorouracil: both increases (21–47%) and decreases (10%) in the AUC of fluorouracil. With CYP2B6 and CYP2C8 substrates: Sorafenib inhibits CYP2B6 and CYP2C8 with ↑ AUC of substrates. With CYP3A4 inducers: 37% ↓ Sorafenib AUC.	PO daily: 400 mg b.i.d. without food. **Warning** 3 days break to be considered.	Very common: 43% diarrhea (2% G 3), 40% erythema, 40% increased lipase-amylase (9% G 3), 37% asthenia (5% G 3), 45% hypophosphatemia (13% G 3), 27% alopecia, 19% pruritus, 17% hypertension, 15% hemorrhage, 12% thrombocytopenia, 10% arthralgia. Uncommon: hypertensive crisis, myocardial ischemia and/or infarction, CHF, folliculitis.
With CYP3A4 inhibitors and inducers: ↑ or ↓ Sunitinib concentrations of ~50%. Dose increase or reduction to be considered by 12.5 mg.	For GIST and RCC: PO: 50 mg daily. 4 wk on/2 wk off (Schedule 4/2). Dose modifications of 12.5 mg according safety. **Warning** Discontinue permanently if CHF. Monitoring for BP and thyroid function; baseline LVEF and thyroid function required.	Very common (≥20%): 58% fatigue (49% G 3–4), 58% diarrhea (6% G 3–4), 49% N, 43% mucositis/stomatitis, 28% V, 30% hypertension, 27% rash, 21% hand-foot syndrome, 30% skin discoloration, 44% altered taste, 38% anorexia, 18% myalgia, 30% bleeding. Serious adverse reactions: left ventricular dysfunction, dose dependent QT prolongation (11% in GIST), hemorrhage, hypertension (30% in RCC), and adrenal function.
With cisplatin: ↑ exposure to CDDP by 30%. No PK interactions with docetaxel, pemetrexed, FOLFIRI, FOLFOX, gemcitabine, vinorelbine.	PO: 300 mg daily o.i.d.	*Most common (>10%):* QT prolongation, hypertension, headache, constipation, diarrhea, nausea, thrombocytopenia, rash, fatigue, weight loss, anorexia, anxiety, depression, insomnia.
With antihypertensive agents: ↑ hypotension with infusion. With DDP: renal failure, use with caution. With live vaccines: ↑ risk of systemic viral infection. Do not mix or dilute with other drugs.	Weekly IV infusion: 375 mg/m^2 on days 1, 8, 15, and 22. *1st infusion rate:* 50 mg/hr with 50 mg/hr increments every 30 min up to 400 mg/hr. *Subsequent infusion rate:* 100 mg/hr initial rate with 100 mg/hr increments every 30 min up to 400 mg/hr. Premedication: analgesic/antipyretic always, consider steroids. **Warning** Close observation for 24 hr after 1st for severe reactions (See Toxicity). Infusion related events: interrupt infusion, give paracetamol and antihistamines, resume infusion at 50% rate once symptoms have resolved.	*Most common* infusion-related events (77% 1st inf., 30% subsequent ones, 14% at 8th inf.): fever, chills/rigor, urticaria, headache, pruritus, hypotension and flushing: 1% HSR with angioedema and bronchospasm, onset within 2 hr; hemic and lymphatic system 67% (48% G 3–4), mainly lymphopenia (G 3–4 40%); 44% skin and appendages (2% G 3–4): 17% rash, night sweats, pruritus, urticaria; musculoskeletal (26% arthralgia, 10% myalgia); *GI* 23% N, 10% V, 10% diarrhea; Others: 40% fatigue, 38% pulmonary events (rarely bronchiolitis and interstitial pneumonitis up to 3–6 mo after treatment), 31% infections (19% bacterial, 10% viral, 1% fungine), 19% headache, 14% abdominal pain, 10% dizziness. 5% cardiotoxicity, supraventricular tachycardia. Immunogenicity HACA not documented.

Name, chemistry, relevant features	Mechanism of action	Pharmacology and dose modifications
Tositumomab Bexxar® Radioimmunotherapeutic murine IgG2a lambda MAB against CD 20, covalently bound to iodine 131.	Binds to CD20 (human B-lymphocyte-restricted differentiation Ag expressed on pre-B cells, mature B cells, and in 90% NHL B cells. CD20 is not internalized upon binding, neither shed nor found in the blood. Mechanisms of action not fully elucidated, may include triggering of apoptosis (with the contribution of ^{131}I), CDC, and ADCC. Still recovering of CD20+ cells after at least 12 wk.	After predosing with unlabeled MAB $\downarrow$ splenic targeting and $\uparrow$ terminal $T_{\frac{1}{2}}$. CL 68 mg/hr. In pts with high tumor burden, splenomegaly, or BM involvement, $\uparrow$ CL, V_d, and $\downarrow$ terminal $T_{\frac{1}{2}}$; elimination by decay and urinary excretion (98%). <u>Special populations</u> *Renal impairment* Not studied; ^{131}I CL might be $\downarrow$ leading to $\uparrow$ exposure.
Ibritumomab tiuxetan In-111 Ibritumomab tiuxetan (In111-I) Y-90 Ibritumomab tiuxetan (Y90-I). Zevalin® Immunoradiotherapeutic agent. Immunoconjugate from a stable thiourea covalent bond between Ibritumomab (murine IgG_1 k MAB anti-CD20) and the linker-chelator tiuxetan, which provides chelation site for Indium-111 or Yttrium-90.	Against CD20 B-lymphocyte antigen (See Tositumomab). Induces apoptosis in vitro. Tiuxetan is covalently linked to the amino groups of exposed lysines and arginines of the MAB. The radioisotopes (^{111}In or ^{90}Y) linked to the MAB can be targeted directly to B-cell lymphoma: In111-I for bioimaging, Y90-I as radioimmunotherapeutic. The beta emission from ^{90}Y induces cellular damage by free radicals in the target and neighboring cells.	When preceded by unlabeled Ibritumomab, ^{111}In Ibritumomab detected 56% and 92% of known disease sites, respectively. Effective $T_{\frac{1}{2}}$ for ^{90}Y activity 30 hr; area under the fraction of injected activity (FIA) vs. time curve 39 hr, 7.2% of the injected activity excreted in 7 days urine.

10.1.5 Other moAb

Alemtuzumab Campath® Recombinant, humanized IgG1k MAB anti-CD52	Against CD52 antigen, cell surface glycoprotein in normal and malignant B and T lymphocytes, some CD34+ cells, NK cells, monocytes, macrophages, and tissues of male reproductive system. Mechanism of action not fully elucidated, possibly ADCC.	Non-linear elimination kinetics. V_{dss}: 0.18 l/kg. CL $\downarrow$ with repeated administrations due to $\downarrow$ receptor-mediated clearance. $T_{\frac{1}{2}}$: 11 hr after the first 30 mg dose, 6 days after the last of 12 wk period. <u>Special populations</u> Liver and renal impairment not studied, no need of dose adjustments according to age.

Drug interactions	Route, schedule, and recommendations	Toxicity
<u>Anticoagulants and drugs affecting Pt function</u>: potential pharmacological interaction with ↑ of bleeding. <u>Vaccines</u>: not studied, but caution is recommended.	Two-step regimen: step 1 dosimetry, followed after 7–14 days by the therapeutic step. <u>Dosimetry</u>: Tositumomab <u>IV (inf. 60 min)</u>: 450 mg, followed by <u>IV (inf. 20 min)</u>: ^{131}I Tositumomab monitor post infusion with SPECT at 1 hr, 2–4 and 7–10 days. If acceptable biodistribution proceed to <u>therapy (single course)</u>: Tositumomab 450 mg IV (inf. 60 min) followed by ^{131}I Tositumomab (35 mg Tositumomab) at therapeutic doses according to Pt count mm^3. Do <u>not</u> treat if Pt < 100,000/mm^3. <u>Maximum dose of</u> ^{131}I Tositumomab: 75 cGy. <u>Thyroid protective therapy</u>: initiate 24 hr before and for 14 days after. Assess thyroid status before treatment and monitor annually. <u>Premedication</u> with acetominophene and antihistamine suggested but value not known. <u>HSR</u>: discontinue treatment and treat appropriately. **Warning** Resuscitation equipment available.	*Most common*: 46% asthenia, 36% N (with V 15%); 29% infusion related effects (chills, fever, rigor, hypotension, dyspnea, bronchospasm, sweating), during or within 48 hr from therapy; 9–17% hypothyroidism, 15% abdominal pain, 14% anorexia. *Most serious*: <u>pancytopenia</u> severe (G 3–4), prolonged: 63% neutropenia, 53% thrombocytopenia, 29% anemia; nadir 4–7 wk, recovering in 30 days (90 days in 5% of pts); 45% infections, 12% hemorrhage; 6% *HSR* (bronchospasm and angioedema), risk ↑ in pts with HAMA. <u>Secondary malignancies</u>: 4.2% and 10.7% AML and myelodysplasia at 2 and 4 yr respectively, onset average 27 mo; other malignancies 5%.
<u>Anticoagulants and drugs affecting Pt function</u>: potential pharmacological interaction with ↑ of bleeding.	The therapeutic regimen is administered in two steps: Step 1 includes one infusion of rituximab preceding In-111 and Step 2 follows Step 1 by 7–9 days and consists of a 2nd infusion of rituximab followed by Y90-I. *Step 1*: Rituximab <u>IV</u> 250 mg/m^2 single infusion followed by In111-I IV push 5.0 mCi (1.6 mg total antibody dose) for dosimetry and biodistribution. *Biodistribution*: post-infusion SPECT at 2–24 hr, 48–72 hr, and 90–120 hr. If acceptable biodistribution proceed <u>after 7–9 days</u> to Step 2. *Step 2*: Rituximab 250 mg/m^2 single infusion, followed by Y90-I IV push doses according to Pt counts (mm^3). Do <u>not</u> treat if Pt < 100,000/mm^3. <u>Maximun dose Y90-I</u>: 32.0 mCi/kg.	*Common*: 43% asthenia, 31% N, 27% CNS (dizziness, insomnia), 18% musculoskeletal, 12% V, 12% headache, 9% diarrhea, 8% rash. *Most serious* <u>prolonged severe pancytopenia</u>: 57% ≥G 2 neutropenia (30% severe), nadir between 7–9 wk, recovering within 3 wk; 95% thrombocytopenia (61% severe), nadir 53 days, recovering in 4–5 wk; 61% anemia (17% severe), nadir 68 days; hemorrhage (1% severe); 29% infections (5% severe); <u>allergic reactions</u> [1–5% G 4, all grades: 24% chills, 17% fever, 14% dispnea, 5% HSR (bronchospasm and angioedema, <1% G 4)]. <u>Secondary malignancies</u> 2%. <u>Immunogenicity</u> within 90 days, 4% HAMA or HACA.
	<u>IV (2 hr inf.)</u>: start at 3 mg daily; if well tolerated (e.g., inf. related toxicities <G2), escalate to 10 mg daily, if well tolerated go to maintenance dose 30 mg/day, three times per week on alternate days (i.e., Monday, Wednesday, and Friday) for up to 12 wk. <u>Premedication</u>: 30 min before, diphenhydramine PO 50 mg, acetaminophen PO 1000 mg. <u>Anti-Herpes and PCP prophylaxis</u>: start with therapy and continue for 2 mo after completion or up to ≥200/mm^3 CD4. <u>Infusion related events</u>: interrupt infusion, give hydrocortisone IV 200 mg. **Warning** *Absolute contraindications*: Active systemic infections; immunodeficiencies. Do <u>not</u> exceed single dose of 30 mg and/or cumulative weekly doses of 90 mg. Do <u>not</u> administer as an IV push or bolus.	*Common*: 86% <u>infusion-related events</u> with: 16% severe chills/rigor, 19% fever, 5% fatigue, 4% V, 3% back pain; <u>infections</u>: 15% sepsis, 10% severe pneumonitis, 17% opportunistic infections; <u>hematological</u>: 64% severe neutropenia lasting 28 days, 38% anemia, 50% thrombocytopenia, profound lymphopenia lasting 6 mo after treatment.

Name, chemistry, relevant features	Mechanism of action	Pharmacology and dose modifications
Gemtuzumab ozogamycin Mylotarg® Recombinant humanized IgG4 k MAB (Gemtuzumab) conjugated to calicheamycin, a semisynthetic cytotoxic antibiotic (ozogamycin).	Against CD33, a sialic acid-dependent adhesion protein, expressed on leukemic blasts in >80% of AML pts, on normal and leukemic myeloid colony-formation cells, but not on pluripotent hematopoietic stem cells or non-hematopoietic cells. After binding, the complex is internalized and ozogamycin released by hydrolysis within the lysosomes of the myeloid cell; the cytotoxic binds to the minor groove of DNA, with DNA-DSB and cell death.	After a dose of 9 mg/m² (2 hr inf.): elimination $T_{1/2}$ of total and unconjugated calicheamycin 45 and 100 hr, respectively; after a second 9 mg/m² dose: $T_{1/2}$ of total calicheamycin 60 hr and AUC twice that after 1st dose. PK of unconjugated calicheamycin not changed. Isoenzyme involved in ozogamycin metabolism not determined. Special populations: *Age* >60 yr pts, ↑ incidence of ↑ LFTs. *Liver impairment* Not studied in pts with bilirubin > 2 mg/dl. Extra caution in pts with ↑ LFTs (See Toxicity). *Renal impairment* No information. *High tumor burden:* WBC count > 30,000/mm³, ↑ risk of TLS, severe infusion related reactions, pulmonary events.

10.2 BCR/ABL

Imatinib mesylate Gleevec® 4-[(4-Methyl-1-piperazinyl) methyl]-N-[4-methyl-3-[[4-(3-pyridinyl)-2-pyrimidinyl] amino]-phenyl]benzamide methanesulfonate.	Competitive inhibitor of Bcr-Abl TK, constitutively activated in Ph+ CML. Inhibits also TK of c-Kit, PDGF, and SCF. Inhibits proliferation and induces apoptosis in vitro and in vivo Ph+ CML cells.	95% protein bound mostly to albumin and AAG; F 98%, T_{max} 2–4 hr, high fat meals ↓ absorption; linear and dose-dependent PK (25–1000 mg). Accumulation at C_{ss} when giveno.i.d., $T_{1/2}$ parent and major active metabolite, 18 and 40 hr respectively. Metabolized mainly by CYP3A4, CYP2D6, and others, N-demethylated piperazine derivative main active human metabolite with potence similar to imatinib; eliminated 13% in 7 days urine and 68% in feces (mostly as metabolites); CL < 40% interpt. variability. Special populations *Age* Edema more frequent in elderly; no pediatric data. *Liver impairment* No guidelines, suggested: bilirubin > 3 × NV and AST 5 × NV: withhold, then if bilirubin < 1.5 × NV and AST < 2.5 × NV: resume at ↓ doses.
Dasatinib Sprycel® N-(2-chloro-6-methylphenyl)-2-[[6-[4-(2-hydroxyethyl)-1-piperazinyl]-2-methyl-4-pyrimidinyl] amino]-5-thiazolecarboxamide, monohydrate.	Inhibition of: BCR-ABL, SRC family (SRC, LCK, YES, FYN), c-KIT, EPHA2, and PDGFRβ. Active in CML tesistant to imatinib because of secondary Bcr-Abl mutations.	>90% human plasma proteins binding of Dasatinib and its active metabolite. Primarily metabolized by CYP3A4 to an active equipotent metabolite corresponding 5% of Dasatinib AUC. Elimination: 85% excreted in feces, 4% in urine. T_{max}: 0.5–6 hr. pH dependent absorption, oral absorption ↑ with food. Linear PK up to 240 mg/day. $T_{1/2}$: 3–5 hr. Extensive tissue distribution. Special populations Data not available with hepatic and renal impairment.
Nilotinib Tasigna® 4-methyl-N-[3-(4-methyl-1H-imidazol-1-yl)-5-(trifluoromethyl) phenyl]-3-[[4-(3-pyridinyl)-2-pyrimidinyl]amino]-benzamide, monohydrochloride, monohydrate.	Bcr-Abl kinase inhibitor, binds and stabilizes inactive conformation of Abl TK domain, able to overcome imatinib resistance due to Bcr-Abl kinase mutations. IC50: Bcr-Abl < PDGFR < c-Kit.	Human protein binding: ~98%. $T_{1/2}$: ~17 hr. C_{ss} achieved by day 8. Metabolized to inactive species through CYP3A4 system. >90% eliminated in feces (69% as parent compound). T_{max}: 3 hr. F affected by food.

Drug interactions	Route, schedule, and recommendations	Toxicity
	<u>IV (2 hr inf.):</u> 9 mg/m² on day 1 and on day 14 (two doses total). <u>Premedication:</u> diphenhydramine PO 50 mg, acetaminophen PO 650–1000 mg followed by two additional doses every 4 hr. <u>Close observation</u> for severe reactions for at least 4 hr (See Toxicity). <u>Leukoreduction with HU or leukapheresis:</u> consider in pts with WBC count > 30,000/mm³. <u>HSR or infusion related events:</u> interrupt infusion, give paracetamol and antihistamines, resume infusion at 50% rate once symptoms are resolved. **Warning** Do <u>not</u> administer as IV push or bolus.	*Most common:* <u>infusion reactions</u> (≥ G 3 in ≤10% of pts): 30–60% chills, fever, N&V, headache, 5–10% hypotension, hypertension, hypoxia, dyspnea, 2% hyperglycemia; <u>hematologic:</u> 98% ≥G 3 myelosuppression (recovery ANC > 500/mm³ 40 days post 1st dose), 15% bleeding, including 2% cerebral intracranial hemorrhage, 2% DIC; <u>others:</u> 28% infection, 35% mucositis, 23% ≥G 3 ↑ bilirubin generally transient. *Most severe:* <u>VOD,</u> ↑ risk in pts either before or after SCT or with ↑ LFT. <u>Pulmonary events:</u> dyspnea, infiltrates, pleural effusion, non-cardiogenic pulmonary edema, ARDS. <u>TLS.</u>
<u>With CYP3A4 inhibitors:</u> (ketoconazole, grapefruit juice, erythromycin, etc.) 40% ↑ AUC. <u>With CYP3A4 inducers:</u> (DXM, St. John's Wort, rifampicin, phenytoin, etc.) ↓ AUC. <u>With CYP3A4 substrates:</u> (cyclosporine, triazolo benzodiazepine, etc.) ↑ plasma concentration of substrate. <u>With CYP2D6 substrates:</u> (CTX, β blockers, morphine, etc.) ↑ plasma concentration of substrate. <u>With warfarin:</u> ↑ anticoagulant effects. <u>With acetaminophen:</u> potential ↑ hepatotoxicity.	<u>PO</u> daily. <u>CML</u> *Chronic phase:* 400 mg daily; *accelerated phase and blastic crisis:* 600 mg daily. ↑ to 600 mg and 800 mg (400 mg × 2 mg) respectively daily, in absence of severe toxicity, if: disease progression or failure to achieve hematological response after 3 mo, or failure to achieve cytogenetic response after 6–12 mo, or loss of previous hem or cytogenetic response. <u>GIST:</u> 400–600 mg daily.	*Very common (>10%):* ↑ weight, neutropenia, thrombocytopenia, anemia, headache, nausea, vomiting, diarrhea, periorbital edema, rash, muscular pain, arthralgia, myalgia, joint pain, fluid retention, fatigue. *Common (>1%):* ↑ AST, ALT, paresthesia, conjunctivitis, gastritis, pruritus, night sweats, photosensitivity, joint swelling, fever. *Uncommon (<1%):* ↑ creatinine, palpitations, tachycardia, CHF, somnolence, neuropathy, stomatitis, esophagitis, pancreatitis, urticaria, purpura, insomnia, gynecomastia, ↑ bilirubin, hypophosphatemia, hyponatremia, chest pain.
With CYP3A4 inhibitors: consider dose ↓. *With CYP3A4 inducers:* consider dose ↑. *With CYP3A4 substrates:* ↑ AUC of substrates. Avoid concomitant antacids and H2 antagonists/proton pump inhibitors. If needed at least 2 hr interval.	<u>CML-CP:</u> PO 100 mg o.i.d. <u>CML-AP and Ph+ ALL:</u> PO 70 mg b.i.d.	<u>Most common:</u> myelosuppression. In CML-CP: 46% neutropenia, 41% thrombocytopenia, 18% anemia. In CML-AP: 68% neutropenia, 71% thrombocytopenia, 55% anemia. 37% fluid retention events (8% G 3), 31% diarrhea (3% G 3–4), 24% headache, 22% skin rash, 22% N, 21% hemorrhage, 21% fatigue, 20% dyspnea, 19% anorexia, hypocalcemia, hypophosphatemia. <u>Most serious:</u> 4% gastrointestinal bleeding, 2% CHF.
Competitive inhibitor of CYP3A4, CYP2C8, CYP2C9, CYP2D6, and UGT1A1. <u>With CYP3A4 strong inhibitors or inducers:</u> significant modification of AUC. If strong CYP3A4 inhibitors cannot be avoided: monitor QT values regularly. **Warning** Hypokalemia or hypomagnesemia must be corrected before starting and should be regularly monitored.	<u>PO:</u> 400 mg b.i.d. continuously (no food for at least 2 hr before and 1 hr after dosing).	In CML-chronic phase: *Most common (>10%):* 33% rash (2% G 3–4), 29% pruritus, 31% nausea, 28% fatigue, 31% headache, 22% diarrhea, 18% arthralgia, 17% cough, 14% myalgia, 11% edema. In CML-accelerated phase (>10%): 28% rash, 20% pruritus, 18% N, 16% fatigue, 19% diarrhea, 16% arthralgia, 13% cough, 14% myalgia, 11% edema. G 3–4 lab abnormalities (chronic/accelerated phase): neutropenia (28%/37%), thrombocytopenia (28%/17%), anemia (8%/23%), ↑ lipase (15%/17%). Rare: 2% QT > 60 msec.

Name, chemistry, relevant features	Mechanism of action	Pharmacology and dose modifications

10.3 mTOR

| **Temsirolimus** Torisel®

 Rapamycin, 42-[3-hydroxy-2-(hydroxymethyl)-2-methylpropanoate]. | Inhibitor of mTOR. Binds to an intracellular protein (FKBP-12), and the protein-drug complex inhibits the activity of mTOR with inhibition of phosphorylation of p70S6k, downstream of mTOR.
 Antiangiogenetic effect through ↓ HIF1 levels. | Metabolized by CYP3A4 to five metabolites of which sirolimus is the principal and the only active metabolite. 14% interpts. CV of AUC.
 Extensive tissue distribution and retention in blood components.
 Elimination primarily via the feces (82% within 14 days).
 $T_{1/2}$ of Temsirolimus and Sirolimus: 17.3 and 54.6 hr respectively.

 Dose modifications: Temsirolimus should be held for ANC <1000/mm^3, pt count <75,000/mm^3, or NCI CTCAE ≥ grade 3 adverse reactions. Once toxicities have resolved to grade ≤2 Temsirolimus may be restarted with the dose reduced by 5 mg/wk to a dose of at least 15 mg/wk. |
| **Everolimus** RAD001

 Oral rapamycin derivative. | Inhibits mTOR through binding to FMBP-12 protein with ↓ phosphorylation of S6K and p-4E-BP1.
 Antiangiogenetic effect through ↓ HIF-1 levels. | Unbound fraction: 26%.
 Extensively metabolized in the liver mainly by CYP3A4 and eliminated in the bile. Major metabolites are inactive. Bioavailability: 30%.
 Linear PK up to 20 mg.
 T_{max} 1–2 hr.
 V_d: 342 l. $T_{1/2}$ ~30 hr.

 <u>Special population</u>
 Liver impairment
 RAD dose to be reduced to half the normal. |

10.4 Others

| **Tretinoin (all-trans-retinoic acid, ATRA)** Vesanoid®

 Natural retinoid; related to retinol (vitamin A); differentiating agent. | Differentiating effect through binding to cytosolic and nuclear receptors (RARs) with induction of transcription of genes involved in growth inhibition and differentiation. ATRA most active among natural retinoids in reversing changes of epithelial derived malignancies. | >95% protein bound; T_{max} 1–2 hr; F 50% affected by biliary pH and high-fat meal; high interpt. variability of absorption and plasma levels. $T_{1/2}$ < 1 hr, undetectable after 10 hr; metabolized by CYP450 to 4-OXO-ATRA then glucuronidated; 60% excretion in urine, 30% in feces.
 Induces its own metabolism: ↑ CL after 2 wk chronic dosing due to ↑ catabolism and ↑ tissue sequestration. |
| **Vorinostat** Zolinza®

 N-hydroxy-*N*'-phenyloctanediamide. | Inhibitor of HDAC1, HDAC2, and HDAC3 (Class I) and HDAC6 (Class II). | 71% human protein binding.
 The major metabolic pathway involve glucuronidation and hydrolysis to inactive species.
 Elimination: >5% dose in urine.
 $T_{1/2}$ ~2.0 hr.
 T_{max} 4 (0.5–14) hr. |

Drug interactions	Route, schedule, and recommendations	Toxicity
<u>CYP3A4 inhibitors:</u> should be avoided. Grapefruit juice may also increase plasma concentrations of Sirolimus and should be avoided. Otherwise a dose reduction to 12.5 mg/wk should be considered.	<u>IV (30–60 min inf.):</u> 25 mg weekly. Premedication: IV antihistamines 30 min before the administration.	*Most common (≥10%):* 47% rash (5% G 3), 41% mucositis (3% G 3), 35% edema (3% G 3), 20% infections, 20% back pain (3% G 3), 14% nail disorders, 11% dry skin. *Most common (≥30%) lab abnormalities:* 94% anemia, 89% hyperglycemia (16% G3), 87% hyperlipemia, 83% hypertriglyceridemia, 53% lymphopenia, 49% hypophosphatemia (18% G 3–4), 40% thrombocytopenia, 21% hypokalemia.
<u>With CYP3A4 and P-gp substrates:</u> competitive inhibition. Coadministration with strong CYP3A inhibitors and strong inducers to be avoided (e.g., Grapefruit and grapefruit juice). <u>With Imatinib:</u> ↑ AUC. RAD001 may affect the response to vaccinations making the response less effective.	<u>PO</u> Weekly: 50–70 mg. Daily: 5–10 mg. With or without food.	*Most common:* 40% stomatitis/oral mucositis (3% G3), 37% fatigue (3% G 3), 25% rash, 16% anorexia, 12% V, 10% edema, 10% infection, 8% polmonitis (3% G 3), 8% dyspnea (1% G 3). 77% hypertriglyceridemia, 76% hypercholesterolemia (3% G 3–4), 50% hyperglycemia (12% G3–4), 46% ↑ creatinine, 32% hypophosphatemia, 20% ↑ AST and ALT, 20% thrombocytopenia, 11% neutropenia.
<u>With CYP450 inducers:</u> ↑ catabolism; unproven clinical relevance. <u>With CYP450 inhibitors:</u> (e.g., ketoconazole) ↑ T$_{1/2}$ of unproven clinical relevance.	<u>Maintenance regimen only.</u> <u>Intermittent PO schedule[a]:</u> 45 mg/m^2 daily, in two divided doses, on days 1–14 every 3 mo. [a]to overcome metabolic induction. <u>Administer in fed conditions.</u> <u>Monitor LFTs:</u> temporary withdrawal if >5 × NV. <u>RA-APL syndrome:</u> HD IV steroids at first suspicion.	86% headache in 50% due to ↑ intracranial pressure (pseudotumor cerebri, especially in children), early signs: papilledema, N&V, visual disturbances; 77% skin and mucosal toxicity (dryness, itching, peeling, cheilitis); 70% bone pain, arthralgia; 50% ↑ LFTs slowly reversible; 25% edema, fatigue, fever, and rigors; 17% ocular disorders; 25% RA-APL syndrome (usually during 1st month) with leukocytosis, fever, hypotension, dyspnea, RX lung infiltrates, fluid retention, CHF, DIC-like syndrome (differential diagnosis with APL). Teratogenic: avoid pregnancy.
Vorinostat is not an inhibitor of CYP metabolizing systems. <u>With anticoagulants:</u> prolongation of PT and INR.	<u>PO:</u> 400 mg with food o.i.d. continously. ↓ to 300 mg o.i.d. according to tolerability. **Warning** Complete CBC, electrolytes, creatinine to be checked every 2 wk, then monthly. Regular ECG control.	*Most common (≥20%):* gastrointestinal symptoms (52% diarrhea, 41% N, 24% anorexia, 21% weight decrease, 15% V, 15% constipation), constitutional symptoms (52% fatigue, 16% chills). Hematologic abnormalities: 26% thrombocytopenia (6% G 3), 14% anemia (2% G 3), and taste disorders (30% dysgeusia, 16% dry mouth). *Most serious:* 5% PE.

Name, chemistry, relevant features	Mechanism of action	Pharmacology and dose modifications
Thalidomide Thalomid® a-(*N*-phtalimido) glutarimide.	Immunomodulatory with anti-inflammatory and antiangiogenic activity. Mechanism of action not fully understood: in humans ↓ of excessive TNFα production and down modulation of selected adhesion molecules involved in leukocytes migration. ↑ NK cells. In MM ↑ in plasma levels of IL-2, IFN-γ. Antiangiogenic through ↓ proliferation of endothelial cells.	55–66% protein bound. Dose-linear PK. 90% bioavailability; T_{max} 3–6 hr, distribution unknown, crosses BBB; metabolism unknown, liver metabolism minimal, undergoes non-enzymatic hydrolysis to multiple metabolic species; mechanism of excretion mostly unknown: $T_{\frac{1}{2}}$ 5–7 hr, CL 1.1 ml/min, 0.7% of dose excreted unchanged in urine. Special populations No need of dose adjustment.
Lenalidomide Revlimid® Thalidomide analogue 3-(4-amino-1-oxo 1,3-dihydro-2H-isoindol-2-yl) piperidine-2,6-dione.	Same mechanism of action of thalidomide.	30% protein bound. 66% eliminated unchanged in urine. Human metabolism unknown. No accumulation after repeated doses. T_{max} 1.5 hr. $T_{\frac{1}{2}}$ 3 hr. Linear PK. Special populations Mild renal impairment: 15% ↑ AUC.
Bortezomib Velcade® Modified dipeptidyl boronic acid derived from leucine and phenylalanine. Hydrolyzed in water to the biologically active boronic form.	Reversible and specific inhibitor of chymotrypsin like activity site of proteasome B 20S subunit with block of NF-κB activation, induction of apoptosis, ↓ adhesion in MM cells to stromal cells, block of intracellular production of IL6, direct cytotoxic effect, production and expression of proangiogenic mediators.	83% protein bound; linear PK with $T_{\frac{1}{2}}\alpha$ < 10 min, $T_{\frac{1}{2}}\beta$ 76–108 hr with extensive tissue distribution (V_d 400–600 L) also in RBC. Maximum PD effect (inhibition of catalytic proteolytic core 20S in whole blood) within 5 min lasting for 24 hr, 10–30% inhibition up to 72 hr, 90% metabolized to small amount of inactive deboronated species by CYP3A4 and 2C19; elimination pathway not characterized in humans. 60% proteasome activity inhibition in pts for plasma levels of 1–2 ng/ml. Special populations *Renal impairment* Even severe does not affect.
Bexarotene Targretin® 4-[1-(5,6,7,8-tetrahydro-3,5,5,8,8-pentamethyl-2-naphthalenyl) ethenyl] benzoic acid.	Mechanism of action on CTCL unknown. Binds selectively RXR subtypes (RXRα, RXRβ, RXRγ), can form heterodimers with other RARs, vitamin D receptor, and PPARs. Activated receptors function as transcription factors for cellular differentiation and proliferation. Induces growth inhibition in vitro, and tumor regression in vivo in some animal models.	>99% protein bound; after topical application plasma concentration usually low (<5 ng/ml). Tissue uptake not studied. After PO metabolized by CYP3A4 to two active oxidative metabolites then glucuronidated; <1% renal excretion. Special populations *Renal impairment* Caution: PK might be altered because of high protein binding. *Liver impairment* Not studied, but expected greatly ↓ CL.

Drug interactions	Route, schedule, and recommendations	Toxicity
None known; avoid concomitant sedatives.	<u>PO daily</u> MM: initial dose 200 mg, after 14 days in absence of severe side effects increase to 400 mg daily. <u>Admnister at bedtime to minimize dizziness and somnolence, at least 1 hr after meal.</u> **Warning** ↑ <u>risk of TEE</u>, pts may benefit of an anticoagulant prophylaxys. <u>Do not start</u> if ANC <750/mm³. <u>Discontinue</u> at earliest symptoms of SPN effects, if clinically appropriate. **Teratogen** Can cause severe defects in humans, male and female contraception must be implemented.	*In combination with dexamethasone:* *Most common:* 79% fatigue (17% severe), 57% peripheral edema (6% severe), 55% constipation (8% severe), 42% dyspnea (12% severe), 30% generalized skin rash (8% severe) (pruritic, macular, erythematous, not dose related, reversible, can be rechallenged at lower doses); 28% dizziness, 28% anorexia (4% severe), 28% confusion (9% severe), 28% N (5% severe), 25% incoordination (1% severe), 23% fever, 22% TE (22% severe), 20% tremor (1% severe), 17% myalgia, 15% anxiety (1% severe). 77% anemia (16% severe), 43% hyponatremia (13% severe), 31% neutropenia (13% severe), 22% hypokalemia (5% severe), 14% hyperbilirubinemia (2% severe). *Most severe:* 90% neurotoxicity (22% severe). <u>SNP</u> (up to 54%) can be irreversible after chronic use (cumulative dose not known) or if severe; starts with symmetrical paresthesias of hands and feet, progresses to cramps, postural tremor, ↓ muscle reflexes.
No known interactions.	<u>Myelodisplastic syndromes:</u> PO daily: 10 mg with water. <u>MM:</u> <u>PO daily:</u> 25 mg days 1–21 every 4 wk. **Warning** Monitor renal function. **Teratogen as thalidomide** Females of childbearing potential should be advised to avoid pregnancy, they must use at least one effective contraceptive method.	*In MDS pts (10 mg):* *Most common:* 61% thrombocytopenia (50% severe), 58.8% neutropenia, 5% febrile neutropenia. 48% diarrhea (4% severe), 42% pruritus (2% severe), 36% rash, 31% fatigue (5% severe), 24% constipation, 24% N (4% severe), 21% pyrexia (4% severe), 20% edema, 22% arthralgia (2% severe), 21% back pain (5% severe), 20% dizziness (3% severe), 20% headache (2% severe), 12% abdominal pain, 10% insomnia. *In MM (25 mg):* 8% DVT (7% G 3–4).
<u>With CYP3A4 strong inhibitors:</u> ↑ AUC.	<u>IV</u> bolus 2 per week for 2 wk every 3 wk: 1.3 mg/m². Dose modified for neuropathic pain and/or SPN according to NCI CTC.	*Common:* 61% asthenia (12% G 3), 57% N (2% G 3), 57% diarrhea (7% G 3), 47% SPN (14% G 3–4), 42% constipation (2% G 3), 35% V (3% G 3), 35% thrombocytopenia (30% G 3–4), 35% fever, 34% anorexia, 26% anemia (9% G 3), 23% headache, 21% cough, 20% dyspnea (5% G 3), 18% insomnia, 18% rash (1% G 3), 14% G 3–4 neutropenia, 19% dysesthesia with partial improvement up to 8 wk after discontinuation (6% G 3), 16% abdominal pain (2% G 3), 15% respiratory infections (4% G 3), 14% dizziness, 14% back pain (3% G 3), 13% herpes zoster (2% G 3), 12% myalgia.
<u>With CYP3A4 substrates:</u> not studied but potential. <u>With gemfibrozil:</u> ↑ bexarotene (oral) plasma concentration. <u>With DEET</u> (*N,N*-diethyl-m-toluamide) containing products (insect repellents): animal studies showed ↑ topical toxicity. **Warning** Limit vitamin A supplementation. Potential photosensitizer.	*Topical gel* 1st week: one application every other day, then ↑ frequency, at weekly intervals, to o.i.d., b.i.d., and t.i.d. daily. ↑ response with ≥b.i.d. *Duration:* optimal unknown, use until benefit, maximum experienced length 172 wk. <u>Wait</u> at least 20 min before bathing. <u>Avoid</u> use of occlusive dressing and contact with healthy skin and mucosa. *Oral form* PO daily: *Dose:* initial 300 mg/m², if not tolerated, decrease by 100 mg/m² decrement until tolerated, then re-escalate to 300 mg/m², if response not achieved after 8 wk and well tolerated escalate to 400 mg/m². *Duration:* optimal unknown, use until benefit, maximum experienced length 97 wk.	72% rash (56% at application site), 36% pruritus (18%), 30% pain (16%), 6% paresthesia (6%), 14% contact dermatitis (8%). *Common:* 70% reversible hypercholesterolemia and hyperlipidemia (G 3–4 30–40%), 45% asthenia, 41% headache (G 3–4 10%), 41% diarrhea (G 3–4 5%), 28% exfoliative dermatitis (G 3–4 8%), 22% infections (G 3–4 4%), 11% alopecia; <u>hematological:</u> 47% leukopenia (G 4 10%), 38% anemia (including hypochromic 13%). *Less frequent:* ↑ LFTs, pancreatitis, hypothyroidism. Severity and incidence ↓ with <300 mg/m².

Name, chemistry, relevant features	Mechanism of action	Pharmacology and dose modifications

11 RADIOCHEMOPROTECTANTS

Dexrazoxane
Zinecard®

Bispiperazinedione; cyclic derivative of EDTA.

Indication: continuation of DOX after ≥300 mg/m² cumulative dose in pts in whom continued therapy is indicated.

Cardioprotection: intracellular hydrolysis to ring-opened chelating agent with removal of Fe^{2+} and Cu^{2+} from DOX-complexes and ↓ of O_2^- free radicals generation.

2% protein bound; minimal tissue binding; $T_{1/2}\alpha$ 15 min, $T_{1/2}\beta$ 140 min; 42% excreted in urine.
Cardioprotection observed in >65 yr old and in pts with LVEF normal.

Amifostine
Ethyol®

Cytoprotective thiophosphate compound.

Indications:
(1) to ↓ the cumulative renal toxicity associated with repeated administrations of DDP in pts with ovarian and NSCL cancers;
(2) to ↓ incidence of moderate to severe xerostomia in pts with H&N receiving post-surgery RT (1.8–2 Gy) to >75% both parotid glands.

Prodrug; selectively dephosphorylated in normal tissues by AP to free thiol which acts (a) by binding to reactive molecules of DDP; (b) as free radical scavenger of free radicals generated by DDP and RT.
Higher uptake and metabolism in normal cells due to higher pH and AP concentration.

Cleared from plasma in 10 min; retained in normal tissues; $T_{1/2}$ 9 min; 4% urinary excretion. High concentration of free thiol in BM, declining within 2.5 hr.

---

12 ENDOCRINE THERAPIES

12.1 Hormones/Estrogens/Progesterones

Estramustine phosphate
(Estracyt®, Emcyt®)

Combination of estradiol phosphate and HN_2 by a carbamate link.

Weak estrogenic effect on hormonally dependent tissues; the metabolites promote microtubule disassembly by binding to tubulin, directly or via microtubular-associated proteins; block P-gp.

Prodrug, rapidly dephosphorylated in the gastric wall to estramustine; produces estradiol plasma levels comparable to those achieved with conventional estradiol (active metabolite), subsequently oxidized to estradiol and estrone; 75% F; selective accumulation in prostate by binding to specific protein.
$T_{1/2}$: 20–24 hr; main biliary excretion.

Special populations
Liver impairment
Guidelines not available, but ↓ dose.

Medroxyprogesterone acetate (MPA)
Provera® (PO only)
Farlutal® (PO/IM)

Megestrol acetate (MGA)
Megace®

Binding to specific cytosol receptors; antiestrogenic effects due decrease of ER, and decrease of Gn secretion; direct cytotoxic activity.

MPA: 95% protein bound; good F; 70% first-pass effect with conjugation. PO: action duration 16 days; IM: 4–6 wk with C_{ss} after 10 days and high interpt. variability, $T_{1/2}$ 60 hr; 40% urinary excretion.
MGA: T_{max} 2–5 hr, 1–3 days of duration of action; $T_{1/2}$ 15–20 hr; 56–78% renal excretion (5–8% metabolites).

Special populations
Liver impairment
HD not advisable; guidelines not available.

Drug interactions	Route, schedule, and recommendations	Toxicity
<u>With DOX:</u> ↓ incidence and severity of DOX cardiomyopathy. Does not influence PK of DOX.	<u>IV</u> (15 min inf.): a maximum of 30 min. Should elapse within the start of infusion and DOX administration. Dosage ratio to DOX: 10:1 (500 mg/m²: 50 mg/m²). **Warning** Cardiac function must be monitored serially. Do <u>not</u> mix with other drugs during infusion.	May add to chemotherapy myelotoxicity: serial CBC monitoring. 7% pain on injection site, 2% urticaria.
<u>With antihypertensives:</u> hypotension, to be interrupted at least 24 hr before Amifostine. **Caution** In pts with pre-existing cardiovascular/cerebrovascular conditions.	<u>With CT:</u> <u>IV</u> (15 min inf.): 910 mg/m² 30 min before DDP (≥100 mg/m²) (keep pts in supine position during and after treatment). <u>With RT:</u> <u>IV</u> (15 min inf.): 200 mg/m² 15–30 min before RT (keep pts in supine position during and after treatment). <u>Antiemetic prophylaxis</u> with steroids and 5HT3 antagonists.	DL toxicities: 92% emesis and 62% hypotension at the end of infusion, lasting 5 min. Less frequent: sneezing, warm flush, mild somnolence, hypocalcemia. Rare (<1%): HSR, serious cutaneous reactions, more frequent in pts receiving RT. **Warning** <u>Incidence</u> of side effects ↑ with longer infusion. <u>HSR, severe cutaneous reaction</u> Discontinue treatment.
In vitro additive effects with VLB and paclitaxel.	<u>PO:</u> 140 mg/10 kg BW in 3–4 divided doses daily (1 hr before meal with water only; avoid milk and dairy products). Lower doses at start. Treat pts for at least 30 up to 90 days before tumor reassessment. **Warning** In pts with metabolic bone disease: treatment associated with hypercalcemia or renal insufficiency. **Absolute contraindications** Active thrombophlebitis or TE disorder, severe liver or cardiac impairment; <u>relative:</u> hypertension, diabetes, cerebro-vascular or coronary artery disease.	↑ risk of TE disorders; 19% fluid retention; acute N&V; 12% diarrhea (first 2 wk of treatment); ↓ glucose tolerance; 70% gynecomastia; 31% ↑ LFT.
	MPA <u>PO:</u> 200–400 mg daily continuously. <u>IM:</u> 500 mg once or twice per week according to tumor type and protocol. *MGA* <u>PO:</u> 160 mg daily continously. **Warning** **Absolute contraindications:** previous TE.	Hot flashes, vaginal bleeding, weight gain, depression, mild fluid retention, acne, ↑ LFTs. Adrenal insufficiency after chronic use (hypotension, N&V, dizziness, weakness): assess with stress doses of rapidly acting glucocorticoids. <u>After MPA:</u> tremor, cramps, headache, dizziness, insomnia, cushingoid facies, thrombophlebitis, glucose intolerance, hypertension. <u>After IM MPA:</u> gluteal abscess.

Name, chemistry, relevant features	Mechanism of action	Pharmacology and dose modifications

12.2 Hormone Antagonists
12.2.1 Antiestrogens

Tamoxifen (TAM) Non-steroidal analogue of clomiphene; trans isomer of a triphenylethylene derivative.	First-generation SERM; binding to ER blocking E action with tissue-specific effects. Antiestrogenic effects in mammary gland; estrogenic effects in bone, liver, heart, and uterus. Inhibitor of P-gp.	T_{max} 5 hr. C_{ss} after 4 wk for TAM and 8 wk for main metabolite N-desmethyl TAM; $T_{1/2}\beta$ of TAM and main metabolite 7 and 14 days. Substrate of CYP450 3A, CYP450 2C9, and CYP450 2D6. Extensive liver metabolism with 6% of dose excreted in bile; long-term tissue retention. ↑ TAM and metabolites levels in liver obstruction. Falsely-negative tumor ER determinations by binding assay within 4–6 wk from the end of TAM. Special populations No age effect.
Toremifene (TOR) Fareston® Nonsteroidal Triphenylethylene derivative.	First-generation SERM. Same effects of TAM; cytotoxic effect at high doses independent of ER binding. Less carcinogenic in animals.	100% protein bound; T_{max} 4 hr; C_{ss} after 2 wk. $T_{1/2}\gamma$ 5 days; extensive tissue distribution and metabolism with 70% excretion in feces. Special populations Renal impairment No dose modification. Liver impairment ↓ dose by 50%.
Raloxifene Evista® Non-steroidal benzothiophene.	Second-generation SERM; binding of the raloxifene-ER complex to unique area of DNA, with block of the E-dependent transcription at the level of α (uterus, breast) and β ER in humans. Anti-estrogenic effects in mammary gland and uterus; estrogenic effects in bone, liver, heart with ↓ bone resorption and ↓ total cholesterol.	98% protein bound; 60% F, $T_{1/2}$ 27.7 hr due to enterohepatic circulation. Important first-pass effect, glucuronidation with main biliary excretion, 6% urinary excretion. Special populations Liver impairment >2.5 fold ↑ plasma concentrations in pts with Childs-Pugh A cirrhosis. Renal impairment Caution in severe impairment.
Fulvestrant Faslodex® Alkyl side chain substituted in 7α of 17β-estradiol.	Pure steroidal antiestrogen; high affinity for ER without agonist activity. In vitro and in vivo activity in TAM resistant cell lines and human breast xenografts; no uterine stimulatory activity.	Long-acting IM administration, T_{max} 7–9 days, $T_{1/2}$ 40 days; accumulation after multiple dosing. Rapidly cleared from plasma with extensive tissue distribution and hepatic metabolism with biliary excretion. Special population No difference in geriatric pts. Liver impairment No dose modification in case of mild ↑ LFT.

12.2.2 Antiandrogens—Nonsteroidal

| **Flutamide**
Flucinom® | Pure A antagonists; A receptor antagonist with binding competition with testosterone and dihydrotestosterone. | 90% protein bound; prodrug, activated to α-hydroxyflutamide, with longer $T_{1/2}$ and higher C_{ss}; absorption within 3 hr with C_{ss} after 5 days of therapy, $T_{1/2}$ 8 hr, 45% urinary excretion in 48 hr, 2% in feces. |

Drug interactions	Route, schedule, and recommendations	Toxicity
↓ cytotoxicity of 5-FU and DOX, ↑ hepatic toxicity of allopurinol; reversal of MDR phenotype <u>in vitro</u> at concentrations achieved in humans after very high dose. Inhibition of CYP450 oxidases of unknown clinical relevance. Monitor PT in pts on coumarins.	<u>PO:</u> 20 mg daily; higher doses of unproven benefit. <u>Contraindications:</u> Prior history of DVT or PE.	<u>Antiestrogenic effects</u> (mainly premenopause): 64% hot flushes; 32% fluid retention, 25% irregular menses; 23% weight loss, 19% skin changes, 16% amenorrhea, 4% edema. Induction of ovulation (use barrier contraception). Rare: ocular disturbances, ↑ cataracts. <u>Estrogenic effects</u> (at lower concentrations and in postmenopause): maintain bone density; ↑ HDL/LDL ratio; ↓ total and LDL cholesterol; acute flare if bone disease (pain and hypercalcemia); ↓ 10% antithrombin III levels; 1% TE disorders; ↑ relative risk (3–5-fold) of endometrial cancer (regular gynecological control, vaginal ultrasound, and endometrial sampling if bleeding).
Block of P-gp by pharmacologic levels of TOR and metabolites. <u>With coumarin-derivative anticoagulants:</u> ↑ PT. <u>With CYP3A4 inducers:</u> (phenytoin, phenobarbital, carbamazepine). ↑ metabolism. <u>With CYP3A4 inhibitors:</u> (ketoconazole, erythromycin). ↓ metabolism.	<u>PO:</u> 60 mg daily on an empty stomach. <u>Contraindications:</u> Prior TE, endometrial hyperplasia.	20% hot flushes, 14% sweating, 8% nausea, 8% vaginal discharge, bone pain, weight gain. Tumor flare and hypercalcemia in pts with bone metastases during the first weeks of treatment; ↓ antithrombin III levels.
<u>With benzodiazepines, coumarin derivative, NSAID:</u> ↑ toxicity because of protein displacement binding.	<u>PO:</u> 60 mg daily.	↑ risk of TE event. 24% vasodilation. 7% legs cramps. 6% constipation. 5% peripheral edema.
<u>With CYP450 inducers:</u> PK not affected.	<u>IM</u> long-acting formulation: 250 mg every 4 wk.	*Common* (all mild intensity): 30% cardiovascular, 26% nausea, 17% hot flushes, 15% headache, 13% vomiting, 12% diarrhea, 12% abdominal pain, 11% injection site reactions, 9% peripheral edema, 7% dizziness.
In combination with LHRH analogue to prevent flare; combined androgen blockade to ↓ A production in surrenal glands. Increase of PT with concomitant coumarin derivatives.	<u>PO:</u> 250 mg daily t.i.d., 30 min before meals. Recommended maximal duration of combined treatment with LHRH ± RT: 16 wk.	<u>In combination with LHRH analogues:</u> 70% hot flushes, 36–81% loss of libido and impotence, 22% gynecomastia, 12% diarrhea. <u>Single agent:</u> 25% gynecomastia; pain in nipple; rarely, transient ↑ LFTs, rare hemolytic anemia, cholestasis.

Name, chemistry, relevant features	Mechanism of action	Pharmacology and dose modifications
Bicalutamide Casodex®	Pure A antagonist; same as that of Flutamide; effect reversible at the end of treatment.	96% protein bound; racemic mixture with active R forms corresponding to 99% of plasma levels. Well absorbed, T_{max} 30 hr, $T_{1/2}$ 6 days. Extensive liver metabolism with glucuronidation with 43% and 36% of the dose excreted through liver and kidney. Special populations *Liver impairment* ALT/AST >2 × NV: discontinue treatment. No modification in mild impairment.
Nilutamide Nilandron®	Pure A antagonist; same as that of flutamide.	84% protein binding; rapid complete absorption, extensive liver metabolism through microsomal oxidation system with main renal excretion (62% in urine within 5 days), $T_{1/2}$ 56 hr; check liver enzymes every 3 mo. Special populations *Liver impairment* ALT/AST >2 × N: discontinue treatment.

12.3 Gonadotrophin-Releasing Hormone Analogues (GnRH, LHRH Analogues)

Goserelin acetate Zoladex® Synthetic decapeptide.	Inhibition of steroid hormone synthesis by binding and downregulating pituary LR-RH receptors, followed by suppression of LH secretion within 2–4 wk. Initial ↑ sex steroids levels with flare, then ↓ up to values comparable to surgical castration after 3–4 wk; effect reversible at the end of treatment.	25% protein bound; metabolized and excreted in urine; effective concentrations lasting for 4 wk. No accumulation with monthly doses. Special population No dose modification in case of renal or liver impairment.
Leuprolide acetate Lupron®, Lucrin **Triptorelin acetate** Decapeptyl Retard® D-amino acid substituted peptide linked to dextran or copolymer.	Same as that of Goserelin acetate; castrate levels of testosterone and estrogens stabilized after 3 wk following the first injection.	46% protein bound; 20% of dose released weekly from IM site; C_{ss} reached in 8 wk; no accumulation with monthly doses: eliminated by metabolism through peptidase and renal excretion.

12.4 Aromatase Inhibitors
12.4.1 Type I Steroidal (Covalent and Irreversible Binding to Aromatase with Enzyme Inactivation)

Exemestane Aromasin® Androstenedione derivative.	Potent AI, 90% ↓ estrone and estradiol levels; 98% in vivo inhibition of peripheral aromatization; does not affect adrenal steroidogenesis after 25 mg.	90% protein bound; well absorbed, T_{max} 2 hr, $T_{1/2}$ 24 hr, extensive tissue distribution, extensively metabolized by CYP3A4; 42% dose excreted as metabolites in feces and in urine. Special population No dose adjustment in pts with moderate renal/liver impairment. No age effect.

12.4.2 Type II Nonsteroidal (Reversible Binding with the P450 Moiety of the Enzyme Complex)

Aminoglutethimide (AG) Orimeten® Derivative of glutethimide; inhibits conversion from androstenedione to estrone.	Peripheral inhibition of aromatase system with 50% ↓ estrone and estradiol in postmenopause; inhibition of other enzymes in steroidogenesis (desmolase, 11β-hydroxylase). Inhibition of thyroxine synthesis, with ↑ of TSH.	25% protein bound; well absorbed with T_{max} 1.5 hr; $T_{1/2}\beta$ 13 hr. Acetylated to *N*-acetyl AG with 20% inhibitory activity; 40% excreted in urine.

Drug interactions	Route, schedule, and recommendations	Toxicity
In combination with LHRH analogues to prevent flare; displacement of coumarin from binding sites: monitor PT in pts on coumarins. Check regularly LFT; longer $T_{1/2}$ only if severe liver disease.	<u>PO:</u> 50 mg daily (start at the same time of LHRH analogue). 150 mg daily for chemical castration for locally advanced disease. **Caution** Cardiac disease.	<u>In combination with LHRH</u> analogues: 49% hot flushes, 27% generalized pain, 17% constipation, 15% asthenia, 11% N, 10% diarrhea, 9% skin rash, 7% impotence and 5% gynecomastia, 7% transient ↑ LFTs. *Rare:* dizziness, dyspnea, diabetes.
Inhibition of CYP450; delayed elimination of vitamin K antagonists and phenytoin; monitor PT in pts on coumarins. Disulfiram-like reaction with alcohol with flushing, headache, nausea, dizziness.	<u>PO:</u> 100 mg t.i.d. for 4 wk (loading dose), then 150 mg daily (maintenance).	In combination with surgical castration: 28% hot flushes; single: 44% gynecomastia, 27% visual disturbances with 13% delay in adaptation to dark, 10% nausea, 8% ↑ AST/ALT (1% severe), 7% dizziness, 6% dyspnea, 2% interstitial pneumonitis (within 3 mo from start, with progressive dyspnea, chest pain, fever, interstitial changes on X ray, reversible).
	<u>SC:</u> 3.6 mg every 4 wk. Coadministration of anti-A to prevent flare.	Initial flare reactions with bone pain and uterine bleeding, possible hypercalcemia if bone metastases (in prostate cancer: spinal cord compression, urinary retention). Male pts: 48% hot flushes, 61% ↓ libido; female pts: 89% hot flushes, 55% headache, 49% depression, 40% gynecomastia; amenorrhea within 1–2 mo, 59% amenorrhea, <10 % fluid retention 3. Both: skin rashes, rash at injection site. No ↓ antithrombin III levels.
Same as that of Goserelin acetate.	<u>IM:</u> 3.75 mg every 4 wk. **Warning** Hematoma at injection site in pts under anticoagulants.	In female and male pts: 30% hot flashes; 10% sweating, gynecomastia, ↑ LFTs; in female pts: 100% reversible amenorrhea after 3 mo, 10% CNS effects, acneiform rash, and hirsutism. *Rare:* headache, insomnia, asthenia, weight changes, visual disturbances, blood pressure changes.
<u>With CYP3A4 inhibitors:</u> uncertain clinical relevance.	PO 25 mg daily. Continuously.	Mild to moderate: 13% hot flushes, 13% depression, 9% N, 8% fatigue, 8% dizziness, 8% headache, 8% weight gain, 4% sweating; ↑ frequency of adverse events at doses >25 mg/day.
AG ↑ metabolism of DXM, TAM, theophylline. <u>With alcohol:</u> ↑ drowsiness.	<u>PO:</u> 250 mg b.i.d. daily with cortisone acetate 37.5 mg total (divided into two doses). Start at 125 mg b.i.d. daily for 1 wk, then ↑ to full dose. Give hydrocortisone (20–40 mg) to overcome ↑ ACTH due to ↓ glucocorticoids (occasional at 500 mg). **Warning** Monitor cortisol levels until plasma suppression achieved. Monitor INR in pts with coumarin derivative anticoagulants.	Dose-related incidence of side effects: 26% early maculopapular rash, self-limiting in 5–8 days; 40% lethargy; 20% dizziness; 5% hypoaldosteronism with postural hypotension; 10% mild N&V. *Rare:* hypothyroidism, ↑ LFTs, renal insufficiency.

Name, chemistry, relevant features	Mechanism of action	Pharmacology and dose modifications
Letrozole Femara® Triazole derivative. Synthetic achiral benzydryltrizole derivative.	75–95% $\downarrow$ estrone, estradiol, and estrone sulfate levels. 10,000-fold more potent than AG in inhibiting aromatase in vivo; does not affect adrenal steroidogenesis.	60% protein bound; 100% F within 1 hr, not influenced by meals; $T_{1/2}$ 75–110 hr; rapid tissue sdistribution, C_{ss} achieved within 2–6 wk; eliminated by CYP3A4-dependent metabolism, no accumulation after repeated dosing. <u>Special populations</u> No influence of renal or liver impairment.
Anastrozole Arimidex®	Potent, highly selective. After 1 mg 70% $\downarrow$ estradiol within 24 hr; does not affect adrenal steroidogenesis.	40% protein bound; 100% F, T_{max} 2 hr not affected by meals. Linear PK, $T_{1/2}$ 40–50 hr. C_{ss} achieved within 7 days. Extensively metabolized in liver with 10% and 60% of unchanged drug and metabolite, respectively, in 72 hr urine. <u>Special populations</u> No age, race effect, no dose modification for renal or severe liver impairment.

13 GROWTH FACTORS AND SUPPORTIVE TREATMENT

Recombinant human erythropoietin (rHuEPO) Glycoprotein hormone for erythropoiesis, produced primarily in peritubular interstitial cells of kidney; $\uparrow$ production due to $\uparrow$ gene transcription if kidney/liver hypoxia. Recombinant made by gene-modified mammalian cells with human gene.	Binds to specific receptors on committed erythroid progenitor cells, stimulates proliferation and differentiation of erythroid cells with negative feedback on hypoxic stimulus. Inverse correlation between erythropoietin plasma levels and Hb concentration if kidney function is normal.	Delayed incomplete absorption with sustained levels after SC. $T_{1/2}$ 3–10 hr, detectable in plasma up to 24 hr; T_{max} between 5–24 hr after SC dosing; hepatic metabolism with desialylation, 10% excretion in urine.
Darbepoetin alfa (Aranesp) Differs from rHuEPO for a five chain, instead of a three chain oligosaccharide, with $\uparrow$ molecular weight.	Same mechanism as endogenous erythropoietin with $\uparrow$ Hb within 2–6 wk after starting.	Linear PK within 0.45–4.5 µg/kg with no accumulation. After SC administration slow rate-limiting absorption with $T_{1/2}$ 49 hr (27–89 hr), C_{max} between 71 and 123 hr; 37% bioavailability in chronic renal failure pts. <u>Special populations</u> No age effect.
Filgrastim Neupogen® G-CSF Recombinant glycoprotein hormone necessary to maintain adequate numbers of circulating PMN; produced by *E.Coli*-inserted G-CSF gene.	By binding to specific receptors induces proliferation of granulocyte progenitor cells, $\uparrow$ PMN chemotaxis, phagocytosis, and intracellular killing.	$T_{1/2}\beta$: 3.5 hr; T_{max}: 2–8 hr; distributed into plasma and BM, metabolized in liver and kidney.

Drug interactions	Route, schedule, and recommendations	Toxicity
	PO: 2.5 mg/day.	Mild to moderate: 20% bone pain, 18% hot flushes, 15% N, 11% fatigue, 8% headache, 5% peripheral edema.
In vitro inhibition of CYP450 3A4 at high concentrations; no evidence of clinically significant inhibition; 27% ↓ anastrozole plasma levels when given with TAM.	PO: 1 mg/day.	Mild to moderate: 26% hot flushes, 19% N, 16% asthenia, 11% bone pain , 9% headache, 10% rash, 4% TE, 2% weight gain, 1% vaginal hemorrhage.
Not known.	SC *CT-associated anemia*: 150–300 mU/kg three times a week for 8 wk. *Zidovudine-associated anemia*: 100 mU/kg three times a week. Supplemental iron if serum ferritin <100 µg/l or serum transferrin saturation <20%. Check hematocrit (Ht) weekly, 25% dose titration up or down, discontinue if Ht >35%. **Warning** EPO likely to be ineffective if erythropoietin plasma levels >500 mU/ml. **Absolute contraindications:** uncontrolled hypertension, severe cardiac/peripheral arteriopathies, recent TIA, DVT.	Exacerbation of pre-existent hypertension with need of weekly monitoring of BP; mild arthralgia, local pain injection, pure red cell aplasia due to neutralizing Ab to native erythropoietin; ↑ incidence of CVC thrombosis; potential stimulation of growth of some tumors.
Not known.	SC: start with 2.25 µg/kg once a week; check Hb once a week, increase to 4.5 µg/kg once a week for ↑ Hb <1 g/dl after 4 wk; discontinue after 4 wk for ↑ Hb still <1 g/dl. Keep Hb around 12 g/dl; ↓ dose for ↑ Hb >1 g/dl over 2 wk; discontinue if Hb >14 g/dl, then restart at 50% dose. Supplemental iron if serum ferritin <100 µg/l or serum transferrin saturation <20%. **Warning** EPO likely to be ineffective if erythropoietin plasma levels >500 mU/ml. **Absolute contraindications:** Uncontrolled hypertension, known hypersensitivity.	↑ risk of cardiovascular events, exacerbation of pre-existing hypertension with need of weekly monitoring of BP; rare: severe allergic reaction requiring discontinuation. *Most common* 23% hypertension, 21% myalgia, 16% headache, 15% diarrhea, 11% edema, 11% arthralgia, 11% fluid retention, 10% back pain, 9% fatigue, 9% fever, 8% CNS, 8% rash, 6% TE, 3% PE.
With lithium: ↑ ANC release, ↑ frequency CBC.	SC *CT-induced neutropenia* 5 µg/kg daily (or 300 µg), starting 1–5 days after CT for 14 days or up to ANC 5'–10'000 mm³; check counts biweekly. *PBPC mobilization* 10 µg/kg (or 480 µg/day) daily. *PBPC reinfusion* 5 µg/kg daily starting up to 5 days after, up to ANC 10,000/mm³. *Autologous or allogenic BMT and in AML:* start the day of BM infusion, >24 hr after CT, >12 hr after total body irradiation, up to ANC 1,500/mm³ for 3 days. Paracetamol to control bone pain.	20% bone pain, mainly medullary and iliac, due to ANC expansion in BM, leg pain, musculoskeletal pain; transient ↑ AP/LDH. *Rare:* HSR, ARDS in neutropenic septic pts; sickle cell crises in pts with sickle cell disease. Exacerbation of pre-existing inflammatory conditions.

Name, chemistry, relevant features	Mechanism of action	Pharmacology and dose modifications
Pegfilgrastim Neulasta® Covalent conjugate of filgrastim and monomethoxypolyethylene glycol.	Same as filgrastim.	$\downarrow$ CL and prolonged persistence; as compared to filgrastim larger intrapt. variability with $T_{1/2}\beta$ of 15–80 hr. Non-linear PK, $\downarrow$ CL for $\uparrow$ dose, serum clearance related to ANC count and body weight. Long-lasting effect. Special populations No age effect.
IL-11 (Oprelvekin) Neumega® Recombinant polypeptide, thrombopoietic growth factor for prevention of severe thrombocytopenia and reduction of transfusions need after myelosuppressive CT.	Stimulation of proliferation of HSC and megakaryocyte progenitor cells, induction of megakaryocyte maturation. Stimulation of osteoclastogenesis.	After SC administration 80% bioavailability. T_{max} 3 ± 2 hr, $T_{1/2}\gamma$ 7 hr with no accumulation after repeated administrations; low urinary excretion. Dose-dependent effect, beginning 5–9 days after start, continuing up to 7 days from end, recovering to baseline within 14 days. **Warning** In pts with CrCL <15 ml/min, doubling of C_{max}, AUC and $\uparrow$ >20% mean plasma volume, with $\downarrow$ RBC volume resulting in dilutional anemia, primarily due to Na and water retention (beginning after 3–5 days, reversible within 1 wk after discontinuation).
Biphosphonates Pamidronate Aredia® Zoledronic acid Zometa®	Inhibition of bone resorption due to: (1) direct inhibition of osteoclastic activity; (2) binding to Ca phosphate crystals in bone blocking its dissolution and bone/cartilage resorption; (3) inhibition of tumor factors activating osteoclasts and bone resorption.	Pamidronate: not metabolized but exclusively eliminated through renal excretion (46%); CL_R closely correlated to renal function. Zoledronic acid: 56% protein bound; 44 ± 18% dose as parent compound in 24 hr urine; triphasic plasma disappearance with $T_{1/2}\alpha$ 0.23 hr, $T_{1/2}\beta$ 1.75 hr, $T_{1/2}\gamma$ 167 hr. Special populations *Renal impairment* Withhold treatment: if Cr baseline normal and Cr $\uparrow$ by 0.5 mg/dl; if Cr baseline abnormal and Cr $\uparrow$ by 1 mg/dl. Re-introduce only if recovery to 10% baseline. **Caution** No data in pts with Cr >3 mg/dl or >245 µmol/l: $\uparrow$ infusion time. If renal impairment after long-term use, discontinue treatment until recovery, repeat examinations every 3–4 wk.

Drug interactions	Route, schedule, and recommendations	Toxicity
<u>With lithium:</u> ↑ ANC release, ↑ frequency CBC.	<u>Approved indication:</u> ↓ incidence of infection. <u>SC:</u> *Adult and children ≥45 kg:* 6 mg once per cycle. *Children <45 kg:* dose not defined (<6 mg). **Warning** Must be given: at least <u>24 hr after</u> CT; at least <u>14 days prior</u> subsequent CT. Avoid use in weekly or <3 wk CT schedules. **Absolute contraindication:** known hypersensitivity.	26% mild to moderate medullary bone pain, 12% requiring non-opioid analgesics, 19% ↑ LDH, 9% ↑ AP. *Rare:* splenic rupture, ARDS, sickle cell crises, HSR.
No interaction with filgrastim.	**SC daily** *Adults:* 50 µg/kg, start 6–24 hr after completion of CT, continue up to post-nadir value of 50,000/mm³ Pt (usually for 10–21 days). *Children:* recommended dose not defined, higher doses used with ↑ side effects, mainly papilledema. See Toxicity. **Warning** Discontinue at least 2 days before restarting CT. Monitor periodically pt count, fluid balance, and electrolytes. <u>Caution in pts with:</u> pre-existing papilledema, prior/concomitant CHF, aggressive hydration, atrial arrhythmias. Safety of chronic dosing not established. **Absolute contraindication:** Prior hypersensitivity.	*Adults:* 59% peripheral edema due to fluid retention, 48% dyspnea, 41% headache, 36% fever; 25% skin rash; <u>cardiac:</u> 14% palpitation, 20% tachycardia, 15% arrhythmia; 1% papilledema. *Children:* ↑ incidence due to ↑ doses up to 125 µg/kg. <u>Cardiac:</u> 84% tachycardia, 24% radiographic evidence of cardiomegaly; 58% conjunctival injection, 16% papilledema after repeated courses, 11% periosteal changes. *Rare(all pts):* HSR including anaphylaxis, after first or subsequent doses.
Warning <u>Do not mix</u> with Ca containing solution, administer through a separate line. *Pamidronate:* none known. *Zoledronic acid:* <u>With loop diuretics, aminoglycosides, thalidomide:</u> possible ↑ renal damage.	*Pamidronate* (P) <u>IV</u> <u>Ostelytic lesions</u> 90 mg every 4 wk. Infusion duration: 2 hr infusion (diluted in 250 ml NS 0.9%); 4 hr infusion (diluted in 500 ml NS 0.9%). <u>Hypercalcemia:</u> Hydrate → daily diuresis 2 l/day. Titrate dose to serum Ca values. Maximum effect within 3–7 days, at least 7 days within retreatments if no activity. *Zoledronic acid* (Z): <u>IV</u> <u>Ostelytic lesions</u> 15 min infusion. 4 mg every 4 wk. <u>Hypercalcemia:</u> Hydrate → daily diuresis 2 l/day. Titrate dose to serum Ca values. **Warning** Tooth extractions and dental surgery major risk for ONJ. Screening of oral cavity and dental care as mandatory preventive measures.	<table><tr><td>Gr 3-4 (%)</td><td>P</td><td>Z</td></tr><tr><td>Hypocalcemia</td><td>2</td><td>1</td></tr><tr><td>Hypophosphatemia</td><td>38</td><td>53</td></tr><tr><td>Hypomagnesemia</td><td>1</td><td>0</td></tr><tr><td>Renal deterioration</td><td><1</td><td><1</td></tr><tr><td>Nausea</td><td>45</td><td>43</td></tr><tr><td>Vomiting</td><td>30</td><td>30</td></tr><tr><td>Fatigue</td><td>37</td><td>36</td></tr><tr><td>Diarrhea</td><td>25</td><td>32</td></tr><tr><td>Pyrexia</td><td>28</td><td>30</td></tr><tr><td>Myalgia</td><td>24</td><td>21</td></tr><tr><td>Paresthesia</td><td>14</td><td>12</td></tr><tr><td>Rash</td><td>11</td><td>11</td></tr></table> *Rare:* scleritis within 6 hr to 2 days after P. <u>ONJ:</u> the incidence of ONJ is estimated to be 1–10/100 oncology patients, risk lower in patients receiving oral bisphosphonate for osteoporosis, with an estimated incidence of 1/10,000 to 1/100,000 patient treatment years. Mandible more commonly affected than maxilla (2:1).

Index

Note: Page numbers in *italics* indicate figures or tables.